Transplantation Pathology

Transplantation Pathology

Second Edition

Edited by
Phillip Ruiz
University of Miami School of Medicine

CAMBRIDGE
UNIVERSITY PRESS

CAMBRIDGE
UNIVERSITY PRESS

University Printing House, Cambridge CB2 8BS, United Kingdom

One Liberty Plaza, 20th Floor, New York, NY 10006, USA

477 Williamstown Road, Port Melbourne, VIC 3207, Australia

314–321, 3rd Floor, Plot 3, Splendor Forum, Jasola District Centre,
New Delhi – 110025, India

79 Anson Road, #06–04/06, Singapore 079906

Cambridge University Press is part of the University of Cambridge.

It furthers the University's mission by disseminating knowledge in the
pursuit of education, learning, and research at the highest international
levels of excellence.

www.cambridge.org
Information on this title: www.cambridge.org/9781107443280
DOI: 10.1017/9781139828581

© Cambridge University Press 2018

This publication is in copyright. Subject to statutory exception
and to the provisions of relevant collective licensing agreements,
no reproduction of any part may take place without the written
permission of Cambridge University Press.

First edition published 2009
Second edition published 2018

Printed in the United Kingdom by Clays, St Ives plc

A catalogue record for this publication is available from the British Library.

Library of Congress Cataloging-in-Publication Data
Names: Ruiz, Phillip, 1954– editor.
Title: Transplantation pathology / edited by Phillip Ruiz, University of
Miami School of Medicine.
Description: University Printing House : Cambridge, United Kingdom ;
New York, NY, 2017. | Includes bibliographical references.
Identifiers: LCCN 2017022979| ISBN 9781107619685 (hardback) | ISBN
9781139828581 (Cambridge core) | ISBN 9781107443280 (mixed media)
Subjects: LCSH: Transplantation of organs, tissues, etc. – Complications. |
Transplantation immunology.
Classification: LCC RD120.78 .T742 2017 | DDC 617.9/54–dc23
LC record available at https://lccn.loc.gov/2017022979

ISBN 978-1-107-44328-0 Mixed Media
ISBN 978-1-107-61968-5 Hardback
ISBN 978-1-139-82858-1 Cambridge Core

Cambridge University Press has no responsibility for the
persistence or accuracy of URLs for external or third-party
internet websites referred to in this publication and does
not guarantee that any content on such websites is, or will
remain, accurate or appropriate.

....

Every effort has been made in preparing this book to provide accurate
and up-to-date information that is in accord with accepted standards
and practice at the time of publication. Although case histories are drawn
from actual cases, every effort has been made to disguise the identities
of the individuals involved. Nevertheless, the authors of the individual
chapters (who are responsible for the scientific content within each one),
editors, and publishers can make no warranties that the information
contained herein is totally free from error, not least because clinical
standards are constantly changing through research and regulation.
The authors, editors, and publishers therefore disclaim all liability
for direct or consequential damages resulting from the use of material
contained in this book. Readers are strongly advised to pay careful
attention to information provided by the manufacturer of any drugs
or equipment that they plan to use.

This book is dedicated to my family, without whom none of this would be possible, and to the transplant patients, whose courage continues to fortify my drive to succeed.

Contents

List of Contributors viii
Preface xi

1 **Immunopathology of Organ Transplantation** 1
Phillip Ruiz

2 **The Pathology of Kidney Transplantation** 25
Phillip Ruiz, George Burke, Gaetano Ciancio, Giselle Guerra, David Roth, Linda Chen, Warren Kupin, and Adela Mattiazzi

3 **Histopathology of Liver Transplantation** 64
Heather L. Stevenson, Marta I. Minervini, Michael A. Nalesnik, Parmjeet S. Randhawa, Eizaburo Sasatomi, and A. J. Demetris

4 **The Pathology of Heart Transplantation** 133
E. Rene Rodriguez and Carmela D. Tan

5 **The Pathology of Lung Transplantation** 156
Carol Farver and W. Dean Wallace

6 **The Pathology of Intestinal and Multivisceral Transplantation** 183
Phillip Ruiz, Jennifer Garcia, Ji Fan, Seigo Nishida, Thiago Beduschi, Akin Tekin, and Rodrigo Vianna

7 **Pancreas and Islet Transplantation Pathology** 216
Cinthia B. Drachenberg and John C. Papadimitriou

8 **Pathology of Hematopoietic Stem Cell Transplantation** 260
Lazaros J. Lekakis and Krishna V. Komanduri

9 **Dermatological Complications in Transplant Patients and Composite Tissue Allotransplant Pathology** 294
Emma Lanuti, Mohammed Sharaf, Brian Keegan, Ingrid Wolf, Marco Romanelli, Phillip Ruiz, and Paolo Romanelli

10 **Malignancies of Transplantation** 312
Michael A. Nalesnik

11 **Laboratory Medicine in Transplantation** 342
Phillip Ruiz, Ana Hernandez, Emilio Margolles-Clark, Alexandra Amador, Valia Bravo, Jennifer McCue, and Casiana Fernandez-Bango

Index 373

Contributors

Alexandra Amador, MS, MT
Department of Pathology
University of Miami Miller School of Medicine
Miami, FL USA

Thiago Beduschi, MD
Department of Surgery
University of Miami Miller School of Medicine
Miami Transplant Institute
Miami, FL USA

Valia Bravo, PhD, ABHI, MBA
Department of Immunogenetics
Children's Hospital of Philadelphia
Philadelphia, PA USA

George Burke, MD
Department of Surgery
University of Miami Miller School of Medicine
Miami Transplant Institute
Miami, FL USA

Linda Chen, MD
Department of Surgery
University of Miami Miller School of Medicine
Miami Transplant Institute
Miami, FL USA

Gaetano Ciancio, MD
Department of Surgery
University of Miami Miller School of Medicine
Miami Transplant Institute
Miami, FL USA

A. J. Demetris, MD
Division of Transplantation and Hepatic Pathology
Montefiore Hospital
University of Pittsburgh Medical Center
Pittsburgh, PA USA

Cinthia B. Drachenberg, MD
Department of Pathology
University of Maryland School of Medicine
Baltimore, MD USA

Ji Fan, MD
Department of Surgery
University of Miami Miller School of Medicine
Miami Transplant Institute
Miami, FL USA

Carol Farver, MD
Department of Anatomic Pathology
Cleveland Clinic
Cleveland, OH USA

Casiana Fernandez-Bango, MS, MT
Department of Surgery, Transplant Labs
University of Miami Miller School of Medicine
Miami, FL USA

Jennifer Garcia, MD
Department of Surgery
University of Miami Miller School of Medicine
Miami Transplant Institute
Miami, FL USA

Giselle Guerra, MD
Department of Medicine-Nephrology
University of Miami Miller School of Medicine
Miami Transplant Institute
Miami, FL USA

Ana Hernandez, PhD
Department of Surgery, Transplant Labs
University of Miami Miller School of Medicine
Miami, FL USA

Brian Keegan, MD
Department of Dermatology
New York University School of Medicine
New York, NY USA

Krishna V. Komanduri
Department of Medicine, Microbiology and Immunology
University of Miami Miller School of Medicine
Miami, FL USA

Warren Kupin, MD
Department of Medicine-Nephrology
University of Miami Miller School of Medicine
Miami Transplant Institute
Miami, FL USA

Emma Lanuti, MD
Department of Dermatology
Anne Arundel Medical Center
Annapolis, MD USA

Lazaros J. Lekakis
Adult Stem Cell Transplant Program,
University of Miami Sylvester Cancer Center
Miami, FL USA

Emilio Margolles-Clark, PhD
Department of Surgery, Transplant Labs
University of Miami Miller School of Medicine
Miami, FL USA

Adela Mattiazzi, MD
Department of Medicine-Nephrology
University of Miami Miller School of Medicine
Miami Transplant Institute
Miami, FL USA

Jennifer McCue, MS, MT
Department of Surgery, Transplant Labs
University of Miami Miller School of Medicine
Miami, FL USA

Marta I. Minervini, MD
Division of Transplantation and Hepatic Pathology
Montefiore Hospital
University of Pittsburgh Medical Center
Pittsburgh, PA USA

Michael A. Nalesnik, MD
Division of Transplantation and Hepatic Pathology
Montefiore Hospital
University of Pittsburgh Medical Center
Pittsburgh, PA USA

Seigo Nishida, MD
Department of Surgery
University of Miami Miller School of Medicine
Miami Transplant Institute
Miami, FL USA

John C. Papadimitriou, MD, PhD
Department of Pathology
University of Maryland School of Medicine
Baltimore, MD USA

Parmjeet S. Randhawa, MD
Division of Transplantation and Hepatic Pathology
Montefiore Hospital
University of Pittsburgh Medical Center
Pittsburgh, PA USA

E. Rene Rodriguez, MD
Department of Anatomic Pathology
The Cleveland Clinic
Cleveland, OH 44195 USA

Marco Romanelli, MD
Department of Clinical and Experimental Medicine
University of Pisa
Pisa PI, Italy

Paolo Romanelli, MD
Department of Dermatology
University of Miami Miller School of Medicine
Miami, FL USA

David Roth, MD
Department of Medicine-Nephrology
University of Miami Miller School
of Medicine
Miami Transplant Institute
Miami, FL USA

Phillip Ruiz, MD, PhD
Department of Surgery, Transplant Labs
University of Miami Miller School of Medicine
Miami, FL USA

Eizaburo Sasatomi, MD, PhD
Department of Pathology and Laboratory
Medicine
UNC School of Medicine
Chapel Hill, NC USA

Mohammed Sharaf, MD
Department of Dermatology
UC Health
Cincinnati, OH USA

Heather L. Stevenson-Lerner MD, PhD
Department of Pathology
University of Texas Medical Branch
Galveston, TX USA

Carmela D. Tan, MD
Department of Anatomic Pathology
The Cleveland Clinic
Cleveland, OH 44195 USA

Akin Tekin, MD
Department of Surgery
University of Miami Miller School of Medicine
Miami Transplant Institute
Miami, FL USA

Rodrigo Vianna, MD
Department of Surgery
University of Miami Miller School of Medicine
Miami Transplant Institute
Miami, FL USA

W. Dean Wallace, MD
Department of Pathology
Ronald Reagan UCLA Health
Los Angeles, CA USA

Ingrid Wolf, MD
Division of General Dermatology
Medical University of Graz
Graz, Austria

Preface

Since the First Edition of Transplantation Pathology, there has continued to be a steady and critical growth in our knowledge base in all areas of the field of transplantation. Central in this progress is our basic understanding of the pathophysiology of the critical cellular and molecular interactions between the allograft and the recipient that dictate the success or failure of the graft. Indeed, improved targeted intervention of specific cellular pathways is enabling scenarios of reduced drug-induced complications while maintaining graft function. In spite of these successes, solid organ and stem cell transplantation remain fraught with potential complications and require, as mentioned in the First Edition, "the unending and indispensable collaboration of, among many others, basic scientists, clinicians, and physicians of all disciplines." As such, there continues to be an evolution in the role(s) that pathologists potentially play in transplantation that now clearly ranges from the classical (but evolving) morphological interpretation of the histological changes of the graft that help determine whether the transplant is a success to the complex clinical laboratory testing needed to monitor these patients. In modern day transplant patient management, it is apparent now more than ever that the transplant pathologist should provide an amalgamation of specific anatomic *and* clinical pathology skills in order to provide the latest and most precise information to the clinical team.

The basic histopathology of transplant biopsies often remains a challenge to general pathologists, since these cases are only rarely seen in most pathology practices, are constantly evolving as clinical protocols are adjusted, and often coexist with other changes that can occur in the native organ counterpart. As in the First Edition, the Second Edition of this textbook assembles a wide range of pathological changes present in numerous types of transplants now commonly performed, and often describes alterations seen in several critical native organs (e.g., skin, gastrointestinal tissue, and lymphoid organs). Incorporating more than basic morphology is now clearly critical in evaluating the status of the transplant patient and thus, an updated chapter on lab medicine and transplantation has again been provided. In particular, molecular biological-based testing continues to grow in importance as a means of assessing the transplant patient; numerous examples are present throughout this textbook.

Lastly, this edition of *Transplantation Pathology* continues to provide some of the critical clinical information and correlates that the pathologist must have, as with many other types of medical biopsies, in order to provide the most comprehensive and relevant information from the biopsied material of the transplant patient.

The production and writing of this Second Edition of Transplantation Pathology would not have been possible without the contribution and cooperation of several of my esteemed friends and collaborators, who are recognized experts in this subdiscipline of pathology. As with the First Edition, I remain grateful to these coauthors for considering and donating their valuable time and effort to this endeavor and delivering what I consider to be wonderful compilations of different areas of the pathology of transplantation. Cambridge University Press continues to be an amazing (and patient!) partner who constantly encouraged me to continue going forward, when many times there were so many impediments to the completion of the sequel. In particular, Neil Ryan, Kirsten Bot, and Nisha Doshi from Cambridge were wonderful in their support and in facilitating the entire process. I am honored and humbled to have been so many years at the University of Miami and with all of the amazing superstars in the Immune Monitoring Laboratory (IML), as well as all of my Miami Transplant Institute friends and colleagues. Also, being the lab director of Auxilio Mutuo Hospital (HAM) in Puerto Rico for now six years has provided me an opportunity to personally grow and contribute to an amazing and dedicated transplant program that has only good things on the horizon. I as well look for many wonderful experiences with my newest partner at the University of Puerto Rico. I remain particularly and deeply indebted to Cristina Hersh and Nicole Lergier (at the University of Miami) and Myriam Centeno (at HAM) for their tireless support and for facilitating my day-to-day operations that allowed me to organize and put this work together.

My inspiration for pursuing and incorporating clinical, research, and educational aspects of transplantation as the major component of my academic life comes from the numerous colleagues and mentors whom I have had the pleasure of working alongside over the years in this field. There are too many of these people to mention who have influenced me, but several stand out as landmarks in my development, most notably, Juan Scornik, Andreas Tzakis, and the late Wayne Streilein. Their dedication, novel insight, and enthusiasm for transplantation and immunology fueled my passion for this field. I am likewise grateful to the devoted assemblage of physicians, nurses, lab technologists, and support staff comprising the outstanding transplant team at the University of Miami and Auxilio Mutuo – their illimitable enthusiasm, energy, and compassion for our patients have always inspired me and make coming to work a labor of love. Importantly, compiling this book or any of my other efforts in my career would not have been possible without the continuous and loving support and sacrifices of my family – they have never questioned the long hours, always provided me encouragement, and were critically important to my success in this field of medicine. Finally, I recognize those patients who have entrusted their lives to our transplant team, and are awaiting or have received this beautiful gift of life. The courage and extraordinary sacrifices of these remarkably strong individuals allows them to possess the marvel of a functioning organ from another person, and their willingness to undertake novel and often extreme new therapies or procedures permits us to acquire the necessary scientific foundation that will benefit future transplant populations.

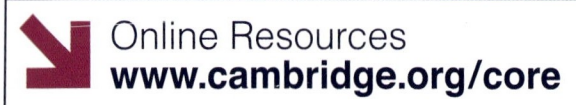

Online Resources
www.cambridge.org/core

- Fully searchable HTML text of the whole book
- Expandable figures and tables

Chapter 1

Immunopathology of Organ Transplantation

Phillip Ruiz

I Introduction

The History of Transplantation

Attempts to exchange tissues within and between species have been documented since the dawn of man, prior to a true scientific comprehension of the principles governing this practice. The ancient history of transplantation is conceptualized from anecdotes and folklore. For example, the Saints Cosmas and Damian allegedly treated a white patient by removing one of his legs and by grafting that of a black man who had died the same day in the third century [1] (see Figure 1.1) and the Chinese physician Bian Que "exchanged hearts" between individuals with different levels of strength. However, it wasn't until modern day medicine when progress was made with the likes of pioneers such as Carrel [2], Jaboulay, and Voronoy. Early on in the 20th century, the pathophysiological basis of organ transplant rejection was not understood, but critical technological and surgical advances were made that allowed the next wave of transplant physicians to attempt these procedures.

From the shaping work of Sir Peter B. Medawar emerged the hypothesis that the failure of organ transplantation is due to reactions seeded and controlled by the host's immune system. Medawar and colleagues described cases of patients with severe burns whereby autologous skin grafts healed in, but not allogeneic grafts, which were rejected, and in an accelerated fashion when taken repeatedly from the same donor [3]. These observations led to broad animal experimentations in this area. Consequently, a number of central tenets about organ transplantation became apparent – (i) a graft may be recognized as antigenic, and it may also be a source of immune cells, (ii) this two-way immune response between recipient and donor necessitates the need for immunosuppression for the survival of the graft and the host, and (iii) the ultimate goal of many of our efforts should be the induction and maintenance of immunological tolerance.

Transplanted grafts were further established to differ in their immunogenicity. Critical to this concept was the development by George Snell of inbred mice, by consecutive brother-sister mating for studying tumor genetics. He observed that tumor grafts and normal tissues were accepted between inbred animals, but not between animals of different strains [4]. Snell, in collaboration with Peter A. Gorer, termed the underlying gene locus most controlling this incompatibility between strains as histocompatibility 2, or H-2. This multifaceted gene locus was found to be remarkably complex, and the concept of the major histocompatibility complex (MHC)

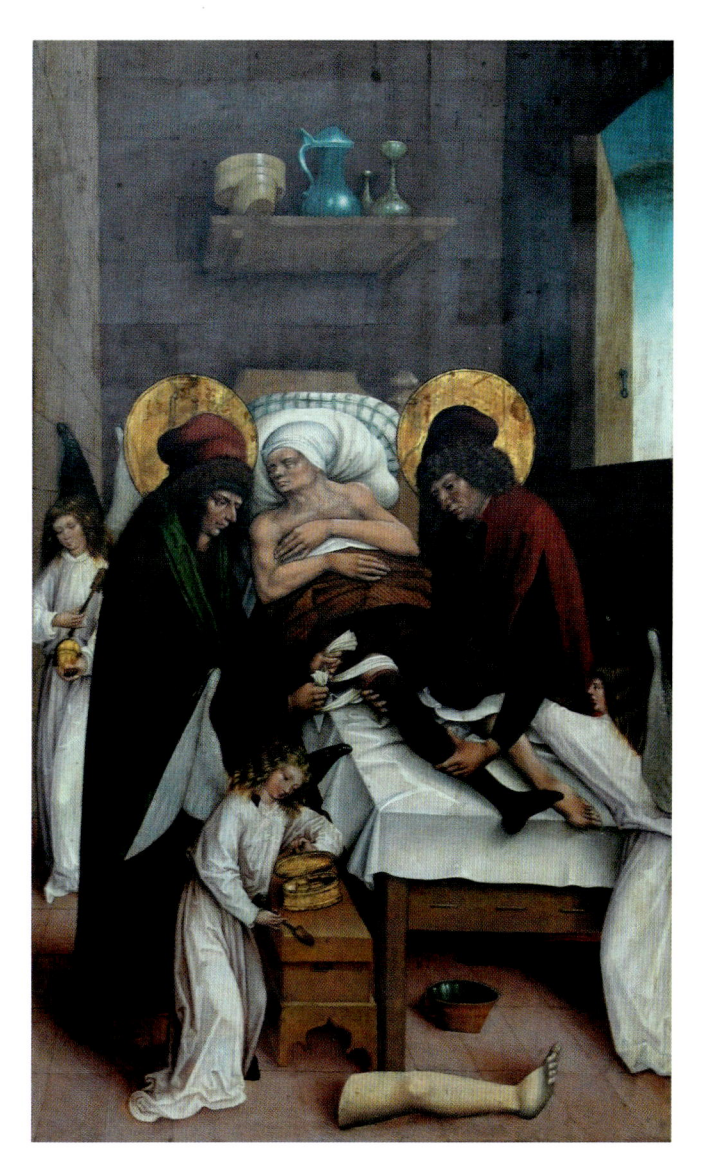

Figure 1.1 Saints Cosmas and Damian. Attributed to the Master of Los Balbases (ca. 1495).

was born, providing the basis for transplantation immunology and immunogenetics [5]. The human MHC was delineated in the beginning of the 1950s from findings in immunohematology. Jean Dausset observed that patients that had received many blood transfusions produced antibodies which could agglutinate white blood cells from donors, but not the patient's own cells [6]. Subsequent family studies suggested a genetically determined system, termed human leukocyte

Table 1.1 Representative Classes of Molecules Involved in Alloimmunity

Antigens and mediators
- Major Histocompatibility Complex, Minor Histocompatibility Antigens, ABO
- Cytokines (immune, inflammatory, regulatory), chemokines
- Various lipid mediators (e.g., leukotrienes, prostaglandins)

Immune receptors
- T cell receptor (TCR), B cell receptor (BCR), killer Ig-like receptor (KIR)

Immunological accessory and signaling molecules
- Adhesion molecules, Fc receptors, tetraspanins
- Cytokine receptors, chemokine receptors
- Costimulatory molecules: Positive Signal transducers
- Inhibitory molecules: Negative Signal transducers
- Pattern-recognition receptors

Signaling molecules

Transcription, Translation Process regulatory molecules (e.g., microRNA)

Antigen processing and presentation

Effector molecules
- Complement, granzyme B, perforin, apoptosis

antigens (HLA), and were found to be analogous with H-2 in the mouse. The MHC research in mice and humans were mutually complementary and the Nobel Prize was awarded to Dausset in 1980, together with Snell. A slew of investigators then began attributing functionality to the MHC that often was connected with the development and control of immune reactions. For example, Rolf Zinkernagel and Peter Doherty, among others, revealed that MHC gene region products are vital in the regulation of immune responses since the coded surface, transmembrane protein products are required for the presentation of peptide antigens to T cell receptors – a phenomenon termed MHC restriction [7]. However, these same molecules, in the context of transplantation between individuals, became the most important markers of biological incompatibility and were defined as the principal transplantation antigens. Numerous molecules maintain a critical role in transplantation and the generation of alloimmunity (see Table 1.1); however, it can be contended that histocompatibility molecules remain among the most critical.

II Basis of Alloreactivity – Histocompatibility Antigens, Non-MHC; Graft Immunogenicity

There are a variety of solid organ allografts, as well as hematopoietic grafts, that can be introduced into a host (see Figure 1.2). As such, there are inherent differences in the immunogenicity between these different types of grafts, as well as distinctive types of cells targeted by the conglomeration of the innate and adaptive immune responses known collectively as *alloimmunity* (see Figure 1.2). At a molecular level, the basis for alloreactive responses is genetic incompatibilities of components of tissue that then represent antigenic disparity between the donor and the recipient. These moieties can be classified into three broad categories: the major histocompatibility complex antigens, minor histocompatibility antigens, and non-MHC or tissue-specific antigens.

a Major Histocompatibility Antigens (MHC)

The MHC of humans encodes two major classes of proteins: HLA class I (HLA -A, -B, and -C), and HLA class II (HLA -DP, -DQ, and -DR) [8, 9]. *Class I transmembrane molecules* are expressed on the surface of virtually all nucleated cells at varying densities. *Class II molecules* are expressed primarily by B lymphocytes, macrophages, and dendritic cells; however, immunomodulatory molecules such as interferon-gamma (IFN-γ) can upregulate class II expression on a variety of cell types, including endothelium, epithelium, and T lymphocytes.

The archetypal function of MHC molecules is to present *antigenic peptides* from proteins generated inside the cell or from an extracellular pool to T cells [10]. MHC class I molecules on antigen-presenting cells (APCs) present endogenous antigens produced within the cell such as viruses and oncogenic products in the form of short (eight to ten amino acids) peptides. These MHC-peptide complexes are then recognized by specific cytotoxic $CD8^+$ T lymphocytes, which become activated, proliferate, and ultimately eliminate virally infected cells and tumor cells. Under normal circumstances, MHC class II on the APC present exogenous antigens as peptide fragments to $CD4^+$ helper T cells (see Figure 1.3). There may also be cross-presentation of extracellular antigen on class I antigens to $CD8^+$ [11]. Generally, two pathways for presenting peptides are determined by the mode of antigen uptake by the APC. For class I restricted presentation, there is the peptide-loading complex, a collection of endoplasmic reticulum proteins in the (ER) that incorporates newly synthesized MHC class I-beta-2 microglobulin heterodimers, and that facilitates peptide loading along with MHC class I assembly [12]. By comparison, external antigen is guided to the lysosomal compartment for presentation by class II MHC. As such, APCs activate and modulate distinctive arms of the T cell response. Activated T helper cells produce cytokines and other molecules that enhance T cell activity and lead to the secretion of antibodies by B cells, which can eliminate extracellular antigens.

The MHC is distinctly *polymorphic*, a mechanism that permits a species to have a superior collective immunity versus constantly mutating pathogens. Regrettably, transplant rejection is a direct outcome of this polymorphic diversity, since the chances of randomly getting an unrelated recipient and donor to be genetically compatible at HLA class I and class II are exceedingly small. As noted before, the MHC molecules themselves act as the primary antigens responsible for the induction of the alloimmune response, via different pathways discussed below.

b Minor Histocompatibility Antigens

Another group of antigens, the minor histocompatibility antigens (MiHA) were discovered somewhat inadvertently. The

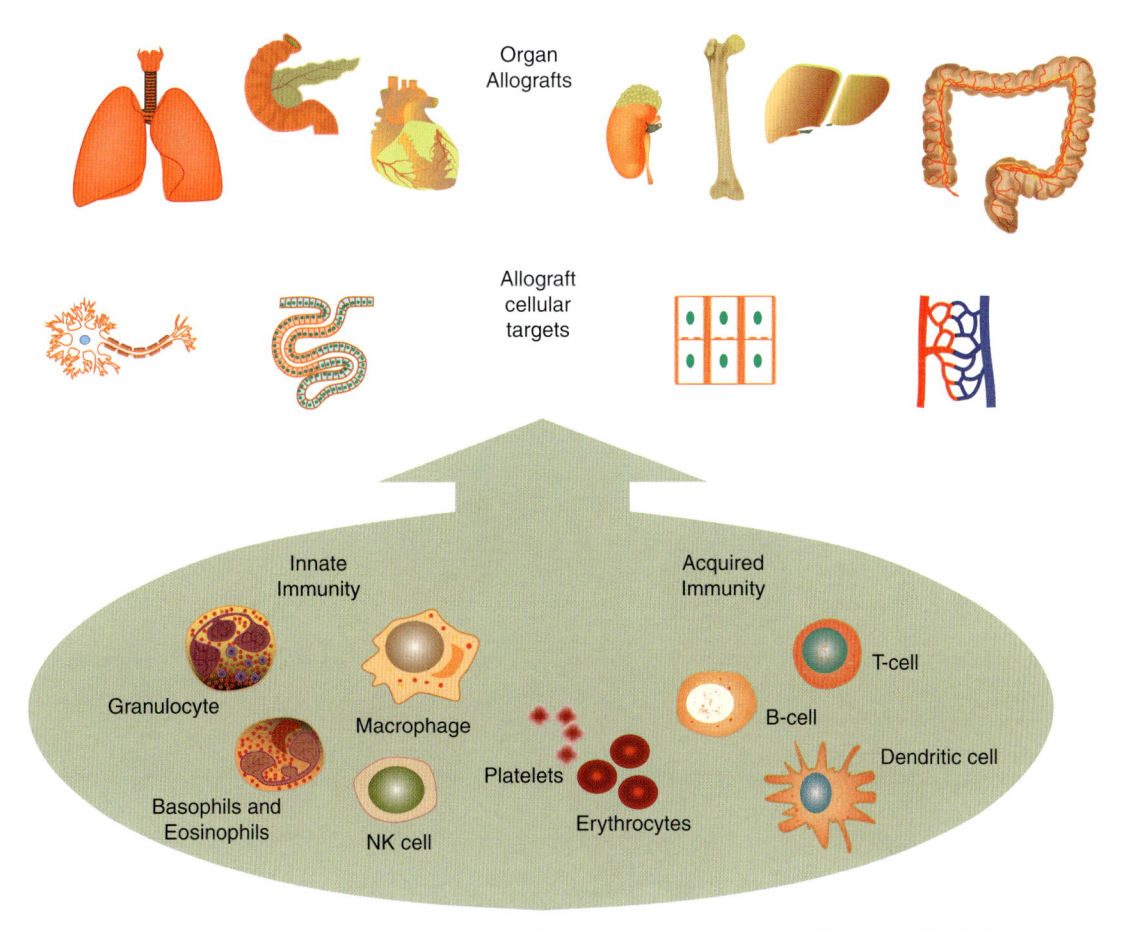

Figure 1.2 Antigen presentation mechanisms operative in allograft recognition and rejection. CD4-positive T cells (donor or recipient, depending upon the organ allograft) upon recognition of alloantigen with APC become activated and serve as central hub for the generation of alloantibodies, cytolytic cell generation, and potentiation of the innate immune response.

first report on the possible influence of MiHAs on the outcome of Hematopoietic Stem Cell Transplantation (HSCT) was observed in a female aplastic anemia patient who rejected the BM transplanted from her HLA-identical brother. Cytotoxic T cells (CTLs) isolated from the patient's blood lysed cells that were HLA matched and of male origin [13, 14]. The T cell reactivity observed in the host-versus-graft (HVG) direction in this case was restricted to male cells, thus indicating that the target structures had to be encoded by a gene on the Y chromosome. Similarly, CTLs isolated from a patient suffering from severe Graft-versus-Host Disease (GVHD) after HLA-identical HSCT lysed patient's hematopoietic cells collected before HSCT, but not those of the donor [14]. The MiHA reactivity in this patient was directed against an antigen encoded by an autosomal gene. Various biochemical and molecular approaches have subsequently been used to characterize human MiHAs. A moderate number of autosomal and Y-chromosome-encoded (e.g., H-Y antigen) MiHAs have been identified in humans and they are polymorphic within the species, thus making them capable of eliciting host response [15] or HVG/GVHD when there is recipient-donor disparity [16, 17]. The MiHAs can be presented as peptides on the cell surface (sometimes exclusively on hematopoietic cells) primarily by MHC class I and occasionally by class II molecules [18, 19].

c Tissue-specific Antigens (TSA)

As has been known for some time, the regulation of central tolerance to self-antigens is a tightly controlled thymic process [20] that, when disrupted, can lead to self-immunity and the ultimate development of autoimmune disease. It is also known that autoimmunity can sometimes develop or be exacerbated following solid organ transplantation or HSCT, presumably via deregulation of self-antigen tolerance processes [21]. As such, molecules that are typically not immunogenic can sometimes elicit powerful responses to the grafted tissue and this is, in a way, *rejection*. These *tissue-specific antigens*, as the name implies, are restricted in their expression to various tissues and organs. As compared to cancer immunology and autoimmunity, TSA remain poorly understood insofar as their role in transplantation immunobiology. Their role(s) may potentially be both as elicitors of anti-graft immune responses or as facilitators of graft acceptance. Some well-characterized molecules, such as myosin, become immunogenic only after injury to the grafted tissue and thereafter perpetuate an organ-specific response [22]. Other molecules are poorly characterized and remain speculative since there are only collections of individual reports with no comprehensive study of these antigens. An intriguing possibility is that TSA possess varying degrees of

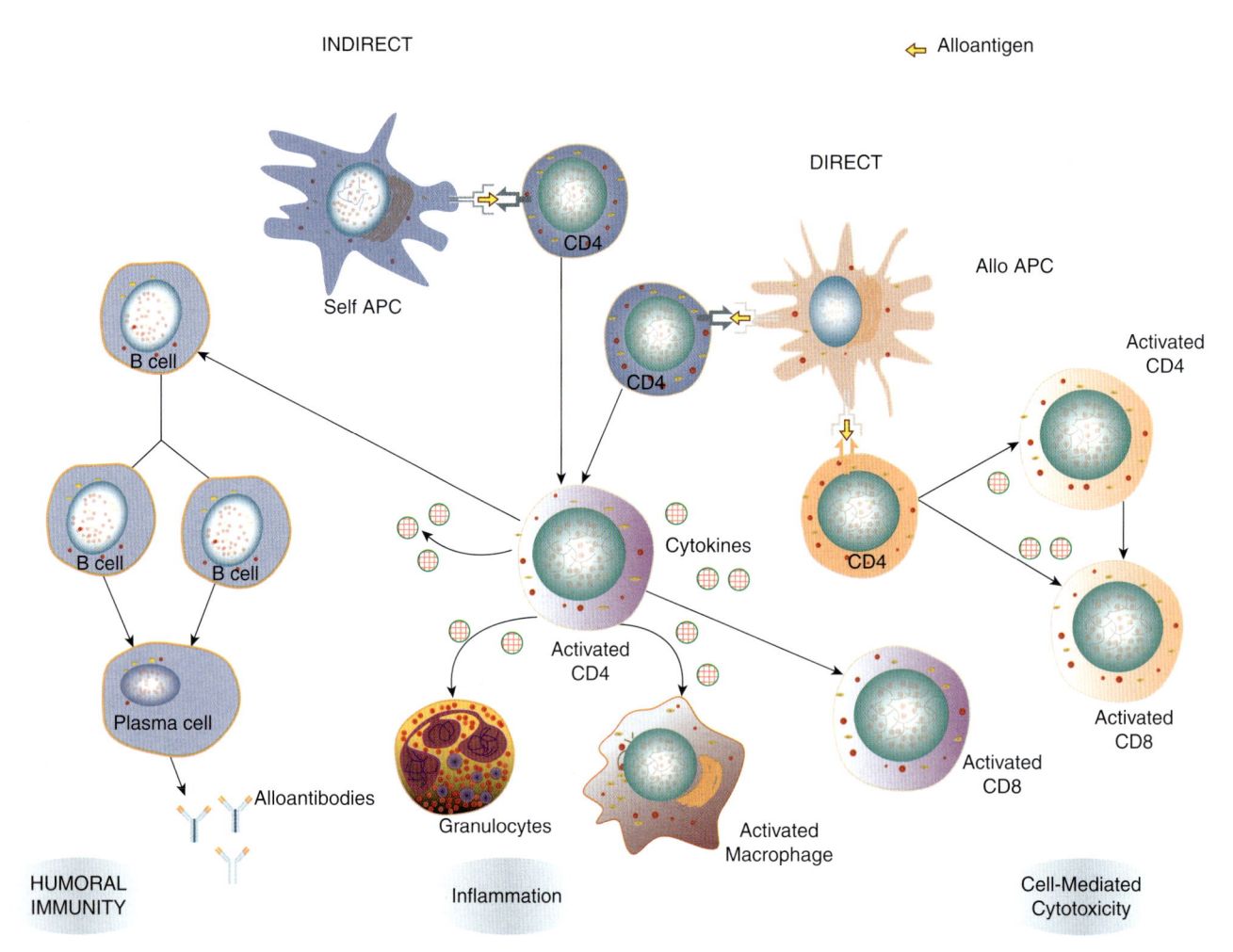

Figure 1.3 Different cell types involved in allograft rejection are involved in organ allograft rejection, comprising both the adaptive general inflammatory responses. A variety of cell types can be targeted, including (from left) neurological cells, epithelial cell structures such as glands, and hepatocytes, as well as veins and arteries. The character of the immune response and types of targeted cells depends upon many variables, including the level of antigen disparity, the immune capacity of the host, and the cellular and physiological composition of the various types of transplanted organs, examples depicted in the top row.

polymorphism [23] among individuals due to variations in their primary or secondary structures. These dissimilarities are potential stimulators or regulators of alloreactivity.

III Immune Networks Involved in Alloreactivity; HVG and GVH, Immune Tolerance

The MHC, MiHA, and TSA differences between the donor and recipient bear the potential to elicit destructive or "effector" alloreactive responses that are manifested clinically as host-versus-graft (HVG) or as graft-versus-host (GVH) responses. If these effector types of responses are of sufficient severity and duration, these reactions can result in the loss of the graft or GVHD that can contribute to the demise of the patient. However, there also sometimes exist initial means to prevent the development of these effector cells and/or there may be expansion of regulatory alloimmune cell populations that may promote graft acceptance and help implement true immunological tolerance.

a Host-versus-Graft (HVG) Reactivity

Following organ transplantation, the recipient recognizes the donor-derived polymorphic MHC, MiHAs, or TSA as foreign and an immune response is then mounted that will destroy the transplanted organ unless effective immunosuppressive measures are taken. *Organ rejection has generally been classified clinically as hyperacute, acute, subclinical, and chronic* [24]. Hyperacute responses occur rapidly (e.g., within minutes to hours), are mediated by high titers of preformed antibody, and depending upon the solid organ being transplanted, tend to be unalterable. Acute and subclinical responses generally are cell-mediated and/or antibody-mediated in nature, occur over the course of days to months, and are often reversible with a variety of immunosuppressive reagents. Chronic rejection occurs in the span of months to years, is typically unresponsive to current therapy, and has emerged as a major impediment to long-term graft survival.

Donor alloantigens are capable of being presented to the recipient immune system via either direct or indirect antigen presentation pathways (see Figure 1.3). In the *direct pathway*, intact donor class I and II MHC molecules present on the

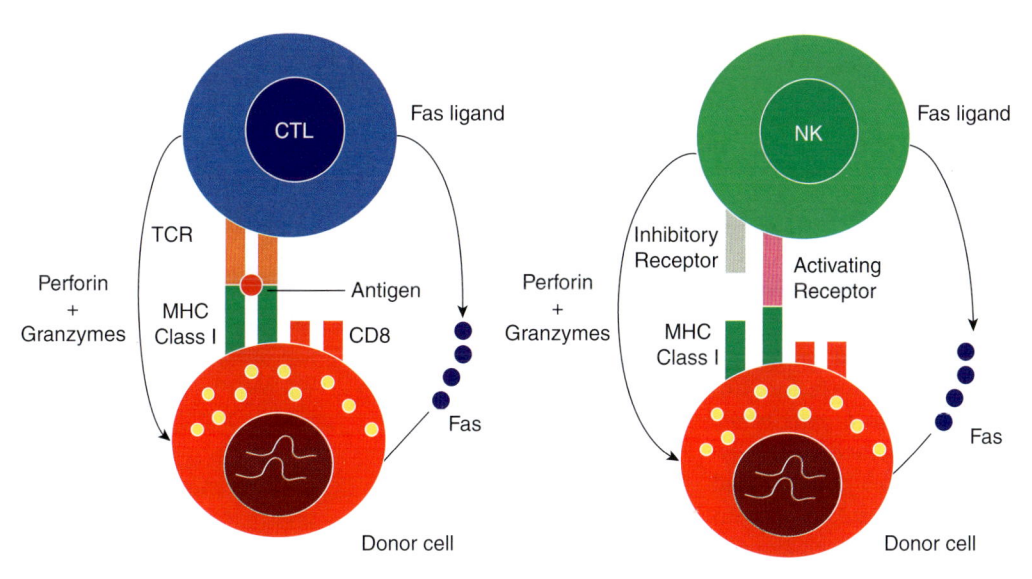

Figure 1.4 Depiction of cytotoxic T cell and NK cell mechanisms of inflicting injury on donor cells.

surface of *donor APC* are recognized directly *by recipient* CD8+ and CD4+ T cells, respectively. In the *indirect pathway*, donor allopeptides are taken up, processed, and presented in the context of *recipient MHC* molecules to *recipient* CD8+ and CD4+ T cells [25, 26]. The T cell receptor repertoire displays a high precursor frequency of alloreactive T cells in the direct pathway and a relatively low frequency in the indirect pathway. This accounts for the vigorous response seen after direct allorecognition and this is responsible for early rejection episodes; the lower number of precursor alloreactive cells present after indirect allorecognition accounts for the more tempered and protracted late rejection events. This is consistent with the notion that donor-derived "passenger" leucocytes in the transplanted organ steadily disappear with time, making the direct pathway progressively inoperative. On the other hand, the acquisition, processing, and presentation of donor antigens by recipient APC is a slower process that is more efficient during later stages after transplantation; the acute rejection derived from the indirect pathway tends to persist and likely underlies chronic rejection, ostensibly by promoting alloantibody production as well as delayed-type hypersensitivity. With the description of these pathways, this advances the query of how directly and indirectly activated T cells interrelate to each other. A third pathway has also been proposed, the *semi-direct pathway* [26] linking the two previous pathways. In this pathway, recipient dendritic cells (DCs) can acquire intact MHC molecules from donor cells and undertake direct presentation to recipient T cells. There is a growing body of evidence suggesting that alloreactive CD4+ and CD8+ T cells with specificity for both direct and indirect pathways contribute to graft rejection [27].

Following the recognition of transplantation antigens in the allograft, recipient or donor T lymphocytes and other effector cell populations are activated to proliferate, differentiate, and secrete a variety of immunomodulatory cytokines. Among their various effects, these cytokines are capable of increasing baseline expression of HLA molecules on engrafted tissues, such as vascular endothelium – this effect can ultimately increase the immunogenicity of the graft. These mediators can also promote B lymphocytes to secrete high affinity and high titer antibodies against the allograft, and can potentiate cytotoxic T cells, macrophages, and natural killer cells to develop cytotoxicity against the graft (see Figure 1.2). To this end, it is important to note that NK and NKT cells are also critical cells in solid organ and bone marrow transplantation since they also have the ability to distinguish allogeneic MHC molecules, and due to their potent cytolytic potential (see Figure 1.4), they participate in the alloimmune response solid organ graft rejection as well as Graft-versus-Host Disease (GVHD) (see Section b, Graft-versus-Host Disease). The participation of NK cells in HVG, GVHD, and allograft tolerance is at least partially mediated by inhibitory and/or activating Killer Ig-like Receptor (KIR) and KIR ligands [28]. This polymorphic gene family expressed on NK cells, γδ T cells, and αβ T cells can influence the activity of these cells depending on the matching KIR/KIR ligand haplotypes between the recipient and donor [29, 30].

b Graft-versus-Host Disease (GVHD)

Graft-versus-Host Disease (GVHD), a common complication of allogeneic hematopoietic stem cell transplantation (HSCT), can also occur, although at a relatively lower frequency after solid organ transplantation [31]. The first case of GVHD following solid organ transplantation was reported in 1988 [32] and the incidence of GVHD in adult liver transplant recipients is estimated to be 1%–2% [33–36]. The frequency of GVHD in other (non-hepatic) solid organ transplant recipients varies, although it remains a complication and it should always be considered when there is a suspicious clinical presentation [37]. In some organs with massive hematopoietic cell inoculums (e.g., multivisceral transplantation), GVHD is a relatively frequent and often fatal complication [38]; by comparison, recipients of kidney, combined kidney–pancreas, and pancreas–spleen allografts, and recipients of heart, lung, or combined heart–lung allografts tend to have GVHD post-transplant less often, likely due to reduced infusion of donor lymphocytes in the graft [39, 40]. These donor cells can potentially be regulatory cells via chimeric influence on reducing immunity [41, 42] or they can evolve to effector immune cells that mediate a vigorous and often protracted assault on host tissues. The mortality of patients diagnosed with GVHD can be very high for the transplant patients experiencing this complication. Risk factors suggested for GVHD in liver transplant recipients include close HLA match between donor and recipient [43], and advanced recipient age [44, 45] and underlying recipient immunodeficiency may be a contributing factor [46].

Graft-versus-Host Disease occurs in both *acute and chronic forms*, each with different kinetics and distinctive pathology. Skin, liver, gut, lung, and lymphoid tissues are the principal target organs of acute GVHD. Historically, acute GVHD can be considered in a framework of *three sequential phases*: conditioning (phase 1), donor T cell activation (phase 2), and cellular and inflammatory effectors (phase 3) [47] [48]. Donor T cells infused into a host that has been profoundly damaged by underlying disease, infection, and the transplant-conditioning regimen result in substantial proinflammatory changes in endothelial and epithelial cells. Thereafter, antigen presentation and the subsequent activation, proliferation, and differentiation of donor T cells result in *alloreactivity* within secondary lymphoid organs [47, 49]. Direct and indirect antigen presentations are both involved, i.e., donor T cells can be directly activated *by host-derived APCs or donor-derived APCs* which cross-present host antigens [47]. Changes in phase 1 dramatically influence antigen presentation. Host DCs can be maturated and activated [50] by (i) inflammatory cytokines such as tumor necrosis factor-alpha (TNF-α) and interleukin-1 (IL-1); (ii) by microbial products such as lipopolysaccharide (LPS) and CpG oligonucleotides entering systemic circulation from intestinal mucosa damaged by conditioning; and (iii) by necrotic cells that were damaged by conditioning. This activation enhances the recognition of MHC antigens or MiHAs by mature donor T cells. As mentioned above, NK and NKT cells are also important in the generation and sustaining of GVHD. The NK cell role in GVHD is affected by the type of KIR/KIR ligand haplotype matching between host and recipient [51] and thus, in addition to HLA matching, it is recommended the KIR matching between donor and recipient be also considered.

Interestingly, genome-wide scans of patients undergoing HSCT have now demonstrated that there may be predisposing genetic associations with GVHD [52]; validation studies will be necessary to establish these molecules as risk factors for the development of GVHD after solid organ transplantation or HSCT.

c Immune Tolerance

Tolerance is the *specific absence of an immune response to a given antigen* and is the long-sought "Holy Grail" of clinical transplantation [53]. Current immunosuppressive protocols in clinical organ transplantation have not typically allowed the development of true immunological tolerance, but rather, on occasion, *operational tolerance*, an occurrence whose underlying

Table 1.2 Tolerance Mechanisms in Transplantation

Tolerance	Mediated by	Mechanism
Central	Deletion	Reactive clones deleted in the thymus by positive or negative selection. Reviewed in [68].
Peripheral	Regulation	Regulatory cell subsets of T, NK, dendritic, and B cell lineages actively inhibiting the responses of reactive clones.
	Anergy	Incomplete activation of clones by the binding of the primary receptor (TCR or BCR) by cognate antigen in the absence of the second signal.
	Clonal exhaustion	Prolonged and sustained stimulation results in the overexertion of the clones, which in turn makes them incapable of further response.
	Deletion	Removal of the reactive clones by active killing, antibody-dependent cellular cytotoxicity (ADCC), apoptosis, cytokine starvation, etc.

mechanisms are only partly understood [54, 55]. The preferred situation with tolerance in transplantation is the lack of a specific *pathogenic* response. Though tolerance can be achieved in animal models through appropriately timed disruption of numerous immune mechanisms, applications of the same methodologies to clinical organ transplantation are promising, but as of yet, have not led to similar levels of success [56]. As such, any meaningful discussion on true immune tolerance can only be made based mostly on studies in animal models. Tolerance is the default response to a multitude of self and environmental antigens, and many of the mechanisms that maintain self-tolerance may *also* be capable of promoting allograft tolerance. Generally, tolerance mechanisms can be broadly classified as either central or peripheral [57]. Peripheral tolerance, the process by which self-reactive T cells that have escaped negative selection in the thymus, are rendered anergic or deleted in the periphery can involve several mechanisms, including ignorance [58, 59], anergy [60, 61], regulation or suppression [62, 63], and apoptosis or peripheral deletion [64, 65] (see Table 1.2). This is all controlled and likely mediated in the periphery by resident dendritic cells and lymph node stroma [66].

i) **Central Tolerance:** Central tolerance refers to the deletion within the thymus of T cells whose affinity for self-antigens is inappropriately high and thus likely to result in autoimmunity [67–69]. The tolerance displayed by neonatal mice to a transplanted organ [70] or mice displaying mixed hematopoietic chimerism following bone marrow transplantation [57] are examples of the central deletional mechanisms. In addition to central deletion, a number of mechanisms operating in the periphery have been reported to contribute to the tolerant state.

ii) **Ignorance**: Immune ignorance is a purported mechanism mediating tolerance that relates to a failure of the immune response to recognize the presence of antigen that does not reach organized lymphoid tissue. For example, mice lacking secondary lymphoid organs can accept skin or heart allografts indefinitely [71]. Impaired rejection in this model results from the failure of T cells to be primed when they encountered donor antigens outside of lymphoid organs. However, later observations of examples where recipient T cells can be primed by alloantigens encountered within the allograft [72] and that memory T cells can be reactivated after encountering antigen outside of secondary lymphoid organs [73, 74] raise the possibility that the role of this mechanism may be limited.

iii) **Suppression**: Active, antigen-specific suppression of immune responses was first described approximately four decades ago [75, 76] and though interest in this phenomenon diminished, the demonstration that an elimination of $CD4^+CD25^+$ T cells in murine models could result in autoimmune disorders [77, 78] revitalized the field. A growing body of experimental and clinical evidence suggests a role for regulatory T cells in the induction and maintenance of tolerance [62, 63]. There is heterogeneity among regulatory immune T cells and it is known that natural Treg cells develop in the thymus or there can be inducible CD4+ Treg cells in the periphery [79]. Although surface CD4/CD25 coexpression is often used to characterize Treg or induce Tregs, to date, the default marker of true regulatory T cells is the intracellular forkhead/winged-helix transcription factor (FoxP3) [80]. The control of FoxP3 expression is complex and critical to the induction of regulatory T cells that govern activity of effector immune cell populations; the Nr4a family of transcription factors appears vital to being the gatekeeper for FoxP3 expression [81].

There are a variety of other regulatory cell populations aside from $CD4^+CD25^+$/FoxP3+ T cells. These include T_R1 cells (FoxP3+ cells that develop in the presence of IL10) [82], CD8+ Treg cells [83], NKT cells [84], CD4-/CD8-/TCRαβ+/CD3+ cells [85], regulatory B cells [86], plasmacytoid dendritic cells (DC) [87], myeloid-derived suppressor cells (MDSC) [88], regulatory macrophages [89], and mesenchymal stem cells (MSC) [90].

With so many potential regulatory cell populations, there are also, predictably, a notable number of potential mechanisms by which tolerance is mediated. For example, production of the *cytokines* IL-10 [91] and TGF-β [92], as well as contact-dependent regulatory effects by the cell surface molecules GITR [93, 94] and CTLA4 [95, 96], are among many purported mechanisms. Understandably, the orchestration of the numerous regulatory cell types and mechanisms in providing the overall comprehensive "suppressive" phenotype has not been dissected.

Although regulatory T cells have been extensively studied in experimental animal models, there is less known about their role in clinical transplantation tolerance. Salama et al. reported that $CD25^+$ regulatory cells developed as early as three months after renal transplantation and persisted for years [97], as well as other studies [98, 99]. However, the presence of clinical tolerance in solid organ transplantation is uncommon and it remains clear that although Treg cells are present, their influence following organ transplantation is insufficient to be able to create and sustain tolerance under current immunosuppressive regimens. Currently, clinical tolerance approaches pertaining to regulatory cells are likely to require interventions that purposely produce regulatory cells and these include infusions and clinical use of *in vitro*-generated regulatory T cells [100]. Alternatively, modification of immunosuppressive agent regimens appears to have an effect on regulatory cells. Delay or sparing of calcineurin inhibitors (known to inhibit the development of tolerance by preventing the activation or function of regulatory T cells) [101], the use of rapamycin [102], and lymphocyte depleting regimens (e.g., alemtuzumab) [103] all may hold promise in facilitating regulatory cell presence. These protocols may be used in the presence of the infusion protocols.

iv) **Anergy and Deletion**: In addition to ignorance and regulation, peripheral deletion of immune cells may contribute to tolerance [104, 105]. This can occur in the setting of chronic alloantigen stimulation or when alloantigen is encountered under suboptimal conditions for T cell activation. For example, *clonal exhaustion* after liver transplantation is due to chronic stimulation induction of peripheral T cell deletion [106]. Suboptimal antigen presentation or an induction of chimerism may facilitate clonal exhaustion. The blockade of costimulatory signals such as CD28 or CD154 at the time T cells encounter alloantigens can result in incomplete T cell activation, anergy, and apoptosis [107, 108]. Potentially, prolonged and sustained anergy can result in the deletion of the reactive clones; the latter can be mediated by apoptosis and this can contribute to long-term allograft acceptance [109, 110]. *Apoptosis* of T cells can be brought about either by cell surface death receptors or cytokine withdrawal. The death receptors mediating apoptosis are comprised of TNF receptor superfamily members that have a cytoplasmic death domain that binds cell-signaling proteins such as TRADD, FADD, FLICE, and caspase-3 [111–113].

v) **Molecular Phenotype of Operational Tolerance**: As mentioned above, to date, the acquisition of "tolerance" in solid organ recipients has involved scenarios where the transplant recipient is no longer taking immunosuppressive medication, but there remains normal functioning of the allograft and no clinical evidence of ongoing rejection. This has been termed "operational tolerance" [54, 55], since there may still be an enduring specific alloimmune response in the host (a situation not seen in true experimental immune tolerance). These relatively rare transplant patients have come about either because of recipient non-compliance with medications, necessary cessation of immunosuppression due to ongoing infectious or malignancy complications, "weaning" protocols in liver transplant patients [114], and some patients that selectively received tolerance induction protocols [115]; at times, these patients manifest acute rejection late in their course, further verifying that indeed the effector portion of their immune response to the donor remains intact. A molecular analysis of these unique operationally tolerant liver and renal transplant recipients has yielded interesting results that to date have confirmed that multiple mechanisms are likely contributing to the clinical phenotype in these patients. For example, liver transplant patients with operational tolerance show peripheral gene signatures that differ from patients that were on immunosuppression, most surprisingly being natural killer-related transcripts [116] and iron homeostasis [117]. By comparison, renal transplant patients with operational tolerance to date have had different molecular signatures from the tolerant liver patients, notably including perturbation of B cell gene profiles [118]. While these initial studies are exciting, they do emphasize that there are not currently any unifying mechanisms in operational tolerance between different organ transplants. At this point, the predisposing (e.g., genetic) factors among transplant recipient populations that incline some persons to becoming operationally tolerant are undetermined. Additionally, the readout of "tolerance" to date in clinical transplantation is far from perfect; clinical and pathological (i.e., biopsy) evidence remain the best indicators of absence of rejection, but do nothing to address the underlying immunological potential of the host to manifest donor-specific alloimmunity. Though there has been some progress in developing specific immune tests, there still remain no unifying and validated laboratory assays or biomarkers that can be clinically utilized to evaluate the presence of immune tolerance [119, 120].

IV Mechanisms of Graft Injury

The principal causes of graft injury can be summarized as those resulting from ischemia, innate immune activation, protracted inflammation with accompanying elaboration of soluble factors, followed by acute and then chronic rejection episodes that are mediated by donor-specific antibodies and/or active cellular infiltrations. It is important to note that a variety of cell types (see Figure 1.2) and mediators can inflict injury to an organ allograft. Infections and recurrent/de novo immune diseases may also produce concomitant tissue damage (see Table 1.3).

a The Effects of Ischemia and Innate Immune Activation

The absence of appropriate blood flow to harvested organs (ischemia) and the return of blood supply to the allograft (reperfusion) can result in a wide variety of inflammatory and oxidative changes that can influence short- and long-term graft function (see Figure 1.5). In addition to ischemia/reperfusion injury (I/R injury), infections and various genetic polymorphisms in the recipient can also contribute to activation of innate immune mechanisms that may then amplify antigen-specific (i.e., allospecific) acquired immune responses. Activation of the innate immune system by these forms of injury typically is more pronounced in cadaveric donors, although it may also be seen to a lesser degree in living

Table 1.3 Mechanisms of Graft Injury

Cell Pathway or Pathological Process	Mediators	Mechanism
Innate Immune Activation	Toll-like receptors, inflammatory, cytokines, and chemokines	Injuries, trauma of death, ischemia, and other insults result in non-cognate inflammation and activation of antigen presenting cells. This can be directly injurious and also may initiate adaptive immunity.
Acute Rejection	Antibody-mediated	Preformed and de novo antibodies to MHC, ABO, MiHAs, and tissue-specific antigens bind to their cognate receptors in the graft and cause injury via activation of the complement pathway or by other means.
	Cell-mediated	Chemokines and cytokines attract and upregulated adhesion molecules retain immune cells, predominantly activated CD4 and CD8 T cells and a mixture of monocytes, B cells, and NK cells, resulting in tissue damage.
Chronic Rejection	Cellular infiltration, TH1/inflammatory cytokines secretion, and antibody deposition	The actions of the immune mediators occur late and for extended duration in the post-transplant period. May result in the fibrosis of various structures of the allograft.
Infection	Viral – CMV, EBV, Polyoma, Hepatitis-C, etc.	Direct pathogenic effects and indirect anti-infection immunity may cause inflammation, arteriosclerosis, or cirrhosis of the allograft.
Recurrent/de novo immune diseases	Recurrence of the original disease for which the native organ needed to be transplanted.	

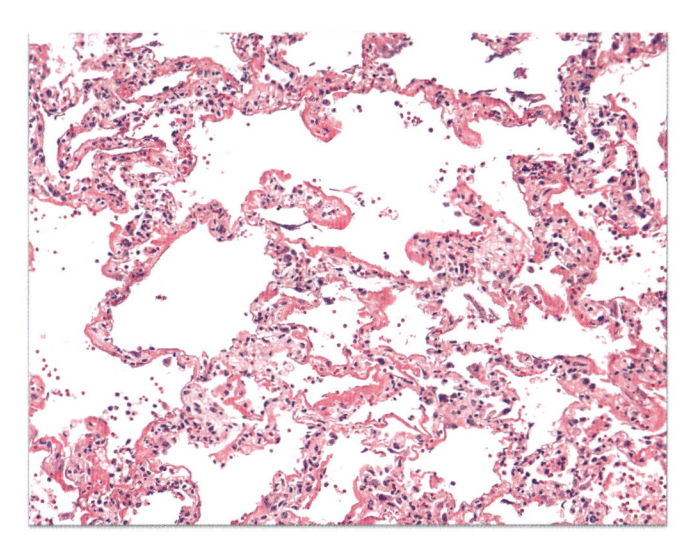

Figure 1.5 Lung undergoing ischemia/reperfusion injury with primary graft failure due to ischemia-reperfusion injury: hyaline membranes line alveolar septa and minimal inflammatory infiltrate is noted (H&E, 400x).

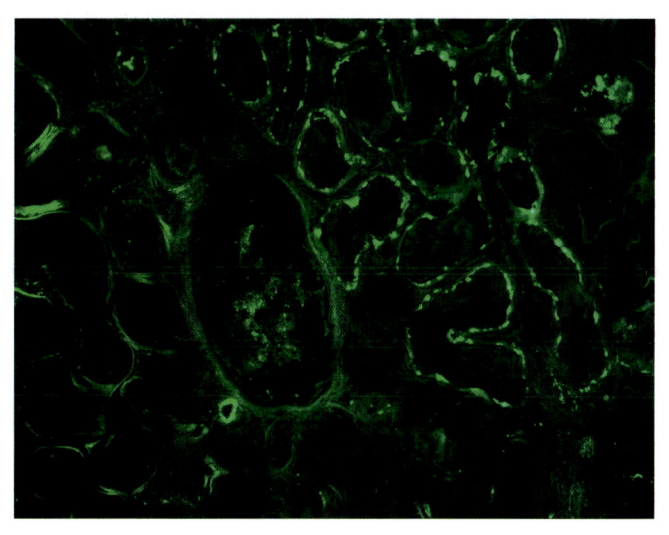

Figure 1.6 C3 in kidney following ischemic reperfusion injury (immunofluorescence, 200x).

donors, depending on the situation [121]. The effects of I/R injury and infections in the newly transplanted organ, aside from innate immune activation, result in the increased appearance of a variety of molecules that potentially contributes to an initiation of acute rejection and thus may also contribute to long-term allograft injury via a potentiation of chronic rejection [122]. Among the molecules that are modified by early nonspecific graft injury are HLA antigens, adhesion molecules, various complement molecules, and mediators involved in the activation of the innate immune response (see Figure 1.6); the early presence of these molecules [123–125] may identify patients at higher risk for early graft dysfunction.

Among the effects of I/R injury to the allograft can be an increased but unpredictable expression of allostimulatory major and minor histocompatibility molecules in a variety of cell types in the transplant. Increased MHC class I, major histocompatibility class I-related chain A (MIC-A) and MIC-B, and *de novo* MHC class II have all been described to increase in allografts following ischemic injury [126–128] [129, 130]. Allografts that have aberrant class II expression on certain parenchymal structures (e.g. tubular cells) may be predisposed to increased risk from inflammatory injury [131, 132]. Atypical class II expression can be immediate following initial injury, but it can also be sustained for an extended period (e.g., up to a year post-transplant), thus serving as continual graft epithelial and endothelial antigenic stimulation to immune cells [133, 134].

All arms of the adaptive immune response can be influenced by initial nonspecific I/R injury and innate immune activation. For example, antibody-mediated allograft rejection is partially mediated and influenced by the presence of complement proteins; these molecules can also be induced following nonspecific injury in the early post-transplant period [135]. Allografts experiencing preservation injury can demonstrate C3 and other split products on many structures of the viscera. If the patient is already allosensitized, this bears the potential of facilitating and accelerating humoral as well as cellular immunity to the graft. Among the many other molecules initiated following innate immunity activation, as well as I/R injury, are Toll-like receptors (TLRs). These membrane-spanning receptors recognize structurally conserved molecules derived from microbes; upon their recognition, these molecules may activate immune cell responses via the innate immune system. TLRs have been demonstrated on harvested organs exposed to ischemia reperfusion injury. Simultaneously, "endogenous" innate immune ligands may be released during inflammation. Such putative ligands include heat shock proteins (HSP), uric acid, hyaluronan, fibrinogen, and chromatin [136–138]. Some of these ligands have been found to signal via TLRs, predominantly TLR 4.

Heat shock proteins (HSPs) are cytoplasmic chaperone proteins that have a variety of functions and that are inducible under stress conditions such as heat and injury [136]. Organ transplants, I/R injury, and infections can induce the expression of this family of molecules with variable expression according to the type of allograft and the extent of injury. Ultimately, the role(s) that HSPs play in graft injury remains undetermined – it is possible that these proteins may contribute to potentiating the alloimmune response and/or they may be cytoprotective and behave as chaperone proteins that allow the cells to survive biochemical insults [139, 140].

All transplanted organs inherently possess a system of innate immune defenses, and a number of the above mentioned molecules and stimuli contribute to an activation of this form of immunity. What remains uncertain is the importance of innate immunity in the context of affecting the specific adaptive immune response to the allograft. The boundary between innate and adaptive immune cells is also more blurred with the discovery of type 1 innate lymphoid cells [141]. APCs, essential regulators of the innate immune response, also play a vital role to connect innate and adaptive immune responses [142]. In addition, the epithelial cell components of these grafts contribute within this complex interplay to induce, perpetuate, and be affected by the activated innate immune system [143, 144]. Future studies will continue to address this critical relationship between these two facets of the immune system and how this contributes to graft injury or acceptance.

b Acute Rejection

The mechanisms by which allografts may experience acute rejection (AR) are complex and can involve almost all components of the immune system. The humoral arm of the immune response (antibody-mediated), the cellular or cell-mediated arm, or a combination of both processes is the general way that alloimmune responses are manifested in the recipient towards the graft. Furthermore, "nonspecific" cell populations, including natural killer cells, eosinophils, and macrophages, are also present within the milieu of inflammation that occurs during acute rejection and they also contribute to the overall inflammation and injury that ensues.

i Acute Antibody-mediated Rejection (AAMR)

Acute rejection can develop from underlying anti-donor antibody that is formed *de novo* following the implantation of the graft or from performed antibody that was present prior to transplantation. Preformed anti-HLA alloantibodies may be present in recipients that had transfusions, pregnancies, or prior transplants [145, 146]. ABO antibodies can also be involved in AAMR, primarily in hyperacute or accelerated acute forms of rejection [147].

Alloantibody causes injury to the transplant via mechanisms similar to how antibody affects other pathogens (e.g., bacteria) confronting the host. The alloantibody is generally either class IgM or IgG and binds specifically to allopeptides present on the structures such as vasculature of the graft (see Figure 1.7) [148, 149, 150], thereby activating the endothelium and resulting in altered cell signaling and increased transcription factors [151]. It also appears that integrin beta 4 may be an important molecule on the targeted endothelial cell (in addition to membrane HLA molecules) that serves to initiate intracellular pathways that lead to cell proliferation [152]. The binding may be high or low affinity in nature and following this specific interaction, there can be fixation of complement. An elaborate series of events then ensues with activation of the complement cascade, including chemokine-driven attraction and activation of cells such as allospecific T cells and monocytes. This results in vascular injury (often because of endothelial cell targeting and injury), hemorrhage, thrombosis, and secondary inflammation throughout many areas of the allograft. Some of the complement components remain bound in covalent fashion to cell structures and this feature has been utilized to help identify the occurrence of humoral alloimmunity in tissue specimens. For example, C4d, and to a lesser extent C3d, are split products that have been identified in tissue sections as "markers" of antibody-antigen interactions [153, 154] (see Figure 1.8). For example, C4d staining can be a valuable criterion to classify antibody-mediated rejection in kidneys, although the staining patterns may change over time [155] and there now appear to be antibody-mediated rejections that are negative for C4d in kidney and other allografts [156, 157]. In addition to injury via complement, long-standing inflammation due to AAMR can result in cell proliferation (e.g., endothelial cells), and architectural alterations in organs such as basement membrane duplication, splitting, and multi-layering [158] in kidneys. Molecular gene profiling of grafts undergoing AAMR has also yielded distinct gene sets that ultimately are useful not only for understanding the pathways and molecules involved in the different variants of AAMR [159], but also could provide biomarkers that could facilitate rapid identification of alloantibody-mediated injury to the graft. Regardless, the presence of antibody-mediated acute rejection in allografts, as identified by typical morphology, immunostaining, or particular cellular constituents (e.g., monocytes) [160, 161] in association with peripheral donor-specific antibodies, generally correlates with reduced graft survival.

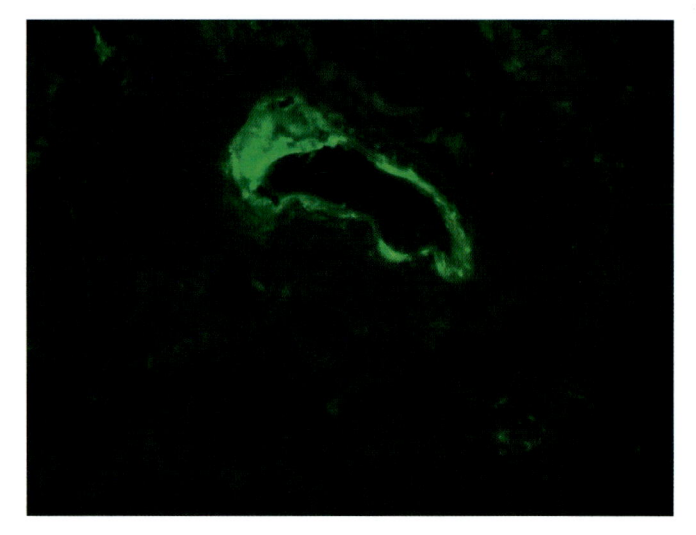

Figure 1.7 IgG along vessel in kidney undergoing humoral acute rejection (immunofluorescence, 400x).

ii Cell-mediated Acute Rejection (CMAR)

Cell-mediated acute rejection is the most common form of rejection in allografts and can markedly fluctuate in intensity, depending upon numerous factors such as the degree of histocompatibility, the timing of the rejection, the level of immunosuppression, and the type of allograft in question [162]. There are not typically pathognomonic or unique lesions, but rather a constellation of morphological changes. The unifying characteristic that most grafts undergoing CMAR demonstrate is a diffuse accumulation of chronic inflammatory cells (e.g., lymphocytes, macrophages) among the connective tissue elements of interstitial spaces. These cells, orchestrated most prominently by T cells, then infiltrate and cause injury to epithelial (e.g., kidney tubules, liver bile ducts, intestinal crypts) and vascular structures (see Figure 1.9). Although not as critical as T cells, there are also varying numbers of other cell populations, including NK/NKT cells, plasma cells, eosinophils, monocytes/macrophages, and B cells, each contributing to the overall inflammatory phenotype of cell-mediated acute rejection [72] [163, 164, 165]. In addition to enacting further injury to graft structures, the roles of these alternate non-T cell populations include antigen presentation [166] [161], cell lysis, and recruitment/activation of inflammatory cells and inflammatory molecule cascades [167, 168]. An identification of the cell populations causing cell-mediated rejection can be achieved via routine histology, immunohistochemistry, cyto-fluorographic analysis, and molecular techniques. The relative

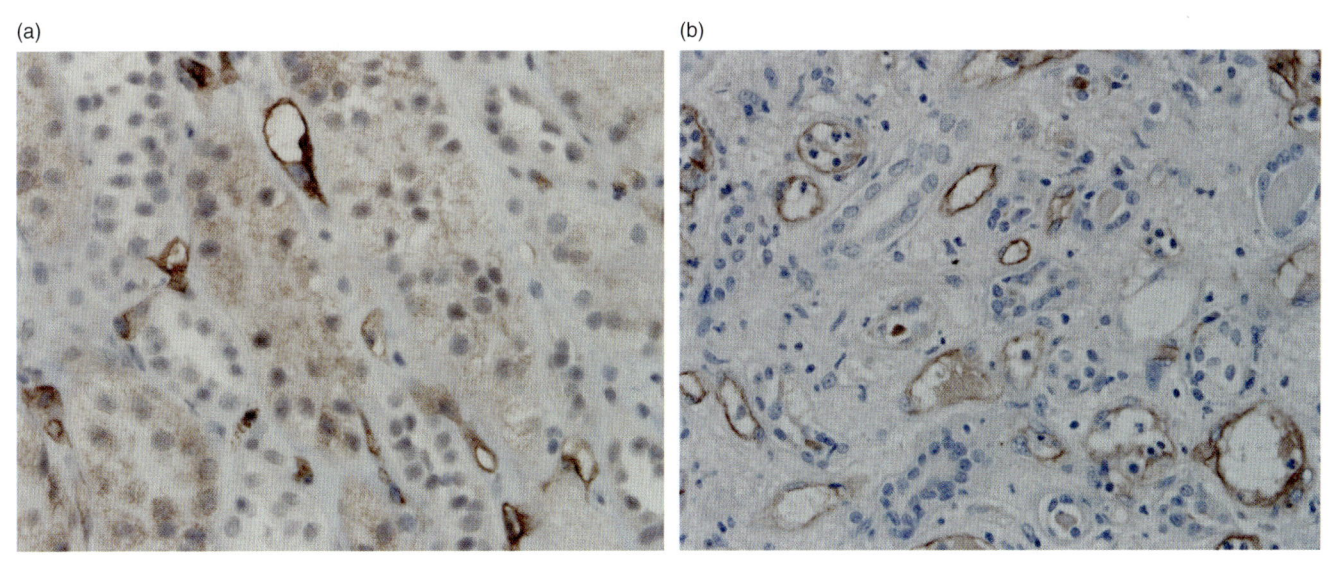

Figure 1.8 C4d (a) and C3d (b) along peritubular capillaries in kidney undergoing acute antibody-mediated rejection (immunohistochemistry, 400x).

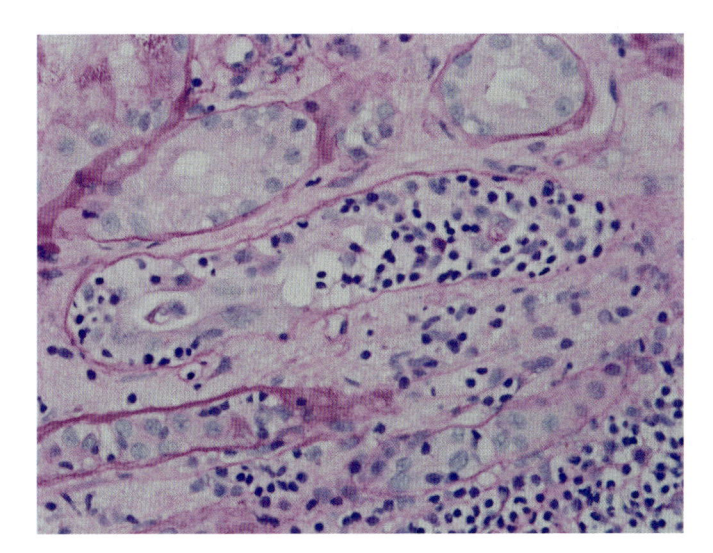

Figure 1.9 Acute T cell-mediated rejection in a kidney with extensive tubulitis (PAS, 400x).

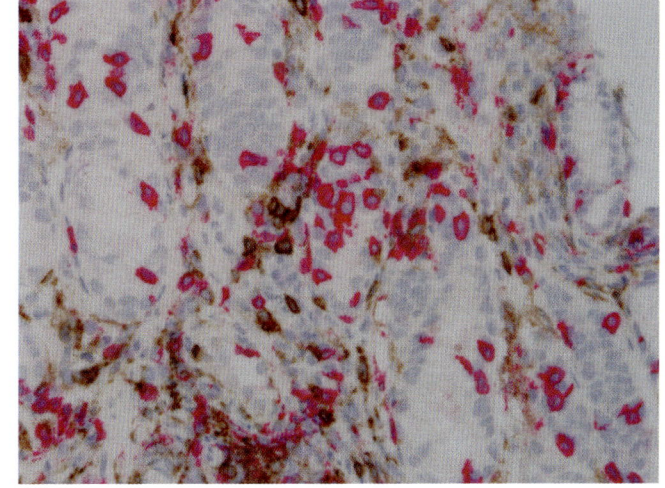

Figure 1.10 Stomach allograft undergoing acute T cell-mediated rejection (moderate). Brown stained cells – CD4; red stained cells CD8 (Two-color immunohistochemistry, 400x).

composition of the different T cell subtypes within rejecting allografts has been extensively examined and appears to have a relationship to the extent and severity of rejection [169] [170–172] (see Figure 1.10). Whole-genome microarray expression profiling of rejecting and stable organ allografts has yielded a plethora of information as to potential mechanisms, concurrent molecular processes, and possible prognostic markers during CMAR [173, 174]. Not surprisingly, histologically similar patterns on biopsies can reveal significant differences in gene expression. It is assumed that characterization of cell subtypes, along with the varying molecular phenotypes in these organs, will ultimately yield tools by which responses to therapy and the ability to be weaned from immunosuppression can be predicted.

The means by which T cells identify and localize to solid organ allografts during CMAR is better comprehended, but there are mechanisms unique with different allografts. For example, CD103 appears to serve as a receptor on epithelium of kidney transplants [175, 176] (see Figure 1.11) for particular cells such as alphaE (CD103) beta7 integrin-positive T cells [177]. Corresponding mechanisms are almost certainly present in other solid organ allografts such as non-suppurative lymphocytic cholangitis in liver allografts [178] and CMAR-induced enterocyte apoptosis in bowel rejection [179]. Inducible lymphocyte costimulatory molecules such as CD40 L and CTLA-4 present in the allograft cell infiltrates are also vitally important in the migration and differentiation of potent alloreactive cell populations [180, 181] [182]. The means by which specific (e.g., T cells) and nonspecific (e.g., NK cells) effector cells cause injury and apoptosis to graft cells are varied, but one prominent system is the perforin/granzyme family of molecules. These enzymatic proteins expressed by effector CD8+ T cells and NK cells can cause lysis of cells and thus the presence of these molecules in the allograft can be indicative of an active and ongoing cell-mediated acute rejection [183, 184]. The measurement of these two molecules can be performed *in situ* by immunohistochemistry [185, 186] or by

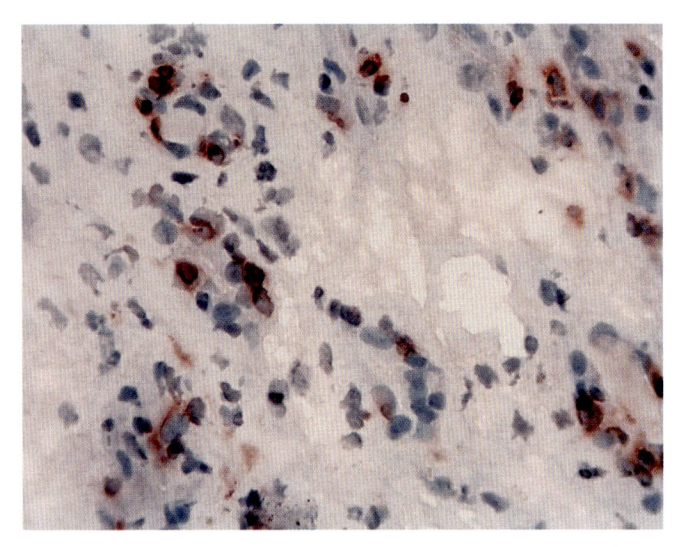

Figure 1.11 CD103+ cells in kidney tubules from allograft undergoing rejection (Immunohistochemistry, 400x).

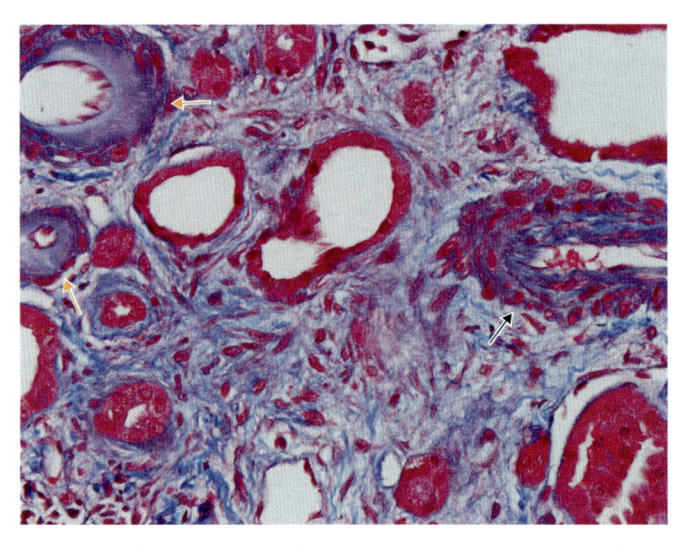

Figure 1.12 Photomicrograph of kidney allograft, showing characteristic vascular lesion in chronic rejection with fibrointimal thickening and medial hyperplasia in artery (white arrow), thickening and hyalinosis in arterioles (orange arrows), interstitial fibrosis, and tubular atrophy (Trichrome, 400x).

molecular techniques such as PCR, where the mRNA levels of perforin and granzyme in tissue and fluids such as urine [187] may be heralding an acute cell-mediated rejection episode. In addition, NK cells and NKT cells can also affect acute rejection of an allograft indirectly by shaping the alloreactivity of T cells or by killing antigen-presenting cells (APCs).

As mentioned before, aberrant expression of histocompatibility molecules occurs with there is "stress" such as ischemia-reperfusion injury. Likewise, CAMR can also upregulate HLA class I and class II expression within allografts, thereby perpetuating the acute rejection [188–190]. Adhesion molecules are also influenced and affected by the presence of rejection and their differential expression, especially the selectins, VLA4-VCAM and LFA1-ICAM [191–193]. Chemokines are among the families of molecules appearing vital to the recruitment of leukocytes into allografts [194, 195]. As with most other studies of molecules involved in graft rejection, chemokines have been identified by immunohistochemical and molecular means. In particular, CXCR3 and CCR5 appear vitally important in the progression of acute rejection [196] [197–199] and their blockade may attenuate graft rejection [197–200].

c Chronic Rejection

Chronic rejection of organ allografts remains as a principal source of recipient morbidity and mortality and presents as the principal challenge to the successful attainment of long-term graft function and survival [201, 202]. Though the treatment of acute rejection over the past two decades has improved, it remains that many solid organ transplants experience unrelenting deposition of fibroelastic material in many compartments of the organ as a result of obliterative vascular injury typical of chronic rejection (see Figure 1.12). This continual alteration of interstitial space, as well as vascular and epithelial structures in transplants, is one of the principal causes for the fact that long-term graft survival has not notably improved as compared to twenty years ago [203]. The underlying causes of chronic rejection are varied and appear to involve interplay of immunological and non-immunological variables in the recipient. Alloimmune processes associated with acute or subclinical rejection, ischemia/reperfusion injury, donor and recipient variables, and as-yet determined variables all simultaneously contribute to the overall injury characterized as chronic rejection.

The principal and most significant lesion in chronic rejection is the progressive arteriopathy affecting small and large muscular arterial vessels. This lesion differs from atherosclerotic lesions in that it is diffusely distributed, has minimal lipid deposition, and has concentric lamination due to intimal hyperplasia and adventitial scarring. This lesion ultimately leads to the downstream chronic injury in the graft that involves the interstitium and other parenchymal structures [204]. Alloimmune responses appear central to the development of the graft arteriopathy, since it is not seen in syngeneic models of transplantation. Antibody-mediated rejection emerges as the predominant form of alloimmunity necessary to develop this vasculopathy as based on experimental and clinical evidence [205–207], although cell-mediated immunity also plays a role. Graft endothelial cells and smooth muscle cells are targeted by alloantibodies and cytotoxic T cells – injury to these cells results in their undergoing apoptosis and removal, as well as proliferative changes of "repair" cell populations. There is also upregulation of molecules within the allograft and release of cytokines by injured endothelial and smooth muscle cells that facilitate the influx of cell populations such as activated macrophages and lymphocytes into the vessel [208, 209]. This culminates in matrix synthesis and cell proliferation. Finally, *host* precursor smooth muscle cells continue to add to the concentric lesion as it progresses [210].

The development of graft fibrosis within the interstitial regions centrally engages the inflammatory cell populations that are identifiable with acute rejection, including T lymphocytes and monocytes/macrophages [211, 212]. Matrix proteins and fibrogenic factors increase principally in perivascular areas [213] and evolve to the diffuse fibrosis manifested in end-stage

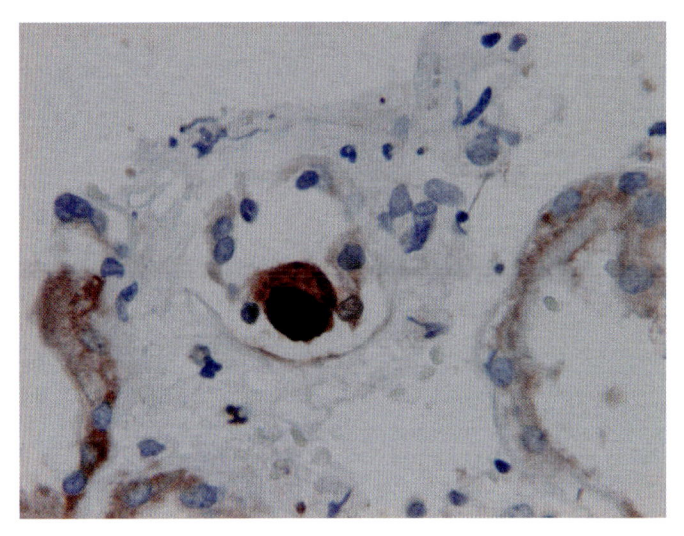

Figure 1.13 CMV inclusion in bowel allograft (600x, immunoperoxidase).

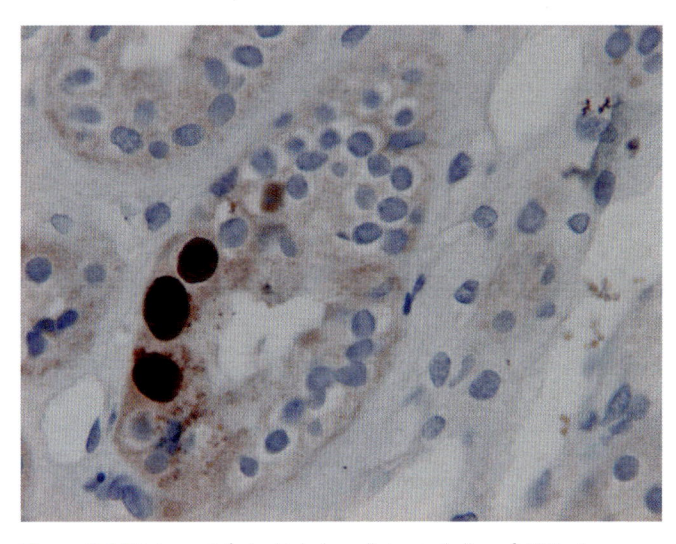

Figure 1.14 Polyoma infected tubular cells in renal allograft (400x, immunoperoxidase, SV-40 antibody).

chronically rejected organs. The mechanisms involved in the development of graft fibrosis are comparable to fibrosis present in other disorders (e.g., pulmonary fibrosis, scleroderma), involving native organs and thus, the targets for the prevention of fibrosis may ultimately be similar between transplants and native fibrogenic processes [214]. Briefly, there is a regenerative phase and fibroplasia phase [215] where simultaneous inflammatory, repair, and tissue remodeling processes occur. Injury to graft tissue vessels and other components exposes tissue determinants to platelets and an entire series of events ensues, including platelet degranulation and production of matrix metalloproteinases (MMP) – this further compromises basement membranes and allows inflammatory cell influx with their production of cytokines and growth factors [223, 224]. Endothelial cells then enclose the injured areas and profibrotic mediators promote differentiation of fibroblasts into myofibroblasts that lay down extracellular matrix (collagen) components. This process tends not to be well-regulated and results in an excess ECM deposition and ineffectual remodeling, ultimately culminating in fibrosis. Chemokines can help regulate this process, as well as the composition of the innate and adaptive immune cell populations involved in these pathways [216, 217]; isoforms of transforming growth factor β (TGF-β) [218, 219] play a critical role in graft fibrogenesis, as well as angiotensin II [220], and plasminogen activator inhibitor [221].

d Infection

As a consequence of the substantial and prolonged interruption of the host's immune system, all transplant recipients are at increased risk for the development of infections. This complication is not only the most common problem facing transplanted patients, but also the most frequent source of serious morbidity and mortality. Significant advances in the prophylaxis and treatment of infections following transplantation has decreased the rate of these complications [222, 223], although the problem remains a notable barrier to success. The range of infections is wide and dependent on various factors that include type of transplant, recipient characteristics, pre-transplant and coexisting disease, degree and type of immunosuppression, timing post-transplant, iatrogenic variables, and environmental conditions. All organs and body cavities can be involved and the scope of infections includes bacterial, viral, protozoal, and fungal, many often in coexistence. Aside from their direct toxicity to the host, the presence of infections also indirectly potentiates acute and chronic rejection processes and on occasion, triggers autoimmune inflammation in the recipient.

Several specific infections are prominent in transplant patient populations. Of the herpes viruses, Cytomegalovirus (CMV) remains a frequent source of infection in transplantation [222, 224, 225] (see Figure 1.13). CMV, a β-herpes-virus, can have life-long latency or persistence within the host. There is a rise of CMV-specific antibodies, often within the first three months of post-transplantation. CMV-seronegative recipients of an organ from a CMV-seropositive donor are at highest risk for disease. Patients can present with a viral syndrome that includes fever, myalgia, and organ disease, often within the transplanted organ, but it can involve many other sites (e.g., central nervous system, eye, urogenital, gastrointestinal tracts) [226]. CMV may potentiate graft rejection by priming immune cell populations [227]. Moreover, CMV also possesses the potential to augment allograft vasculopathy [228], a feature ascribed to several other viruses such as enterovirus, parvovirus, and adenovirus [229]. Aside from CMV and EBV (discussed below), other members of the herpes virus family are also important infections in transplantation. For example, herpes simplex virus (HSV) and VZ can initiate severe disease; as well, human herpes virus 6 (HHV-6), human herpes virus 7 (HHV-7), and human herpes virus 8 (HHV-8) have all been found to cause infectious complications following the receipt of an organ allograft [230].

Polyoma virus (PPV) is a noteworthy pathogen in the renal allograft population [231] and its identification has been associated with the implementation of newer immunosuppressive drugs [232]. The polyoma viruses, which include BK virus, JC virus, and SV40 virus, are members of the retrovirus family and they can infect urothelium and be associated with the development of nephritis (see Figure 1.14). Most nephritis

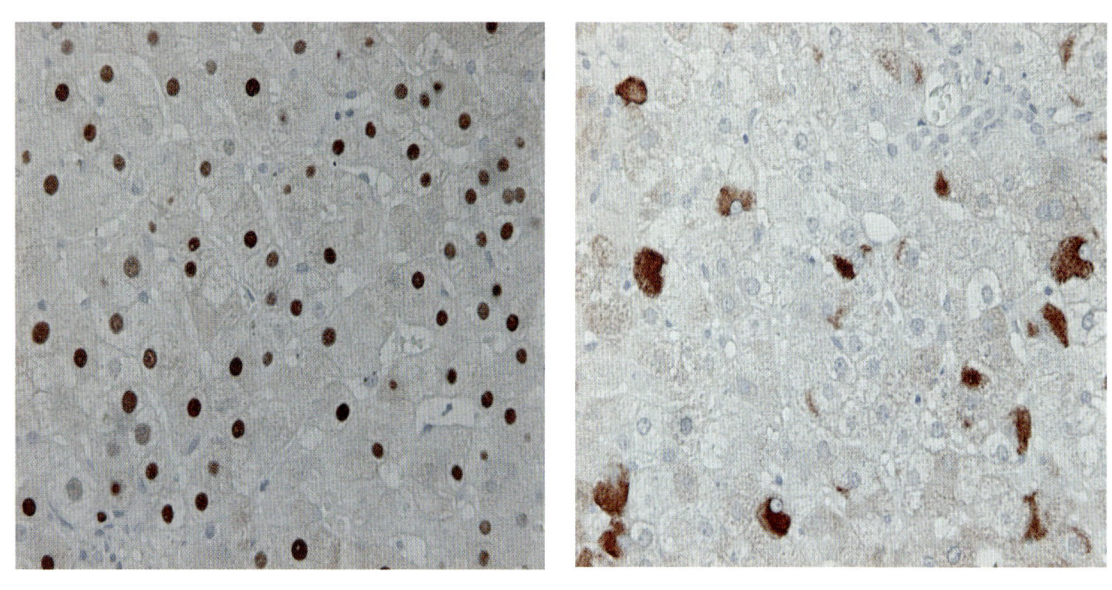

Figure 1.15 Recurrent Hepatitis B infection in a liver allograft. Left: Hepatitis core antigen-positive cells; right: Hepatitis B surface antigen-positive cells (immunoperoxidase, 400x).

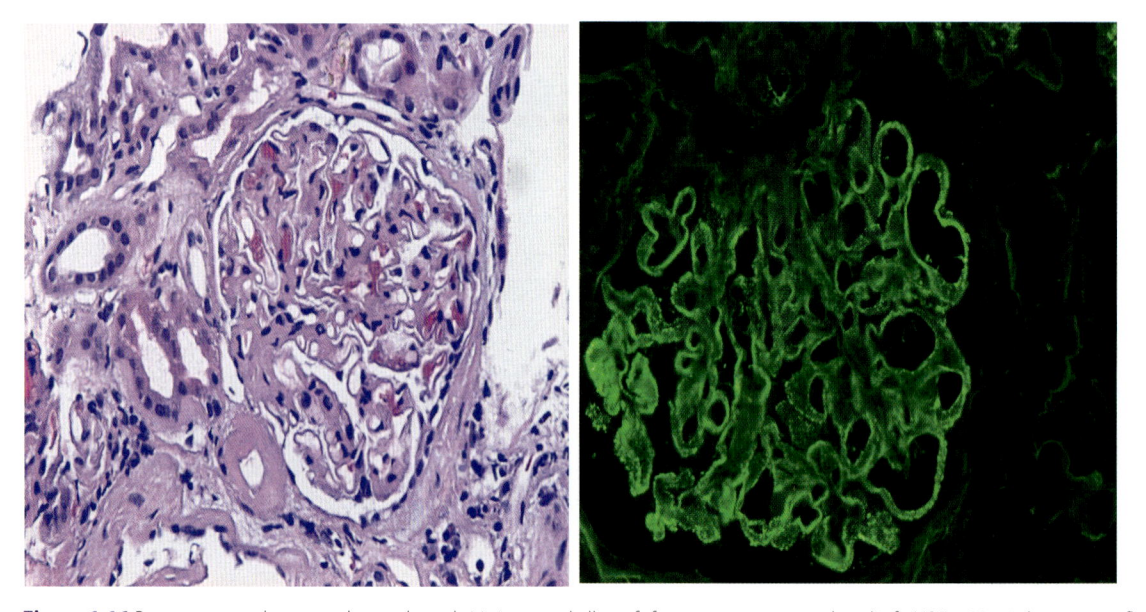

Figure 1.16 Recurrent membranous glomerulonephritis in a renal allograft four years post-transplant (Left: H&E, 400x; right: immunofluorescence, IgG, 400x).

cases are due to BK virus, some with co-infection with JC virus [233]. Light microscopy, immunostaining, and molecular methods are used for the diagnosis and to determine extent of infection by PPV [234, 235].

Hepatitis C infection, and especially as recurrent disease, is a major problem in liver allografts; there is a high incidence of recurrence post-transplant [236, 237] and this reemergence of the virus can be aggressive and quick in some cases [238, 239]. Unfortunately, there are currently no reliable immunoprobes to identify hepatitis C in tissues, although there have been notable advances in identifying genetic predisposition to recurrence of Hepatitis C, including genotypes of IL28 [240]. Hepatitis B infection tends to be less of problem in recent years in liver transplantation due to improved therapies and the presence of vaccines for this virus; this virus can be diagnosed by immunostaining for any of several virus-associated antigens [241] (see Figure 1.16) and by molecular analysis of allograft tissue.

Post-transplant lymphoproliferative disorder (PTLD) (see chapter) is a frequent complication following organ transplantation and is often [242] but not exclusively associated [243] with Epstein-Barr virus (EBV), another herpes virus. EBV bears the potential for a varied number of acute and chronic effects on the transplant recipients aside from PTLD. Aside from classical histopathological changes, immunohistochemistry, in situ hybridization, and other molecular means are utilized in helping identify and distinguish this virus from other processes (e.g., rejection) that may appear similar in presentation and appearance. The management of EBV infection may be a cessation of immunosuppression treatment; thus, careful identification of the virus (as with many other viruses in transplant patients) must be achieved from rejection processes that require additional immunosuppression.

e Recurrent/de Novo Immune Diseases

All solid organ allografts may experience de novo disease associated with that organ. In particular, the kidney transplant is particularly susceptible to development of recurrent or de novo renal maladies such as Focal Segmental Glomerulosclerosis (FSGS), IgA nephropathy, membranoproliferative glomerulonephritis (MPGN), membranous nephropathy (see Figure 1.16), fibrillary glomerulopathy, dense deposit disease, anti-glomerular basement membrane disease, and lupus nephritis. These entities can lead to graft loss and significant morbidity [244–246]. Recurrence of amyloidosis in organ allografts may occur. Finally, as mentioned, recurrent hepatitis B and C infections of the liver allograft are commonly encountered.

f Drug Toxicity

The wide array of immunosuppressive reagents and other medications administered to transplant patients bear the potential of direct or indirect injury to the transplant, as well as to the host in general. Although beyond the scope of this chapter, it should be noted that particular entities such as long-term steroid usage morbidity, calcineurin inhibitor renal (see Figure 1.17) and other organ toxicity, mycophenolate-associated gastrointestinal injury, hepatotoxicity due to a variety of various drugs, and cardiotoxicity can all significantly contribute to the demise of the allograft. Therefore, various treatment algorithms have been developed to try to minimize the effects of these compounds on the recipient.

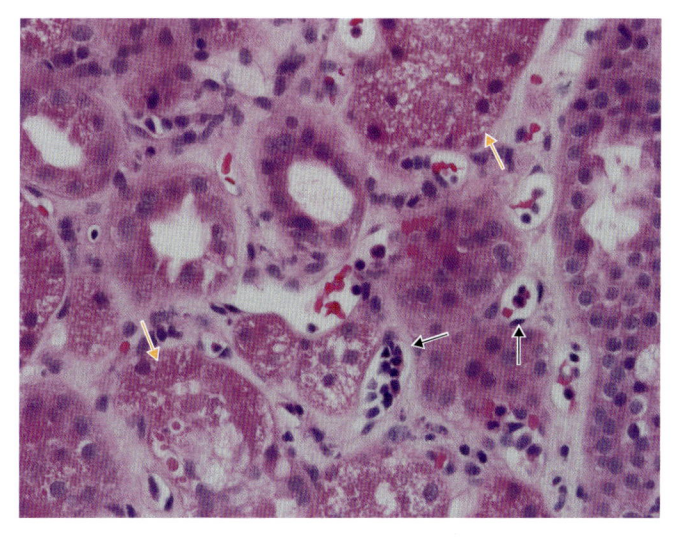

Figure 1.17 Renal allograft experiencing tacrolimus-associated nephropathy with characteristic tubular vacuolization (orange arrows), acute tubular necrosis, and hyalinization of arterioles (not shown). This kidney was also simultaneously experiencing acute antibody-mediated rejection, and peritubular capillaritis is also present (white arrows).

V Summary

The organ allograft is unceasingly confronted with numerous potential pathological processes for its survival. From the initial trauma and injury associated with the procurement from the donor, to the host immune response and other complications, the graft has to sustain normal function for the host in the face of often-severe acute or chronic injurious developments. Immunosuppressive agents and other drugs that inhibit some of the above mentioned mediators are crucial to allowing the transplant to survive, but can often themselves be the source of injury to the graft or other organ sites. As such, only the ability to induce donor-specific immune tolerance will allow the recipient to enjoy the benefits of the transplanted organ without the morbidity associated with current pharmaceutical therapies.

References

1. Rinaldi E. The First Homoplastic Limb Transplant According to the Legend of Saint Cosmas and Saint Damian. Italian Journal of Orthopedics and Traumatology. 1987;**13**(3):393–406.

2. Dutkowski P, De Rougemont O, Clavien PA. Alexis Carrel: Genius, Innovator and Ideologist. American Journal of Transplantation. 2008;**8**(10):1998–2003.

3. Billingham RE, Brent L, Medawar PB. Actively Acquired Tolerance of Foreign Cells. Nature. 1953 Oct 3;**172**(4379):603–6. PubMed PMID: 13099277.

4. Snell GD. The Genetics of Transplantation. Ann N Y Acad Sci. 1957 Dec 16;**69**(4):555–60. PubMed PMID: 13488312.

5. Gorer PA, Boyse EA. Pathological Changes in F1 Hybrid Mice Following Transplantation of Spleen Cells from Donors of the Parental Strains. Immunology. 1959 Apr;**2**(2):182–93. PubMed PMID: 13653737.

6. Dausset J, Rapaport FT, Colombani J, Feingold N. A Leucocyte Group and Its Relationship to Tissue Histocompatibility in Man. Transplantation. 1965 Nov;**3**(6):701–5. PubMed PMID: 5324831.

7. Doherty PC, Zinkernagel RM. A Biological Role for the Major Histocompatibility Antigens. Lancet. 1975 Jun 28;**1**(7922):1406–9. PubMed PMID: 49564.

8. Petersdorf E. The HLA Complex in Biology and Medicine: A Resource Book. Bone Marrow Transplant. 2011 04//print;**46**(4):625.

9. Marsh SGE, Albert ED, Bodmer WF, Bontrop RE, Dupont B, Erlich HA, et al. Nomenclature for Factors of the HLA System, 2010. Tissue Antigens. 2010;**75**(4):291–455.

10. Hennecke J, Wiley DC. T Cell Receptor-MHC Interactions up Close. Cell. 2001 Jan 12;**104**(1):1–4. PubMed PMID: 11163234.

11. Burgdorf S, Kautz A, Bohnert V, Knolle PA, Kurts C. Distinct Pathways of Antigen Uptake and Intracellular Routing in CD4 and CD8 T Cell Activation. Science. 2007 Apr 27;**316**(5824):612–6. PubMed PMID: 17463291.

12. Cresswell P, Ackerman AL, Giodini A, Peaper DR, Wearsch PA. Mechanisms

of MHC Class I-restricted Antigen Processing and Cross-presentation. Immunol Rev. 2005 Oct;207:145–57. PubMed PMID: 16181333. Epub 2005/09/27. English.

13. Goulmy E. Human Minor Histocompatibility Antigens. Current Opinion in Immunology. 1996 Feb;8(1):75–81. PubMed PMID: 8729449.

14. Goulmy E. Minor Histocompatibility Antigens: From Transplantation Problems to Therapy of Cancer. Human Immunology. 2006 Jun;67(6):433–8. PubMed PMID: 16728266.

15. Nielsen HS. Secondary Recurrent Miscarriage and H-Y Immunity. Human Reproduction Update. 2011 July 1, 2011;17(4):558–74.

16. Dierselhuis M, Goulmy E. The Relevance of Minor Histocompatibility Antigens in Solid Organ Transplantation. Curr Opin Organ Transplant. 2009 Aug;14(4):419–25. PubMed PMID: 19444105. Epub 2009/05/16. English.

17. Mutis T, Gillespie G, Schrama E, Falkenburg JH, Moss P, Goulmy E. Tetrameric HLA Class I-minor Histocompatibility Antigen Peptide Complexes Demonstrate Minor Histocompatibility Antigen-specific Cytotoxic T Lymphocytes in Patients with Graft-versus-Host Disease. Nat Med. 1999 Jul;5(7):839–42. PubMed PMID: 10395333. Epub 1999/07/08. English.

18. Spierings E, Vermeulen CJ, Vogt MH, Doerner LEE, Falkenburg JHF, Mutis T, et al. Identification of HLA Class II-restricted H-Y-specific T-helper Epitope Evoking CD4+ T-helper Cells in H-Y-mismatched Transplantation. Lancet. 2003 Aug 23;362(9384):610–5. PubMed PMID: 12944060.

19. van Els CA, Zantvoort E, Jacobs N, Bakker A, van Rood JJ, Goulmy E. Graft-versus-Host Disease Associated T Helper Cell Responses Specific for Minor Histocompatibility Antigens Are Mainly Restricted by HLA-DR Molecules. Bone Marrow Transplantation. 1990 Jun;5(6):365–72. PubMed PMID: 2142441.

20. Anderson MS, Su MA. Aire and T Cell Development. Current Opinion in Immunology. 2011;23(2):198–206. PubMed PMID: 21163636. Pubmed Central PMCID: NIHMS259332 PMC3073725.

21. Boros P, Bromberg JS. De Novo Autoimmunity after Organ Transplantation: Targets and Possible Pathways. Human Immunology. 2008;69(7):383–8. PubMed PMID: 18638653.

22. Veillette GR, Sahara H, Meltzer AJ, Weiss MJ, Iwamoto Y, Kim KM, et al. Autoimmune Sensitization to Cardiac Myosin Leads to Acute Rejection of Cardiac Allografts in Miniature Swine. Transplantation. 2011;91(11):1187–91. PubMed PMID: 21512437. Pubmed Central PMCID: NIHMS339140 PMC3232060.

23. Takase H, Yu CR, Mahdi RM, Douek DC, Dirusso GB, Midgley FM, et al. Thymic Expression of Peripheral Tissue Antigens in Humans: A Remarkable Variability among Individuals. International Immunology. 2005;17(8):1131–40. PubMed PMID: 16030131. PubMed Central PMCID: NIHMS44922 PMC2366090.

24. Suthanthiran M, Strom TB. Renal Transplantation. New England Journal of Medicine. 1994 Aug 11;331(6):365–76. PubMed PMID: 7832839.

25. Krensky AM. The HLA System, Antigen Processing and Presentation. Kidney International – Supplement. 1997 Mar;58:S2–7. PubMed PMID: 9067934.

26. Jiang S, Herrera O, Lechler RI. New Spectrum of Allorecognition Pathways: Implications for Graft Rejection and Transplantation Tolerance. Current Opinion in Immunology. 2004 Oct;16(5):550–7. PubMed PMID: 15341998.

27. Brown K, Sacks SH, Wong W. Coexpression of Donor Peptide/Recipient MHC Complex and Intact Donor MHC: Evidence for a Link between the Direct and Indirect Pathways. Am J Transplant. 2011 Apr;11(4):826–31. PubMed PMID: 21401861. Epub 2011/03/16. English.

28. Hsu KC, Chida S, Geraghty DE, Dupont B. The Killer Cell Immunoglobulin-like Receptor (KIR) Genomic Region: Gene-order, Haplotypes and Allelic Polymorphism. Immunol Rev. 2002 Dec;190:40–52. PubMed PMID: 12493005. Epub 2002/12/21. English.

29. Beksac M, Dalva K. Role of Killer Immunoglobulin-like Receptor and Ligand Matching in Donor Selection. Bone Marrow Research. 2012;2012:271695. PubMed PMID: 23193479. PubMed Central PMCID: PMC3502759. Epub 2012/11/30. English.

30. Nowak I, Magott-Procelewska M, Kowal A, Miazga M, Wagner M, Niepieklo-Miniewska W, et al. Killer Immunoglobulin-like Receptor (KIR) and HLA Genotypes Affect the Outcome of Allogeneic Kidney Transplantation. PLoS One. 2012;7(9):e44718. PubMed PMID: 23028591. PubMed Central PMCID: PMC3441441. Epub 2012/10/03. English.

31. Zhang Y, Ruiz P. Solid Organ Transplant-associated Acute Graft-versus-Host Disease. Arch Pathol Lab Med. 2010 Aug;134(8):1220–4. PubMed PMID: 20670147. Epub 2010/07/31. English.

32. Burdick JF, Vogelsang GB, Smith WJ, Farmer ER, Bias WB, Kaufmann SH, et al. Severe Graft-versus-Host Disease in a Liver-transplant Recipient. New England Journal of Medicine. 1988 Mar 17;318(11):689–91. PubMed PMID: 3278235.

33. Chan EY, Larson AM, Gersheimer TB, Kowdley KV, Carithers RL, Jr., Reyes JD, et al. Recipient and Donor Factors Influence the Incidence of Graft-vs.-Host Disease in Liver Transplant Patients. Liver Transplantation. 2007 Apr;13(4):516–22. PubMed PMID: 17394149.

34. Ghali MP, Talwalkar JA, Moore SB, Hogan WJ, Menon KVN, Rosen CB. Acute Graft-versus-Host Disease after Liver Transplantation. Transplantation. 2007 Feb 15;83(3):365–6. PubMed PMID: 17297417.

35. Olszewski WL. Donor DNA Is Present in Recipient Tissues after Grafting also in Graft-versus-Host Disease-free Individuals. Transplantation. 2007 Jan 15;83(1):107–8. PubMed PMID: 17220809.

36. Perri R, Assi M, Talwalkar J, Heimbach J, Hogan W, Moore SB, et al. Graft vs. Host Disease after Liver Transplantation: A New Approach Is Needed. Liver Transplantation. 2007 Aug;13(8):1092–9. PubMed PMID: 17663410.

37. Assi MA, Pulido JS, Peters SG, McCannel CA, Razonable RR. Graft-vs.-Host Disease in Lung and Other Solid Organ Transplant Recipients. Clinical Transplantation. 2007 Jan–Feb;21(1):1–6. PubMed PMID: 17302584.

38. Wu G, Selvaggi G, Nishida S, Moon J, Island E, Ruiz P, et al. Graft-versus-Host Disease after Intestinal and Multivisceral Transplantation. Transplantation. 2011 Jan 27;91(2):219–24. PubMed PMID: 21076376. Epub 2010/11/16. English.

39. Klingebiel T, Schlegel PG. GVHD: Overview on Pathophysiology, Incidence, Clinical and Biological Features. Bone Marrow

40. Triulzi DJ, Nalesnik MA. Microchimerism, GVHD, and Tolerance in Solid Organ Transplantation. Transfusion. 2001 Mar;41(3):419–26. PubMed PMID: 11274601.

41. Flesland O, Pfeffer PF, Solheim BG, Mellbye OJ. Donor Lymphocytes Transferred with the Graft to Kidney Recipients. Potential for Establishing Microchimerism. Transfusion & Apheresis Science. 2003;28(2):125–8. PubMed PMID: 12679115.

42. Wiebe BM, Mortensen SA, Petterson G, Svendsen UG, Andersen CB. Macrophage and Lymphocyte Chimerism in Bronchoalveolar Lavage Cells from Human Lung Allograft Recipients. APMIS. 2001;109(6):435–40. PubMed PMID: 11506475.

43. Petersdorf EW, Malkki M. Genetics of Risk Factors for Graft-versus-Host Disease. Seminars in Hematology. 2006 Jan;43(1):11–23. PubMed PMID: 16412785.

44. Fraser CJ, Scott Baker K. The Management and Outcome of Chronic Graft-versus-Host Disease. British Journal of Haematology. 2007 Jul;138(2):131–45. PubMed PMID: 17593020.

45. Holler E. Progress in Acute Graft versus Host Disease. Current Opinion in Hematology. 2007 Nov;14(6):625–31. PubMed PMID: 17898566.

46. Rodriguez V, Anderson PM, Trotz BA, Arndt CAS, Allen JA, Khan SP. Use of Infliximab-Daclizumab Combination for the Treatment of Acute and Chronic Graft-versus-Host Disease of the Liver and Gut. Pediatric Blood & Cancer. 2007 Aug;49(2):212–5. PubMed PMID: 16261610.

47. Ferrara JLM, Reddy P. Pathophysiology of Graft-versus-Host Disease. Seminars in Hematology. 2006 Jan;43(1):3–10. PubMed PMID: 16412784.

48. Blazar BR, Murphy WJ, Abedi M. Advances in Graft-versus-Host Disease Biology and Therapy. Nature Reviews Immunology. 2012;12(6):443–58. PubMed PMID: 22576252.

49. Copelan EA. Hematopoietic Stem-cell Transplantation. New England Journal of Medicine. 2006 Apr 27;354(17):1813–26. PubMed PMID: 16641398.

50. Steinman RM. Dendritic Cells: Understanding Immunogenicity. European Journal of Immunology. 2007 Nov;37 Suppl 1:S53–60. PubMed PMID: 17972346.

51. Ludajic K, Balavarca Y, Bickeboller H, Rosenmayr A, Fae I, Fischer GF, et al. KIR Genes and KIR Ligands Affect Occurrence of Acute GVHD after Unrelated, 12/12 HLA Matched, Hematopoietic Stem Cell Transplantation. Bone Marrow Transplant. 2009 01/26/online;44(2):97–103.

52. Chien JW, Zhang XC, Fan W, Wang H, Zhao LP, Martin PJ, et al. Evaluation of Published Single Nucleotide Polymorphisms Associated with Acute GVHD. Blood. 2012;119(22):5311–9. PubMed PMID: 22282500. PubMed Central PMCID: PMC3369619.

53. Schwartz RH. Historical Overview of Immunological Tolerance. Cold Spring Harbor Perspectives in Biology. 2012;4(4):a006908. PubMed PMID: 22395097.

54. Szabolcs P, Burlingham WJ, Thomson AW. Tolerance after Solid Organ and Hematopoietic Cell Transplantation. Biology of Blood & Marrow Transplantation. 2012;18(1 Suppl):S193–200. PubMed PMID: 22226107. PubMed Central PMCID: NIHMS379899 PMC3374726.

55. Levitsky J. Operational Tolerance: Past Lessons and Future Prospects. Liver Transplantation. 2011;17(3):222–32.

56. Bluestone JA, Auchincloss H, Nepom GT, Rotrosen D, St. Clair EW, Turka LA. The Immune Tolerance Network at 10 Years: Tolerance Research at the Bedside. Nat Rev Immunol. 2010 11//print;10(11):797–803.

57. Sykes M. Immune Tolerance: Mechanisms and Application in Clinical Transplantation. Journal of Internal Medicine. 2007 Sep;262(3):288–310. PubMed PMID: 17697153.

58. Starzl TE. Chimerism and Tolerance in Transplantation. Proceedings of the National Academy of Sciences of the United States of America. 2004;101 Suppl 2:14607–14. PubMed PMID: 15319473. PubMed Central PMCID: PMC521985.

59. Perales MA, Blachere NE, Engelhorn ME, Ferrone CR, Gold JS, Gregor PD, et al. Strategies to Overcome Immune Ignorance and Tolerance. Seminars in Cancer Biology. 2002;12(1):63–71. PubMed PMID: 11926414.

60. Macian F, Im S-H, Garcia-Cozar FJ, Rao A. T-cell Anergy. Current Opinion in Immunology. 2004 Apr;16(2):209–16. PubMed PMID: 15023411.

61. Brennan PJ, Saouaf SJ, Greene MI, Shen Y. Anergy and Suppression as Coexistent Mechanisms for the Maintenance of Peripheral T Cell Tolerance. Immunologic Research. 2003;27(2–3):295–302. PubMed PMID: 12857976.

62. Wood KJ, Bushell A, Hester J. Regulatory Immune Cells in Transplantation. Nat Rev Immunol. 2012 06//print;12(6):417–30.

63. Shuiping J. Recent Advances in Regulatory T Cells. Seminars in Immunology. 2011;23(6):399–400.

64. Franck E, Bonneau C, Jean L, Henry J-P, Lacoume Y, Salvetti A, et al. Immunological Tolerance to Muscle Autoantigens Involves Peripheral Deletion of Autoreactive CD8+ T Cells. PLoS ONE. 2012;7(5):e36444.

65. Gurung P, Kucaba TA, Schoenberger SP, Ferguson TA, Griffith TS. TRAIL-expressing CD8+ T Cells Mediate Tolerance Following Soluble Peptide-induced Peripheral T Cell Deletion. Journal of Leukocyte Biology. 2010;88(6):1217–25. PubMed PMID: 20807702. PubMed Central PMCID: PMC2996898.

66. Cohen JN, Guidi CJ, Tewalt EF, Qiao H, Rouhani SJ, Ruddell A, et al. Lymph Node–Resident Lymphatic Endothelial Cells Mediate Peripheral Tolerance via Aire-independent Direct Antigen Presentation. The Journal of Experimental Medicine. 2010 April 12, 2010;207(4):681–8.

67. Gallegos AM, Bevan MJ. Central Tolerance: Good but Imperfect. Immunological Reviews. 2006 Feb;209:290–6. PubMed PMID: 16448550.

68. Kyewski B, Klein L. A Central Role for Central Tolerance. Annu Rev Immunol. 2006;24:571–606. PubMed PMID: 16551260.

69. Mathis D, Benoist C. Back to Central Tolerance. Immunity. 2004 May;20(5):509–16. PubMed PMID: 15142520.

70. Ruiz P, Streilein JW. Evidence that I-E-negative Mice Resistant to Neonatal H-2 Tolerance Induction Display Ubiquitous Thymic Clonal Deletion of Donor-reactive T Cells. Transplantation. 1993 Feb;55(2):321–8. PubMed PMID: 8434383. Epub 1993/02/01. English.

71. Lakkis FG, Arakelov A, Konieczny BT, Inoue Y. Immunologic 'Ignorance' of Vascularized Organ Transplants in the Absence of Secondary Lymphoid Tissue. Nature Medicine. 2000 Jun;6(6):686–8. PubMed PMID: 10835686.

72. Alegre M-L, Florquin S, Goldman M. Cellular Mechanisms Underlying Acute Graft Rejection: Time for Reassessment.

Current Opinion in Immunology. 2007 Oct;**19**(5):563–8. PubMed PMID: 17720467.

73. Trambley J, Bingaman AW, Lin A, Elwood ET, Waitze SY, Ha J, et al. Asialo GM1+ CD8+ T Cells Play a Critical Role in Costimulation Blockade-resistant Allograft Rejection. Journal of Clinical Investigation. 1999;**104**(12):1715–22.

74. Neujahr DC, Chen C, Huang X, Markmann JF, Cobbold S, Waldmann H, et al. Accelerated Memory Cell Homeostasis during T Cell Depletion and Approaches to Overcome It. Journal of Immunology. 2006;**176**(8):4632–9.

75. Gershon RK. A Disquisition on Suppressor T Cells. Transplantation Reviews. 1975;**26**:170–85. PubMed PMID: 1101469.

76. Gershon RK, Cohen P, Hencin R, Liebhaber SA. Suppressor T Cells. Journal of Immunology. 1972 Mar;**108**(3):586–90. PubMed PMID: 4401006.

77. Takahashi T, Kuniyasu Y, Toda M, Sakaguchi N, Itoh M, Iwata M, et al. Immunologic Self-tolerance Maintained by CD25+CD4+ Naturally Anergic and Suppressive T Cells: Induction of Autoimmune Disease by Breaking Their Anergic/Suppressive State. Int Immunol. 1998 December 1, 1998;**10**(12):1969–80.

78. Sakaguchi S, Sakaguchi N, Asano M, Itoh M, Toda M. Immunologic Self-tolerance Maintained by Activated T Cells Expressing IL-2 Receptor Alpha-chains (CD25). Breakdown of a Single Mechanism of Self-tolerance Causes Various Autoimmune Diseases. Journal of Immunology. 1995 Aug 1;**155**(3):1151–64. PubMed PMID: 7636184.

79. Josefowicz SZ, Lu LF, Rudensky AY. Regulatory T Cells: Mechanisms of Differentiation and Function. Annu Rev Immunol. 2012;**30**:531–64. PubMed PMID: 22224781. Epub 2012/01/10. English.

80. Tang Q, Bluestone JA. The Foxp3+ Regulatory T Cell: A Jack of all Trades, Master of Regulation. Nat Immunol. 2008;**9**(3):239–44.

81. Bandukwala HS, Rao A. 'Nurr'ishing Treg Cells: Nr4a Transcription Factors Control Foxp3 Expression. Nat Immunol. 2013 03//print;**14**(3):201–3.

82. Pot C, Apetoh L, Kuchroo VK. Type 1 Regulatory T Cells (Tr1) in Autoimmunity. Semin Immunol. 2011 Jun;**23**(3):202–8. PubMed PMID: 21840222. PubMed Central PMCID: PMC3178065. Epub 2011/08/16. English.

83. Burlingham WJ, Goulmy E. Human CD8+ T-regulatory Cells with Low-avidity T-cell Receptor Specific for Minor Histocompatibility Antigens. Hum Immunol. 2008 Nov;**69**(11):728–31. PubMed PMID: 18812197. PubMed Central PMCID: PMC2665292. Epub 2008/09/25. English.

84. Monteiro M, Almeida CF, Caridade M, Ribot JC, Duarte J, Agua-Doce A, et al. Identification of Regulatory Foxp3+ Invariant NKT Cells Induced by TGF-beta. J Immunol. 2010 Aug 15;**185**(4):2157–63. PubMed PMID: 20639482. Epub 2010/07/20. English.

85. Fischer K, Voelkl S, Heymann J, Przybylski GK, Mondal K, Laumer M, et al. Isolation and Characterization of Human Antigen-specific TCRαβ+ CD4-CD8- Double-negative Regulatory T Cells. Blood. 2005 April 1, 2005;**105**(7):2828–35.

86. DiLillo DJ, Matsushita T, Tedder TF. B10 Cells and Regulatory B Cells Balance Immune Responses during Inflammation, Autoimmunity, and Cancer. Ann N Y Acad Sci. 2010;**1183**(1):38–57.

87. Morelli AE, Thomson AW. Tolerogenic Dendritic Cells and the Quest for Transplant Tolerance. Nat Rev Immunol. 2007 08//print;**7**(8):610–21.

88. Haile LA, von Wasielewski R, Gamrekelashvili J, Kruger C, Bachmann O, Westendorf AM, et al. Myeloid-derived Suppressor Cells in Inflammatory Bowel Disease: A New Immunoregulatory Pathway. Gastroenterology. 2008 Sep;**135**(3):871–81, 81 e1–5. PubMed PMID: 18674538. Epub 2008/08/05. English.

89. Fleming BD, Mosser DM. Regulatory Macrophages: Setting the Threshold for Therapy. Eur J Immunol. 2011 Sep;**41**(9):2498–502. PubMed PMID: 21952805. Epub 2011/09/29. English.

90. English K, French A, Wood KJ. Mesenchymal Stromal Cells: Facilitators of Successful Transplantation? Cell Stem Cell. 2010 Oct 8;**7**(4):431–42. PubMed PMID: 20887949. Epub 2010/10/05. English.

91. Kim HJ, Hwang SJ, Kim BK, Jung KC, Chung DH. NKT Cells Play Critical Roles in the Induction of Oral Tolerance by Inducing Regulatory T Cells Producing IL-10 and Transforming Growth Factor Beta, and by Clonally Deleting Antigen-specific T Cells. Immunology. 2006 May;**118**(1):101–11. PubMed PMID: 16630027.

92. Carrier Y, Yuan J, Kuchroo VK, Weiner HL. Th3 Cells in Peripheral Tolerance. I. Induction of Foxp3-positive Regulatory T Cells by Th3 Cells Derived from TGF-beta T Cell-transgenic Mice. Journal of Immunology. 2007 Jan 1;**178**(1):179–85. PubMed PMID: 17182553.

93. Biagi E, Di Biaso I, Leoni V, Gaipa G, Rossi V, Bugarin C, et al. Extracorporeal Photochemotherapy Is Accompanied by Increasing Levels of Circulating CD4+CD25+GITR+Foxp3+CD62 L+ Functional Regulatory T-cells in Patients with Graft-versus-Host Disease. Transplantation. 2007 Jul 15;**84**(1):31–9. PubMed PMID: 17627234.

94. Hilchey SP, De A, Rimsza LM, Bankert RB, Bernstein SH. Follicular Lymphoma Intratumoral CD4+CD25+GITR+ Regulatory T Cells Potently Suppress CD3/CD28-costimulated Autologous and Allogeneic CD8+CD25- and CD4+CD25- T Cells. Journal of Immunology. 2007 Apr 1;**178**(7):4051–61. PubMed PMID: 17371959.

95. Ferretti G, Felici A, Pino MS, Cognetti F. Does CTLA4 Influence the Suppressive Effect of CD25+CD4+ Regulatory T Cells? Journal of Clinical Oncology. 2006 Dec 1;**24**(34):5469–70; author reply 70–1. PubMed PMID: 17135653.

96. Quezada SA, Peggs KS, Curran MA, Allison JP. CTLA4 Blockade and GM-CSF Combination Immunotherapy Alters the Intratumor Balance of Effector and Regulatory T Cells. Journal of Clinical Investigation. 2006 Jul;**116**(7):1935–45. PubMed PMID: 16778987.

97. Salama AD, Najafian N, Clarkson MR, Harmon WE, Sayegh MH. Regulatory CD25+ T Cells in Human Kidney Transplant Recipients. Journal of the American Society of Nephrology. 2003 Jun;**14**(6):1643–51. PubMed PMID: 12761267.

98. Cirocco RE, Carreno MR, Mathew JM, Garcia-Morales RO, Fuller L, Esquenazi V, et al. FoxP3 mRNA Transcripts and Regulatory Cells in Renal Transplant Recipients 10 Years after Donor Marrow Infusion. Transplantation. 2007 Jun 27;**83**(12):1611–9. PubMed PMID: 17589345.

99. Dijke IE, Weimar W, Baan CC. Regulatory T Cells after Organ Transplantation: Where Does Their Action Take Place? Human Immunology. 2008;**69**(7):389–98.

100. Brunstein CG, Miller JS, Cao Q, McKenna DH, Hippen KL, Curtsinger J, et al. Infusion of Ex Vivo Expanded T Regulatory Cells in Adults Transplanted

with Umbilical Cord Blood: Safety Profile and Detection Kinetics. Blood. 2010 October 15.

101 Farkas SA, Schnitzbauer AA, Kirchner G, Obed A, Banas B, Schlitt HJ. Calcineurin Inhibitor Minimization Protocols in Liver Transplantation. Transplant International. Official Journal of the European Society for Organ Transplantation. 2009 Jan;**22**(1):49–60. PubMed PMID: 19121146. Epub 2009/01/06. English.

102 Moreira-Teixeira L, Resende M, Devergne O, Herbeuval J-P, Hermine O, Schneider E, et al. Rapamycin Combined with TGF-β Converts Human Invariant NKT Cells into Suppressive Foxp3+ Regulatory Cells. The Journal of Immunology. 2012 January **15**, 2012;**188**(2):624–31.

103 Ciancio G, Burke GW. Alemtuzumab (Campath-1 H) in Kidney Transplantation. American Journal of Transplantation. Official Journal of the American Society of Transplantation and the American Society of Transplant Surgeons. 2008 Jan;**8**(1):15–20. PubMed PMID: 18093269. Epub 2007/12/21. English.

104 Chiffoleau E, Walsh PT, Turka L. Apoptosis and Transplantation Tolerance. Immunological Reviews. 2003 Jun;**193**:124–45. PubMed PMID: 12752677.

105 Sohn SJ, Thompson J, Winoto A. Apoptosis during Negative Selection of Autoreactive Thymocytes. Current Opinion in Immunology. 2007 Oct;**19**(5):510–5. PubMed PMID: 17656079.

106 Dresske B, Lin X, Huang D-S, Zhou X, Fandrich F. Spontaneous Tolerance: Experience with the Rat Liver Transplant Model. Human Immunology. 2002 Oct;**63**(10):853–61. PubMed PMID: 12368037.

107 Vincenti F, Luggen M, Vincenti F, Luggen M. T cell Costimulation: A Rational Target in the Therapeutic Armamentarium for Autoimmune Diseases and Transplantation. Annual Review of Medicine. 2007;**58**:347–58. PubMed PMID: 17020493.

108 Vincenti F, Larsen C, Durrbach A, Wekerle T, Nashan B, Blancho G, et al. Costimulation Blockade with Belatacept in Renal Transplantation. The New England Journal of Medicine. 2005 Aug 25;**353**(8):770–81. PubMed PMID: 16120857. Epub 2005/08/27. English.

109 Bonfoco E, Stuart PM, Brunner T, Lin T, Griffith TS, Gao Y, et al. Inducible Nonlymphoid Expression of Fas Ligand Is Responsible for Superantigen-induced Peripheral Deletion of T Cells. Immunity. 1998 Nov;**9**(5):711–20. PubMed PMID: 9846492.

110 Kurts C, Heath WR, Kosaka H, Miller JF, Carbone FR. The Peripheral Deletion of Autoreactive CD8+ T Cells Induced by Cross-presentation of Self-antigens Involves Signaling through CD95 (Fas, Apo-1). Journal of Experimental Medicine. 1998 Jul 20;**188**(2):415–20. PubMed PMID: 9670055.

111 Dempsey PW, Doyle SE, He JQ, Cheng G. The Signaling Adaptors and Pathways Activated by TNF Superfamily. Cytokine & Growth Factor Reviews. 2003 Jun–Aug;**14**(3–4):193–209. PubMed PMID: 12787559.

112 Feng X. Regulatory Roles and Molecular Signaling of TNF Family Members in Osteoclasts. Gene. 2005 Apr 25;**350**(1):1–13. PubMed PMID: 15777737.

113 Sheikh MS, Huang Y. Death Receptor Activation Complexes: It Takes Two to Activate TNF Receptor 1. Cell Cycle. 2003 Nov–Dec;**2**(6):550–2. PubMed PMID: 14504472.

114 Tryphonopoulos P, Tzakis AG, Weppler D, Garcia-Morales R, Kato T, Madariaga JR, et al. The Role of Donor Bone Marrow Infusions in Withdrawal of Immunosuppression in Adult Liver Allotransplantation. American Journal of Transplantation. 2005 Mar;**5**(3):608–13. PubMed PMID: 15707417.

115 Leventhal J, Abecassis M, Miller J, Gallon L, Ravindra K, Tollerud DJ, et al. Chimerism and Tolerance without GVHD or Engraftment Syndrome in HLA-mismatched Combined Kidney and Hematopoietic Stem Cell Transplantation. Science Translational Medicine. 2012 March 7, 2012;**4**(124):124ra28.

116 Martinez-Llordella M, Puig-Pey I, Orlando G, Ramoni M, Tisone G, Rimola A, et al. Multiparameter Immune Profiling of Operational Tolerance in Liver Transplantation. American Journal of Transplantation. 2007 Feb;**7**(2):309–19. PubMed PMID: ISI:000243440100008. eng.

117 Bohne F, Martínez-Llordella M, Lozano J-J, Miquel R, Benítez C, Londoño M-C, et al. Intra-graft Expression of Genes Involved in Iron Homeostasis Predicts the Development of Operational Tolerance in Human Liver Transplantation. The Journal of Clinical Investigation. 2012;**122**(1):368–82.

118 Newell KA, Asare A, Kirk AD, Gisler TD, Bourcier K, Suthanthiran M, et al. Identification of a B Cell Signature Associated with Renal Transplant Tolerance in Humans. The Journal of Clinical Investigation. 2010;**120**(6):1836–47.

119 Newell KA, Larsen CP. Tolerance Assays: Measuring the Unknown. Transplantation. 2006 Jun 15;**81**(11):1503–9. PubMed PMID: 16770237.

120 Londono MC, Danger R, Giral M, Soulillou JP, Sanchez-Fueyo A, Brouard S. A Need for Biomarkers of Operational Tolerance in Liver and Kidney Transplantation. Am J Transplant. 2012 Jun;**12**(6):1370–7. PubMed PMID: 22486792. Epub 2012/04/11. English.

121 Nankivell BJ, Chapman JR. Chronic Allograft Nephropathy: Current Concepts and Future Directions. Transplantation. 2006 Mar 15;**81**(5):643–54. PubMed PMID: 16534463.

122 Wood KJ, Goto R. Mechanisms of Rejection: Current Perspectives. Transplantation. 2012;**93**(1):1–10.1097/TP.0b013e31823cab44.

123 Huang Y, Rabb H, Womer KL. Ischemia-reperfusion and Immediate T Cell Responses. Cellular Immunology. 2007 Jul;**248**(1):4–11. PubMed PMID: 17942086.

124 Kupiec-Weglinski JW, Busuttil RW. Ischemia and Reperfusion Injury in Liver Transplantation. Transplantation Proceedings. 2005 May;**37**(4):1653–6. PubMed PMID: 15919422.

125 Ysebaert DK, De Greef KE, De Beuf A, Van Rompay AR, Vercauteren S, Persy VP, et al. T cells as Mediators in Renal Ischemia/Reperfusion Injury. Kidney International. 2004 Aug;**66**(2):491–6. PubMed PMID: 15253695.

126 Andersen CB, Ladefoged SD, Larsen S. Acute Kidney Graft Rejection. A Morphological and Immunohistological Study on "Zero-hour" and Follow-up Biopsies with Special Emphasis on Cellular Infiltrates and Adhesion Molecules. APMIS. 1994;**102**(1):23–37.

127 Devouassoux G, Pison C, Drouet C, Pin I, Brambilla C, Brambilla E. Early Lung Leukocyte Infiltration, HLA and Adhesion Molecule Expression Predict Chronic Rejection. Transplant

128. van der Woude FJ, Deckers JG, Mallat MJ, Yard BA, Schrama E, van Saase JL, et al. Tissue Antigens in Tubulointerstitial and Vascular Rejection. Kidney International – Supplement. 1995 Dec;**52**:S11–3. PubMed PMID: 8587271.

129. Hengstenberg C, Hufnagel G, Haverich A, Olsen EGJ, Maisch B. De Novo Expression of MHC Class I and Class II Antigens on Endomyocardial Biopsies from Patients with Inflammatory Heart Disease and Rejection Following Heart Transplantation. European Heart Journal. 1993 January 2;**14**(6):758–63.

130. Farr AG, Mannschreck JW, Anderson SK. Expression of Class II MHC Antigens in Murine Pancreas after Streptozocin-induced Insulitis. Diabetes. 1988 October 1;**37**(10):1373–9.

131. Hasegawa S, Becker G, Nagano H, Libby P, Mitchell RN. Pattern of Graft- and Host-specific MHC Class II Expression in Long-term Murine Cardiac Allografts: Origin of Inflammatory and Vascular Wall Cells. American Journal of Pathology. 1998 Jul;**153**(1):69–79. PubMed PMID: 9665467.

132. Haverty TP, Watanabe M, Neilson EG, Kelly CJ. Protective Modulation of Class II MHC Gene Expression in Tubular Epithelium by Target Antigen-specific Antibodies. Cell-surface Directed Down-regulation of Transcription Can Influence Susceptibility to Murine Tubulointerstitial Nephritis. J Immunol. 1989 August 15;**143**(4):1133–41.

133. Adoumie R, Serrick C, Giaid A, Shennib H, Adoumie R, Serrick C, et al. Early Cellular Events in the Lung Allograft. Annals of Thoracic Surgery. 1992 Dec;**54**(6):1071–6; discussion 6–7. PubMed PMID: 1449289.

134. Denton MD, Davis SF, Baum MA, Melter M, Reinders ME, Exeni A, et al. The Role of the Graft Endothelium in Transplant Rejection: Evidence that Endothelial Activation May Serve as a Clinical Marker for the Development of Chronic Rejection. Pediatric Transplantation. 2000 Nov;**4**(4):252–60. PubMed PMID: 11079263.

135. Baldwin WM, Larsen CP, Fairchild RL. Innate Immune Responses to Transplants: A Significant Variable with Cadaver Donors. Immunity. 2001;**14**(4):369–76.

136. Borges TJ, Wieten L, van Herwijnen MJ, Broere F, van der Zee R, Bonorino C, et al. The anti-inflammatory Mechanisms of Hsp70. Front Immunol. 2012;**3**:95. PubMed PMID: 22566973. PubMed Central PMCID: PMC3343630. Epub 2012/05/09. English.

137. Jiang W, Hu M, Rao J, Xu X, Wang X, Kong L. Over-expression of Toll-like Receptors and Their Ligands in Small-for-Size Graft. Hepatology Research: The Official Journal of the Japan Society of Hepatology. 2010 Apr;**40**(4):318–29. PubMed PMID: 20070394. Epub 2010/01/15. English.

138. Pockley AG, Muthana M. Heat Shock Proteins and Allograft Rejection. Contrib Nephrol. 2005;**148**:122–34. PubMed PMID: 15912031. Epub 2005/05/25. English.

139. Hiratsuka M, Yano M, Mora BN, Nagahiro I, Cooper JD, Patterson GA, et al. Heat Shock Pretreatment Protects Pulmonary Isografts from Subsequent Ischemia-Reperfusion Injury. Journal of Heart & Lung Transplantation. 1998 Dec;**17**(12):1238–46. PubMed PMID: 9883766.

140. Squiers EC, Bruch D, Buelow R, Tice DG, Squiers EC, Bruch D, et al. Pretreatment of Small Bowel Isograft Donors with Cobalt-Protoporphyrin Decreases Preservation Injury. Transplantation Proceedings. 1999 Feb-Mar;**31**(1-2):585–6. PubMed PMID: 10083247.

141. Bernink JH, Peters CP, Munneke M, te Velde AA, Meijer SL, Weijer K, et al. Human Type 1 Innate Lymphoid Cells Accumulate in Inflamed Mucosal Tissues. Nat Immunol. 2013 03//print;**14**(3):221–9.

142. Ito T, Connett JM, Kunkel SL, Matsukawa A. The Linkage of Innate and Adaptive Immune Response during Granulomatous Development. Frontiers in Immunology. 2013 January 31;**4**. eng.

143. Penfield JG, Wang Y, Li S, Kielar MA, Sicher SC, Jeyarajah DR, et al. Transplant Surgery Injury Recruits Recipient MHC Class II-positive Leukocytes into the Kidney. Kidney International. 1999 Nov;**56**(5):1759–69. PubMed PMID: 10571784.

144. Olszewski WL, Olszewski WL. Innate Immunity Processes in Organ Allografting–Their Contribution to Acute and Chronic Rejection. Ann Transplant. 2005;**10**(2):5–9. PubMed PMID: 16218025.

145. Akalin E, Watschinger B. Antibody-mediated Rejection. Seminars in Nephrology. 2007 Jul;**27**(4):393–407. PubMed PMID: 17616272.

146. Truong LD, Barrios R, Adrogue HE, Gaber LW. Acute Antibody-mediated Rejection of Renal Transplant: Pathogenetic and Diagnostic Considerations. Archives of Pathology & Laboratory Medicine. 2007 Aug;**131**(8):1200–8. PubMed PMID: 17683182.

147. Horie K, Kanou Y, Sato M, Tsuyuki M, Ishida S, Shimoji T, et al. A Case of Early Graft Loss Due to Hyperacute Rejection after ABO-incompatible Renal Transplantation. Clinical Transplantation. 2008 //;**22**(s19):42–6.

148. Baldwin WM. Samaniego-Picota M, Kasper EK, Clark AM, Czader M, Rohde C, et al. Complement Deposition in Early Cardiac Transplant Biopsies Is Associated with Ischemic Injury and Subsequent Rejection Episodes. Transplantation. 1999 Sep 27;**68**(6):894–900. PubMed PMID: 10515392.

149. Shimizu A, Colvin RB. Pathological Features of Antibody-mediated Rejection. Current Drug Targets – Cardiovascular & Haematological Disorders. 2005 Jun;**5**(3):199–214. PubMed PMID: 15975034.

150. Akalin E, Watschinger B, Akalin E, Watschinger B. Antibody-mediated Rejection. Seminars in Nephrology. 2007 Jul;**27**(4):393–407. PubMed PMID: 17616272.

151. Naemi FM, Ali S, Kirby JA. Antibody-mediated Allograft Rejection: The Emerging Role of Endothelial Cell Signalling and Transcription Factors. Transpl Immunol. 2011 Sep;**25**(2-3):96–103. PubMed PMID: 21782944. Epub 2011/07/26. English.

152. Zhang X, Rozengurt E, Reed EF. HLA Class I Molecules Partner with Integrin Beta4 to Stimulate Endothelial Cell Proliferation and Migration. Science Signaling. 2010;**3**(149):ra85. PubMed PMID: 21098729. Epub 2010/11/26. English.

153. Feucht HE, Felber E, Gokel MJ, Hillebrand G, Nattermann U, Brockmeyer C, et al. Vascular Deposition of Complement-split Products in Kidney Allografts with Cell-mediated Rejection. Clinical & Experimental Immunology. 1991 Dec;**86**(3):464–70. PubMed PMID: 1747954.

154. Feucht HE, Schneeberger H, Hillebrand G, Burkhardt K, Weiss M, Riethmuller G, et al. Capillary Deposition of C4d Complement Fragment and Early Renal Graft Loss. Kidney International. 1993;43(6):1333–8.

155. Banasik M, Boratynska M, Nowakowska B, Halon A, Koscielska-Kasprzak K, Drulis-Fajdasz D, et al. C4D Deposition and Positive Posttransplant Crossmatch Are Not Necessarily Markers of Antibody-mediated Rejection in Renal Allograft Recipients. Transplantation Proceedings. 2007 Nov;39(9):2718–20. PubMed PMID: 18021967.

156. Seemayer CA, Gaspert A, Nickeleit V, Mihatsch MJ. C4d Staining of Renal Allograft Biopsies: A Comparative Analysis of Different Staining Techniques. Nephrology Dialysis Transplantation. 2007 Feb;22(2):568–76. PubMed PMID: 17164320.

157. Sun Q, Liu ZH, Ji S, Chen J, Tang Z, Zeng C, et al. Late and Early C4d-positive Acute Rejection: Different Clinico-histopathological Subentities in Renal Transplantation. Kidney International. 2006 Jul;70(2):377–83. PubMed PMID: 16760909.

158. Roufosse CA, Shore I, Moss J, Moran LB, Willicombe M, Galliford J, et al. Peritubular Capillary Basement Membrane Multilayering on Electron Microscopy: A Useful Marker of Early Chronic Antibody-mediated Damage. Transplantation. 2012 Aug 15;94(3):269–74. PubMed PMID: 22790448. Epub 2012/07/14. English.

159. Sis B, Halloran PF. Endothelial Transcripts Uncover a Previously Unknown Phenotype: C4d-negative Antibody-mediated Rejection. Curr Opin Organ Transplant. 2010 Feb;15(1):42–8. PubMed PMID: 20009933. Epub 2009/12/17. English.

160. Mengel M, Sis B, Haas M, Colvin RB, Halloran PF, Racusen LC, et al. BANFF 2011 Meeting Report: New Concepts in Antibody-mediated Rejection. American Journal of Transplantation. 2012;12(3):563–70.

161. Hammond ME, Stehlik J, Snow G, Renlund DG, Seaman J, Dabbas B, et al. Utility of Histologic Parameters in Screening for Antibody-mediated Rejection of the Cardiac Allograft: A Study of 3,170 Biopsies. J Heart Lung Transplant. 2005 Dec;24(12):2015–21. PubMed PMID: 16364843.

162. Nankivell BJ, Alexander SI. Rejection of the Kidney Allograft. New England Journal of Medicine. 2010;363(15):1451–62. PubMed PMID: 20925547.

163. Jukes J-P, Wood KJ, Jones ND. Natural Killer T Cells: A Bridge to Tolerance or a Pathway to Rejection? Transplantation. 2007 Sep 27;84(6):679–81. PubMed PMID: 17893598.

164. Kitchens WH, Uchara S, Chasc CM, Colvin RB, Russell PS, Madsen JC. The Changing Role of Natural Killer Cells in Solid Organ Rejection and Tolerance. Transplantation. 2006 Mar 27;81(6):811–7. PubMed PMID: 16570001.

165. Goldman M, Le Moine A, Braun M, Flamand V, Abramowicz D. A Role for Eosinophils in Transplant Rejection. Trends Immunol. 2001 May;22(5):247–51. PubMed PMID: 11323281. Epub 2001/04/27. English.

166. Chantranuwat C, Qiao JH, Kobashigawa J, Hong L, Shintaku P, Fishbein MC. Immunoperoxidase Staining for C4d on Paraffin-embedded Tissue in Cardiac Allograft Endomyocardial Biopsies: Comparison to Frozen Tissue Immunofluorescence. Appl Immunohistochem Mol Morphol. 2004 Jun;12(2):166–71. PubMed PMID: 15354744.

167. Aguilar P, Mathieu CP, Clerc G, Ethevenot G, Fajraoui M, Mattei S, et al. Modulation of Natural Killer (NK) Receptors on NK (CD3-/CD56+), T (CD3+/CD56-) and NKT-like (CD3+/CD56+) Cells after Heart Transplantation. Journal of Heart & Lung Transplantation. 2006 Feb;25(2):200–5. PubMed PMID: 16446221.

168. McNerney ME, Lee KM, Zhou P, Molinero L, Mashayekhi M, Guzior D, et al. Role of Natural Killer Cell Subsets in Cardiac Allograft Rejection. American Journal of Transplantation. 2006 Mar;6(3):505–13. PubMed PMID: 16468959.

169. Sanfilippo F, Kolbeck PC, Vaughn WK, Bollinger RR. Renal Allograft Cell Infiltrates Associated with Irreversible Rejection. Transplantation. 1985 Dec;40(6):679–85. PubMed PMID: 3907043.

170. Azzawi M, Hasleton PS, Geraghty PJ, Yonan N, Krysiak P, El-Gammal A, et al. RANTES Chemokine Expression Is Related to Acute Cardiac Cellular Rejection and Infiltration by CD45RO T-lymphocytes and Macrophages. Journal of Heart & Lung Transplantation. 1998 Sep;17(9):881–7. PubMed PMID: 9773860.

171. Erren M, Arlt M, Willeke P, Schluter B, Junker R, Deng MC, et al. Predictive Value of the CD45RO Positive T-helper Lymphocyte Subset for Acute Cellular Rejection during the Early Phase after Kidney Transplantation. Transplantation Proceedings. 1999 Feb–Mar;31(1–2):319–21. PubMed PMID: 10083125.

172. Wang P, Zhu L, Liu T, Zhang X, Qiu Y. Intragraft CD45 RO Gene Expression Is an Early Marker to Detect Small Bowel Allograft Rejection in Rats. Microsurgery. 1999;19(7):348–50. PubMed PMID: 10586202.

173. Mueller TF, Einecke G, Reeve J, Sis B, Mengel M, Jhangri GS, et al. Microarray Analysis of Rejection in Human Kidney Transplants using Pathogenesis-based Transcript Sets. Am J Transplant. 2007 Dec;7(12):2712–22. PubMed PMID: 17941957. Epub 2007/10/19. English.

174. Sarwal M, Chua MS, Kambham N, Hsieh SC, Satterwhite T, Masek M, et al. Molecular Heterogeneity in Acute Renal Allograft Rejection Identified by DNA Microarray Profiling. The New England Journal of Medicine. 2003 Jul 10;349(2):125–38. PubMed PMID: 12853585. Epub 2003/07/11. English.

175. Hadley G. Role of Integrin CD103 in Promoting Destruction of Renal Allografts by CD8 T Cells. American Journal of Transplantation. 2004 Jul;4(7):1026–32. PubMed PMID: 15196058.

176. Wang D, Yuan R, Feng Y, El-Asady R, Farber DL, Gress RE, et al. Regulation of CD103 Expression by CD8+ T Cells Responding to Renal Allografts. Journal of Immunology. 2004 Jan 1;172(1):214–21. PubMed PMID: 14688328.

177. Al-Hamidi A, Pekalski M, Robertson H, Ali S, Kirby JA. Renal Allograft Rejection: The Contribution of Chemokines to the Adhesion and Retention of AlphaE(CD103)Beta7 Integrin-expressing Intratubular T Cells. Mol Immunol. 2008 Sep;45(15):4000–7. PubMed PMID: 18649941. Epub 2008/07/25. English.

178. Adams DH, Afford SC. Effector Mechanisms of Nonsuppurative Destructive Cholangitis in Graft-versus-Host Disease and Allograft Rejection. Seminars in Liver Disease. 2005 Aug;25(3):281–97. PubMed PMID: 16143944. Epub 2005/09/07. English.

179. Delacruz V, Garcia M, Mittal N, Nishida S, Levi D, Selvaggi G, et al.

Immunoenzymatic and Morphological Detection of Epithelial Cell Apoptotic Stages in Gastrointestinal Allografts from Multivisceral Transplant Patients. Transplantation Proceedings. 2004 Mar;36(2):338–9. PubMed PMID: 15050151.

180 Alegre M, Fallarino F, Zhou P, Frauwirth K, Thistlethwaite J, Newell K, et al. Transplantation and the CD28/CTLA4/B7 Pathway. Transplantation Proceedings. 2001 Feb–Mar;33(1–2):209–11. PubMed PMID: 11266782.

181 Clarkson MR, Sayegh MH, Clarkson MR, Sayegh MH. T-cell Costimulatory Pathways in Allograft Rejection and Tolerance. Transplantation. 2005 Sep 15;80(5):555–63. PubMed PMID: 16177624.

182 Kitchens WH, Haridas D, Wagener ME, Song M, Ford ML. Combined Costimulatory and Leukocyte Functional Antigen-1 Blockade Prevents Transplant Rejection Mediated by Heterologous Immune Memory Alloresponses. Transplantation. 2012 May 27;93(10):997–1005. PubMed PMID: 22475765. Epub 2012/04/06. English.

183 Ho J, Wiebe C, Gibson IW, Rush DN, Nickerson PW. Immune Monitoring of Kidney Allografts. Am J Kidney Dis. 2012 Oct;60(4):629–40. PubMed PMID: 22542291. Epub 2012/05/01. English.

184 Hodge G, Hodge S, Li-Liew C, Reynolds PN, Holmes M. Increased Natural Killer T-like Cells Are a Major Source of Pro-inflammatory Cytokines and Granzymes in Lung Transplant Recipients. Respirology. 2012 Jan;17(1):155–63. PubMed PMID: 21995313. Epub 2011/10/15. English.

185 Clement MV, Haddad P, Soulie A, Benvenuti C, Lichtenheld MG, Podack ER, et al. Perforin and Granzyme B as Markers for Acute Rejection in Heart Transplantation. International Immunology. 1991 Nov;3(11):1175–81. PubMed PMID: 1760412.

186 Griffiths GM, Namikawa R, Mueller C, Liu CC, Young JD, Billingham M, et al. Granzyme A and Perforin as Markers for Rejection in Cardiac Transplantation. European Journal of Immunology. 1991 Mar;21(3):687–93. PubMed PMID: 2009911.

187 Madsen CB, Norgaard A, Iversen M, Ryder LP. Elevated mRNA Levels of CTLA-4, FoxP3, and Granzyme B in BAL, but Not in Blood, during Acute Rejection of Lung Allografts. Transpl Immunol. 2010 Oct;24(1):26–32. PubMed PMID: 20633650. Epub 2010/07/17. English.

188 Ahmed-Ansari A, Tadros TS, Knopf WD, Murphy DA, Hertzler G, Feighan J, et al. Major Histocompatibility Complex Class I and Class II Expression by Myocytes in Cardiac Biopsies Posttransplantation. Transplantation. 1988 May;45(5):972–8. PubMed PMID: 3285544.

189 Barrett M, Milton AD, Barrett J, Taube D, Bewick M, Parsons VP, et al. Needle Biopsy Evaluation of Class II Major Histocompatibility Complex Antigen Expression for the Differential Diagnosis of Cyclosporine Nephrotoxicity from Kidney Graft Rejection. Transplantation. 1987 Aug;44(2):223–7. PubMed PMID: 3307046.

190 Belitsky P, Miller SM, Gupta R, Lee S, Ghose T. Induction of MHC Class II Expression in Recipient Tissues Caused by Allograft Rejection. Transplantation. 1990 Feb;49(2):472–6. PubMed PMID: 2305472.

191 Briscoe DM, Cotran RS. Role of Leukocyte-endothelial Cell Adhesion Molecules in Renal Inflammation: In Vitro and in Vivo Studies. Kidney International – Supplement. 1993 Jul;42:S27–34. PubMed PMID: 8361125.

192 Heemann UW, Tullius SG, Azuma H, Kupiec-Weglinsky J, Tilney NL. Adhesion Molecules and Transplantation. Annals of Surgery. 1994 Jan;219(1):4–12. PubMed PMID: 8297174.

193 Kirby JA. The Role Played by Adhesion Molecules during Allograft Rejection. Transplant Immunology. 1994 Jun;2(2):129–32. PubMed PMID: 7953308.

194 Mulligan MS, McDuffie JE, Shanley TP, Guo RF, Vidya Sarma J, Warner RL, et al. Role of RANTES in Experimental Cardiac Allograft Rejection. Experimental & Molecular Pathology. 2000 Dec;69(3):167–74. PubMed PMID: 11115358.

195 Schroppel B, Fischereder M, Lin M, Marder B, Schiano T, Kramer BK, et al. Analysis of Gene Polymorphisms in the Regulatory Region of MCP-1, RANTES, and CCR5 in Liver Transplant Recipients. Journal of Clinical Immunology. 2002 Nov;22(6):381–5. PubMed PMID: 12462338.

196 Miura M, Morita K, Kobayashi H, Hamilton TA, Burdick MD, Strieter RM, et al. Monokine Induced by IFN-gamma Is a Dominant Factor Directing T Cells into Murine Cardiac Allografts during Acute Rejection. Journal of Immunology. 2001 Sep 15;167(6):3494–504. PubMed PMID: 11544343.

197 Schnickel GT, Bastani S, Hsieh GR, Shefizadeh A, Bhatia R, Fishbein MC, et al. Combined CXCR3/CCR5 Blockade Attenuates Acute and Chronic Rejection. J Immunol. 2008 April 1, 2008;180(7):4714–21.

198 Merani S, Truong WW, Hancock W, Anderson CC, Shapiro AMJ. Chemokines and Their Receptors in Islet Allograft Rejection and as Targets for Tolerance Induction. Cell Transplantation. 2006;15(4):295–309. PubMed PMID: 16898223.

199 Smith RN, Ueno T, Ito T, Tanaka K, Shea SP, Abdi R. Chemokines and Chronic Heart Allograft Rejection. Transplantation. 2007 Aug 15;84(3):442–4. PubMed PMID: 17700176.

200 Stasikowska O, Wagrowska-Danilewicz M. Chemokines and Chemokine Receptors in Glomerulonephritis and Renal Allograft Rejection. Medical Science Monitor. 2007 Feb;13(2):RA31–6. PubMed PMID: 17261994.

201 Smith RN, Colvin RB. Chronic Alloantibody Mediated Rejection. Semin Immunol. 2012 Apr;24(2):115–21. PubMed PMID: 22051115. Epub 2011/11/05. English.

202 Takeda A, Horike K, Ohtsuka Y, Inaguma D, Goto N, Watarai Y, et al. Current Problems of Chronic Active Antibody-mediated Rejection. Clin Transplant. 2011 Jul;25 Suppl 23:2–5. PubMed PMID: 21623906. Epub 2011/06/03. English.

203 Arias M, Seron D, Moreso F, Bestard O, Praga M. Chronic Renal Allograft Damage: Existing Challenges. Transplantation. 2011 May 15;91(9 Suppl):S4–25. PubMed PMID: 21519213. Epub 2011/04/29. English.

204 Hayry P. Chronic Allograft Vasculopathy: New Strategies for Drug Development. Transplantation proceedings. 1998 Dec;30(8):3989–90. PubMed PMID: 9865271.

205 Lachmann N, Terasaki PI, Schonemann C, Lachmann N, Terasaki PI, Schonemann C. Donor-specific HLA Antibodies in Chronic Renal Allograft Rejection: A Prospective Trial with a Four-year Follow-up. Clinical Transplants. 2006:171–99. PubMed PMID: 18365377.

206 Takahashi H, Kato T, Mizutani K, Terasaki P, Delacruz V, Tzakis AG,

et al. Simultaneous Antibody-mediated Rejection of Multiple Allografts in Modified Multivisceral Transplantation. Clinical Transplants. 2006:529–34. PubMed PMID: 18365419.

207 Terasaki P, Lachmann N, Cai J. Summary of the Effect of de Novo HLA Antibodies on Chronic Kidney Graft Failure. Clinical Transplants. 2006:455–62. PubMed PMID: 18365403.

208 Denton MD, Davis SF, Baum MA, Melter M, Reinders ME, Exeni A, et al. The Role of the Graft Endothelium in Transplant Rejection: Evidence that Endothelial Activation May Serve as a Clinical Marker for the Development of Chronic Rejection. Pediatric Transplantation. 2000 Nov;**4**(4):252–60. PubMed PMID: 11079263.

209 Kauppinen H, Soots A, Krogerus L, Brummer T, Ahonen J, Lautenschlager I. Different Expression of Adhesion Molecules ICAM-1 and VCAM-1 and Activation Markers MHC Class II and IL-2 R in Acute and Chronic Rejection of Rat Kidney Allografts. Transplantation Proceedings. 1997 Nov;**29**(7):3150–1. PubMed PMID: 9365703.

210 Grimm PC, Nickerson P, Jeffery J, Savani RC, Gough J, McKenna RM, et al. Neointimal and Tubulointerstitial Infiltration by Recipient Mesenchymal Cells in Chronic Renal-allograft Rejection. The New England Journal of Medicine. 2001 July 12;**345**(2):93–7.

211 Allan JS, Madsen JC. Recent Advances in the Immunology of Chronic Rejection. Current Opinion in Nephrology & Hypertension. 2002 May;**11**(3):315–21. PubMed PMID: 11981262.

212 Ozdemir BH, Ozdemir FN, Gungen Y, Haberal M. Role of Macrophages and Lymphocytes in the Induction of Neovascularization in Renal Allograft Rejection. American Journal of Kidney Diseases. 2002 Feb;**39**(2):347–53. PubMed PMID: 11840376.

213 Ravalli S, Albala A, Ming M, Szabolcs M, Barbone A, Michler RE, et al. Inducible Nitric Oxide Synthase Expression in Smooth Muscle Cells and Macrophages of Human Transplant Coronary Artery Disease. Circulation. 1998 Jun 16;**97**(23):2338–45. PubMed PMID: 9639378.

214 de Andrade JA, Thannickal VJ. Innovative Approaches to the Therapy of Fibrosis. Curr Opin Rheumatol. 2009 Nov;**21**(6):649–55. PubMed PMID: 19667993. Pubmed Central PMCID: PMC2862988. Epub 2009/08/12. English.

215 Wynn TA. Cellular and Molecular Mechanisms of Fibrosis. Journal of Pathology. 2008 Jan;**214**(2):199–210. PubMed PMID: 18161745.

216 Nadeau KC, Azuma H, Tilney NL. Sequential Cytokine Dynamics in Chronic Rejection of Rat Renal Allografts: Roles for Cytokines RANTES and MCP-1. Proceedings of the National Academy of Sciences of the United States of America. 1995 Sep 12;**92**(19):8729–33. PubMed PMID: 7568006.

217 Russell ME, Wallace AF, Hancock WW, Sayegh MH, Adams DH, Sibinga NE, et al. Upregulation of Cytokines Associated with Macrophage Activation in the Lewis-to-F344 Rat Transplantation Model of Chronic Cardiac Rejection. Transplantation. 1995 Feb 27;**59**(4):572–8. PubMed PMID: 7533347.

218 Csencsits K, Wood SC, Lu G, Faust SM, Brigstock D, Eichwald EJ, et al. Transforming Growth Factor Beta-induced Connective Tissue Growth Factor and Chronic Allograft Rejection. American Journal of Transplantation. 2006 May;**6**(5 Pt 1):959–66. PubMed PMID: 16611331.

219 Rintala JM, Savikko J, Rintala SE, von Willebrand E. The Effect of Leflunomide Analogue FK778 on Development of Chronic Rat Renal Allograft Rejection and Transforming Growth Factor-BETA Expression. Transplantation Proceedings. 2006 Dec;**38**(10):3239–40. PubMed PMID: 17175234.

220 Barocci S, Ginevri F, Valente U, Torre F, Gusmano R, Nocera A. Correlation between Angiotensin-converting Enzyme Gene Insertion/Deletion Polymorphism and Kidney Graft Long-term Outcome in Pediatric Recipients: A Single-center Analysis. Transplantation. 1999 Feb 27;**67**(4):534–8. PubMed PMID: 10071023.

221 Ikegami M, Nagano T, Hara Y, Negita M, Imanishi M, Ishii T, et al. [Tissue Type Plasminogen Activator (t-PA) and Plasminogen Activator Inhibitor (PAI) in Transplanted Kidneys]. Nippon Hinyokika Gakkai Zasshi – Japanese Journal of Urology. 1995 May;**86**(5):991–5. PubMed PMID: 7596085.

222 Legendre C, Pascual M. Improving Outcomes for Solid-organ Transplant Recipients at Risk from Cytomegalovirus Infection: Late-onset Disease and Indirect Consequences. Clinical Infectious Diseases. 2008 Mar 1;**46**(5):732–40. PubMed PMID: 18220478.

223 Grossi PA, Costa AN, Fehily D, Blumberg EA, Kuehnert MJ, Fishman JA, et al. Infections and Organ Transplantation: New Challenges for Prevention and Treatment—A Colloquium. Transplantation. 2012;**93**: S4–S39 10.1097/ TP.0b013e3182481347.

224 Egli A, Binggeli S, Bodaghi S, Dumoulin A, Funk GA, Khanna N, et al. Cytomegalovirus and Polyomavirus BK Posttransplant. Nephrology Dialysis Transplantation. 2007 Sep;**22** Suppl 8:viii72–viii82. PubMed PMID: 17890268.

225 Steininger C. Clinical Relevance of Cytomegalovirus Infection in Patients with Disorders of the Immune System. Clinical Microbiology & Infection. 2007 Oct;**13**(10):953–63. PubMed PMID: 17803749.

226 Watkins RR, Lemonovich TL, Razonable RR. Immune Response to CMV in Solid Organ Transplant Recipients: Current Concepts and Future Directions. Expert Review of Clinical Immunology. 2012 May;**8**(4):383–93. PubMed PMID: 22607184. Epub 2012/05/23. English.

227 Streblow DN, Orloff SL, Nelson JA. Acceleration of Allograft Failure by Cytomegalovirus. Current Opinion in Immunology. 2007 Oct;**19**(5):577–82. PubMed PMID: 17716883.

228 Potena L, Valantine HA. Cytomegalovirus-associated Allograft Rejection in Heart Transplant Patients. Current Opinion in Infectious Diseases. 2007 Aug;**20**(4):425–31. PubMed PMID: 17609604.

229 Valantine H. Cardiac Allograft Vasculopathy after Heart Transplantation: Risk Factors and Management. J Heart Lung Transplant. 2004 May;**23**(5 Suppl): S187–93. PubMed PMID: 15093804.

230 Carratala J, Montejo M, Perez-Romero P. Infections Caused by Herpes Viruses Other than Cytomegalovirus in Solid Organ Transplant Recipients. Enferm Infecc Microbiol Clin. 2012 Mar;**30**

231. Bennett SM, Broekema NM, Imperiale MJ. BK Polyomavirus: Emerging Pathogen. Microbes and infection / Institut Pasteur. 2012 Aug;14(9):672–83. PubMed PMID: 22402031. PubMed Central PMCID: PMC3568954. Epub 2012/03/10. English.

232. Acott P, Babel N. BK Virus Replication Following Kidney Transplant: Does the Choice of Immunosuppressive Regimen Influence Outcomes? Ann Transplant. 2012 Jan–Mar;17(1):86–99. PubMed PMID: 22466913. Epub 2012/04/03. English.

233. Delbue S, Ferraresso M, Ghio L, Carloni C, Carluccio S, Belingheri M, et al. A Review on JC Virus Infection in Kidney Transplant Recipients. Clinical & Developmental Immunology. 2013;2013:926391. PubMed PMID: 23424601. PubMed Central PMCID: PMC3569895. Epub 2013/02/21. English.

234. Hirsch HH, Drachenberg CB, Steiger J, Ramos E. Polyomavirus Associated Nephropathy in Renal Transplantation: Critical Issues of Screening and Management. In: Ahsan N, editor. Polyomaviruses and Human Diseases. Advances in Experimental Medicine and Biology, vol. **577**. 1st ed. New York, N.Y. Georgetown, T.X.: Springer Science+Business Media, Landes Bioscience / Eurekah.com; 2006. p. 160–73.

235. Nishi S. Polyomavirus Nephropathy – Recent Pathological Diagnostic Problems and the Report from the 2011 BANFF Meeting. Clin Transplant. 2012 Jul;**26** Suppl 24:9–12. PubMed PMID: 22747469. Epub 2012/07/07. English.

236. Duvoux C, Firpi R, Grazi GL, Levy G, Renner E, Villamil F. Recurrent Hepatitis C Virus Infection Post Liver Transplantation: Impact of Choice of Calcineurin Inhibitor. Transpl Int. 2013 Feb 18. PubMed PMID: 23413991. Epub 2013/02/19. English.

237. Manzia TM, Angelico R, Toti L, Lai Q, Ciano P, Angelico M, et al. Hepatitis C Virus Recurrence and Immunosuppression-free State after Liver Transplantation. Expert Review of Clinical Immunology. 2012 Sep;**8**(7):635–44. PubMed PMID: 23078061. Epub 2012/10/20. English.

238. Dixon LR, Crawford JM. Early Histologic Changes in Fibrosing Cholestatic Hepatitis C. Liver Transpl. 2007 Feb;**13**(2):219–26. PubMed PMID: 17205558.

239. Neff GW, Shire N, Ruiz P, O'Brien C, Garcia M, Dela Garza J, et al. The Importance of Clinical Parameters when Differentiating Cholestatic Hepatitis C Virus from Allograft Rejection. Transplantation Proceedings. 2005 Dec;**37**(10):4397–402. PubMed PMID: 16387130.

240. Ge D, Fellay J, Thompson AJ, Simon JS, Shianna KV, Urban TJ, et al. Genetic Variation in IL28B Predicts Hepatitis C Treatment-induced Viral Clearance. Nature. 2009;**461**(7262):399–401.

241. Nayak NC, Sachdeva R. Localization of Hepatitis B Surface Antigen in Conventional Paraffin Sections of the Liver. Comparison of Immunofluorescence, Immunoperoxidase, and Orcein Staining Methods with Regard to Their Specificity and Reliability as Antigen Marker. American Journal of Pathology 1975 **81**(3):479–92.

242. Green M, Michaels MG. Epstein-Barr Virus Infection and Posttransplant Lymphoproliferative Disorder. Am J Transplant. 2013 Feb;**13** Suppl 3:41–54; quiz PubMed PMID: 23347213. Epub 2013/02/01. English.

243. Morscio J, Dierickx D, Ferreiro JF, Herreman A, Van Loo P, Bittoun E, et al. Gene Expression Profiling Reveals Clear Differences between EBV-positive and EBV-negative Posttransplant Lymphoproliferative Disorders. Am J Transplant. 2013 Mar 14. PubMed PMID: 23489474. Epub 2013/03/16. English.

244. Kennedy C, Obilana A, O'Brien F, O'Kelly P, Dorman A, Denton M, et al. Glomerular Disease Recurrence in Second and Subsequent Kidney Transplants. Clin Nephrol. 2013 Jan;**79**(1):31–6. PubMed PMID: 23073068. Epub 2012/10/18. English.

245. Moroni G, Casati C, Quaglini S, Gallelli B, Banfi G, Montagnino G, et al. Membranoproliferative Glomerulonephritis Type I in Renal Transplantation Patients: A Single-center Study of a Cohort of 68 Renal Transplants Followed up for 11 Years. Transplantation. 2011 Jun 15;**91**(11):1233–9. PubMed PMID: 21502910. Epub 2011/04/20. English.

246. Pham PT, Pham PC. Graft Loss Due to Recurrent Lupus Nephritis in Living-related Kidney Donation. Clin J Am Soc Nephrol. 2011 Sep;**6**(9):2296–9. PubMed PMID: 21799149. Pubmed Central PMCID: PMC3359005. Epub 2011/07/30. English.

Chapter 2

The Pathology of Kidney Transplantation

Phillip Ruiz, George Burke, Gaetano Ciancio, Giselle Guerra, David Roth, Linda Chen, Warren Kupin, and Adela Mattiazzi

I Introduction

The successful implementation of kidney transplantation more than 50 years ago has been one of the most remarkable medical achievements of the past century [1]. Transplant surgery quickly evolved in the 1960s, and the development of powerful immunosuppressive medications permitted transplantation to be performed between non-identical individuals, including unrelated living or deceased donors. This has allowed numerous patients relegated to dialysis to attain the ultimate substitute and to date, there have been greater than 100,000 renal transplants performed, averaging more than 10,000 per year [2]. A majority of the causes of end-stage renal disease (ESRD) are treatable with kidney transplantation with relatively few exceptions, such as the presence of cancer and active infections. Although there may be complications associated with renal transplantation (as described herein), when functional, it provides the most desirable substitute to renal dialysis. Unfortunately, a marked shortage of donor organs relegates numerous ESRD patients to wait in anticipation for their chance at this remarkable therapy.

The advancement in pharmaceutical and biological immunosuppressive therapies has affected graft and patient survival in renal transplantation such that first-year acute rejection is now notably improved compared to years past [3, 4]. However, acute rejection in all of its forms, as well as other complications within the initial post-transplant period, remains a frequent issue. Moreover, the incidence and severity of chronic allograft injury in renal transplantation has not been notably altered despite the advent of more effective and specific immunosuppression. As with any other solid organ transplant, kidney transplantation is affected by a variety of immunological and non-immunological variables present within the donor, as well as the recipient. For example, HLA matching has a notable impact upon graft survival, but other variables including donor or recipient age, clinical status, or native disease state have significant impact upon whether there will be optimal graft survival in both the short or long-term periods. In addition, the actual acquisition and sustenance of the donor allograft can have a prominent impact upon how the explanted organ will function in the new host [5, 6]. Alongside all of these better-described variables is our understanding of the basic pathophysiologic processes involved in the alloreactivity between donor and recipient. As cell-mediated rejection and humoral rejection become better defined, transplant pathologists now have improved tools to identify and define the occurrence of these complications. These tools (e.g., C4d, DSA information) are primarily utilized within and related to the renal allograft biopsy. This in combination with the application of uniform criteria between centers (e.g., BANFF) has helped to standardize how biopsies are interpreted and compared between different centers. As additional biomarkers obtained in the periphery (e.g., serum/cells) improve in their diagnostic specificity, it may be that they will be used in conjunction with and applied to the findings present within tissue obtained from the graft. However, to date, the renal allograft biopsy remains as an initial "gold standard" in describing the status and/or presence of complications occurring within the kidney transplant. As evidence to this, clinical diagnoses and therapy are frequently changed because of the findings present within the biopsy.

II Varieties of Biopsies and Technical Features

Though the Kidney Donor Risk Index [7] and other systems are used to assess donor kidney quality, it is a frequent practice of many institutions (including ours) to routinely biopsy prospective donor kidneys. Recently, the Organ Procurement and Transplantation Network in the United States sanctioned a new national deceased donor kidney allocation (Kidney Allocation System, i.e., KAS) policy that introduces the kidney donor profile index (KDPI) [8], which gives scores of 0%–100% based on a variety of donor factors. Kidneys with lower KDPI scores are associated with better post-transplant survival and most centers will biopsy any donor with KDPI >85%.

The procurement of renal biopsies from potential kidney donors and from implanted kidney allografts are done at most centers with a similar approach and equipment as utilized for native kidneys. Donor biopsies can be either wedge or needle biopsies with the critical point here being that a sufficient number of glomeruli from cortical areas (e.g., optimally at least 20 glomeruli in our center) must be obtained in order to provide the transplant pathologist adequate material to be able to delineate any donor associated acute or chronic injury. Biopsies from vascularized, implanted allografts tend to be needle biopsies – these generally fall into two categories of either protocol/study or indication biopsies.

Needle biopsies (for either protocol or indication purposes) are acquired with the appropriate needle gauge and optimally two to three tissue cores are obtained, most often by a trained interventional radiologist, surgeon, or nephrologist [9–12]. An important aspect of this process is that the pathologist or trained renal histotechnologist is present in the procedure room to visualize with zoom microscopy the adequacy of the freshly procured material. Renal cortex and the presence of glomeruli are needed and communicated to clinician performing the procedure. If adequate, the tissue is then separated into pieces for light microscopy, immunofluorescence, and electron microscopy. If inadequate, the tissue typically is submitted entirely for light microscopy at our institution, since many newer procedures can now be performed with formalin-fixed paraffin-embedded (FFPE) material. The 1997 BANFF criteria outlines that an "optimal"/adequate biopsy consists of one that has ten or more glomeruli and at least two arteries, three glomeruli for immunofluorescence, and one glomerulus for electron microscopy [13]; marginal and unsatisfactory categories consists of biopsies that have seven to ten glomeruli and one artery, and <7 glomeruli with no arteries, respectively. The purpose of having these categories of adequacy for the renal biopsies is that the sensitivity of identifying various processes such as acute rejection improves as the amount of tissue is optimized [14, 15].

Donor, protocol, and *indication* biopsies are obtained for different reasons. *Donor biopsies* provide a description of possible underlying injury in the tissue that may be grafted. With the shortage of donors, there has been an evolution in the types of organs that are now being considered; also contributing is that the population is aging and there are older transplant candidates, as well as older potential donors of kidneys. Extended criteria donors (ECD) are now quite commonly being considered (17%–20% of transplants now being performed use ECD donors) and they are defined as any donor aged 60 or over, or any donor from 50 to 59 years of age that contains at least two of three criteria: terminal serum creatinine >1.5 mg/dL, hypertension history, or cerebrovascular death. With such a potential for containing chronic injury, ECD donors are frequently biopsied for evaluation by pathologists. Although the histopathologic changes in the biopsy are critical in determining whether the organ will be utilized, other factors also play a role. It is important to note that there are no well-defined "standard" criteria for evaluation of suitable histology in donor biopsies at this time.

Protocol biopsies are not routinely performed in most centers, but are increasingly being recognized as useful predictors of problems that the graft will eventually display, as well as being able to define acute and chronic inflammatory and parenchymal injury that is not being manifested at a clinical level (e.g., subclinical rejection) [16, 17]. The phenomenon of subclinical rejection will be discussed in the sections of acute rejection in this chapter. Protocol biopsies can be useful in identifying the underlying etiology of delayed graft function (DGF) and in some institutions with ABO incompatible kidney transplant monitoring. There are variations in the schedule of protocol biopsies from center to center [18].

The obtaining of *indication biopsies* is done based on clinical alterations in the patient that include minor or abrupt changes in creatinine and BUN from the baseline, abnormal urinalysis, the presence of donor-specific alloantibodies, proteinuria, or acute renal failure. It has long been recognized that these clinical symptoms are nonspecific and that the biopsy provides useful information pertaining to the causation of the symptoms. In general, indication biopsies can identify rejection processes, infections, tubular injury, drug toxicities, de novo, and recurrent disease, among other pathologic entities.

The processing of donor, protocol, or indication biopsies is typically done in similar fashion with formalin fixation and routine processing for the light microscopy. Protocol and indication biopsies are usually performed with H&E (at least three), PAS [1–3], trichrome [1], and silver [1] stains; donor biopsies often only have H&E, as well as a connective tissue stain such as trichrome. Immunofluorescence (IgG, IgA, IgM, fibrinogen, C3, C4, C1q, albumin) and electron microscopy are often performed for protocol and indication biopsies, whereas donor biopsies tend to not have these ancillary techniques as part of the evaluation. Immunohistochemistry is becoming more frequently utilized particularly for stains such as C4d. Immunophenotypic analysis for immune effector populations on occasion can be useful, such as analysis of subpopulations of T cells.

III Donor Organs and Implantation Biopsies

The assessment of pre-implantation tissue from kidneys destined for transplant, also known as donor organ biopsies, is relatively common and as noted above, critical for the evaluation of extended criteria donors [19]. Typically, these donor biopsies are procured at the time of harvest, up until vascularization of the graft. Biopsies may also be taken after the graft has been anastomosed. At our institution, wedge biopsies from potential donor organs are the most common biopsies that are obtained, although core biopsies can also be obtained. Our preference at this point remains the wedge biopsies, due to the large number of glomeruli and tissue available for evaluation; if sufficient numbers of glomeruli are obtained, then accurate percentages for the percentage of changes seen can be provided. The biopsies are immediately placed in a buffered formalin solution; we then institute a rapid processing method (non-microwave based) and obtain permanent sections for evaluation roughly two hours after the biopsy is obtained in the laboratory. Of course, frozen sections may be obtained in certain scenarios, but we have found that there is marked improvement in the consistency of assessment of potential grafts using this method.

The intention of evaluating donor kidneys by these biopsies is to assess a particular collection of acute or chronic lesions pre-existing in the individual donating the organs. More often than not, these pre-existing lesions were clinically silent, but could have marked impact on the behavior of the organ once grafted. The most common lesions seen in donor kidneys are arteriosclerosis changes within arteries and arterioles (see Figure 2.1). These vascular lesions are typically graded in non-standardized, semiquantitative fashion, from mild to severe, and characteristics such as hyalinosis are also described [20]. Classic arteriosclerosis lesions within the mid- and large-sized arteries that include intimal thickening (as well as medial thickening in more severe cases) are often eccentric in pattern. Arteriosclerosis varies in intensity often between vessels within the biopsy, and we grade these changes from mild to severe

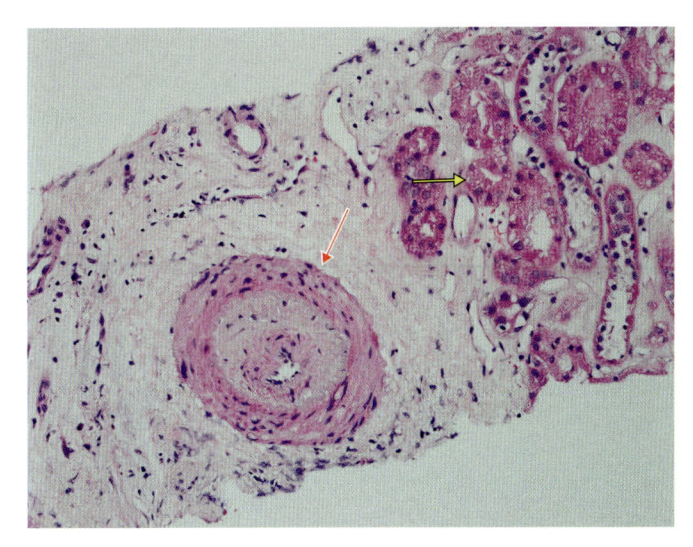

Figure 2.1 Severe arteriosclerosis in donor kidney biopsy (orange arrow) associated with chronic tubulointerstitial injury. Coexisting acute tubular injury (yellow arrow) is present. This organ was evaluated by rapid permanent sections and based on this information was not utilized for transplant (H&E, 200x).

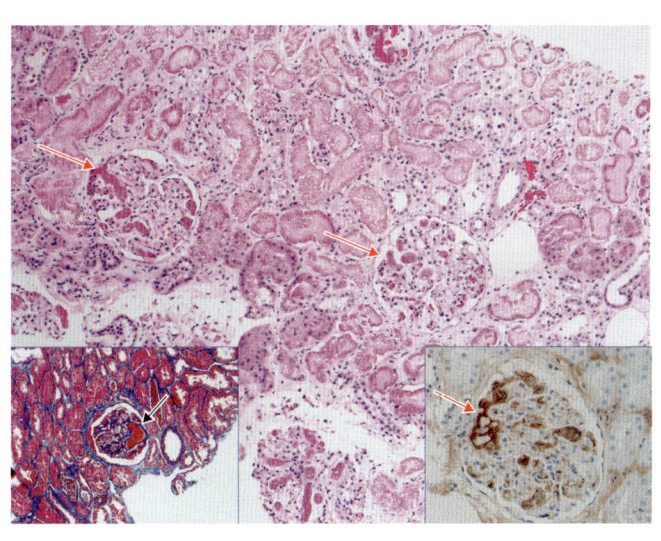

Figure 2.2 Disseminated intravascular coagulation (DIC) in donor kidney. The H&E slide (background slide, 200x) displays several glomeruli that contain impacted, hyalinotic material in the capillary loops (see arrows). The trichrome stain (lower left, 200x) and fibrinogen immunohistochemistry stain (lower right, 400x) highlight the thrombi within the capillary loops.

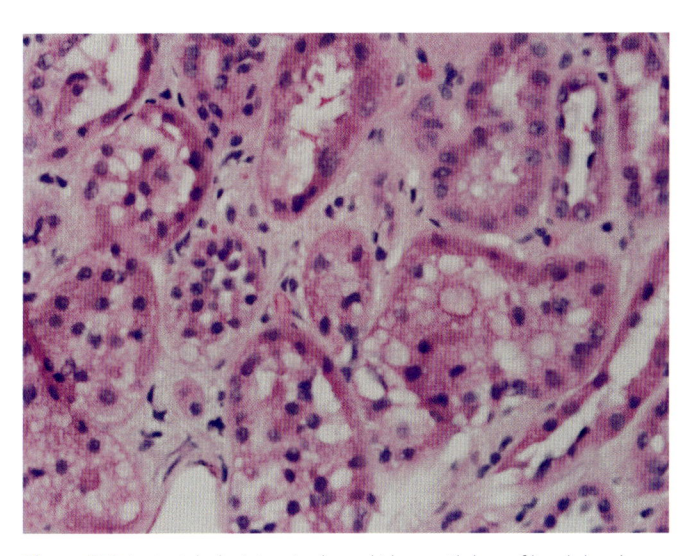

Figure 2.3 Acute tubular injury in donor kidney with loss of brush borders, nonisometric vacuolization, and some cell sloughing (H&E, 400x).

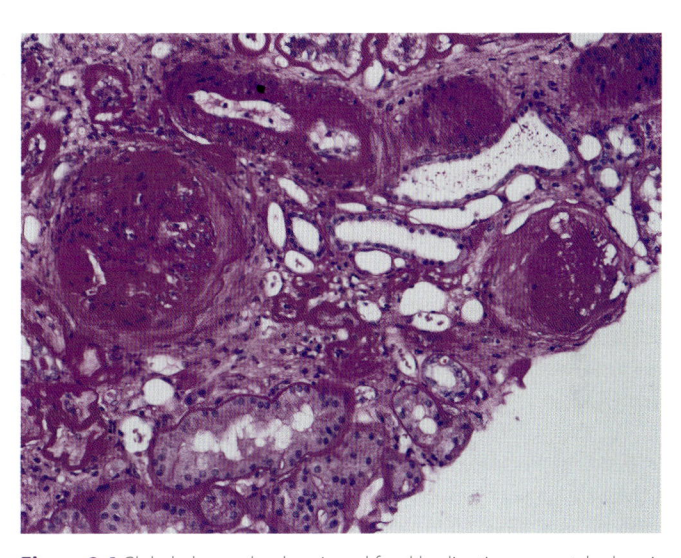

Figure 2.4 Global glomerulosclerosis and focal hyalinotic segmental sclerosis in a donor kidney. The donor had diabetes (PAS, 200x).

based on the vessels that show the most significant changes. Other chronic changes may also typically be present when the primary vascular arteriosclerosis lesions are seen, including chronic tubular interstitial injury, and glomerulosclerosis [21]. Severe arterial sclerosis can be associated with a high risk of delayed graft function in recipients of ECD organs [19, 22]. One of the most common "acute" vascular lesions seen is microthrombi within the glomerular capillaries (see Figure 2.2). The most common cause of these microthrombi is Disseminated Intravascular Coagulation (DIC) present during the terminal events of the donor [23]; rare subclinical Thrombotic Thrombocytopenic Purpura (TTP) may also be the cause. Vasculitis and cholesterol emboli are extremely rare lesions to see within vessels. Acute tubular injury (see Figure 2.3), glomerular thrombi, interstitial inflammation, and fibrosis tend to be relatively common and can coincide and be relational with the extent of arterio-arteriolosclerosis.

The presence of glomerular sclerosis (see Figure 2.4) that is global is one of the most common pathological changes observed in donor biopsies. While there are no firm guidelines for the percentage of global glomerulosclerosis that would prevent usage of the donor [24, 25], it is relatively common for there to be a cutoff of 20% when potential grafts are not utilized. A variety of studies have demonstrated variability between different centers as to the implications of the 20% cut off – several studies suggest no significant difference between <20% and >20%, while others do not recommend using kidneys that have >20% [26–28]. In our experience, global glomerulosclerosis does not tend to be an isolated lesion; it is typically associated with chronic tubulointerstitial injury and arteriosclerosis. Of course, other subclinical glomerular disease may also be present, including FSGS, diabetic nephropathy, IgA nephropathy, and early membranous glomerulonephritis. In our experience, diabetic nephropathy tends to be the most common among these latter lesions.

Acute tubular injury (ATI) and acute tubular necrosis (ATN) are relatively common lesions, particularly ATI. Tubules experiencing ATI have a loss of brush borders with tubular epithelial cell nuclei being dropped out and there may be some mild sloughing into the tubular lumen. ATN is a more severe lesion and involves frank necrosis of the tubular epithelial cells with more extensive sloughing and denuding. ATN can be a notable problem and may be a contributor to delayed graft function [28, 29].

The presence of a limited set of tumors involving the kidney may also be apparent. Grossly evident lesions on the capsular surface noted during procurement are often separately biopsied. Some of the lesions that can be evident in these suspicious nodules include renal cell carcinoma (RCC) (malignant) (see Figure 2.5) [30, 31], angiomyolipoma (a benign lesion) [32], and neurofibroma (benign) [33]. We have also frequently identified clear cell lesions that resemble RCC, but are actually benign adrenal rests. Since we do rapid processing for permanent sections, we also are now capable of rapidly performing immunohistochemistry and all clear cell lesions are subjected to a brief panel of RCC, CD10, and inhibin [34] – we have found this very useful for distinguishing ectopic adrenal rest tissue, since the inhibin is uniformly positive in the latter lesion. The implication of the size of the renal cell carcinoma is becoming critical as several centers, including our own, may decide to excise the lesion since there is now evidence showing minimal possibility for transmission of the lesion to the recipient [35].

At this point, there is no grading scheme ubiquitously utilized by pathologists for assessing potential donor kidneys, although several have been proposed. In general, transplant centers have developed their own guidelines and the communication between the transplant pathologist and the surgeons, along with experience of both individuals, is critical in order to establish a consistent system for evaluation of these donor organs.

IV Post-transplant Pathological Entities

Protocol and indication biopsies are capable of identifying an array of potential complications in the post-transplant period following kidney transplantation. As noted above, protocol biopsies in general will reveal only a limited number of these complications, since patients are typically clinically stable. Indication biopsies comprise the majority of biopsies that are performed.

a Ischemia Reperfusion Injury

Ischemia Reperfusion (IR) injury is the phenomenon where following varying periods of ischemia to an organ, blood supply

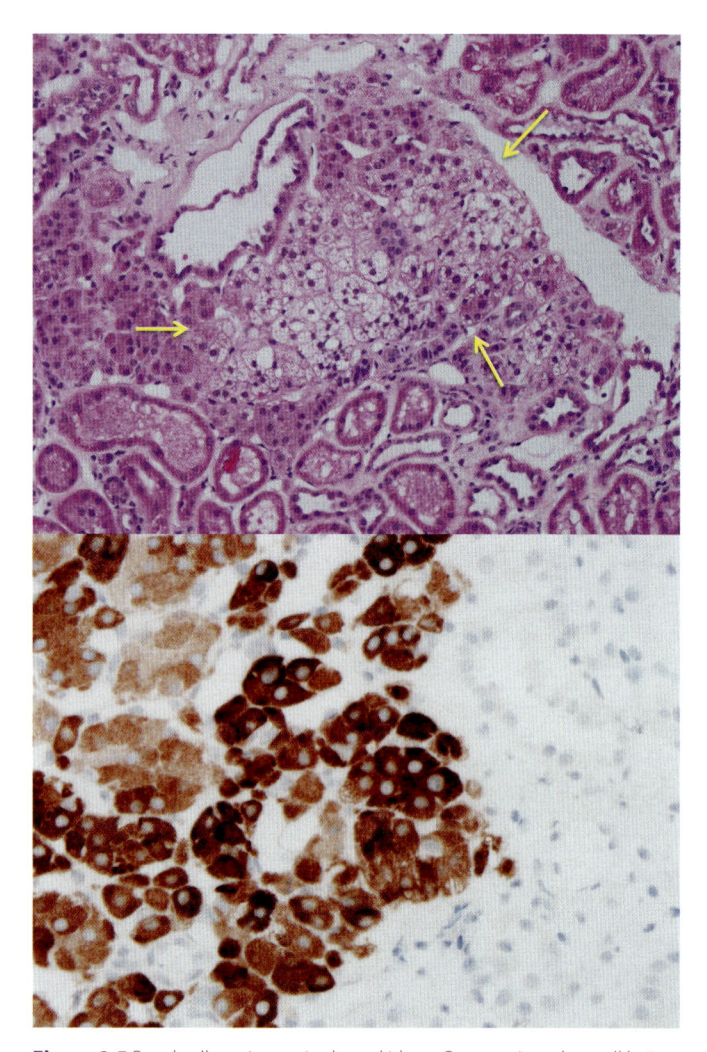

Figure 2.5 Renal cell carcinoma in donor kidney. On occasion, clear cell lesions are discovered within donor kidneys that are morphologically benign, but must be pursued. A small immunohistochemical panel of markers helps to rapidly distinguish renal cell carcinoma; in this example, there is a clear cell lesion present.

is returned and upon re-exposure, there are various types of cellular and structural injury that can take place, depending upon the period without oxygen [36, 37]. There can be multicellular dysfunction leading up to cell death, including endothelial cells, the latter leading to microvascular injury. An excessive production quantity of reactive oxygen species is a critical mechanism of reperfusion injury, among others described below.

Thus, on occasion, IR injury following the implantation of a diseased donor organ, and rarely organs from living donors [38, 39], results in Delayed Graft Function – if the DGF is more severe and it is a graft that never produces urine, this is termed "Primary Non-function" [40–42]. DGF can become an unfortunately common occurrence when kidneys of non-heart beating donor origin are used (e.g., 33%–84% of cases), compared to between 15% and 23% in kidneys from heart beating donors; primary non-function in kidneys from non-heart beating donors can be as high as 7%–18% [19, 38, 39, 43, 44]. A majority (e.g., 95%–98%) of grafts functionally recover [40].

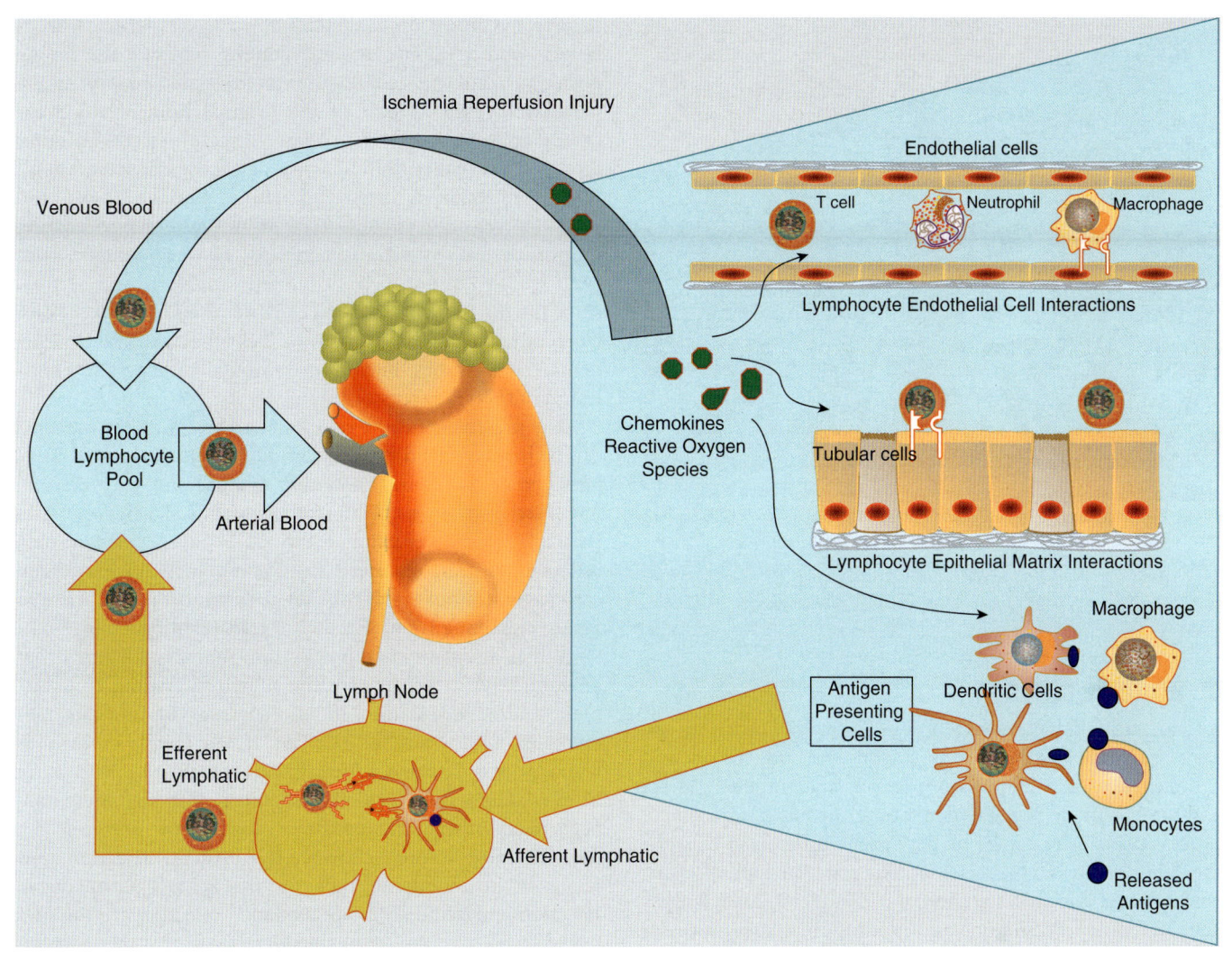

Figure 2.6 Diagram of Ischemia Reperfusion injury and the kidney.

The underlying precipitating factors sometimes associable with DGF include surgical complications, ischemic tubular injury, drug induced toxicity (e.g., calcineurin inhibitor, rapamycin), hyperkalemia, accelerated antibody or cellular-mediated rejection, and significant donor organ arteriosclerosis. Indication and sometimes protocol biopsies are typically done to assist in identifying the injury underlying the DGF.

CD4+ T cells, natural killer cells, and IFN-γ participate in the development of IR injury likely due to interaction of activated T lymphocytes with adhesion molecules on vascular endothelium of the microvasculature [45, 46] (see Figure 2.6). Numerous gene changes [47–51] take place and there are transient changes in the level of several critical membrane molecules following IR injury; this is one of the reasons why ischemia is known to promote acute rejection. At this point, isolated IR injury as an independent risk factor (i.e., excluding other causes of delayed graft function such as early rejection episodes, surgical complications) is not clearly associable with poorer long-term graft survival [52, 53]. Rather, it appears that I-R injury promotes alloreactive processes and this negatively impacts graft survival, as evidenced by increased acute rejection in protocol biopsies early post-transplant in patients with delayed graft function [52–54].

On biopsy, a majority of kidney grafts displaying DGF histologically demonstrate acute ischemic injury, so-called "acute tubular injury" (ATI) (see Figure 2.7). The morphological changes include loss of the tubular brush border, intra-tubular proteinaceous debris and altered tubular epithelial cell morphology that includes tubular dilatation and/or flattening, and mitotic figures. Intra-tubular neutrophils may also be present, although not to the density evident in pyelonephritis. Tubules may also display non-isometric vacuolization.

ATI may also concomitantly be associated with interstitial edema and occasional neutrophils; the presence of a "capillaritis" such that peritubular capillaries contain neutrophils and mononuclear cells is unusual in our experience, but is sporadically seen. This may present a mild diagnostic dilemma if the patient is far enough post-transplant and also has a donor-specific alloantibody (DSA); in the latter scenario, capillaritis could also represent acute antibody-mediated rejection (AAMR), particularly if there is C4d staining along the capillary lumens. C4d tends to be absent with ischemia reperfusion injury, although C4d-negative AAMR is well-described. Clinical correlation with graft symptomatology and other morphological changes needs to be considered.

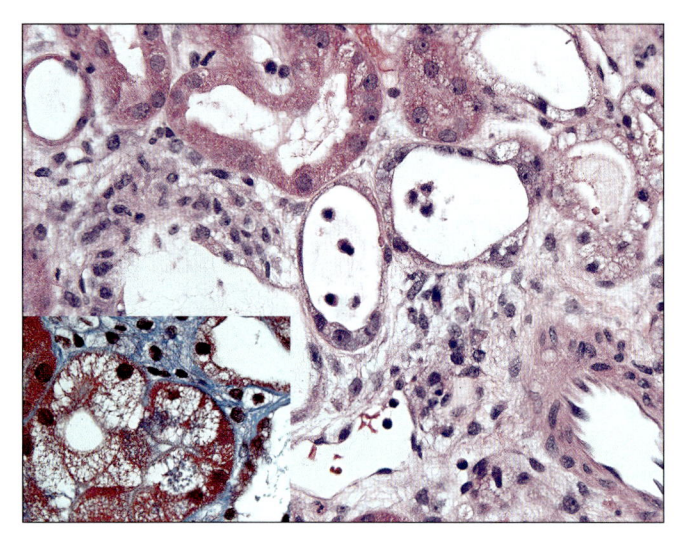

Figure 2.7 Renal graft (eight days post-transplant) with delayed function ischemic tubular injury with tubular dilatation and epithelial flattening, as well as scattered inflammatory cells. The interstitium revealed moderate edema, scattered mononuclear inflammatory cells, and focal dilatation of peritubular capillaries. There was no evidence of rejection (H&E, 200x). The lower left insert of this case (trichrome stain, 400x) highlights non-isometric vacuolization of the cytoplasm.

b   Acute Rejection

As with native kidneys, a variety of inflammatory processes can also affect transplanted kidneys. However, one broad and complex class of inflammatory lesions that uniquely affect and are specific to renal allografts is termed *acute rejection*, a process principally driven by the genetic differences between the donor organ and the recipient. The principles and mechanisms of acute rejection are covered in Chapter 1. Essentially, a conglomeration of immune and non-immune host processes stimulated by donor/recipient disparity at HLA and non-HLA loci, initiates a vigorous cell-mediated and antibody-mediated onslaught on the donor organ that, left untreated, can damage the organ and lead to its demise. Immunosuppressive therapy, a stalwart of the medications given to solid organ transplant recipients since the beginning, has been done to prevent primarily acute rejection. Present immunosuppressive drug regimens including tacrolimus, mycophenolate-mofetil, and sirolimus, often combined with potent induction protocols, have lessened the frequency of acute rejection episodes from a couple of decades past. As such, it is roughly estimated that rejection episodes affect 12%–18% of living donor kidneys and 14%–30% of cadaveric organs during the first six months post-grafting. Acute rejection currently accounts for 11%–16% of graft losses in the first year [55, 56]. These numbers are improved, but still represent a notable proportion of the post-transplant complications that present in these patients; in addition, this speaks primarily to clinically apparent acute rejection. Subclinical rejection [57–60] is a more frequent lesion believed to bear the potential to cause long-term graft injury, possibly in the form of chronic rejection.

The pathological classification of acute rejection has had a history of being influenced from several generations of clinicians, pathologists, and scientists that have recommended a multiplicity of schemes that were loosely (and sometimes incorrectly) based on available knowledge, experience, technology, and opinions. In some grading schemes, the timing post-transplant when some variants of rejection *most often* take place were used as part of the original nomenclature; for example, "hyperacute" or "accelerated acute" rejection denotes a very early event (within hours or days post-transplantation), "acute" rejection is diagnosed within days or weeks, and "chronic" rejection is considered to be a late event occurring months or years after transplantation. These terms have since been recognized not to be accurate in categorizing rejection, since the time frames ascribed can and often have exceptions. Currently, "acute" and "chronic" changes are not sharply demarcated entities, but rather represent a range and continuum of several processes [61, 62].

The presence of acute rejection can be clinically suspected on the basis of rapid rises of serum creatinine, elevated BUN levels, graft tenderness, retaining of fluid and, on occasion, increased proteinuria. Unfortunately, clinical parameters, in particular serum creatinine and BUN levels, inadequately reflect intra-graft disease. Graft injury, including rejection, can occur without significant renal dysfunction and a rise in serum creatinine is not specific for transplant rejection.

When discussing acute rejection, one should know that anatomically, it can involve the tubulo-interstitial compartment and/or vasculature, its etiology may be immune cell-mediated and/or antibody driven, it can appear as early as few days or as late as decades after transplantation, and it can be overlaid on other types of graft injury. Although there have been many other terms used to describe acute rejection [63, 64], the most favored classification of acute rejection now relates to the underlying *etiology* so that acute T cell-mediated rejection and acute antibody-mediated rejection are the preferred terms. An important consideration is that the morphological interpretation as to the etiology and type of acute rejection that is present is based upon morphological, immunohistochemical, and laboratory parameters seen in the biopsy. However, molecular analysis of various gene sets promises to refine and possibly redefine the origins of the acute (and chronic) rejection present. We are very close to having adjunct molecular assays being performed [65] as a means of enhancing our accuracy of diagnosis and ultimately our prognosticating capacity associated with the interpretation.

As mentioned above, there has been a variety of grading scoring systems that have been utilized and proposed for evaluating acute rejection in renal allograft biopsies. The two most common proposed grading schemes were the Cooperative Clinical Trials in Renal Transplantation (CCTT) [66] and the BANFF schemes [67]. Fortunately, there was a merger of the BANFF and CCTT schemes in 1997 [13], and since that point, there has been biannual updating of the BANFF criteria. The BANFF schemes tend to be etiology-driven and are the most utilized; we will be using BANFF as our classification categories and will use their terminology.

i   Acute T Cell-mediated Rejection (TCMR)

This form of acute rejection has also been known as "Acute Cellular Rejection" or "Acute Tubulointerstitial Rejection" and

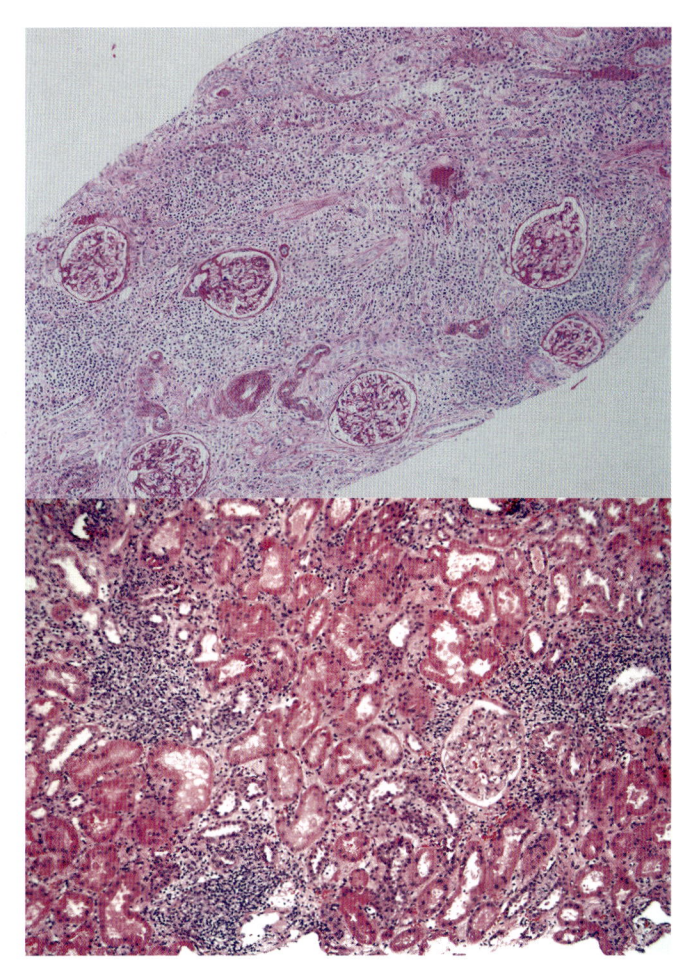

Figure 2.8 Acute T cell-mediated rejection in the early post-transplantation period. The tubulointerstitial compartment demonstrates intense, diffuse, mononuclear inflammatory cell infiltrates and edema. PAS, 40x (top), H&E, 100x (bottom).

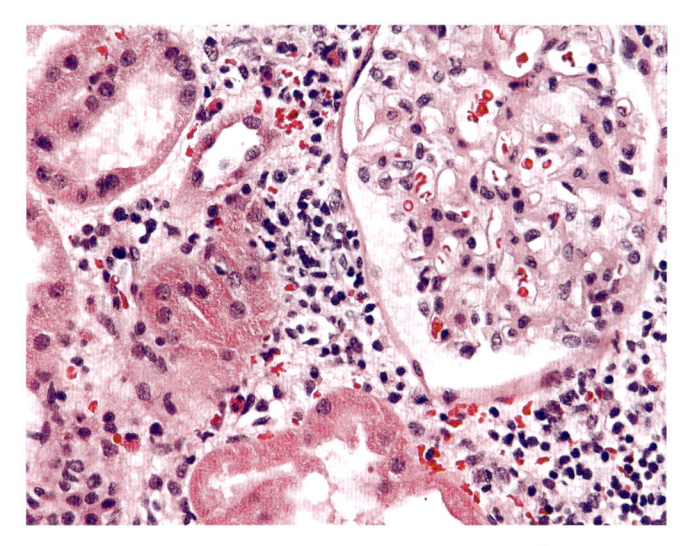

Figure 2.9 Acute T cell-mediated rejection showing mixed inflammatory infiltrate with plasma cells, mononuclear cells, and eosinophils (H&E, 400x, 200x).

is in general characterized by varying degrees of mononuclear cell-rich inflammatory infiltrates principally localized in the interstitial compartment accompanied in the presence of edema and tubulitis (i.e., permeation of inflammatory mononuclear cells into non-atrophic tubules). While we tend to view acute TCMR in isolated fashion, the reality is that this entity frequently occurs in the context of other complicating issues occurring with the renal allograft, including acute antibody-mediated rejection (AAMR). The coexistence of acute TCMR and AAMR is also known as "mixed acute rejection" and is in our experience relatively common.

As the name implies, T cells have experimentally been demonstrated to be the driving force and principal etiology of TCMR [68]. However, that does not translate to an isolated, monomorphic population of cells present within the graft – in fact, it is the heterogeneous, mixed chronic inflammatory cell infiltrate that is characteristic of TCMR. Numerous studies have shown that there is additional heterogeneity within the T cell subsets that are participating in initiating and maintaining the alloreactive response. However, depending upon the genetic disparity, type and level of immunosuppressive therapy, and other factors, the composition of the *effector* T cell population can widely vary. In addition, *regulatory* T cell populations also participate and are at varying levels within different individuals. If the proportion of effector cells to regulatory cells varies, then an "inflammatory" population may be present, but there may not be end organ injury since a dampening by the regulatory population may be taking place [69]. While these particular issues are beyond the scope of this chapter, it is important to consider that eventual in situ and/or gene profile measurements of these different T cell subpopulations may eventually be a common, ancillary tool used in addition to the biopsy. This may provide information as to the potential for graft injury to occur in the presence of an inflammatory infiltrate.

There are a few gross pathology evaluations of kidneys undergoing acute TCMR, but when this occurs, the organs are often enlarged pale, yellow-brown, with the medulla slightly darker on cross section, especially along the corticomedullary junction.

There is a notable degree of variability in the histological appearance of TCMR, but the typical appearance is that of a renal cortical predominant, focal, and/or diffuse mononuclear inflammatory cell infiltrate, characteristically complemented by interstitial edema; the medulla is sometimes involved in more severe rejection episodes (see Figures 2.8–2.11). The appearance of the mixed lymphocytic, macrophage, and plasma cell inflammatory cells includes resting and activated cells (e.g., class II, IL25 receptor-positive), often displaying mitotic figures, and exhibiting markers of cell proliferation, such as KI-67. The cells tend to loosely associate among non-atrophic tubules, but there are also infiltrates present in fibrotic areas with atrophic tubules. This latter point is important since the scoring of one of the principal lesions for TCMR, tubulitis (see Figures 2.10 and 2.11), is considered only on non-atrophic tubules. Immunophenotypic evaluations both experimentally and clinically have revealed that the inflammatory infiltrate is primarily composed of activated T-lymphocytes (CD3, CD4, CD8) (see Figure 2.12), abundant and sometimes dominant

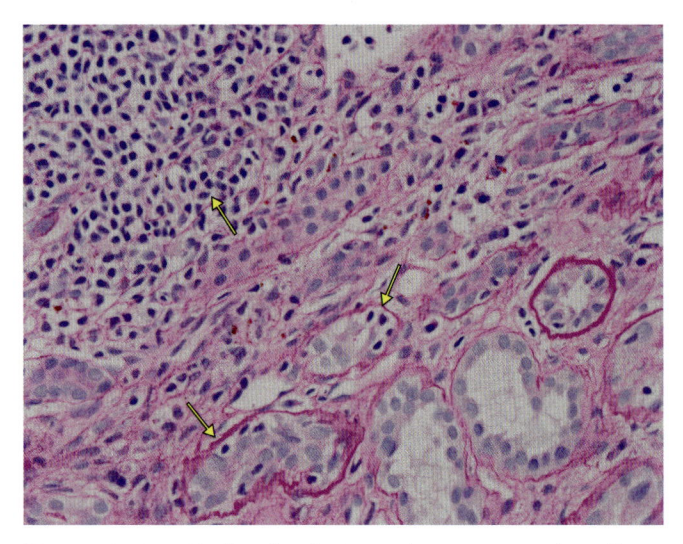

Figure 2.10 Acute T cell-mediated rejection showing mononuclear infiltrate with foci of tubulitis ranging from mild to severe (arrows) (PAS, 200x).

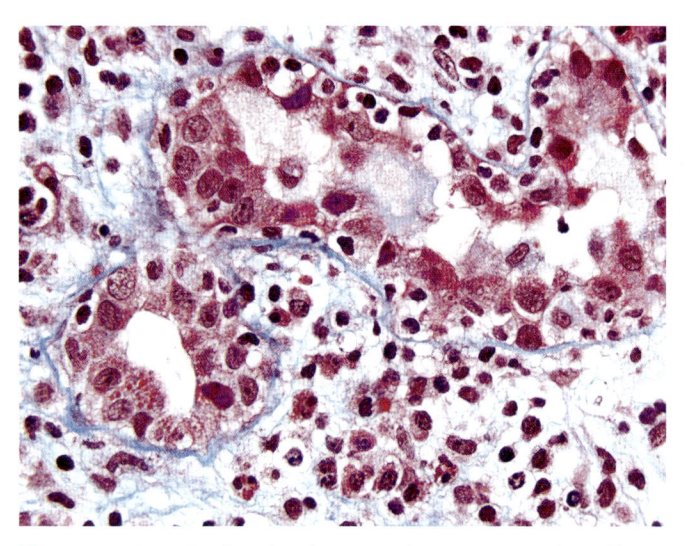

Figure 2.11 Acute T cell-mediated rejection showing mononuclear infiltrate with foci of tubulitis with prominent perinuclear halos (Trichrome, 400x).

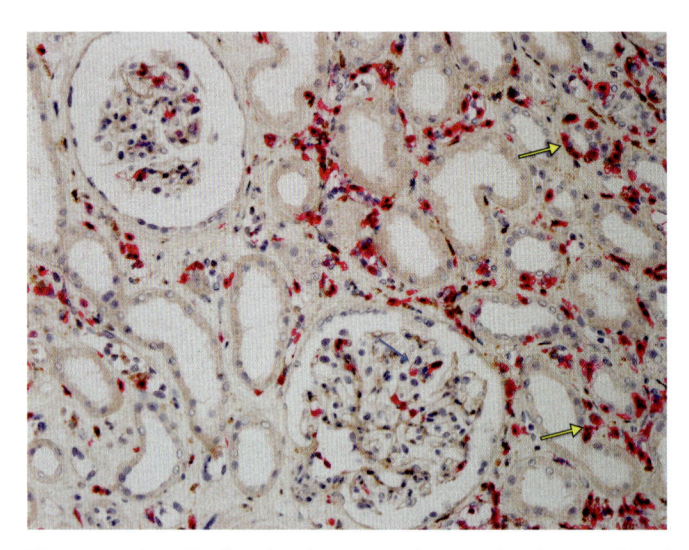

Figure 2.12 Acute T cell-mediated rejection – showing CD4+ (brown cells) and CD8+ (red cells) mononuclear infiltrate with foci of tubulitis (yellow arrows) and coexisting glomerulitis (blue arrow). Two-color immunohistochemistry to CD4/CD8, 400x.

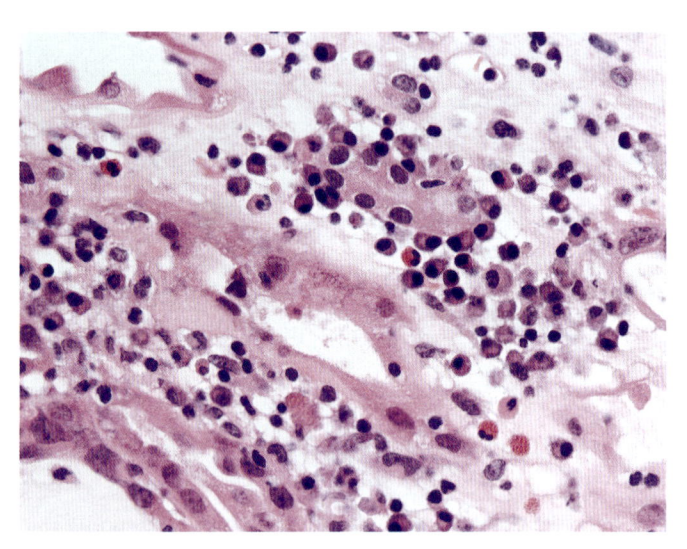

Figure 2.13 Acute T cell-mediated rejection, plasma cell-rich with many plasma cells surrounding tubules without overt tubular injury (H&E, 400x).

macrophages/histiocytes (CD68) [70–74], as well as varying numbers of plasma cells (CD138-positive) sometimes mounting "plasma cell-rich" rejection episodes [75, 76] (see Figures 2.13 and 2.14). In addition, CD20-positive B cells, eosinophilic leukocytes, and polymorphonuclear leukocytes can be detected. CD20-positive lymphocytes can infiltrate the cortex diffusely, form small nodules (see Figure 2.15), and occasionally even germinal centers (e.g., tertiary germinal centers); when their numbers generally exceed more than 50% of the inflammatory reaction [71, 77–80], then we consider that other B cell processes may be contributing to the inflammation (e.g., PTLD) and pursue further evaluation of this possibility. Many other cell types contribute to the inflammatory response in tubulo-interstitial cellular rejection, such as natural killer cells, mast cells, or dendritic cells [81–83]. Polymorphonuclear leukocytes are commonly seen in or adjacent to severely injured tubules; they can be abundant adjacent to infarcts. The presence of eosinophils and edema could be heralding a more "active" phase of the TCMR, but the possibility of a concomitant allergic etiology/allergic interstitial nephritis must always be considered. The presence of inflammation within peritubular capillaries [84, 85] (see Figure 2.16) could be foreshadowing a migration from the capillaries into the interstitium and tubules, but the presence of "capillaritis" is also an important component of acute antibody-mediated rejection (discussed below). In general, the response of the different forms of TCMR to immunosuppression shows that the "lower" or less severe forms (e.g., BANFF categories Borderline, IA, IB) do have an improved response and therefore better clinical outcomes and fewer incidents of recurrence.

Tubulitis is illustrated by mononuclear cells (one or more T lymphocytes and/or macrophages) located inside the basement membrane and under or in-between epithelial cells; although recognizable on the H&E stain (see Figure 2.16), it is best

The Pathology of Kidney Transplantation

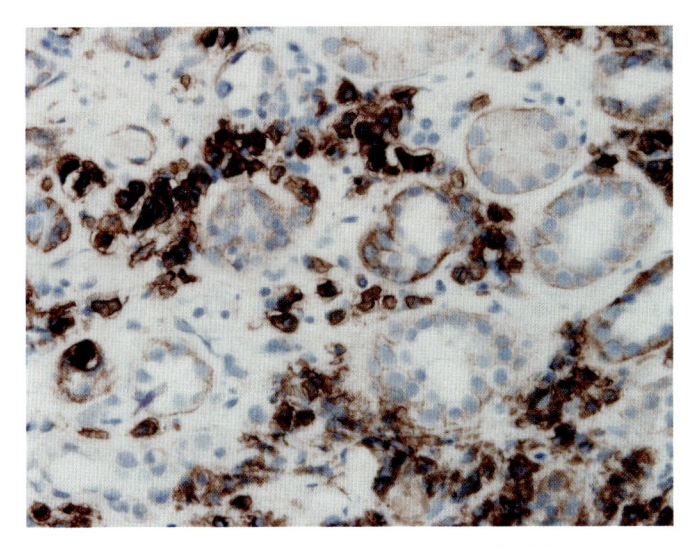

Figure 2.14 Acute T cell-mediated rejection, plasma cell-rich (same case as Figure 2.13, but separate area) showing focal accumulations of CD138+ plasma cells. Immunohistochemistry to CD138, 400x.

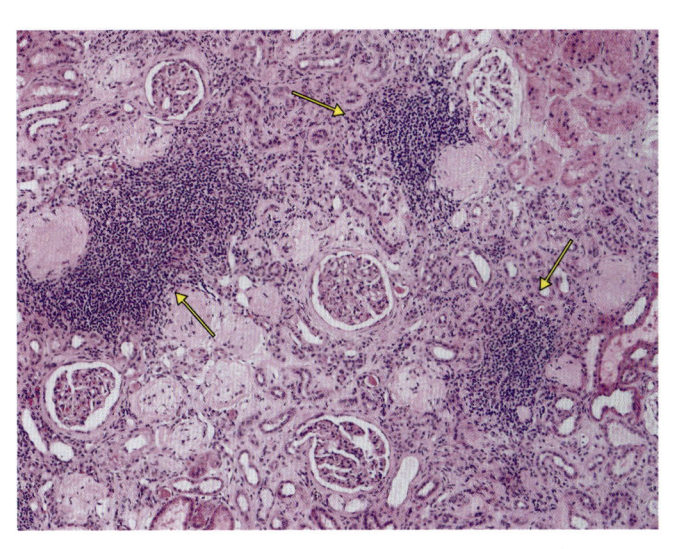

Figure 2.15 Lymphocyte aggregates in kidney allograft (predominantly B cells; IHC not shown) and shown by the arrows. These cell accumulations tend to occur in long-standing kidney grafts with repeated history of acute rejection (H&E, 200x).

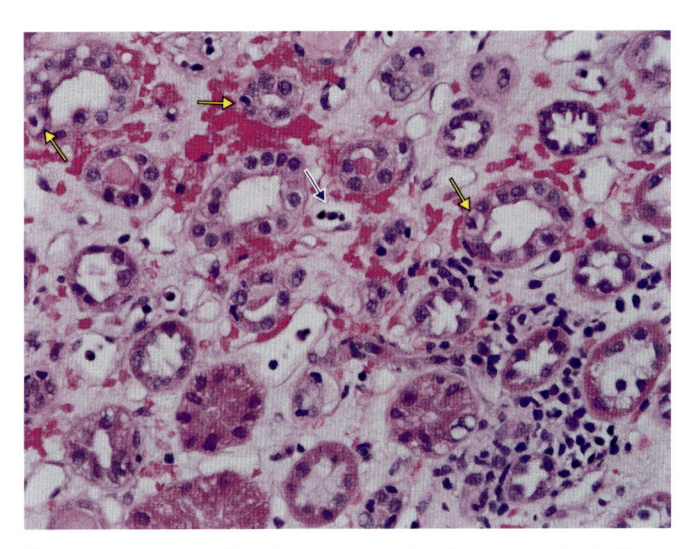

Figure 2.16 Acute T cell-mediated rejection showing mononuclear infiltrate with foci of tubulitis (yellow arrows) and capillary collections of inflammatory cells (blue arrow) sometimes seen in TCMR (H&E, 200x).

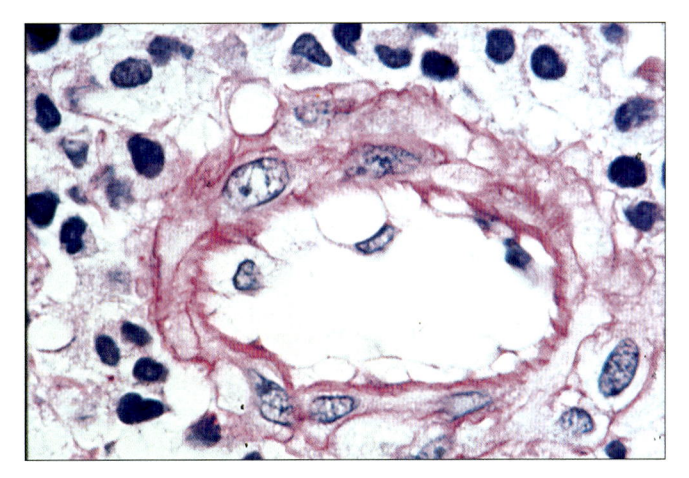

Figure 2.17 Endothelial cell activation in a small arterial branch with only rare inflammatory cells (H&E, 400x).

visualized by the PAS or trichrome stains. Inflammatory cells exhibiting tubulitis often show a perinuclear halo (see Figures 2.10 and 2.11). One useful distinguishing feature is that tubular epithelial cell nuclei are normally larger than the infiltrating inflammatory cells, often contain small nucleoli, and show a less dense, often finely granular chromatin structure. Eosinophils and polymorphonuclear leukocytes tend not to be involved in rejection tubulitis. Tubulo-interstitial inflammation in TCMR can be in combination with rejection phenomena in other tissue compartments, including endarteritis. The extent of distribution and severity of tubulointerstitial inflammation and tubulitis comprise the most essential criteria for BANFF categories "Borderline," IA, and IB (see Table 2.1).

Arteritis is inflammation present within the arterial tree from large arteries to arterioles; inflammation can also be present within venules and lymphatics [86], but these latter two sites do not tend to be incorporated into grading criteria for acute rejection [87, 88]; endothelial reactivity is also present in most cases of arteritis (see Figure 2.17), but must be accompanied by inflammation to be considered as arteritis. This type of inflammatory change within vessels tends to be relatively infrequent in acute rejection as compared to interstitial inflammation with tubulitis. There are varieties of forms of arteritis, all that are incorporated into the BANFF criteria – IIA (see Figure 2.18), IIB (see Figure 2.19), and III (see Figure 2.20) for acute T cell-mediated rejection (see Table 2.1). For example, there may be endothelialitis, which is an accumulation of mononuclear inflammatory cells beneath the endothelial layer of arterial branches within the kidney (see Figure 2.18) and there may be relatively small numbers of these cells, which tend to be lymphocytes (see Figure 2.18) or macrophages. There may

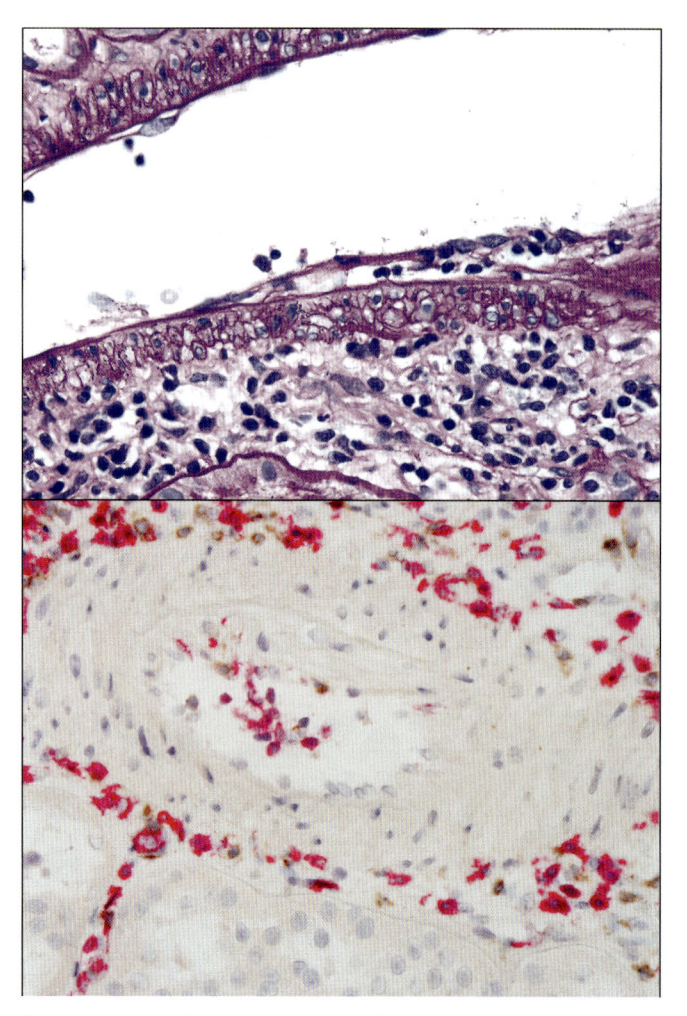

Figure 2.18 Arteritis with inflammatory cells in-between and under activated endothelial cells along one segment of an interlobular artery (Top, PAS, 400x), BANFF IIA. Two-color immunohistochemistry to CD4/CD8 showing CD4+ (brown cells) and CD8+ (red cells) mononuclear infiltrate within artery with BANFF IIA (Bottom, 400x).

be more extensive and severe forms of arteritis, including focal inflammatory changes within the vascular wall, sometimes with fibrinoid changes (see Figure 2.20). This may be also associated with necrosis. If there is inflammation throughout the arterial wall, it is termed as transmural arteritis and is a relatively rare lesion. BANFF criteria for vascular forms of acute T cell-mediated rejection incorporate these various lesions from endothelialitis to transmural arteritis, although these forms tend to be much less frequently found than the tubulointerstitial forms of acute T cell-mediated rejection. Although they are documented, the presence of arteritis does not appear to have an effect on graft survival compared with the absence of arteritis [89].

Other lesions seen in TCMR can include lymphocytic aggregates and tubulitis adjacent to sclerotic glomeruli, in the arterial adventitia layer, and at the cortico-medullary junction. Lymphocytes may be present with interstitial fibrosis and tubulitis may be seen in atrophic tubules with thickened basement membranes. At present, these changes are considered to be non-diagnostic for rejection [78, 90, 91], but should be described. In addition to the tubulointerstitial inflammation and tubulitis lesions, TCMR may also manifest itself with other lesions that are not necessarily specific to TCMR, but should be described. For example, glomerulitis and arteritis can be a component of TCMR, but may also be a component of AAMR.

Glomerulitis or endocapillary hypercellularity with mononuclear and/or polymorphonuclear cells inside dilated capillary loops can be evident in TCMR, but is not common with a "pure" T cell-mediated process. Glomerulitis is not used in the BANFF criteria for acute T cell-mediated rejection and, in fact, glomerulitis is typically associable with AAMR and, if present (along with the other criteria for AAMR described below), is considered a "mixed" rejection. This form of inflammation often is the precursor process of glomerular remodeling (e.g., transplant glomerulopathy), but must be distinguished from other potential

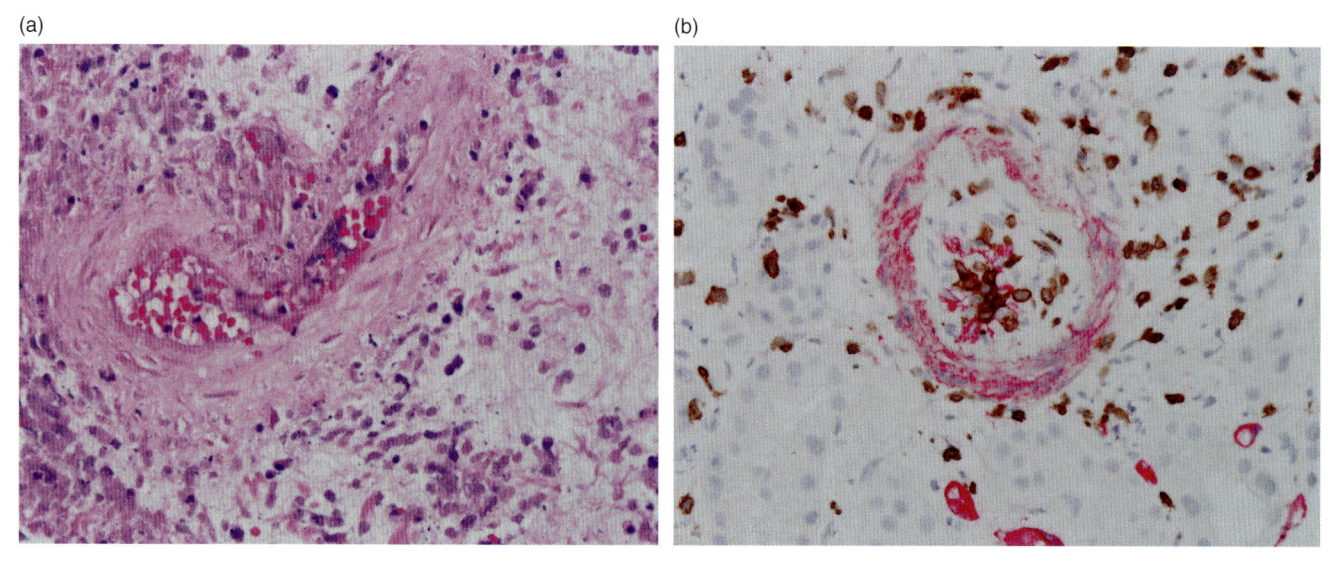

Figure 2.19 BANFF IIB lesions. 19A – Section of artery with arteritis involving entire interior of vessel (H&E, 400x). 19B – Two-color immunohistochemistry of an artery showing a BANFF IIB lesion, with CD3+ T cells (brown cells) circumferentially lining the arterial intima that has endothelial cells highlighted in red after being stained with CD34 (Two-color immunohistochemistry to CD3/CD34, 400x).

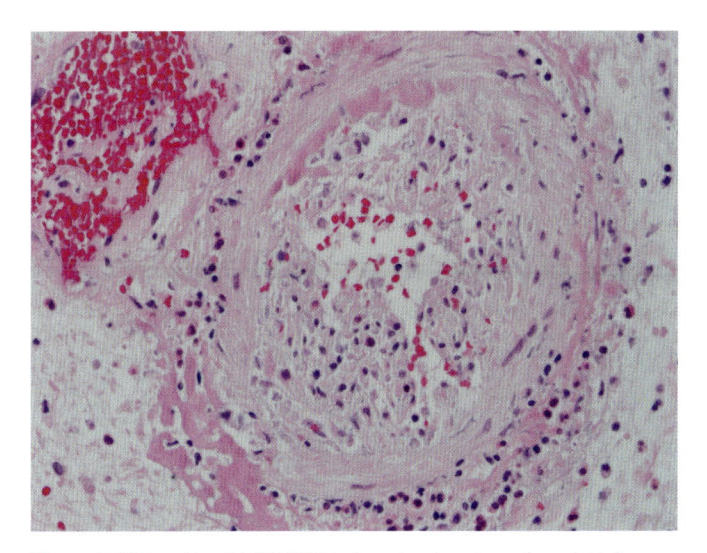

Figure 2.20 Arteritis with BANFF III lesion, showing circumferential inflammation along intima and within vessel wall. Fibrinous material is also present (H&E, 400x).

glomerular diseases, including immune complex-mediated glomerulonephritides or thrombotic microangiopathies. Transplant glomerulitis commonly affects capillary tufts in a focal and segmental pattern; diffuse and global lesions are uncommon. The affected glomerular loops are characteristically dilated and contain three or more mononuclear cells – lymphocytes, monocytes, activated endothelial cells – and/or polymorphonuclear leukocytes (see Figures 2.21 and 2.22). BANFF scoring for glomerulitis or "g score" is based upon the *percentage of involved glomeruli*: 1–25, 26–50, and more than 50% for g1, g2, and g3, respectively. This is particularly used in AAMR (described below). Glomerulitis with or without alloantibody formation and associated with T cell rejection does portend a poorer prognosis for graft survival [92]. "Plasma cell-rich" acute rejection (PCAR) is an uncommon form of acute rejection that likely has a component of T cell-mediated alloreactivity [75, 76]. In general, PCAR is defined as cellular rejection with >10% plasma cells in the infiltrating population (see Figure 2.14). It is not currently classified separately in the BANFF criteria. The clinical significance of PCAR has been minimally addressed, but it has been described that PCAR may be resistant to intensified steroid pulse therapy with some response to antithymocyte globulins or OKT3 [93].

ii Acute Antibody-mediated Rejection

Acute Antibody-mediated Rejection (AAMR) is also known as humoral acute rejection and is based upon the identification of antigenic allodeterminants on the transplant tissue by pre-existing or de novo alloantibodies or isoantibodies. There are a variety of forms of AAMR.

Hyperacute rejection is AAMR that occurs when there are high levels of preformed antibodies in the recipient and that are directed to ABO or HLA antigens on the transplanted graft. Thankfully, this potentially devastating form of AAMR is rare in modern times due to the tremendous success of pretransplant crossmatching and the use of ABO compatible donors in solid organ transplantation [94]. This form of antibody-mediated rejection tends to be dramatic and occurs within hours of vascular anastomosis of the graft, often leading to irreversible injury, particularly in renal transplantation. Typically, during surgery, the grafts swell and turn reddish-blue, mottled, and develop infarcts. The histopathology of hyperacute rejection is based upon the underlying pathology of most variants of AAMR, that being microvascular injury and inflammation, with margination of neutrophils and monocytes/macrophages. In hyperacute rejection/AAMR, there is a graft arteriopathy with massive thrombosis and the presence of occlusive thrombi in all caliber arteries and capillaries due to deposition of preformed antibodies and severe endothelial injury (see Figure 2.23). There are fibrin thrombi in large- and small-caliber arteries, as well as glomerular capillaries. Arterial thrombi can show a polymorphonuclear leukocyte reaction along the endothelial cell surface. Despite intravascular thrombosis, vascular walls often remain viable, even in areas of infarction. If renal allografts survive the initial rejection phase, then subsequent biopsies may show surprisingly few thrombi in some arteries only. This focality is due to the unaltered fibrinolytic activity in the recipient resulting in thrombolysis in the allograft. Thrombus formation causes severe acute ischemic injury, focal hemorrhage, polymorphonuclear leukocyte infiltration, and in most severe cases, frank infarcts. Polymorphonuclear leukocytes are found in the interstitium either as a demarcation phenomenon between viable and infarcted areas or adjacent to tubules with severe ischemic injury (see Figure 2.23). Significant lymphocytic infiltrates, i.e., signs of cellular rejection in the interstitium and arteries, are generally lacking, although they can evolve if grafts survive for a few weeks. Immunofluorescence evaluations during the early phases of rejection often reveal linear deposits of IgG and IgM together with complement factors including C4d along the endothelium of arteries, glomeruli, and peritubular capillaries. Transplant arteriopathy episodes with massive thrombosis are generally C4d-positive (in particular in the renal medulla since capillaries in the cortex may be severely damaged).

Accelerated Acute Rejection is another form of AAMR [63, 95] that is also relatively rare and is a term used to describe AAMR beyond rejection within hours from implementation of the allograft. In general, accelerated acute rejection also demonstrates the same dramatic fibrin thrombi within vessels with secondary ischemic injury. This form of rejection is also due to preformed antibodies.

In general, the most ubiquitous form of *Acute Antibody-mediated Rejection* or AAMR tends to be acute graft injury due to either preformed or developing antibodies, but without the dramatic and devastating presentation as the two forms described above. Aside from hyperacute rejection and accelerated acute rejection, both of whose timing is rapid, including hours or days, the more common and "garden-variety" forms of AAMR can occur in a variety of histological patterns and importantly, at any time following transplant. Although the incidence of AAMR is less than TCMR, it has become much more recognizable in recent years due to the marked

Table 2.1 2013 Update of the BANFF Classification Scheme

1 Normal

2 Antibody-mediated changes (may coincide with categories 3, 4, 5, and 6)

Acute/active ABMR; all three features must be present for diagnosis

    1 Histologic evidence of acute tissue injury, including one or more of the following:

        Microvascular inflammation (g>0 and/or ptc>0)

        Intimal or transmural arteritis (v>0)

        Acute thrombotic microangiopathy, in the absence of any other cause

        Acute tubular injury, in the absence of any other apparent cause

    2 Evidence of current/recent antibody interaction with vascular endothelium, including at least one of the following:

        Linear C4d staining in peritubular capillaries (C4d2 or C4d3 by IF on frozen sections, or C4d>0 by IHC on paraffin sections)

        At least moderate microvascular inflammation ([g + ptc] >2)

        Increased expression of gene transcripts in the biopsy tissue indicative of endothelial injury, if thoroughly validated

    3 Serologic evidence of donor-specific antibodies (DSAs) (HLA or other antigens)

Chronic, active ABMR; all three features must be present for diagnosis

    1 Morphologic evidence of chronic tissue injury, including one or more of the following:

        Transplant glomerulopathy (TG) (cg>0), if no evidence of chronic thrombotic microangiopathy

        Severe peritubular capillary basement membrane multilayering (requires EM)

        Arterial intimal fibrosis of new onset, excluding other causes

    2 Evidence of current/recent antibody interaction with vascular endothelium, including at least one of the following:

        Linear C4d staining in peritubular capillaries (C4d2 or C4d3 by IF on frozen sections, or C4d>0 by IHC on paraffin sections)

        At least moderate microvascular inflammation ([g + ptc] >2)

        Increased expression of gene transcripts in the biopsy tissue indicative of endothelial injury, if thoroughly validated

    3 Serologic evidence of DSAs (HLA or other antigens)

C4d staining without evidence of rejection; all three features must be present for diagnosis

    1 Linear C4d staining in peritubular capillaries (C4d2 or C4d3 by IF on frozen sections, or C4d>0 by IHC on paraffin sections)

    2 g=0, ptc=0, cg=0 (by light microscopy and by EM if available), v=0; no TMA, no peritubular capillary basement membrane multilayering, no acute tubular injury (in the absence of another apparent cause for this)

    3 No acute cell-mediated rejection (BANFF 97 type 1A or greater) or borderline changes

3 Borderline changes: 'Suspicious' for acute T cell-mediated rejection (may coincide with categories 2, 5, and 6)

    This category is used when no intimal arteritis is present, but there are foci of tubulitis (t1, t2, or t3) with minor interstitial infiltration (i0 or i1) or interstitial infiltration (i2 or i3) with mild (t1) tubulitis

4 T cell-mediated rejection (TCMR, may coincide with categories 2 and 5)

    Acute T cell-mediated rejection (Type/Grade:)

        IA Cases with significant interstitial infiltration (>25% of parenchyma affected, i2 or i3) and foci of moderate tubulitis (t2)

        IB Cases with significant interstitial infiltration (>25% of parenchyma affected, i2 or i3) and foci of severe tubulitis (t3)

        IIA Cases with mild-to-moderate intimal arteritis (v1)

        IIB Cases with severe intimal arteritis comprising >25% of the luminal area (v2)

        III Cases with 'transmural' arteritis and/or arterial fibrinoid change and necrosis of medial smooth muscle cells with accompanying lymphocytic inflammation (v3)

Table 2.1 (cont.)

Chronic active T cell-mediated rejection

"chronic allograft arteriopathy" (arterial intimal fibrosis with mononuclear cell infiltration in fibrosis, formation of neo-intima)

5 Interstitial fibrosis and tubular atrophy, no evidence of any specific etiology

(may include nonspecific vascular and glomerular sclerosis, but severity graded by tubulointerstitial features)

Grade

I Mild interstitial fibrosis and tubular atrophy (<25% of cortical area)

II Moderate interstitial fibrosis and tubular atrophy (26%–50% of cortical area)

III Severe interstitial fibrosis and tubular atrophy/loss (>50% of cortical area)

6 Other: changes not considered to be due to acute or chronic rejection

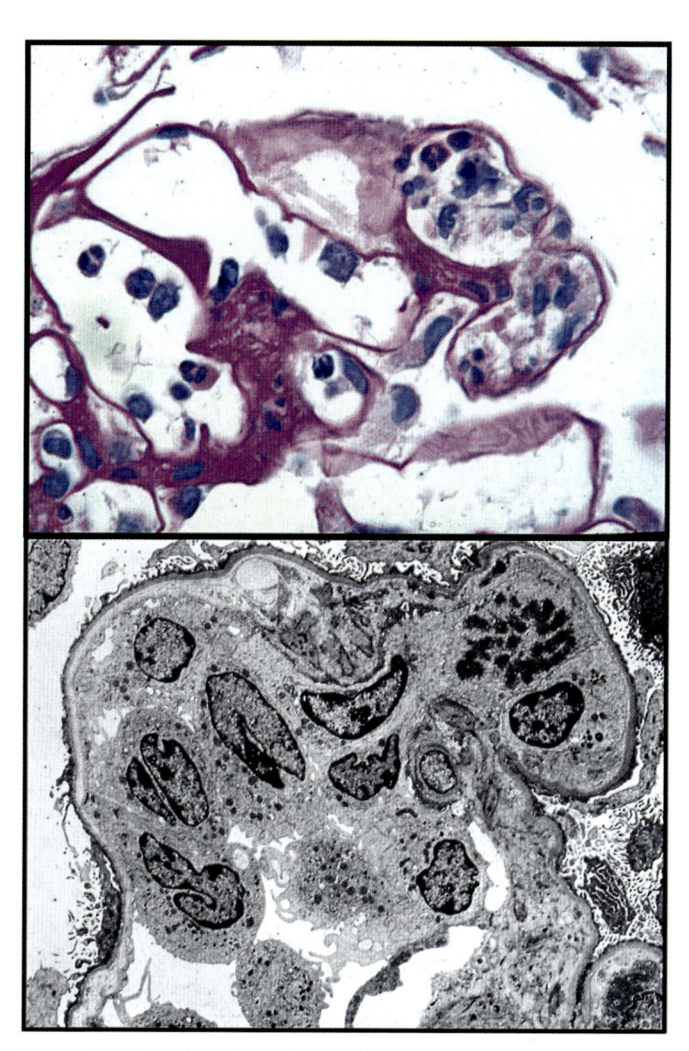

Figure 2.21 Transplant glomerulitis. Top figure shows dilated glomerular capillaries segmentally occluded by inflammatory cells, i.e., the glomeruli showed transplant glomerulitis (PAS, 400x). Electron microscopy (bottom figure) demonstrated abundant intra-capillary mononuclear cells with one mitotic figure (upper right corner) (electron microscopy, x6000 original magnification).

advancements in histocompatibility laboratory measurements of these alloantibodies, as well as in the histopathologic tools now used in allograft biopsies. AAMR is demonstrable in a variety of forms and can show many potential histological changes. Overall, AAMR tends to have poorer responses to standard immunotherapies and as such, grafts with AAMR veer towards a reduced capacity to ultimately survive and function as compared to long-term TCMR. There is no specific clinical symptomatology that can separate AAMR from TCMR or other graft complications, but generally there is also oliguria, rapid rise in creatinine, and laboratory measurements of DSA can show upward shifts. However, these changes are nonspecific and biopsies are extremely useful in helping to nail down the identification of this entity.

There are varieties of morphological presentations for typical AAMR and they are described in the BANFF criteria. Mild forms of AAMR can manifest as acute tubular necrosis (ATN) (see Figure 2.24); in our experience, this form occurs, but at less frequency than forms containing capillaritis or glomerulitis. More severe forms of AAMR show capillaritis, which is an accumulation of monocytes/macrophages in peritubular capillaries and/or glomerulitis, where these cells become impacted within the glomerular vasculature (see Figure 2.25). There can also be thrombotic microangiopathy (TMA) and fibrinoid necrosis of the microvasculature (see Figure 2.19). Intimal, non-necrotizing arteritis has also now been demonstrated to not only be a component of acute Type II TCMR, but also AAMR. Unfortunately, these morphological findings are not specific for antibody-mediated acute rejection and can be found with calcineurin inhibitor toxicity or other causes of TMA. As such, it is very useful to have morphological evidence via ancillary techniques to identify the presence of alloantibody within the graft biopsy. Some years ago, the identification of C4d as a biomarker helped to revolutionize our means of identifying antibody within the graft. C4d as visualized by immunofluorescence (see Figure 2.26) or immunohistochemistry (see Figures 2.24 and 2.25) has evolved and clearly been more successful in identifying alloantibody than previously utilized testing by immunofluorescence for immunoglobulins. The fact that C4d is covalently bound within the tissue has aided in this improved detection within biopsies. The BANFF criteria consequently implemented C4d identification along with suitable morphological changes and clinical evidence of DSA as the basis for identification of AAMR (see Figures 2.24,

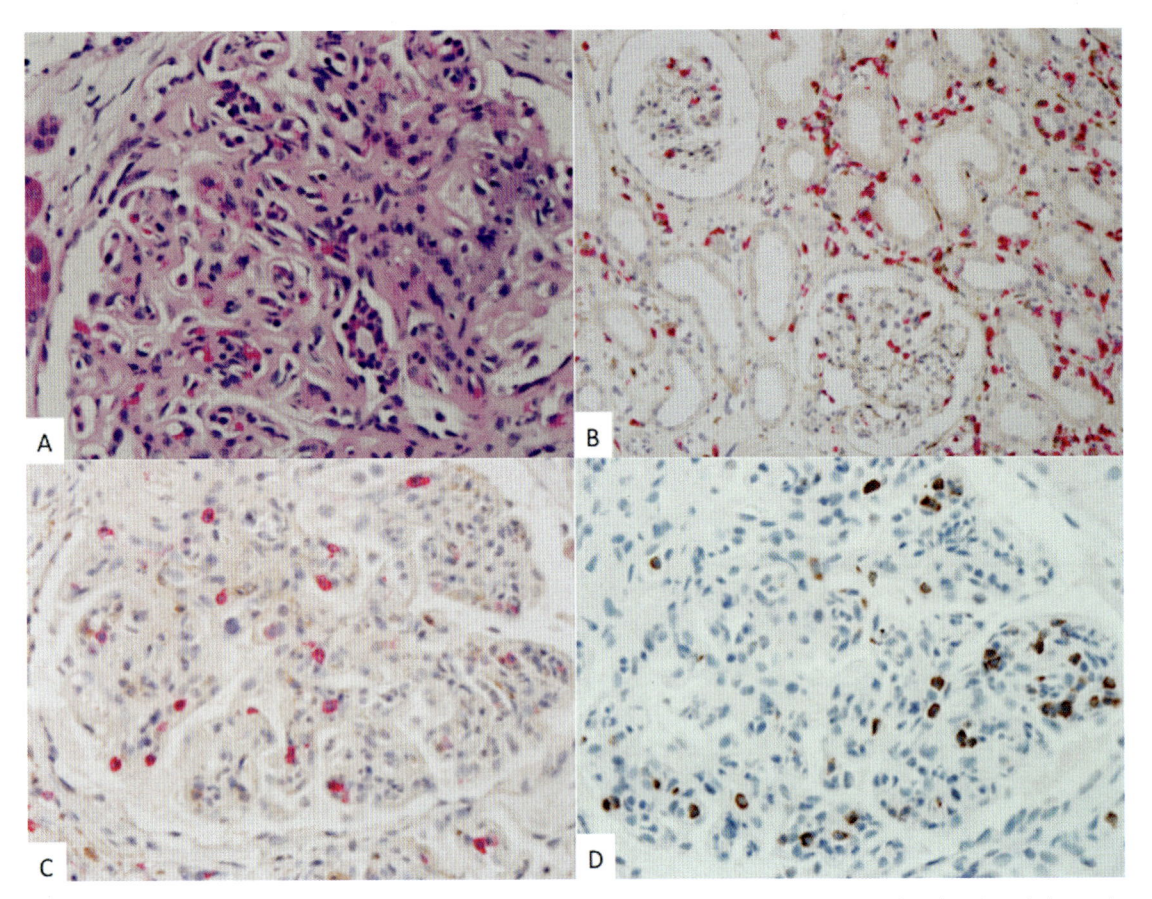

Figure 2.22 Transplant glomerulitis. Composite showing high magnification ("A" – H&E, 400x) micrograph with enlarged glomerulus containing numerous inflammatory cells within the capillary loops. "B" and "C" are the same case showing CD4+ (brown cells) and CD8+ (red cells) T cells within the glomeruli, as well as within the interstitium, thereby demonstrating TCMR (Two-color immunohistochemistry to CD4/CD8, 200x, 400x (B and C respectively)). This case was also C4d-positive and the patient had donor-specific antibody so there was simultaneous antibody-mediated rejection. This is a case of "Mixed Rejection." "D" is the same case, showing the presence of perforin-positive cells within the glomeruli (Immunohistochemistry to perforin, 400x).

2.25, and 2.26). Since these changes, there have now been documented cases showing that the presence of DSA can be associated with microvascular injury within renal biopsies, but in the absence of C4d deposition [96]. Therefore, C4d-negative AAMR is now recognized and a modification of the BANFF AAMR criteria has been submitted [97]. Now, C4d staining is not a prerequisite for identification of AAMR if there is at least moderate microvascular inflammation (based on the scoring criteria) or genetic transcripts for endothelial genes. The latter finding is somewhat controversial since "standardization" of these assays remains elusive. Nevertheless, "validated" identification of endothelial gene upregulation will likely become an acceptable supplement if there is no C4d staining seen within the biopsy. In summary, the identification of AAMR involves characteristic morphological changes (e.g., microvascular injury), clinical documentation of DSA alloantibody, and evidence of antibody interaction with vascular endothelium (e.g., C4d deposition) (Table 2.1).

As noted above, AAMR can occur at any time, even years post-transplantation. The histological findings, along with documentation of antibody/endothelium interaction and the presence of DSA, are still maintained as essential criteria in order to designate the entity as AAMR. It is not uncommon that these late-occurring AAMR cases are clinically silent ("subclinical"). These patients should still be treated since they are at higher risk of developing graft injury and chronic rejection.

There is also a form of antibody-mediated rejection that displays chronic injury and is classified in the BANFF criteria as chronic, active antibody-mediated rejection (Table 2.1). This is covered in the section below, Chronic Rejection.

c Chronic Rejection

The phenomenon of "chronic rejection" or "chronic allograft nephropathy" is actually an accumulation of varying amounts of different tissue injury characterized by nondescript tissue remodeling and sclerosis. It is a relentlessly progressive form of injury that frequently occurs in all solid organ allografts, including kidneys, and is a common cause of graft failure [98, 99]. This "chronic" scarring injury of the interstitial, tubular, glomerular, and vascular compartments of the kidney are the result of a protracted interplay of immune (e.g., smoldering rejection episodes) and non-immune (e.g., recruitment of "non-classical" inflammatory cell elements such as myofibroblasts) factors [98, 99]. The end result of this fibrosing injury is

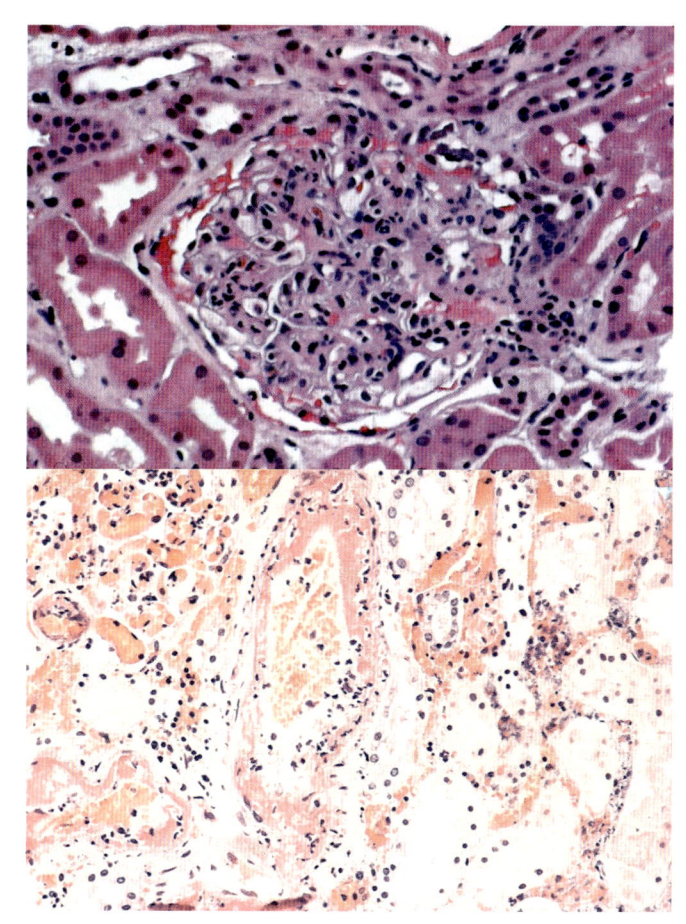

Figure 2.23 Hyperacute rejection occurring within hours after vascular anastomosis in a sensitized patient with high level of donor-specific alloantibody. The top micrograph represents changes within the glomeruli minutes after vascularization (post-implantation biopsy) with capillary congestion and the presence of neutrophils (H&E, 400x). The bottom micrograph represents changes hours later with diffuse necrosis, arteritis, extensive vascular congestion, and interstitial hemorrhage (H&E, 400x).

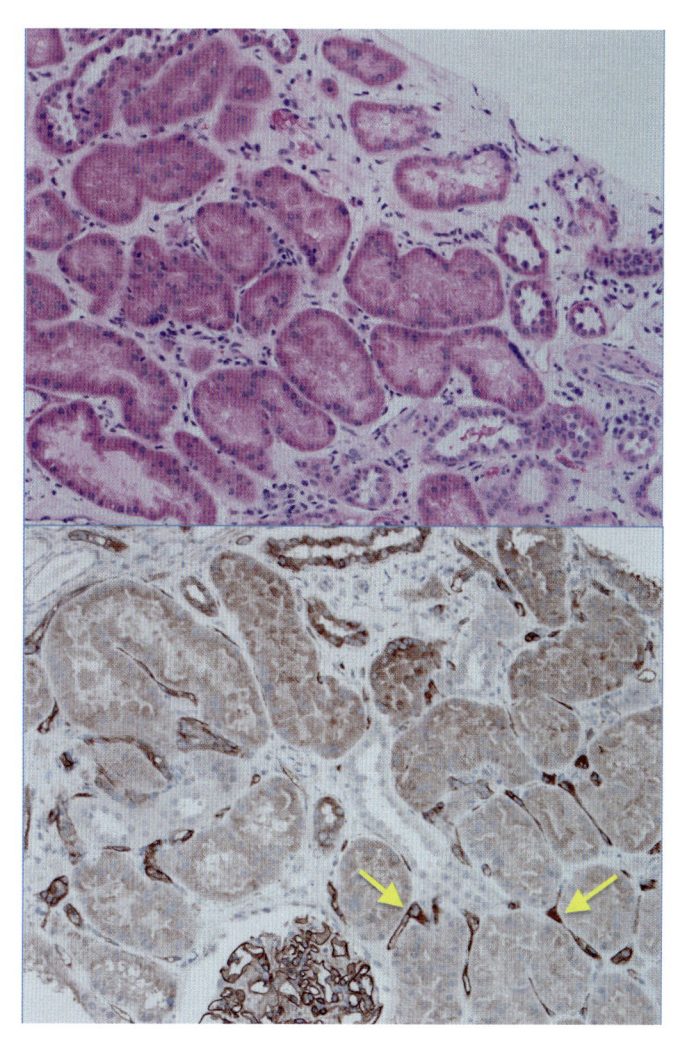

Figure 2.24 AAMR with ATN. The top micrograph is a renal graft biopsy from a patient with rising DSA and increased creatinine. No significant capillaritis and only minimal glomerulitis were observed. Tubules show a loss of brush borders (mild acute tubular injury) without notable interstitial inflammation (H&E, 200x). The lower micrograph shows immunohistochemical deposition of C4d along peritubular capillaries (arrows) and lining glomerular capillaries (Immunohistochemistry to C4d, 200x).

sclerosis with varying degrees of "burnt-out" scar formation [61, 62], grossly apparent as a fibrosed, often hemorrhagic and shrunken kidney with extensive loss of function (see Figure 2.27).

When considering the *tubulointerstitial* compartment, it is useful, if possible, to distinguish rejection-induced graft *interstitial* fibrosis from other types of graft injury and scar formation, e.g. pre-existing donor disease, de novo hypertension induced arteriolosclerosis, calcineurin inhibitor induced structural toxicity, and various recurrent or de novo kidney diseases. Though inadequately treated and smoldering cellular rejection episodes can lead to increasing levels of interstitial fibrosis and tubular atrophy [78, 100, 101] (see Figure 2.28), if the likely cause of graft sclerosis cannot be determined, then the descriptive term "interstitial fibrosis and tubular atrophy, not otherwise specified (NOS)" is appropriate when describing interstitial compartment injury. The term "chronic allograft nephropathy" (CAN) is no longer used in pathological diagnoses [102]. The different disease entities that can result in interstitial scarring (mentioned above) often do so in combination with persistent rejection, thus distinguishing an exact etiology of the interstitial injury is often difficult.

Changes within the *vascular* and *glomerular* compartments in chronic rejection of the kidney can show distinct chronic induced tissue remodeling that is not evident within the tubulo-interstitial compartment. In *arteries*, transplant endarteritis can progress from the inflammatory phases (e.g., transplant endarteritis) (see Figure 2.29) where there is a subendothelial intimal accumulation of one or more lymphocytes or histiocytes into the proliferative stage which contains subendothelial mononuclear cell elements, but also by proliferating spindle-shaped cells (i.e. myofibroblasts [62, 103]). As myofibroblasts increase, there is a reduction in inflammatory cells within the vessel [62, 103] (see Figure 2.30). Foam cells typically persist (see Figure 2.31) and transplant endarteritis is commonly accompanied by acute T Cell-Mediated Rejection (TMCR) and/or antibody-mediated acute rejection [104–108] (see Figure 2.29). The accumulation of C4d along the endothelium of arteries is a non-diagnostic phenomenon, also detected in native kidneys. Transplant endarteritis is limited to arteries in approximately 5%–10% of cases. Glomeruli

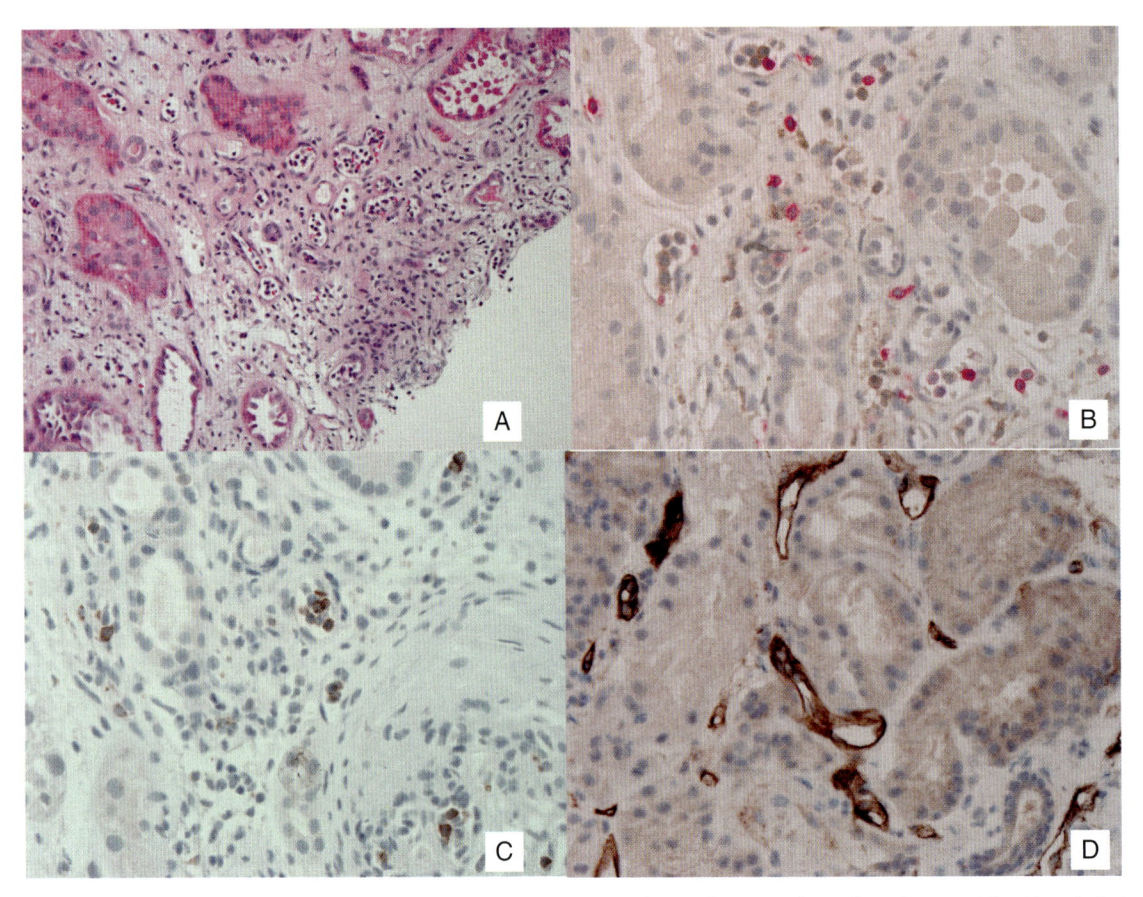

Figure 2.25 AAMR with capillaritis. "A" is a micrograph showing an accumulation of mononuclear cells and neutrophils with peritubular capillaries in a patient with high cPRA and DSA (H&E, 200x). "B" is same case showing CD4+ (brown cells) and CD8+ (red cells) T cells within the capillaries (Two-color immunohistochemistry to CD4/CD8, 400x). "C" is the same case showing the presence of perforin-positive cells within the capillaries (Immunohistochemistry to perforin, 400x). "D" is the same case showing diffuse C4d staining of peritubular capillaries (Immunohistochemistry to C4d, 400x).

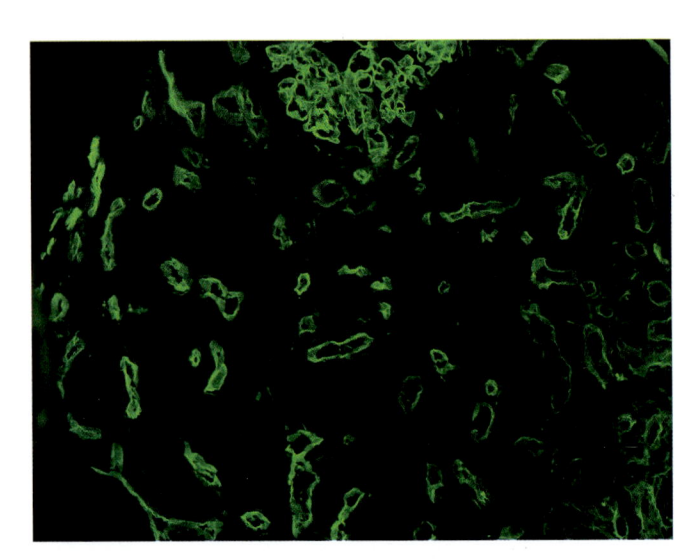

Figure 2.26 C4d by immunofluorescence. C4d is detected with strong, linear staining intensity along the walls of peritubular capillaries in non-fibrotic areas (Indirect immunofluorescence with monoclonal antibody to C4d, fresh frozen tissue, 100x).

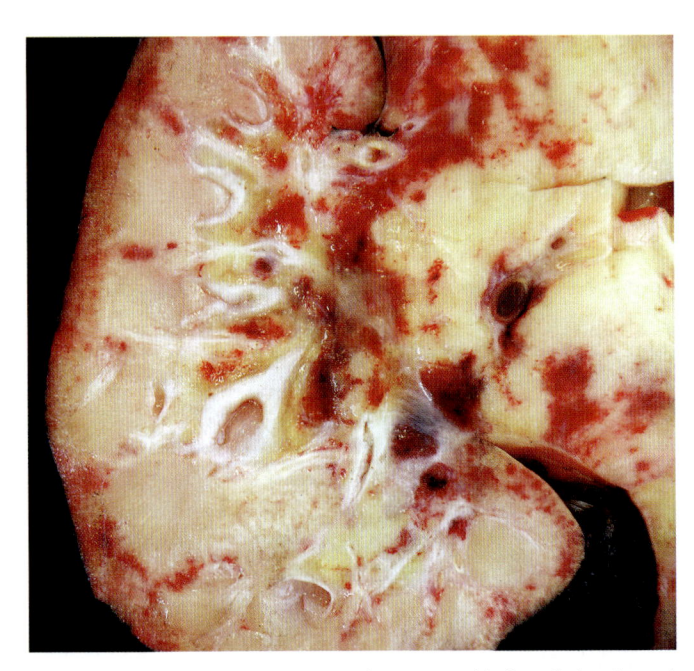

Figure 2.27 Transplant nephrectomy of a ten-year-old allograft that showed severe (active) sclerosing transplant arteriopathy with focal occlusive thrombosis, transplant glomerulopathy, and marked parenchymal fibrosis. Multiple foci of hemorrhage are also present.

The Pathology of Kidney Transplantation

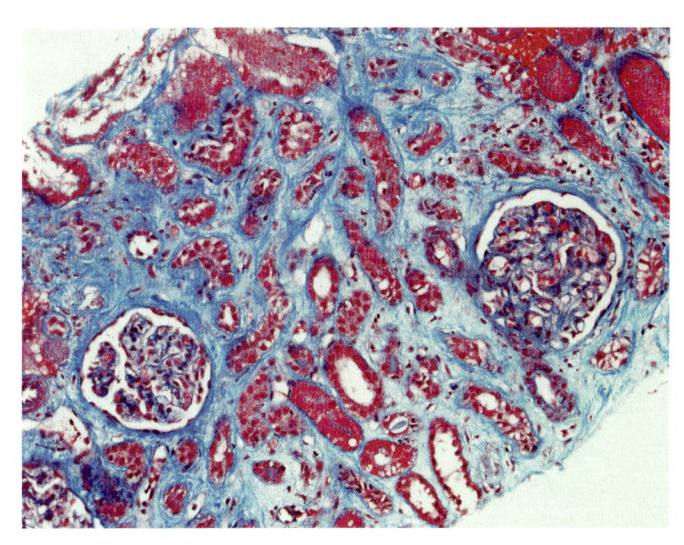

Figure 2.28 Interstitial fibrosis and tubular atrophy in a renal transplant biopsy two years post-transplant with widened collagen-containing spaces between tubules (Trichrome stain, 200x).

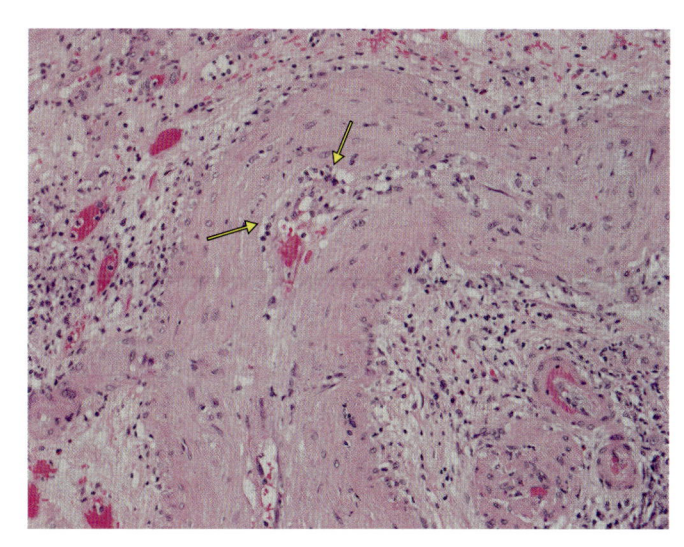

Figure 2.29 Chronic allograft arteriopathy with prominent inflammatory component along intimal area (arrows), superimposed upon significant chronic injury to intimal, medial, and adventitial layers of a larger muscular artery. Smaller arterial branches also show inflammatory changes (H&E, 400x).

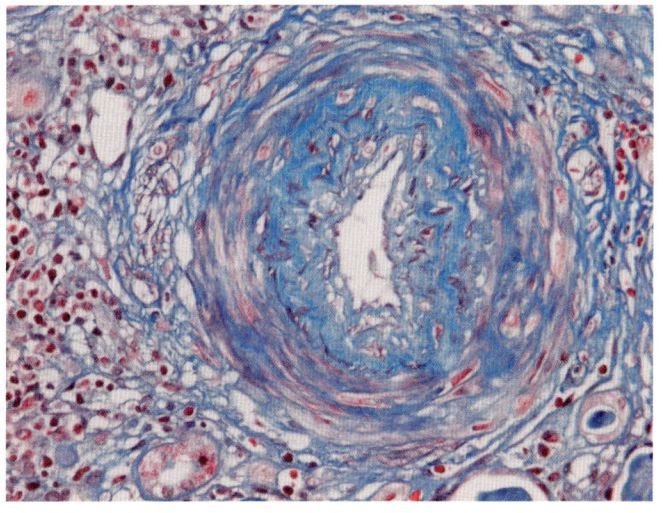

Figure 2.30 Chronic allograft arteriopathy with minimal inflammatory component showing concentric fibrointimal proliferation, increased myoblasts, and progressive occlusion of vessel lumen (Trichrome, 400x).

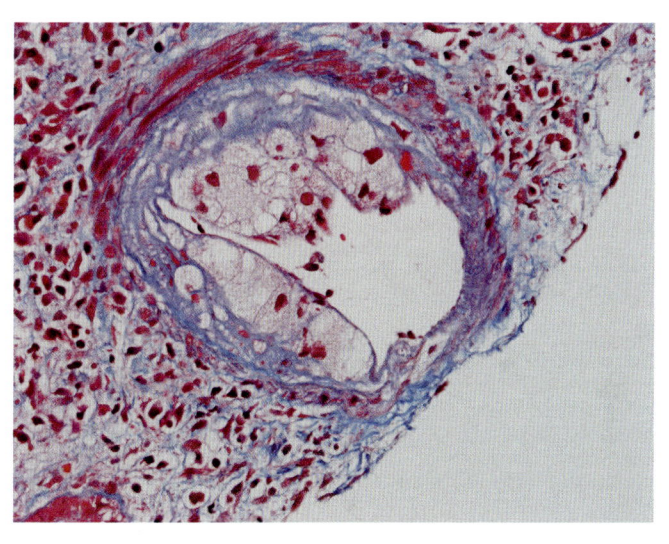

Figure 2.31 Chronic allograft arteriopathy with foam cells along intimal surface (Trichrome, 400x).

can be normal, or show transplant glomerulitis in approximately 30% of cases. Many cells infiltrating the intima of arteries are CD68-positive monocytes/macrophages along with CD8+ and CD4+ T cells (about 2:1) [62, 103] (see Figure 2.32). Immunofluorescence microscopy with a standard antibody panel of antibodies does not reveal a specific staining pattern in arteries or glomeruli.

As the arterial inflammation dissipates (i.e., "smoldering") there is myofibroblast activation (for collagen types 1 and 3 production and intimal scar formation) and ultimately progressive intimal sclerosis or *sclerosing transplant arteriopathy* (BANFF category 4 chronic active T cell-mediated rejection or BANFF category 2 chronic active antibody-mediated rejection). This entity, often named chronic vascular rejection, is characterized by rejection-induced variable arterial intimal thickening due to types I/III collagen deposition, without fibroelastosis and minimal to marked intimal inflammation (see Figure 2.30). The intimal scar formation is often accentuated at arterial branching points. There are varying numbers of irregularly arranged myofibroblasts and occasional foam cells. The presence of mononuclear inflammatory cells, i.e. lymphocytes and histiocytes, allows a designation of "active" chronic allograft arteriopathy (see Figure 2.29). Sclerosing or sclerosed transplant arteriopathy can have concomitant pre-existing donor disease (e.g., hypertension-induced arteriolosclerosis, which tends to have more elastosis), transplant glomerulopathy, glomerulitis, or tubulo-interstitial rejection. As the transplant arteriopathy progresses, there can be arterial stenosis with secondary ischemia, tubular atrophy, and interstitial fibrosis (see Figure 2.30). A glassy-appearing interstitial fibrosis that develops in cases of persistent and severe interstitial

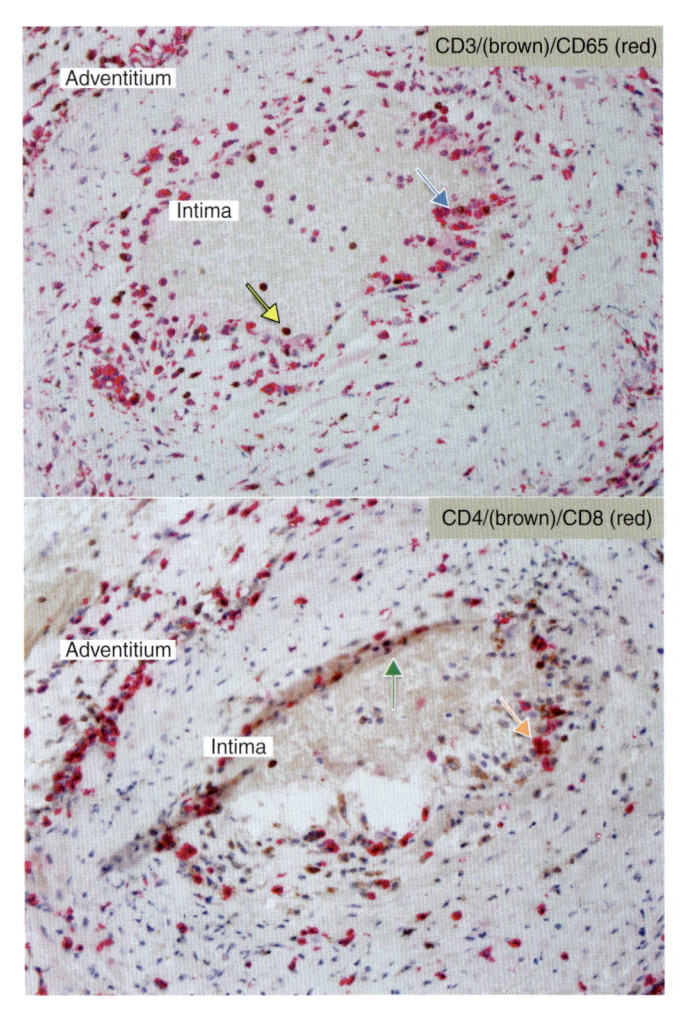

Figure 2.32 Chronic "active" allograft arteriopathy with prominent inflammatory component involving intimal and periadventitial areas; the separate slides showed this inflammation was superimposed upon significant chronic injury to intima, medial, and adventitial layers of this artery. The top photograph shows a prominence of macrophages (CD68-positive, blue arrow) in the inflammation with a smaller component of CD3+ T cells (yellow arrow) (Two-color immunohistochemistry, 400x, CD3-brown, CD68-red). The bottom photograph shows a mixture of CD4+ (green arrow) and CD8+ (orange arrow) T cells in the intimal inflammation (Two-color immunohistochemistry, 400x, CD4-brown, CD8-red).

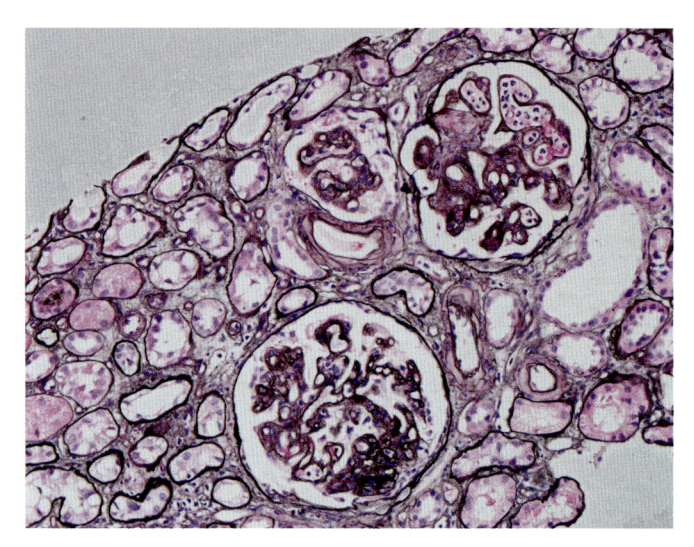

Figure 2.33 Example of ongoing transplant glomerulopathy as demonstrated in a silver stain. Note the widened mesangial areas and thickened basement membranes with frequent dual contour formation. Adhesions to Bowman's capsule are present and occasional inflammatory cells are found within the capillary lumens. The surrounding smaller vessels are laminated with chronic injury (Silver stain, 400x).

edema (aka "scleredema") implies an underlying severe vascular stenosis and impaired blood flow. Immunohistochemistry and immunofluorescence are nonspecific in their patterns, including C4d deposition [103, 107].

Thrombotic microangiopathies that are sclerosing can resemble rejection-induced transplant arteriopathies with both cases having myofibroblast proliferation lacking fibroelastosis in the intimal layers. The former tend to affect small arteries, arterioles, and glomerular vascular poles, whereas rejection-induced changes are predominately found in arcuate caliber vessels. Sclerosing thrombotic microangiopathies tend to be without significant inflammation.

Transplant glomerulopathy (or chronic transplant glomerulopathy) signifies glomerular basement membrane duplication without significant cell interposition, i.e. thrombotic microangiopathy-like glomerular remodeling. It is an inflammation-driven process resulting in variable capillary wall remodeling [61, 62, 109, 110], best seen in PAS or silver stains [111] (see Figure 2.33). Mesangial cell interposition is usually absent though mesangiolysis, as seen in protracted cases of thrombotic microangiopathy (see Figure 2.33). Mesangial regions are generally expanded and segmental glomerulosclerosis (i.e., secondary FSGS), global glomerular sclerosis, and nephron loss are also commonly apparent.

Ultrastructural evaluation by electron microscopy is useful in the diagnosis of transplant glomerulopathy [112]. It reveals endothelial cell activation, loss of fenestration, and associated widening of the lamina rara interna early in transplant glomerulopathy. As the process progresses with continual endothelial cell activation, there can be deposition of subendothelial basement membrane/lamina densa like material and GBM duplication [113] (see Figure 2.34). Dotted, electron-dense deposits may be found along the lamina rara interna, often associated with the interposition of endothelial cell processes, though this is not characteristic of a membranoproliferative, immune complex-mediated glomerulonephritis [114]. Peritubular capillaries can also show basement membrane laminations by electron microscopy that can be used to establish a diagnosis in some cases [115]. Transplant glomerulopathy often has concurrent evidence of glomerulitis and/or acute cell-mediated rejection [62, 111] along with transplant endarteritis, sclerosing, or sclerosed arteriopathy [62, 109, 113].

Immunohistochemistry can show glomerular C4d, IgM, and complement factor C3, followed by minimal deposits of IgG or fibrin. C4d is often found with moderate-to-strong linear staining intensity along the duplicated peripheral glomerular capillaries.

Transplant glomerulopathy, which represents rejection induced glomerular injury and the remodelling stage of transplant glomerulitis, shows an increasing prevalence reaching 25% in kidney transplants older than ten years in one series [109]. As mentioned, it closely resembles thrombotic microangiopathies with GBM duplications [61, 62, 109] and can

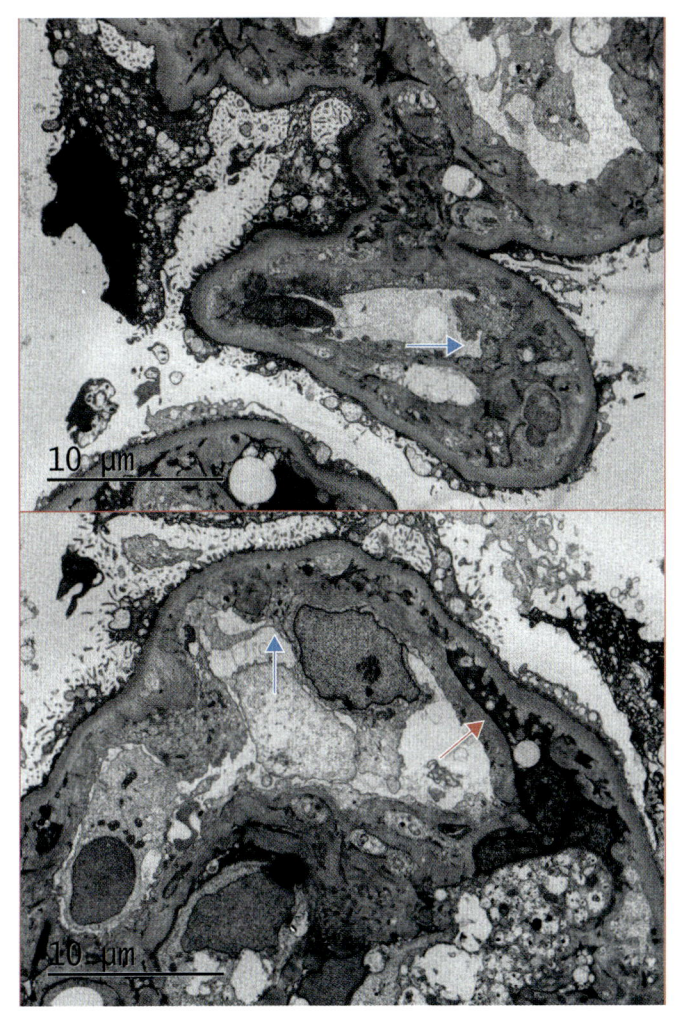

Figure 2.34 Transmission electron microscopy of glomeruli of patient with transplant glomerulopathy. Note the thickened basement membranes with endothelial cell activation (blue arrows) and GBM duplication (red arrow) (Electron microscopy, top and bottom, 7000x).

clinically mimic primary glomerulopathies (e.g., FSGS), since patients usually present with varying degrees of hematuria and proteinuria that can reach nephrotic range in cases of marked GBM duplication [109].

i Molecular Assays of Acute and Chronic Rejection

The molecular assessment of a variety of molecules in nephrology is expanding and rapidly assuming prominent importance in lab medicine. Both individual and groups of biomarkers are now being measured peripherally and *in situ* in regards to infectious, neoplastic, metabolic, and inflammatory processes occurring in patients with native renal disorders and kidney transplants. Though "molecular lab medicine" is an enormous subject and well beyond the scope of this book, it is worth briefly mentioning that molecular assessment of inflammatory aspects of acute and chronic rejection complications is being actively pursued as an adjunct and refining addition to the renal biopsy.

A variety of approaches have been employed to discover which molecules play a role in the various forms of alloreactive processes occurring in "rejecting" vs. "stable" kidney grafts; among the many goals of this exercise is to be able to measure particular molecules that can accurately discriminate to what degree different inflammatory and immunological changes are taking place, as defined by the changes from baseline of the selected genes (and their products). Laborious but fruitful techniques such as whole genome sequencing and screening have revealed numerous potential molecule sets that appear to *specifically* change during various forms of rejection. While this has been very useful, what has also resulted is that the co-existence of different types of rejection (as well as other complications) is now apparent from these studies. Hence, as shown in biopsies, it is not unusual to have both antibody and cell-mediated forms of acute rejection simultaneously, and to be superimposed on fibrogenic processes as seen in chronic rejection. What has yet to be defined is the *degree* of changes that can be accurately measured solely with molecular assays. Moreover, numerous other variables can clearly influence the final outcome of the measurement of these gene sets, including the methodology utilized, the source of the sample (i.e., blood, urine vs. intragraft measurements), the fixation state of the sample, the tremendous heterogeneity of different clinical variables (e.g., age, transplant time, drug profiles, histocompatibility differences, etc.), and the interpretation of the measurements (e.g., change in levels vs. presence/absence).

In spite of these limitations, tremendous progress has been made.

d Drug Toxicities

i Calcineurin inhibitors

Calcineurin inhibiting pharmaceutical agents (CNI), chiefly cyclosporine-A (CsA) [116] and tacrolimus (FK506) [117], have transformed and significantly improved outcomes in organ transplantation [118]. Both CsA and tacrolimus bind to immunophilins that are intracytoplasmic receptor proteins [119–124] and thereafter, the immunophilin/CsA or tacrolimus complexes bind to and inhibit a phosphatase, calcineurin. Calcineurin typically promotes T cell activation by dephosphorylating intracytoplasmic nuclear regulatory proteins and facilitates their translocation into the nucleus and activation as intranuclear [125] transcription factors for various mediators (e.g. IL-2, IL-4, interferonγ, and TNF-α).

Calcineurin inhibitors play a major role in the immunosuppression of allograft recipients, though their complications are significant [126, 127]. There is an important problematic nephrotoxic side effect, which can be seen as functional toxicity and as structural toxicity (with various early or late histologic alterations, typically associated with functional toxicity). These complications are dose-dependent and though often seen with high levels, can be evident with idiosyncratic reactions at optimal therapeutic concentrations. Both CsA and tacrolimus demonstrate indistinguishable structural toxicity chiefly involving tubules, arterioles, and glomeruli in native and transplanted kidneys, known as "calcineurin inhibitor induced toxicity (CNIT)" [128–131].

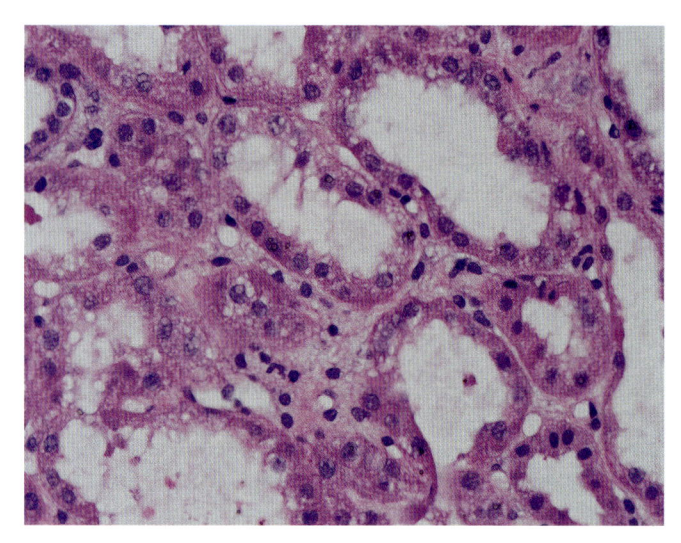

Figure 2.35 Calcineurin inhibitor induced early tubulopathy. The patient presented 20 days post-transplantation on tacrolimus based immunosuppression with impaired graft function. Tubular epithelial cells showed "osmotic nephrosis," i.e., isometric vacuolization of the cytoplasm suggestive of calcineurin inhibitor induced toxic changes (H&E, 400x).

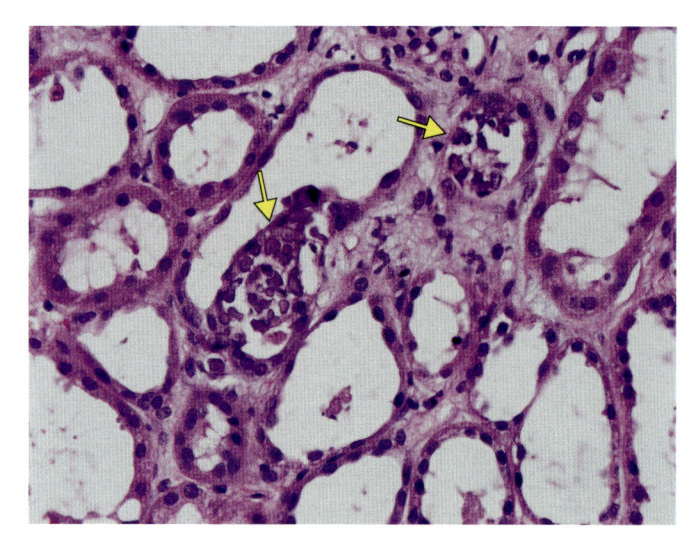

Figure 2.36 Calcineurin inhibitor induced toxicity. Microcalcifications (arrows) present within tubules as part of spectrum of calcineurin inhibitor induced toxic changes (H&E, 400x).

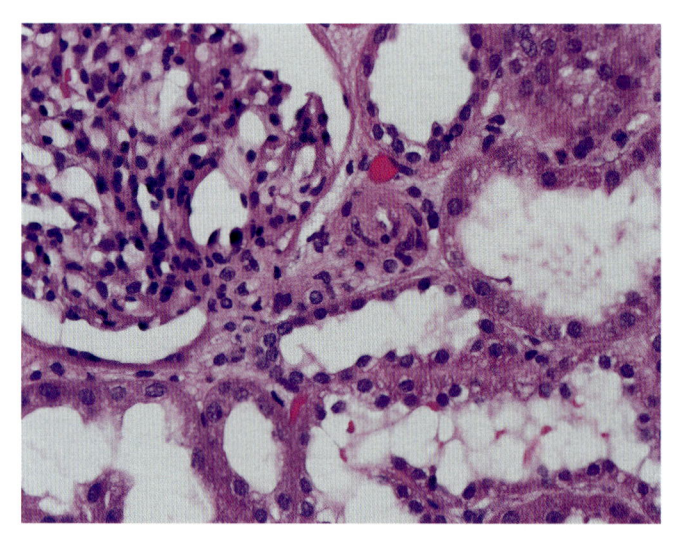

Figure 2.37 Calcineurin inhibitor induced early tubulopathy. The patient presented several weeks post-transplantation on tacrolimus based immunosuppression with impaired graft function. Tubular epithelial cells showed "osmotic nephrosis," i.e., isometric vacuolization of the cytoplasm suggestive of calcineurin inhibitor induced toxic changes (H&E, 400x). Early arterial thickening with minimal hyalinosis is also present.

CsA and tacrolimus can contribute to deterioration of renal function over many years (likely in association with other contributing factors such as hypertension or hyperlipidemia) [132, 133], sometimes with end-stage renal failure [134]. Patients displaying calcineurin inhibitor "functional toxicity" commonly show a markedly decreased glomerular filtration rate (due to arteriolar vasospasms) and evidence of arterial hypertension, sometimes with acute renal failure and oliguria. Morphologically, these allograft biopsies lack characteristic structural changes. Extended functional CNIT can show signs of acute tubular injury (ATI), dilatation, mononuclear cells containing peritubular capillaries, and mild interstitial edema [131, 135]. Functional toxicity typically reverses upon dose reduction [136].

Structural changes induced by calcineurin inhibitors can primarily be seen in tubules, arterioles, and glomeruli and are generally associated with a component of functional toxicity. The proximal tubules generally show the greatest morphologic changes, whereas ducts in the medulla typically remain unaffected. Three morphologic changes in the tubular compartment have been linked to calcineurin inhibitor induced toxicity: i) isometric vacuolization (see Figure 2.35), ii) tubular calcifications (see Figure 2.36), and iii) giant mitochondria. They may occur alone or in combination in the same biopsy sample and can be detected by light and electron microscopy. Isometric vacuolization (see Figures 2.35–2.37), (uniformly sized small vacuoles) is found in tubular epithelial cell cytoplasm and often associated with brush border loss [137] and, by electron microscopy, represents dilated and empty-appearing portions of the endoplasmic reticulum [137]. Isometric vacuolization of tubular epithelial cells is not pathognomonic for CNIT, since they may be evident in fatty changes in the setting of the nephrotic syndrome and "osmotic nephrosis" following therapy with mannitol, dextran, radiolabeled contrast media,+ or sucrose-rich hyperimmune globulin and IVIG solutions [138–140]. These latter entities typically demonstrate dilated lysosomes by electron microscopy. Giant mitochondria and tubular microcalcifications have been also been described as signs of CNIT [131] (see Figure 2.36); both isometric vacuolization and giant mitochondria are reversible on dose, and dystrophic calcifications likely persist.

Structural CNIT in arterioles and glomeruli is characterized as a "thrombotic microangiopathy" ranging from common, very mild and limited variants (i.e., CNIT arteriolopathies or glomerulopathies) to fully developed forms of the hemolytic uremic syndrome [130]. The afferent arteriolar lesions include marked "ballooning," or swelling of medial smooth muscle cells.

CNIT *arteriolopathy* (see Figures 2.37–2.38) may also have nodular protein deposits (hyaline deposits) within smooth muscle cells of the media or the adventitial layer, and are

The Pathology of Kidney Transplantation

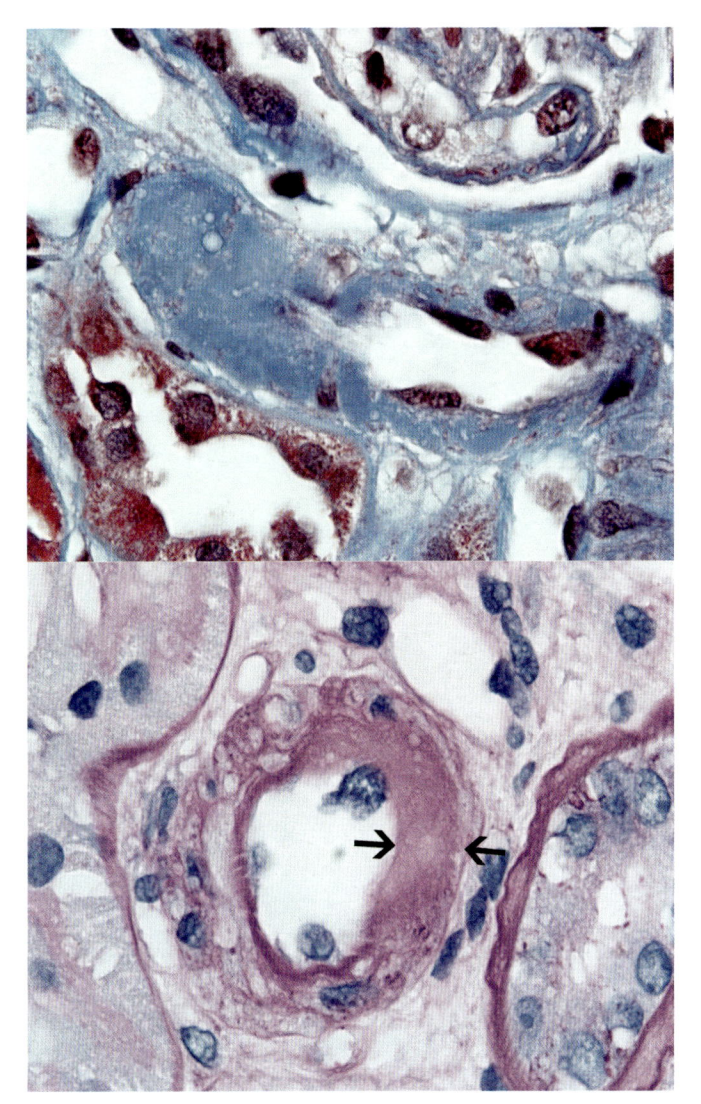

Figure 2.38 Calcineurin inhibitor induced arteriolopathy. The afferent arterioles show segmental transmural hyaline deposits replacing medial smooth muscle cells (aah2, arrows in bottom picture). Note: hypertension (not shown) most often induces subendothelial hyaline deposits that can occasionally protrude into the medial layer without significant replacement of smooth muscle cells. (Top) Trichrome stain, and (Bottom) PAS stain, x350.

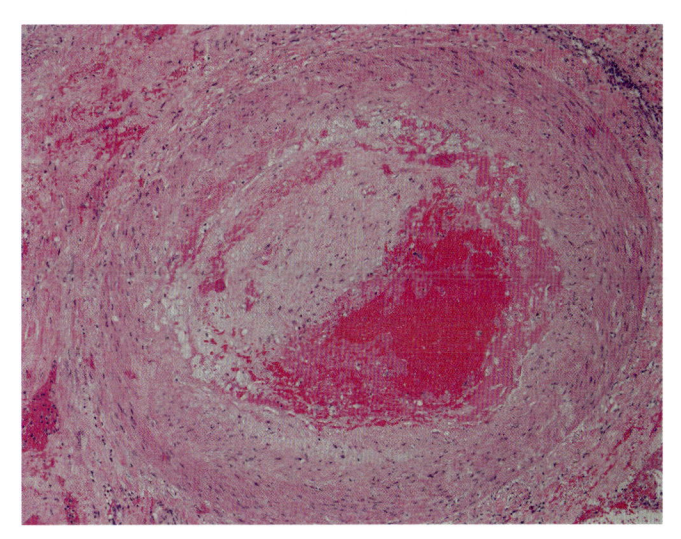

Figure 2.39 Thrombosed renal artery (with underlying chronic injury) in patient with longstanding calcineurin inhibitor toxicity and antibody mediate rejection (H&E, 200x).

PAS-positive (see Figure 2.38). There may be considerable differences in the severity of CNIT arteriolopathy even in the same biopsy. Some vessels might show mild changes, whereas others can demonstrate transmural hyalinosis, complete loss of medial smooth muscle cells, and stenosis. Immunofluorescence microscopy is nonspecific with the accumulation of IgM and the complement factors C1q, C3, C5b-9, and C4d in foci of hyaline deposits. There is no widely accepted scheme for scoring the severity and degree of CNIT arteriolopathies. BANFF scoring [91] has introduced an alternative quantitative scoring scheme of CNIT arteriolopathies.

On dose reduction or discontinuation, there may be regression of arteriolopathies [141, 142] with resolution of hyaline deposits and arteriolar wall remodeling. Arteriolar hyalinosis may also be seen in patients suffering from long-standing arterial hypertension or diabetes mellitus. Arteriolosclerosis associated with arterial hypertension presents predominantly showing subendothelial hyaline deposits with medial and transmural hyaline deposits being less common. Arteriolosclerosis can develop post-grafting, but can also be donor-derived. Arteriolar hyalinosis in cases of diabetic nephropathy, in native or transplanted kidneys, is very similar to CNIT arteriolopathy and a distinction cannot be simply made based on morphologic grounds [131]. Larger arteries are rarely affected though longstanding CNIT in conjunction with other complications such as antibody-mediated rejection, which can sometimes result in large vessel thrombosis, particularly if there is underlying chronic injury to the artery (see Figure 2.39).

There are a variety of *glomerular alterations* associable with CNIT. Focal and segmental intraglomerular fibrin thrombi are most often found in cases of calcineurin inhibitor induced thrombotic microangiopathies or may occur as isolated events [143] (see Figure 2.40). Glomerular endothelial cell injury and activation, without fibrin thrombi, are frequently seen (see Figure 2.40). Protracted calcineurin inhibitor induced glomerular endothelial cell injury can result in remodeling phenomena with widening of the lamina rara interna and subendothelial new basement membrane formation ("splitting") resulting in the duplication of capillary walls, i.e., CNIT glomerulopathy (see Figure 2.41). Mesangial regions are often slightly expanded due to matrix deposition (see Figure 2.40). The glomerular capillary lumens can contain scattered rare mononuclear cell elements, including lymphocytes, although conspicuous intracapillary inflammatory cell aggregates as well as prominent cell interpositions along duplicated capillary walls are not features of structural glomerular toxicity. There may be occasional small (non-diagnostic) electron-dense deposits. Nonspecific IgM and complement factor C1q, C3, and C5b-9 glomerular deposits are present by immunofluorescence microscopy (see Figure 2.40).

Thrombotic microangiopathy (hemolytic-uremic-syndrome) with arteriolar and glomerular capillary thrombi represents the most severe form of CNIT. Calcineurin inhibitor induced TMA is

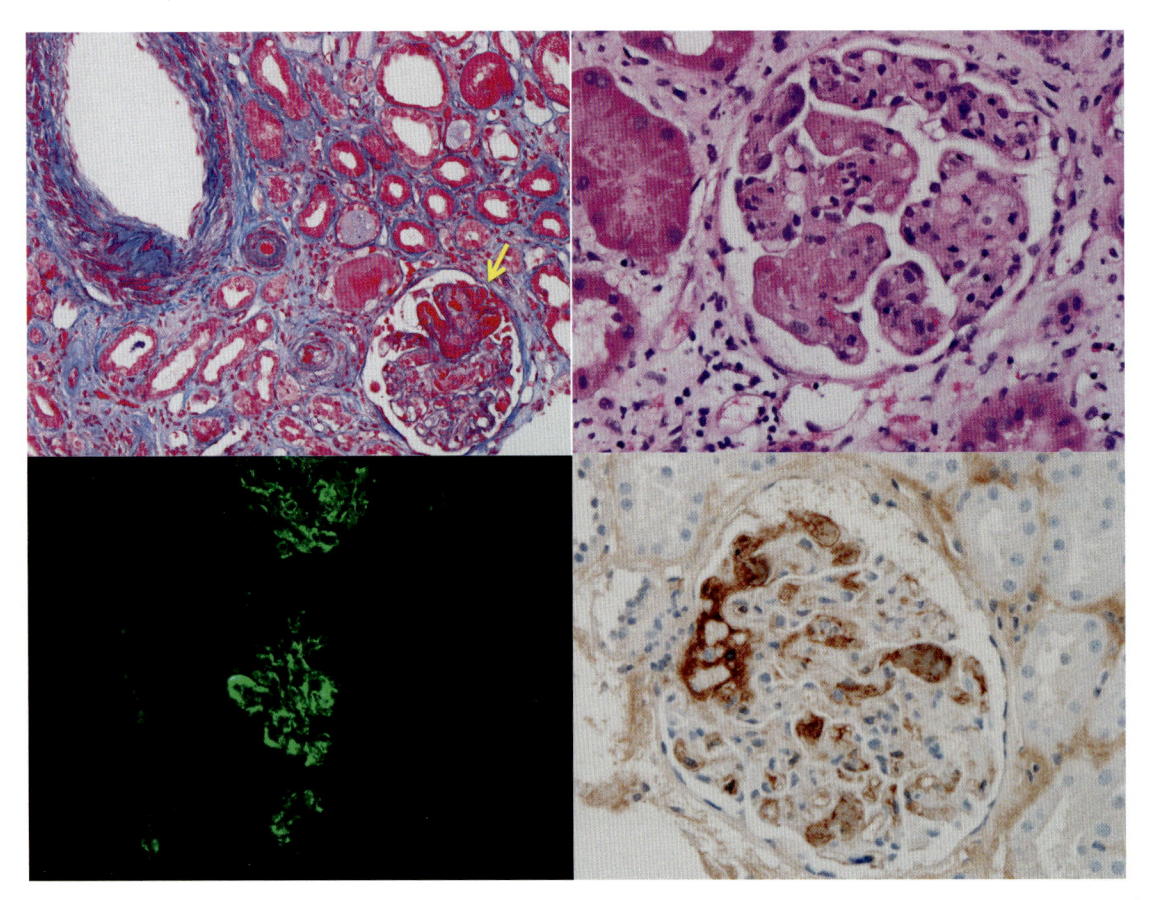

Figure 2.40 Calcineurin inhibitor induced thrombotic glomerulopathy. This occurred within the first year post-transplant with a renal transplant patient showing elevated tacrolimus levels. In some areas, the glomeruli displayed frank and florid intracapillary thrombi (arrow, upper left, trichrome, 200x) within glomeruli. There was also arteriolar injury and a toxic tubulopathy. The lower left picture is the positive IgM seen in the same case (200x, IgM, Immunofluorescence); C3 was also positive; all other immunoreactants were negative. Other areas showed dissolution of mesangial areas (lysis) (upper right, H&E, 400x) within the glomeruli. Immunohistochemistry to fibrinogen confirmed the presence within the glomerular capillaries (lower right, 400x).

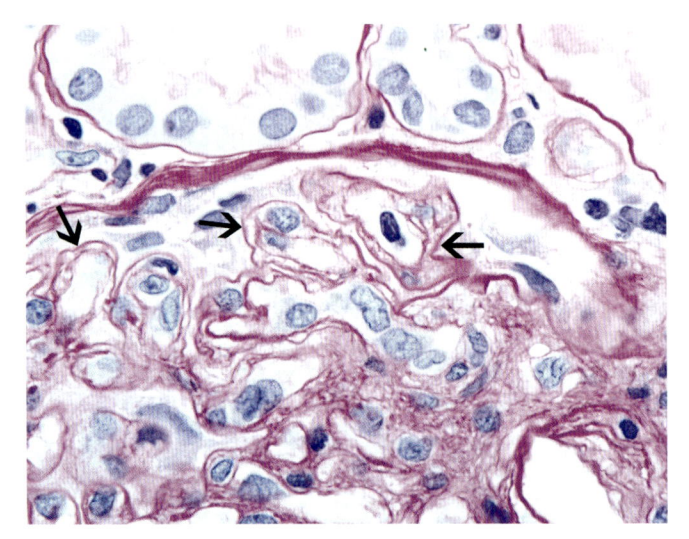

Figure 2.41 Calcineurin inhibitor induced late glomerulopathy. The patient presented six years post-transplantation on tacrolimus monotherapy with glomeruli showing global thickening of capillary walls with duplications (arrows) (PAS stain, x250 oil original magnification).

generally an early event occurring within the first few weeks to months post-grafting [144, 145]. Severe forms of CNIT induced TMA show typical systemic signs with thrombocytopenia, microangiopathic hemolytic anemia, elevated lactic dehydrogenase, and hyperbilirubinemia. Arterioles are focally affected and often with fibrin and platelet thrombi at the glomerular vascular poles. Medial smooth muscle layers can show single-cell necrosis [143]. As with other types of TMA, vascular lesions can undergo "onion skin" remodelling with intimal sclerosis. Glomerular remodelling following the lysis of thrombi and endothelial cell injury can result in mesangiolysis and segmental duplication of peripheral basement membranes.

Calcineurin inhibitor therapy contributes to interstitial scarring, although "striped" interstitial fibrosis is a secondary phenomenon solely reflecting nephron loss that lacks diagnostic specificity [146].

ii Drug-induced Acute Tubulo-interstitial Nephritis

An assorted number of drugs can induce allergic types of interstitial nephritides, often with changes indistinguishable from those seen in cases of tubulo-interstitial rejection. However, acute allergic interstitial nephritides seem uncommon after renal transplantation [147]; this may be due to a lack of clinical suspicion, to their morphologic similarity to other inflammatory complications, and possibly due to steroid-based immunosuppression preventing the development of interstitial inflammation in many cases. Allergic type interstitial nephritides and tubulo-interstitial rejection both can demonstrate patchy mononuclear

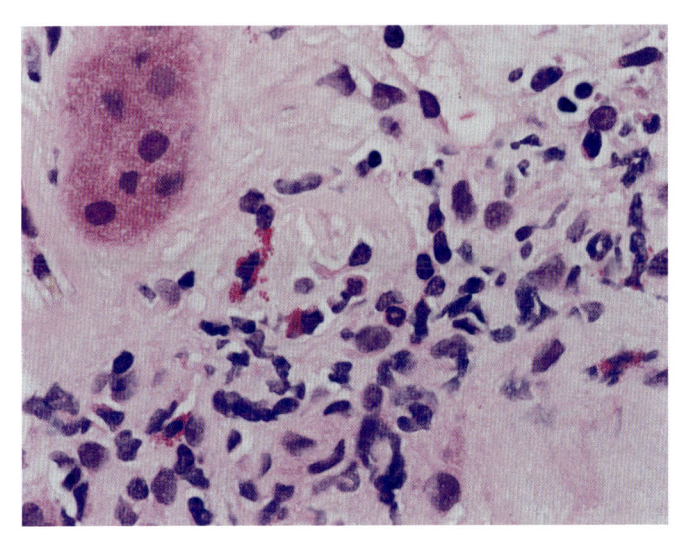

Figure 2.42 Acute interstitial nephritis with eosinophils occurring in a renal transplant primarily in medullary area that ultimately resolved with drug discontinuance (H&E, 1000x).

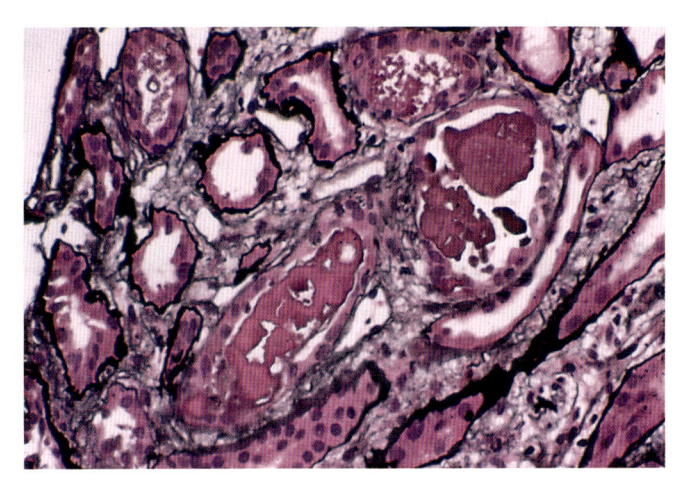

Figure 2.43 Tubulopathy present in kidney of patient with sirolimus therapy. Amorphous, proteinaceous material (granular or casts with fracture lines) (Methenamine silver, x160 original magnification).

cell infiltrates, often with small clusters of plasma cells, eosinophils in variable numbers, edema, focal tubulitis, and tubular injury (see Figure 2.42). Acute rejection sporadically has a prominent eosinophilic infiltrate [148–153], while drug-induced interstitial nephritis on the other hand may have no eosinophils [154]. One potential distinction is if the inflammatory cells predominate at the cortico-medullary junction/outer medulla and spare the cortex, then a diagnosis of allergic interstitial nephritis should be considered [147]. However, medullary inflammation by itself does not help to distinguish "allergic nephritis" from "rejection." Small, non-necrotizing granulomas may serve as a further diagnostic clue in some cases. Drug discontinuance in allergic interstitial nephritides often ameliorates the inflammation [147]. Since both diseases can involve the cortex and medulla, it is often impossible to make a clear distinction based on morphologic criteria.

iii Sirolimus and Everolimus (Mammalian Target of Rapamycin [mTOR] Inhibitors)

Sirolimus (or rapamycin, Rapamune) [155–160] and everolimus (Zortress) [161, 162] bind to the same cytoplasmic receptor proteins as tacrolimus, though this drug: receptor binding inhibits mTOR instead of calcineurin, leading to inhibition of lymphocyte activation and proliferation [163]. They also block via mTOR, the production of vascular endothelial growth factor (VEGF), and can induce endothelial cell death and thrombosis in tumor vessels [164–166]. In theory, the mTOR inhibitors may prevent the development of graft sclerosis [167–169]. They are metabolized by CYP3A and p-glycoprotein. As compared with CNIs, mTOR inhibitors were originally thought to be less nephrotoxic, but they can still delay recovery from acute tubular necrosis following renal transplantation [170], and concomitant administration of mTOR inhibitors and standard-dose CNIs potentiate nephrotoxicity [162, 171]. *De novo* or exaggeration of pre-existing proteinuria is common [162, 172] and thrombocytopenia and dyslipidemia are common, especially when combined with other immunosuppressive medication causing such side effects [155]. Fluid retention, pneumonia, and delayed wound healing are occasionally observed. Because of its antitumor properties, higher-dose everolimus may be used for certain neoplastic diseases – mTOR inhibitors may be of value in transplant patients with or at high risk for post-transplant neoplasms (e.g., skin cancer) [173, 174].

These drugs can in a dose-dependent manner increase the frequency [175] and duration of delayed graft function [176–178]. Smith and colleagues described early after transplantation how tubules can show "myeloma-cast-like" changes with fractured, eosinophilic, proteinaceous material, histiocytes, and multi-nucleated giant cells (see Figure 2.43) [175]. These changes are most pronounced in biopsies taken more than two weeks into the course of delayed graft function from patients treated with sirolimus and often a calcineurin inhibitor. The mTOR inhibitors can potentially injure small vessels [179–182] and thrombotic microangiopathies have been described [182, 183]. Sirolimus also stimulates proteinuria and possibly the development of focal and segmental glomerulosclerosis [184–187].

e Infections

An unfortunate consequence of the powerful immunosuppression administered in transplantation is the occurrence of a large number of infections, which can present systemically or in limited fashion. Several infections affecting the allograft are discussed herein; however, a comprehensive evaluation of all renal infections is beyond the scope of this chapter.

i Polyoma BK-virus Nephropathy (PVN)

The polyomavirus family consists of double stranded, non-encapsulated DNA viruses with different strains, among which the BK- and JC-virus strains are pathogenic in humans and can cause renal allograft infections (the SV40 strain only seems to play a very minor role). Typically, PVN is nearly always caused by a productive infection with the BK-virus strain. Disease triggered by polyomaviruses is predominantly seen in profoundly immunosuppressed patients. Polyomavirus

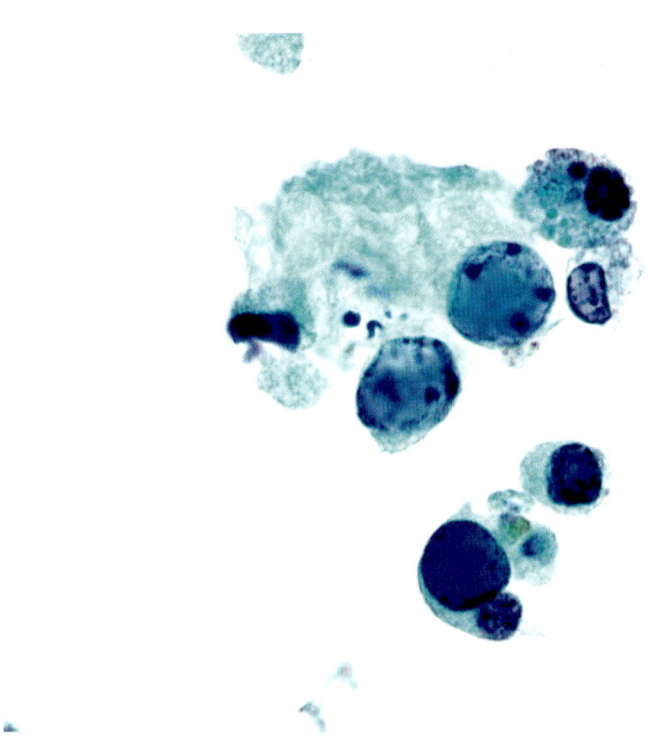

Figure 2.44 Urine sample showing "Decoy Cells," a morphologic sign of polyomavirus activation (Liquid-based urine cytology preparation, Papanicolaou stain, x600 oil original magnification).

allograft nephropathy (PVN) post-kidney transplantation was first described by Mackenzie [188] and has been mostly an iatrogenic complication due to "over immunosuppression" [189–195] with poorly defined risk factors [196, 197]. Presently, PVN has a prevalence of 1%–10% and a reported graft failure rate of more than 50% in some series [194, 198–203]. Specific and potent antiviral drugs to treat productive polyomavirus infections are not available.

PVN is caused by the re-activation of latent donor-derived polyomaviruses (located typically in the urothelium) [204] under intense immunosuppression. This activation is illustrated by the detection of free viral particles in the urine (by electron microscopy or PCR techniques) and viral inclusion bearing cells, so-called "decoy cells" in urine cytology specimens (see Figure 2.44). Transient, asymptomatic viral activation can also be detected in by PCR assays in serum, not necessarily accompanied by PVN, although PVN is always associated and preceded by polyomavirus activation [191, 205–210]. The typical timing of PVN-associated allograft dysfunction is 10–14 months post-transplantation, although this has wide variation [201, 208]. In general, PVN persists for months or even years.

PVN is best diagnosed histologically in a graft biopsy, which additionally provides relevant information on other contemporaneous complications. PVN focally affects the kidney so adequate samples are needed to guarantee an optimal diagnostic yield. The diagnosis may be missed if only one small core of renal cortex is sampled [200, 211] and ancillary techniques (immunohistochemistry, in-situ hybridization) help establish a definitive diagnosis [212]. Polyomavirus infection changes in the kidney are found in epithelial cells lining collecting ducts, tubules, and Bowman's capsule (parietal epithelial cells), including intra-nuclear inclusion bodies, cell injury, and lysis [190–192, 213, 214], without cytoplasmic inclusions. Four types of virally induced nuclear changes exist and hybrid forms are common [213–215] (see Figure 2.45): *type 1* (the most frequent form) – an amorphous basophilic ground-glass inclusion body; *type 2* – a central, eosinophilic, granular inclusion surrounded by a mostly complete halo (CMV like); *type 3* – a finely granular variant without a halo; and *type 4* – a vesicular variant with clumped, irregular chromatin and large viral aggregates; nucleoli may be found. PVN typically involves renal tubules and collecting ducts in a focal fashion. Severely injured tubules containing many inclusion-bearing epithelial cells are typically located adjacent to normal ducts. Viral inclusion bodies are often most abundant in the renal medulla. Viral inclusion bodies are also found in the transitional cell layer lining the renal pelvis, the (graft) ureter, and potentially even the recipient's urinary bladder [213, 216]. Rare histologic features of PVN include pseudo-crescents in glomeruli [213, 217, 218], non-necrotizing small epithelioid granulomas [219], and immune complex type deposits in tubular basement membranes [220].

In tissue sections, polyomavirus is readily detected with antibodies directed against the SV-40 T antigen (large T antigen) that cross-react with all polyomaviruses pathogenic in humans (see Figure 2.46). T antigen expression is associated with the initial phase of polyomavirus replication and precedes the formation of intra-nuclear viral inclusion bodies. Polyomaviruses can also be identified by in-situ hybridization or with antibodies directed against viral capsid proteins.

PCR techniques can be utilized to demonstrate viral DNA or RNA in tissue samples [221–223]. PVN is diagnosed by PCR, however, only when there are positive results (large number of copies) in the setting of histologically or immunohistochemically demonstrable virally induced cytopathic changes [221, 222, 224–228]. Positive PCR of viral RNA in the absence of histological or immunohistochemical changes is likely identifying non-PVN associated viral replication.

In PVN, standard immunofluorescence microscopy generally does not show any diagnostic staining pattern in tubules, glomeruli, or blood vessels. In some patients, PVN is associated with a type III hypersensitivity reaction, resembling "anti-TBM disease" in native kidneys. These cases are characterized by granular immune deposits along thickened tubular basement membranes that are easily discernible by immunofluorescence microscopy (using various antibodies directed against immunoglobulins and complement factors) or by electron microscopy [229].

By electron microscopy, polyomaviruses present as viral particles of 30 to 50 nm in diameter that occasionally form crystalloid aggregates [206, 209]. Polyomaviruses are ultrastructurally identified by size and their icosahedral capsid structure; polyomavirus strains cannot be distinguished. Virions are primarily found in the nucleus, rarely in the cytoplasm.

PVN is sub-grouped into four disease stages: early "A," fully developed "B," fibrosing "C," and burnt-out "D" [200, 206, 211,

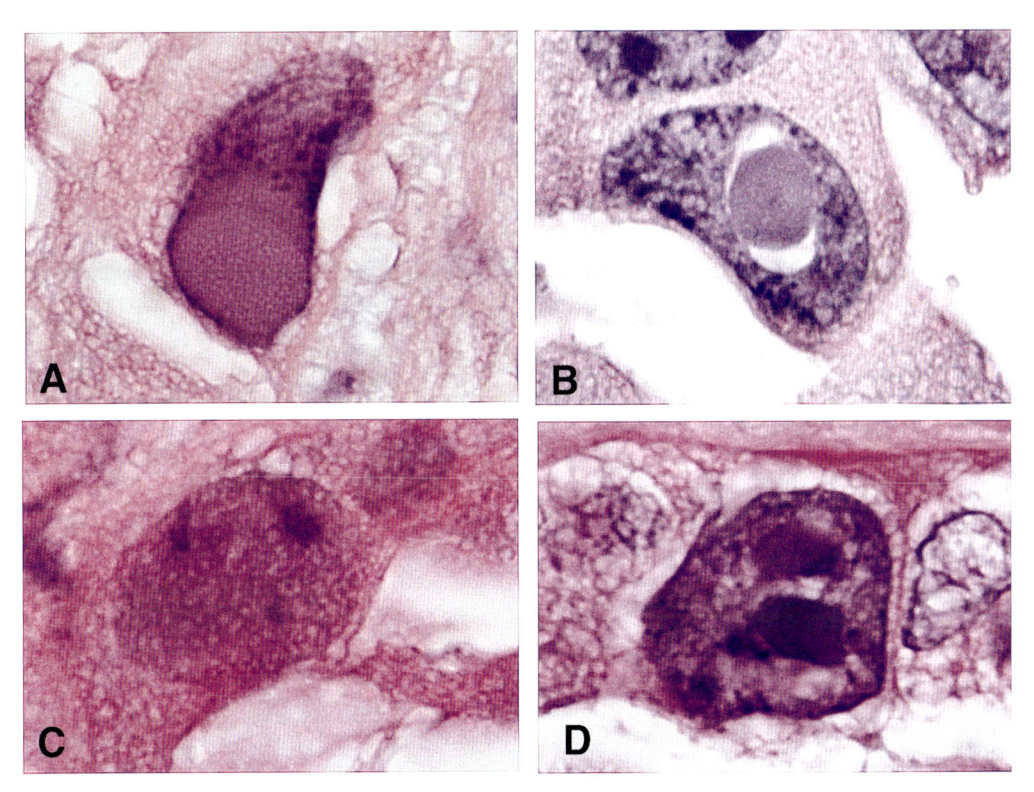

Figure 2.45 Polyomavirus nephropathy (A-D) showing different nuclear alterations: (A) amorphous, ground-glass type of inclusion body (type 1); (B) central intranuclear inclusion body surrounded by a halo (type 2); (C) nuclear enlargement and finely granular changes (type 3); (D) vesicular, clumped changes (type 4) (H&E stain, x400 oil original magnification).

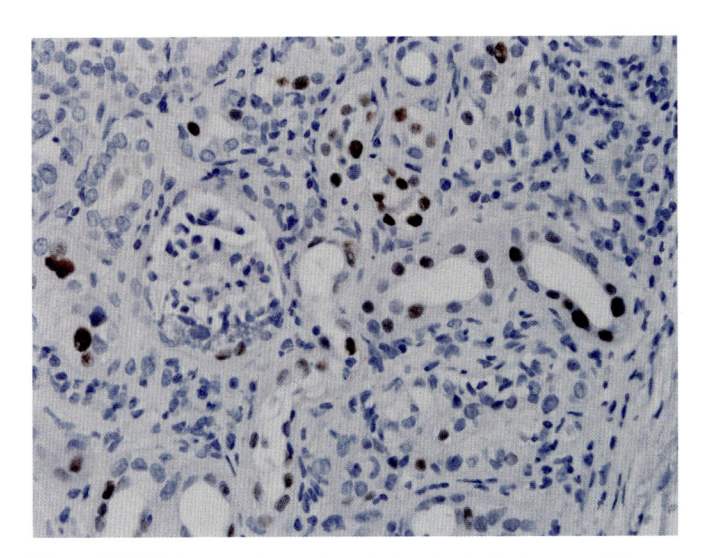

Figure 2.46 BK virus-positive tubular cells in patient with polyoma (BK) nephropathy (Immunohistochemistry to SV-40, 400x).

230–234]. Rather than the extent of interstitial inflammation, the virally induced epithelial cell injury, interstitial fibrosis, and tubular atrophy are pertinent to staging, with stages often progressing from one to another [199, 233]. The inflammation detectable in Stages B, C, and D varies and can represent "virally induced" interstitial nephritis with neutrophils located adjacent to severely injured tubules, plasma cells, and rarely plasma cell tubulitis [191, 206, 208, 234]. Patchy inflammatory cell infiltrates in the medulla and associated with tubular epithelial cell atypia are more often present with PVN. *Concurrent acute allograft rejection* with tubulitis, glomerulitis, and/or arteritis can often be evident, thereby preventing a singular diagnosis or separation of the two entities. The earliest disease phase with minimal "non-lytic" viral replication and denudation of tubular basement membranes is known as *PVN stage A*. The interstitium is normal or with minimal inflammation and fibrosis. The detection of one or more intra-nuclear viral inclusion bodies or by immunohistochemistry is needed. *PVN stage B* is characterized by marked virally induced tubular injury and epithelial cell lysis, abundant denudation of tubular basement membranes, and interstitial edema with a mixed, mild-to-marked inflammatory cell infiltrate. *PVN stage C* shows marked interstitial fibrosis (>50%) and tubular atrophy with varying degrees of inflammation and viral replication. *PVN stage D* demonstrates nonspecific chronic changes with varying degrees of interstitial fibrosis and tubular atrophy (ranging from minimal to marked), and occasionally mild lymphocytic inflammation in areas of parenchymal scarring. There are no signs of polyomavirus replication by light microscopy and immunohistochemistry/in-situ hybridization.

ii Cytomegalovirus (CMV)

Cytomegalovirus (CMV) is a common herpes virus pathogen in kidney transplantation. CMV can cause a symptomatic infection in the first months post-transplantation, generally

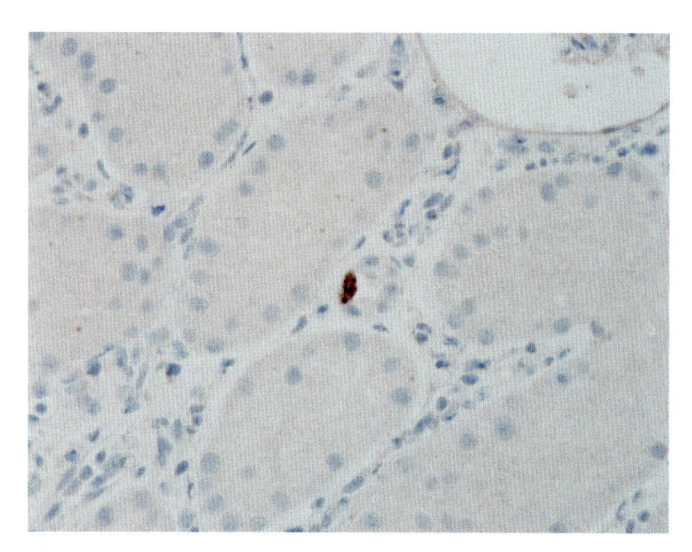

Figure 2.47 Cytomegalovirus infection in a kidney allograft. Immunohistochemistry to CMV demonstrates infected cell within tubules (Immunohistochemistry, 400x).

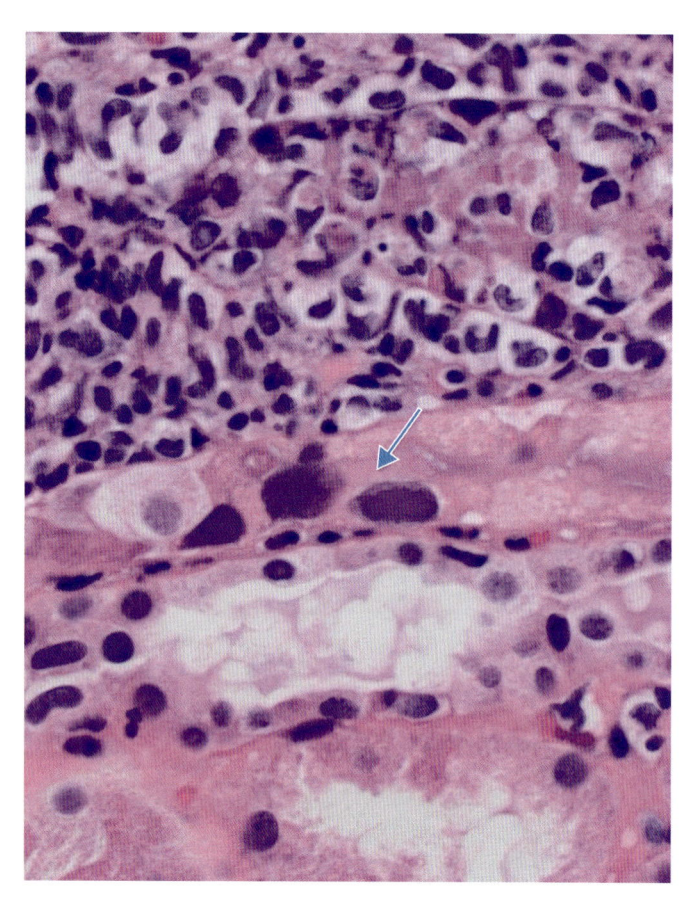

Figure 2.48 Adenovirus infection in kidney allograft. Arrow points out infected tubular epithelial cells with smudgy, "ground-glass" type inclusions (H&E, oil immersion, 1000x).

characterized by fever, leukopenia, hepatitis, or pneumonitis, and viremia [235] with kidneys involved in approximately 25% of patients [236, 237]. Productive CMV infections of renal transplants are rare.

Lesions induced by the replication of CMV in the kidneys have been described both in native organs and transplants [236, 237]. Viral cytopathic changes are typically focal and seen in the nuclei and cytoplasm of tubular epithelial cells, endothelial cells, and occasionally in mononuclear inflammatory cells [236, 237]. CMV-infected cells can show the typical "owls-eye" appearance with nuclei containing a central round inclusion body surrounded by a halo. Homogenous smudgy-appearing intranuclear inclusions and small basophilic "lumpy" cytoplasmic viral inclusions can also be evident [236]. Occasionally, granulomatous-appearing mononuclear inflammatory cell inflammation is present [237]. Foci of necrosis and micro abscesses can occur, but are uncommon [237]. Rarely, CMV infects glomerular cells and causes an acute glomerulonephritis with crescents [238–241].

Ancillary diagnostic techniques are important to confirm the diagnosis of a productive CMV infection; these include immunohistochemistry (see Figure 2.47), in-situ hybridization, and rarely by electron microscopy. Ultrastructurally, virions of approximately 150 nanometers are found in nuclei and the cytoplasm. The pattern of immunofluorescence microscopy with a standard panel of antibodies detecting immunoglobulins and complement factors is typically not specific [236]. A useful adjunct test is the quantitative measurement of CMV DNA from the biopsy. Since CMV DNA can be found in the absence of cytopathic changes, PCR studies for viral DNA do not clearly distinguish between productive and latent infections [242]; however, it remains useful to establish that CMV copies are present in the graft [243]. In summary, CMV nephritis is best diagnosed when there are cytopathic changes, along with demonstration of CMV proteins and/or DNA. Morphologically, CMV nephropathy can resemble other types of viral infections, mainly caused by polyomaviruses or adenovirus. Since CMV (in contrast to polyomavirus and adenovirus) often replicates in endothelial and inflammatory cells, a distinction between rejection-induced changes and infection-driven inflammation is difficult. What was known as "CMV-glomerulopathy" [244] is now classified as rejection-induced transplant glomerulitis. Indeed, CMV infections, along with other infectious pathogens, can stimulate indirect effects on the kidney graft by modulating the immune response and promoting acute and chronic rejection episodes [245–247].

iii Adenovirus

Adenovirus infections of renal allografts are relatively rare [248, 249]. Morphologically, productive infections can show intranuclear viral inclusions in epithelial cells, interstitial hemorrhage, tubular injury with necrosis, interstitial inflammation, and intra-tubular red blood cell casts [250, 251]. The intranuclear cytopathic changes in tubular cells and in parietal epithelial cells are smudgy, "ground-glass" types of inclusion bodies (similar to polyomavirus type 1 changes) with rare viral inclusion bodies surrounded by a halo (i.e. CMV-like) [252, 253] (see Figure 2.48). The inflammatory cell infiltrates primarily have mononuclear and plasma cells with areas of necrosis and tubular disruption showing abundant polymorphonuclear leukocytes. Glomeruli and blood vessels are generally not affected. Immunohistochemistry reveals strong nuclear and less intense cytoplasmic staining in epithelial cells. Ultrastructural virions of approximately 75–80 nm are found in nuclei and the cytoplasm, but EM is infrequently used for detecting. Immunofluorescence microscopy to immunoglobulins and complement factors are nonspecific.

Infections can be asymptomatic, localized (e.g., enteritis, cystitis, or nephritis), or as disseminated. Adenovirus subgroup B, serotypes 7, 11, 34, and 35 cause the most renal transplant infection, including hemorrhagic cystitis and necrotizing interstitial nephritis [252–256]. Adenovirus-induced nephritis most often presents within the first three months after transplantation, with possible symptoms including renal failure, hematuria, dysuria, hemorrhagic cystitis, and a generalized infection. Disseminated adenovirus infections tend to have high mortality [252, 253, 257–259].

iv Epstein-Barr Virus/Post-transplant Lymphoproliferative Disorders

Post-transplant Lymphoproliferative Disorder, or PTLD, represents a lymphoid proliferation or lymphoma involving many organ sites and that develops as a consequence of immunosuppression in a recipient of a solid organ or bone marrow allograft. Briefly, PTLDs range from early Epstein-Barr virus (EBV) driven polyclonal proliferations resembling infectious mononucleosis to EBV-positive or EBV-negative lymphomas of predominantly B cell or less often T cell types [260]. There is a progression from polymorphism to clonality and subsequent oncogene mutations [261]. The PTLD stages of plasmacytic hyperplasia, polymorphic B cell hyperplasia and lymphoma, and immunoblastic lymphoma or multiple myeloma are discussed in more detail in other chapters. The development of PTLD is associated with intense immunosuppression, with the more rapid onset of PTLD often being associated with the higher levels of immunosuppression. The recipient's and donor's EBV serological status, i.e., sero-positive transplant into a sero-negative recipient, is linked with an elevated risk for PTLD [262]. A majority of PTLD cases are EBV-positive [260, 263, 264], though EBV-negative cases are present among renal allograft recipients [260, 265]. PTLDs originate from B cells in the majority of transplant recipients [266, 267]. PTLD has a low prevalence among renal allograft recipients as compared to other solid organ grafts [268] [269].

PTLD involving the kidneys are often of the polymorphic variant [270, 271] and can resemble acute cell-mediated rejection [271–283]. The interstitial accumulation of hematopoietic cells compartment typically shows nodular, expansile aggregates of mononuclear cell elements often plasma cell-rich with varying numbers of activated lymphocytes and "blastoid" cell elements containing prominent nucleoli (see Figure 2.49). There are mitotic figures, sometimes with focal necrosis. The neoplastic (and reactive) mononuclear cells can be amid tubulitis and endarteritis; no viral inclusion bodies

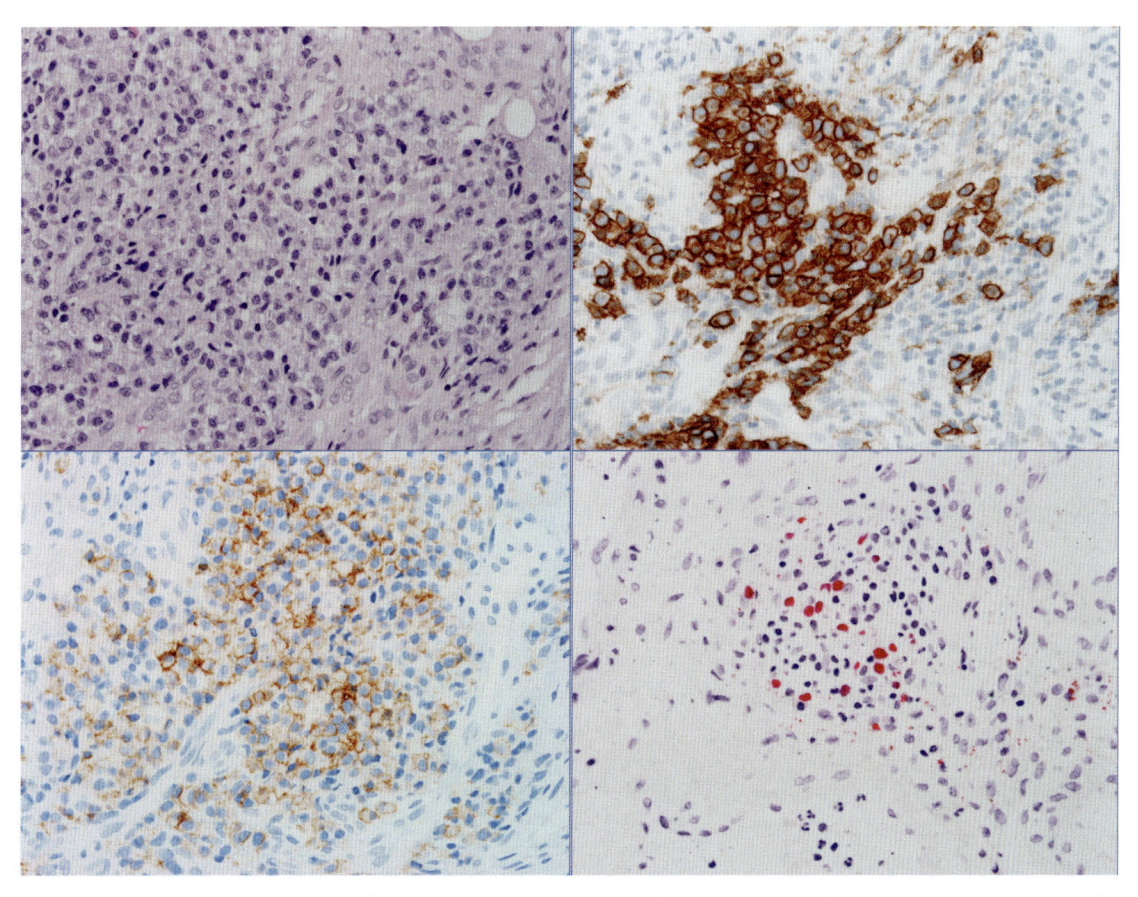

Figure 2.49 Post-transplant Lymphoproliferative Disease (PTLD) in a renal allograft. The upper-left photomicrograph (H&E, 200x) shows a heterogeneous infiltrate with plasma cells, atypical blasts, and lymphocytes. The upper-right picture (immunohistochemistry to CD138, 400x) highlights the presence of plasma cells, and the lower-left picture (immunohistochemistry to CD20, 400x) reveals the presence of CD20+ B cells with mild surface staining. In situ hybridization to EBV (lower right, 400x) shows the presence of EBV+ cells.

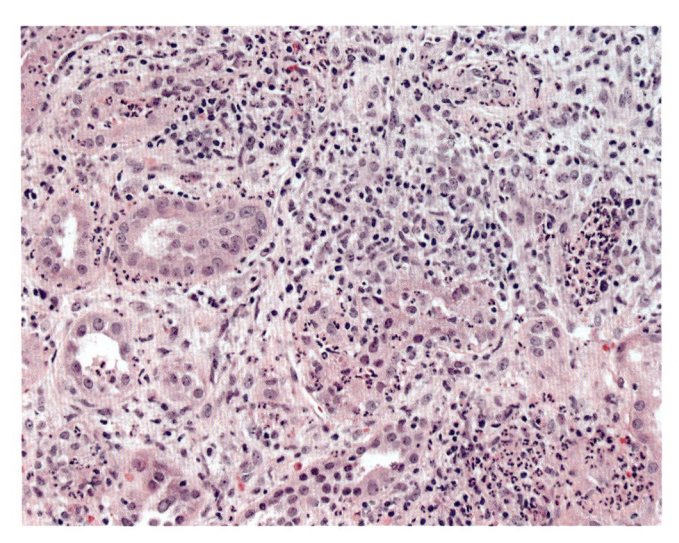

Figure 2.50 Bacterial pyelonephritis in an allograft with an inflammatory cell infiltrate containing numerous neutrophils that infiltrate tubules (H&E, 400x).

are seen. Thus, there are several features present both in rejection and PTLD. The presence of dense, nodular, expansile sheets of activated lymphoid cell elements without interstitial edema raises the likelihood of PTLD, though rejection can co-exist with PTLD [271].

Ancillary diagnostic techniques are critical to help identify PTLD. Since a majority of PTLDs are of B cell lineage and integrated with the replication of EBV, immunohistochemistry to B lineage antigens (e.g., CD20, CD19 and/or CD79a) as well as in-situ hybridization for EBV-encoded nuclear RNA (EBER) (see Figure 2.49) can be very useful in helping diagnosing PTLD [260].

The number of positive B cells and EBER+ cells can be highly variable. Tests to detect clonality (e.g., B or T antigen receptor rearrangement) help to confirm the presence of a monomorphic PTLD. Elevated plasma EBV viral load levels (by PCR) may further help confirm the diagnosis of PTLD.

v Pyelonephritis

Acute bacterial pyelonephritis can occur in transplanted kidneys (as in native kidneys); predictably, the diagnosis in kidney transplants can be challenging (see Figure 2.50). Morphologically, there is mixed interstitial inflammatory cell infiltrate with polymorphonuclear leukocytes, as well as tubular polymorphonuclear leukocyte casts. Pyelonephritis is often a patchy inflammatory process with accentuation in the medulla. In severe cases, (e.g., associated with bacteremia or urosepsis), microabscesses can be seen. C4d is characteristically absent and not detected along peritubular capillaries. Several other entities may partially mimic pyelonephritis, including acute ischemic tubular injury (ATI), or an antibody-mediated rejection episode. ATI typically reveals marked and diffuse tubular injury with tubular epithelial cell vacuolization and scattered polymorphonuclear leukocytes. Antibody-mediated rejection tends to have microvascular injury (as described above), along with C4d positivity in many cases.

f Recurrent Disease

A frequent primary cause of end-stage renal disease leading to renal transplantation is glomerulonephritis, which occurs in 30%–50% of kidney transplant recipients. In addition, recurrence of the initial glomerular disease is an important determinant of long-term graft outcome after transplantation in 30%–40% of these patients [284, 285], although the actual incidence is often difficult to discern due to a lack of information on the primary disease (i.e., an end-stage kidney disease with no biopsy diagnosis). Thus, de novo glomerulonephritis cannot be distinguished from a recurrent glomerulonephritis since the original disease is sometimes unknown. There is a variation in the frequency of recurrence rate depending upon the type of original glomerular disease and predictably, the incidence of recurrent glomerulopathies rises as the post-transplant period increases. The most common recurrent glomerulonephritis is FSGS [286, 287] followed by IgA nephropathy [288, 289]; a variety of other glomerular entities follow thereafter, including diabetic nephropathy, MPGN, lupus nephritis, and light chain nephropathy, among others. We will briefly describe several recurrent entities.

In our experience and others [286, 287], *Focal Segmental Glomerulosclerosis (FSGS)* is the most common recurrent and de novo glomerulopathy present following renal transplantation. The biopsies morphologically demonstrate, in identical fashion, the wide spectrum of FSGS changes seen in native kidneys (see Figure 2.51), including the variants (i.e., cellular perihilar, collapsing, not otherwise specified [NOS] and cellular) described by the Columbia group [290, 291]. The recurrence can rapid (e.g., within days) and aggressive. Differentiation from a de novo or donor-transmitted (very rare) FSGS is not sometimes possible, though biopsies of the original diseased native kidney of the recipient often are extremely useful in identifying the origin of the FSGS in the transplant. Recurrence of FSGS occurs mainly in primary forms and is only infrequently described in secondary varieties. However, calcineurin inhibitors and sirolimus [292] have clearly been shown to be associated with de novo FSGS in kidney allografts. There are some risk factors affecting the rate of primary FSGS recurrence that should be considered, including age and the original type of FSGS present [293].

Membranoproliferative Glomerulonephritis (MPGN) is a glomerulopathy that can be Type I, Type II, or secondary in affecting renal demise. Patients receiving renal transplants for this entity can show recurrence of any of these forms, with morphological features comparable to the native kidney lesions [294–297]. Type I MPGN has a typical recurrence rate of approximately 20% and is a risk for graft failure. A variety of factors may influence the risk of recurrence, including the class II MHC genotype of the recipient [294]. Proteinuria is a common presenting symptom. Type II MPGN has a very high recurrence rate [298] and can be confused with transplant glomerulopathy.

arteriolar hyalinosis. Nodular mesangial lesions (Kimmelstiel-Wilson nodules) and characteristic ultrastructural findings can also be seen [301]; these lesions can be displayed in recurrent diabetic nephropathy. The recurrence of diabetic nephropathy tends faster than the more protracted course that occurs in native kidneys [287, 299]. Transmission from donors is unlikely and risk factors for recurrence of DN vary and include race, age, and donor-recipient HLA disparity, among others.

Recurrent *lupus nephritis* is another glomerulopathy that can become a post-transplant complication, with a recurrence rate that has been reported from approximately 10%–30% [302], although the overall impression is that unless you are looking for it, it will not be found [303]. In our experience, lupus tends to recur several years from transplantation and all histological subtypes may be evident, including mesangial, proliferative, and membranous patterns. Immunofluorescence and electron microscopy are clearly valuable to the diagnosing pathologist in order to document the presence of immune complexes. Graft loss tends to be rare due to recurrent lupus nephritis.

Thrombotic microangiopathy (TMA), a post-transplant complication that can occur due to several *de novo* causes (e.g., calcineurin inhibitors – see drug toxicity section [304]; Shiga toxin), can also be present in the kidney transplant from recurrent disease, including *Hemolytic Uremic Syndrome* (HUS), anti-phospholipid syndrome [305], familial HUS [306, 307], and several viral diseases such as HIV and CMV [308]. There is significant variability in the recurrence of these entities leading to TMA; the incidence of recurrent TMA tends to be low and the timing of TMA post-transplant ranges from days to years. Morphologically, TMA due to recurrent disease is morphologically identical to de novo TMA.

Finally, there are other entities that may recur in renal transplants, including ANCA vasculitis [309, 310], Membranous Glomerulonephritis [311], anti-GBM disease, and Oxalosis.

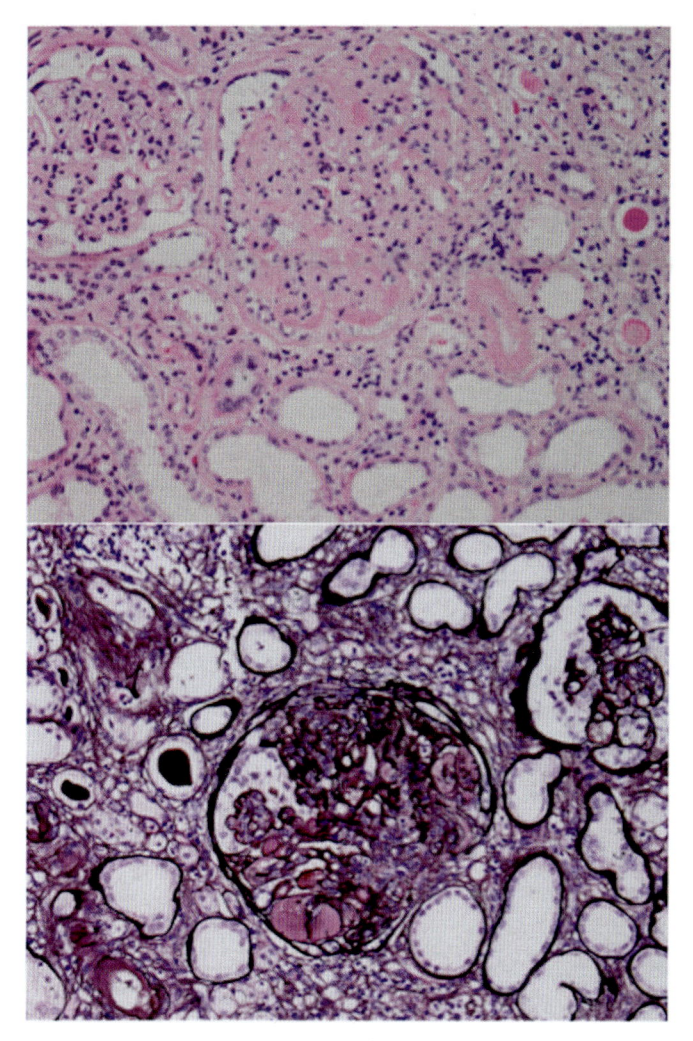

Figure 2.51 Recurrent Focal Segmental Glomerulosclerosis (FSGS) in a kidney allograft, two years post-transplant. The top photograph shows a glomerulus with sclerosing changes in the tuft with hyalinosis and podocyte hyperplasia. A hyalinotic arteriole is also present (H&E, 400x). The bottom photo shows a silver stain that highlights a separate area of the same kidney with adhesion to Bowman's capsule, hyalinosis, and sclerosis without collapsing (Jones silver, 400x).

Diabetic Nephropathy (DN) is among the more common recurring renal diseases in kidney transplants [287, 299] with up to 30% recurrence rate. The lesions in diabetic nephropathy [300] include thickened glomerular basement membranes, mild to severe mesangial expansion and repair, and

Acknowledgements

I wish to thank Dr. Volker Nickeleit for his generous sharing of some figures and for allowing an editing of his original chapter.

References

1. Stefoni S, Campieri C, Donati G, Orlandi V. The History of Clinical Renal Transplant. J Nephrol. 2004;**17**(3):475–8.
2. Cecka JM. The OPTN/UNOS Renal Transplant Registry. Clin Transpl. 2005:1–16.
3. Dharnidharka VR, Fiorina P, Harmon WE. Kidney Transplantation in Children. New England Journal of Medicine. 2014;**371**(6):549–58.
4. Cohen DJ, St Martin L, Christensen LL, Bloom RD, Sung RS. Kidney and Pancreas Transplantation in the United States, 1995–2004. Am J Transplant. 2006;**6**(5 Pt 2):1153–69.
5. de Vries DK, Wijermars LG, Reinders ME, Lindeman JH, Schaapherder AF. Donor Pre-treatment in Clinical Kidney Transplantation: A Critical Appraisal. Clin Transplant. 2013;**27**(6):799–808.
6. Catena F, Coccolini F, Montori G, Vallicelli C, Amaduzzi A, Ercolani G, et al. Kidney Preservation: Review of Present and Future Perspective. Transplantation Proceedings. 2013;**45**(9):3170–7.
7. Lee AP, Abramowicz D. Is the Kidney Donor Risk Index a Step Forward in the Assessment of Deceased Donor Kidney Quality? Nephrol Dial Transplant. 2014.
8. Friedewald JJ, Samana CJ, Kasiske BL, Israni AK, Stewart D, Cherikh W, et al. The Kidney Allocation System. Surg Clin North Am. 2013;**93**(6):1395–406.

9. Nicholson ML, Wheatley TJ, Doughman TM, White SA, Morgan JD, Veitch PS, et al. A Prospective Randomized Trial of Three Different Sizes of Core-cutting Needle for Renal Transplant Biopsy. Kidney International. 2000;58(1):390–5.

10. Jennette JC, Kshirsagar AV. How Can the Safety and Diagnostic Yield of Percutaneous Renal Biopsies Be Optimized? Nat Clin Pract Nephrol. 2008;4(3):126–7.

11. Manno C, Strippoli GF, Arnesano L, Bonifati C, Campobasso N, Gesualdo L, et al. Predictors of Bleeding Complications in Percutaneous Ultrasound-guided Renal Biopsy. Kidney Int. 2004;66(4):1570–7.

12. Song JH, Cronan JJ. Percutaneous Biopsy in Diffuse Renal Disease: Comparison of 18- and 14-gauge Automated Biopsy Devices. J Vasc Interv Radiol. 1998;9(4):651–5.

13. Racusen LC, Solez K, Colvin RB, Bonsib SM, Castro MC, Cavallo T, et al. The BANFF 97 Working Classification of Renal Allograft Pathology. Kidney International. 1999;55(2):713–23.

14. Colvin RB, Cohen AH, Saiontz C, Bonsib S, Buick M, Burke B, et al. Evaluation of Pathologic Criteria for Acute Renal Allograft Rejection: Reproducibility, Sensitivity, and Clinical Correlation. J Am Soc Nephrol. 1997;8(12):1930–41.

15. Sorof JM, Vartanian RK, Olson JL, Tomlanovich SJ, Vincenti FG, Amend WJ. Histopathological Concordance of Paired Renal Allograft Biopsy Cores. Effect on the Diagnosis and Management of Acute Rejection. Transplantation. 1995;60(11):1215–9.

16. Pegas KL, Michel K, Garcia VD, Goldani J, Bittar A, Seelig D, et al. Histopathological Analysis of Pre-implantation Donor Kidney Biopsies: Association with Graft Survival and Function in One Year Post-transplantation. Jornal brasileiro de nefrologia: 'orgao oficial de Sociedades Brasileira e Latino-Americana de Nefrologia. 2014;36(2):186–93.

17. Eccher A, Boschiero L, Fior F, Casartelli Liviero M, Zampicini L, Ghimenton C, et al. Donor Kidneys with Miliary Papillary Renal Cell Neoplasia: The Role of the Pathologist in Determining Suitability for Transplantation. Ann Transplant. 2014;19:362–6.

18. Chapman JR. Do Protocol Transplant Biopsies Improve Kidney Transplant Outcomes? Curr Opin Nephrol Hypertens. 2012;21(6):580–6.

19. Saidi RF, Elias N, Kawai T, Hertl M, Farrell ML, Goes N, et al. Outcome of Kidney Transplantation Using Expanded Criteria Donors and Donation after Cardiac Death Kidneys: Realities and Costs. Am J Transplant. 2007;7(12):2769–74.

20. Patel SK, Pankewycz OG, Weber-Shrikant E, Zachariah M, Kohli R, Nader ND, et al. Graft Arteriosclerosis and Glomerulosclerosis Correlate with Flow and Resistance to Machine Perfusion in Kidney Transplantation. Transplantation Proceedings. 2012;44(7):2197–201.

21. Gaber LW, Moore LW, Alloway RR, Amiri MH, Vera SR, Gaber AO. Glomerulosclerosis as a Determinant of Posttransplant Function of Older Donor Renal Allografts. Transplantation. 1995;60(4):334–9.

22. Karpinski J, Lajoie G, Cattran D, Fenton S, Zaltzman J, Cardella C, et al. Outcome of Kidney Transplantation from High-risk Donors Is Determined by Both Structure and Function. Transplantation. 1999;67(8):1162–7.

23. Wang CJ, Shafique S, McCullagh J, Diederich DA, Winklhofer FT, Wetmore JB. Implications of Donor Disseminated Intravascular Coagulation on Kidney Allograft Recipients. Clin J Am Soc Nephrol. 2011;6(5):1160–7.

24. De Vusser K, Lerut E, Kuypers D, Vanrenterghem Y, Jochmans I, Monbaliu D, et al. The Predictive Value of Kidney Allograft Baseline Biopsies for Long-term Graft Survival. J Am Soc Nephrol. 2013;24(11):1913–23.

25. Singh P, Farber JL, Doria C, Francos GC, Gulati R, Ramirez CB, et al. Peritransplant Kidney Biopsies: Comparison of Pathologic Interpretations and Practice Patterns of Organ Procurement Organizations. Clin Transplant. 2012;26(3):E191–9.

26. Kasiske BL, Stewart DE, Bista BR, Salkowski N, Snyder JJ, Israni AK, et al. The Role of Procurement Biopsies in Acceptance Decisions for Kidneys Retrieved for Transplant. Clin J Am Soc Nephrol. 2014;9(3):562–71.

27. Toft BG, Federspiel BH, Sorensen SS, Bagi P, Nielsen HB, Andersen CB. A Histopathological Score on Baseline Biopsies from Elderly Donors Predicts Outcome 1 Year after Renal Transplantation. APMIS. 2012;120(3):182–6.

28. Sulikowski T, Tejchman K, Zietek Z, Urasinska E, Domanski L, Sienko J, et al. Histopathologic Evaluation of Pretransplantation Biopsy as a Factor Influencing Graft Function after Kidney Transplantation in 3-Year Observation. Transplantation Proceedings. 2010;42(9):3375–81.

29. Hall IE, Reese PP, Weng FL, Schroppel B, Doshi MD, Hasz RD, et al. Preimplant Histologic Acute Tubular Necrosis and Allograft Outcomes. Clin J Am Soc Nephrol. 2014;9(3):573–82.

30. Yu N, Fu S, Fu Z, Meng J, Xu Z, Wang B, et al. Allotransplanting Donor Kidneys after Resection of a Small Renal Cancer or Contralateral Healthy Kidneys from Cadaveric Donors with Unilateral Renal Cancer: A Systematic Review. Clin Transplant. 2014;28(1):8–15.

31. Musquera M, Perez M, Peri L, Esforzado N, Sebastia MC, Paredes D, et al. Kidneys from Donors with Incidental Renal Tumors: Should They Be Considered Acceptable Option for Transplantation? Transplantation. 2013;95(9):1129–33.

32. Lappin DW, Hutchison AJ, Pearson RC, O'Donoghue DJ, Roberts IS. Angiomyolipoma in a Transplanted Kidney. Nephrol Dial Transplant. 1999;14(6):1574–5.

33. Buob D, Lionet A. The Case | Peculiar Fibrous Nodules in a Renal Transplant Biopsy. Kidney Int. 2014;85(2):483–4.

34. Sangoi AR, Fujiwara M, West RB, Montgomery KD, Bonventre JV, Higgins JP, et al. Immunohistochemical Distinction of Primary Adrenal Cortical Lesions from Metastatic Clear Cell Renal Cell Carcinoma: A Study of 248 Cases. Am J Surg Pathol. 2011;35(5):678–86.

35. Nicol D, Fujita S. Kidneys from Patients with Small Renal Tumours Used for Transplantation: Outcomes and Results. Current Opinion in Urology. 2011;21(5):380–5.

36. Eltzschig HK, Eckle T. Ischemia and Reperfusion – From Mechanism to Translation. Nat Med. 2011;17(11):1391–401.

37. Carden DL, Granger DN. Pathophysiology of Ischaemia-Reperfusion Injury. J Pathol. 2000;190(3):255–66.

38. Rudich SM, Kaplan B, Magee JC, Arenas JD, Punch JD, Kayler LK, et al. Renal Transplantations Performed Using Non-Heart-Beating Organ Donors: Going back to the Future? Transplantation. 2002;74(12):1715–20.

39. Nicholson ML, Metcalfe MS, White SA, Waller JR, Doughman TM, Horsburgh T, et al. A Comparison of the Results of

Renal Transplantation from Non-Heart-Beating, Conventional Cadaveric, and Living Donors. Kidney Int. 2000;58(6):2585-91.

40. Perico N, Cattaneo D, Sayegh MH, Remuzzi G. Delayed Graft Function in Kidney Transplantation. Lancet. 2004;364(9447):1814-27.

41. Dittrich S, Groneberg DA, von Loeper J, Lippek F, Hegemann O, Grosse-Siestrup C, et al. Influence of Cold Storage on Renal Ischemia Reperfusion Injury after Non-Heart-Beating Donor Explantation. Nephron Exp Nephrol. 2004;96(3):e97-102.

42. Arias-Diaz J, Alvarez J, del Barrio MR, Balibrea JL. Non-Heart-Beating Donation: Current State of the Art. Transplantation Proceedings. 2004;36(7):1891-3.

43. Renkens JJ, Rouflart MM, Christiaans MH, van den Berg-Loonen EM, van Hooff JP, van Heurn LW. Outcome of Nonheart-Beating Donor Kidneys with Prolonged Delayed Graft Function after Transplantation. Am J Transplant. 2005;5(11):2704-9.

44. Sanchez-Fructuoso A, Prats Sanchez D, Marques Vidas M, Lopez De Novales E, Barrientos Guzman A. Non-Heart Beating Donors. Nephrol Dial Transplant. 2004;19 Suppl 3:iii26-31.

45. Molitoris BA, Sutton TA. Endothelial Injury and Dysfunction: Role in the Extension Phase of Acute Renal Failure. Kidney Int. 2004;66(2):496-9.

46. Bonventre JV, Zuk A. Ischemic Acute Renal Failure: An Inflammatory Disease? Kidney Int. 2004;66(2):480-5.

47. Di Y, Lei Y, Yu F, Changfeng F, Song W, Xuming M. MicroRNAs Expression and Function in Cerebral Ischemia Reperfusion Injury. Journal of Molecular Neuroscience: MN. 2014;53(2):242-50.

48. Cai Y, Xu H, Yan J, Zhang L, Lu Y. Molecular Targets and Mechanism of Action of Dexmedetomidine in Treatment of Ischemia/Reperfusion Injury. Molecular Medicine Reports. 2014;9(5):1542-50.

49. Li YF, Jing Y, Hao J, Frankfort NC, Zhou X, Shen B, et al. MicroRNA-21 in the Pathogenesis of Acute Kidney Injury. Protein & Cell. 2013;4(11):813-9.

50. Cooper JE, Wiseman AC. Acute Kidney Injury in Kidney Transplantation. Curr Opin Nephrol Hypertens. 2013;22(6):698-703.

51. Eltzschig HK, Eckle T. Ischemia and Reperfusion-From Mechanism to Translation. Nat Med. 2011;17(11):1391-401.

52. Troppmann C, Gillingham KJ, Gruessner RW, Dunn DL, Payne WD, Najarian JS, et al. Delayed Graft Function in the Absence of Rejection Has No Long-term Impact. A Study of Cadaver Kidney Recipients with Good Graft Function at 1 Year after Transplantation. Transplantation. 1996;61(9):1331-7.

53. Benedetti E, Najarian JS, Gruessner AC, Nakhleh RE, Troppmann C, Hakim NS, et al. Correlation between Cystoscopic Biopsy Results and Hypoamylasuria in Bladder-drained Pancreas Transplants. Surgery. 1995;118(5):864-72.

54. Howard RJ, Pfaff WW, Brunson ME, Scornik JC, Ramos EL, Peterson QS. Increased Incidence of Rejection in Patients with Delayed Graft Function. Clinical Transplantation. 1994;8(6):527-31.

55. Kasiske BL, Gaston RS, Gourishankar S, Halloran PF, Matas AJ, Jeffery J, et al. Long-term Deterioration of Kidney Allograft Function. Am J Transplant. 2005;5(6):1405-14.

56. Cecka JM. The OPTN/UNOS Renal Transplant Registry. Clinical Transplants 2003. Los Angeles: UCLA Immunogenetics Center; 2004. p. 1.

57. Haas M. Subclinical Acute Antibody-mediated Rejection in Positive Crossmatch Renal Allografts. Am J Transplant. 2007;7:576-85.

58. Moreso F, Ibernon M, Goma M, Carrera M, Fulladosa X, Hueso M, et al. Subclinical Rejection Associated with Chronic Allograft Nephropathy in Protocol Biopsies as a Risk Factor for Late Graft Loss. American Journal of Transplantation. 2006;6(4):747-52.

59. Rush D, Winnipeg Transplant G. Insights into Subclinical Rejection. Transplantation Proceedings. 2004;36(2 Suppl):71S-3S.

60. Roberts IS, Reddy S, Russell C, Davies DR, Friend PJ, Handa AI, et al. Subclinical Rejection and Borderline Changes in Early Protocol Biopsy Specimens after Renal Transplantation. Transplantation. 2004;77(8):1194-8.

61. Mihatsch MJ, Nickeleit V, Gudat F. Morphologic Criteria of Chronic Renal Allograft Rejection. Transplantation Proceedings. 1999;31(1-2):1295-7.

62. Wieczorek G, Bigaud M, Menninger K, Riesen S, Quesniaux V, Schuurman HJ, et al. Acute and Chronic Vascular Rejection in Nonhuman Primate Kidney Transplantation. Am J Transplant. 2006;6(6):1285-96.

63. Colvin RB. Kidney. In: Colvin RB, Bhan AK, McCluskey RT, editors. Diagnostic Immunopathology. 2 ed. New York: Raven Press; 1995. p. 329-65.

64. Mauiyyedi S, Colvin RB. Pathology of Kidney Transplantation. In: Morris PJ, editor. Kidney Transplantation. 5th ed. Philadelphia: W. B. Saunders Co.; 2001. p. 243-376.

65. Halloran PF. An Integrated View of Molecular Changes, Histopathology and Outcomes in Kidney Transplants. Am J Transplant. 2010;10:2223-30.

66. Murine OKT4A Immunosuppression in Cadaver Donor Renal Allograft Recipients: A Cooperative Pilot Study (Report 1). Cooperative Clinical Trials in Transplantation (CCTT) Research Group. Transplantation Proceedings. 1995;27(1):863.

67. Solez K, Racusen LC. The BANFF Classification Revisited. Kidney Int. 2013;83(2):201-6.

68. Nankivell BJ, Alexander SI. Rejection of the Kidney Allograft. New England Journal of Medicine. 2010;363(15):1451-62.

69. Wood KJ, Bushell A, Hester J. Regulatory Immune Cells in Transplantation. Nature Reviews Immunology. 2012;12(6):417-30.

70. Hiki Y, Leong AS, Mathew TH, Seymour AE, Pascoe V, Woodroffe AJ. Typing of Intraglomerular Mononuclear Cells Associated with Transplant Glomerular Rejection. Clin Nephrol. 1986;26(5):244-9.

71. Bishop GA, Hall BM, Duggin GG, Horvath JS, Sheil AG, Tiller DJ. Immunopathology of Renal Allograft Rejection Analyzed with Monoclonal Antibodies to Mononuclear Cell Markers. Kidney Int. 1986;29(708):708-17.

72. Zhang PL, Malek SK, Prichard JW, Lin F, Yahya TM, Schwartzman MS, et al. Monocyte-mediated Acute Renal Rejection after Combined Treatment with Preoperative Campath-1H (Alemtuzumab) and Postoperative Immunosuppression. Ann Clin Lab Sci. 2004;34(2):209-13.

73. Hancock WW, Thomson NM, Atkins RC. Composition of Interstitial Cellular Infiltrate Identified by Monoclonal Antibodies in Renal Biopsies of Rejecting Human Renal Allografts. Transplantation. 1983;35(5):458-63.

74. Hancock WW, Atkins RC. Immunohistological Analysis of Sequential Renal Biopsies from Patients with Acute Renal Rejection. J Immunol. 1985;**136**(2416):2416–20.

75. Charney DA, Nadasdy T, Lo AW, Racusen LC. Plasma Cell-rich Acute Renal Allograft Rejection. Transplantation. 1999;**68**(6):791–7.

76. Meehan SM, Domer P, Josephson M, Donoghue M, Sadhu A, Ho LT, et al. The Clinical and Pathologic Implications of Plasmacytic Infiltrates in Percutaneous Renal Allograft Biopsies. Human Pathology. 2001;**32**(2):205–15.

77. Martins HL, Silva C, Martini D, Noronha IL. Detection of B Lymphocytes (CD20+) in Renal Allograft Biopsy Specimens. Transplantation Proceedings. 2007;**39**(2):432–4.

78. Mengel M, Gwinner W, Schwarz A, Bajeski R, Franz I, Brocker V, et al. Infiltrates in Protocol Biopsies from Renal Allografts. Am J Transplant. 2007;**7**(2):356–65.

79. Bagnasco SM, Tsai W, Rahman MH, Kraus ES, Barisoni L, Vega R, et al. CD20-positive Infiltrates in Renal Allograft Biopsies with Acute Cellular Rejection Are Not Associated with Worse Graft Survival. Am J Transplant. 2007;**7**(8):1968–73.

80. Hippen BE, DeMattos A, Cook WJ, Kew CE, 2nd, Gaston RS. Association of CD20+ Infiltrates with Poorer Clinical Outcomes in Acute Cellular Rejection of Renal Allografts. Am J Transplant. 2005;**5**(9):2248–52.

81. Loverre A, Capobianco C, Stallone G, Infante B, Schena A, Ditonno P, et al. Ischemia-Reperfusion Injury-induced Abnormal Dendritic Cell Traffic in the Transplanted Kidney with Delayed Graft Function. Kidney Int. 2007;**72**(8):994–1003.

82. Woltman AM, de Fijter JW, Zuidwijk K, Vlug AG, Bajema IM, van der Kooij SW, et al. Quantification of Dendritic Cell Subsets in Human Renal Tissue under Normal and Pathological Conditions. Kidney Int. 2007;**71**(10):1001–8.

83. Lajoie G, Nadasdy T, Laszik Z, Blick KE, Silva FG. Mast Cells in Acute Cellular Rejection of Human Renal Allografts. Mod Pathol. 1996;**9**(12):1118–25.

84. Gibson IW, Gwinner W, Brocker V, Sis B, Riopel J, Roberts IS, et al. Peritubular Capillaritis in Renal Allografts: Prevalence, Scoring System, Reproducibility and Clinicopathological Correlates. Am J Transplant. 2008.

85. Fahim T, Bohmig GA, Exner M, Huttary N, Kerschner H, Kandutsch S, et al. The Cellular Lesion of Humoral Rejection: Predominant Recruitment of Monocytes to Peritubular and Glomerular Capillaries. Am J Transplant. 2007;**7**(2):385–93.

86. Jurcic V, Jeruc J, Maric S, Ferluga D. Histomorphological Assessment of Phlebitis in Renal Allografts. Croat Med J. 2007;**48**(3):327–32.

87. Torbenson M, Randhawa P. Arcuate and Interlobular Phlebitis in Renal Allografts. Human Pathology. 2001;**32**(12):1388–91.

88. Stuht S, Gwinner W, Franz I, Schwarz A, Jonigk D, Kreipe H, et al. Lymphatic Neoangiogenesis in Human Renal Allografts: Results from Sequential Protocol Biopsies. Am J Transplant. 2007;**7**(2):377–84.

89. Salazar IDR, López MM, Chang J, Halloran PF. Reassessing the Significance of Intimal Arteritis in Kidney Transplant Biopsy Specimens. Journal of the American Society of Nephrology. 2015.

90. Colvin RB. Eye of the Needle. Am J Transplant. 2007;**7**(2):267–8.

91. Solez K, Colvin R, Racusen L, Haas M, Sis B, Mengel M, et al. BANFF 07 Classification of Renal Allograft Pathology: Updates and Future Directions. Am J Transplant. 2008;**8**(4):753–60.

92. Nabokow A, Dobronravov VA, Khrabrova M, Gröne H-J, Gröne E, Hallensleben M, et al. Long-term Kidney Allograft Survival in Patients With Transplant Glomerulitis. Transplantation. 2015;**99**(2):331–9.

93. Desvaux D, Le Gouvello S, Pastural M, Abtahi M, Suberbielle C, Boeri N, et al. Acute Renal Allograft Rejections with Major Interstitial Oedema and Plasma Cell-rich Infiltrates: High Gamma-Interferon Expression and Poor Clinical Outcome. Nephrol Dial Transplant. 2004;**19**(4):933–9.

94. Lobo PI, Spencer CE, Isaacs RB, McCullough C. Hyperacute Renal Allograft Rejection from Anti-HLA Class 1 Antibody to B Cells–Antibody Detection by Two Color FCXM Was Possible Only after Using Pronase-digested Donor Lymphocytes. Transpl Int. 1997;**10**(1):69–73.

95. Racusen LC, Solez K, Colvin RB, Bonsib SM, Castro MC, Cavallo T, et al. The BANFF 97 Working Classification of Renal Allograft Pathology. Kidney Int. 1999;**55**(2):713–23.

96. Haas M. C4d-negative Antibody-mediated Rejection in Renal Allografts: Evidence for Its Existence and Effect on Graft Survival. Clin Nephrol. 2011;**75**(4):271–8.

97. Haas M. An Updated BANFF Schema for Diagnosis of Antibody-mediated Rejection in Renal Allografts. Current Opinion in Organ Transplantation. 2014;**19**(3):315–22.

98. LeBleu VS, Taduri G, O'Connell J, Teng Y, Cooke VG, Woda C, et al. Origin and Function of Myofibroblasts in Kidney Fibrosis. Nat Med. 2013; advance online publication.

99. Pascual J, Pérez-Sáez MJ, Mir M, Crespo M. Chronic Renal Allograft Injury: Early Detection, Accurate Diagnosis and Management. Transplantation Reviews. 2012;**26**(4):280–90.

100. Shimizu A, Yamada K, Sachs DH, Colvin RB. Persistent Rejection of Peritubular Capillaries and Tubules Is Associated with Progressive Interstitial Fibrosis. Kidney Int. 2002;**61**(5):1867–79.

101. Rush D, Nickerson P, Gough J, McKenna R, Grimm P, Cheang M, et al. Beneficial Effects of Treatment of Early Subclinical Rejection: A Randomized Study. J Am Soc Nephrol. 1998;**9**(11):2129–34.

102. Solez K, Colvin RB, Racusen LC, Sis B, Halloran PF, Birk PE, et al. BANFF '05 Meeting Report: Differential Diagnosis of Chronic Allograft Injury and Elimination of Chronic Allograft Nephropathy ('CAN'). Am J Transplant. 2007;**7**(3):518–26.

103. Alpers CE, Gordon D, Gown AM. Immunophenotype of Vascular Rejection in Renal Transplants. Modern Path. 1990;**3**(2):198–203.

104. Nickeleit V, Zeiler M, Gudat F, Thiel G, Mihatsch MJ. Detection of the Complement Degradation Product C4d in Renal Allografts: Diagnostic and Therapeutic Implications. J Am Soc Nephrol. 2002;**13**(1):242–51.

105. Herzenberg AM, Gill JS, Djurdjev O, Magil AB. C4d Deposition in Acute Rejection: An Independent Long-term Prognostic Factor. J Am Soc Nephrol. 2002;**13**(1):234–41.

106. Wang X, Smith KD, Nicosia RF, Alpers CE, Kowalewska J. Associations of C4d Deposition, Transplant Glomerulopathy and Rejection in Renal Allograft Biopsies Performed 10 or More Years after Transplantation. Modern Path. 2008;**21** (supplement 1):296A (abstract).

107 Mauiyyedi S, Pelle PD, Saidman S, Collins AB, Pascual M, Tolkoff-Rubin NE, et al. Chronic Humoral Rejection: Identification of Antibody-mediated Chronic Renal Allograft Rejection by C4d Deposits in Peritubular Capillaries. J Am Soc Nephrol. 2001;12(3):574-82.

108 Collins AB, Schneeberger EE, Pascual MA, Saidman SL, Williams WW, Tolkoff-Rubin N, et al. Complement Activation in Acute Humoral Renal Allograft Rejection: Diagnostic Significance of C4d Deposits in Peritubular Capillaries. J Am Soc Nephrol. 1999;10(10):2208-14.

109 Habib R, Broyer M. Clinical Significance of Allograft Glomerulopathy. Kidney International – Supplement. 1993;43:S95-8.

110 Axelsen RA, Seymour AE, Mathew TH, Canny A, Pascoe V. Glomerular Transplant Rejection: A Distinctive Pattern of Early Graft Damage. Clinical Nephrology. 1985;23(1):1-11.

111 Gloor JM, Sethi S, Stegall MD, Park WD, Moore SB, DeGoey S, et al. Transplant Glomerulopathy: Subclinical Incidence and Association with Alloantibody. Am J Transplant. 2007;7(9):2124-32.

112 Ivanyi B, Kemeny E, Szederkenyi E, Marofka F, Szenohradszky P. The Value of Electron Microscopy in the Diagnosis of Chronic Renal Allograft Rejection. Mod Pathol. 2001;14(12):1200-8.

113 Maryniak RK, First MR, Weiss MA. Transplant Glomerulopathy: Evolution of Morphologically Distinct Changes. Kidney International. 1985;27(5):799-806.

114 Zollinger HU, Mihatsch MJ. Renal Pathology in Biopsy. 1 ed. Berlin, Heidelberg, New York: Springer Verlag; 1978. 684.

115 Drachenberg CB, Steinberger E, Hoehn-Saric E, Heffes A, Klassen DK, Bartlett ST, et al. Specificity of Intertubular Capillary Changes: Comparative Ultrastructural Studies in Renal Allografts and Native Kidneys. Ultrastruct Pathol. 1997;21(3):227-33.

116 Borel JF, Kis ZL. The Discovery and Development of Cyclosporine (Sandimmune). Transplantation Proceedings. 1991;23(2):1867-74.

117 Danovitch GM. Cyclosporin or Tacrolimus: Which Agent to Choose? Nephrol Dial Transplant. 1997;12(8):1566-8.

118 Tanabe K. Calcineurin Inhibitors in Renal Transplantation: What Is the Best Option? Drugs. 2003;63(15):1535-48.

119 Fischer G, Wittmann-Liebold B, Lang K, Kiefhaber T, Schmid FX. Cyclophilin and Peptidyl-Prolyl Cis-Trans Isomerase Are Probably Identical Proteins. Nature. 1989;337(6206):476-8.

120 Takahashi N, Hayano T, Suzuki M. Peptidyl-Prolyl Cis-Trans Isomerase is the Cyclosporin A-binding Protein Cyclophilin. Nature. 1989;337(6206):473-5.

121 Borel JF, Baumann G, Chapman I, Donatsch P, Fahr A, Mueller EA, et al. In Vivo Pharmacological Effects of Ciclosporin and Some Analogues. Advances in Pharmacology. 1996;35:115-246.

122 Kapturczak MH, Meier-Kriesche HU, Kaplan B. Pharmacology of Calcineurin Antagonists. Transplantation Proceedings. 2004;36(2 Suppl):25S-32S.

123 Wiederrecht G, Hung S, Chan HK, Marcy A, Martin M, Calaycay J, et al. Characterization of High Molecular Weight FK-506 Binding Activities Reveals a Novel FK-506-binding Protein as Well as a Protein Complex. J Biol Chem. 1992;267(30):21753-60.

124 Maki N, Sekiguchi F, Nishimaki J, Miwa K, Hayano T, Takahashi N, et al. Complementary DNA Encoding the Human T-cell FK506-binding Protein, a Peptidylprolyl Cis-Trans Isomerase Distinct from Cyclophilin. Proceedings of the National Academy of Sciences of the United States of America. 1990;87(14):5440-3.

125 Dudek RW, Lawrence IE, Jr., Hill RS, Johnson RC. Induction of Islet Cytodifferentiation by Fetal Mesenchyme in Adult Pancreatic Ductal Epithelium. Diabetes. 1991;40(8):1041-8.

126 Wong W, Venetz JP, Tolkoff-Rubin N, Pascual M. Immunosuppressive Strategies in Kidney Transplantation: Which Role for the Calcineurin Inhibitors? Transplantation. 2005;80(3):289-96.

127 Halloran PF. Immunosuppressive Drugs for Kidney Transplantation. The New England Journal of Medicine. 2004;351(26):2715-29.

128 Mihatsch MJ, Theil G, Spichtin HP, Oberholzer M, Brunner FP, Harder F, et al. Morphological Findings in Kidney Transplants after Treatment with Cyclosporine. Transplantation Proc. 1983;15 [Suppl 1]:2821-35.

129 Mihatsch MJ, Ryffel B, Gudat F. The Differential Diagnosis between Rejection and Cyclosporine Toxicity. Kidney International – Supplement. 1995;52:S63-9.

130 Mihatsch MJ, Morozumi K, Strom EH, Ryffel B, Gudat F, Thiel G. Renal Transplant Morphology after Long-term Therapy with Cyclosporine. Transplantation Proceedings. 1995;27(1):39-42.

131 Mihatsch MJ, Gudat F, Ryffel B, Thiel G. Cyclosporine Nephropathy. In: Tisher CC, Brenner BM, editors. Renal Pathology – With Clinical and Functional Correlations. 2nd ed. Philadelphia: J.B. Lippincott; 1994. p. 1641-81.

132 Stratta P, Canavese C, Quaglia M, Balzola F, Bobbio M, Busca A, et al. Posttransplantation Chronic Renal Damage in Nonrenal Transplant Recipients. Kidney Int. 2005;68(4):1453-63.

133 Ojo AO, Held PJ, Port FK, Wolfe RA, Leichtman AB, Young EW, et al. Chronic Renal Failure after Transplantation of a Nonrenal Organ. The New England Journal of Medicine. 2003;349(10):931-40.

134 English RF, Pophal SA, Bacanu SA, Fricker J, Boyle GJ, Ellis D, et al. Long-term Comparison of Tacrolimus- and Cyclosporine-induced Nephrotoxicity in Pediatric Heart-transplant Recipients. Am J Transplant. 2002;2(8):769-73.

135 Mihatsch MJ, Thiel G, Basler V, Ryffel B, Landmann J, von Overbeck J, et al. Morphological Patterns in Cyclosporine-treated Renal Transplant Recipients. Transplantation Proceedings. 1985;17(4 Suppl 1):101-16.

136 Hall BM, Tiller DJ, Duggin GG, Horvath JS, Farnsworth A, May J, et al. Post-transplant Acute Renal Failure in Cadaver Renal Recipients Treated with Cyclosporine. Kidney International. 1985;28(2):178-86.

137 Mihatsch M, Thiel G, Ryffel B. Cyclosporine Nephrotoxicity. Advances in Nephrology. 1988;17:303-20.

138 Tsinalis D, Dickenmann M, Brunner F, Gurke L, Mihatsch M, Nickeleit V. Acute Renal Failure in a Renal Allograft Recipient Treated with Intravenous Immunoglobulin. Am J Kidney Dis. 2002;40(3):667-70.

139 Haas M, Sonnenday CJ, Cicone JS, Rabb H, Montgomery RA. Isometric Tubular Epithelial Vacuolization in

Renal Allograft Biopsy Specimens of Patients Receiving Low-dose Intravenous Immunoglobulin for a Positive Crossmatch. Transplantation. 2004;78(4):549–56.
140. Moreau JF, Droz D, Sabto J, Jungers P, Kleinknecht D, Hinglais N, et al. Osmotic Nephrosis Induced by Water-soluble Triiodinated Contrast Media in Man. A Retrospective Study of 47 Cases. Radiology. 1975;115(2):329–36.
141. Collins BS, Davis CL, Marsh CL, McVicar JP, Perkins JD, Alpers CE. Reversible Cyclosporine Arteriolopathy. Transplantation. 1992;54(4):732–4.
142. Morozumi K, Thiel G, Albert FW, Banfi G, Gudat F, Mihatsch MJ. Studies on Morphological Outcome of Cyclosporine-associated Arteriolopathy after Discontinuation of Cyclosporine in Renal Allografts. Clin Nephrol. 1992;38(1):1–8.
143. Bren A, Pajek J, Grego K, Buturovic J, Ponikvar R, Lindic J, et al. Follow-up of Kidney Graft Recipients with Cyclosporine-associated Hemolytic-Uremic Syndrome and Thrombotic Microangiopathy. Transplantation Proceedings. 2005;37(4):1889–91.
144. Rangel EB, Gonzalez AM, Linhares MM, Araujo SR, Franco MF, de Sa JR, et al. Thrombotic Microangiopathy after Simultaneous Pancreas-Kidney Transplantation. Clin Transplant. 2007;21(2):241–5.
145. Karthikeyan V, Parasuraman R, Shah V, Vera E, Venkat KK. Outcome of Plasma Exchange Therapy in Thrombotic Microangiopathy after Renal Transplantation. Am J Transplant. 2003;3(10):1289–94.
146. Lewis RM, Verani RR, Vo C, Katz SM, Van BCT, Radovancevic B, et al. Evaluation of Chronic Renal Disease in Heart Transplant Recipients: Importance of Pretransplantation Native kidney Histologic Evaluation. Journal of Heart & Lung Transplantation. 1994;13(3):376–80.
147. Josephson MA, Chiu MY, Woodle ES, Thistlethwaite JR, Haas M. Drug-induced Acute Interstitial Nephritis in Renal Allografts: Histopathologic Features and Clinical Course in Six Patients. Am J Kidney Dis. 1999;34(3):540–8.
148. Kormendi F, Amend W. The Importance of Eosinophil Cells in Kidney Allograft Rejection. Transplantation. 1988;45(3):537–9.
149. Weir MR, Hall-Craggs M, Shen SY, Posner JN, Alongi SV, Dagher FJ, et al. The Prognostic Value of the Eosinophil in Acute Renal Allograft Rejection. Transplantation. 1986;41(6):709–12.
150. Hongwei W, Nanra RS, Stein A, Avis L, Price A, Hibberd AD. Eosinophils in Acute Renal Allograft Rejection. Transplant Immunology. 1994;2(1):41–6.
151. Almirall J, Campistol JM, Sole M, Andreu J, Revert L. Blood and Graft Eosinophilia as a Rejection Index in Kidney Transplant. Nephron. 1993;65(2):304–9.
152. Hallgren R, Bohman SO, Fredens K. Activated Eosinophil Infiltration and Deposits of Eosinophil Cationic Protein in Renal Allograft Rejection. Nephron. 1991;59(2):266–70.
153. Ten RM, Gleich GJ, Holley KE, Perkins JD, Torres VE. Eosinophil Granule Major Basic Protein in Acute Renal Allograft Rejection. Transplantation. 1989;47(6):959–63.
154. Colvin RB, Fang LS-T. Interstitial Nephritis. In: Tisher CC, Brenner BM, editors. Renal Pathology. 2nd ed. Philadelphia, PA: JB Lippincott; 1994. p. 723–68.
155. Groth CG, Backman L, Morales JM, Calne R, Kreis H, Lang P, et al. Sirolimus (Rapamycin)-based Therapy in Human Renal Transplantation: Similar Efficacy and Different Toxicity Compared with Cyclosporine. Sirolimus European Renal Transplant Study Group. Transplantation. 1999;67(7):1036–42.
156. Flechner SM, Goldfarb D, Modlin C, Feng J, Krishnamurthi V, Mastroianni B, et al. Kidney Transplantation without Calcineurin Inhibitor Drugs: A Prospective, Randomized Trial of Sirolimus versus Cyclosporine. Transplantation. 2002;74(8):1070–6.
157. Larson TS, Dean PG, Stegall MD, Griffin MD, Textor SC, Schwab TR, et al. Complete Avoidance of Calcineurin Inhibitors in Renal Transplantation: A Randomized Trial Comparing Sirolimus and Tacrolimus. American Journal of Transplantation: Official Journal of the American Society of Transplantation and the American Society of Transplant Surgeons. 2006;6(3):514–22.
158. Kahan BD, Julian BA, Pescovitz MD, Vanrenterghem Y, Neylan J. Sirolimus Reduces the Incidence of Acute Rejection Episodes Despite Lower Cyclosporine Doses in Caucasian Recipients of Mismatched Primary Renal Allografts: A Phase II Trial. Rapamune Study Group. Transplantation. 1999;68(10):1526–32.
159. Kahan BD. Efficacy of Sirolimus Compared with Azathioprine for Reduction of Acute Renal Allograft Rejection: A Randomised Multicentre Study. The Rapamune US Study Group. Lancet. 2000;356(9225):194–202.
160. MacDonald AS. A Worldwide, Phase III, Randomized, Controlled, Safety and Efficacy Study of a Sirolimus/Cyclosporine Regimen for Prevention of Acute Rejection in Recipients of Primary Mismatched Renal Allografts. Transplantation. 2001;71(2):271–80.
161. Vitko S, Margreiter R, Weimar W, Dantal J, Viljoen HG, Li Y, et al. Everolimus (Certican) 12-month Safety and Efficacy versus Mycophenolate Mofetil in de Novo Renal Transplant Recipients. Transplantation. 2004;78(10):1532–40.
162. Lorber MI, Mulgaonkar S, Butt KM, Elkhammas E, Mendez R, Rajagopalan PR, et al. Everolimus versus Mycophenolate Mofetil in the Prevention of Rejection in de Novo Renal Transplant Recipients: A 3-year Randomized, Multicenter, Phase III Study. Transplantation. 2005;80(2):244–52.
163. Kahan BD. Sirolimus: A Comprehensive Review. Expert Opinion on Pharmacotherapy. 2001;2(11):1903–17.
164. Bruns CJ, Koehl GE, Guba M, Yezhelyev M, Steinbauer M, Seeliger H, et al. Rapamycin-induced Endothelial Cell Death and Tumor Vessel Thrombosis Potentiate Cytotoxic Therapy against Pancreatic Cancer. Clin Cancer Res. 2004;10(6):2109–19.
165. Guba M, Yezhelyev M, Eichhorn ME, Schmid G, Ischenko I, Papyan A, et al. Rapamycin Induces Tumor-specific Thrombosis via Tissue Factor in the Presence of VEGF. Blood. 2005;105(11):4463–9.
166. Guba M, von Breitenbuch P, Steinbauer M, Koehl G, Flegel S, Hornung M, et al. Rapamycin Inhibits Primary and Metastatic Tumor Growth by Antiangiogenesis: Involvement of Vascular Endothelial Growth Factor. Nat Med. 2002;8(2):128–35.
167. Kahan BD. Sirolimus. In: Morris PJ, editor. Kidney Transplantation: Principles and Practice. 5th ed.

Philadelphia, London, New York: W.B. Saunders Company; 2001. p. 279–88.

168. Fellstrom B. Cyclosporine Nephrotoxicity. Transplantation Proceedings. 2004;36(2 Suppl):220S–3S.

169. Stallone G, Infante B, Schena A, Battaglia M, Ditonno P, Loverre A, et al. Rapamycin for Treatment of Chronic Allograft Nephropathy in Renal Transplant Patients. J Am Soc Nephrol. 2005;16(12):3755–62.

170. McTaggart RA, Gottlieb D, Brooks J, Bacchetti P, Roberts JP, Tomlanovich S, et al. Sirolimus Prolongs Recovery from Delayed Graft Function after Cadaveric Renal Transplantation. Am J Transplant. 2003;3(4):416–23.

171. Ciancio G, Burke GW, Gaynor JJ, Ruiz P, Roth D, Kupin W, et al. A Randomized Long-term Trial of Tacrolimus/Sirolimus versus Tacrolimums/Mycophenolate versus Cyclosporine/Sirolimus in Renal Transplantation: Three-year Analysis. Transplantation. 2006;81(6):845–52.

172. Buchler M, Caillard S, Barbier S, Thervet E, Toupance O, Mazouz H, et al. Sirolimus versus Cyclosporine in Kidney Recipients Receiving Thymoglobulin, Mycophenolate Mofetil and a 6-month Course of Steroids. American Journal of Transplantation: Official Journal of the American Society of Transplantation and the American Society of Transplant Surgeons. 2007;7(11):2522–31.

173. Stallone G, Schena A, Infante B, Di Paolo S, Loverre A, Maggio G, et al. Sirolimus for Kaposi's Sarcoma in Renal-transplant Recipients. The New England Journal of Medicine. 2005;352(13):1317–23.

174. Campistol JM, Eris J, Oberbauer R, Friend P, Hutchison B, Morales JM, et al. Sirolimus Therapy after Early Cyclosporine Withdrawal Reduces the Risk for Cancer in Adult Renal Transplantation. Journal of the American Society of Nephrology: JASN. 2006;17(2):581–9.

175. Smith KD, Wrenshall LE, Nicosia RF, Pichler R, Marsh CL, Alpers CE, et al. Delayed Graft Function and Cast Nephropathy Associated with Tacrolimus Plus Rapamycin Use. J Am Soc Nephrol. 2003;14(4):1037–45.

176. McTaggart RA, Tomlanovich S, Bostrom A, Roberts JP, Feng S. Comparison of Outcomes after Delayed Graft Function: Sirolimus-based versus Other Calcineurin-inhibitor Sparing Induction Immunosuppression Regimens. Transplantation. 2004;78(3):475–80.

177. McTaggart RA, Gottlieb D, Brooks J, Bacchetti P, Roberts JP, Tomlanovich S, et al. Sirolimus Prolongs Recovery from Delayed Graft Function after Cadaveric Renal Transplantation. Am J Transplant. 2003;3(4):416–23.

178. Boratynska M, Banasik M, Patrzalek D, Szyber P, Klinger M. Sirolimus Delays Recovery from Posttransplant Renal Failure in Kidney Graft Recipients. Transplantation Proceedings. 2005;37(2):839–42.

179. Reynolds JC, Agodoa LY, Yuan CM, Abbott KC. Thrombotic Microangiopathy after Renal Transplantation in the United States. Am J Kidney Dis. 2003;42(5):1058–68.

180. Hardinger KL, Cornelius LA, Trulock EP, 3rd, Brennan DC. Sirolimus-induced Leukocytoclastic Vasculitis. Transplantation. 2002;74(5):739–43.

181. Pasqualotto AC, Bianco PD, Sukiennik TC, Furian R, Garcia VD. Sirolimus-induced Leukocytoclastic Vasculitis: The Second Case Reported. Am J Transplant. 2004;4(9):1549–51.

182. Sartelet H, Toupance O, Lorenzato M, Fadel F, Noel LH, Lagonotte E, et al. Sirolimus-induced Thrombotic Microangiopathy Is Associated with Decreased Expression of Vascular Endothelial Growth Factor in Kidneys. Am J Transplant. 2005;5(10):2441–7.

183. Novick AC, Hwei HH, Steinmuller D, Streem SB, Cunningham RJ, Steinhilber D, et al. Detrimental Effect of Cyclosporine on Initial Function of Cadaver Renal Allografts Following Extended Preservation. Results of a Randomized Prospective Study. Transplantation. 1986;42(2):154–8.

184. van den Akker JM, Wetzels JF, Hoitsma AJ. Proteinuria Following Conversion from Azathioprine to Sirolimus in Renal Transplant Recipients. Kidney Int. 2006;70(7):1355–7.

185. Letavernier E, Bruneval P, Mandet C, Van Huyen JP, Peraldi MN, Helal I, et al. High Sirolimus Levels May Induce Focal Segmental Glomerulosclerosis de Novo. Clin J Am Soc Nephrol. 2007;2(2):326–33.

186. Letavernier E, Pe'raldi MN, Pariente A, Morelon E, Legendre C. Proteinuria Following a Switch from Calcineurin Inhibitors to Sirolimus. Transplantation. 2005;80(9):1198–203.

187. Merkel S, Mogilevskaja N, Mengel M, Haller H, Schwarz A. Side Effects of Sirolimus. Transplantation Proceedings. 2006;38(3):714–5.

188. Mackenzie EF, Poulding JM, Harrison PR, Amer B. Human Polyoma Virus (HPV)–A Significant Pathogen in Renal Transplantation. Proc Eur Dial Transplant Assoc. 1978;15:352–60.

189. Binet I, Nickeleit V, Hirsch HH, Prince O, Dalquen P, Gudat F, et al. Polyomavirus Disease under New Immunosuppressive Drugs: A Cause of Renal Graft Dysfunction and Graft Loss. Transplantation. 1999;67(6):918–22.

190. Drachenberg CB, Beskow CO, Cangro CB, Bourquin PM, Simsir A, Fink J, et al. Human Polyoma Virus in Renal Allograft Biopsies: Morphological Findings and Correlation with Urine Cytology. Human Pathology. 1999;30(8):970–7.

191. Nickeleit V, Hirsch HH, Zeiler M, Gudat F, Prince O, Thiel G, et al. BK-virus Nephropathy in Renal Transplants-tubular Necrosis, MHC-class II Expression and Rejection in a Puzzling Game. Nephrol Dial Transplant. 2000;15(3):324–32.

192. Randhawa PS, Finkelstein S, Scantlebury V, Shapiro R, Vivas C, Jordan M, et al. Human Polyoma Virus-associated Interstitial Nephritis in the Allograft Kidney. Transplantation. 1999;67(1):103–9.

193. Howell DN, Smith SR, Butterly DW, Klassen PS, Krigman HR, Burchette JL, Jr., et al. Diagnosis and Management of BK Polyomavirus Interstitial Nephritis in Renal Transplant Recipients. Transplantation. 1999;68(9):1279–88.

194. Cosio FG, Amer H, Grande JP, Larson TS, Stegall MD, Griffin MD. Comparison of Low versus High Tacrolimus Levels in Kidney Transplantation: Assessment of Efficacy by Protocol Biopsies. Transplantation. 2007;83(4):411–6.

195. Mengel M, Bogers JP, Bosmans JL, Seron D, Gwinner W, Haller H. Incidence of C4d Staining and Morphology of Acute Humoral Rejection in Protocol Biopsies of Renal Allografts: A Multicenter Study. Journal of the American Society of Nephrology. 2003;14:11A.

196. Nickeleit V, Singh HK, Mihatsch MJ. Polyomavirus Nephropathy: Morphology, Pathophysiology, and Clinical Management. Curr Opin Nephrol Hypertens. 2003;12:599–605.

197. Khamash HA, Wadei HM, Mahale AS, Larson TS, Stegall MD, Cosio FG, et al. Polyomavirus-associated Nephropathy

198. Ramos E, Drachenberg C, Hirsch HH, Munivenkatappa R, Papadimitriou J, Nogueira J, et al. BK Polyomavirus Allograft Nephropathy (BKPVN): Eight-fold Decrease in Graft Loss with Prospective Screening and Protocol Biopsy. Am J Transplant (supplement). 2006;WTC 2006 congress abstracts:121.

199. Gaber LW, Egidi MF, Stratta RJ, Lo A, Moore LW, Gaber AO. Clinical Utility of Histological Features of Polyomavirus Allograft Nephropathy. Transplantation. 2006;82(2):196–204.

200. Nickeleit V, Mihatsch MJ. Polyomavirus Nephropathy in Native Kidneys and Renal Allografts: An Update on an Escalating Threat. Transpl Int. 2006;19(12):960–73.

201. Sachdeva MS, Nada R, Jha V, Sakhuja V, Joshi K. The High Incidence of BK Polyoma Virus Infection among Renal Transplant Recipients in India. Transplantation. 2004;77(3):429–31.

202. Nada R, Sachdeva MU, Sud K, Jha V, Joshi K. Co-infection by Cytomegalovirus and BK Polyoma Virus in Renal Allograft, Mimicking Acute Rejection. Nephrol Dial Transplant. 2005;20(5):994–6.

203. Mindlova M, Boucek P, Saudek F, Jedinakova T, Voska L, Honsova E, et al. Kidney Retransplantation Following Graft Loss to Polyoma Virus-associated Nephropathy: An Effective Treatment Option in Simultaneous Pancreas and Kidney Transplant Recipients. Transpl Int. 2008;21(4):353–6.

204. Nickeleit V, Gordon J, Thompson D, Romeo C. Antibody Titers and Latent Polyoma-BK-Virus (BKV) Loads in the General Population: Potential Donor Risk Assessment for the Development of BK-Virus Nephropathy (BKN) Post Transplantation. J Am Soc Nephrol (abstracts issue). 2004;15:524A

205. Hirsch HH, Knowles W, Dickenmann M, Passweg J, Klimkait T, Mihatsch MJ, et al. Prospective Study of Polyomavirus Type BK Replication and Nephropathy in Renal-transplant Recipients. The New England Journal of Medicine. 2002;347(7):488–96.

206. Nickeleit V, Hirsch HH, Binet IF, Gudat F, Prince O, Dalquen P, et al. Polyomavirus Infection of Renal Allograft Recipients: From Latent Infection to Manifest Disease. J Am Soc Nephrol. 1999;10(5):1080–9.

207. Nickeleit V, Klimkait T, Binet IF, Dalquen P, DelZenero V, Thiel G, et al. Testing for Polyomavirus Type BK DNA in Plasma to Identify Renal Allograft Recipients with Viral Nephropathy. The New England Journal of Medicine. 2000;342(18):1309–15.

208. Nickeleit V, Steiger J, MJ M. BK Virus Infection after Kidney Transplantation. Graft. 2002;5(December suppl):S46–S57.

209. Singh HK, Bubendorf L, Mihatsch MJ, Drachenberg CB, Nickeleit V. Urine Cytology Findings of Polyomavirus Infections. In: Ahsan N, editor. Polyomaviruses and Human Diseases. Advances in Experimental Medicine and Biology, vol. 577. 1st ed. New York, N.Y. Georgetown,TX.: Springer Science+Business Media, Landes Bioscience / Eurekah.com; 2006. p. 201–12.

210. Singh HK, Madden V, Shen YJ, Thompson D, Nickeleit V. Negative Staining Electron Microscopy of Urine for the Detection of Polyomavirus Infections. Ultrastruct Pathol. 2006:(in press).

211. Drachenberg CB, Papadimitriou JC, Hirsch HH, Wali R, Crowder C, Nogueira J, et al. Histological Patterns of Polyomavirus Nephropathy: Correlation with Graft Outcome and Viral Load. Am J Transplant. 2004;4(12):2082–92.

212. Drachenberg CB, Hirsch HH, Papadimitriou JC, Gosert R, Wali RK, Munivenkatappa R, et al. Polyomavirus BK versus JC Replication and Nephropathy in Renal Transplant Recipients: A Prospective Evaluation. Transplantation. 2007;84(3):323–30.

213. Nickeleit V, Hirsch HH, Binet IF, Gudat F, Prince O, Dalquen P, et al. Polyomavirus Infection of Renal Allograft Recipients: From Latent Infection to Manifest Disease. Journal of the American Society of Nephrology. 1999;10(5):1080–9.

214. Nickeleit V, Steiger J, Mihatsch MJ. BK Virus Infection after Kidney Transplantation. Graft. 2002;5(December suppl):S46–S57.

215. Nickeleit V, Hirsch HH, Zeiler M, Gudat F, Prince O, Thiel G, et al. BK-virus Nephropathy in Renal Transplants-tubular Necrosis, MHC-class II Expression and Rejection in a Puzzling game. Nephrology, Dialysis, Transplantation. 2000;15(3):324–32.

216. Singh D, Kiberd B, Gupta R, Alkhudair W, Lawen J. Polyoma Virus-induced Hemorrhagic Cystitis in Renal Transplantation Patient with Polyoma Virus Nephropathy. Urology. 2006;67(2):423 e11–e12.

217. Celik B, Randhawa PS. Glomerular Changes in BK Virus Nephropathy. Human Pathology. 2004;35(3):367–70.

218. Nair R, Katz DA, Thomas CP. Diffuse Glomerular Crescents and Peritubular Immune Deposits in a Transplant Kidney. Am J Kidney Dis. 2006;48(1):174–8.

219. Nickeleit V, Thompson B, Latour M, Chan G, Shingh HK. Tubulo-centric Granulomatous Interstitial Nephritis in Renal Allograft Recipients with Polyomavirus Nephropathy. Lab Invest. 2007;87 (suppl 1):274A (abstract).

220. Bracamonte ER, Furmanczyk PS, Smith KD, Nicosia RF, Alpers CE, Kowalewska J. Tubular Basement Membrane Immune Deposits Associated with Polyoma Virus Nephropathy in Renal Allografts. Lab Invest. 2006;86 (suppl 1):259A (abstract).

221. Randhawa PS, Vats A, Zygmunt D, Swalsky P, Scantlebury V, Shapiro R, et al. Quantitation of Viral DNA in Renal Allograft Tissue from Patients with BK Virus Nephropathy. Transplantation. 2002;74(4):485–8.

222. Schmid H, Burg M, Kretzler M, Banas B, Grone HJ, Kliem V. BK Virus Associated Nephropathy in Native Kidneys of a Heart Allograft Recipient. Am J Transplant. 2005;5(6):1562–8.

223. Schmid H, Nitschko H, Gerth J, Kliem V, Henger A, Cohen CD, et al. Polyomavirus DNA and RNA Detection in Renal Allograft Biopsies: Results from a European Multicenter Study. Transplantation. 2005;80(5):600–4.

224. Nickeleit V, Singh HK, Gilliland MGF, Thompson D, Romeo C. Latent Polyomavirus Type BK Loads in Native Kidneys Analyzed by TaqMan PCR: What Can Be Learned to Better Understand BK Virus Nephropathy? (abstract). Journal of the American Society of Nephrology. 2003;14:424A.

225. Boldorini R, Veggiani C, Barco D, Monga G. Kidney and Urinary Tract Polyomavirus Infection and

225. Distribution: Molecular Biology Investigation of 10 Consecutive Autopsies. Arch Pathol Lab Med. 2005;**129**(1):69–73.
226. Randhawa P, Shapiro R, Vats A. Quantitation of DNA of Polyomaviruses BK and JC in Human Kidneys. J Infect Dis. 2005;**192**(3):504–9.
227. Chesters PM, Heritage J, McCance DJ. Persistence of DNA Sequences of BK Virus and JC Virus in Normal Human Tissues and in Diseased Tissues. J Infect Dis. 1983;**147**(4):676–84.
228. Limaye AP, Smith KD, Cook L, Groom DA, Hunt NC, Jerome KR, et al. Polyomavirus Nephropathy in Native Kidneys of Non-renal Transplant Recipients. Am J Transplant. 2005;**5**(3):614–20.
229. Bracamonte E, Leca N, Smith KD, Nicosia RF, Nickeleit V, Kendrick E, et al. Tubular Basement Membrane Immune Deposits in Association with BK Polyomavirus Nephropathy. Am J Transplant. 2007:(in press).
230. Colvin RB, Nickeleit V. Renal Transplant Pathology. In: Jennette JC, Olson JL, Schwartz MM, Silva FG, editors. Pathology of the Kidney. 2. 6 ed. Philadelphia, Baltimore, New York, London: Lippincott Williams & Wilkins; 2007. p. 1347–490.
231. Nickeleit V, Mihatsch MJ. Polyomavirus Nephropathy: Pathogenesis, Morphological and Clinical Aspects. In: Kreipe HH, editor. Verh Dtsch Ges Pathol, 88 Tagung. Muenchen, Jena: Urban & Fischer; 2004. p. 69–84.
232. Hirsch HH, Brennan DC, Drachenberg CB, Ginevri F, Gordon J, Limaye AP, et al. Polyomavirus-associated Nephropathy in Renal Transplantation: Interdisciplinary Analyses and Recommendations. Transplantation. 2005;**79**(10):1277–86.
233. Drachenberg RC, Drachenberg CB, Papadimitriou JC, Ramos E, Fink JC, Wali R, et al. Morphological Spectrum of Polyoma Virus Disease in Renal Allografts: Diagnostic Accuracy of Urine Cytology. Am J Transplant. 2001;**1**(4):373–81.
234. van Gorder MA, Della Pelle P, Henson JW, Sachs DH, Cosimi AB, Colvin RB. Cynomolgus Polyoma Virus Infection: A New Member of the Polyoma Virus Family Causes Interstitial Nephritis, Ureteritis, and Enteritis in Immunosuppressed Cynomolgus Monkeys. Am J Pathol. 1999;**154**(4):1273–84.
235. Rubin RH, Colvin RB. Impact of Cytomegalovirus Infection on Renal Transplantation. In: L.C. R, Solez K, Burdick JF, editors. Kidney Transplant Rejection: Diagnosis and Treatment. 3rd ed. NY: Marcel Dekker; 1998. p. 605–25.
236. Battegay EJ, Mihatsch MJ, Mazzucchelli L, Zollinger HU, Gudat F, Thiel G, et al. Cytomegalovirus and Kidney. Clinical Nephrology. 1988;**30**(5):239–47.
237. Joshi K, Nada R, Radotra BD, Jha V, Sakhuja V. Pathological Spectrum of Cytomegalovirus Infection of Renal Allograft Recipients – An Autopsy Study from North India. Indian J Pathol Microbiol. 2004;**47**(3):327–32.
238. Cozzutto C, Felici N. Unusual Glomerular Change in Cytomegalic Inclusion Disease. Virchows Arch A Pathol Anat and Histol. 1974;**364**:365–9.
239. Beneck D, Greco MA, Feiner HD. Glomerulonephritis in Congenital Cytomegalic Inclusion Disease. Human Pathol. 1986;**17**:1054–9.
240. Onuigbo M, Haririan A, Ramos E, Klassen D, Wali R, Drachenberg C. Cytomegalovirus-induced Glomerular Vasculopathy in Renal Allografts: A Report of Two Cases. Am J Transplant. 2002;**2**(7):684–8.
241. Detwiler RK, Singh HK, Bolin P, Jr., Jennette JC. Cytomegalovirus-induced Necrotizing and Crescentic Glomerulonephritis in a Renal Transplant Patient. 1998;32(5):820–4.
242. Kadereit S, Michelson S, Mougeno tB, Thibault P, Verroust PJ, Mignon F, et al. Polymerase Chain Reaction Detection of Cytomegalovirus Genome in Renal Biopsies. Kidney International. 1992;**42**:1012–6.
243. Liapis H, Storch GA, Hill DA, Rueda J, Brennan DC. CMV Infection of the Renal Allograft Is Much More Common Than the Pathology Indicates: A Tetrospective Analysis of Qualitative and Quantitative Buffy Coat CMV-PCR, Renal Biopsy Pathology and Tissue CMV-PCR. Nephrol Dial Transplant. 2003;**18**(2):397–402.
244. Richardson WP, Colvin RB, Cheeseman SH, Tolkoff-Rubin NE, Herrin JT, Cosimi AB, et al. Glomerulopathy Associated with Cytomegalovirus Viremia in Renal Allografts. New Engl J Med. 1981;**305**(2):57–63.
245. Streblow DN, Orloff SL, Nelson JA. Acceleration of Allograft Failure by Cytomegalovirus. Current Opinion in Immunology. 2007;**19**(5):577–82.
246. Fateh-Moghadam S, Bocksch W, Wessely R, Jager G, Hetzer R, Gawaz M. Cytomegalovirus Infection Status Predicts Progression of Heart-transplant Vasculopathy. Transplantation. 2003;**76**(10):1470–4.
247. Reinke P, Fietze E, Ode-Hakim S, Prosch S, Lippert J, Ewert R, et al. Late-acute Renal Allograft Rejection and Symptomless Cytomegalovirus Infection. Lancet. 1994;**344**(8939-8940):1737–8.
248. Emovon OE, Chavin J, Rogers K, Self S. Adenovirus in Kidney Transplantation: An Emerging Pathogen? Transplantation. 2004;**77**(9):1474–5.
249. Asim M, Chong-Lopez A, Nickeleit V. Adenovirus Infection of a Renal Allograft. Am J Kidney Dis. 2003;**41**(3):696–701.
250. Nickeleit V. Critical Commentary To: Acute Adenoviral Infection of a Graft by Serotype 35 Following Renal Transplantation. Pathol Res Pract. 2003;**199**:701–2.
251. Singh HK, Nickeleit V. Kidney Disease Caused by Viral Infections. Curr Diag Pathol. 2004;**10**:11–21.
252. Ito M, Hirabayashi N, Uno Y, Nakayama A, Asai J. Necrotizing Tubulointerstitial Nephritis Associated with Adenovirus Infection. Human Pathology. 1991;**22**(12):1225–31.
253. Bruno B, Zager RA, Boeckh MJ, Gooley TA, Myerson DH, Huang ML, et al. Adenovirus Nephritis in Hematopoietic Stem-cell Transplantation. Transplantation. 2004;**77**(7):1049–57.
254. Mazoyer E, Daugas E, Verine J, Pillebout E, Mourad N, Molina JM, et al. A Case Report of Adenovirus-related Acute Interstitial Nephritis in a Patient with AIDS. Am J Kidney Dis. 2008;**51**(1):121–6.
255. Mathur SC, Squiers EC, Tatum AH, Szmalc FS, Daucher JW, Welker DM, et al. Adenovirus Infection of the Renal Allograft with Sparing of Pancreas Graft Function in the Recipient of a Combined Kidney-Pancreas Transplant. Transplantation. 1998;**65**(1):138–41.
256. Friedrichs N, Eis-Hubinger AM, Heim A, Platen E, Zhou H, Buettner R. Acute Adenoviral Infection of a Graft by Serotype 35 Following Renal

257 Seidemann K, Heim A, Pfister ED, Koditz H, Beilken A, Sander A, et al. Monitoring of Adenovirus Infection in Pediatric Transplant Recipients by Quantitative PCR: Report of Six Cases and Review of the Literature. Am J Transplant. 2004;**4**(12):2102–8.

258 Lion T, Baumgartinger R, Watzinger F, Matthes-Martin S, Suda M, Preuner S, et al. Molecular Monitoring of Adenovirus in Peripheral Blood after Allogeneic Bone Marrow Transplantation Permits Early Diagnosis of Disseminated Disease. Blood. 2003;**102**(3):1114–20.

259 Myerowitz RL, Stalder H, Oxman MN, Levin MJ, Moore M, Leith JD, et al. Fatal Disseminated Adenovirus Infection in a Renal Transplant Recipient. Am J Med. 1975;**59**(4):591–8.

260 Harris NL, Swerdlow SH, Frizzera G, Knowles DM. Post-transplant Lymphoproliferative Disorders. In: Jaffe ES, Harris NL, Stein H, Vardiman JW, editors. Pathology and Genetics of Tumours of Haematopoietic and Lymphoid Tissues World Health Organization Classification of Tumours. Lyon: IARC Press; 2001. p. 264–9.

261 de Silva LM, Bale P, de Courcy J, Brown D, Knowles W. Renal Failure due to BK Virus Infection in an Immunodeficient Child. J Med Virol. 1995;**45**(2):192–6.

262 Mueller-Hermelink HK, Ott G, Kneitz B, Ruediger T. The Spectrum of Lymphoproliferations and Malignant Lymphoma after Organ Transplantation. In: Kreipe HH, editor. Verhandlungen der Deutschen Gesellschaft fuer Pathologie, 88 Tagung. 1. Muenchen, Jena: Urban &Fischer; 2004. p. 63–8.

263 Frank D, Cesarman E, Liu Yf, Michler RE, Knowles DM. Posttransplantation Lymphoproliferative Disorders Frequently Contain Type A and Not Type B Epstein-Barr Virus. Blood. 1995;**85**:1396–403.

264 Lager DJ, Burgart LJ, Slagel DD. Epstein-Barr Virus Detection in Sequential Biopsies from Patients with a Posttransplant Lymphoproliferative Disorder. Mod Pathol. 1993;**6**(1):42–7.

265 Ferry JA, Harris NL. Pathology of Posttransplant Lymphoproliferative Disorders. In: Solez K, Racussen LC, Billingham ME, editors. Solid Organ Transplant Rejection. New York: Marcel Dekker; 1996. p. 277–98.

266 Penn I. The Changing Pattern of Posttransplant Malignancies. Transplantation Proceedings. 1991;**23**:1101–3.

267 Capello D, Rossi D, Gaidano G. Post-transplant Lymphoproliferative Disorders: Molecular Basis of Disease Histogenesis and Pathogenesis. Hematological Oncology. 2005;**23**(2):61–7.

268 Caillard S, Dharnidharka V, Agodoa L, Bohen E, Abbott K. Posttransplant Lymphoproliferative Disorders after Renal Transplantation in the United States in Era of Modern Immunosuppression. Transplantation. 2005;**80**(9):1233–43.

269 Shapiro R, Nalesnik M, McCauley J, Fedorek S, Jordan ML, Scantlebury VP, et al. Posttransplant Lymphoproliferative Disorders in Adult and Pediatric Renal Transplant Patients Receiving Tacrolimus-based Immunosuppression. Transplantation. 1999;**68**(12):1851–4.

270 Koike J, Yamaguchi Y, Hoshikawa M, Takahashi H, Horita S, Tanabe K, et al. Post-Transplant Lymphoproliferative Disorders in Kidney Transplantation: Histological and Molecular Genetic Assessment. Clin Transplant. 2002;**16** Suppl 8:12–7.

271 Randhawa PS, Magnone M, Jordan M, Shapiro R, Demetris AJ, Nalesnik M. Renal Allograft Involvement by Epstein-Barr Virus Associated Post-transplant Lymphoproliferative Disease. American Journal of Surgical Pathology. 1996;**20**(5):563–71.

272 Cockfield SM, Preiksaitis JK, Jewell LD, Parfrey NA. Post-transplant Lymphoproliferative Disorder in Renal Allograft Recipients. Clinical Experience and Risk Factor Analysis in a Single Center. Transplantation. 1993;**56**(1):88–96.

273 Citterio F, Lauriola L, Nanni G, Vecchio FM, Magalini SC, Castagneto M. Polyclonal Lymphoma Confined to Renal Allograft: Case Report. Transplantation Proceedings. 1987;**19**(5):3732–4.

274 Jones C, Bleau B, Buskard N, Magil A, Yeung K, Shackleton C, et al. Simultaneous Development of Diffuse Immunoblastic Lymphoma in Recipients of Renal Transplants from a Single Cadaver Donor: Transmission of Epstein-Barr Virus and Triggering by OKT3. American Journal of Kidney Diseases. 1994;**23**(1):130–4.

275 Denning DW, Weiss LM, Martinez K, Flechner SM. Transmission of Epstein-Barr Virus by a Transplanted Kidney, with Activation by OKT3 Antibody. Transplantation. 1989;**48**:141–4.

276 Nádasdy T, Park CS, Peiper SC, Wenzl JE, Oates J, Silva FG. Epstein-Barr Virus Infection-associated Renal Disease: Diagnostic Use of Molecular Hybridization Technology in Patients with Negative Serology. Journal of the American Society of Nephrology. 1992;**2**(12):1734–42.

277 Weissman DJ, Ferry JA, Harris NL, Louis DN, Delmonico F, Spiro I. Posttransplant Lymphoproliferative Disorders in Solid Organ Recipients Are Predominately Aggressive Tumors of Host Origin. Am J Clin Pathol. 1995;**103**:748–55.

278 Delecluse H-J, Kremmer E, Rouault J-P, Cour C, Bornkamm G, Berger F. The Expression of Epstein-Barr Virus Latent Proteins Is Related to the Pathological Features of Post-transplant Lymphoproliferative Disorders. Am J Pathol. 1995;**146**:1113–20.

279 Thomas JA, Hotchin NA, Allday MJ, Amolot P, Rose M, Yacoub M, et al. Immunohistology of Epstein-Barr Virus-associated Antigens in B Cell Disorders from Immunocompromised Individuals. Transplantation. 1990;**49**:944–533.

280 Renoult E, Aymard B, Gregoire MJ, Bellou A, Hubert J, Hestin D, et al. Epstein-Barr Virus Lymphoproliferative Disease of Donor Origin after Kidney Transplantation: A Case Report. American Journal of Kidney Diseases. 1995;**26**(1):84–7.

281 Hjelle B, Evans HM, Yen TS, Garovoy M, Guis M, Edman JC. A Poorly Differentiated Lymphoma of Donor Origin in a Renal Allograft Recipient. Transplantation. 1989;**47**(6):945–8.

282 Ulrich W, Chott A, Watschinger B, Reiter C, Kovarik J, Radaszkiewicz T. Primary Peripheral T Cell Lymphoma in a Kidney Transplant under Immunosuppression with Cyclosporine A. Human Pathology. 1989;**20**(10):1027–30.

283 Meduri G, Fromentin L, Vieillefond A, Fries D. Donor-related Non-Hodgkin's Lymphoma in a Renal Allograft Recipient. Transplantation Proceedings. 1991;**23**(5):2649–50.

284 Sprangers B, Kuypers DR. Recurrence of Glomerulonephritis after Renal

Transplantation. Pathol Res Pract. 2003;**199**(8):565–70.

285. Marinaki S, Lionaki S, Boletis JN. Glomerular Disease Recurrence in the Renal Allograft: A Hurdle but Not a Barrier for Successful Kidney Transplantation. Transplantation Proceedings. 2013;45(1):3–9.

286. Ulinski T. Recurrence of Focal Segmental Glomerulosclerosis after Kidney Transplantation: Strategies and Outcome. Curr Opin Organ Transplant. 2010;15(5):628–32.

287. Ponticelli C, Moroni G, Glassock RJ. Recurrence of Secondary Glomerular Disease after Renal Transplantation. Clin J Am Soc Nephrol. 2011;6(5):1214–21.

288. van der Boog PJ, de Fijter JW, Bruijn JA, van Es LA. Recurrence of IgA Nephropathy after Renal Transplantation. Annales de medecine interne. 1999;150(2):137–42.

289. Jeong HJ, Huh KH, Kim YS, Kim SI. IgA Nephropathy in Renal Allografts-recurrence and Graft Dysfunction. Yonsei Med J. 2004;45(6):1043–8.

290. D'Agati V. Pathologic Classification of Focal Segmental Glomerulosclerosis. Semin Nephrol. 2003;23(2):117–34.

291. D'Agati VD, Alster JM, Jennette JC, Thomas DB, Pullman J, Savino DA, et al. Association of Histologic Variants in FSGS Clinical Trial with Presenting Features and Outcomes. Clin J Am Soc Nephrol. 2013;8(3):399–406.

292. Letavernier E, Bruneval P, Mandet C, Van Huyen J-PD, Péraldi M-N, Helal I, et al. High Sirolimus Levels May Induce Focal Segmental Glomerulosclerosis De Novo. Clinical Journal of the American Society of Nephrology. 2007;2(2):326–33.

293. Leca N. Focal Segmental Glomerulosclerosis Recurrence in the Renal Allograft. Adv Chronic Kidney Dis. 2014;21(5):448–52.

294. Green H, Rahamimov R, Rozen-Zvi B, Pertzov B, Tobar A, Lichtenberg S, et al. Recurrent Membranoproliferative Glomerulonephritis Type I After Kidney Transplantation: A 17-Year Single-center Experience. Transplantation. 2014.

295. McCaughan JA, O'Rourke DM, Courtney AE. Recurrent Dense Deposit Disease after Renal Transplantation: An Emerging Role for Complementary Therapies. Am J Transplant. 2012;12(4):1046–51.

296. Moroni G, Casati C, Quaglini S, Gallelli B, Banfi G, Montagnino G, et al. Membranoproliferative Glomerulonephritis Type I in Renal Transplantation Patients: A Single-center Study of a Cohort of 68 Renal Transplants Followed up for 11 Years. Transplantation. 2011;91(11):1233–9.

297. Lorenz EC, Sethi S, Leung N, Dispenzieri A, Fervenza FC, Cosio FG. Recurrent Membranoproliferative Glomerulonephritis after Kidney Transplantation. Kidney Int. 2010;77(8):721–8.

298. Ponticelli C, Glassock RJ. Posttransplant Recurrence of Primary Glomerulonephritis. Clin J Am Soc Nephrol. 2010;5(12):2363–72.

299. Canaud G, Audard V, Kofman T, Lang P, Legendre C, Grimbert P. Recurrence from Primary and Secondary Glomerulopathy after Renal Transplant. Transpl Int. 2012;25(8):812–24.

300. Najafian B, Alpers CE, Fogo AB. Pathology of Human Diabetic Nephropathy. Contrib Nephrol. 2011;170:36–47.

301. Tervaert TW, Mooyaart AL, Amann K, Cohen AH, Cook HT, Drachenberg CB, et al. Pathologic Classification of Diabetic Nephropathy. J Am Soc Nephrol. 2010;21(4):556–63.

302. Norby GE, Strom EH, Midtvedt K, Hartmann A, Gilboe IM, Leivestad T, et al. Recurrent Lupus Nephritis after Kidney Transplantation: A Surveillance Biopsy Study. Ann Rheum Dis. 2010;69(8):1484–7.

303. Weng F, Goral S. Recurrence of Lupus Nephritis after Renal Transplantation: If We Look for It, Will We Find It? Nat Clin Pract Neph. 2005;1(2):62–3.

304. Zarifian A, Meleg-Smith S, O'Donovan R, Tesi RJ, Batuman V. Cyclosporine-associated Thrombotic Microangiopathy in Renal Allografts. Kidney Int. 1999;55(6):2457–66.

305. Barbour TD, Crosthwaite A, Chow K, Finlay MJ, Better N, Hughes PD, et al. Antiphospholipid Syndrome in Renal Transplantation. Nephrology (Carlton, Vic). 2014;19(4):177–85.

306. Salameh H, Abu Omar M, Alhariri A, Kisra S, Qasem A, Bin Abdulhak A. Adult Post-kidney Transplant Familial Atypical Hemolytic Uremic Syndrome Successfully Treated with Eculizumab: A Case Report and Literature Review. American Journal of Therapeutics. 2014.

307. Chua S, Wong G, Lim WH. The Importance of Genetic Mutation Screening to Determine Retransplantation Following Failed Kidney Allograft from Recurrent Atypical Haemolytic Ureamic Syndrome. BMJ Case Reports. 2014.

308. Ruggenenti P. Post-transplant Hemolytic-uremic Syndrome. Kidney Int. 2002;62(3):1093–104.

309. Hruskova Z, Geetha D, Tesar V. Renal Transplantation in Anti-neutrophil Cytoplasmic Antibody-associated Vasculitis. Nephrol Dial Transplant. 2014.

310. Berre LL, Dufay A, Cantarovich D, Meurette A, Audrain M, Giral M, et al. Early and Irreversible Recurrence MPO-ANCA-positive Glomerulonephritis after Renal Transplantation. Clin Nephrol. 2014.

311. Kowalewska J. Pathology of Recurrent Diseases in Kidney Allografts: Membranous Nephropathy and Focal Segmental Glomerulosclerosis. Curr Opin Organ Transplant. 2013;18(3):313–8.

Chapter 3: Histopathology of Liver Transplantation

Heather L. Stevenson, Marta I. Minervini, Michael A. Nalesnik, Parmjeet S. Randhawa, Eizaburo Sasatomi, and A. J. Demetris

List of Abbreviations: ADV: adenovirus; AIH: autoimmune hepatitis; ALD: Alcoholic liver disease; AMR: antibody-mediated rejection; AMA: Antimitochondrial antibodies; AS: anastomotic biliary structures; ASH: alcoholic steatohepatitis; BEC: biliary epithelial cells; BSEP: bile salt export pump; CIT: Cold ischemia time; CMV: cytomegalovirus; DBD: donation after brain death; DCD: donated after cardiac death; DILI: drug-induced liver injury; DSA: Donor specific antibodies; EBV: Epstein-Barr virus; ECD: extended criteria donor; FCH: fibrosing cholestatic hepatitis; FFPE: formalin-fixed paraffin-embedded; HAT: Hepatic artery thrombosis; HAV: Hepatitis A virus; HBV: hepatitis B virus; HCC: hepatocellular carcinoma; HCV: Hepatitis C virus; HDV: hepatitis delta virus; HEV: Hepatitis E Virus; HIV: human immunodeficiency virus; HLA: human leukocyte antigen; HSV: herpes simplex virus; IPTH: Idiopathic Post-transplant Hepatitis; IS: immunosuppression; LSEC: liver sinusoidal endothelial cells; MFI: mean fluorescence intensity; NAFLD: non-alcoholic fatty liver disease; NAS: nonanastomotic biliary strictures; NRH: nodular regenerative hyperplasia; PBC: primary biliary cirrhosis; PSC: primary sclerosing cholangitis; PTLD: post-transplant lymphoproliferative disorder; RAI: Rejection activity index; SFSS: Small-for-size syndrome; SVR: sustained viral response; TCMR: T cell-mediated rejection; UDCA: ursodeoxycholic acid; VZ: Varicella-Zoster virus

Introduction

Chronic liver disease is a leading cause of mortality in the United States: an estimated 60,000 people die annually [1, 2]. Orthotopic liver transplantation is currently the only option for patients with end-stage liver disease and an estimated 15% of patients die while on the liver transplant waiting list [3]. Indeed, liver transplantation is now commonplace throughout the world and is used to treat all end-stage liver diseases: chronic necroinflammatory, metabolic, developmental, and neoplastic disorders limited to the liver. Hepatitis C virus (HCV), alcoholic and non-alcoholic fatty liver disease (NAFLD)-induced cirrhosis, and malignancies, often combined with underlying necroinflammatory disease, remain the leading indications in the United States with approximately 6,000 transplants completed in 2013 [4]. Similar profiles exist in Europe and South America. Although hepatitis B virus (HBV)-induced cirrhosis is still the most common cause for transplantation in Asia [5], effective HBV vaccination, anti-HBV [6, 7] and anti-HCV [8–10] medications, and better control of acute T cell-mediated rejection (TCMR) will fundamentally change future disease indications. Unfortunately, original disease recurrence is common and liver allografts are susceptible to a variety of technical complications; therefore, the histopathology of liver transplantation is among the broadest and complex of any solid organ allograft.

Histopathological manifestations of common hepatic diseases and insults are similar or identical to those seen in non-allograft livers and are covered elsewhere in general liver pathology texts. This chapter will emphasize conditions unique to allograft livers (e.g. extra-corporeal perfusion, small-for-size syndrome, T cell and antibody-mediated rejection (AMR), preservation/reperfusion injury, and immunosuppression (IS) minimization).

This work evolved as an update from previous versions of the chapter in this book, as well as chapters from other books and other recent publications and reviews from our group on the same subjects [11–15]. Therefore, similarities naturally exist and specific references are not included at each site to avoid redundancy. We have, however, substantially updated most sections and inserted new sections that illustrate the evolving nature of the field, especially when compared to the first liver transplant conducted in 1963 [16].

The chapter is arranged roughly in the order in which pathology tissue specimens are received for evaluation.

Machine Perfusion in Liver Transplantation

Indications for liver transplantation have increased more than the donor pool, resulting in a major shortage of available organs. This shortage has resulted in less stringent criteria for organs selected as suitable for donation, including those from older donors, livers with higher percentages of steatosis, and those donated after circulatory death (DCD) [17–19]. It is currently estimated that the organ discard rates for standard donors range from 20%–40% and are even higher for DCDs [20–22].

Although extended criteria donor (ECD) use has expanded the donor pool, they have resulted in a ~10% lower one-year graft survival rate when compared to standard criteria donation after brain death (DBD) donors. ECD and DCD usage also resulted in increased ischemia-related injury, particularly non-anastomotic biliary strictures (NAS) and other biliary complications [23–26].

Machine perfusion consists of a complex spectrum of techniques all with the common goal of decreasing ischemia reperfusion injury and increasing the donor pool of livers by increasing their viability and usability for transplantation. Main differences include the phase in which perfusion is implemented and perfusion duration and temperature [23, 27]. Some devices are utilized during the DCD harvesting, *ex situ* at the donor site, during transportation, and pre-implantation. Most strategies still involve at least one static cold storage stage. The main temperature variations are hypothermic (0–10°C), subnormothermic (+/- 21°C), and normothermic (37°C)[23].

Other component variables include perfusate composition and perfusion via the hepatic artery, portal vein, or both. Solution complexity increases with increasing temperature, and calcium is required for proper bile transport [23], but human blood depleted of leukocytes and platelets can also be used for normothermic perfusion. In other systems, optimal oxygen delivery might require artificial oxygen carriers [28]. Ravikumar et al. [29] suggested that organ preservation should: 1) reverse the injury sustained before or during organ retrieval (i.e., resuscitation), 2) avoid ischemia during reperfusion, 3) minimize reperfusion injury, and 4) enable viability testing prior to transplantation.

Proper perfusion through either the portal vein or hepatic artery can be challenging due to temperature and pressure requirements. Although the hepatic artery primarily supplies the bile ducts, the portal vein also contributes to this delicate vascular network [30, 31]. Normothermic oxygenated machine perfusion has shown promising results in protecting the biliary tree from ischemic injury; however, more research is needed in this area to determine if it truly results in better preservation of the biliary epithelium [32, 33].

Predicting the Development of Non-anastomotic Biliary Strictures Post-transplantation

The pathogenesis of biliary strictures after transplantation is currently evolving and supported by several recent studies [32, 34–38]. About 10%-20% (depending on the study) of liver allografts develop non-anastomotic (NAS) or anastomotic (AS) biliary strictures. These were originally attributed to a loss of biliary epithelial cells (BEC), with investigations [34, 35] showing that >80% of donor livers have major BEC loss. Recent evidence, however, suggests that biliary stricture development is related to the depth of bile duct wall injury and vascular and perhaps BEC regeneration insufficiencies from progenitor cells in peribiliary glands [32, 36–38]. Op den Dries et al. [36] confirmed the initial studies [34, 35] and showed that even though most donor livers (91.8% in this study) showed a substantial loss (>50%) of BEC, NAS only occurred in 16.4%. Interestingly, peribiliary gland progenitor cell loss was no different between DBD or DCD donors, but DCD donors showed more injury and small capillary loss within the peribiliary plexus.

Current preservation methods based on donor organ cooling may not optimally preserve the bile ducts or progenitor cells [36]. In addition, preservation fluids designed to protect hepatocytes and LSEC might not be ideal for BEC, bile duct wall, or peribiliary gland integrity.

Normothermic Machine Preservation

Normothermic (37°C) machine perfusion supports normal hepatic physiology, which helps maintain the cellular energy pathways and decreases the buildup of waste products [29, 31]. It can be implemented earliest along the pathway of organ harvesting by using *in situ* in the donor, immediately following circulatory arrest [23]. Normothermia also enables data collection on organ viability (e.g., enzymes, lactate dehydrogenase, bile production) prior to transplantation [29]. Static cold storage, in contrast, uses cooling to decrease the rate of ATP depletion, but in doing so, promotes activation of the ischemia/reperfusion injury cascade when oxygenated blood is resupplied during reperfusion [39].

Experimental normothermic perfusion studies [40–43] showed that it was superior to static cold storage in promoting graft survival with less cellular damage. Some of these studies simulated the parameters of DCD in human liver transplantation. Normothermic machine perfusion has been used in animal models either with or without a cold ischemic period. The best protection of the bile ducts is observed when there is no cooling of the organ; however, this may not be feasible in clinical applications [44]. Studies using porcine models have confirmed that normothermic machine perfusion decreases biliary injury [28, 33, 45] and others have shown that bile production is a critical parameter of viability in the perfused liver and recently, criteria have been established for this assessment [46]. Several randomized controlled clinical trials are currently underway to assess normothermic machine perfusion [23].

Hypothermic Machine Preservation Including Hypothermic Oxygenated Machine Perfusion (HOPE)

Hypothermic (0–10°C) machine perfusion most commonly uses an acellular perfusion solution at low pressures. One advantage of hypothermic machine perfusion is that it defaults to static cold preservation if the perfusion pump fails [23]. However, a major disadvantage, unlike normothermia, is the inability to provide a functional assessment of the liver prior to transplantation. The liver does not produce bile under these conditions, and therefore, there are very few studies that have assessed its effects on preservation of the biliary system [23, 27].

The first clinical study of hypothermic machine perfusion (without oxygenation) showed improved outcomes and decreased biliary strictures compared to controls (subjected to static cold storage) [47]. HOPE has been tested by several studies [48, 49] and can be conducted using single (portal vein) or dual (hepatic artery and portal vein) perfusion. Although neither biliary function nor injury were able to be assessed, one group was able to show preservation of the peribiliary vascular plexus using this technique in a porcine model [50]. In addition, Dutkowski et al. compared eight DCD livers to eight matched DBD donors using HOPE prior to transplantation and showed a similar incidence of biliary complications among the two groups, indicating a possible protective effect of HOPE during DCD.

Subnormothermic Machine Perfusion

Subnormothermic machine combines some of the advantages of both of the above machine perfusion techniques by decreasing the temperature slightly below physiologic temperature (i.e., +/- 21°C), which decreases the metabolic rate by approximately 25%

while still allowing for functional assessment prior to transplantation [51, 52]. This technique has been tested in experimental models, with and without red blood cells or an artificial oxygen carrier [51] and has shown evidence of decreased biliary injury [53, 54]. Kneek et al. showed bile duct histology with preserved bile duct integrity in the subnormothermic machine perfused group when compared to their matched static cold storage group, which showed severe bile duct necrosis in three out of five animals, indicating that subnormothermic conditions are able to reduce bile duct injury after liver transplantation.

Machine Perfusion Devices

A review by Ravikumar et al. [29] described some of the devices currently in clinical or preclinical testing which include the Liver Assist (www.organ-assist.nl/products/liver-assist), OrganOx metra (www.organox.com), and the Transmedics Organ Care System (OCS™) (www.transmedics.com). According to their website, the Liver Assist is a device for *ex vivo* perfusion of donor livers. Two different pump units provide a pulsatile perfusion of the hepatic artery and continuous flow to the portal vein. The oxygenated perfusion is pressure controlled and the temperature can be set from hypothermic to normothermic conditions. This device was recently used with a cell-free oxygen carrier under subnormothermic conditions and showed promising results in a porcine model [20]. Six livers were subjected to machine perfusion with nine hours of cold ischemia time (CIT) and followed for five days after transplantation, and were compared to livers transplanted after normal cold storage conditions. The machine perfused livers had significantly increased survival (100% compared to 33%), superior graft function, eight times higher oxygen delivery than consumption, and significantly greater bile production [20].

The OrganOx metra is a portable normothermic perfusion system that allows for continuous flow through both hepatic artery and portal vein. It is the first and only fully automated normothermic liver perfusion device, and according to their website, has been designed with every step of the organ retrieval, transport, and transplant process in mind, and was designed by transplant surgeons.

Finally, the OCS™ Liver is a portable perfusion and monitoring system that maintains the organ in a near physiologic state. The system enables surgeons to perfuse and monitor the organ between the donor and recipient sites. Their device is in the pre-clinical stage with clinical trials expected to start soon. More clinical trials are needed to determine the best perfusion parameters and techniques to be used for liver transplantation; however, the future looks promising and successful implementation of these devices should significantly increase the donor pool, particularly from ECDs.

Deceased Donor Biopsy Evaluation

An ideal, or reference, donor has been defined as age <40 years, trauma as the cause of death, DBD, hemodynamically stable at the time of procurement, no steatosis or any other underlying chronic liver lesion, and no transmissible disease (reviewed in [55–59]). Frozen section examination is often used in the evaluation of ECDs, which is generally defined by contrast with an ideal or reference donor (reviewed in [55–59]). Common characteristics include increased age (>60 years), hypernatremia (>155 meq/L), macrovesicular steatosis (>40%), CIT exceeding 12 hours, partial-liver allografts (DCD), hemodynamically instable, use of vasopressors, hypernatremia, HBV or HCV infection or anti-HBc antibody positivity, presence of a liver mass, and fibrosis or other focal lesions or history of cancer. A "donor risk index" introduced by Feng et al. [60] differentially weighed and summed scores for: old age (>60 years), anoxic and cerebrovascular causes of death, black race, short height, DCD and split/partial grafts, regional or national sharing, and cold ischemic time; the index independently predicted graft failure[60]. Organs from donors positive for specific serologically diagnosed infections (e.g., HIV, HCV, rabies, etc.) or for a history of a high-risk malignancy are usually disqualified for transplantation [61, 62], which has kept disease transmission from donor to recipient low [63].

Some ECD characteristics potentially have histopathologic manifestations where liver biopsy is justified: advanced age (>60 years), macrovesicular steatosis (>40%), HCV infection, and cardiovascular instability/ischemic injury. Others do not, and biopsy is not justified: black race, short stature, cerebrovascular cause of death, hypernatremia (>155 meq/L), CIT exceeding 12 hours, and partial-liver allografts. DCD represent a donor organ source (approximately 5% of the total donor pool [64]) that is troubled with drawbacks, especially ischemic cholangiopathy that often develops several weeks to months after transplantation. American Society of Transplant Surgeons (ASTS) best practice guidelines suggest [64] limiting warm ischemia <20 minutes, but even under ideal conditions, complications can arise. Peripheral core needle biopsy evaluation of DCD is usually not helpful in predicting future complications.

Deceased donor histopathology requests can be prompted because of: 1) the clinical history or circumstances surrounding donor death or harvesting procedure; 2) the gross appearance, "feel," or color of the donor liver; and 3) known pre-existing donor disease (e.g., HCV). A grossly fatty appearance most commonly precipitates requests for frozen section evaluation. Since experienced donor surgeons are usually able to accurately estimate steatosis severity before biopsy evaluation, any apparent discrepancies should be resolved. Reasons for differences between the gross and microscopic evaluation include suboptimal illumination in the operating room and micro-versus-macrovesicular steatosis.

Tissue sampling for frozen section should be obtained fresh, preferably with the pathologist's assistance to assure representative sampling. Routine sampling includes two 2.0 cm, 16-gauge needle cores, one each from the right and left lobes, and one 2.0 cm^2 subcapsular right lobe wedge biopsy. Needle cores enable a "deeper" view of the liver, whereas the wedge is helpful for evaluating arterial/arteriolar disease and more accurately estimating the severity of steatosis.

The liver tissue should be quickly triaged to the frozen section room, avoiding storage in "physiologic" saline, air drying, and placement of the tissue sample on an absorbent substrate. Absorbent substrates blot fat out of the tissue, resulting in an underestimation of the extent of fatty infiltration, which can lead to disturbing consequences. Air drying and storage in physiologic saline can cause hepatocytes to appear shrunken/necrotic, leading to overestimation of ischemic injury.

Biopsy findings that usually disqualify organs include widespread hepatocyte necrosis, severe (>30%) *macro*vesicular steatosis (defined below), advanced intra-hepatic atherosclerosis, and definite evidence of bridging fibrosis [65–67]. Recognition of hepatocytes in various stages of injury/necro-apoptosis because of ischemic damage can be enhanced by staining several sections for increasing lengths of time in eosin, which enhances contrast between viable and damaged/nonviable hepatocytes: the latter are more hypereosinophilic and often show early nuclear karyorrhexis. Polarization microscopy can be used to assess fibrosis in the frozen section setting.

In fatty donor liver evaluation, it is important to determine whether the steatosis is macro or microvesicular because severe (>30%) *macrovesicular* steatosis, defined as large fat globules (>2X nuclear diameter) that usually displace the nucleus to the cell periphery, increases susceptibility to preservation/reperfusion injury, impairs regeneration, and is associated with decreased graft survival (reviewed in [58, 59, 68]). In contrast, *microvesicular* steatosis presents as multiple small fat globules (<nuclear diameter) usually associated with a centrally-placed nucleus. Relatively short (approximately 60 min) periods of warm ischemia and other insults can cause microvesicular steatosis and usually does not adversely affect outcome, except in one study where "high-grade" microvesicular steatosis was associated with delayed graft function [69]. We estimate the severity of macrovesicular steatosis to the nearest 10% based on H&E stained slides alone. Making the macro-versus microvesicular distinction can be problematic because of a spectrum of fat globule sizes and nuclear displacement often seen.

Others and we scale macrovesicular steatosis [58, 70] as follows: *mild* (<10%) does not usually influence organ triage, whereas *moderate* (10%–30%) prompts considerations of other factors (e.g., ECD characteristics) to determine whether the organ is utilized. Donor livers with *severe* steatosis (>30%) are usually discarded or utilized only under very special circumstances and all or nearly all other characteristics are those of an ideal donor (see above). Other groups, however, apply an evenly distributed macrovesicular steatosis scoring range: mild <30%; moderate = 30%–60%; and severe >60% [71]. Although some centers are more aggressive, most disqualify donor livers with >50% *macrovesicular* steatosis because of the high risk of early dysfunction and failure (reviewed in [18, 58, 59, 68]). Some centers question the practice of discarding fatty livers [18, 69, 72], especially if other donor risk factors (e.g., age, cold ischemia time) have been mitigated because the outcome in such situations can be comparable to non-steatotic donor livers [72, 73].

Donor macrovesicular steatosis assessment by pre-transplant frozen section evaluation is reproducible [74, 75], but cutoff values lower than 30% can decrease reproducibility [74, 75]. The merits of various non-invasive modalities, such as the preferred method of unenhanced CT, as well as ultrasound and MR imaging, have been reviewed in comparison to biopsy [76].

A standardized scoring system for necrosis in donor biopsies has not been developed, which might account for some [71, 77], but not other [69, 75], studies reporting a negative impact on recipient outcome. Regardless, necrosis should *not* be assessed in the subcapsular location alone: necrosis is commonly seen at this site due to surgical manipulation. We roughly estimate the total percentage of necrotic hepatocytes on H&E stains throughout all tissue specimens and correlate the findings with trends in liver injury tests. If necrotic hepatocytes account for >10% of all hepatocytes, diffusely distributed throughout the biopsy, and liver injury tests are rising, the liver is usually disqualified. However, if necrosis is <10% and liver injury tests are trending downward, other characteristics are considered in the decision-making process. Extra-corporeal perfusion of donor liver with necrosis will likely change this approach.

Utilization of young HCV+ donors yields recipient graft and patient survival rates comparable to HCV -donors (reviewed in [78]). Historically, bridging fibrosis (3/6, using the Ishak scale) was used as a cutoff, but others have demanded less fibrosis (<2/6) [79]. Although more rapid progression of fibrosis can occur [79], emergence of newer and more effective anti-HCV therapies with fewer side effects will further enable this approach with the biological "point of no return" yet to be determined [78].

HBV can be transmitted from anti-HBc+ donors to naïve and unvaccinated recipients [80]; the risk for transmission is lower in vaccinated and anti-HBc+ recipients and can be further reduced by anti-HBV medications and passive administration of antibodies [81]. Donor biopsy evaluation is usually not helpful because the vast majority of biopsies from anti-HBc+ livers are normal in the absence of other diseases.

A number of neoplastic, infectious, and metabolic diseases have been inadvertently transferred from donors to recipients (reviewed in [62, 63]). Some of these diseases are potentially detectable by pathologists. Included are cancers, amyloidosis, hemochromatosis, and fungal, viral, and parasitic diseases (reviewed in [62, 63]). Metabolic diseases, such as familial amyloid polyneuropathy [82], oxalosis [83], and possibly α-1-anti-trypsin deficiency [84] can be intentionally transferred with the donor organ in so-called "domino" transplants: the rationalization is that the latency period between transplantation and recipient disease onset improves overall survival. Inadvertent transmission can also occur (reviewed in [62, 63]).

The final critical step in donor biopsy evaluation is to correlate the findings with donor history, laboratory values, and agonal, including organ harvesting, events. Donor biopsies are but one tool used to assess the donor. Pathologists should not work in isolation, as they are unable to guarantee organ function after transplantation based on donor liver frozen section light microscopic evaluation in the absence of obvious findings.

Living Donor Biopsy Evaluation

Living donors accounted for 211/5921 (3.6%) of liver transplants performed in 2013 in the United States [4], but represent most liver transplants in Asia [85]. Right lobes are most often used [4], which represents a major donor liver resection with 0.2% mortality and 24% morbidity rates [86, 87]. Biopsies are routinely conducted in potential living donors to further minimize donor risk and disease transmission, but the yield is relatively low, resulting in an unfavorable risk-benefit ratio [88–92].

Most potential living donor biopsies are either entirely normal or show mild steatosis; 20%–50% show usually mild abnormalities (reviewed in [93]) with macrovesicular steatosis being the most common (14%–53%) reason for donor disqualification [88–90, 93–95]. Most programs disqualify donors with >30% macrovesicular steatosis because of the potential for post-surgical complications in either donor or recipient [86, 90]; other programs are more conservative, requiring <10%–20% [95, 96]. Disqualification rates based on biopsy findings alone vary from 3% to 21% [93].

The range of biopsy findings include low-grade chronic hepatitis/portal inflammation of undetermined etiology [97], granulomas, and a variety of other unexpected findings (e.g., unexpected early-stage primary biliary cirrhosis (PBC) [93]). Mild (1–2+ on a scale of 0–4) periportal hepatocellular iron deposits are present in approximately 17% of mostly male potential donors. Unexplained portal tract eosinophilia can also be occasionally seen and did not adversely affect the post-operative donor or recipient clinical course in two cases [93].

Determination of Causes of Graft Dysfunction after Transplantation

Understanding the Operation and Timing of Causes of Dysfunction

Familiarity with donor and recipient operations facilitates biopsy evaluation since many causes of dysfunction are attributable to surgical complexities and/or agonal donor events. Donor and recipient are usually matched for size and usually ABO blood groups. Deceased donor organs usually utilize end-to-end anastomoses connecting the recipient and donor portal vein, hepatic artery, bile duct, and vena cava [98], but there are numerous surgical variations (e.g., variant biliary anastomoses, reduced-size livers, alternate vena caval anastomoses) that are important to understand, but beyond the scope of this chapter. Reduced-size grafts (living donors, splits, etc.) are substantially more complicated and technically demanding operations that deviate from reconstruction of normal anatomy and increase the risk of both vascular and biliary tract complications.

An understanding of basic transplant immunology, IS management, and technical complications facilitates accurate biopsy interpretation. Certain complications occur during characteristic times after transplantation (Table 3.1). Knowledge of the original disease, time after transplantation, liver injury test profile, DSA status, and technical complications usually provides enough information to generate a reasonably accurate differential diagnosis. Since more than one cause of liver injury is often present, listing the diagnoses in order after thorough clinicopathological correlation helps patient management.

Post-transplant Allograft Needle Biopsies

Liver allograft biopsies are invasive and expensive, but provide hard-to-replace information, including: 1) determining the cause of dysfunction, if present; 2) monitoring the effect of therapy and/or progression of disease; 3) documenting the immunologic and/or architectural status to help guide chronic immunosuppressive therapy; and 4) research. Tissue triage depends on the reason for biopsy, clinical differential diagnosis, and time after transplantation. The American Association for the Study of Liver Disease (AASLD) has recommended two passes with a 16 gauge needle for adequate assessment of fibrosis because staging is subject to sampling error for thin (<16 gauge) and small (<20 mm long) biopsies. Biopsies containing <11 portal tracts might not be representative (reviewed in [99]). The same guidelines were recommended for liver allografts by the BANFF Working Group [100].

Two H&E-stained slides each containing 2–4-step sections of routinely processed, formalin-fixed paraffin-embedded (FFPE) stains provide most information. We do not routinely conduct special stains unless clinically indicated because of the need to preserve tissue for investigative studies. Commonly helpful special stains include trichrome and reticulin stains for fibrosis and architectural distortion, C4d for AMR (AMR) monitoring (see below), glutamine synthetase for assessment of architecture, CK7 [101] and copper for monitoring of biliary drainage (ductular metaplasia of hepatocytes and chronic cholestasis, respectively), and a variety of immunohistochemical stains for viral antigens or nucleic acids (CMV, adenovirus (ADV), EBV, etc.). C4d staining on frozen tissue is ideal, but can be difficult to interpret [11].

Optimal information needed for biopsy assessment includes the original disease, ABO compatibility, donor specific antibodies (DSA) status, time after transplantation, liver injury test profile, and type of transplant (i.e., standard whole organ deceased, DCD livers, reduced-size deceased, living related, etc.). A clinical differential diagnosis is also very valuable. Microscopic findings can be scored according to a standardized template that can be later harvested for translational research studies. Since awareness of clinical information before biopsy review can bias the interpretation, it is preferable to first complete the slide review. Then the findings should be correlated with the clinical, serological, and radiographic profile and a differential diagnosis should be generated. Comparison of current findings to those in previous biopsies is routine. Re-review of all liver allograft biopsies at a weekly clinicopathological conference can be a useful quality assessment tool.

Failed Allograft Evaluations

Gross examination of failed allograft specimens should follow a standardized approach similar to that used for native hepatectomy specimens. Special attention should be paid to dissection and inspection of anastomotic biliary, hepatic artery, portal, and hepatic vein sites [102]. Assistance of the operative surgeon to explain the surgical anatomy might be required. Routine tissue sampling for microscopy should include: 1) anastomoses, if present; 2)

Table 3.1 Approximate Timing of Common Allograft Syndromes (Adapted from [606] and [314]).

Syndrome	Clinical Associations/Observations	Peak Time Period
"Preservation" reperfusion injury	Long cold (>12 hrs.) or warm (>120 minutes) ischemic time; older (>60 yrs.), hemodynamically unstable, DCD, "re-do" of anastomoses; poor bile production; prolonged cholestatic phase predisposes to biliary sludge syndrome	Recognized primarily in post-reperfusion biopsies and biopsies obtained within the first several weeks after OLTx; changes can persist for several months depending on the severity of the initial injury
AMR	ABO-incompatible donor; high titer (>1:32) lymphocytotoxic crossmatch DSA; presents with persistently low platelet counts and complement levels during first several weeks of transplantation	First several weeks to months after transplantation; later onset less common and not well-defined
Acute cellular rejection	Younger, "healthier," female, and inadequately immunosuppressed recipients, long cold ischemic times, and those with disorders of dysregulated immunity (e.g., PSC, AIH, PBC)	Peak dependent on IS regimen; usually between 3–40 days; later onset usually associated with inadequate IS
Chronic rejection	Usually occurs in inadequately immunosuppressed patients (e.g., infections, tumors, PTLD) and patients have a history of moderate, severe, or persistent acute rejection episodes, or are non-compliant	Bimodal distribution; early peak during first year and later increase in non-compliant and inadequately immunosuppressed patients
Hepatic artery thrombosis (HAT)	Suboptimal anastomosis; pediatric/small caliber vessels; donor and/or recipient atherosclerosis; suboptimal or difficult arterial anastomosis; large difference in vessel caliber across anastomosis; hypercoagulopathy; suboptimal arterial flow (vasospasm from SFSS)	Bimodal distribution; early peak between 0–4 weeks and later peak between 18–36 months (see text)
Biliary tract obstruction or stricturing	Arterial insufficiency or thrombosis; long cold ischemia, DCD, difficult biliary anastomosis; AMR; original disease of PSC	Variable, but timing can be used to determine etiology: <6 months usually mechanical, preservation/reperfusion injury (ischemic cholangiopathy) or AMR; >6 months recurrent disease, mechanical
Venous outflow obstruction	Difficult "piggyback" hepatic vein reconstruction; cardiac failure	Usually during the first several months
"Opportunistic" viral (CMV, EBV, ADV, etc.) and fungal infections (see text)	Seropositive donors to seronegative recipients (often pediatric); over-IS	0–8 weeks, much less common thereafter except for EBV-related PTLDs and other EBV-related tumors (See text)
Recurrent or new onset of viral hepatitis (e.g., HBV, HCV, HEV).	Original disease HBV, HCV, or acquired HEV-induced hepatitis in patients with contact with animals or culinary inconsistencies	Usually first becomes apparent 4–6 weeks after transplantation and persists thereafter; earlier onset (within two weeks) in aggressive cases
Recurrent AIH, PBC, and PSC	Original disease of AIH, PBC, or PSC; see text for risk factors	Usually more than six months after transplantation; incidence of recurrence increases with time after transplantation
Alcohol abuse	Psychiatric co-morbidity/social instability; non-compliance with treatment protocols; GGTP:ALP ratio >1.4; see text for risk factors	Usually >6 months
Non-alcoholic steatohepatitis	Original disease non-alcoholic steatohepatitis or cryptogenic cirrhosis; persistent or worsening risk factors for NASH in general population	Usually >3–4 weeks and increases with time if risk factors persist.

superficial and deep sections of the right and left lobe; 3) at least one deep hilar section with cross sections of the medium-sized bile ducts and arteries; and 4) any grossly obvious defects.

Causes of allograft failure vary according to the time after transplantation. "Preservation/reperfusion" injury or primary non-function, vascular thrombosis, and patient death are the leading causes of early (<3 months) allograft failure; few allografts fail because of TCMR during this time period [103–107]. Recurrent disease, delayed manifestations of technical complications such as vascular thrombosis or biliary sludge syndrome, and patient death are most commonly responsible for late graft failures occurring >1 year after transplantation. Classically defined chronic rejection is relatively uncommon as a cause of graft failure [107, 108], but newly recognized manifestations of chronic injury related to DSA might change this impression. Recurrent HCV-induced cirrhosis has been a leading cause for allograft failure [109], but newer, more effective anti-HCV therapy should prevent many of these graft failures [8–10].

Special Considerations in Reduced Size and Living-related Liver Allografts

Reduced-size allografts (living donors, splits, etc.) usually compromise, at least focally, one or more of the afferent or efferent vascular or biliary conduits, especially near the parenchymal surgical margin. This creates a significant potential for sampling errors: localized vascular or biliary obstructive changes can be misinterpreted as a global change and there may be a lack of correlation between substantial graft pathology and normal liver injury test profiles. Since more than one biliary anastomosis might be functional, and biopsy from one lobe might show obstructive cholangiopathy, whereas the other lobe might be normal, complete clinicopathological and laboratory correlation should be carried out before rendering a final diagnosis.

Reduced-size/living donor allografts usually undergo rapid growth shortly after transplantation and are more susceptible to damage from needle biopsies [110] and acute AMR [111]. Late after transplantation, portal venopathy, low-grade ductular reactions, and nodular regenerative hyperplasia (NRH) changes are also common findings in reduced-size and living donor liver allografts [112].

Preservation/Reperfusion Injury

"Preservation/reperfusion" injury generally refers to damage sustained during agonal events in the donor, cold preservation, and reperfusion in the recipient, including recipient cardiovascular instability [113, 114]. "Cold ischemia" refers to damage occurring when the donor organ is stored in preservation fluid and immersed in an ice bath; it preferentially damages LSEC causing them to lift from the underlying matrix. "Warm ischemia" occurs when the organ is suboptimally perfused with blood because of hypotension or death, which preferentially damages hepatocytes [113, 114]. A series of complex and interrelated interactions among various cell populations including Kupffer cells, LSEC, hepatocytes, leukocytes, and platelets is divided into damage occurring during ischemic injury and damage precipitated as a consequence of blood reperfusion. Microcirculatory compromise is an important final common pathway of injury (reviewed in [113, 114]). Steatosis, starvation, and advanced donor age increase susceptibility to both warm and cold ischemic injury (reviewed in [113, 114]). Preservation-reperfusion injury in DCD donors is inextricably linked with ischemic cholangiopathy [24, 115–117]; this occurs when extended warm ischemia and platelet and leukocyte sludging compromises peribiliary plexus patency.

Clinical Presentation

Reliable early signs of severe preservation/reperfusion injury after complete revascularization include poor bile production, persistent elevation of serum lactate, and marked (>2500 IU/ml) elevations of serum ALT and AST during the first few days after transplantation [118]. This is usually followed by rapid ALT/AST normalization during the first week and a prolonged "cholestatic phase" characterized by persistent elevation of total bilirubin and γ-GTP. Cases that recover from early significant injury show a gradual resolution of abnormal liver injury tests, but these grafts remain at risk for ischemic cholangiopathy [119, 120].

Histopathologic Findings

Post-reperfusion, also referred to as "time-0" needle biopsies, obtained within several hours of complete revascularization, can reliably gauge the extent of preservation/reperfusion injury and predict one-year graft loss [118, 121–123]. Mild damage, present in most liver allografts, includes microvesicular steatosis, which is usually attributable to warm ischemia, hepatocellular cytoaggregation (i.e., detachment of individual hepatocytes from each other and "rounding up" of the cytoplasm), hepatocellular swelling, and occasional neutrophils [102, 118, 122, 123]. Severe injury is characterized by zonal or confluent coagulative necrosis, particularly if it is periportal or bridging, and combined with severe neutrophilic inflammation [102, 118, 122, 123]. "Surgical hepatitis" characterized by perivenular sinusoidal neutrophilia without necrosis, or manipulation injury, manifests as necrosis and neutrophilia in immediate subcapsular parenchyma in wedge biopsies, and should not be interpreted as preservation/reperfusion injury.

Regenerative/reparative responses usually begin after one to two days and are proportional to preservation/reperfusion injury severity. Response to mild injury includes hepatocellular mitosis and plate thickening, which can later be accompanied by mild centrilobular hepatocellular swelling and hepatocanalicular cholestasis, which can persist for several weeks. Response to severe preservation/reperfusion injury usually includes marked centrilobular hepatocellular swelling and hepatocanalicular and cholangiolar cholestasis [102, 118] that often persist for one or two months. Cholangiolar proliferation is also usually present, triggered by periportal and confluent bridging necrosis or by increased endotoxin in the portal circulation, or co-existent sepsis [102, 114, 118] (see Figure 3.1). The graft parenchyma usually recovers, but such patients are at risk for ischemic cholangiopathy [24, 26]. Apoptotic hepatocytes or coagulative necrosis occurring more than several days after transplantation should arouse the suspicion of another, usually ischemic, insult [124].

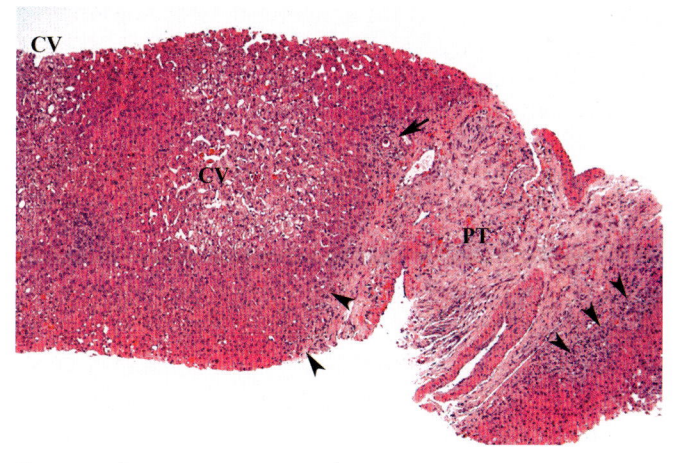

Figure 3.1 Severe preservation/reperfusion injury is usually seen during the first several weeks after transplantation and characterized by centrilobular hepatocellular swelling, cholangiolar proliferation (arrowhead), and mild, neutrophilic, or mixed portal inflammation without significant eosinophilia or blastic lymphocytes. Note the absence of edema around the true bile duct (arrow), which helps to distinguish severe preservation/reperfusion injury from biliary tract obstruction/stricturing (PT = portal tract; CV = central vein).

Macrosteatotic donor livers have increased susceptibility to preservation/reperfusion injury. Death of a fraction of fat-containing hepatocytes releases lipid droplets into the sinusoids [113, 114] where they coalesce into larger globules. This triggers local fibrin deposition, neutrophilia, local sinusoidal obstruction, and red blood cell congestion [65]. Macrophages eventually surround and resorb the large fat globules over a period of several weeks if the grafts survive.

Differential Diagnosis

Biliary obstruction/pancreatitis, sepsis, acute AMR, and cholestatic hepatitis can all produce histopathological changes that resemble preservation/reperfusion injury. A detailed clinical and laboratory correlation is needed to sort through the possibilities. Information about the donor (e.g., age and type (e.g., ECD, DCD), cold and warm ischemic times), recipient (operative difficulties, and clinical profile), laboratory (blood culture and crossmatch and DSA results), and C4d staining results help to determine the likely source of injury [125].

Preservation/reperfusion injury and biliary tract obstruction/stricturing can be distinguished from each other by examining the true bile ducts (not cholangioles) contained within the original portal tract stroma and the interface zone (see Figure 3.1). Periductal lamellar edema surrounding the true bile ducts or stellate-shaped septal bile duct lumens often accompanied by neutrophils within the lumen or infiltrating between BEC and foam cells at the interface zone are more common with suboptimal biliary drainage. In contrast, neutrophils surrounding interface zone cholangioles, acute cholangitis, periductal edema, and interface foam cells are less common in preservation/reperfusion injury. Centrilobular, hepatocanalicular, cholangiolar cholestasis, and intralobular neutrophil clusters are common to both insults and acute cholangitis/biliary sludge syndrome can complicate severe preservation/reperfusion injury.

Cholestatic hepatitis shares some features with preservation/reperfusion injury, but the clinical context, history, and laboratory profile differ substantially. Cholestatic hepatitis (e.g., HBV, HCV, and drug-related) is unusual before three to four weeks after transplantation and usually worsens with time unless the patient is specifically treated, whereas preservation/reperfusion usually improves gradually.

TCMR superimposed on preservation injury is recognized by the appearance of blastic and smaller lymphocytes and especially eosinophils in portal and perivenular regions combined with convincing lymphocytic cholangitis, and lymphocytic or eosinophilic central perivenulitis.

Distinguishing preservation injury from AMR is discussed in the AMR section.

Portal Hyperperfusion or "Small-for-Size" Syndrome

Introduction and Clinical Presentation

The "hyperdynamic" splanchnic circulation in cirrhotic patients with portal hypertension exposes reduced-size liver grafts (e.g., living donor, split, etc.) to portal hyperperfusion. When this exceeds a certain threshold, the "small-for-size" or portal hyperperfusion syndrome can occur, which Dahm et al. defined as at least two of the following complications, on three consecutive days, within the first several weeks after transplantation: elevated bilirubin (>100 µmol/L), INR >2, and grade 3 or 4 encephalopathy after exclusion of technical, immunological, or infectious complications [126]. SFSS occurs more frequently when a reduced size/living donor allograft is <30% of expected recipient liver volume or <0.8% recipient body weight. However, SFSS is not based solely on the size of the graft, but on the combination of portal hypertension severity and graft size.

SFSS occurs, at least partly, because the donor liver fragment is unable to accommodate the significantly increased portal inflow, especially if the hepatic venous drainage is also compromised [127, 128]. The hyperdynamic portal circulation injures portal venous and periportal sinusoidal endothelium [112, 129] and triggers the arterial buffer response [130, 131], which refers to portal venous blood flow regulation of arterial flow, independent of innervation [130, 131]. When portal flow is diminished, arterial resistance decreases and arterial flow increases. Conversely, when portal vein flow increases, as during portal hyperperfusion in reduced-size livers, arterial resistance increases and flow decreases [112, 131, 132]. This response appears to be mediated primarily by adenosine, an arterial vasodilator that is "washed out" during high venous flow causing arterial constriction. However, nitric oxide, carbon monoxide, and H_2S are also likely contributors [130, 131]. Since portal vein flow is regulated by splanchnic venous return, changes in hepatic artery flow do not precipitate a reciprocal reaction in portal vein flow. SFSS has been successfully ameliorated by reducing portal venous inflow using transient portal-caval shunting, banding, splenic artery ligation, and pharmacologic manipulation [127, 131, 132], all of which enable smaller graft use [133].

Adequate liver regeneration [112, 134] is dependent on optimal portal venous flow: too much causes SFSS; too little can impair regeneration and cause graft steatosis [135, 136]. Portal pressure elevation after partial hepatectomy is dependent upon graft size [137] and the regeneration rate is directly proportional to increased portal pressure and flow and inversely correlated with residual volume [138, 139]. Failure of liver regeneration is generally not a major clinical problem unless there is co-existent suboptimal hepatic venous drainage [140].

Surgeons are usually aware of the potential for SFSS because of the surgical setting and operative observations. However, a SFSS diagnosis can be difficult to establish with certainty. Some clinical manifestations are not entirely specific and potentially caused by other insults. In addition, the SFSS probably also contributes to so-called "technical" complications, which are also found with increased frequency in reduced-size allografts (e.g., arterial vasospasm predisposing to thrombosis [112]).

Histopathologic Findings

Early SFSS events are most reliably observed in experimental animal models [129, 138, 141, 142] and in post-reperfusion or early post-transplant allograft biopsies obtained within the first several days in humans.

Focal denudation of portal vein and periportal sinusoidal endothelium can occur within five minutes after revascularization [112, 129, 138, 141, 142]. When severe microvascular rupture at portal vein-sinusoidal junctions occurs, there can be hemorrhage into the portal and periportal connective tissue with dissection into the hepatic parenchyma [143, 144].

Reparative changes are triggered if the allograft survives the initial insult. Endothelial cell hypertrophy and subendothelial edema are accompanied by an in-growth of myofibroblasts into the subendothelial space, which eventually result in fibrointimal hyperplasia/intimal thickening and luminal obliteration or re-canalization of thrombi. Typical venous findings are uncommonly detected in peripheral core needle biopsies. Instead, a constellation of nonspecific findings are often found, including variable centrilobular, hepatocanalicular cholestasis, centrilobular hepatocyte steatosis or hepatocyte atrophy with sinusoidal dilatation, and/or centrilobular hepatocyte necrosis and a low-grade ductular reaction. If the graft recovers, portal hypertension and ascites resolve over a period of several weeks accompanied by restoration of the normal architecture. Severely affected grafts, however, can develop nodular regenerative hyperplasia (NRH) changes, most likely as a result of portal venopathy [112].

Peri-hilar sections of allografts that fail from SFSS frequently show changes of traumatic injury to larger portal vein endothelium, focal portal vein branch fibrointimal hyperplasia, evidence of arterial vasospasm, most commonly involving medium-sized peri-hilar arteries, and in some cases, ischemic cholangitis, particularly if accompanied by HAT [112].

Differential Diagnosis

Suboptimal arterial flow because of arterial thrombosis or stricturing, sepsis, hypotension, biliary tract obstruction/stricturing, ischemic cholangitis, and preservation/reperfusion injury can cause histopathologic changes similar to SFSS. Biliary tract obstruction/stricturing and ischemic cholangitis alone, however, are not usually accompanied by either portal tract connective tissue hemorrhage or centrilobular hepatocyte ischemic changes. Since SFSS can compromise arterial flow because of arterial vasospasm, arterial thrombosis can occur as a complication.

Vascular Complications

General Considerations

Most vascular complications occur during the first several months after transplantation and are related to anatomic complexity (e.g., small caliber vessels and/or abnormal anatomy), anastomotic imperfections (e.g., iatrogenic narrowing or dramatic caliber reductions, intimal flaps), pre-existing atherosclerotic disease, operative manipulation, abnormal tortuosity, devitalized vessel wall, and/or thrombogenic metabolic or physiologic abnormalities, or a combination of these factors.

Hepatic Artery Thrombosis

Introduction, Pathophysiology, and Clinical Presentation

Allografts are more susceptible to arterial ischemia than native livers because they are devoid of arterial collaterals, at least early after transplantation. The hepatic artery supplies primarily the extra- and intra-hepatic bile ducts, hilar and portal tract connective tissue, and hilar lymph nodes; these structures are preferentially damaged by inadequate arterial flow or after arterial thrombosis resulting in "ischemic cholangitis" [102, 119] or "ischemic cholangiopathy" [120], frank bile duct necrosis, poor biliary wound/anastomotic healing resulting in biliary leaks, or cholangitic abscesses, resulting in the biliary sludge syndrome.

HAT occurs in 2%–20% of transplants usually within 30 days (early) of transplantation (reviewed in [145, 146]). Risk factors for early HAT include the pediatric age group, CMV mismatch re-transplantation, arterial conduit use, long operation time, variant arterial anatomy, and low volume transplantation centers (reviewed in [145]). Most early HAT presents as fever, leukocytosis, marked liver injury test elevations, and septic shock (reviewed in [145, 146]). Late HAT can be asymptomatic or present insidiously with cholangitis, relapsing fevers, and sepsis related to hepatic infarcts, abscesses, and ischemic cholangiopathy (reviewed in [145, 146]). Risk factors for late HAT include CMV infection and accessory hepatic artery anastomosis [146, 147].

Histopathologic Findings

Structures most susceptible to arterial ischemic injury (e.g., peri-hilar tissue and large bile ducts) are not routinely sampled in peripheral core needle biopsies, leading to sampling issues [102, 148, 149]. When present, changes include centrilobular coagulative necrosis or marked centrilobular hepatocyte swelling combined with changes of ischemic cholangiopathy: portal/periportal edema, ductular reaction, and acute cholangitis. HAT can occasionally present as spotty acidophilic necrosis and mitosis of hepatocytes or so-called "ischemic hepatitis" and mimics acute viral hepatitis [150]. Chronic arterial narrowing and suboptimal flow can also cause centrilobular hepatocellular atrophy/perivenular sinusoidal dilatation.

Allografts that failed because of HAT often show necrosis of extra-hepatic bile ducts with bile extravasation, biliary stones/sludge, biliary abscesses superinfected with fungi and bacteria, and patchy parenchymal ischemic necrosis (see Figure 3.2 and Figure 3.3).

Differential Diagnosis

Arterial insufficiency can mimic many, mostly non-inflammatory, causes of liver allograft dysfunction, such as viral hepatitis and cholestatic drug-induced liver injury (DILI), and be complicated by ischemic cholangiopathy. Therefore, hepatic arterial patency should be examined when biliary tract complications are encountered if no other cause is apparent.

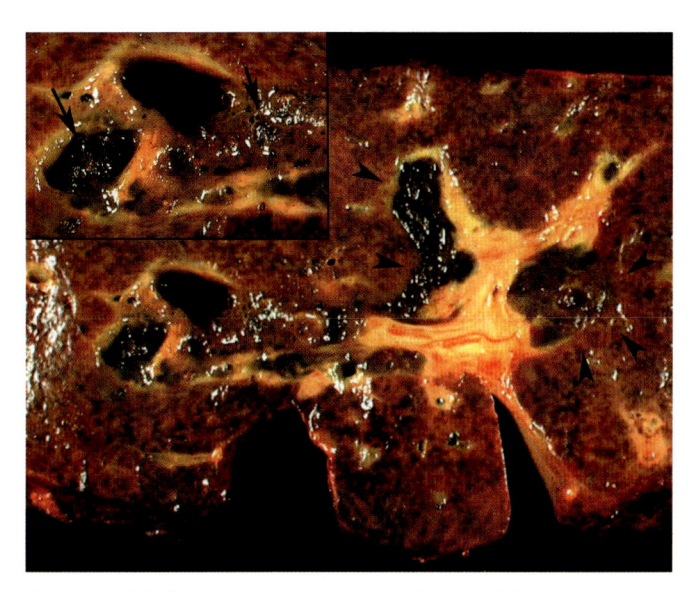

Figure 3.2 HAT frequently results in necrosis of the large bile ducts and formation of biliary sludge and casts (arrows in left upper inset). The peri-hilar bile ducts show focal necrosis with bile staining and extravasation of bile (arrowheads). This gross image illustrates why biopsies obtained from the periphery of the liver are not a good method to establish the diagnosis of HAT; they can show various changes, or even be misleading.

Portal Vein Thrombosis

Introduction and Clinical Presentation

Large portal vein abnormalities, such as thrombosis, stenosis, and suboptimal flow, are unusual and involve approximately 1%–2% of recipients (reviewed in [151, 152]). Risk factors include reduced-size donor organs, small portal vein diameter/pediatric recipients, caliber differences between donor and recipient, previous portal vein thrombosis, surgical shunting before transplantation, splenectomy (reviewed in [151, 152]), and use of cryopreserved venous interposition grafts [153].

Portal vein thrombosis early after transplantation can present with fulminant hepatic failure and later with bleeding varices, portal hypertension with massive ascites, and edema (reviewed in [151]).

Histopathologic Findings

Histopathologic findings depend on the severity of compromised flow, time after transplantation, and the condition/structure of the allograft. Early after transplantation, complete portal venous thrombosis often causes widespread necrosis (see Figure 3.4). Bacterial seeding of a non-occlusive portal vein thrombus can result in septic phlebitis and small miliary intra-hepatic abscesses. Suboptimal portal vein flow because of stenosis, kinks, or persistent collateral circulation can cause periportal and/or midzonal hepatocyte atrophy, coagulative necrosis (see Figure 3.5), and unexplained zonal or panlobular steatosis [154]. Chronically suboptimal portal flow can cause NRH.

Differential Diagnosis

Linear zones of either ischemic necrosis and/or hepatocellular atrophy favor the suboptimal portal vein inflow; red blood cell congestion within central veins and centrilobular sinusoids and obliterative central venopathy favors suboptimal hepatic venous drainage; centrilobular hepatocyte ballooning or necrosis without congestion favors suboptimal hepatic arterial flow. Imaging studies are needed to specifically characterize vascular abnormalities.

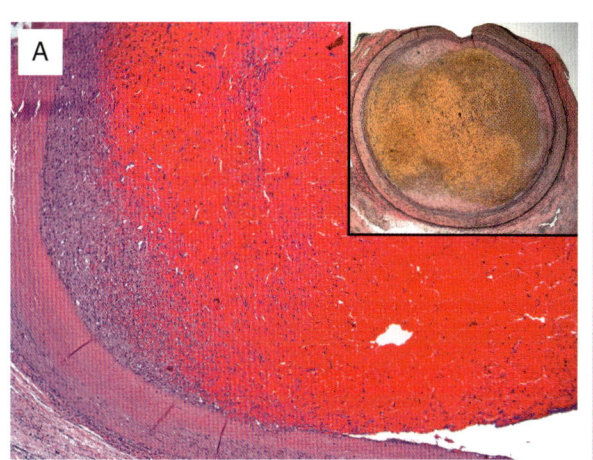

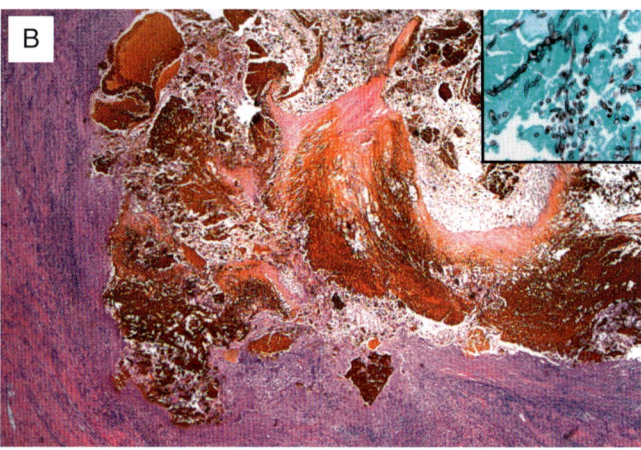

Figure 3.3 Sections through the hilum of a failed allograft with HAT (A) (Verhoeff-Van Gieson elastic stain in right upper inset) shows necrosis of the large bile duct with leakage of bile into the surrounding connective tissue (B). This necrotic tissue frequently becomes seated with bacteria and fungi (right upper inset).

Histopathology of Liver Transplantation

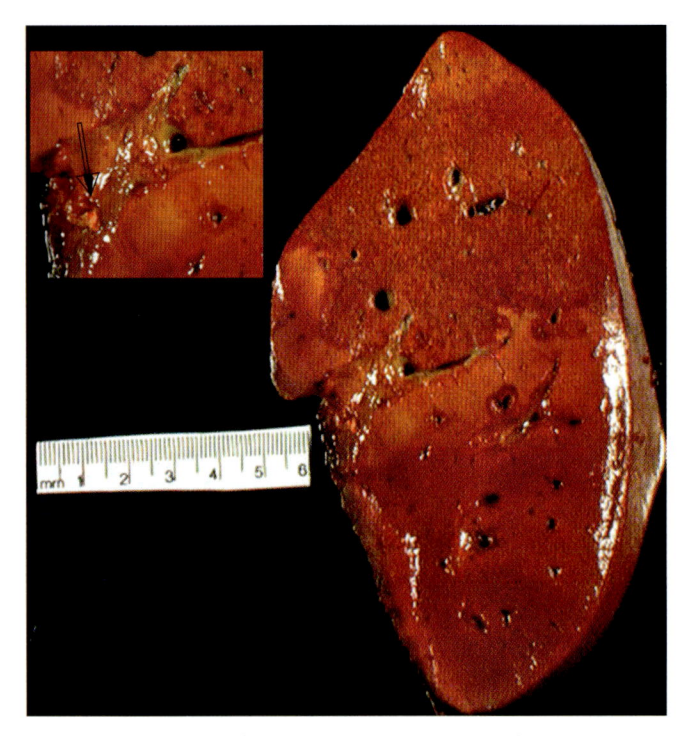

Figure 3.4 Thrombosis of the large extrahepatic portion of the portal vein (arrow in left upper inset) in a noncirrhotic allograft is relatively uncommon early after transplantation. When it does occur, it frequently results in large areas of necrosis and in zones of hepatocyte atrophy and/or necrosis represented by the mottled areas in this image.

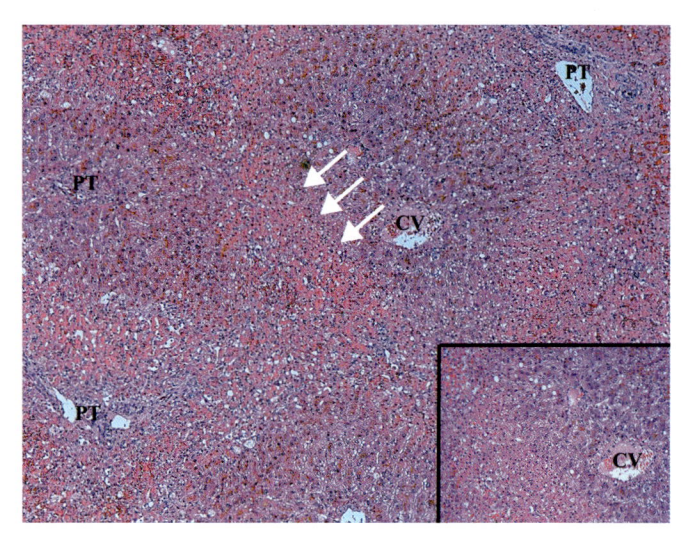

Figure 3.5 Microscopic examination of a liver with portal vein thrombosis often shows linear zones of ischemic hepatocytes, which can manifest as hepatocyte atrophy or coagulative necrosis (outlined by arrowheads) that are often periportal or mid zonal in distribution (lower right inset) (PT = portal tract; CV = central vein).

Hepatic Vein and Vena Caval Complications

Introduction and Clinical Presentation

Hepatic venous outflow complications are relatively uncommon. Risk factors include reduced-size/living donor allografts without inclusion of the middle hepatic vein [127, 155] and difficulties reconstructing the venous outflow tract [156].

Clinical presentation depends on the severity of outflow tract compromise: severe stenosis or thrombosis can present as the Budd-Chiari syndrome (e.g. hepatic enlargement, tenderness, and ascites with edema). Less severe stenosis might initially result only in histopathologic manifestations, or an increase in the portal vein/vena cava pressure gradient.

Histopathologic Findings

Perivenular sinusoidal congestion with or without focal hemorrhage, usually without perivenular lymphocytic inflammation, are the most reliable histopathologic findings. Bland centrilobular hepatocyte necrosis and dropout signal high-grade outflow compromise. Chronically suboptimal drainage changes include NRH, perivenular fibrosis, central vein occlusion, and veno-centric cirrhosis accompanied by a prominent ductular reaction at the interface zone and perivenular areas.

Differential Diagnosis

Centrilobular congestion and hemorrhage combined with significant lymphocytic, histiocytic, and/or lymphoplasmacytic inflammation suggests an immunologically mediated cause of injury, such as TCMR, autoimmune hepatitis (AIH), and drug-induced liver injury. However, perivenular inflammation might be only transiently present, rendering an immunological from mechanical cause indistinguishable [157]. Review of the clinical history and previous biopsies can help distinguish between these causes.

Bile Duct Complications

Introduction

Hepatic parenchymal health depends on biliary tree patency: complications occur in approximately 20% of recipients [37, 158–161] in whole cadaveric donors and a higher percentage in reduced-size allografts (reviewed in [37, 160, 161]). Biliary tract reconstruction varies considerably (reviewed in [160]); the most common types used in cadaveric whole organs are end-to-end, duct-to-duct, or donor biliary-recipient enteric anastomosis. Ischemic, traumatic, and immunologic injury [162, 163], especially when combined with abnormal anatomy, predispose to poor biliary tree wound healing [160, 164], biliary sludge, strictures/obstruction, anastomotic breakdown and bile leakage, cholangitic abscesses, ascending cholangitis, bile casts, ampullary dysfunction, and biliary-vascular fistulas (reviewed in [160, 165–168]).

Strictures are the most common complication. They are categorized according to time after transplantation and location: early and late, and anastomotic or non-anastomotic (intra-hepatic) (reviewed in [37, 158, 161, 165–168]). Intra-hepatic strictures are further categorized into peri-hilar versus peripheral.

Anastomotic strictures usually appear within the first several months after transplantation, but continue to occur, albeit less frequently, for the life of the allograft (reviewed in [158, 165, 166]). Risk factors include postoperative bile leaks, female donor-male recipient, and recent transplant year [158, 160, 165]. Anastomotic strictures are usually more amenable to treatment and less negatively impact both long-term graft and patient survival than non-anastomotic strictures [37, 158, 161, 165–168].

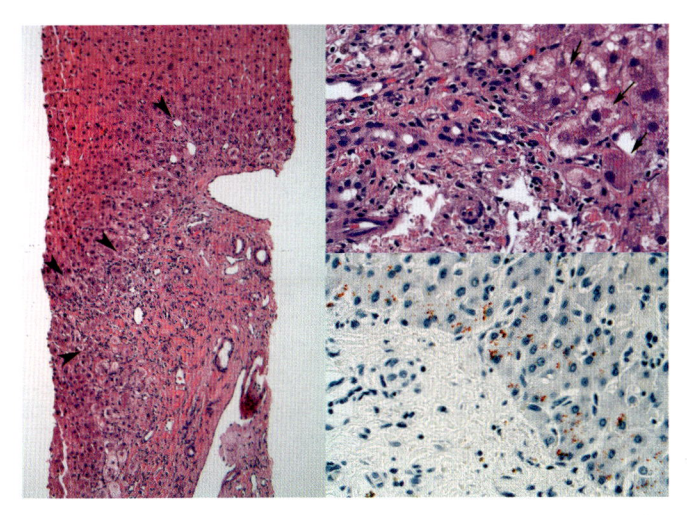

Figure 3.6 Chronic biliary tract strictures can show predominantly mononuclear inflammation with interface activity resembling late onset acute rejection and chronic hepatitis. This particular biopsy, obtained from a recipient fourteen years after transplantation, showed mild predominantly lymphoplasmacytic portal inflammation with interface activity (arrowheads, left panel). However, ductular reaction, periportal edema, periportal Mallory's hyaline (arrow, upper right panel), and deposition of copper in periportal hepatocytes (lower right panel) were the changes that pointed toward chronic biliary tract strictures.

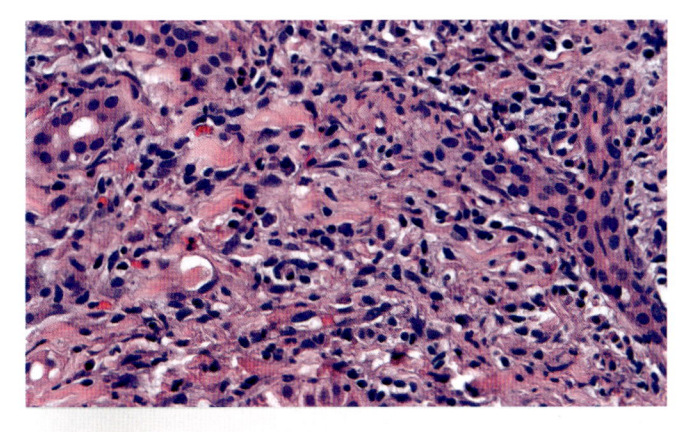

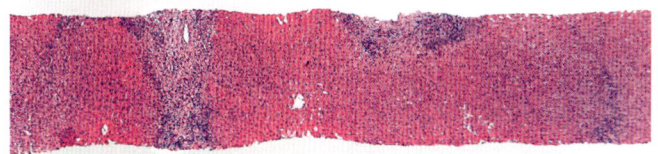

Figure 3.7 This example of obstructive cholangiopathy was detected eleven months after liver transplantation. Features used to establish the diagnosis included the prominent portal edema, ductular reaction, and predominantly acute portal inflammation. Note the significant portal eosinophilia (upper panel). In contrast to early after transplantation, late after transplantation, portal edema with eosinophilia should suggest obstructive cholangiopathy, especially in a patient with adequate immunosuppressive drug levels.

Conversely, non-anastomotic strictures usually occur later after transplantation, are more difficult to treat, cause progressive graft damage, and more negatively impact long-term graft and patient survival than anastomotic strictures [37, 158, 161, 165–168]. Risk factors include use of high viscosity preservation solution, primary sclerosing cholangitis (PSC) original disease, Roux-en-Y biliary anastomoses, CMV infection, and AMR [11, 37, 160–163, 165, 167–169]. Early (<1 year) non-anastomotic strictures are often associated with preservation-related injury [168, 170] and are usually located in peri-hilar bile ducts. As expected, risk factors include long cold and warm ischemic times, high viscosity preservation solution, older recipient age, a duct-to-duct biliary anastomosis, and bile leaks [168]. Late (>1 year) non-anastomotic strictures are usually located peripherally and associated with immunological risk factors, such as PSC as the original disease.

The peribiliary capillary plexus is susceptible to preservation/reperfusion damage during operative manipulation [171]. DCD donors predispose to leukocyte and platelet sludging and thrombosis in the peribiliary plexus, especially when combined with the viscous University of Wisconsin preservation solution [172, 173], which prevents adequate reperfusion (reviewed in [160]). Peribiliary plexus perfusion using thrombolytic agents and/or less viscous preservation solutions (e.g., HTK) [172, 173] before reperfusion with blood (reviewed in [160, 164, 174]), can mitigate these insults. Arterial and peribiliary capillary plexus can also be affected by: 1) severe spasm in the small-for-size syndrome [112]; 2) prolonged cold ischemia; 3) donor atherosclerotic disease; and 4) preformed or de novo anti-donor antibodies (e.g., ABO isoagglutinin or anti-HLA antibodies [160, 169, 175, 176]).

Clinical Presentation

Minor biliary tract complications, such as strictures and stones, usually first come to clinical recognition because of routine monitoring of liver injury tests that show selective elevation of γ-glutamyl transpeptidase and alkaline phosphatase. More serious biliary tract complications, such as obstruction, bacterial cholangitis, and biliary abscesses usually present with fever, jaundice, upper right quadrant pain, and intermittent bacteremia. Cholangiography (MRCP, ERCP (duct-to-duct) or percutaneous transhepatic cholangiography (PTC)) is needed to confirm the diagnosis and localize the defect(s) [158, 165, 177–179]. T-tube stents provide ready access for cholangiograms during the first three months after transplantation [160].

Histopathologic Findings

As in native livers, portal/periductal edema, predominantly neutrophilic portal inflammation, intra-epithelial and intra-luminal neutrophils within true bile ducts, varying severity ductular reaction, centrilobular hepatocanalicular cholestasis, and small neutrophils clusters spread randomly throughout the lobules are typical findings. Mixed or predominantly lymphocytic portal inflammation, biliary epithelial cell senescence changes, and low-grade ductopenia often evolve over time in recipients with chronic biliary tract strictures, mimicking chronic hepatitis (see Figure 3.6); later than one year after transplantation, portal eosinophilia can replace the neutrophilia (see Figure 3.7).

Biliary-vascular fistulas are rare complications recognized by red blood cells in lumen of bile ducts or bile casts surrounded by macrophages in portal vein branches. Inordinate conjugated serum bilirubin elevations beyond normal pathophysiologic ranges (>40 mg/dl), similar to that seen with renal failure, can also be seen. Transhepatic cholangiography can cause periductal hemorrhage surrounding small interlobular bile ducts for several days after the procedure [180].

Differential Diagnosis

Recurrent PSC cannot be reliably distinguished from other causes of biliary tract stricturing on peripheral needle biopsy evaluation. Features that favor biliary tract obstruction/stricturing over TCMR include neutrophilic-predominant portal infiltrate, periductal edema, and retention of the normal nuclear-to-cytoplasmic ratio in BEC, and an absence of perivenular mononuclear inflammation. TCMR is more likely when the portal infiltrate consists of blastic and small lymphocytes, plasma cells, eosinophils, lymphocytic cholangitis, and increased nuclear-to-cytoplasmic ratio in BEC and perivenular inflammation are seen. Portal eosinophilia early after transplantation favors TCMR, especially in patients treated with "steroid-sparing" IS regimens [181]. When portal capillary dilation accompanies the edema, acute AMR should also be considered, especially if accompanied by microvascular endothelial cell hypertrophy and monocyte/macrophage capillaritis [182].

Low-grade late onset and/or chronic biliary tract complications can occasionally present with predominantly mononuclear portal inflammation with variable, but usually low-grade, ductopenia [13, 15, 183] and can mimic TCMR, chronic viral and AIH (see Figure 3.6). Classically defined chronic rejection can also be especially difficult to distinguish from biliary strictures (especially recurrent PSC) (reviewed in [184]). Clinically at-risk populations are similar: both show "cholestatic" liver injury test elevations, and on biopsy, intra-hepatic cholestasis, biliary epithelial cell senescence changes, and small bile duct loss. Examination of the clinical history and serial biopsies are needed [13–15, 184, 185].

A history of biliary tract complications and/or PSC original disease, periductal lamellar edema involving septal ducts, stellate portal expansion, portal neutrophilia, and a ductular reaction, and, importantly, deposition of copper or copper-associated protein in periportal hepatocytes or ductular metaplasia of hepatocytes on CK7 staining favor biliary strictures/recurrent PSC. A previous history of TCMR, inadequate IS, lymphoplasmacytic portal inflammation, small portal tracts, absence of a ductular reaction, active central perivenulitis or perivenular fibrosis, and absence of periportal copper deposition favor TCMR and/or chronic rejection.

Findings in failed allografts used to distinguish between biliary strictures/recurrent PSC and classically defined chronic rejection are reviewed in [184]. Chronically rejected livers are usually of normal or slightly increased weight, lymph nodes are usually atrophic and/or fibrotic; hepatic artery branches show foam cell or concentric fibrointimal hyperplasia, and large bile ducts are uncommonly ulcerated. In contrast, failed allografts with obstructive cholangiography are usually enlarged, lymph nodes show bile-pigmented sinus histiocytosis, artery branches are either normal or show mild and focal eccentric fibrointimal hyperplasia, and extra-hepatic bile ducts often show focal ulceration, periductal lymphoplasmacytic inflammation, and fibrosis. Recurrent or de novo IgG4 sclerosing disease should also be considered when plasma cells are abundant [186].

Angiography and cholangiography also help distinguish obstructive cholangiopathy and classically-defined chronic rejection. "Pruning" of the peripheral arterial and biliary trees and poor peripheral filling are seen in chronic rejection, whereas some intra-hepatic duct dilation is observed with obstructive cholangiopathy and arterial changes are either not present or not significant.

Cholangitis favors a biliary tract complication whereas cholangiolitis, lobular disarray, and mononuclear inflammation favor chronic viral or AIH. The cholestatic liver injury tests profile favors obstructive cholangiopathy, except for patients with cholestatic variants of viral hepatitis or DILI. Review of HBV and/or HCV nucleic acid levels and drug history helps to distinguish among these possibilities. Cholestatic viral hepatitis is variably associated with very high levels of viral replication (e.g., >30 million IU/mL HCV RNA) [187]. Deposits of copper or copper-associated protein and/or ductular metaplasia of periportal hepatocytes on CK7 staining point toward obstructive cholangiopathy.

Rejection

General Considerations

Liver allograft rejection can be categorized into acute AMR, TCMR, and chronic rejection similar to other solid organ allografts. Chronic AMR is an emerging diagnosis that is currently incompletely defined (reviewed in [11, 209]). Isolated acute AMR is rare and usually occurs within the first several weeks after transplantation in ABO-incompatible allografts and in recipients usually showing polyspecific and high mean fluorescence intensity (MFI) DSA in solid phase assays and strongly positive lymphocytotoxic crossmatch in cell-based assays [175, 182, 188, 189]. Effective IS has made "classical" TCMR and chronic rejection uncommon-to-rare causes of allograft failure [108, 190, 191], but other morphological manifestations of chronic rejection are emerging, discussed below [11, 192].

Antibody-mediated Rejection (AMR)

General Considerations

ABO incompatible (ABO-I) recipients harboring high titer iso-agglutinins (≥1:64) predictably experience severe liver allograft injury shortly after transplantation [163, 169, 193–196]. Consequently, ABO-I transplants are generally avoided in most North American and European countries because of the potential for acute AMR and availability of an alternative donor source. Asian programs, however, more often utilize ABO-I and accept the penalty of increased biliary strictures ([163, 169, 193–195]) – the major risk of ABO-I AMR [175, 195, 196].

Liver allografts are resistant to, but not exempt from, anti-HLA class I and II antibody-related acute AMR when compared to heart and kidney allografts (reviewed in [11, 125, 162, 192]). DSA status, therefore, does not: a) usually influence organ triage/recipient selection at the vast majority of centers [125, 175, 197]; or b) routinely influence short-term survival [125, 197–199]; but c) can be associated with increased rejection rates, fibrosis progression, and decreased survival at some centers [188, 192, 200–202].

The presence pre-transplant of antibodies associated with a positive complement-dependent cytotoxicity (CDC+) crossmatch are encountered in approximately 10%–15% of recipients with a female and autoimmune predilection [125, 175, 198, 199, 203–206]; current solid phase assays yield similar results (reviewed in [192]). Approximately 96% of cell-based CDC- recipients are DSA-, but >50% of class I or II DSA+ patients were also CDC- [203]. Risk factors for acute AMR include polyspecific and high-titer (or high MFI (MFI >5000) after dilution runs) by single antigen bead testing, but only 5%–20% of DSA+ recipients have high enough titers to cause clinically significant liver injury [11, 125, 175, 188, 192].

Clinical Presentation

Hyperacute AMR occurring in the operating room is rare because of pre-transplant ABO isoagglutinin titer and anti-HLA DSA testing. When it has rarely occurred (reviewed in [162]), initial signs of problems emerged immediately after complete revascularization, including uneven reperfusion, swelling, dusky appearance, cessation of bile flow, difficulty in achieving hemostasis and coagulopathy, and inordinate need for platelets and other blood products [163].

Acute AMR more commonly presents with increased serum bilirubin and ALT/AST during the first several days to weeks, associated with persistence of high titer isoagglutinins or DSA, unexplained and refractory thrombocytopenia, and low serum complement activity [11, 175, 205, 207]. Hepatic angiograms often show segmental narrowing indicative of immunologically mediated arterial vasospasm and diffuse luminal narrowing with poor peripheral filling (reviewed in [162]).

Histopathologic Features

Acute AMR (Table 3.2) defined in the era of solid phase DSA testing [11, 182, 188, 208] depends on biopsy timing and the (sub-) class, titer, and specificity of the anti-donor antibodies (ABO, DSA, etc.) (reviewed in [11, 162, 188]), though there are now BANFF criteria for diagnosing Acute AMR [209]. Isoagglutinins generally cause more red blood cell congestion and necrosis than anti-HLA antibodies [11] (see Figures 3.8, 3.9, and 3.10).

Post-reperfusion biopsies from recipients harboring high titer (>1:32–64) isoagglutinins usually show sinusoidal and portal vein sludging with platelet-fibrin thrombi, neutrophils, and red blood cells, often accompanied by focal Disse's space and portal connective tissue hemorrhage and spotty hepatocellular apoptosis/necrosis [163]. In patients that develop ABO-I AMR, the following findings often appear during the first week: portal microvascular endothelial cell hypertrophy, focal fibrin deposition, portal edema, small, often periportal, clusters of hepatocytes showing coagulative necrosis [163, 196], mild neutrophilic portal inflammation accompanied by a ductular reaction, acute cholangitis, with or without small portal artery fibrinoid necrosis.

Portal stromal C4d deposition is said to be characteristic of acute ABO-I AMR during the first weeks [210]. Microvascular endothelial cell C4d deposition does not necessarily correlate with other features of acute AMR in those with low-titer (<1:32–64) isoagglutinins [193]. Untreated ABO-I acute

Table 3.2

Criteria for diagnosis of acute AMR (all four are required): Adapted from O'Leary et al. 2014 [182, 209]

1 Histopathological pattern of injury consistent with acute AMR
    - Marked portal microvascular endothelial cell hypertrophy
    - Monocytic, eosinophilic, and neutrophilic portal microvasculitis
    - Portal edema, ductular reaction, and variable cholestasis

2 Diffuse microvascular C4d deposition (on frozen or formalin-fixed or paraffin-embedded tissue)
3 Circulating DSA in serum samples measured within two weeks of biopsy (>5000 MFI on a single antigen bead test or positive lymphocytotoxic crossmatch)
4 Reasonable exclusion of other insults that might cause a similar pattern of injury

AMR can progress to hemorrhagic infarction and organ failure; patients successfully treated for ABO-I AMR can later develop biliary strictures [162, 169, 211–213].

Post-reperfusion biopsies from patients with high titer/high MFI (>15,000) despite serial dilutions of anti-HLA DSA can show platelet aggregates in portal and/or central veins [118, 175] and diffuse portal microvasculature C4d staining [188, 204]. The following histopathological findings appear within days to several weeks in those developing acute DSA-AMR: portal microvascular endothelial hypertrophy and cytoplasmic eosinophilia; microvascular dilatation and capillaritis mediated by macrophages, eosinophils, and neutrophils involving portal vein branches; inlet venules, portal capillaries, peribiliary plexus capillaries, and occasionally central veins; periportal edema and a ductular reaction; and spotty hepatocyte necrosis, centrilobular hepatocellular swelling, and hepatocanalicular cholestasis. Focal bile duct necrosis and arterial changes strongly suggestive of arterial vasospasm or lymphocytic arteritis can rarely appear in severe cases (see Figure 3.10), but these are diagnostic of acute AMR when seen in conjunction with diffuse C4d deposits and DSA [175, 182, 188, 214]. Superimposed TCMR is frequently also present [175].

The current diagnostic criteria (Table 3.2) needed to establish an acute AMR diagnosis include: 1) histopathological changes consistent with AMR; 2) exclusion of other insults causing a similar injury pattern; 3) serum DSA; and 4) strong and diffuse complement (C4d) deposition (see Figures 3.11 and 3.12) [125, 182, 188, 207, 215, 216] defined as strong portal vein and capillary and usually periportal sinusoidal endothelial staining involving a majority of portal tracts.

Differential Diagnosis

Distinguishing AMR from preservation/reperfusion injury and biliary strictures can be quite difficult, but pre-sensitization (high titer/MFI after dilution of isoagglutinins, DSA, etc.), persistence of serum antibodies after transplantation, diffuse microvascular endothelial C4d staining [125], and

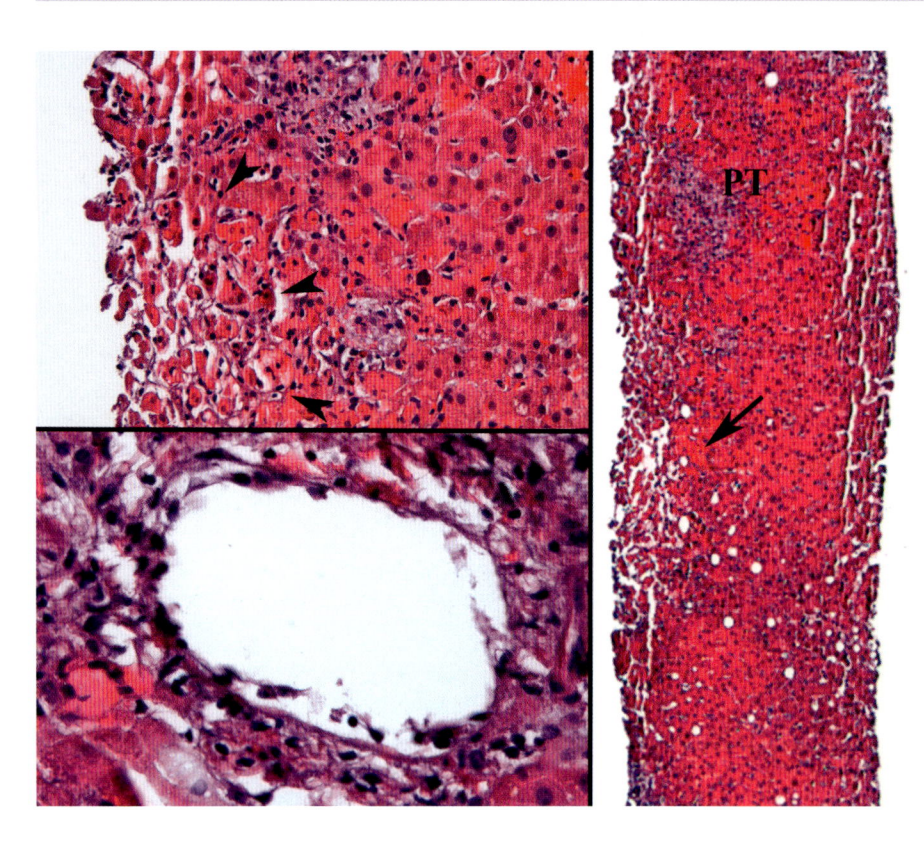

Figure 3.8 AMR of an ABO-incompatible liver allograft usually causes significantly more damage than lymphocytotoxic antibodies. This biopsy was obtained eight days after transplantation of an ABO-incompatible liver. Note the mild, predominantly neutrophilic portal inflammation (upper left panel) and patchy areas of coagulative necrosis (arrow), which are illustrated at higher magnification in the upper left inset. Note also the endothelial cell reactivity of the central vein illustrated at higher magnification in the lower left inset (PT = portal tract). Follow-up tissue samples from this particular patient are illustrated in Figures 3.9 and 3.10.

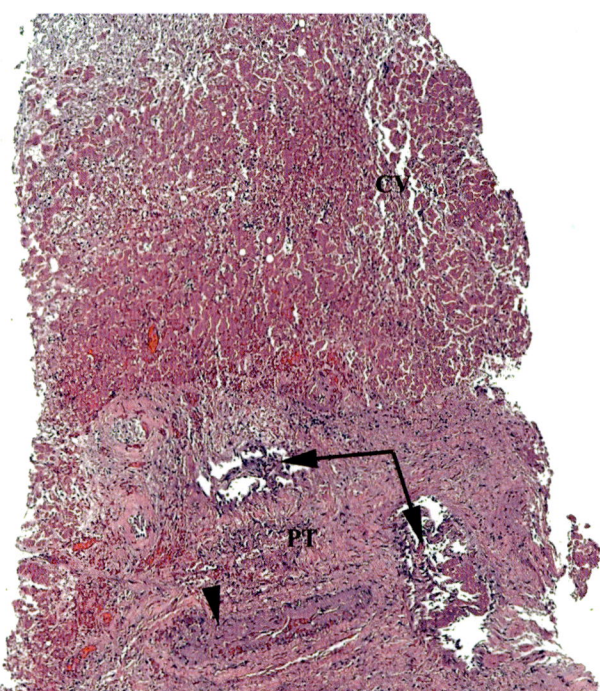

Figure 3.9 Follow-up biopsy at fourteen days after liver transplantation of the same patient illustrated in Figure 3.8. The biopsy now shows widespread coagulative necrosis, flame-shaped portal vein thrombi (arrows), and focal fibrinoid necrosis of a hepatic artery branch (arrowhead) (PT = portal tract; CV = central vein).

Figure 3.10 Follow-up failed allograft specimen from the patient whose biopsy specimens were illustrated in Figures 3.8 and 3.9, obtained at eighteen days after transplantation. This ABO-incompatible liver allograft showed findings typical of severe AMR, such as fibrointimal hyperplasia of the peri-hilar hepatic artery branches (arrowhead). When viewed at higher magnification (lower right inset), significant neutrophilic and lymphocytic intimal inflammation were easily detectable. Note also that the large bile duct is totally necrotic and bile has leaked into the surrounding connective tissue, which is severely inflamed. This illustrates that AMR is an important cause of ischemic cholangitis. Note also the bacterial colonies in the necrotic bile duct wall (left lower inset).

post-transplant clinical and laboratory profiles provide discriminating information. DSA+ acute AMR should be suspected in female liver allograft recipients with high titer DSA who show DSA persistence after transplantation and develop graft dysfunction, refractory and otherwise unexplained thrombocytopenia, and circulating low complement levels [11, 125, 175, 182, 188, 205, 207].

Histopathology of Liver Transplantation

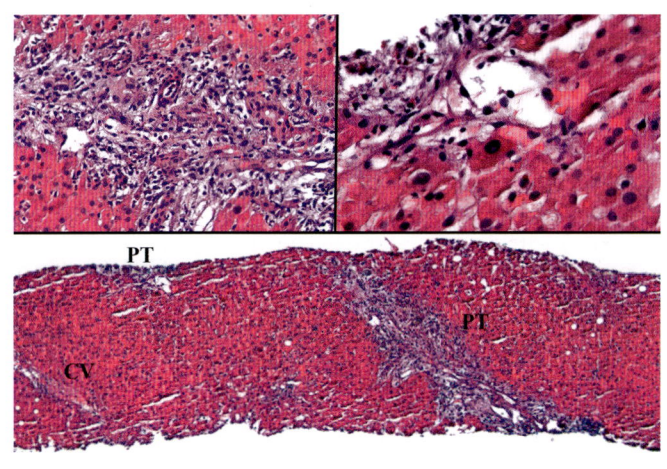

Figure 3.11 AMR in a recipient with a strong (usually >1:32–64) lymphocytotoxic cross-match is usually detected within the first week after transplantation and closely resembles preservation/reperfusion injury. Features include mild, predominantly neutrophilic portal inflammation and mild cholangiolar proliferation (upper left inset), sinusoidal leukocytosis, and reactive-appearing endothelial cells in the portal and/or central veins (upper right inset). These changes, however, can be subtle, are not entirely specific, and require clinical pathological correlation (see text) and demonstration of immunoglobulin and complement in the tissues (see Figure 3.12) (PT = portal tract; CV = central vein).

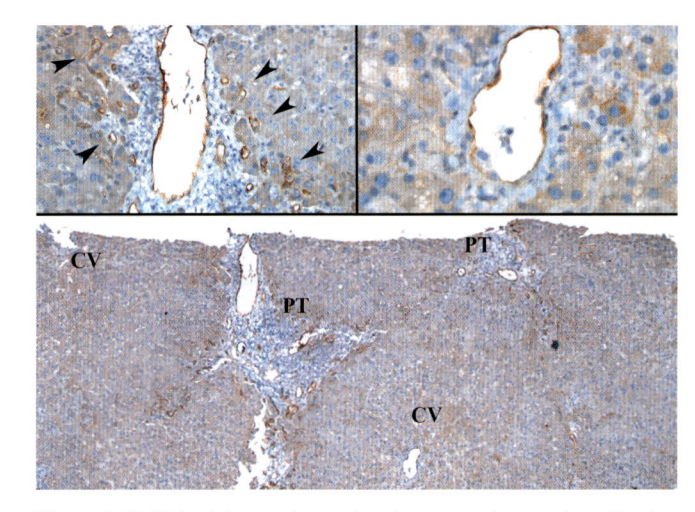

Figure 3.12 C4d staining can be used to detect complement deposition in FFPE tissue samples. This biopsy is the same biopsy as illustrated in Figure 3.11, obtained from a recipient with a strongly positive lymphocytotoxic crossmatch six days after liver transplantation. Note the strong staining in the portal vein (upper left inset), hepatic artery, sinusoidal (upper left inset, arrowheads), and central vein endothelium (upper right inset) (PT = portal tract; CV = central vein).

AMR should be histopathologically favored over preservation/reperfusion injury and biliary stricturing when the following findings are detected in biopsies: 1) portal capillary dilatation combined with endothelial cell hypertrophy and reactivity; 2) margination of macrophages, eosinophils, neutrophils, and to a lesser extent, lymphocytes, along the luminal aspect of the portal microvasculature and central veins; and 3) diffuse microvascular endothelial C4d staining. Portal/periportal edema, necrosis, and congestion and hemorrhage should raise the possibility of ABO-I acute AMR.

Chronic Antibody-mediated Injury

Candidate histopathological lesions of chronic AMR are emerging primarily from studies of: 1) long-term follow-up of pediatric liver allograft recipients [217–223]; 2) suboptimally immunosuppressed recipients, some included in IS minimization trials [11, 203, 217, 222–225]; and 3) long-term survival that includes protocol serum and biopsy sampling [226].

Histopathological changes observed in Japanese pediatric IS weaning trials were the first to suggest a chronic AMR phenotype that included: increased periportal and perivenular fibrosis with or without co-existent lymphocytic inflammation. These changes were either directly or indirectly attributed to IS minimization [222, 227, 228] and associated with anti-HLA class II DSA (esp. anti-DQ), endothelial and stromal C4d, and CD20+ perivenular infiltrates [222]. Peribiliary capillary plexus and sinusoidal endothelial cell HLA-DR upregulation was spatially linked with nearby inflammation, which was most prominent in patients with co-existent TCMR with or without perivenular fibrosis [223]. Re-institution or increasing IS decreased C4d deposits and stabilized or reversed perivenular fibrosis [228].

Only a few studies exist of protocol follow-up biopsy findings after sustained lowering or withdrawal of IS [100, 229–231, 232] Stellate and Endothelial Phenotype Monitoring in ITN029ST Tolerance Pediatric Liver Transplant Recipients over 5+ Years of Follow-up). However, not all patients that develop de novo or recurrent DSA after weaning experience significant liver inflammation, TCMR, fibrosis, architectural deterioration, or changes in sinusoidal endothelial (CD34- to CD34+) or stellate cell phenotype (SMA- to SMA+) within five years [232].

Since most original pediatric diseases do not recur following transplantation, recognizing potential chronic AMR changes has been less challenging than in adults where disease recurrence is common. Included is a spectrum of relatively potentially associated histopathological findings: non-inflammatory portal/periportal, sinusoidal, and perivenular fibrosis, portal tract collagenization, low-grade portal inflammation ± necro-inflammatory-type interface activity, plasma cell hepatitis, portal venopathy/NRH, and variable but usually positive microvascular endothelial C4d staining, have been associated with chronic DSA [11, 217, 219, 220, 222, 226, 232]. Except for obliterative arteriopathy, many candidate lesions can also be caused by technical complications [100, 229, 233].

Differential Diagnosis for Chronic AMR

Three proposed criteria used for establishing a chronic AMR diagnosis: (1) A high cAMR score, which includes weighted clinical and histopathological variables: 0.226 (HCV) + 0.7748 (Lobular inflammation severity) + 0.3901 (interface hepatitis) + 0.3561 (portal tract collagenization) + 0.2886 (portal venopathy) + 0.116 (sinusoidal fibrosis) × 10. The HCV status is scored as no=0; yes=1. The histopathological variables are scored as 0: none; 1: minimal; 2: mild; 3: moderate; and 4: severe. (2) Serum DSA (>10,000 MFI). (3) Other potential causes of a similar injury pattern should be reasonably excluded. Most cases are also some C4d-positivity, but, as in renal allografts with chronic AMR [234], C4d staining can wax and wane [226]. A cAMR score >27.5, optimized to 80% sensitivity and specificity predicted a 50% ten-year allograft failure rate [226].

Many features, listed above, are also seen with recurrent viral, autoimmune, and idiopathic post-transplant hepatitis (IPTH); portal tract collagenization is less common and not widely recognized. In addition, the lobular inflammation is often perivenular, as noted in earlier IS weaning studies [222, 227, 228]. Negative serological studies for hepatitis A, B, C, and E infection with positive serum DSA and C4d staining favor chronic AMR. Banff criteria for chronic AMR have now been established [209]; however, more work is needed in this area.

Interpretation of C4d Staining

IgG, IgM, C3, and C4 can be detected by immunofluorescence staining in frozen sections in sinusoids, peri-hilar arteries, portal veins, and peribiliary plexus in association with high titer DSA+ recipients with acute AMR, but these deposits are present only transiently [163, 175, 207]. C4d staining improves detection of complement deposition in liver allografts with AMR because it: a) persists for several days after deposition; b) survives in FFPE tissues; and c) usually correlates with serum DSA [11, 125, 189, 216, 235, 236].

No studies of liver allografts have directly compared frozen versus immunoperoxidase staining on FFPE C4d staining. Frozen tissue can be more sensitive for kidney allograft C4d staining [237, 238], but frozen liver tissue can be difficult to interpret. Sinusoidal C4d labeling is also more often detected in frozen tissue. Immunoperoxidase staining of FFPE tissue affects sensitivity; pressure cooker and high-pH (pH = 9.0 vs. 6.0) antigen retrieval often yield more sensitive results, but background staining can be problematic [210, 235, 239–245].

Liver allograft biopsies without significant pathology are usually negative for endothelial cell C4d staining, but nonspecific C4d staining can be seen in arterial elastic laminas, portal and perivenular elastic fibers, necrotic and steatotic hepatocytes, and areas of sinusoidal fibrosis. Portal vein and capillary, sinusoidal, central vein, arterial endothelium, lymphoid nodules, and periductal and portal stromal cell C4d staining have been described in *native pediatric livers* with hepatitis B (HBV) and C (HCV), and AIH [246] and in allografts when other insults are thought to be the primary cause of allograft dysfunction, such as biliary obstruction [235], recurrent HBV [239] or HCV [241], and plasma cell hepatitis (*de novo* AIH) [247]. However, endothelial C4d deposits in rejection-*un*related allograft disorders are reportedly less prevalent and intense than in acute AMR [204, 208, 216, 240, 248, 249]. In addition, AMR can be superimposed on other causes of liver allograft dysfunction when the diagnosis is based on H&E stains alone.

Regardless, microvascular endothelial C4d staining of portal veins, capillary and artery branches, and sinusoids has been significantly associated with anti-HLA DSA [243] in recipients with isolated AMR [207, 245]. C4d staining has also been observed in association with macrophage and plasma cell infiltrates [240], microvasculitis [175, 188], and TCMR [125, 210, 215, 235, 239–245], which, in some studies, was directly proportional to BANFF grade [210, 235, 239–245]. Portal microvascular and sinusoidal endothelial cell C4d staining appears to be most specific for *acute AMR*, but "portal C4d stromal" staining has also been described in ABO-incompatible AMR [210], ACR [243], and chronic rejection [215, 250].

Microvascular endothelial cell HLA class II expression can vary depending on co-existent pathology [226]. The pattern of C4d staining, however, can be contextual: central perivenulitis associated with TCMR locally upregulates HLA class II, leading to preferential C4d deposition in central vein and perivenular sinusoidal endothelium.

T Cell-mediated Rejection (TCMR)

Introduction and Clinical Presentation

TCMR has been defined as, "inflammation of the allograft, elicited by a genetic disparity between the donor and recipient, primarily affecting interlobular bile ducts and vascular endothelia, including portal and hepatic veins and occasionally the hepatic artery and its branches" [251]. *Early (≤6 months) TCMR* usually presents between 5–30 days after transplantation and currently affects approximately 30% of recipients [252]. Risk factors include the IS regimen, young and "healthy" recipients (normal serum creatinine, Child's classification, etc.), HLA-DR mismatch, recipient dysregulated immune syndromes (e.g., PSC, AIH and PBC), prolonged cold ischemia, older donor, and HLA-C genotype (reviewed in [252, 253]). It rarely leads to allograft failure or permanent allograft damage, and is usually amenable to treatment [108, 254].

Clinical findings are often absent in early or mild TCMR, but fever, allograft enlargement, cyanosis, and tenderness are often seen with severe TCMR; non-selective elevations of standard liver injury tests, leukocytosis, and eosinophilia are also frequently present [251]. Decreased bile flow, thin and pale bile, ascites, liver swelling, and increased lymph production can occasionally occur [251]. A variety of proteins (e.g., interleukins, neopterin, amyloid A protein, etc.) are increased in the peripheral blood, but none are routinely used to monitor recipients (reviewed in [255]). Sensitized patients and those suboptimally immunosuppressed can experience earlier TCMR, while recipients treated with lymphocyte-depleting antibodies can have later presentations.

Late onset (≥1 year) TCMR is often associated with inadequate IS, development of DSA [226], and is more frequently treatment-resistant and causes allograft failure (reviewed in [253, 256, 257]). Histopathologically late onset TCMR more closely resembles chronic hepatitis, and more often results in fibrosis and architectural distortion, possibly related to a treatment delay [229, 252, 257, 258].

Histopathologic Findings and Grading

Early TCMR features include: a) predominantly mononuclear but mixed portal inflammation containing blastic or activated lymphocytes, neutrophils, and eosinophils; b) subendothelial inflammation of portal and/or terminal hepatic venules; and c) bile duct inflammation and damage [251, 259]. *Minimal diagnostic criteria needed to establish the diagnosis of TCMR include at least two of the above histopathologic findings.* The diagnosis is

Histopathology of Liver Transplantation

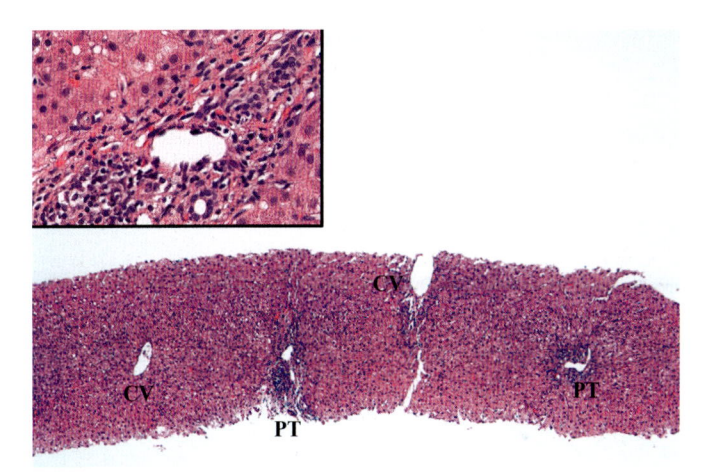

Figure 3.13 This biopsy shows histopathological evidence of mild acute cellular rejection. Only two portal tracts shown in this biopsy, which contains ten other portal tracts were inflamed. The upper left inset shows the characteristic "rejection-type" portal infiltrate comprised of blastic and small lymphocytes and eosinophils and focal bile duct inflammation and damage (PT = portal tract; CV = central vein).

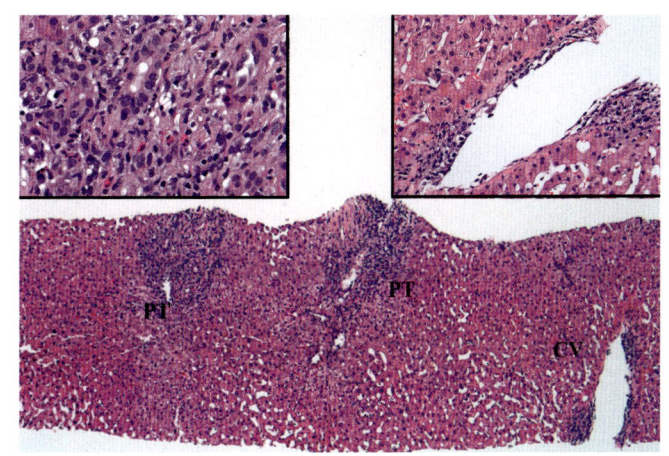

Figure 3.14 In moderate acute cellular rejection, a rejection type infiltrate noticeably expands most or all of the portal tracts, as shown in this photomicrograph. The upper right inset illustrates classic "endothelialitis," or infiltration of inflammatory cells into the subendothelial space. The upper left inset nicely illustrates the pleomorphic, typical, "rejection-type" infiltrate comprising blastic and small lymphocytes, eosinophils, and neutrophils (PT = portal tract; CV = central vein).

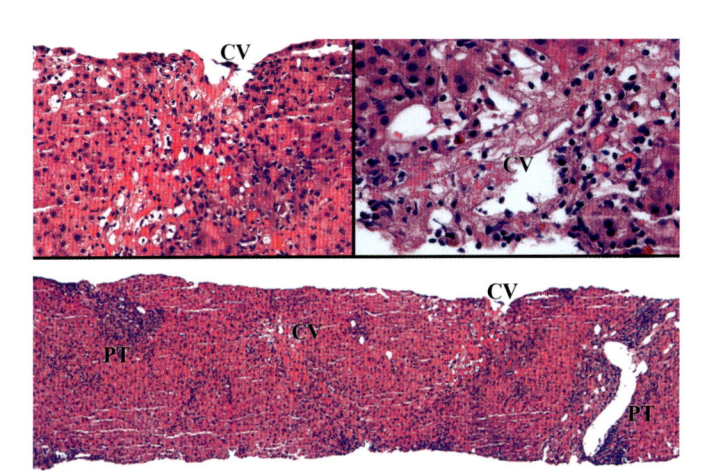

Figure 3.15 This example, a moderate-to-severe acute cellular rejection, shows noticeable expansion of most or all of the portal tracts by a significant infiltrate. In addition, this biopsy shows a similar infiltrate in the perivenular regions (upper right inset) in some areas with congestion and hemorrhage (upper left inset) in other areas (PT = portal tract; CV = central vein).

strengthened if greater than 50% of the ducts or terminal hepatic veins are damaged or if unequivocal endothelialitis of portal or terminal hepatic vein branches can be identified. Histopathologic evidence of severe injury includes perivenular inflammation, centrilobular necrosis, arteritis, and inflammatory, usually central-to-central, bridging inflammation/necrosis [251, 254].

Early TCMR "rejection-type" infiltrates, described above, preferentially involve portal tracts (see Figure 3.13), but also surround central veins in severe episodes. "Endothelialitis" or infiltration of lymphocytes underneath the portal and central vein endothelium is a characteristic feature that can also be seen with other causes of allograft dysfunction [260] (see Figure 3.14). Immunophenotypic analysis of TCMR infiltrates usually shows a predominance of T-lymphocytes with CD8+ cells surrounding and invading bile ducts [261, 262] with far fewer B cells. Macrophages and other leukocytes usually predominate in severe early TCMR [261–263]. Immunophenotypic analysis of graft infiltrating lymphocytes has not proven to be prognostically useful, except for distinguishing TCMR (T cell predominant) from most PTLD (B cell predominant; also See Differential Diagnosis).

Lymphocytes inside the ductal basement membrane of small interlobular bile ducts (<100 μm shortest diameter) is an important diagnostic feature and associated with BEC injury and repair, including perinuclear vacuolization, apoptosis, and increased nuclear-to-cytoplasmic ratio, mitoses, and nucleoli. Breaks in the basement membrane signify severe bile duct damage. Cytoplasmic eosinophilia and multinucleation signal senescence-related changes [183].

Inflammatory and/or necrotizing arteritis is a feature of severe TCMR, but is rarely detected in needle biopsies because affected arteries are rarely sampled [264]. Interface necroinflammatory activity is not seen with typical early mild and moderate TCMR, but spillover of portal infiltrates into periportal sinusoids can be seen with severe TCMR [229].

Early TCMR-type infiltrates can also be seen around terminal hepatic venules and sublobular veins – so-called "central perivenulitis" [229]. This feature is present in up to 30% of TCMR episodes, especially late (>100 days) after transplantation, when it is more commonly seen. *Severe TCMR should be diagnosed only when typical portal changes of TCMR are accompanied by perivenular inflammation and zonal centrilobular congestion, hemorrhage, and hepatocyte necrosis and dropout* (see Figures 3.15 and 3.16).

The BANFF Grading schema for TCMR and chronic rejection (Table 3.3A and 3.3B) [259, 209] is widely utilized [265], simple and easy to apply, reproducible [266], scientifically correct, and has been shown to have prognostic significance in prospective [254] and retrospective studies [267]. Descriptive grades of indeterminate, mild, moderate, and severe rejection (Table 3.3A) are with a semi-quantitative rejection activity index (RAI) (Table 3.3B) [259] – a remnant of the European

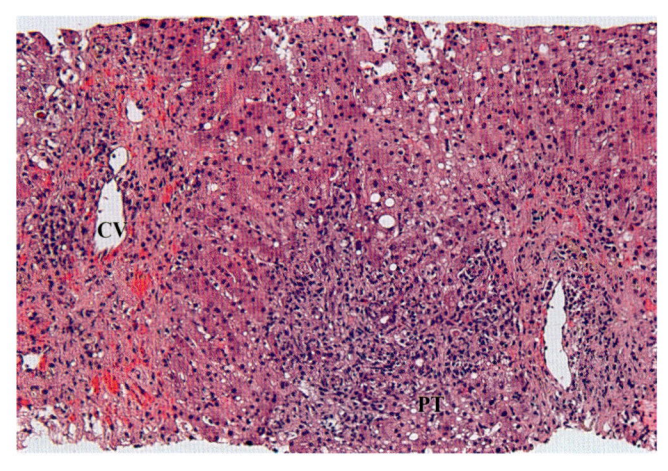

Figure 3.16 Severe acute cellular rejection shows noticeable expansion of most or all portal tracts by a rejection-type infiltrate, as in moderate acute cellular rejection. Note, however, that there is also prominent central perivenulitis associated with perivenular hepatocyte necrosis and dropout. Biopsy showing only the perivenular changes, without the portal tract changes, should not be diagnosed as "severe" acute cellular rejection (PT = portal tract; CV = central vein).

Table 3.3A BANFF Grading of Acute Liver Allograft Rejection [259, 209]

Global Assessment	Criteria
Indeterminate	Portal inflammatory infiltrate that fails to meet the criteria for the diagnosis of acute rejection (see text)
Mild	Rejection infiltrate in a minority of the triads, generally mild and confined within the portal spaces
Moderate	Rejection infiltrate, expanding most or all of the triads
Severe	As above for moderate, with spillover into periportal areas and moderate-to-severe perivenular inflammation that extends into the hepatic parenchyma and is associated with perivenular hepatocyte necrosis

NOTE: Global assessment of rejection grade is made on review of the entire biopsy, and only after the diagnosis of rejection has been established. It is inappropriate to provide a "rejection grade" when the diagnosis of rejection is uncertain.
*Verbal description of mild, moderate, or severe acute rejection could also be labeled as Grade I, II, and III, respectively.

grading system [268] and conceptual equivalent of the hepatitis activity index [269]. RAI semi-quantitatively scores the prevalence and severity of three separate histopathologic features on a scale of 0 to 3: portal inflammation, bile duct damage, and subendothelial inflammation. Individual components are added together for a total possible RAI score of "9," which is rarely achieved [254].

Total RAI scores directly correlate with descriptive grading and an increased risk of persistent/recurrent TCMR, chronic rejection, and graft failure [254]. Usual ranges of RAI scores are indeterminate [1–2], mild [3–4], moderate [5–7], and severe TCMR (>7). Most isolated episodes of early TCMR are graded as "mild," have a total RAI <6, respond to increased IS, and rarely lead to permanent scarring, bile duct loss, arteriopathy, or allograft failure [254].

Additional IS given before a biopsy specimen is obtained alters the histopathological appearance, making interpretation more difficult. Potential treatment-related changes include loss of subendothelial infiltration, decreased inflammation, increased centrilobular hepatocyte swelling, and hepatocanalicular cholestasis. Complete resolution of changes after treatment generally requires seven to ten days or more.

Late onset TCMR (>1 year) appears similar to early TCMR, as described above, but evolution of the response is also frequently seen (reviewed in [229]): fewer blastic lymphocytes, more necro-inflammatory type interface activity, less venous subendothelial inflammation, a higher incidence of perivenular inflammation, and slightly more lobular activity, which cause these biopsies to more closely resemble chronic hepatitis (reviewed in [229]). Indeed, late onset TCMR often presents exclusively or predominantly as perivenular lymphocytic inflammation and hepatocyte dropout with minimal or no portal tract changes (so-called "central perivenulitis") [270–272]. Isolated central perivenulitis can evolve into typical or classical chronic rejection with ductopenia and perivenular fibrosis, presenting with Budd-Chiari or a veno-occlusive-like clinical syndrome when severe [157, 273]. BANFF criteria grading of central perivenulitis is shown below [229]:

"Minimal" and "mild" cases, as described above, may resolve spontaneously [271], but sampling errors cannot be excluded. Moderate and severe perivenular changes probably warrant more aggressive treatment to avoid progressive fibrosis, but randomized trials have not been carried out.

Differential Diagnosis

Distinguishing among TCMR, preservation injury, and obstructive cholangiopathy/cholangitis was discussed above. Late onset TCMR needs to be distinguished from all of the various causes of allograft hepatitis (viruses, drugs, autoimmunity), chronically suboptimal biliary drainage, and various causes of perivenular fibrosis.

TCMR and chronic hepatitis show predominantly lymphohistiocytic portal inflammation, lymphocytic cholangitis, and acidophilic necrosis of hepatocytes. The severity and prevalence of bile duct damage, interface activity, lobular changes, and perivenular inflammation can be used to correctly categorize most cases [187]. Features favoring TCMR include lymphocytic cholangitis and perivenular inflammation involving a majority of the ducts and central veins, respectively, and low-grade or absent lobular and interface necro-inflammatory activity. Conversely, interface and lobular necro-inflammatory activity predominating over bile duct damage and perivenular changes favor chronic hepatitis.

Table 3.3B Acute RAI [259, 209]

Category	Criteria	Score
Portal Inflammation	Mostly lymphocytic inflammation involving, but not noticeably expanding, a minority of the triads	1
	Expansion of most or all of the triads, by a mixed infiltrate containing lymphocytes with occasional blasts, neutrophils, and eosinophils	2
	Marked expansion of most or all of the triads by a mixed infiltrate containing numerous blasts and eosinophils with inflammatory spillover into the periportal parenchyma	3
Bile Duct Inflammation Damage	A minority of the ducts are cuffed and infiltrated by inflammatory cells and show only mild reactive changes, such as increased nuclear:cytoplasmic ratio of the epithelial cells	1
	Most or all of the ducts infiltrated by inflammatory cells. More than an occasional duct shows degenerative changes such as nuclear pleomorphism, disordered polarity, and cytoplasmic vacuolization of the epithelium	2
	As above for 2, with most or all of the ducts showing degenerative changes or focal luminal disruption	3
Venous Endothelial Inflammation	Subendothelial lymphocytic infiltration involving some, but not a majority, of the portal and/or hepatic venules	1
	Subendothelial infiltration involving most or all of the portal and/or hepatic venules	2
	As above for 2, with moderate or severe perivenular inflammation that extends into the perivenular parenchyma and is associated with perivenular hepatocyte necrosis	3

NOTE: Total RAI Score = Sum of all component scores for portal inflammation, bile duct inflammation/damage, and venous endothelial inflammation.

Table 3.3C BANFF Criteria of Central Perivenulitis

Descriptor	Findings
Minimal/Indeterminate	Perivenular inflammation involving a minority of terminal hepatic veins with patchy perivenular hepatocyte loss without confluent perivenular necrosis.
Mild	As above, but involving a majority of terminal hepatic veins.
Moderate	As above, with at least focal confluent perivenular hepatocyte dropout and mild-to-moderate inflammation, but without bridging necrosis (see Figure 3.17).
Severe	As above, with confluent perivenular hepatocyte dropout and inflammation involving a majority of hepatic venules with central-to-central bridging necrosis.

Chronic Rejection

General Considerations

Classically defined or typical chronic rejection usually evolves from severe or persistent TCMR, and results in potentially irreversible damage to bile ducts, arteries, and veins (reviewed in [274]). "Chronic" implies a time parameter; however, this is not always applicable since [251] historically, it often occurred within the first year after transplantation (reviewed in [274]).

Classically defined chronic rejection (e.g., ductopenia, obliterative arteriopathy, and perivenular fibrosis) affects about 3%–5% of liver allograft recipients by five years after transplantation, which is a dramatic decrease since the 1980s when the incidence was 15%–20% [274]. Classically defined chronic rejection also does not appear to increase with time after transplantation. However, features associated with chronic rejection are expanding to those associated with chronic AMR, discussed below.

Chronic rejection, regardless the definition, remains an important cause of late liver allograft dysfunction and failure, seen mostly in non-compliant patients, HCV+ recipients treated with an immune activating drug, such as alpha interferon [275, 276], and recipients who have IS lowered because of medication adverse side effects, such as lymphoproliferative disorders [277].

Risk factors for chronic rejection have generally been divided into two general categories: 1) non-alloantigen-dependent and 2) alloantigen-dependent or rejection-related factors. Non-alloantigen-dependent or "non-immunological" risk factors include donor age >40 years [278]. Alloantigen-dependent risk factors include the number and severity of TCMR episodes (reviewed in [253, 274, 279]). Late onset TCMR, younger recipient age, male-to-female sex mismatch, a primary diagnosis of AIH or biliary disease, baseline IS, interactions between HLA-DR3, TNF-2 status, and CMV infection are risk factors for the development of chronic rejection in cyclosporine-treated cohorts [280], non-Caucasian recipient race (reviewed in [274]), use of interferon alpha to treat recurrent HCV [275, 276]. The effects of histocompatibility differences and CMV infection are controversial. Most

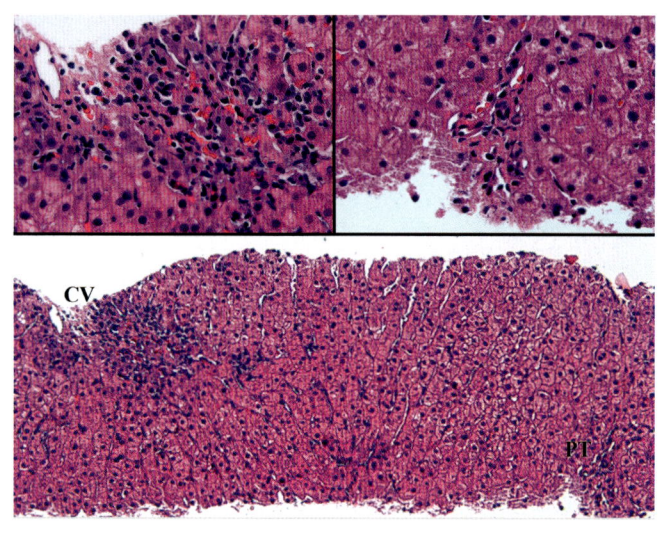

Figure 3.17 Acute rejection can occasionally present as "isolated central perivenulitis" without, or with minimal, accompanying portal tract changes (PT = portal tract; shown at higher magnification in the upper right inset). Severe acute rejection should not be diagnosed in such cases. Similar changes can be seen with new onset and recurrent AIH. In this case of "moderate" central perivenulitis, note the prominent perivenular inflammation and hepatocyte dropout (CV = central vein; shown at higher magnification in the upper left inset). The changes are less prominent in "mild" but "severe" central perivenulitis changes similar to those seen here, but with at least focal central-to-central bridging necrosis.

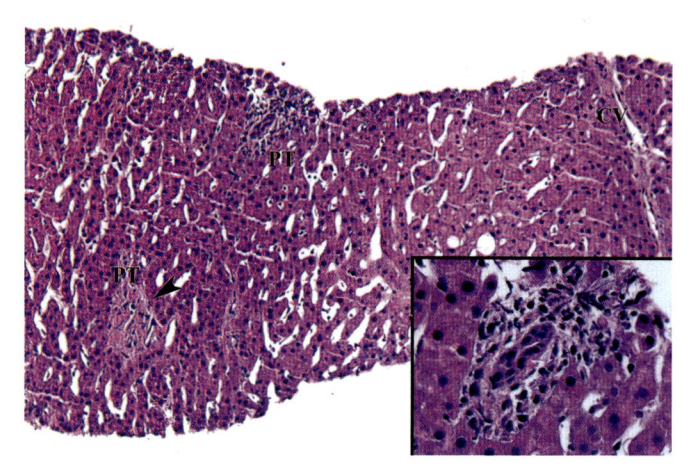

Figure 3.18 Early chronic rejection is characterized by mild, predominantly mononuclear inflammation with variable bile duct loss (arrowhead) and biliary epithelial senescence changes (lower right inset) involving a majority of bile ducts. The senescence changes include eosinophilic transformation of the cytoplasm, an increased nuclear: cytoplasmic ratio, uneven nuclear spacing, and multinucleation (PT = portal tract).

matching factors described for cyclosporine-treated recipients were eliminated as significant risk factors, but the influence of the number and severity of TCMR episodes remained in a large Tacrolimus-treated cohort [278]. Recent studies suggest that persistent and high MFI (>10,000) DSA is associated with rejection-related late graft loss and show that Tacrolimus more effectively controls de novo DSA development than cyclosporine [11, 200, 203, 225, 226, 281].

Clinical Presentation

Classically defined chronic rejection usually occurs in patients with a history of significant TCMR, who develops progressive cholestasis and an increase in canalicular enzymes, or becomes unresponsive to anti-rejection treatment [251]. However, fibrosis and low-grade necro-inflammatory-type interface activity can develop in otherwise stable recipients with normal liver injury tests [226]. Two typical clinical settings include: 1) the culmination of multiple and/or unresolved/persistent TCMR, 2) an indolent presentation without preceding clinically recognizable episodes of TCMR. The first scenario was historically the most common, but the latter is becoming more common with recognition of chronic AMR [226]. Risk factors include inadequately immunosuppressed patients, either as a result of non-compliance or because of infectious, neoplastic, or toxic complications of chronic IS [278].

Standard liver injury tests usually show a cholestatic or "biliary" pattern with preferential elevation of γ-glutamyl transpeptidase and alkaline phosphatase in those with classically defined chronic rejection with ductopenia [251, 282, 283]. Persistent elevation of ALT and total bilirubin usually marked the transition from acute to chronic rejection and can presage allograft failure [278, 284, 285]. Clinical symptoms, if present, resemble those of TCMR until dysfunction becomes significant enough to cause jaundice. Alternatively, indolently developing fibrosis can present initially as portal hypertension. Biliary sludging, biliary strictures, hepatic infarcts, and loss of hepatic synthetic function, manifest as coagulopathy and malnutrition, are other late findings that often occur immediately before allograft failure [251]. Hepatic angiograms, in a typical case with obliterative arteriopathy, show pruning of the intra-hepatic arteries with poor peripheral filling and segmental narrowing [251, 286]. The early phase of chronic rejection is potentially reversible [183, 284, 287–289], which depends on preservation of ductules and surrounding microvasculature [290].

Histopathologic Findings and Staging

The BANFF Schema divides classically defined chronic rejection findings into portal tracts and perivenular regions and "early" (see Figure 3.18) and "late" (see Figure 3.19) stages (Table 3.4) [290, 291]. Early chronic rejection is characterized by mild portal inflammation, lymphocytic cholangitis, and biliary epithelial cell senescence changes involving a majority of small bile ducts, and variable small bile duct loss usually involving <50% of portal tracts (see Figure 3.18). Compared to TCMR, chronic rejection usually has less severe inflammation and the inflammation consists primarily of lymphocytes, plasma cells, and mast cells [292]. A diagnosis of classically defined chronic rejection should be based on a combination of the clinical, laboratory, and histopathological findings that can be supported by radiographic findings. *In a biopsy specimen, the minimal diagnostic criteria for chronic rejection are:* a) senescent changes, affecting a majority of the bile ducts, with or without bile duct loss; or b) convincing foam cell obliterative arteriopathy; or c) bile duct loss affecting greater than 50% of the portal tracts [291].

Histopathology of Liver Transplantation

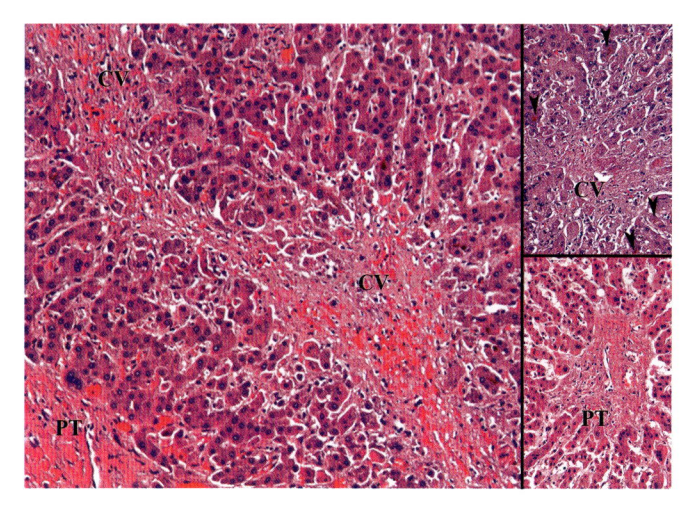

Figure 3.19 The typical case of late chronic rejection is characterized by small bile duct loss involving a majority of the portal tracts and/or severe perivenular fibrosis with at least focal central-to-central bridging, as illustrated in this photomicrograph. Many cases of late chronic rejection show loss of both small bile ducts and hepatic artery branches in the portal tracts (lower right inset), such that it is difficult to distinguish between portal tracts and central veins. However, the cholestasis in late chronic rejection is centrilobular, which helped to identify the fibrotic central veins (upper right inset) (PT = portal tract; CV = central vein).

Table 3.4 Features of Early and Late Chronic Liver Allograft Rejection (Adapted from [291]).

Structure	Early CR	Late CR
Small bile ducts (<60 μm)	Bile duct loss in <50% of portal tracts	Loss in ≥50% of portal tracts.
	Degenerative change involving a majority of ducts:	Degenerative changes in remaining bile ducts
	eosinophilic transformation of the cytoplasm; nuclear hyperchromasia; uneven nuclear spacing; ducts only partially lined by BEC.	
Terminal hepatic venules and zone 3 hepatocytes	Intimal/luminal inflammation	Focal obliteration
	Lytic zone 3 necrosis and inflammation	Variable inflammation
	Mild perivenular fibrosis	Severe perivenular fibrosis, defined as central-to-central bridging fibrosis
Portal tract hepatic arterioles	Occasional loss involving <25% of portal tracts.	Loss involving >25% of portal tracts
Other	So-called "transitional*" hepatitis with spotty necrosis of hepatocytes	Sinusoidal foam cell accumulation; marked cholestasis
Large peri-hilar hepatic artery branches	Intimal inflammation, focal foam cell deposition without luminal compromise	Luminal narrowing by subintimal foam cells
		Fibrointimal proliferation
Large peri-hilar bile ducts	Inflammation damage and focal foam cell deposition	Mural fibrosis

*"Transitional" hepatitis: Mild lobular disarray and spotty acidophilic necrosis of hepatocytes that can occur during evolution or transition from early to late stages of chronic rejection [607].

Histopathological features attributable to chronic rejection are expanding and are likely to undergo formal re-classification. Included are non-inflammatory portal/periportal, sinusoidal, and perivenular fibrosis, and otherwise unexplained low-grade portal inflammation ± necro-inflammatory-type interface activity, plasma cell hepatitis, and portal venopathy/NRH, accompanied by variable microvascular endothelial C4d positivity [11, 217, 219, 220, 222, 226, 232]. Except for obliterative arteriopathy, most candidate lesions are also caused by technical complications [100, 229, 233] and therefore are not specific requiring reasonable exclusion of other insults.

Biliary epithelial cell senescence changes [183] include: nuclear enlargement, hyperchromasia, uneven spacing resembling cytological dysplasia, syncytia formation, eosinophilic transformation of the cytoplasm, and bile ducts only partially lined by BEC (see Figure 3.18). Immunohistochemical markers of senescence, such as p16 [293] and $p21^{WAF1/Cip1}$, without co-existent Ki-67 expression, becomes upregulated in cells under severe stress and inhibit cell cycle progression [183]. Downregulation of epithelial junctional proteins from combined upregulation of mesenchymal proteins can also be seen, perhaps in response to injury [294]). Late-stage chronic rejection portal changes include bile duct loss involving >50% of portal tracts, portal capillary, and occasionally arteriolar loss.

Terminal portal tracts are defined as "foci within the parenchyma containing connective tissue and at least two luminal structures embedded in the connective tissue mesenchyme, each with a continuous connective tissue circumference [295]." In normal native livers, bile ducts and hepatic artery branches are detectable in 93 ± 6% and 91 ± 7% of portal tracts, respectively [295]. Fewer bile ducts were found by others using larger tissue samples [296]. Bile duct loss is considered present when <80% of portal tracts contain bile ducts (>2 standard deviations from normal). Arterial loss is considered present when <77% of terminal portal tracts contain hepatic artery branches. Alternatively, ductopenia has also been defined by at least one unpaired artery in >10% of all portal tracts or two unpaired arteries in different portal tracts [297]. Unpaired arteries are defined as arteries without an accompanying bile duct within a radius of ten hepatic artery diameters from the artery edge. Cytokeratin 19 and 7 staining can be used to help substantiate bile duct loss. The latter stain can also detect ductular metaplasia of periportal hepatocytes [101].

Late chronic rejection can cause both bile duct and arterial loss [296, 298] making it difficult to apply morphometric analyses (see Figure 3.19). In such cases, cholestasis is centrilobular. A ductular reaction at the interface zone is unusual in chronic rejection, unless the liver is recovering from chronic rejection [284, 287, 288].

Early perivenular chronic rejection is characterized by subendothelial and/or perivenular mononuclear inflammation (see Figure 3.18), consisting of lymphocytes, pigment-laden macrophages, and plasma cells [291, 299] often accompanied by perivenular hepatocyte dropout and mild perivenular fibrosis [291]. Late findings include severe (bridging) perivenular fibrosis with at least focal central-to-central or central-to-portal bridging and occasional obliteration of terminal hepatic venules (see Figure 3.19) [291]. Perivenular hepatocyte ballooning and dropout, centrilobular hepatocanalicular cholestasis, NRH changes, and intrasinusoidal foam cell clusters are other common findings in late chronic rejection (see Figure 3.19). Well-developed cirrhosis, attributable to classically defined chronic rejection, is unusual until the very late stages when venous obliteration leads to areas of parenchyma extinction and veno-centric cirrhosis [300].

Additional features of chronic rejection identified in *failed allografts* include obliterative arteriopathy in at least some of the peri-hilar arteries, except in cases characterized by bile duct loss and/or perivenular fibrosis alone. Foamy macrophage accumulation first occurs in the intima and eventually causes intimal thickening/luminal narrowing and medial thinning as arteries attempt to dilate and compensate for reduced arterial flow. Compensatory mechanisms eventually fail and foam cells replace the entire wall. Foamy macrophages can also deposit around bile ducts, veins, and in connective tissue. Large peri-hilar bile ducts can also show focal sloughing of the epithelium, papillary hyperplasia, mural fibrosis, and acute and chronic inflammation.

Chronic rejection staging assumes the diagnosis has been correctly established [291]. *Early chronic rejection* implies that a significant potential for recovery exists if the source/cause of immunologic can be controlled or reversed. *Late chronic rejection* implies a reduced potential for recovery and re-transplantation should be considered. However, it is not well-established that all patients proceed sequentially in an orderly fashion from the early to late chronic rejection. Some patients appear to persist in the acute/early-stage for months or years, while others rapidly develop severe fibrosis and late changes within the first year after transplantation or within weeks or months after the first onset. Some cases show predominantly or exclusively either bile duct loss or arteriopathy alone, but usually both features occur together [291].

Biopsy staging of chronic rejection, however, does not define a point of no return, but provides information about the likelihood of recovery and should be correlated with other clinical and laboratory parameters. Persistently elevated serum bilirubin >20 mg/dl, progressive decline in synthetic function, superimposed HAT, and bile duct necrosis or biliary sludging are poor prognostic findings [291].

Differential Diagnosis

Review of prior biopsies and correlation with the histopathologic findings is the best approach to establishing a diagnosis of chronic rejection. There is usually a history of severe or unresolved TCMR preceding the development of small bile duct damage and loss and perivenular fibrosis. Arteries with pathognomonic changes are rarely present in needle biopsy specimens [279]. Duct injury and ductopenia can also occur because of non-rejection-related complications, such as obstructive cholangiopathy, hepatic artery stricturing or thrombosis, "cholangitic" DILI, CMV infection, or can be idiopathic. Perivenular fibrosis can be caused by suboptimal hepatic venous drainage and other causes of perivenular injury. Therefore, *a diagnosis of chronic rejection based on biliary epithelial senescence or loss or isolated perivenular fibrosis alone should first exclude other non-rejection-related causes of ductal injury and loss or perivenular fibrosis.*

Chronic rejection is very difficult to distinguish from biliary tract obstruction or stricturing, including recurrent PSC (reviewed in [184]). Features favoring obstructive cholangiopathy include: 1) bile duct loss in some portal tracts accompanied by a ductular reaction in others; 2) neutrophil clusters within the lobules; 3) bile infarcts; 4) deposition of copper/copper-associated protein in periportal hepatocytes; and 5) hepatocanalicular cholestasis out of proportion ductopenia (<50%). Features that favor chronic rejection include: 1) cholangiopathic changes combined with central changes; and 2) absence of changes typical of obstructive cholangiopathic changes, described above. Cholangiography and/or angiography may be required to distinguish between chronic rejection and obstructive cholangiopathy. "Pruning" and poor peripheral filling favor chronic rejection. A prominent ductular reaction signals either regrowth of bile ducts [284, 287, 289] or biliary strictures that are often associated with prominent ductular metaplasia of hepatocytes and periportal hepatocyte copper deposits. Otherwise unexplained perivenular fibrosis can also be caused by mechanical outflow obstruction, adverse drug reactions and veno-occlusive disease, and Budd-Chiari syndrome.

Infections: Bacterial and Fungal

Stress, tissue damage from operations, and IS needed to prevent TCMR within the first two months after transplantation places recipients at highest risk for serious "opportunistic" fungal and viral infections [301]. Therefore, infections should always be suspected when reviewing tissue specimens from liver allograft patients. More than six months after transplantation, more typical bacterial infections occur. Fever, anastomotic or wound dehiscence, persistent abdominal pain, and vascular thrombosis are typical clinical signs and symptoms that should arouse suspicion [302]. The patient's immune status depends on many factors, including the IS regimen, immune senescence, and their underlying immune deficiencies (e.g., comorbidities such as diabetes, HIV, etc.) [303, 304].

Bacterial and fungal infections often arise in non-viable tissue; therefore, necrotic tissue should be routinely stained for bacteria and fungi. Co-existent acute and chronic inflammation and granulomas are always good surrogate markers of infection, but might not appear because of heavy IS [305]. Histopathologic recognition of deep fungal and bacterial infections familiar to most pathologists is beyond the intended scope of this chapter. The transplant pathologist, however, should be aware of the possibility of bacterial infections, as they are most common in organ recipients and represent about 70% of cases, followed by viral (20%) and fungal (8%) causes [305].

Infections: "Opportunistic" Hepatitis Viruses

CMV, EBV, Herpes Simplex (HSV) or Varicella-Zoster (VZV), and ADV infections are considered "opportunistic" and do not usually cause clinically significant acute hepatitis in immunocompetent individuals. However, they can do so in immunologically naïve recipients and in patients with compromised immune systems who receive organs from seropositive donors [306, 307]. These opportunistic viruses do not cause chronic hepatitis. Most adults have community acquired immunity that keeps viral replication in check after transplantation, while children, depending on age, are usually naïve and susceptible to primary infection.

However, vigorous IS therapy renders all liver allograft recipients vulnerable to acute hepatitis caused by opportunistic viruses. Patients with latent infections develop "reactivation" infection/disease, whereas "naïve" recipients develop primary infection/disease, which in general is more severe. Periodic viral shedding into the peripheral circulation is an important aspect of latent infection where it can be monitored by measuring viral antigen or nucleic acid shedding. When viral markers surpass empirically set thresholds, preemptive lowering of IS and/or treatment with specific anti-viral agents is often used to prevent active disease [307–309]. Monitoring and preemptive antiviral therapy has dramatically reduced the incidence of, but has not eliminated, diseases caused by these viruses. Therefore, a tissue diagnosis of CMV, EBV, HSV, and VZ hepatitis is becoming increasingly rare in routine adult and uncommon in pediatric clinical practice.

Cytomegalovirus Hepatitis

Introduction

CMV is the most common viral infection that affects the outcome of liver transplantation [310]. Prophylactic and preemptive therapy have greatly decreased the incidence and impact of symptomatic viral hepatitis. However, if used in all patients, including those that are seronegative, prophylaxis has also been associated with suboptimal long-term outcome (reviewed in [306, 307, 311, 312]). Even though clinically significant CMV disease is uncommon, it has been associated with increased risk of acute and chronic rejection, biliary strictures, vascular thrombosis, accelerated HCV recurrence, other opportunistic infections, and decreased patient and graft survival (reviewed in [306, 311, 312]).

Risk factors for CMV disease include seronegativity before transplantation, TCMR, viral replication (usually associated with over IS), mycophenolate mophetil, anti-leukocyte antibody therapy, HHV-6, HHV-7, TLR gene polymorphisms, mannose binding lectin deficiency, chemokine and cytokine defects (IL-10, MCP-1, CCR5), and deficiency of viral-specific T cells (reviewed in [311, 312]). Compartmentalized disease is an emerging challenge, detectable in tissue biopsies, but not in various serologic assays (reviewed in [311, 312]). Thus, CMV-specific immunohistochemical stains in seronegative recipients or low virus levels by quantification assays should be considered in the face of suspicious histopathological findings, described below.

Clinical Presentation

The most common clinical presentation of CMV infection is fever with bone marrow suppression, termed the CMV syndrome [306]. Any organ system can be involved depending on the extent of viral dissemination. The most common tissue-invasive disease is gastrointestinal involvement characterized by fever, diarrhea and gastrointestinal ulcers, leukopenia, and low-grade hepatitis with modestly elevated liver injury tests (reviewed in [306, 311, 312]). Respiratory insufficiency/pneumonia and retinitis are signs of severe disseminated disease [313]. CMV can also occasionally cause a syndrome that mimics EBV-associated PTLD with lymphadenopathy, fever, and atypical lymphocytosis (reviewed in [314]).

Histopathologic Findings

CMV hepatitis incidence has greatly decreased because of prophylactic therapy, serologic monitoring for antigenemia, and preemptive anti-viral therapy (reviewed in [306, 311, 312]). Common CMV-hepatitis histopathologic features, when they occur, include spotty lobular necrosis, Kupffer cell hypertrophy, mild lobular disarray, and patchy lobular inflammation. Under current management schemes, infected hepatocytes rarely contain diagnostic nuclear and/or cytoplasmic inclusions. Instead, inclusions are limited to patients who are over-immunosuppressed and not adequately monitored or treated. Therefore, if any features, described below, are observed, CMV-specific immunohistochemical stains should be performed. Any cell type can be infected. Diagnostic features include large eosinophilic intra-nuclear inclusions surrounded by a clear halo accompanied by small basophilic or amphophilic cytoplasmic inclusions. In severe cases (largely of historical significance), numerous cells containing CMV inclusions can be seen, but CMV alone does not cause submassive or massive necrosis (reviewed in [314]). Instead, microabscesses, or clusters of macrophages (microgranulomas) and lymphocytes surrounded by neutrophils, are usually observed. CMV hepatitis can also be associated with mild lymphoplasmacytic portal inflammation and lymphocytic cholangitis that can superficially resemble

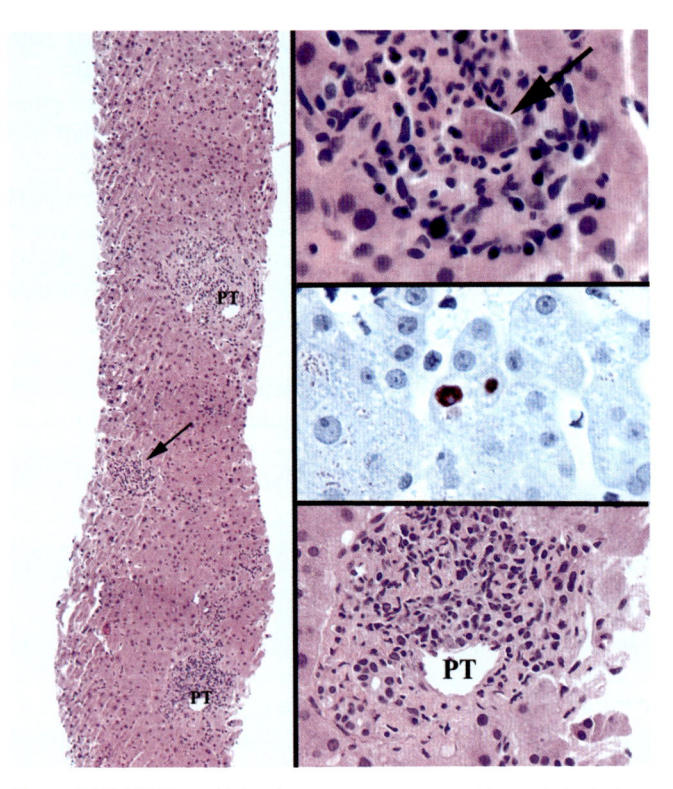

Figure 3.20 CMV hepatitis has become an uncommon histopathological diagnosis because of peripheral blood monitoring and preemptive adjustments in IS and/or antiviral drug therapy. The typical case usually shows variable lymphoplasmacytic portal inflammation (lower right inset), minimal lobular disarray, and microgranulomas or microabscesses (arrow, and upper right inset) scattered throughout the lobules. A CMV-infected cell is shown at higher magnification in the upper right inset (arrow). Immunostaining for CMV antigens is diagnostic when viral inclusions are not seen (right middle inset) (PT = portal tract).

acute or early chronic rejection (see Figure 3.20). Bile duct loss and chronic rejection have been associated with persistent allograft CMV infection (reviewed in [311, 312]).

Since characteristic inclusions are now rare, CMV hepatitis often presents with the parenchymal alterations, described above, but without characteristic or classical inclusions. Medical therapy often causes "fragmented" nuclear CMV inclusions, which are difficult to categorize without immunoperoxidase staining to detect viral antigens or in situ hybridization to detect nucleic acids. Rapidly dividing tissues such as young granulation tissue, proliferating cholangioles, edges of infarcts, abscesses, or other intraparenchymal defects are fertile soil for CMV growth [102]. CMVpp65 matrix protein immunostaining generally requires frozen tissue and might be more sensitive; therefore, it is used less frequently than routinely used antibodies directed at CMVp52 and an immediate early nuclear protein that works in FFPE specimens [311, 315].

Differential Diagnosis

CMV hepatitis can be difficult to distinguish from the early or lobular phase of HBV or HCV recurrence, especially when CMV inclusions are not detected and mononuclear portal inflammation is present. CMV can also be difficult to distinguish from HSV-induced hepatitis because both can cause multinucleation and intra-nuclear eosinophilic inclusions surrounded by halos. CMV inclusion-containing cells, however, can also show small basophilic or amphophilic cytoplasmic inclusions, which distinguish them from HSV-infected cells. Circumscribed foci of coagulative necrosis characteristic of HSV are not a feature of CMV hepatitis [314, 315].

Subtle clues in cases without characteristic inclusions that suggest CMV enabling distinction from HBV or HCV hepatitis include less lobular disarray and hepatocyte swelling and the presence of microabscesses or microgranulomas. A definitive CMV diagnosis requires either rarely present characteristic inclusions or positive staining for viral antigens or nucleic acids [315].

CMV hepatitis can be confused with EBV hepatitis because they share mild lymphoplasmacytic portal and lobular inflammation and can elicit intra-hepatic blastic and atypical-appearing lymphocyte responses. However, these changes are usually more florid with EBV, and CMV more commonly causes characteristic microgranulomas or microabscesses. Proper work-up includes examination of deeper levels and immunohistochemical or in situ hybridization for EBV and CMV viral antigens or nucleic acids, respectively [316].

Patients recently treated with increased IS are most susceptible to CMV hepatitis. It can also be difficult to determine whether liver inflammation and injury are attributable to residual CMV hepatitis, residual acute TCMR, or development of chronic rejection. An association between CMV infection and chronic rejection by some [317, 318], but not others [319] further complicates the issue. In our opinion, CMV inclusions or antigens/nucleic acid should be given priority and treated appropriately.

Epstein-Barr Virus

Introduction

EBV infection "immortalizes" B lymphocytes in vitro, but lies dormant in B lymphocytes and some epithelial cells in vivo, controlled by T cell surveillance, which checks EBV replication and B cell proliferation following a primary infection (reviewed in [320–322]). Primary EBV infections occur in children; ~90% of adults are infected. Reactivation, therefore, likely accounts for pathology in adult recipients [323]. A recent study has shown that the donor replication status for EBV does not impact recipient viral replication [324].

IS enhances EBV replication and increases the risk of various EBV disease manifestations, ranging from self-limited EBV-like syndromes to aggressive PTLD similar to lymphoma (reviewed in [320–322]). Disease incidence is higher in seronegative, typically pediatric recipients, but varies from 1%–5% of all liver allograft recipients, and increases with time after transplantation (reviewed in [320–322]). Risk factors for acquiring PTLD include primary EBV infection, primary CMV infection, and high IS levels [325]. Underlying liver diseases such as viral hepatitis, autoimmune liver disease, or alcoholic liver cirrhosis also contribute to an increased risk of developing PTLD (reviewed in [326]). A recent study shows a decreasing incidence of EBV-related diseases, including PTLD, in pediatric recipients that correlates with decreased IS usage in this vulnerable population [327].

Histopathology of Liver Transplantation

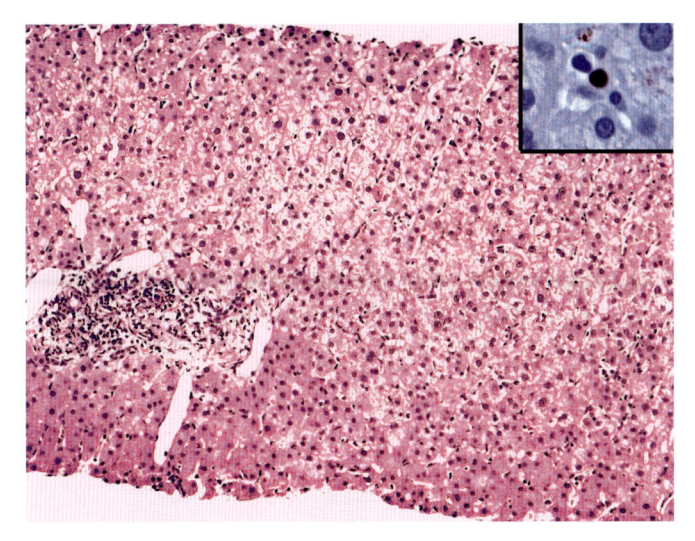

Figure 3.21 EBV hepatitis is characterized by variable, but usually mild, mononuclear portal inflammation without bile duct damage, accompanied by mild sinusoidal lymphocytosis and low-grade hepatocyte apoptosis. In situ hybridization for EBV RNA in occasional portal and/or sinusoidal lymphocytes is confirmatory (upper right inset).

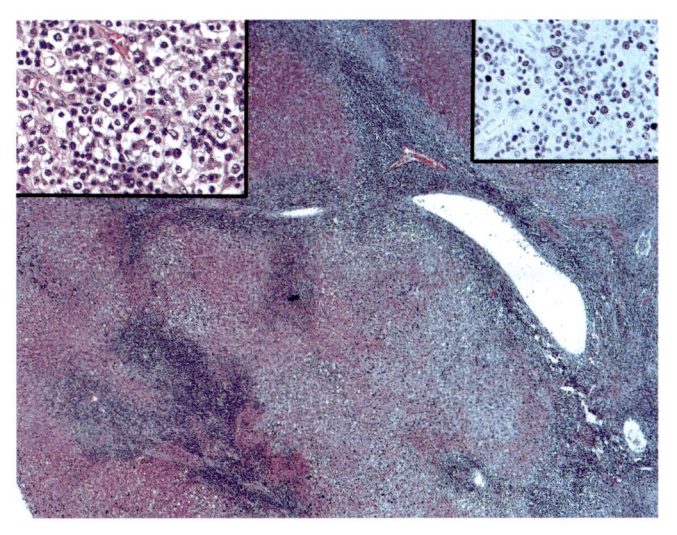

Figure 3.22 Uncontrolled EBV replication results in the development of PTLDs. Characteristic features include a dense portal infiltrate comprised of a relatively monomorphic population of lymphocytes and plasmacytoid lymphocytes (upper left inset) that overrun the normal portal architecture or landmarks. In contrast to CMV, PTLDs can cause confluent or even larger map-like areas of necrosis. Compare this infiltrate with that seen in acute rejection from Figure 3.14. In situ hybridization for EBV RNA (upper right inset) confirmed the diagnosis.

Clinical Presentation

Highly variable clinical manifestations [328] include hepatitis, gastroenteritis, B, T, and NK cell PTLDs, Hodgkin's disease, smooth muscle stromal tumors, and a variety of cancers (e.g., nasopharyngeal, gastric, etc.) (reviewed in [320–322, 329]). Clinically evident EBV-related syndromes often resemble classical infectious mononucleosis presenting with fever, malaise, lymphadenitis, pharyngitis, atypical lymphocytosis, and/or thrombocytopenia. Jaundice has also been described. Atypical signs and symptoms include jaw pain, arthralgia, joint space effusions, diarrhea, encephalitis, pneumonitis, mediastinal lymphadenopathy, and ascites. Liver allograft hepatitis or PTLD involvement usually shows mildly elevated ALT and AST and circulating atypical lymphocytes; pancytopenia is noted on occasion [330–332]. A serious and often fatal PTLD presentation is the hemophagocytic syndrome, but a recent report had a good outcome with prompt diagnosis by PCR and treatment with rituximab [333].

Risk factors for serious EBV-associated disease include primary infection, heavy IS, underlying Langerhans cell histiocytosis, and co-existent CMV disease. Risk of developing PTLD late after transplantation does not appear to be influenced by the type of IS agents, but by IS duration and intensity [320, 321, 334].

Peripheral blood EBV nucleic acids monitoring by PCR is used to follow viral replication [320]; when elevated, the patient is examined for lymphadenopathy and other signs of EBV-related disease(s) and preemptive IS reductions are usually made before more serious EBV-related disease occurs (reviewed in [335]). Monitoring is critical in pediatric recipients where increased viral nucleic acids have been successfully detected several weeks before the onset of clinical manifestations [336]. The therapeutic approach for EBV-related disease depends on the clinicopathological presentation and clonality: polyclonal infectious mononucleosis-like syndromes usually respond to lowering of IS, whereas monomorphic PTLD resembling lymphomas often require more aggressive immune- and/or chemotherapy (reviewed in [320–322, 329]).

Histopathologic Findings

Histopathologic EBV manifestations are also highly variable and can show acute EBV-hepatitis characterized by mild nonspecific portal and sinusoidal lymphocytosis to PTLDs resembling diffuse large B cell lymphomas [330–332, 337]. Even patients with enhanced EBV replication/viremia show increased intra-graft T and B cells [338], the latter occasionally containing evidence of EBV replication sequences (by the EBER-1 gene) [331, 332]. In patients without overt disease, EBER+ cells can be admixed among other inflammatory cells associated with other causes of allograft dysfunction [337]. The assertion that EBV might cause chronic hepatitis or recurrent acute relapses is controversial [339].

EBV hepatitis usually manifests as mild portal lymphoplasmacytic inflammation combined with sinusoidal lymphocytosis (lining up" of lymphocytes) comprised of small or mildly atypical lymphocytes. Lobular changes include focal hepatocellular swelling, low-grade hepatocyte apoptosis, and mild lobular disarray/regenerative activity (see Figure 3.21).

PTLD usually presents as cytologically atypical lymphoplasmacytic portal infiltrates. In early polymorphic lesions, atypical cells are usually intermixed with small and blastic lymphocytes, plasmacytoid lymphocytes, and plasma cells. Atypical cells predominate in monomorphic lesions, similar to immunoblastic lymphoma, manifesting as map-like portal tract enlargement by sheets of atypical immunoblastic cells. Similarly atypical cells can be seen in the sinusoids. Some cases are accompanied by significant hepatocyte necrosis. Hodgkin's-like lymphoma PTLDs with classical Reed-Sternberg cells can also occur and is associated with bile duct loss. Subendothelial localization of lymphocytes in portal and/or central veins can mimic acute rejection (see Figure 3.22) [330].

Extrahepatic PTLD usually presents in lymph nodes and intestines and should also be categorized according to the WHO classification scheme [340]: 1) Early lesions (reactive plasmacytic hyperplasia and infectious mononucleosis-like); 2) polymorphic (hyperplasia and lymphoma); 3) monomorphic (T and B cell subtypes); and 4) Hodgkin and Hodgkin-like lesions [341].

In situ hybridization for EBV RNA (EBER sequence) is needed to diagnose any EBV-related disorder and should be liberally employed to evaluate suspicious infiltrates. Immunohistochemical stains or in situ hybridization for kappa and lambda light chains, and CD20 to determine possible responsiveness to anti-CD20 antibodies should also be included. We also occasionally examine EBV antigen expression, and if enough fresh tissue is available, flow cytometric and molecular analyses, which enable detailed phenotyping and immunoglobulin gene rearrangements studies [322].

Differential Diagnosis

The most difficult challenge is distinguishing EBV hepatitis/PTLD from severe TCMR. Features favoring TCMR include pleomorphic, "rejection-type" portal and/or perivenular inflammatory infiltrates, including conspicuous eosinophils, and severe bile duct damage that correlates with the severity of the inflammation. Features favoring EBV include relatively monomorphic portal infiltrates that consist primarily of activated and immunoblastic mononuclear cells, some of which are atypical and/or show features of plasmacytic differentiation, and only focal mild bile duct damage, less than would be expected based on lymphocytic infiltrate severity [328, 337].

EBV hepatitis also needs to be distinguished from nonspecific, acute HBV, HCV or CMV. HCV and EBV can show sinusoidal lymphocytosis, but EBV-related disorders usually contain at least occasional atypical cells, whereas lymphocytes associated with HCV hepatitis are usually small, round, and inactive-appearing and often form portal-based nodular aggregates [330–332, 337]. Clinical suspicion and increased peripheral blood EBV nucleic acid levels also point toward the correct diagnosis.

The final diagnosis of any EBV-related disorder is heavily dependent on in situ hybridization for EBV RNA (EBER probing), but results should be interpreted with caution [342]: rare EBER+ cells are not uncommon amongst lymphocyte populations. EBV+ cells are found with slightly increased frequency in allograft recipients, the significance of which is open to debate [342]. In our opinion, clustering of EBER+ cells into aggregates, or EBER+ cells in tissues showing other histopathologic features of EBV-associated disease, is indicative of enhanced EBV replication; such patients are at increased risk of developing EBV-related disease. Closer follow-up and cautious IS management are warranted.

EBV-negative PTLDs occur. They are similar to non-Hodgkin's lymphoma in the general population and should be worked-up accordingly [341, 343]. Gene expression profiling has shown that these are truly two different entities with unique pathogenic mechanisms [344].

Herpes Simplex and Varicella-Zoster Viral Hepatitis

Introduction

Routine antiviral prophylaxis use have rendered Herpes Simplex (type I and II) Virus (HSV) and Varicella-Zoster (VZ) hepatitis relatively rare occurrences, but when they occur (reviewed in [314, 345]), fever, oral or genital mucositis, vesicular skin rashes, fatigue and body pain, and elevated liver injury tests are frequent manifestations. If undetected, HSV hepatitis can rapidly lead to submassive or massive hepatic necrosis, hypotension, disseminated intravascular coagulation, metabolic acidosis, and death [346]. Fulminant cases occur more often as a result of a primary infection. VZ-induced hepatitis is also becoming rare because of effective vaccines and anti-VZ immunoglobulin [347]. Vulnerable recipients exposed to Varicella-Zoster are routinely given prophylaxis with Varicella-Zoster immunoglobulin. Since the vaccine is an attenuated live virus, it is not recommended after transplantation [348]. HSV and VZ hepatitis can be fatal – prompt recognition and communication with the clinical team is crucial because effective antiviral treatment is available [349] [350].

Histopathologic Findings

Two histopathologic patterns of HSV hepatitis, localized and diffuse, have been described. Both patterns cause characteristic circumscribed areas of coagulative-type necrosis, showing no respect for the lobular architecture (reviewed in [314, 351]). Necrotic zone centers are occupied by hepatocyte ghosts, intermixed with neutrophils and nuclear debris, whereas more viable hepatocytes rimming the periphery usually contain recognizable HSV/VZ inclusions, if present. Infected cells are usually slightly enlarged and contain "smudgy," ground-glass nuclei or characteristic Cowdry type A eosinophilic inclusions. Multi-nucleate cells are occasionally present, but similar to other viruses, diagnostic inclusions are often absent.

Immunoperoxidase stains for HSV antigens are confirmatory and should be conducted in all cases. Antibody preparations used to detect HSV I and II show can show cross reactivity with each other and with VZ, making it difficult to distinguish among these viruses. Anti-VZ antibodies directed against precursor and mature glycoprotein are more discriminating.

Differential Diagnosis

Effective antiviral therapy can be discontinued if the diagnosis is not confirmed by immunostaining, which is an essential part of the workup, especially in cases without diagnostic inclusions. Necrotic lesions of HSV/VZ hepatitis are distinguished from infarcts by examining viable cells at the edge of the necrotic lesions for characteristic viral inclusions. In our experience, over-calling HSV hepatitis on H&E sections is preferable to missing this diagnosis. The histopathologic differential diagnosis of CMV and HSV hepatitis has been discussed above.

Human Herpes Virus-6 (HHV-6)

HHV-6, a member of the β-Herpesviridae subfamily of human herpes viruses, is a ubiquitous virus that usually first infects humans during the first two years of life and then lies dormant in a vast majority (>90%) of adults. Reactivation infection occurs in 15%–80% of liver allograft recipients, usually during the first 2–8 weeks after transplantation, often precipitated by heavy IS (reviewed in [352]). HHV-6 is thought to have synergistic effects with other latent viruses [353]. A clinical diagnosis of HHV-6 is difficult, as PCR results may detect latent infections and result in over diagnosis. However, the same anti-viral agents (ganciclovir, foscarnet, and cidofovir) used against CMV are effective treatment [354].

There are two recognized variants (A and B); the B variant is thought to cause most infections in transplant patients. Reactivation infections usually occur two to eight weeks post-transplantation [353] and manifest as fever with or without a rash, myelosuppression, hepatitis, interstitial pneumonitis, and neurological dysfunction. Indirect HHV-6 effects include exacerbation of CMV disease, increased severity of HCV recurrence, increased risk of other opportunistic infections, allograft dysfunction, and TCMR (reviewed in [352]).

Histopathologic findings of HHV-6 liver infection/hepatitis are variable and include moderate lymphocytic portal and patchy lobular inflammation, microabscesses [355, 356], and syncytial giant cell hepatitis [357]. Concurrent TCMR has also been reported [355, 356]. Immunoperoxidase stains for HHV-6 viral antigens localize primarily to mononuclear inflammatory cells [355] and to hepatocyte syncytial giant cells in a single case report [357].

Human Herpes Virus-8 (HHV-8)

HHV-8, also called KS-associated herpesvirus (KSHV), is a lymphotropic gamma herpes virus family member exerting a pathogenic role in Kaposi's sarcoma (KS), multi-centric Castleman's disease, and primary-effusion lymphoma in the general population and in liver allograft recipients (reviewed in [358–360]). HHV-8 is prevalent (>50%) in sub-Saharan Africa and up to 18% in Southern Italy and less prevalent elsewhere.

Primary and re-activation infections trigger antibody and nucleic acid production. Primary infection might be more severe and can result in variable manifestations: liver dysfunction, multiorgan failure, multi-centric Castleman's disease, and Kaposi's sarcoma (reviewed in [358–360]), including purplish nodular skin lesions, systemic KS-like involvement, or a post-transplant lymphoproliferative-like disease [361–363].

Liver biopsy findings are typical for an acute viral hepatitis and include lobular disarray, ballooning, hepatocyte swelling and apoptosis, and a variable ductular reaction. Follow-up in one patient showed widespread necrosis, but connection to HHV-8 is uncertain, as the patient had multi-organ failure. Regardless, when multicentric Castleman's disease, Kaposi's sarcoma, or an unexplained acute hepatitis are recognized, one should include HHV-6 and HHV-8 in the differential diagnosis [354, 362].

Adenovirus (ADV) Hepatitis

Introduction and Pathophysiology

ADV-related disease is largely restricted to pediatric recipients with primary infections [364, 365], although occasional cases have been reported in adults [366, 367] and mimic those seen in the general population (reviewed in [368]). Infections in adult solid organ transplant recipients, although rare, are associated with high mortality [369]. ADV is a double-stranded DNA virus comprised of 51 different serotypes that cause a substantial number of respiratory infections in children <5 years, including conjunctivitis, pharyngitis, croup, bronchiolitis, bronchitis, and pneumonia and diarrhea. Immune compromised patients can present with fulminant hepatitis, usually within six months of transplantation. The diagnosis is usually made by liver biopsy [364–367, 370]. Diagnosis can be life-saving because of successful treatment of ADV hepatitis infection in pediatric [371] and adult liver transplant patients with cidofovir and intravenous immunoglobulin [369].

The liver is the most common site of invasive disease (reviewed in [368, 370]) usually presenting within 50–100 days after transplantation with fever, respiratory distress, elevated liver injury tests, diarrhea, and leukocytosis. Viral subtypes 1, 2, and 5 have been isolated from the lung and gastrointestinal tract [364, 365, 372]. Allograft hepatitis is most often caused by viral subtype 5, but in the general population, hepatitis has also been caused by subtypes 2, 11, and 16 and might also be expected to infect and cause hepatitis in liver allografts [364, 365].

Histopathologic Findings

Typical ADV hepatitis causes "pox-like" granulomas, consisting of macrophages without neutrophils spread randomly throughout the parenchyma (see Figure 3.23); in other cases, the granulomas surround small map-like areas of necrosis [364–366]. ADV inclusions are usually found in nuclei of viable hepatocytes near the edge of the necrotic zones and/or

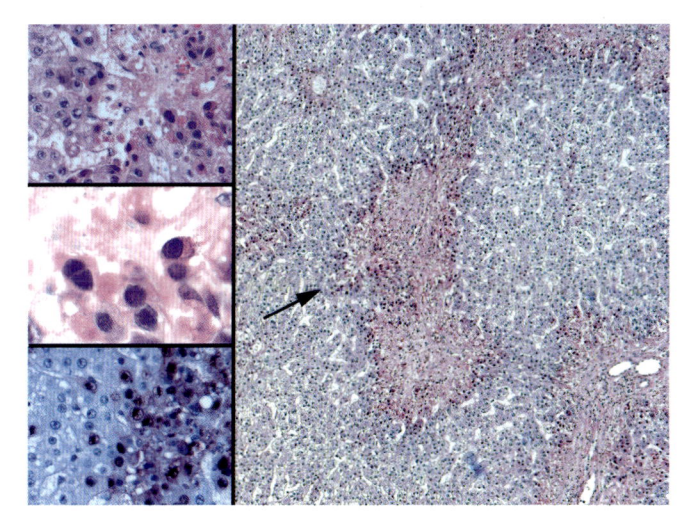

Figure 3.23 Adenoviral hepatitis is characterized by map-like areas of necrosis, which are sometimes surrounded by macrophages and/or neutrophils. But in this case, the widespread necrosis is accompanied only by a few neutrophils. The area highlighted by the arrow is shown at higher magnification in the upper right inset; note the inclusion-containing cells located at the edge of the necrotic zone. The middle left inset shows characteristic adenoviral nuclear inclusions under oil immersion. Note the "baked-muffin" appearance of the nuclear inclusions and the smudgy appearance of infected cells. As with all other opportunistic viruses, immunostaining for viral antigens confirms the diagnosis (case courtesy of Dr. Ron Jaffe; Children's Hospital of Pittsburgh).

granulomas: "smudgy"-appearing infected cells show chromatin margination toward the nuclear membrane, which makes the nucleus look like a "baked muffin." Immunohistochemical staining is required to confirm the diagnosis (see Figure 3.23) and given the 52 serotypes, it seems prudent to employ antibodies reactive with the hexon protein common to all serotypes of ADV (e.g., MAB805, blend of clones 20/11 and 2/6; CHEMICON International Inc., Temecula, California, USA) [367].

Differential Diagnosis

Recognizing typical ADV inclusions distinguishes ADV hepatitis from other causes of focal necrosis and hepatic granulomas such as HSV/VZ, infarcts, and deep fungal or mycobacterial infections. HSV/VZ and CMV hepatitis also cause granulomatous infiltrates and focal necrosis, respectively. ADV, however, usually causes less necrosis than either Herpes Simplex or Varicella-Zoster hepatitis [364–366]. ADV-associated granulomas are much larger than typical CMV "micro-granulomas" and multinucleated giant cells are rare in ADV hepatitis. CMV cell infection, in contrast, causes cytomegaly and produces eosinophilic intra-nuclear inclusions, surrounded by a clear halo, and basophilic or amphophilic small *cytoplasmic* inclusions. ADV does not cause cytomegaly, the nucleus assumes a "smudgy" appearance, and cytoplasmic inclusions are absent [364–366]. Ultimately, immunostaining and/or in situ hybridization for ADV are needed to confirm the diagnosis, often in conjunction with stains to exclude HSV/VZ and CMV viral antigens and/or nucleic acids [373].

Recurrent Diseases in Liver Allografts

Recurrence of the original disease is the major cause of late liver allograft injury and dysfunction in adults, whereas chronic IS decreases long-term morbidity-free survival due to extra-hepatic complications (e.g., renal toxicity). Classes of native liver diseases include: 1) infectious (viral hepatitis A, B, C, D, E, etc.); 2) dysregulated immunity (AIH, PBC, PSC, and overlap syndromes); 3) neoplastic (hepatocellular and cholangiocarcinomas); 4) toxic insults, such as alcohol abuse and DILI; and 5) hepatic-based metabolic and developmental diseases such as α-1-antitrypsin deficiency, Wilson's disease and extra-hepatic-based metabolic disorders (e.g., metabolic syndrome, hemochromatosis, Gaucher's disease, etc.), and extra- and intra-hepatic biliary atresia. Neither hepatic-based metabolic diseases nor developmental disorders recur after transplantation.

Hepatic transplantation for hepatocellular carcinoma (HCC) is based on disease stage. Potential recipients whose tumor(s) fulfill Milan criteria (one lesion ≤5 cm, or two to three lesions ≤3 cm) are given added priority for wait listing, but recent data suggests that these criteria are too stringent (reviewed in [374, 375]). Several options for treating recurrent HCC exist, which are similar to those recommended for native livers [376].

Careful patient selection and extensive perioperative treatment by neoadjuvant radiochemotherapy recently produced impressive survival data in specialized transplant centers (reviewed in [377]). Regardless, transplantation should be considered for early-stage (I and II) cholangiocarcinomas, particularly in PSC patients, and might again become an option instead of resection for patients with localized, node-negative, hilar cholangiocarcinoma (reviewed in [378]).

Several diseases of uncertain etiology (ies) can also recur after liver transplantation and include sarcoidosis [379, 380], idiopathic granulomatous hepatitis [282], post-infantile giant cell hepatitis [381], and Budd-Chiari syndrome [382–384]. Liver transplantation can transmit diseases such as familial amyloidosis polyneuropathy [82] and oxalosis [83] when these genetically diseased, but phenotypically normal, livers are used as "domino" transplants.

Hepatitis Virus Infections (A, B, C, D, and E)

Introduction

HBV and HCV with or without HCC account for a majority of liver transplants worldwide: HBV-induced cirrhosis in Asia [385] and HCV-induced cirrhosis throughout the world [386, 387]. Like the opportunistic viruses, HBV and HCV can remain in the circulation and infect extra-hepatic tissues. If HBV or HCV are capable of replication, they universally re-infect the new liver [388, 389]. Effective screening of blood products and organ donors has dramatically decreased acquisition of new infections during the transplant, but newly acquired infections after transplantation are not rare.

Clinical and histopathologic presentations and evolution of HBV and HCV-induced allograft hepatitis are nearly the same as those observed in the general population, with several important exceptions: 1) viral replication is significantly enhanced because of IS; 2) inflammation might be slightly less, but fibrosis progression definitely occurs more rapidly after, than before, transplantation; 3) in a small percentage of cases, markedly enhanced viral replication results in atypical clinical and histopathologic presentations, described in more detail below [388, 389]. Hepatitis E virus (HEV) has also recently been identified as a cause of chronic hepatitis in liver allograft recipients [390]. However, effective HBV vaccination and introduction of new and highly effective anti-HBV [6, 7] and anti-HCV [8–10] medications may render much of what is written below as only of historical interest.

Hepatitis A

Fulminant hepatic failure induced by Hepatitis A virus (HAV) is a rare indication for liver replacement. Several case reports show that HAV can persist/recur after transplantation, as determined by detection of genomic HAV RNA by RT-PCR in liver tissue, serum, and stool at the time of transient graft dysfunction and one case of apparent HAV-induced allograft failure (reviewed in [391, 392]). Biopsy findings at the time of dysfunction onset showed changes attributable to hepatitis: variable hepatocyte apoptosis, degenerative changes of hepatocytes with cholestasis, mild portal inflammation with variable bile duct damage, and ductular cholestasis (reviewed in [391, 392]). However, HAV RNA can be detected in liver tissue of patients with otherwise typical acute and/or chronic rejection (reviewed in [391–394]). Thus, the diagnosis of recurrent/persistent HAV after transplantation should be based on complete clinicopathological and serological correlation.

Hepatitis B and Delta Hepatitis

Introduction

HBV-induced cirrhosis has dramatically decreased in the western world due to successful preventative measures (e.g., mandatory HBV vaccination), prophylactic regimens (e.g., hepatitis B immune globulin, HBIG), and effective anti-viral medications (e.g., nucleoside analogs) that generally arrest disease progression. Despite this significant progress, HBV is still the leading indication for liver replacement in China [385]. However, decreased prevalence to intermediately endemic from highly endemic indicates a slight decrease since previous 2006 reports [395, 396]. Active viral replication before transplantation, recognized by HBeAg sero-positivity or detection of circulating HBV DNA, almost assures allograft re-infection. Re-infection and recurrent disease are less predictable in patients who had HBV-induced fulminant liver failure or in those with chronic liver disease who had become anti-HBe-positive and serum HBV DNA and HBeAg-negative prior to transplantation co-infected with hepatitis delta virus (HDV) (reviewed in [397–399]).

Donor and blood product screening has largely limited HBV-induced allograft dysfunction to those infected before transplantation, except for a small cohort of naïve recipients who acquire HBV infection during or after transplantation (reviewed in [398, 399]).

Anti-viral treatment of HBV after transplantation has significantly diminished the clinical manifestations and histopathologic lesions attributable to HBV induced allograft dysfunction and greatly improved patient and allograft survival (reviewed in [398, 399]). Unfortunately, treatment modalities cannot entirely prevent allograft re-infection. Included are polyclonal and monoclonal hepatitis B immune globulins, α-interferon, and anti-viral drugs such as lamivudine, and the nucleoside analogs adefovir, entecavir, and tenofovir. These agents effectively control viral replication and limit recurrent disease incidence to less than 10% particularly when anti-HBsAg is combined with lamivudine or other nucleoside analogs (reviewed in [398, 399]). Newer nucleoside analogs, such as entecavir and tenofovir, which have lower resistance rates, are recommended for treating HBV+ transplant recipients [400]. Some studies show that certain oral combinations, for example, tenofovir and emtricitabine, can be used successfully without immunoglobulin after transplantation [6, 400, 401].

Delta hepatitis is not common, but the acute form can result in the most severe form of viral hepatitis. Acute delta hepatitis can occur as a result of coinfection with hepatitis B and delta virus, and currently there is no treatment, except transplantation [402]. Two major patterns of infection occur: coinfection with HBV and HDV; and a carrier of HBsAg and HDV can result in superinfection and result in chronic delta hepatitis, where hepatitis D is the dominant virus. The first type is easily eradicated by treatment for HBV. The second type results in chronic hepatitis D. The only effective treatment for superinfection is conventional or pegylated interferon for a duration of one year, which is contraindicated in patients with decompensated liver disease and effective in only ~20% of patients [403]. Newer strategies using hepatocyte entry inhibitors are under development for chronic delta hepatitis treatment, particularly in endemic areas [402] and for liver transplant recipients [404, 405]. Delta agent co-infection of HBV+ recipients usually results in a lower incidence of recurrent disease compared to HBV+/delta- recipients, particularly in pharmacologically treated recipients [403].

Clinical Presentation

Historical observations are presented below. These are rare-to-non-existent currently because of effective anti-HBV medications. In untreated recipients, historical observations show that HBV liver allograft re-infection occurs immediately after transplantation. Clinical manifestations first become obvious in untreated recipients about six to eight weeks as otherwise unexplained elevations of liver ALT and AST [406, 407]. More significant hepatitis is accompanied by nausea, vomiting, jaundice, and, in rare cases, fulminant hepatic failure. The clinical presentation is quite similar to HBV hepatitis seen in other IS hosts and non-IS patients from the general population. Recipients treated with too much IS can develop severe disease due to fibrosing cholestatic hepatitis (FCH) [408, 409]. In contrast, rapid tapering and/or withdrawal of IS should also be avoided in HBV+ recipients with evidence of active viral replication. This maneuver can cause robust activation of the immune system and result in severe immune-mediated liver injury and fulminant hepatic failure [408, 409].

Histopathologic Findings

Effective anti-HBV medications have largely eliminated the clinical presentations, above, and histopathological observations described below (reviewed in [398, 399]). They are listed primarily for historical interest, inadequately treated recipients, or those who develop drug-resistant viral mutants [6, 400]. The histopathologic manifestations of HBV infection of hepatic allografts in untreated recipients are similar to that seen in native livers, except for the rare occurrence of the fibrosing cholestatic variant (see Figure 3.24) [407, 409, 410].

The acute hepatitis phase is typically first recognizable within four to six weeks after transplantation and can be identified by expression of hepatitis core antigen in the cytoplasm of occasional hepatocytes [406, 407], followed by surface antigen expression [406, 407], spotty hepatocyte apoptosis, lobular inflammation, Kupffer cell hypertrophy, and lobular disarray. Portal inflammation is variable at this time. A small percentage of untreated HBV+ recipients will develop confluent/bridging, and even submassive necrosis, especially if IS is rapidly lowered or withdrawn [406]. Delta antigen can be detected by immunohistochemical staining [404, 411]. In untreated recipients, the histopathologic manifestations of HDV co-infection are similar to those seen in native livers [404].

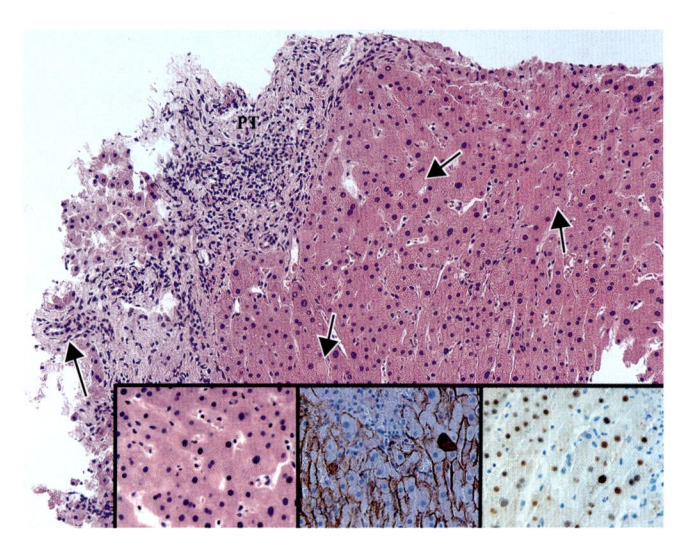

Figure 3.24 Recurrent acute and chronic HBV hepatitis is becoming relatively uncommon because of vaccination and effective antiviral drugs, which inhibit HBV replication and prevent chronic liver inflammation. It is still seen occasionally, however, and the histopathological changes are usually typical of chronic hepatitis as seen in other settings, except perhaps, for enhanced viral replication. Note the abundant expression of hepatitis B core antigen (lower right inset), hepatitis B surface antigen (middle lower inset), and numerous ground-glass hepatocytes (arrowheads and lower left inset). Note also that the portal inflammation is not "bilio-centric"; instead, the bile ducts are intact (arrow).

Rare recipients will show complete resolution of acute disease activity and will immunologically "control" the virus. Most untreated recipients that manifest hepatitis, however, evolve into the chronic phase. Cirrhosis used to develop within 12 to 18 months after transplantation in untreated recipients [406, 407], but there is no effective treatment for liver allograft recipients if chronic delta virus hepatitis is present [405].

Evolution from acute to chronic HBV hepatitis in untreated patients is characterized by lymphoplasmacytic portal inflammation with relative sparing of the bile ducts and portal and hepatic veins. The portal/periportal inflammation is associated with variable interface necro-inflammatory activity. Lobular findings in the chronic phase are usually much less conspicuous than during the acute phase and include ground-glass hepatocytes or hepatocytes with sanded nuclei that stain positively for hepatitis B surface and core antigen, respectively, and mild disarray and low-grade necro-inflammatory activity [407, 409, 410].

Over-IS can lead to massive HBV replication, and MHC non-identity between the liver and recipient can result in FCH. Viral mutants can also cause FCH [407, 412]. Swollen and degenerating hepatocytes usually show massive hepatocellular expression of HB core and/or surface antigen, suggesting that HBV is directly cytopathic under these special circumstances [407, 413]. Effects of HDV on HBV-related pathology in untreated recipients would be expected to be similar to that seen in the general population [414].

Differential Diagnosis

The differential diagnosis for acute HBV should include other causes of acute hepatitis, such as CMV, HCV, and EBV, as well as other causes of spotty hepatocyte apoptosis, such as "ischemic" hepatitis and portal and so-called "transitional" hepatitis that accompanies the transition from TCMR to chronic rejection. In order to properly differentiate among these various entities, careful review of the clinical, histopathological, immunohistochemical, and serologic profile is mandatory [407, 409, 410].

The main differential diagnosis for chronic HBV includes the other causes of chronic hepatitis such as HCV, AIH, and DILIs. Detection of ground-glass hepatocytes or viral antigens and/or nucleic acid in the blood or tissues, and an absence of other causes for chronic hepatitis, favors chronic HBV. Detection of viral antigens and/or nucleic acids in the blood or tissues combined with histologic features of an active lobular hepatitis, and an absence of other causes, favors recurrent HBV, but does not exclude other causes of allograft dysfunction [407]. Therefore, serologic evidence of viral infection or detection of viral antigens or nucleic acid in the liver has to be correlated with the histological pattern of injury.

FCH can appear similar to bile duct obstruction, but has more periportal sinusoidal fibrosis, lobular disarray and hepatocyte swelling, and absence of periportal CK7 positivity [415]. Features used to distinguish between acute rejection and acute or chronic hepatitis have already been discussed above (see "Acute Rejection-Differential Diagnosis").

Hepatitis C Virus (HCV)

Introduction

HCV-induced cirrhosis is a leading indication for liver replacement world-wide. Re-infection and subsequent viremia occurs within days after transplantation in almost all HCV+ recipients and hepatitis eventually develops in a vast majority. New onset HCV infection after transplantation generally reflects that which is seen in the general population [416]. The availability of the newer direct acting antivirals and the elimination of IFN-based regimens has made viral eradication prior to liver transplant possible, although their high cost may limit widespread use. IFN-free regimens show promise in treating mild-to-moderately decompensated liver disease with a greater than 90% sustained viral response (SVR) or "cure"; however, the safety and efficacy data in patients with severely decompensated cirrhosis is limited [416, 417]. Different regimens are recommended depending on the HCV viral genotype, fibrosis stage, presence or absence of comorbidities, and interaction with other medications (including IS) and are thus beyond the scope of this chapter [10].

Most HCV+ recipients develop chronic hepatitis, which evolves slowly in most patients, but fibrosis progression is significantly faster than in native livers and up to 20% are cirrhotic again by five years after transplantation. More aggressive disease progression is very likely attributable to a combination of IS and MHC-mismatching between the donor and recipient, which in turn leads to alloimmune injury and impaired immunologic control of viral replication (reviewed in [418–420]). A small percentage of recipients develop aggressive recurrence, FCH [421], which should also decrease in incidence with antiviral treatment.

Similar to HBV, rapid IS tapering can lead to rapidly progressive recurrent HCV probably related to immune system "re-arming" at a time of high HCV replication [422–424]. Instead, slower IS tapering, particularly in long-surviving recipients, seems more advisable [422–424]. Similar to non-transplant patients [425], nucleotide polymorphisms of IL28B and HCV RNA mutations in liver allograft recipients are predictive of more aggressive disease and less SVR [426, 427].

Any "second hit" to underlying HCV (e.g., co-existent steatosis, high viral replication and oxidative stress, iron deposits, co-existent damage from preservation/reperfusion injury, biliary stricturing, TCMR, or DSA [201]) can accelerate HCV-related disease progression [428]. Fibrosis stage and other factors that accelerate disease progression may be perquisites for treatment with the newer direct-acting antivirals in these patients [10, 429].

The rate of HCV-induced fibrosis progression is initially linear. But once bridging fibrosis develops, subsequent deterioration toward end-stage cirrhosis and decompensation can occur more rapidly [418, 420, 430, 431]. This concept also explains why use of ECDs in HCV+ recipients has offset the recent improvements in medical management of HCV leading to no net improvement in long-term outcomes (reviewed in [418, 420, 428]); however, newer antiviral agents should improve outcomes [386, 417]. For example, obtaining post-transplant SVR is associated with improved histopathology and graft survival [432].

A complex interplay between the immune system, HCV, and IS [433] leads to distinct histopathologic variants of recurrent HCV in transplant patients: 1) usual or conventional; 2) fibrosing cholestatic HCV; 3) plasma cell-rich; and 4) overlap with acute and chronic rejection. Each is discussed in more detail, below.

Clinical Presentation

Post-transplant HCV hepatitis is similar to HCV hepatitis in the general population. Acute hepatitis, which develops in most recipients, is often asymptomatic, and recognized primarily by elevation of ALT and AST four to eight times baseline levels [428]. This usually becomes apparent between three to six weeks after transplantation in routinely monitored liver injury tests; earlier onset within 10–14 days can be associated with more aggressive disease. Symptoms, when present, usually include fatigue and nausea.

Jaundice at initial presentation is unusual unless the recipient is at risk for FCH; fulminant liver failure is not seen outside of this context [421]. FCH HCV is clearly associated with "over IS" and characterized clinically by malaise, jaundice, and marked and preferential elevations of bilirubin, alkaline phosphatase, and gamma glutamyl transpeptidase. This usually occurs within the first year and evolves subacutely over a period of weeks to months. Later onset can also occur, most commonly when recurrent HCV is misdiagnosed as TCMR and the patient is treated vigorously with increased IS. Early FCH HCV recognition relies on a high index of suspicion, recognition of the typical clinical circumstances, and elevated HCV RNA levels.

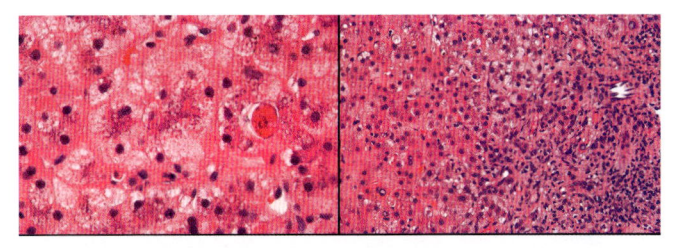

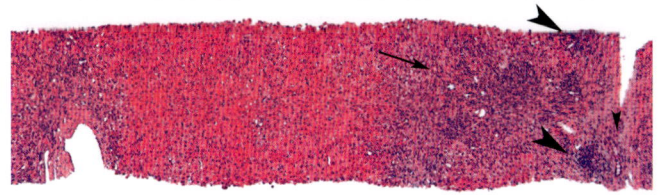

Figure 3.25 Recurrent HCV appears histologically quite similar to that seen in native livers with predominantly mononuclear inflammation, portal-based nodular lymphoid aggregates (large arrowheads), and interface activity. However, in general, when compared to native livers, allografts usually show less inflammation and more often ductular-type interface activity is seen (arrow), which is shown at higher magnification in the upper right inset. Note that the bile ducts are intact (small arrowhead). This particular case is bordering on FCH.

Histopathology

Usual Variant: Most acute phase features are similar to those seen in the general population (see Figure 3.25), but allografts generally show less portal and lobular inflammation. Chronic phase changes include nodular aggregates of portal-based lymphocytes, but usually more ductular-type interface activity than native livers (reviewed in [428, 434]).

The acute or lobular phase usually appears between 4 to 12 weeks, but can be detected as early as 10–14 days. Lobular disarray, Kupffer cell hypertrophy, hepatocyte apoptosis, mild sinusoidal lymphocytosis, usually mild mononuclear portal inflammation, and macrovesicular steatosis involving periportal and midzonal hepatocytes are typical findings. Lymphocytic cholangitis and reactive BEC changes, if present, involve a minority of bile ducts [428]. Transition from acute to chronic HCV is accompanied by waning of lobular changes, an increase in portal inflammation, variable nodular portal-based lymphoid aggregate formation, and emergence of necro-inflammatory and ductular-type interface activity [428].

Chronic HCV, usually evident by 6 to 12 months, is often dominated by portal and periportal changes including chronic portal inflammation, occasional portal-based lymphoid aggregates, and necro-inflammatory and ductular-type interface activity of varying severity. Focal lymphocytic cholangitis can be seen, but it is neither severe nor widespread, and duct loss is not seen. Central perivenulitis can also be seen in a minority of central veins, but it is neither severe nor widespread in recurrent HCV [428].

Some studies show no correlation between viral genotype and/or viral load and the severity of liver damage [435], while others showed that HCV RNA is higher during the acute/lobular phase of hepatitis and progression to chronic hepatitis is associated with significantly decreased liver HCV RNA, probably as a result of immune control of viral replication.

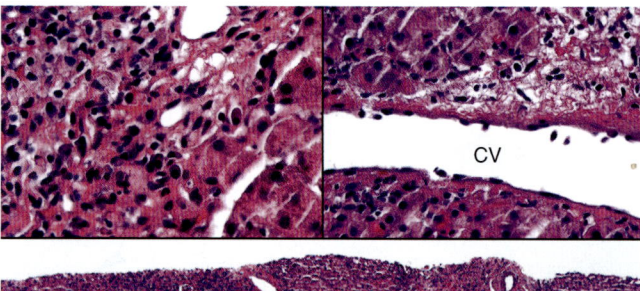

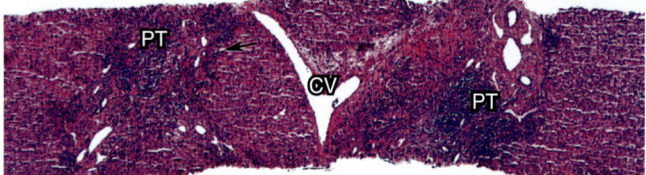

Figure 3.26 Some cases of recurrent HCV show "autoimmune" features such as prominent plasmacytic inflammation (upper left inset), aggressive interface activity (arrow), and plasma cell-rich perivenular inflammation and hepatocyte dropout. This biopsy was obtained about twenty-six months after transplantation from a female recipient who was HCV RNA-positive, but also had serological evidence of coexistent autoimmunity. Bile duct damage was not a prominent feature, but a majority of the central veins showed central perivenulitis. It is difficult to distinguish between centrilobular-based rejection and AIH in such cases. Both will respond to increased IS, but in HCV+ recipients, immunosuppressive therapy can hinder antiviral immunity (PT = portal tract; CV = central vein).

Other studies show that ballooning degeneration and cholestasis at initial presentation correlate with more rapid development of allograft cirrhosis [436, 437]. Another study showed no difference in the histopathologic appearance or rate of progression of recurrent versus de novo HCV, whereas another showed that de novo infection caused more aggressive disease [438].

Plasma Cell-rich or "Autoimmune" Variant of HCV: Recurrent chronic HCV can present with aggressive plasma cell-rich interface and perivenular necro-inflammatory activity resembling AIH (see Figure 3.26) (reviewed in [428, 439–441]. This variant is often first recognized during the transition from acute to chronic hepatitis or after the onset of chronic hepatitis and manifests as severe interface and/or perivenular necro-inflammatory activity mediated by "sheets of plasma cells."

More studies are needed to determine whether this represents an "autoimmune variant of HCV," TCMR, actual AIH, or a combination of these possibilities (reviewed in [428, 439, 440]). Emerging evidence suggests that this presentation most likely represents an overlap between allo- and autoimmunity. Similar changes in non-AIH, HCV patients would be considered as plasma cell-rich TCMR. Fiel et al. [442] favored TCMR because the plasma cell-rich presentation frequently developed association with suboptimal IS, and the patients: a) had a high incidence and propensity to develop TCMR; and b) had a better outcome when they were treated with increased IS. Castillo-Rama et al. showed a high frequency of HLA-DR15, less female predominance than AIH, and increased IgG4 positive plasma cells in afflicted older males [441]. Berardi et al. [443] reported development of "de novo AIH" after successful treatment of HCV with pegylated-interferon alpha-2b and ribavirin for at least six months. Significant graft dysfunction and hepatitis despite HCV-RNA clearance and laboratory, microbiological, imaging, and histological evaluations suggested de novo AIH according to the International AIH scoring system criteria [444]. Anti-viral treatment withdrawal and prednisone therapy resulted in five remissions and four graft failures with two deaths. Recognition of AIH-like features in native liver chronic HCV is based on the presence of significant plasma cells and aggressive interface activity [445, 446], which is often associated with hypergamma-globulinemia, greater frequency of cirrhosis, higher mean Knodell score, a higher frequency of HLA DR3, and a greater occurrence of high-titer smooth muscle antibodies [446]. HCV infection appears to trigger a genetic susceptibility to autoimmune phenomena in some patients that can accelerate the tissue damage. Indeed, plasma cell-rich infiltrates in explant livers is a risk factor for the development of plasma cell-rich allograft HCV recurrence [445–447]. Alternatively, an initially anti-viral immune response might eventually spread to include auto-epitopes (reviewed in [428, 439, 440]).

HCV+ recipients can also develop autoimmune phenomena similar to HCV+ patients from the general population [448]. The outcome in liver allograft recipients appears to be worse than with the usual variant of chronic HCV. A majority of reported cases have died or developed liver failure and/or portal hypertension [442, 447]. Results of these studies, however, are difficult to interpret because of variable treatment with IS and detailed reasons for the deterioration were not provided.

IS therapy with prednisone with or without azathioprine (in addition to the basic IS regimen), can lessen the severity of liver damage in patients with plasma cell-rich HCV in the general population [449] and in allograft recipients with plasma cell-rich interface and perivenular necro-inflammatory activity [439, 440, 442]. This can occur, however, at the expense of enhancing HCV replication and an impeding eventual HCV clearance [449]. Availability of the newer agents might eliminate HCV breaking the cycle [440].

Perivenular necro-inflammatory activity involving a majority of central veins, plasma cell-rich or not, is a feature of TCMR and AIH, but not of recurrent HCV. Central perivenulitis is usually responsive to increased IS, regardless of whether the patient is HCV+ or not, and regardless of whether the patient is an allograft recipient or not (reviewed in [428, 439, 440]). In contrast, perivenular necro-inflammatory activity is not a feature of recurrent HCV alone or of HCV in native livers. Differentiating between HCV and other common diagnoses, such as TCMR, can be facilitated by review of serum HCV viral load; errors can be minimized by strict adherence to specific histopathologic criteria and close clinicopathological correlation, including examination of HCV RNA levels [187]. Like other HCV manifestations, the above presentation is likely to be of historic interest with the advent of effective anti-HCV therapy.

FCH: This potentially fatal manifestation of recurrent HCV usually occurs within the first year after transplantation in the context of over IS and typically characterized by homogeneous viral quasi-species and increased HCV RNA replication in the peripheral circulation (usually

>30–50 million IU/mL). FCH-associated liver damage is likely caused by a direct hepatocyte viral cytopathy. The intrahepatic immune response in HCV-induced FCH is typically TH2-like, in contrast to the TH-1-predominant response in conventional recurrent HCV, and the few infiltrating lymphocytes often lack HCV specificity [450].

FCH results in cholestasis, hepatocyte ballooning degeneration, fibrosis (periportal, portal, and bridging), and a ductular reaction [451]. Spotty apoptosis/necrosis and mild mixed or even neutrophilic-predominant portal inflammation are also often seen. Compared to usual recurrent chronic HCV, the distinctive features are hepatocyte swelling, paucity of mononuclear portal inflammation, and ductular reaction. Similar to HBV, HCV-induced FCH can appear similar to bile duct obstruction, but has more periportal sinusoidal fibrosis, lobular disarray and hepatocyte swelling, and absence of periportal CK7 positivity [415]. FCH HCV occurs as a spectrum of severity: mild cases show only mild hepatocyte swelling, slightly more mononuclear portal inflammation, and only a low-grade or minimal ductular reaction. The diagnosis of severe FCH used to presage impending graft failure, but rapid treatment with the newer anti-viral agents shows promising results [386, 452].

Diagnosing Co-existent Conditions in the Context of Recurrent HCV

The most frequent HCV-related mistake is to over-diagnose TCMR in HCV+ recipients, resulting in unnecessary IS increases (reviewed in [187, 428]). Features attributable to TCMR and chronic rejection include: a) lymphocytic cholangitis and/or biliary epithelial senescence changes, respectively; and b) central perivenulitis and fibrosis, involving a majority of bile ducts or terminal hepatic veins, respectively. Features attributable to recurrent or new onset HCV include: a) lobular necro-inflammatory activity; and b) necro-inflammatory and ductular type interface activity. The key to successfully establishing a final diagnosis and the proper predominant insult is to determine which constellations of findings predominate and to use available additional information, such as HCV RNA level, to guide this distinction [187].

Most clinically significant TCMR episodes occurring in the context of recurrent HCV are graded as "moderate" according to the BANFF criteria [259]. BEC senescence involving a majority of bile ducts leads to a diagnosis of chronic rejection, which is often associated with a reduction in IS and/or treatment with an immune stimulator like alpha-interferon (reviewed in [428, 453]). When either TCMR or chronic rejection is the predominant process, the changes should be obvious.

Differential Diagnosis

Acute and chronic HCV need to be distinguished from acute and chronic rejection, recurrent non-HCV viral hepatitis (e.g., HBV, CMV, EBV), and recurrent or new onset AIH, PBC, and PSC, and biliary tract obstruction or structuring (reviewed in [428, 434]). C4d deposits and HCV protein and nucleic acid expression have been used as adjuvants techniques to assist with the differential diagnosis with limited success (reviewed in [428, 434]). Other causes of injury can also occur in the context of recurrent HCV. The timing of the biopsy is also important: HCV is an uncommon cause of allograft dysfunction during the first several weeks after transplantation except for rare cases that begin as early as 10–14 days. Most cases, however, occur between three and eight weeks after transplantation. Most acute rejection episodes, in contrast, occur within the first 30 days, with a median of eight days [454].

Distinguishing HCV from other causes of chronic hepatitis such as HBV, AIH, and drug-induced hepatitis requires evaluation of the complete clinical, biochemical, and serologic profile. A detailed histopathologic examination, however, can be extremely helpful. Viral antigen and/or nucleic acid detection, ground-glass cells, or sanded nuclei distinguish HBV from HCV. Confluent necrosis is rarely, if ever, seen in HCV alone. Recurrent or de novo AIH is recognized by sheets of plasma cells in the portal and interface areas and causes perivenular inflammation with confluent perivenular necrosis, especially when combined with autoantibodies and hypergammaglobulinemia. In contrast, low-grade periportal and midzonal steatosis and portal lymphoid aggregates favor recurrent HCV [363, 373].

Portal edema and portal versus periportal neutrophilia and periportal foam cells are common in duct obstruction and/or acute cholangitis. A prominent ductular reaction and acute cholangiolitis without portal edema is more characteristic of non-obstructive cholestatic hepatitis. Lobular disarray and marked hepatocellular swelling is usual for viral hepatitis, but uncommon in duct obstruction alone.

Hepatitis E Virus (HEV)

Introduction, Pathophysiology, and Clinical Presentation

HEV is a single-stranded, non-enveloped hepatotropic RNA virus endemic in Southern Asia and Africa with at least five different genotypes, four of which infect humans. HEV genotype 3 is frequently associated with zoonotic infections, whereas HEV genotypes 1 and 2 appear to primarily infect humans [455, 456]. HEV is most often transmitted by a fecal-oral route, but transmission by blood transfusion, contact with pigs and other animals, and consumption of infected and undercooked meat is also suspected [455–461].

HEV is an emerging disease in developed countries and is usually an asymptomatic, self-limited illness [390]. More serious acute disease occurs in pregnant females and chronic infection can occur in immune suppressed individuals (reviewed in [462, 463]). As with other "hepatitic" viruses, acute infection is diagnosed by HEV RNA detection and anti-HEV IgM seroconversion. Convalescence is marked by anti-HEV IgM to IgG seroconversion and HEV nucleic acid clearance [463]. Nucleic acid studies to detect HEV are usually more reliable than serological response studies in IS individuals, as might be expected. HEV infection in liver allograft recipients has been associated with acute and chronic hepatitis in children and adults [390, 455–461, 464]. Genotype 3, perhaps acquired via contact with pigs or animals or eating insufficiently cooked meat, is suspected in some cases.

Manifestations of acute HEV include elevated liver injury tests, fatigue, diffuse arthralgias, weight loss, and myalgias over a period of one to two weeks. Chronic/relapsing disease occurs more commonly in those who acquire a primary infection after transplantation [455–461]. Chronic infection is usually detected using HEV RNA PCR, as the appearance of anti-HEV IgM, and later, anti-HEV IgG seroconversion is often delayed for weeks or months. Some cases spontaneously resolve, but up to 60% of chronically infected (defined as HCV RNA+ in the stool or serum for six months) develop chronic hepatitis and 15% of these progressed toward cirrhosis (reviewed in [457]). Risk factors for chronic hepatitis include Tacrolimus IS and low platelet counts [457]. IS lowering can lead to infection and chronic hepatitis resolution [457], which is of potential importance for drug minimization trials. Peters et al. showed that ribavirin monotherapy was an effective and safe treatment of allograft HEV [465].

Histopathologic Findings and Differential Diagnosis

Similar to the HBV and HCV, acute and chronic phases are described [455, 456, 458, 461, 464]. The acute phase is characterized by predominantly lobular inflammation and spotty hepatocyte necrosis/apoptosis. Portal tracts show mild to moderate expansion by inflammation composed mainly of lymphocytes; mild necro-inflammatory-type interface activity was also observed [461].

Histopathologic features of chronic infection are typical of those in any chronic viral hepatitis and characterized by variable lymphocytic and lymphoplasmacytic portal infiltrates with variable necro-inflammatory-type interface activity and progressive fibrosis [455, 456, 458, 461, 464]. HEV adds yet another possible cause of chronic hepatitis in liver allograft recipients. The same criteria used to distinguish chronic HBV or HCV from acute and chronic rejection can also be used for HEV. Serologic and/or molecular biologic studies for HEV RNA are needed to make a definitive diagnosis, but are still evolving [462, 466].

Disorders of Dysregulated Immunity

Introduction

Reoccurrence of disorders of immune regulation including PBC PSC, AIH, and overlap syndromes is an ongoing challenge. Although the approximate incidence is ~25% by five years after transplantation that increases with time, long-term graft and patient survival, however, has not yet been significantly influenced by recurrent disease. This is at least partly attributable to effective therapy with UDCA, which can delay progression of fibrosis before transplantation and improve liver injury test profiles after transplantation, but survival is not affected to date (reviewed in [467]). Disease recurrence of course will continue, but emerging therapies will likely decrease the need for transplantation and prevent the impact of recurrence on morbidity and mortality [468].

Recurrence diagnosis can be especially problematic because even before transplantation, the diagnosis is based, at least partially, on exclusionary criteria. Additionally, various clinical, serological, histopathological, and radiological findings compatible with recurrent disease also can occur with other causes of allograft dysfunction. For example, there are numerous causes of intra-hepatic biliary strictures other than recurrent PSC that can affect PSC patients. Autoantibodies, such as anti-nuclear antibodies (ANA) and Antimitochondrial antibodies (AMA), used to establish the diagnosis of AIH or PBC before transplantation only transiently disappear and then quickly reappear, albeit at lower titers, even in the absence of clinical or histopathologic evidence of recurrent disease. A set of specific consensus criteria were recently proposed by the BANFF Working Group to suggest a standardized approach to these uncertainties [229].

New approaches show promising results that may potentially be used to differentiate between these diseases that often have an overlap of histopathologic features. For example, Liaskou et al. showed that high-throughput T cell receptor sequencing could potentially be used to differentiate between various chronic liver diseases such as PBC and PSC using distinct disease-associated T cell signatures [469].

Recurrent and New Onset "Autoimmune" Hepatitis

Introduction, Pathophysiology, and Clinical Presentation

AIH is a disease of unknown etiology, characterized by steroid-responsive lymphoplasmacytic liver inflammation that has the potential to progress to cirrhosis. An AIH diagnosis is based on a combination of serological findings (autoantibodies (ANA and SMA) and hypergammaglobulinemia), histopathological evidence of hepatitis, and steroid-responsiveness combined with exclusion of other causes of liver injury (reviewed in [470, 471]).

Establishing a recurrent or de novo AIH diagnosis is even more difficult than before transplantation for several reasons including: a) the above serologic abnormalities either persist or transiently decline and then reappear in the vast majority of recipients without a tight association to disease recurrence, and b) histopathologic evidence of liver injury from other causes of allograft injury can mimic AIH (reviewed in [470, 471]). The BANFF Working Group, therefore, advocated relatively strict criteria [229] to establish the diagnosis of AIH after transplantation.

Recurrent AIH risk factors include suboptimal IS, recipient HLA DR3 and DR4, type I versus type II AIH before transplantation, severe inflammation in the explant/native liver, and longer follow-up (reviewed in [470, 471]). Wozniak et al. showed that DSA (esp. anti-DQ) can also be a risk factor for de novo AIH, late TCMR, and chronic rejection [219].

De novo AIH is an uncommon cause of late (>1 year) graft dysfunction associated with serologic and histologic features that resemble AIH and develops in 3%–5% of recipients transplanted for indications other than AIH. TCMR and steroid-dependence are risk factors for de novo AIH in pediatric recipients [472]. Liver/kidney microsome autoantibodies and anti-glutathione-S-transferase T1 (GSST1) have been associated with de novo AIH (reviewed in [233, 470, 471]). Null GSTT1 genotype recipients of GSTT1+ donor liver triggers antibodies against the allograft that contribute to the development of hepatitis; microvascular C4d deposits have also been described [247]. Other groups have not seen this association (reviewed in [233, 470, 471]). Other autoantibodies include antibodies to cytokeratin 8/18 [473] and atypical LKM antibodies directed at isoforms of carbonic anhydrase III, subunit β1 of proteasome, and members of different glutathione S-transferase (GST) families [474]. Autoantibodies directed at class II HLA antigens play a role in AIH [475].

It is not unreasonable to suggest that "de novo" AIH might simply represent plasma cell-rich TCMR. Most patients with recurrent or new onset AIH are first detected because of elevated liver injury tests, often when an attempt is made to routinely discontinue corticosteroids from the IS regimen. The diagnosis is established on needle biopsy combined with clinicopathologic and serologic correlation [229].

A unique setting in which de novo development of antibodies directed against bile salt export pump (BSEP) proteins occurs in the pediatric population. BSEP proteins are expressed on the canalicular membrane of hepatocytes, and similar to blood group antigens, anti-BSEP antibodies can occur in recipients deficient for these proteins [476–478]. Therefore, proteins missing since birth can trigger immunologic reactions after transplantation, which may occur from months to many years after transplantation [476–478]. The clinical presentation most often includes jaundice, pruritus, and elevated bilirubin and aminotransferases, and an important finding in this setting to distinguish it from other causes of graft intra-hepatic cholestasis is the presence of normal GGTP levels [476–478].

Histopathology and Differential Diagnosis

Histopathologic features of de novo or recurrent AIH are indistinguishable from those observed in native livers and are characterized in the typical case by aggressive, often plasma cell-rich necro-inflammatory-type interface activity with variable perivenular necro-inflammatory activity [479]. This constellation of features is an excellent, but not infallible, histopathologic marker of autoimmunity [445, 446]. Plasma cell-rich central perivenulitis is also common, which can also be a feature of acute TCMR in both adults and pediatric patients [480]. Distinguishing between centrilobular-based acute rejection and AIH can be problematic. A high percentage of plasma cells (>30%) favors AIH, whereas inflammatory bile duct damage or BEC senescence changes involving a majority of ducts favors rejection [479].

Liver recipients that develop de novo anti-BSEP antibodies present histologically with cholestasis, hepatocyte multinucleation/giant cells, prominent interface ductular reaction, and fibrosis, which can all lead to allograft failure. Aggressive plasma cell-rich interface or perivenular necro-inflammatory activity or inflammatory bile duct damage has *not* been described [476–478].

An AIH diagnosis in an allograft needs to be properly correlated with clinicopathologic and serologic profiles. Once a "hepatitic" pattern of injury is morphologically established, examination of the medical record is needed to: a) support an autoimmune etiology (e.g., ANA, ASMA, LKM, serum gamma globulins); and b) reasonably exclude other causes of a chronic hepatitis pattern of injury, such as HBV, HCV, HEV, PBC, and obstructive cholangiopathy (reviewed in [233, 470, 471]).

Distinguishing AIH from conventional acute and chronic rejection uses the same criteria as those used to distinguish acute and chronic rejection from viral hepatitis (see HCV). Distinguishing AIH from obstructive cholangiopathy and PBC has already been discussed in the sections on biliary tract complications and PBC, respectively.

Primary Biliary Cirrhosis (PBC)

Introduction and Pathophysiology

PBC is a rare chronic cholestatic liver disease of unknown etiology [481] characterized by destructive lymphogranulomatous cholangitis, which, if left untreated, progresses toward cirrhosis over a period of 10–30 years (reviewed in [481, 482]). Treatment with UDCA can slow disease progression and has resulted in fewer PBC patients requiring liver replacement (reviewed in [481, 482]).

PBC recurs in approximately 9%–35% of recipients, depending on whether protocol biopsies are conducted or not, with an average time to recurrence from three to five and a half years. Variation in rates among centers is usually attributable to whether biopsies are done by indication or protocol, sampling variation, and histopathologic criteria used to establish the diagnosis (reviewed in [481, 482]). Interestingly, new onset PBC has not been reported. Risk factors for recurrent PBC include recipient age, gender, HLA status and IS, and donor age, gender, and ischemic time, although debate exists for each (reviewed in [481, 482]).

Clinical Presentation

Centers that conduct protocol biopsies most often detect recurrent disease in those biopsies from asymptomatic patients who often have (near) normal liver injury test profiles [482]; jaundice is uncommonly observed. Other symptoms, such as fatigue and metabolic bone disease, can be multifactorial and nonspecific. In the large Mayo experience, only 12% of recurrent PBC patients report disease-related symptoms, with fatigue and pruritus being most common [482]. Centers conducting indication-only biopsies first detect recurrent PBC because of preferential increases in alkaline phosphatase and/or gamma glutamyl transpeptidase during routine serologic monitoring.

Recurrent PBC can progress after liver transplantation, but retransplantation for recurrent PBC is still rare and long-term patient and graft survival results are excellent [482]. AMA are of little additional benefit in establishing the diagnosis because AMA transiently decline shortly after transplantation, but then recur in the vast majority, even without recurrent disease. Allograft needle biopsy is needed to establish the diagnosis with certainty. UDCA treatment of recurrent PBC after transplantation is still undergoing evaluation and has not yet significantly impacted patient or allograft survival [482]. However, a recent study has shown that

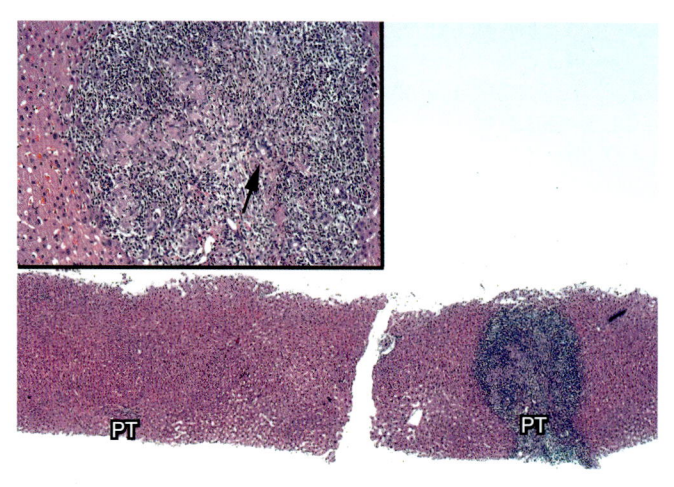

Figure 3.27 Recurrent PBC is diagnosed using the same criteria as in native livers. Usually, there is significant mononuclear inflammation, but it only involves a minority of the portal tracts, at least in the early stages when recurrent disease is most often first discovered. The diagnosis is based on noninfectious, non-caseating, granulomatous duct destructive lesions, as shown in the upper left inset. The arrow highlights the damaged bile duct (PT = portal tract).

preventative UDCA administration reduces the risk of PBC reoccurrence [483].

Histopathologic Findings

Due to the nonspecificity of clinical, serological, and biochemical parameters, the same strict histopathologic criteria are recommended for a recurrent PBC diagnosis as for native livers (see Figure 3.27). Diagnostic lesions include non-infectious, non-caseating, granulomatous, or severe lymphocytic cholangitis producing breaks in the ductal basement membranes, referred to as "florid duct lesions" (reviewed in [482]). Patchy dense portal plasmacytic infiltrates at one year after transplantation presage later development of full-blown disease [484].

Diagnostic bile duct lesions are not always present. Instead, recurrent PBC often presents with patchy mononuclear portal inflammation with focal lymphocytic cholangitis accompanied by portal lymphoid nodules and prominent ductular type interface activity and typical "biliary" changes: interface ductular reaction, periportal "clearing" or edema, cholestasis, accumulation of copper or copper associated pigment in periportal hepatocytes, and patchy small bile duct loss [482]. Such cases are deemed "strongly suggestive" of recurrent PBC if they occur in the proper context, which includes an original disease of PBC with no other reasonable explanation for the biliary pathology and preferential elevation of the γGTP and ALP.

A recurrent PBC diagnosis is less certain in biopsies with only mild changes or without significant lymphocytic cholangitis or a biliary gestalt. For example, "possible" recurrent PBC might first present as unexplained chronic hepatitis [282, 485] because a sampling problem may have missed the bile duct damage or the patient is presenting as an overlap syndrome with AIH [485] or as AIH, alone [486].

Lobular findings in recurrent PBC are usually mild and nonspecific: mild spotty necrosis, slightly increased sinusoidal lymphocytes, mild NRH changes, and Kupffer cell granulomas. More significant lobular findings usually signal another or co-existent insult. Recurrent PBC progression is characterized by development of "biliary-type" fibrosis, cholestasis, and deposition of copper and copper-associated proteins at the edge of the lobules, and portal-to-portal bridging fibrosis.

Differential Diagnosis

Recurrent PBC needs to be distinguished from acute TCMR and chronic rejection, obstructive cholangiopathy, chronic viral, autoimmune or idiopathic hepatitis, and DILI [487]. Other causes of granulomatous cholangitis, such as fungal or acid-fast bacterial infections and HCV, should also be reasonably excluded [488]. These same disorders can also co-exist with recurrent PBC.

Neither acute TCMR nor chronic rejection shows a significant ductular reaction or leads to biliary fibrosis/cirrhosis. Rejection-associated portal inflammation and lymphocytic cholangitis usually involves a majority of portal tracts and preferentially involves small bile ducts (<20 microns in smallest diameter). PBC-associated portal inflammation and lymphocytic cholangitis, in contrast, is typically patchy and preferentially involves medium-sized bile ducts (>40–50 microns in shortest diameter).

PBC patients can also develop de novo AIH or an overlap syndrome after liver transplantation [486, 489]. Clinical, serologic, and histopathologic criteria used to establish the diagnosis of AIH and overlap syndrome before transplantation can also be used after transplantation, but are more difficult to apply. Bhanji et al. showed that patients that received an allograft for end-stage liver disease secondary to overlap syndrome had a higher rate of disease recurrence when compared with transplant recipients with single autoimmune liver disorders [490].

Recurrent PBC can be quite difficult to distinguish from obstructive cholangiopathy because both produce a biliary profile, described above. The clinical history and radiographic findings can be particularly helpful in making this distinction. Any history of biliary tract stricturing, or any factors predisposing to one, should make one favor obstructive cholangiopathy because mechanical problems tend to persist. Histopathologic features that favor obstructive cholangiopathy over recurrent PBC include: 1) edema and/or neutrophilic inflammation in and around the true bile ducts in the middle of the portal connective tissue; 2) centrilobular hepatocanalicular cholestasis; 3) bile infarcts; and 4) intralobular neutrophil clusters. Cholangiography may still be required to exclude a mechanical problem [488, 491].

PBC can be difficult to distinguish from chronic viral and AIH, particularly since some manifestations of recurrent HCV can show a prominent ductular reaction, mimicking a biliary profile, as described above. Careful bile duct examination for evidence of significant lymphocytic or granulomatous duct damage and small bile duct loss can be helpful. In addition, most chronic hepatitis cases do not produce a biliary profile. Portal granulomas have been reported with recurrent chronic

HCV [492]. This observation, however, is uncommon and HCV-associated granulomas rarely cause noticeable or severe ductal damage. Finally, copper and copper-associated protein stains can be used to distinguish between ductular reactions attributable to chronic cholestasis from those related to other insults.

Recurrent PSC

Introduction and Clinical Presentation

PSC is also a disease of dysregulated immunity that usually arises in males (approximately 60%–70%) with co-existent ulcerative colitis (reviewed in [493]). It is the most common indication for liver transplantation in Scandinavian countries (reviewed in [493]) and the cause is unknown. The recurrence rate is approximately 20% by five years, appears to increase with time, and recent data suggest that disease recurrence is beginning to adversely affect long-term patient and allograft survival (reviewed in [493]). However, recurrent PSC can be challenging to diagnose with certainty because of numerous other biliary insults (e.g. ischemic injury from prolonged preservation or non-heart beating donors, imperfect biliary anastomoses, inadequate hepatic arterial flow, acute AMR, and non-anastomotic intra-hepatic biliary strictures). All of these allograft complications can mimic recurrent PSC.

Early-stage recurrent PSC is usually first detected after more than six to nine months because of selective elevation of alkaline phosphatase and gamma glutamyl transpeptidase. The usual cause of these biochemical abnormalities is the development of non-anastomotic intra-hepatic biliary strictures. Occasionally, inadequately followed patients will first present with jaundice and/or signs and symptoms of ascending cholangitis. Non-anastomotic intra-hepatic biliary strictures that develop *before* 90 days after transplantation are usually not attributable to recurrent disease, and therefore, other causes should be sought.

Recurrent PSC risk factors include donor or recipient HLA-DRB1*08, absence of donor HLA DR52, gender mismatch, male recipients, older and younger recipient age [494], intact colon [495], increased body mass index (BMI) [495], related or ECDs, episodes of TCMR, maintenance steroid therapy for ulcerative colitis for >3 months, ulcerative colitis post-transplant [494], co-existent cholangiocarcinoma, and concurrent CMV infection. Conflicting results in the literature likely point toward disease complexity. Most studies have shown that colectomy before or after transplantation is protective. Patients with PSC are also at greater risk for acute and chronic and steroid-resistant rejection.

Recent studies suggest that recurrent disease is beginning to adversely affect long-term patient and allograft survival (reviewed in [493]). A Hungarian study showed that recurrent PSC significantly affects long-term mortality and graft loss and suggested that pre-transplant total colectomy might exert a protective effect [495]. As in native livers, recurrent PSC progresses over a period of years and eventually results in biliary-type fibrosis/cirrhosis. Cholangiographic (PTC, ERCP, MRCP) findings that help distinguish recurrent PSC from other causes of biliary strictures include time after transplantation (>90 days), mural irregularity, diverticulum-like outpouchings, and an overall appearance resembling PSC in native livers [496]. These findings are not specific and PTC and ERCP might be more sensitive than MRCP in detecting early abnormalities.

Histopathologic Findings

Recurrent PSC is histopathologically similar to native disease and cannot be reliably distinguished from other causes of biliary tract stricturing in a needle biopsy [497, 498]. Typical early-stage findings include mild nonspecific acute and chronic "pericholangitis" and a variable, low-grade interface ductular reaction. A "biliary" profile appears as the disease progresses: irregular stellate fibrous expansion of most portal tracts accompanied by variable portal edema, periductal lamellar edema, stellate-shaped lumen of septal bile ducts, intra-epithelial or intra-luminal neutrophils within bile ducts, fibrous cholangitis, focal small bile duct loss, interface foamy macrophages tissue, ductular-type interface activity surrounded by edema, and periportal deposition of golden pigment and copper and copper-associated protein and hepatocyte ductular metaplasia on CK7 staining.

The spatial relationship between expanded portal tracts and central veins remains intact until well-developed cirrhosis appears. Lobular findings in early recurrent PSC include variable cholestasis, lobular neutrophil clusters, and mild NRH [497, 498]. Later stages are characterized by biliary cirrhosis, cholestasis, intra-lobular foam cell clusters, marked deposition of copper and copper-associated protein, and Mallory's hyaline at the edge of the nodules. A recent bioinformatics study of PSC in explanted livers also determined that arterial fibrointimal hyperplasia was a distinctive feature that may aid in diagnosis [499].

Differential Diagnosis

Similar to native liver PSC, extensive clinicopathologic and radiographic correlation is needed to determine whether recurrent PSC or one of the many other causes of biliary tract pathology is responsible for the changes observed. This distinction is not possible based on peripheral core needle biopsy findings alone. Instead, recurrent PSC should be diagnosed only after on a complete analysis of clinical, histopathologic, and radiographic findings, including important exclusionary criteria [497].

Metabolic Diseases and Toxic Insults

Jaffe [500] devised an algorithm to separate metabolic diseases into three categories for the purpose of understanding the impact of liver transplantation on the disease process and the potential for recurrent disease (Table 3.5). As more medical therapies appear, however, the need for liver replacement therapy is decreasing, but still effective when required (reviewed in [501]). Jaffe's classification system is as follows: 1) the liver is the primary site of the defect and causes end-stage liver disease; 2) the liver is the primary site of the defect, but adverse effects manifest primarily extra-hepatically; and 3) the defect is extrahepatic and effects on the liver are secondary.

Table 3.5 Summary of Metabolic Disease Treated by Liver Transplantation Classified According to the System of Jaffe et al. [500] (See Text)

Liver Is the Site of the Primary Metabolic Defect and Liver Is Usually Diseased (See Text)	Liver Is the Site of Primary Metabolic Defect, but Liver Is Usually Normal or Near Normal	Site of Primary Metabolic Defect Is Probably Extra-hepatic and Liver Transplantation Decreases Morbidity and Mortality Associated with Liver Disease
α₁ –Antitrypsin deficiency [501, 608]	Branched chain amino acid deficiencies (reviewed in [501])	Cystinosis [500] does not generally cause liver disease; one patient developed intra-hepatic crystal deposits in liver with perivenular fibrosis and recurrent disease in the allograft [500]
Bile acid synthesis defects [501]	Crigler-Najjar syndrome [609, 610]	Cystic fibrosis; cures liver disease, and if liver transplant is done early, lung function can improve [501]
Carbohydrate metabolism defects (review in [501]	Familial amyloid polyneuropathy (FAP) [611]. Mild liver abnormalities; amyloid deposits in portal tracts and nerve trunks; use of FAP-affected liver is controversial	Porphyria (reviewed in [612, 613])
Familial intra-hepatic cholestasis syndromes (review in [501])	Familial hypercholesterolemia [500]	Hemochromatosis or (inadvertent transplantation of donor with hemochromatosis) reviewed in [614]
Glycogen storage disease, type I and Ib, III, IV [501, 615, 616]	Hemophilia A and B [500]	Niemann-Pick disease [500, 501]
Hemochromatosis, neonatal (review in [501])	Oxaluria, type I [500, 501]	Sea-blue histiocyte syndrome [617]
Mitochondrial defects, limited to liver (reviewed in [501])	Urea cycle enzyme deficiencies [500, 501]	
Tyrosinemia [501, 618]		
Wilson's disease [501, 619]		

Patients in the first group who failed medical or other surgical therapy, if available, are prime candidates for liver transplantation because the cirrhotic liver is replaced by a genetically and structurally normal one that generally cures the disease. Some familial intra-hepatic cholestasis syndromes, however, recur because de novo antibodies develop in response to non-inherited proteins introduced with the donor organ [476–478] (see AIH section).

The liver is structurally normal or near normal in the second group. The goal of liver transplantation is to alleviate the systemic disease burden of abnormal liver physiology. Some *resected native livers* from patients in this group (e.g., familial amyloid polyneuropathy (FAP) [82], oxalosis [83], and perhaps, α-1-anti-trypsin deficiency [84]) are then knowingly or unknowingly transplanted in adult recipients with a different chronic liver disease. These "domino" transplants transfer the structurally normal but genetically abnormal donor liver, and the underlying systemic disease, to the recipient. The rationale is that decades of survival are possible before clinically significant recipient disease manifests.

The liver allograft is vulnerable to recurrent disease in the third group since the metabolic disorder persists after transplantation. Improved survival and/or quality of life issues, however, justify liver replacement [500].

Recurrent Non-alcoholic Steatohepatitis

Introduction and Clinical Presentation

The worldwide obesity epidemic affects every aspect of liver transplantation: an increased need of liver transplants due to NASH; decreased quality of fatty deceased and live donor livers; negative impact of obesity on graft outcomes; and finally, the recurrence or development of de novo NAFLD/NASH [502]. NAFLD is currently the most common cause of chronic liver disease [487], the second most common etiology of liver disease among wait-listed patients (reviewed in [503]), and the third leading indication for liver transplantation in the United States, but is on trajectory to become the most common indication [504]. It is also thought to be the primary cause of cryptogenic cirrhosis, which accounts for another 7%–14% of liver transplants in the United States [505].

Liver replacement for NAFLD is more likely to occur in older, female, and higher BMI recipients. The relatively low rates of advanced fibrosis and NAFLD-associated graft loss when compared with the increased survival rates because of transplantation suggest that although NAFLD can recur, the clinical significance of disease recurrence appears to be small (reviewed in [506]). Fibrosis progression for recurrent NASH versus HCV showed more rapid fibrosis progression in the latter and steroid use increased fibrosis progression in NAFLD recipients [507].

Many NAFLD risk factors, such as obesity, diabetes, metabolic syndrome/insulin resistance, etc. persist, or are made worse after transplantation by the IS [508–513]. Therefore, the incidence of recurrence is high: 70%–100% for steatosis at three to five years and 5%–25% develop steatohepatitis. However, less than 5% patients have developed progressive fibrosis/cirrhosis [508–513]. Progression from steatosis to steatohepatitis and progressive fibrosis in some patients suggest that recurrent NAFLD might become a more important cause of late allograft injury, fibrosis, and failure, although the benefits of transplantation appear to outweigh risks [507].

Recurrent NAFLD is usually first detected on protocol or indicated allograft biopsies in asymptomatic patients with normal or near normal liver injury tests. Many patients have multiple NAFLD risk factors such as obesity, diabetes, and hypertension. A minority of otherwise healthy recipients develop unexplained NALFD; in these patients, metabolic testing for insulin resistance and a search for more esoteric NAFLD causes (see differential diagnosis) is warranted. A significant proportion of patients who underwent liver transplantation for cryptogenic cirrhosis will also develop NAFLD after transplantation [505, 509, 514, 515]. Presumably, these patients had undetected NAFLD before transplantation, but histopathologic features were not obvious in the explant cirrhotic liver.

A variety of treatments have been proposed to treat NAFLD and reduce the manifestations of metabolic syndrome in transplant patients; however, there are no published drug trials that specifically address it in the post-transplant population (reviewed in [503]). The most obvious intervention is lifestyle modifications, including dietary restrictions and exercise. Other supplement treatments and medications such as vitamin E, statins, ACE inhibitors, pentoxifyline, metformin, PPAR agonists, obeticholic acid, SGLT2 inhibitors, and GLP-1 analogs have been proposed (reviewed in [503]). Bariatric surgery has had mixed reviews with some studies showing benefit [516, 517].

Histopathology and Differential Diagnosis

A detailed description of the histopathology of hepatic steatosis and steatohepatitis are known to most pathologists and appear similar to native livers. Readers, therefore, are referred elsewhere for an excellent review [518]. Detailed studies to determine whether the histopathology of NAFLD/NASH in liver allograft recipients differs that seen in native livers have not been conducted.

NAFLD refers to biopsies with greater than 5% of hepatocytes showing steatosis; a NASH diagnosis also requires evidence of hepatocyte injury (ballooning, apoptosis, or lytic necrosis) and lobular inflammation. The presence of fibrosis is not required [518], although it typically begins in perivenular sinusoids.

The differential diagnosis for recurrent alcoholism and NAFLD is extensive and includes all of the disorders known to cause steatosis and steatohepatitis in the general population. Alcoholic liver disease (ALD) is very difficult to distinguish from NASH with certainty. In native livers, steatosis and nuclear vacuoles are more prevalent in the NAFLD group than in the ALD. In contrast, ballooning hepatocytes, lipogranulomas, focal necrosis, acidophilic bodies, and fibrosis and Mallory-Denk bodies are more remarkable in ALD. The steatosis severity and lipogranulomas gradually decrease as the stage of liver fibrosis progresses.

Determining the underlying cause of steatohepatitis in allografts can be particularly difficult in a minority of allografts. Less common causes include poor nutrition, such as protein-calorie malnutrition, starvation, rapid weight loss, and various intestinal bypass or gastric stapling surgeries. Hepatic steatosis and steatohepatitis can also be the result of medications, including amiodarone, perhexiline maleate, glucocorticoids, synthetic estrogens, calcium channel blockers, tamoxifen, methotrexate, valproic acid, cocaine, and anti-viral agents (Zidovudine, Didanosine, and Fialuridine). Metabolic disorders can also cause steatosis and steatohepatitis: hyperlipidemia, Wilson's disease, adult onset citrullinemia (type II), lipodystrophy, dysbetalipoproteinemia, Weber-Christian Disease, Wolman's Disease, cholesterol ester storage disease, and fatty liver of pregnancy. Other less common causes include inflammatory bowel disease, intestinal bacterial overgrowth, and exposure to environmental toxins, including phosphorus, petrochemicals, toxic mushrooms, and organic solvents.

Abnormalities of hepatic blood flow are an important cause of hepatic steatosis and steatohepatitis, especially when it appears in the allograft within several months after transplantation. Examples include porto-systemic shunting because of collaterals that persist after transplantation, pre-hepatic portal hypertension, and patent ductus venosus.

A thorough clinicopathologic correlation is needed to substantiate a suspicion of alcohol relapse or metabolic abnormalities leading to NAFLD. Awareness of the original disease(s), detailed clinical history, including current alcohol use, blood alcohol levels, and the ratio of γ-glutamyl transpeptidase to alkaline phosphatase can be used to distinguish between these possibilities.

Recurrent Alcoholic Liver Disease

Introduction and Pathophysiology

ALD is the second leading indication for liver transplantation in the United States and Europe and is often combined with coexistent conditions such as HCV infection, HCC and metabolic disorders, such as hemochromatosis and alpha one antitrypsin deficiency. The exact incidence of recurrent alcohol use/abuse after transplantation is difficult to determine with certainty, but reported values range from 15%–50% by five years after transplantation (reviewed in [519]).

Recurrent alcohol abuse can directly damage the allograft, or indirectly contribute to allograft dysfunction because of rejection related to non-compliance with IS (reviewed in [519, 520]). Patients transplanted for alcohol-induced liver disease are at increased risk of developing de novo malignancies [521] and

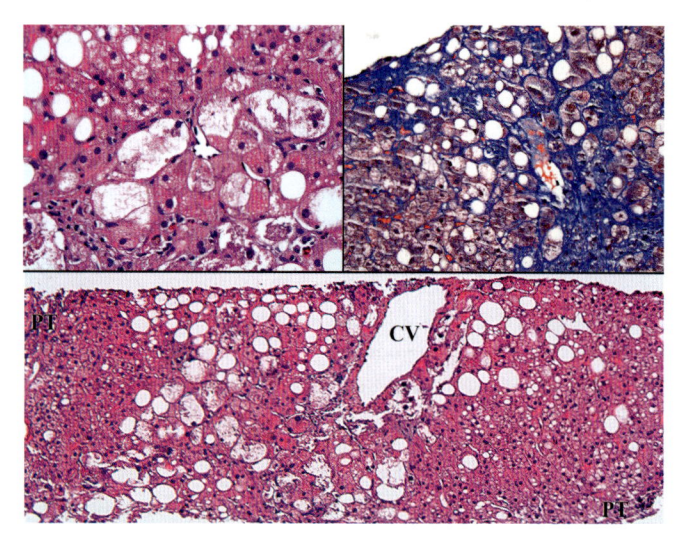

Figure 3.28 Recurrent alcohol abuse is a relatively uncommon cause of significant allograft injury, although it is seen occasionally. In our experience, it is difficult to distinguish alcoholic from NAFLD, but the strict perivenular distribution of mixed steatosis with so-called foamy degeneration of hepatocytes (upper left panel) is typical of recurrent alcohol use. Eventually, this can lead to subsinusoidal fibrosis (upper right inset) (CV = central vein).

cardiovascular diseases, the incidence of which is increased in patients that are smokers (reviewed in [487]).

Clinical Presentation

Problems with alcohol recidivism are usually detected because of elevation of routinely obtained liver injury tests [520], missed medical appointments [522], inappropriate social behavior [282], and non-compliance with IS (reviewed in [519, 520]). A high γ-glutamyl transpeptidase to alkaline phosphatase ratio might provide biochemical evidence of alcohol recurrence [282, 520]. But blood alcohol levels are more definitive proof of relapse. A small minority of recipients experience a rapid downhill course because of recurrent alcoholic or non-alcoholic steatohepatitis [523–525], but in general, this course of events is rare.

Pretransplant screening programs attempt to identify patients who are likely to relapse after transplantation; however, patients, particularly those undergoing transplant evaluation, have been shown to under report evidence of abuse [526]. Since none are entirely successful, a comprehensive psychosocial evaluation is recommended (reviewed in [519, 520, 526]).

Since definition of alcohol relapse varies, a wide range (10%–90%) of estimated recurrence exists (reviewed in [487]). Most alcoholics do not relapse badly enough to cause significant alcoholic liver allograft disease. Rice et al. showed that 16% of patients relapsed, but only 5.3% continued heavy drinking, which was the only type of relapse that increased graft fibrosis and decreased graft survival [527]. Therefore, recurrent ALD minimally impacts long-term patient and allograft survival and is generally a good indication for liver replacement (reviewed in [519, 520]).

Histopathologic Findings and Differential Diagnosis

Alcoholic allograft liver disease causes identical histopathologic changes as those seen in native livers. The most common histopathologic presentation is small and large droplet steatosis involving primarily centrilobular hepatocytes. The zonal distribution pattern of the steatosis is usually distinctive (see Figure 3.28). More significant abuse and injury can lead to so-called "foamy" degeneration of centrilobular hepatocytes, followed by fully developed "alcoholic hepatitis" with Mallory-Denk bodies, ballooning degeneration of hepatocytes, and lobular inflammation or satelliteosis [528, 529]. Persistent abuse can eventually cause perivenular and subsinusoidal fibrosis [520, 523]. In our experience, relapse can also present with increased iron deposition in periportal hepatocytes and the reticular-endothelial cells and hepatocytes without significant steatosis [282]. As in the native livers, alcoholic steatohepatitis (ASH) can co-exist with HCV and any other cause of allograft dysfunction and combined insults can lead to more rapid development of fibrosis [520, 523].

Protocol biopsy follow-up of alcoholic recipients at one, three, five, and ten years after transplantation showed no differences in fibrosis between those known to return to abuse compared to those who apparently did not. Portal inflammation, however, was significantly increased at all-time points examined, but there was only minimal deterioration of allograft structure over time and there was not association with recurrent alcohol abuse, similar to that seen in another study [530].

For the differential diagnosis, please see the above section on non-alcoholic steatohepatitis.

Idiopathic Post-transplant Hepatitis (IPTH)

Introduction, Pathophysiology, and Clinical Presentation

IPTH is a diagnostic term coined by Hubscher [531] to describe patients that show chronic hepatitis changes on allograft biopsy (i.e., mononuclear portal inflammation with variable interface activity) but have no clinical or serologic evidence of viral hepatitis infection, autoimmunity, or adverse drug reaction (reviewed in [100, 229]). According to the definition, features of TCMR, such as bile duct damage and venous endothelial inflammation, are neither severe nor widespread (reviewed in [100, 229]).

The prevalence of IPTH will likely dwindle as the underlying etiology is discovered. Examples re-assigned to other etiologies include chronic HEV infection, discussed above; DSA+ recipients with lymphocytic portal inflammation and low-grade interface activity [217, 219, 226, 236, 532]; and a small subgroup of likely recurrent AIH, although strict criteria might not always be met [531].

Most recipients with IPTH are first detected on protocol allograft biopsy evaluation and are usually asymptomatic with normal or near normal liver tests. Therefore, incidence and prevalence of IPTH is generally higher at centers that conduct protocol biopsies. Lack of a consensus definition, different IS regimens, undiscovered virus(es) (e.g., HEV [461]), and a combination of these reasons probably explain the center variations [533]. More importantly, about 5% of IPTH patients followed up for a minimum of ten years will develop progressive fibrosis/cirrhosis [531]. Figures for IPTH and progressive fibrosis are even higher in children (reviewed in [100, 229]), and nearly 60% of pediatric recipients develop IPTH by ten years and 15% develop significant fibrosis/cirrhosis by ten years (reviewed in [100, 229, 233].

Aini et al. showed that graft aging (measured by TI decline and donor abnormal karyotype ratio) was associated with IPTH in long-surviving allografts [534]. More studies are needed on this topic, but current thinking suggests that a substantial percentage of IPTH cases represent a variant of late onset of TCMR with or without chronic AMR (reviewed in [100, 229, 233, 533]).

Histopathology and Differential Diagnosis

IPTH is characterized by chronic portal inflammation, variable interface, and lobular necro-inflammatory activity, but without prominent or prevalent bile duct damage or central perivenulitis. Prevalent lymphocytic cholangitis and central perivenulitis are more suggestive of active TCMR. Significant plasma cell inflammation comprising greater than 30% of the infiltrates is uncommon and suggests recurrent AIH or plasma cell hepatitis [535]. Other causes of chronic hepatitis, such as HBV, HCV, HEV, and recurrent AIH should be reasonably excluded using a combination of clinical, serologic, and molecular diagnostic parameters.

The differential diagnosis for IBTH is the same as that for hepatitis B or C virus infection or AIH, discussed above.

Long-term Changes Not Readily Explained by Recurrent Disease

Long-surviving allografts may show histopathologic changes that cannot be attributed to disease recurrence or placed into a specific diagnostic category. These changes might represent adverse side effects of medications' long-term engraftment, abnormal graft physiology (reviewed in [229, 233, 282]), and chronic AMR [217, 219, 226, 236, 532]. Included are portal venopathy and NRH, thickening and hyalinization of small hepatic artery branches [282, 536], subsinusoidal fibrosis, and "nonspecific" portal and lobular inflammation (reviewed in [229, 233, 282]).

If NRH changes are detected early (less than four years) after transplantation, progression to portal hypertension can occur [537]. Older livers placed into younger recipients (e.g., parent to child living donation) continue to age at the same or an accelerated rate (unpublished observation) and do not appear to experience any rejuvenation by being placed into a young body [538]. Emerging evidence suggests that late onset TCMR, NRH, de novo AIH, and IPTH may all be part of an overlapping spectrum of immune-mediated injury [233]. As long-term survival after liver replacement is becoming increasingly common, more study on these issues will be needed.

Adverse Drug Reactions and Toxic Injury

Histopathologic manifestations associated with DILI are generally the same as those in native livers. An exception might be drugs that elicit allergic reactions, which might be muted because of potent baseline IS. It is still difficult, however, to distinguish hepatic-based DILI from TCMR, recurrent disease, and other complications. Nevertheless, complaints of DILI after liver replacement are relatively uncommon [539]. Azathioprine use has been associated with centrilobular necrosis and central vein and subsinusoidal fibrosis [540]. NRH has been attributed to chronic toxicity [536], but is also frequently seen in recipients not treated with this medication. Pseudo-ground-glass cells, composed of abnormal glycogen and closely resembling polyglucosan bodies, are seen with increased frequency in liver allografts [541] and might be related to disturbed glycogen metabolism and polypharmacotherapy.

Considerations Involved in the Evaluation of Late Liver Allograft Dysfunction and Protocol Biopsies

Liver allograft biopsy evaluation for late dysfunction is challenging and increasingly important because of excellent short-term survival. A broad spectrum of insults can cause dysfunction and many of them show overlapping clinical, serological, and histopathologic features. These issues were addressed by the BANFF Working Group for liver allograft pathology, who spent several years constructing a consensus document to help guide the interpretation of such biopsies [229].

Recipients are routinely monitored for liver allograft dysfunction using liver injury tests more than one year after transplantation. Late biopsies are obtained in most programs only by indication [229]. Despite differences in recipient pools, immunosuppressive regimens, and study designs, the structural integrity and causes of late liver allograft dysfunction in recipients 1–19 years after transplantation are remarkably similar (reviewed in [233, 282]).

Leading causes of late liver allograft dysfunction include recurrence of the original disease and obstructive cholangiopathy (Tables 3.6 and 3.7) (reviewed in [233, 282]). TCMR and chronic rejection was detected in only 4%–38% of late biopsies. Knowledge of the original disease, changes in IS, previous biopsy findings, the clinical and laboratory profile, and the results of any therapeutic or diagnostic tests or intervention should be incorporated into the final interpretation (reviewed in [229, 233, 282]).

Few programs obtain protocol biopsies in HCV-negative recipients. Obtaining protocol allograft biopsies in asymptomatic long-term survivors with normal or near normal liver tests is controversial [229, 233, 542–544], but resistance is less strong because of changes associated with de novo DSA and putative chronic AMR [217, 219, 226, 236, 532]. Morbidity and mortality, costs, inconvenience, resource utilization, and potential adverse impacts of unexplained histopathologic findings that might precipitate unnecessary therapy are arguments against protocol biopsies. These should be weighed against potential individual and/or societal benefits, such as: 1) early detection of clinically unapparent disease, including chronic AMR; 2) monitoring the effects of IS optimization and weaning (reviewed in [229, 233, 282]); and 3) the impact of chronic low-grade recurrent disease and long-term engraftment.

Table 3.6 Histopathologic Features Most Commonly Detected with Various Causes of Late Liver Allograft Dysfunction;* Adapted from [229].

Histopathologic Features	AIH2	Acute Rejection	Chronic Rejection	Chronic Viral Hepatitis Types B and C	PBC	PSC/BD Strictures
Distribution, severity, and composition of portal inflammation	Usually diffuse predominantly mononuclear of varying intensity; often prominent plasma cell component	Usually diffuse, variable intensity; mixed "rejection-type" (see text) infiltrate	Patchy, usually minimal or mild lymphoplasmacytic	Patchy, variable intensity; predominantly mononuclear; nodular aggregates	Noticeably patchy and variable intensity; predominantly mononuclear; nodular aggregates and granulomas	Usually patchy to diffuse depending on stage; mild neutrophilic, eosinophilic, or occasionally mononuclear predominant
Presence and type of interface activity	Usually prominent and defining feature: necro-inflammatory-type; often plasma cell-rich	Focally present and mild necro-inflammatory type	Minimal to absent	Variable, usually not prominent: necro-inflammatory and (ductular-type)	Important feature later in disease development: ductular and necro-inflammatory-type with copper deposition	Prominent and defining feature: ductular-type with portal and periportal edema
Bile duct inflammation and damage	Variable; if present, involves a minority of bile ducts	Present and usually involves a majority of bile ducts	Focal ongoing lymphocytic bile duct damage; inflammation wanes with duct loss	Variable; if present, involves a minority of bile ducts	Granulomatous or focally severe lymphocytic cholangitis is diagnostic in proper setting	Periductal lamellar edema, "fibrous cholangitis," acute cholangitis, and multiple intra-portal ductal profiles
Biliary epithelial senescence changes and small bile loss	Absent or involves only a minority of ducts/portal tracts, but may be focally severe	Absent or involves only a minority of ducts	Senescence/atrophy/atypia involve a majority of remaining ducts (see text)	Absent or involves only a minority of ducts	Small bile duct loss associated with ductular reaction	Small bile duct loss associated with ductular reaction
Perivenular mononuclear inflammation and/or hepatocyte dropout	Variable, can involve a majority of perivenular regions, similar to rejection (see text); may be plasma cell-rich.	Variable, if defining feature should involve a majority of perivenular regions; may also show subendothelial inflammation of vein (see text)	Usually present, but variable	Variable, but generally mild; if present, involves a minority of perivenular regions	Variable, but generally mild; if present, involves a minority of perivenular regions	Absent

Lobular findings and necro-inflammatory activity	Variable severity; rosettes may be present and/or prominent	Variable; if present, concentrated in perivenular regions	Disarray variable; variable severity; necro-inflammatory activity	Mild disarray, parenchymal granulomas, periportal copper deposition, and cholatestasis are late features	Disarray unusual; neutrophil clusters; ± Cholestasis
Pattern of fibrosis during progression toward cirrhosis	Usually macronodular, post-hepatitic pattern	Rare	Usually macronodular, hepatitic pattern; may be micronodular (see text)	Biliary pattern	Biliary pattern

* The histopathologic findings in this table should be combined with clinical, serological, radiographic, and important exclusionary criteria listed in Table 3.2 to arrive at a final diagnosis.[2] The same findings apply to recurrent and de novo AIH.

Table 3.7 Inclusionary and Exclusionary Criteria for the Diagnosis of Recurrent and New Onset Chronic Necro-inflammatory Diseases after Liver Transplantation and Timing of First Onset and Pattern of Liver Test Elevations.[1] Adapted from [229] and [606].

Diagnosis	Original Disease	Serology/Molecular Testing[2]	Timing[3] and Liver Injury Test Profile[4]	Important Exclusionary Criteria
Recurrent AIH	AIH	- auto-antibodies** (ANA, ASMA, ALKM) usually in high titers (>1:80); raised serum IgG	- >6 months; hepatocellular	- acute and chronic rejection, HBV, HCV, HEV infection, as determined by third-generation ELISA assay and/or by serum or tissue PCR
De novo AIH	Other than AIH	-Same as above	- >6 months; hepatocellular;	- same as above
Recurrent HBV or HCV	HBV- or HCV-induced cirrhosis	- HBV or HCV infection using standard, third-generation serologic criteria and/or positive molecular testing for HBV or HCV nucleic acids	usually 6-8 weeks, but as early as ten days - usually hepatocellular, but may be cholestatic	- acute and chronic rejection; AIH
Recurrent PBC	PBC	- positive AMA, but little additional benefit because AMA remains elevated in the majority of patients after transplantation	>one year; cholestatic	- biliary tract obstruction/strictures
Recurrent PSC	PSC	NA	- usually >1 yr.; cholestatic	- HA thrombosis/stenosis, chronic (ductopenic) rejection, abnormal surgical anatomy, anastomotic strictures alone, non-anastomotic strictures occurring <90 d after OLTx, and ABO incompatibility
Acute rejection	NA (see text for risk factors)	NA	- any time; usually hepatocellular; may be mixed if superimposed on chronic rejection	- inadequate IS usually, but not always present (see text); important exclusions: biliary tract obstruction/strictures, HBV, HCV, AIH
Chronic rejection	NA (see text for risk factors)	NA	- any time, but usually <1 year; cholestatic; rarely hepatocellular in veno-occlusive variant (see text).	- inadequate IS usually, but not always present (see text); important exclusions: biliary tract obstruction/strictures, HBV, HCV, AIH
IPTH	Non-viral and non-AIH	- Negative testing for HBV, HCV, and HEV infection and autoantibodies	>1 year; usually hepatocellular	- acute and chronic rejection, all other causes of chronic hepatitis, and biliary tract obstruction/strictures reasonably excluded; all attempts should be made to determine cause before establishing this diagnosis

[1] See Table 3.5 for compatible histopathologic findings.[2] Timing=usual timing of first onset.[3] ANA=anti-nuclear antibodies; ASMA=anti-smooth muscle antibodies; ALKM=anti-liver-kidney microsomal antibodies.[4] Sustained elevation for more than one month; Hepatocellular=ALT and/or AST >ALP and/or GGTP; Cholestatic=ALP and/or GGTP >AST and/or ALT; Abbreviations: AIH: AIH; PBC: PBC; PSC: PSC

Successful HCV treatment will remove monitoring this disease from consideration.

Most biopsies (~75%) from recipients surviving >1 year with abnormal liver tests or symptoms show significant histopathological abnormalities (reviewed in [229, 233, 282], usually attributable to recurrent disease or biliary tract strictures. Surprisingly, the latter can be clinically and biochemically occult. About 25% of biopsies from long-surviving asymptomatic recipients with normal liver tests also show significant abnormalities, particularly if the original disease is one that commonly recurs (e.g. HCV, PBC, and AIH (reviewed in [229, 233, 282])).

Minor histopathologic abnormalities occur in about 60%–70% of asymptomatic patients with (near) normal liver tests even in the absence of recurrent disease. Common minor abnormalities include portal venopathy and NRH, thickening and hyalinization of small hepatic artery branches, and "nonspecific" portal and lobular inflammation. The pathogenesis and long-term consequences of these otherwise unexplained long-term histopathological findings are currently under more scrutiny because more patients are affected.

Many late post-transplant biopsies show portal-based mononuclear inflammation with variable necro-inflammatory-type interface activity even in patients without recurrence of chronic necro-inflammatory diseases (e.g., hepatitis virus, PBC, PSC [229]). A combination of subtle histopathologic cues, serological studies, and clinical correlation is relied upon to distinguish among several possible specific causes of dysfunction. Recent evidence linked many of these findings with de novo DSA and inadequate IS [217, 219, 226, 236, 532]. However, the underlying cause of the inflammation is not always apparent even after extensive analysis and issuing a definitive diagnosis might not be possible. Hedging the interpretation by using "features suggestive of early" emphasizing a tentative diagnosis is suggested [229].

Laboratory tests used to establish a diagnosis before transplantation may not have the same significance after transplantation [229]. AMA and ANA often transiently disappear, only to re-appear at lower titers after transplantation in patients with PBC or AIH – even without histopathologic evidence of recurrent disease. Patients without AIH before transplantation can develop auto-antibodies either as a complication of otherwise typical rejection.

Late allograft injury can be mediated by a combination of insults and biopsy reviews to prioritize their relative importance, but careful review and clinicopathologic correlation are needed [229]. IS drug levels can also influence the severity of recurrent viral hepatitis, AIH, TCMR, and chronic AMR. Late onset TCMR, for example, is often precipitated by inadequate IS and recipients with disorders of dysregulated immunity are often steroid-dependent (reviewed in [229, 233]).

Criteria used to diagnose various cause(s) of late liver allograft dysfunction can be generalized to evaluate all potential causes [229]: 1) the histopathologic evidence of liver injury and liver injury tests should show patterns consistent with the diagnosis (e.g., ductular proliferation and elevated biliary enzymes with biliary stricturing); 2) the diagnosis should be supported by positive serologic, molecular biologic, immunologic, or radiographic evidence of pathogen or possible cause of injury; and 3) other causes of similar histopathologic changes and elevated liver tests should have been reasonably excluded (summarized in Tables 3.6 and 3.7).

Monitoring fibrosis progression from either recurrent disease, chronic AMR, or other insults is an important aspect of long-term follow-up, which has recently been aided by quantitative morphometry, discussed below. Concern about recurrent HCV evolution, which can now be successfully treated, has been replaced by concern about long-term consequences of de novo DSA [217, 219, 226, 236, 532]. An increasing number of non-invasive assays intent on reducing the number of biopsies, which is certainly reasonable, have not performed as sensitively or accurately as liver biopsy evaluation [545, 546].

Role of the Pathologist in Chronic Immunosuppression Management

Introduction and Clinical Presentation

Allograft biopsy evaluation plays an important role in IS optimization. This includes closely supervised clinical trials that have a goal of complete IS withdrawal in highly selected recipients (reviewed in [100, 229, 233, 547–550]). Complete weaning of IS is made possible by: 1) liver allograft "tolerogenicity" [252, 551]; and 2) if TCMR does occur during or after weaning, it is usually rapidly reversible with current IS regimens and the allografts heal without significant fibrosis or loss of function (reviewed in [100, 229, 233, 547–550]).

Clinical features associated with successful weaning include longer time intervals between transplantation and weaning initiation [552, 553] (preferably >3 years), less DSA [224, 552], lower incidence of previous TCMR episodes, non-autoimmune primary liver disease, already minimized IS [553], HCV-induced immune senescence [550], and perhaps lower recipient age at time of transplantation [554, 555].

Histopathology and Differential Diagnosis

Most biopsies obtained during IS minimization occur under the auspices of closely supervised clinical trials and are considered mandatory (reviewed in [100, 556]). Findings are the same as those reported in protocol biopsies from asymptomatic long-surviving recipients with normal or near normal liver chemistry tests (reviewed in [100, 229, 233]). Baseline or pre-weaning biopsies obtained just before lowering IS document any inflammatory and structural changes that might preclude IS minimization because of a likelihood of progressive pathology if weaning is attempted (reviewed in [100]).

Most IS minimization protocols exclude patients with advanced fibrosis (i.e., ≥3 Ishak scale) because portal/periportal and perivenular fibrosis has been associated with persistent or de novo DSA and might represent chronic AMR that could worsen after weaning [226]. One study involving HCV+ recipients, however, included recipients with advanced fibrosis and did not encounter problems after weaning and might have benefited from better control of viral replication [557] – a moot point in the current era of high HCV cure rates.

Pre-weaning biopsy findings associated with successful weaning include: 1) less portal inflammation [552, 558]; 2) fewer CD3+ and CD8+ lymphocytes, but more CD45RO+ lymphocytes within the lobules [558]; 3) more portal fibrosis in HCV+ recipients [557], and less prevalent microvascular C4d deposits [552]. These observations suggest that chronic portal inflammation in HCV- patients and tissue C4d deposits in those with circulating DSA might represent a latent form of rejection that manifests clinically after the lowering or removal of IS (reviewed in [100]). Indeed, recent studies suggest that otherwise unexplained chronic hepatitis and fibrosis likely represent a manifestation of chronic AMR (see above).

"For-cause" allograft biopsies obtained during and after IS weaning because of elevated liver injury tests, which often occur during the first several months, most often show TCMR (reviewed in [100, 547]). Liver test elevations, however, can be nonspecific in these closely monitored patients (reviewed in [100, 547]). Gamma-glutamyl transpeptidase elevations appear to be the most specific and sensitive indicator of emerging TCMR [559, 560].

TCMR that manifests during weaning from IS most often resembles so-called "classical" TCMR, described above. However, atypical or incomplete presentations are common because: 1) clinical anxiety may initiate biopsies before characteristic histopathological changes have time to develop; 2) late (>1 year) TCMR differs histologically from early (<3 months) TCMR; 3) the allograft and recipient immune system are chimerically different early versus late after transplantation; and 4) TCMR can evolve more slowly late after transplantation (reviewed in [100, 229, 547]). "Atypical" TCMR presentations include: a) less prevalent and severe inflammatory bile duct damage; b) more prevalent and severe interface and lobular necro-inflammatory activity; and c) less portal venous subendothelial inflammation, resembling low-grade chronic hepatitis (reviewed in [100, 547]).

Early rapid IS weaning from HCV+ [424] and some HCV- recipients [424] treated with lymphocyte-depleting antibodies may "rearm" the immune system (immune reconstitution syndrome) [424] and trigger an aggressive hepatitis with rapid fibrosis progression [424]. These potential complications, however, likely will be eliminated with new effective anti-HCV medications.

Few protocol follow-up biopsy studies have been published from patients after sustained lowering or complete withdrawal of IS (reviewed in [100, 229, 547]. Development of progressive fibrosis, with or without inflammation, has been the major concern (reviewed in [100, 229], although a similar course of events has been documented in patients maintained on standard IS regimens (reviewed in [100, 229]). The BANFF Working Group recommended adequate (two passes with a 16 gauge needle >20 mm and >11 portal tracts (reviewed in [99])) protocol biopsies in patients who do not develop elevated liver injury tests at one, three, five, and ten years after major decreases or total withdrawal of IS (reviewed in [100]).

Follow-up biopsy findings that should elicit concern include any new onset or noticeably increased inflammation especially when associated with tissue damage, such as lymphocytic cholangitis or interface or perivenular necro-inflammatory activity, and obliterative or inflammatory arteriopathy. The same rigorous approach to differential diagnosis used in patients maintained on standard IS regimens should be used in patients undergoing adjustments in IS, but with a heightened awareness of potential rejection.

Molecular Phenotyping of Allograft Biopsies

Introduction

Histopathologic evaluation remains the gold standard for diagnosing rejection in transplanted organs, but there are increasing expectations for pathologists to provide more extensive and granular biopsy data. The hope is that specific results can lead to individually-tailored treatment and/or better predict outcomes. Molecular allograft biopsy analysis is rapidly fulfilling this function by providing important additional data about infiltrative cell populations and activation of specific signaling pathways.

Renal and Heart Allografts

Renal and heart allograft biopsies have been the first subjected to molecular platform analyses. Molecular signatures for kidney allografts [561–566] include profiles for TCMR and increased endothelial cell reactivity/injury transcript expression signals in AMR (endothelial activation and injury transcripts (ENDATs)), including factor VIII/von Willebrand factor, melanoma cell adhesion molecule (MCAM), cadherin-5, selectin E, platelet endothelial cell adhesion molecule 1 (PECAM/CD31), CD34, and caveolin 1, combined with the presence of recipient alloantibodies have increased sensitivity for diagnosing active antibody-mediated injury in renal allografts [567]. Indeed, clinical validation of an AMR signature [568] resulted in revised BANFF criteria [569]. However, local ENDATs use requires local validation and correlation to histopathologic findings, DSA testing, and peritubular capillary C4d results [568].

The AlloMap Molecular Expression Testing for cardiac allograft biopsies assesses the mRNA profile of peripheral blood mononuclear cells (PBMC), based on the Cardiac Allograft Rejection Gene Expression Observation (CARGO) study [570–573]. AlloMap Testing is intended identify stable heart transplant recipients with a low probability of moderate/severe acute cellular rejection (≥2 R according to the current ISHLT criteria). Results show an 84% agreement compared to endomyocardial biopsy scoring [571]. While promising, discordant results and the need for validation in patients with infections (besides CMV) and certain histopathologic findings (e.g., quilty effects) require more attention [571]. Some observed discordances might result from PBMCs versus allograft tissue. A large-scale study, "Invasive Monitoring Attenuation through Gene Expression" (IMAGE), has been conducted and the results will

Liver Transplantation

Initial molecular liver allograft studies were based on peripheral blood analysis [576, 577]. Microarray transcriptome profiling using Affymetrix and Agilent platforms identified biomarkers associated with operational liver transplant tolerance [576–578], providing potential insights into genes related to the recipient's immune response, such as γδ T cells and natural killer cells. The plethora of data generated, inability to find similar profiles in other patient cohorts, and lack of correlation with liver tissue immunopathology are weaknesses. These assays are not feasible for large-scale retrospective studies where blood is not readily available. Some found that molecular signatures could differentiate recurrent HCV from TCMR in liver biopsies [579, 580], but the need for fresh frozen tissue limits general applicability. RNA extracted from FFPE tissue sections are often degraded due to oxidation, cross-linking, and other chemical modifications that are enhanced by exposure to air [581, 582], but several recent reports describing successful transcriptome profiling of FFPE tissues, including both freshly cut and archived sections [582], are a reason for optimism.

Molecular Platforms for Use with FFPE Tissues

The Nanostring nCounter Digital Analysis System (Seattle, WA) high throughput gene expression platform has been used to successfully analyze FFPE tissues. Its probe-based technology does not require amplification and can directly measure low concentration, short DNA, RNA, mRNA, or micro RNA (miRNA) fragments [583]. The analyzer quantifies hundreds of targets simultaneously similar to microarray or multiplex PCR. This probe-based technology enables an individual biopsy to be assigned its own molecular signature that, when compared with known genomic or proteomic data, can: a) be correlated with histopathological findings; b) provide insights about immune reactivity; c) assess potential response(s) to IS; and d) quantify risk(s) for developing infections or cancer [583–585].

The Nanostring technology has been used to provide molecular signatures for multiple liver disease processes, including HCV-related prognostic indices [586], individual responses to HCV anti-viral treatments [585], and molecular classification of HCC [584]. Pfeffer et al. [585] showed an interferon response gene signature association with therapeutic responses HCV+ patients. Tan et al. [584] used Nanostring molecular profiling of FFPE tissue to subclassify HCC into: steatohepatitic, macrotrabecular, and high serum AFP hepatomas. These subclasses tightly associated with dysregulation of therapeutically targetable molecular pathways [584]. Few studies, however, have used the Nanostring platform to study liver allograft biopsies [587, 588].

Future Applications of Molecular Signatures

Kidney, heart, and liver allografts display heterogeneous histopathologic features of rejection, but some elegant studies [589, 590] have shown a significant overlap between the molecular signatures in different allograft organs, termed "Immunologic Constant of Rejection," or Common Rejection Modules, demonstrating common TCMR features, despite the organ. Pathologists must keep current with these cutting edge technologies, and incorporate their outputs with biopsy analysis, or their expertise will become obsolete. Since biopsies are invasive and potential morbidity-producing, adding "value" to biopsy interpretation is warranted [591].

Digital Pathology

Ehrlich performed the first liver aspiration in 1883 and the first percutaneous liver biopsy for diagnostic purposes was conducted in 1923 (reviewed in [592]). Needle liver biopsies have been used for close to 100 years and have been considered the gold standard for diagnosing allograft rejection and inflammatory liver diseases. However, they are expensive, invasive, not without complications, and interpretation is subject to interobserver variability and sampling error [542, 544].

New technologies including nucleic acid, protein, and metabolic array analyses of blood, liver tissue, and bile are emerging as powerful tools in the study of hepatic pathophysiology that go beyond using classical H&E staining and light microscopic examination [593]. A detailed review of this approach, which can significantly enhance histopathologic examination of liver tissue and enable quantitative analysis and interpretation of routine liver biopsy results, is highlighted by Isse et al. [593]. Multiplex quantum dot (nanoparticle) staining is combined with high-resolution whole-slide imaging, and FARSIGHT (www.farsight-toolkit.org) and NearCyte (www.nearcyte.org/) image analysis to assist in analyzing the abundant data generated from multiplex staining [593]. Potential clinical applications include in situ phenotypic analysis of immune cells and correlation with responses to treatment and graft outcome.

Another emerging technology enables imaging and quantitative analysis of individual cells, in situ, using laser scanning cytometry using chromogens and fluorophores on FFPE tissues [594, 595]. Similar to flow cytometry, laser scanning cytometry allows for specific labelling of cells with fluorescently labelled antibodies and analysis using built-in WSI to generate both qualitative and quantitative statistical data. Takahashi et al. successfully utilized this technology to quantify and characterize regulatory T cells in situ on FFPE liver allograft biopsies [596]. The ability to detect and analyze cell-cell interactions in situ will significantly advance our understanding of immune pathogenesis and provide novel diagnostic and predictive tools [595].

Quantitative digital morphometric analysis (DMA) can provide a standardized, objective evaluation of liver fibrosis by calculating the collagen proportionate area (CPA). This approach has been successfully implemented for HCV in both native and allograft livers [597–600]. Another group [601] used an automated classifier to detect and quantify macrovesicular steatosis, lobular inflammation, and hepatocellular ballooning in NAFLD liver biopsies, which correlated with expert hepatopathologist observations.

Telepathology can be used to assess liver and kidney biopsies from potential donors when rapid microscopic tissue assessment is needed to determine organ suitability for transplantation. The center in which the donor tissue is obtained needs a slide scanner to create a whole slide image from a frozen section slide that can be uploaded to an online data sharing program [602–605]. HIPAA guidelines, CAP regulations, and licensure issues are already being addressed in the USA, where digital pathology is increasingly being practiced [605]. The advantages of 24-hour access to expert histopathologic consultation could clearly benefit the surgeon who requires help after hours, and might also help general pathologists to obtain a rapid expert opinion when needed. It may also be feasible for the donor biopsy to be evaluated by the transplant team at the receiving institution; an active role for all stakeholders could improve donor organ triage [602].

References

1. Roberts HW, Utuama OA, Klevens M, Teshale E, Hughes E, Jiles R. The Contribution of Viral Hepatitis to the Burden of Chronic Liver Disease in the United States. The American Journal of Gastroenterology. 2014;109(3):387–93; quiz 6, 94.
2. Asrani SK, Larson JJ, Yawn B, Therneau TM, Kim WR. Underestimation of Liver-Related Mortality in the United States. Gastroenterology. 2013;145(2):375–82 e1-2.
3. Kim WR, Therneau TM, Benson JT, Kremers WK, Rosen CB, Gores GJ, et al. Deaths on the Liver Transplant Waiting List: An Analysis of Competing Risks. Hepatology. 2006;43(2):345–51.
4. Kim WR, Lake JR, Smith JM, Skeans MA, Schladt DP, Edwards EB, et al. OPTN/SRTR 2013 Annual Data Report: Liver. Am J Transplant. 2015;15 Suppl 2:1–28.
5. Shukla A, Vadeyar H, Rela M, Shah S. Liver Transplantation: East versus West. J Clin Exp Hepatol. 2013;3(3):243–53.
6. Fung J. Management of Chronic Hepatitis B before and after Liver Transplantation. World J Hepatol. 2015;7(10):1421–6.
7. Ghaziani T, Sendi H, Shahraz S, Zamor P, Bonkovsky HL. Hepatitis B and Liver Transplantation: Molecular and Clinical Features that Influence Recurrence and Outcome. World J Gastroenterol. 2014;20(39):14142–55.
8. Burra P, De Martin E, Zanetto A, Senzolo M, Russo FP, Zanus G, et al. HCV and Liver Transplantation: Where Do We Stand? Transpl Int. 2015.
9. Muir AJ, Naggie S. HCV Treatment: Is It Possible to Cure All HCV Patients? Clin Gastroenterol Hepatol. 2015.
10. Pipili C, Cholongitas E. Treatment of Chronic Hepatitis C in Liver Transplant Candidates and Recipients: Where Do We Stand? World J Hepatol. 2015;7(12):1606–16.
11. Demetris AJ, Zeevi A, O'Leary JG. ABO-compatible Liver Allograft Antibody-mediated Rejection: An Update. Curr Opin Organ Transplant. 2015;20(3):314–24.
12. Demetris AJ, Crawford JM, Isse K, Minervini MI, Nalesnik MA, Rubin E, et al. Pathology of Liver and Hematopoietic Stem Cell Transplantation. In: Odze RD, Goldblum JR, editors. Surgical Pathology of the GI Tract, Liver, Biliary Tract and Pancreas 3rd ed. Philadelphia, PA: Elsevier/Saunders; 2015. p. 1408–61.
13. Demetris AJ, Minervini MI, Nalesnik MA, Randhawa P, Sasatomi E. Histopathology of Liver Transplantation. In: Busuttil RW, Klintmalm GK, editors. Transplantation of the Liver 3rd ed. Philadelphia, PA: Elsevier/Saunders; 2015. p. 1112–70.
14. Demetris AJ, Minervini MI, Nalesnik M, Rubin E, Randhawa P, Sasatomi E. Histopathological Syndromes of Graft Rejection and Recurrent Disease: Liver. In: Kirk A, Knechtle S, Larsen C, Pearson T, Madsen J, Webber S, editors. Textbook of Organ Transplantation. Hoboken, NJ: Wiley-Blackwell; 2014. p. 927–56.
15. Demetris AJ, Minervini MI, Nalesnik MA, Randhawa PS, Sasatomi E. Liver Transplantation. In: McManus LM, Mitchell R, editors. Pathobiology of Human Disease: A Dynamic Encyclopedia of Disease Mechanisms. San Diego, CA: Elsevier; 2014. p. 676–93.
16. Starzl TE, Marchioro TL, Von Kaulla KN, Hermann G, Brittain RS, Waddell WR. Homotransplantation of the Liver in Humans. Surg Gynecol Obstet. 1963;117:659–76.
17. Merion RM, Goodrich NP, Feng S. How Can We Define Expanded Criteria for Liver Donors? Journal of Hepatology. 2006;45(4):484–8.
18. McCormack L, Dutkowski P, El-Badry AM, Clavien PA. Liver Transplantation Using Fatty Livers: Always Feasible? Journal of Hepatology. 2011;54(5):1055–62.
19. Op den Dries S, Sutton ME, Lisman T, Porte RJ. Protection of Bile Ducts in Liver Transplantation: Looking beyond Ischemia. Transplantation. 2011;92(4):373–9.
20. Fontes P, Lopez R, van der Plaats A, Vodovotz Y, Minervini M, Scott V, et al. Liver Preservation with Machine Perfusion and a Newly Developed Cell-free Oxygen Carrier Solution under Subnormothermic Conditions. Am J Transplant. 2015;15(2):381–94.
21. Orman ES, Mayorga ME, Wheeler SB, Townsley RM, Toro-Diaz HH, Hayashi PH, et al. Declining Liver Graft Quality Threatens the Future of Liver Transplantation in the United States. Liver Transpl. 2015;21(8):1040–50.
22. Orman ES, Barritt ASt, Wheeler SB, Hayashi PH. Declining Liver Utilization for Transplantation in the United States and the Impact of Donation after Cardiac Death. Liver Transpl. 2013;19(1):59–68.
23. Weeder PD, van Rijn R, Porte RJ. Machine Perfusion in Liver Transplantation as a Tool to Prevent Non-anastomotic Biliary Strictures: Rationale, Current Evidence and Future Directions. Journal of Hepatology. 2015;63(1):265–75.
24. Foley DP, Fernandez LA, Leverson G, Anderson M, Mezrich J, Sollinger HW, et al. Biliary Complications after Liver Transplantation from Donation after Cardiac Death Donors: An Analysis of Risk Factors and Long-term Outcomes from a Single Center. Ann Surg. 2011;253(4):817–25.
25. Abt P, Crawford M, Desai N, Markmann J, Olthoff K, Shaked A. Liver Transplantation from Controlled Non-Heart-Beating Donors: An Increased Incidence of Biliary Complications. Transplantation. 2003;75(10):1659–63.
26. Jay CL, Lyuksemburg V, Ladner DP, Wang E, Caicedo JC, Holl JL, et al. Ischemic Cholangiopathy after Controlled Donation after Cardiac Death Liver Transplantation: A Meta-analysis. Ann Surg. 2011;253(2):259–64.
27. Schlegel A, Dutkowski P. Role of Hypothermic Machine Perfusion in Liver Transplantation. Transpl Int. 2015;28(6):677–89.

28. Liu Q, Nassar A, Farias K, Buccini L, Baldwin W, Mangino M, et al. Sanguineous Normothermic Machine Perfusion Improves Hemodynamics and Biliary Epithelial Regeneration in Donation after Cardiac Death Porcine Livers. Liver Transpl. 2014;20(8):987–99.

29. Ravikumar R, Leuvenink H, Friend PJ. Normothermic Liver Preservation: A New Paradigm? Transpl Int. 2015;28(6):690–9.

30. Slieker JC, Farid WR, van Eijck CH, Lange JF, van Bommel J, Metselaar HJ, et al. Significant Contribution of the Portal Vein to Blood Flow through the Common Bile Duct. Ann Surg. 2012;255(3):523–7.

31. Barrou B, Billault C, Nicolas-Robin A. The Use of Extracorporeal Membranous Oxygenation in Donors after Cardiac Death. Curr Opin Organ Transplant. 2013;18(2):148–53.

32. Karimian N, Op den Dries S, Porte RJ. The Origin of Biliary Strictures after Liver Transplantation: Is It the Amount of Epithelial Injury or Insufficient Regeneration that Counts? Journal of Hepatology. 2013;58(6):1065–7.

33. Boehnert MU, Yeung JC, Bazerbachi F, Knaak JM, Selzner N, McGilvray ID, et al. Normothermic Acellular ex Vivo Liver Perfusion Reduces Liver and Bile Duct Injury of Pig Livers Retrieved after Cardiac Death. Am J Transplant. 2013;13(6):1441–9.

34. Brunner SM, Junger H, Ruemmele P, Schnitzbauer AA, Doenecke A, Kirchner GI, et al. Bile Duct Damage after Cold Storage of Deceased Donor Livers Predicts Biliary Complications after Liver Transplantation. Journal of Hepatology. 2013;58(6):1133–9.

35. Hansen T, Hollemann D, Pitton MB, Heise M, Hoppe-Lotichius M, Schuchmann M, et al. Histological Examination and Evaluation of Donor Bile Ducts Received during Orthotopic Liver Transplantation–A Morphological Clue to Ischemic-type Biliary Lesion? Virchows Arch. 2012;461(1):41–8.

36. Op den Dries S, Westerkamp AC, Karimian N, Gouw AS, Bruinsma BG, Markmann JF, et al. Injury to Peribiliary Glands and Vascular Plexus before Liver Transplantation Predicts Formation of Non-anastomotic Biliary Strictures. Journal of Hepatology. 2014.

37. Karimian N, Westerkamp AC, Porte RJ. Biliary Complications after Orthotopic Liver Transplantation. Curr Opin Organ Transplant. 2014;19(3):209–16.

38. Karimian N, Weeder PD, Bomfati F, Gouw AS, Porte RJ. Preservation Injury of the Distal Extrahepatic Bile Duct of Donor Livers Is Representative for Injury of the Intrahepatic Bile Ducts. Journal of Hepatology. 2015;63(1):284–7.

39. Clavien PA, Harvey PR, Strasberg SM. Preservation and Reperfusion Injuries in Liver Allografts. An Overview and Synthesis of Current Studies. Transplantation. 1992;53(5):957–78.

40. Schon MR, Kollmar O, Wolf S, Schrem H, Matthes M, Akkoc N, et al. Liver Transplantation after Organ Preservation with Normothermic Extracorporeal Perfusion. Ann Surg. 2001;233(1):114–23.

41. Friend PJ, Imber C, St Peter S, Lopez I, Butler AJ, Rees MA. Normothermic Perfusion of the Isolated Liver. Transplantation Proceedings. 2001;33(7–8):3436–8.

42. Butler AJ, Rees MA, Wight DG, Casey ND, Alexander G, White DJ, et al. Successful Extracorporeal Porcine Liver Perfusion for 72 Hr. Transplantation. 2002;73(8):1212–8.

43. Imber CJ, St Peter SD, Lopez de Cenarruzabeitia I, Pigott D, James T, Taylor R, et al. Advantages of Normothermic Perfusion over Cold Storage in Liver Preservation. Transplantation. 2002;73(5):701–9.

44. Reddy S, Greenwood J, Maniakin N, Bhattacharjya S, Zilvetti M, Brockmann J, et al. Non-Heart-Beating Donor Porcine Livers: The Adverse Effect of Cooling. Liver Transpl. 2005;11(1):35–8.

45. Boehnert MU, Yeung JC, Knaak JM, Selzner N, Selzner M. Normothermic Acellular ex Vivo Liver Perfusion (NEVLP) Reduces Liver and Bile Duct in DCD Liver Grafts. Am J Transplant. 2013;13(12):3290.

46. Sutton ME, op den Dries S, Karimian N, Weeder PD, de Boer MT, Wiersema-Buist J, et al. Criteria for Viability Assessment of Discarded Human Donor Livers during ex Vivo Normothermic Machine Perfusion. PLoS One. 2014;9(11):e110642.

47. Guarrera JV, Henry SD, Samstein B, Reznik E, Musat C, Lukose TI, et al. Hypothermic Machine Preservation Facilitates Successful Transplantation of "Orphan" Extended Criteria Donor Livers. Am J Transplant. 2015;15(1):161–9.

48. Dutkowski P, Furrer K, Tian Y, Graf R, Clavien PA. Novel Short-term Hypothermic Oxygenated Perfusion (HOPE) System Prevents Injury in Rat Liver Graft from Non-Heart Beating Donor. Ann Surg. 2006;244(6):968–76; discussion 76–7.

49. Schlegel A, Graf R, Clavien PA, Dutkowski P. Hypothermic Oxygenated Perfusion (HOPE) Protects from Biliary Injury in a Rodent Model of DCD Liver Transplantation. Journal of Hepatology. 2013;59(5):984–91.

50. Op den Dries S, Sutton ME, Karimian N, de Boer MT, Wiersema-Buist J, Gouw AS, et al. Hypothermic Oxygenated Machine Perfusion Prevents Arteriolonecrosis of the Peribiliary Plexus in Pig Livers Donated after Circulatory Death. PLoS One. 2014;9(2):e88521.

51. Berendsen TA, Bruinsma BG, Lee J, D'Andrea V, Liu Q, Izamis ML, et al. A Simplified Subnormothermic Machine Perfusion System Restores Ischemically Damaged Liver Grafts in a Rat Model of Orthotopic Liver Transplantation. Transplantation Research. 2012;1(1):6.

52. Bruinsma BG, Yeh H, Ozer S, Martins PN, Farmer A, Wu W, et al. Subnormothermic Machine Perfusion for ex Vivo Preservation and Recovery of the Human Liver for Transplantation. Am J Transplant. 2014;14(6):1400–9.

53. Tolboom H, Izamis ML, Sharma N, Milwid JM, Uygun B, Berthiaume F, et al. Subnormothermic Machine Perfusion at Both 20 Degrees C and 30 Degrees C Recovers Ischemic Rat Livers for Successful Transplantation. J Surg Res. 2012;175(1):149–56.

54. Knaak JM, Spetzler VN, Goldaracena N, Boehnert MU, Bazerbachi F, Louis KS, et al. Subnormothermic ex Vivo Liver Perfusion Reduces Endothelial Cell and Bile Duct Injury after Donation after Cardiac Death Pig Liver Transplantation. Liver Transpl. 2014;20(11):1296–305.

55. Routh D, Naidu S, Sharma S, Ranjan P, Godara R. Changing Pattern of Donor Selection Criteria in Deceased Donor Liver Transplant: A Review of Literature. J Clin Exp Hepatol. 2013;3(4):337–46.

56. Harring TR, O'Mahony CA, Goss JA. Extended Donors in Liver Transplantation. Clinics in Liver Disease. 2011;15(4):879–900.

57. Nickkholgh A, Weitz J, Encke J, Sauer P, Mehrabi A, Büchler MW, et al. Utilization of Extended Donor Criteria in Liver Transplantation: A Comprehensive Review of the Literature. Nephrol Dial Transplant. 2007;22 Suppl 8:viii29–viii36.

58. Busuttil RW, Tanaka K. The Utility of Marginal Donors in Liver Transplantation. Liver Transpl. 2003;9(7):651–63.
59. Alkofer B, Samstein B, Guarrera JV, Kin C, Jan D, Bellemare S, et al. Extended-donor Criteria Liver Allografts. Seminars in Liver Disease. 2006;26(3):221–33.
60. Feng S, Goodrich NP, Bragg-Gresham JL, Dykstra DM, Punch JD, DebRoy MA, et al. Characteristics Associated with Liver Graft Failure: The Concept of a Donor Risk Index. Am J Transplant. 2006;6(4):783–90.
61. Nalesnik MA, Woodle ES, Dimaio JM, Vasudev B, Teperman LW, Covington S, et al. Donor-transmitted Malignancies in Organ Transplantation: Assessment of Clinical Risk. American Journal of Transplantation: Official Journal of the American Society of Transplantation and the American Society of Transplant Surgeons. 2011;11(6):1140–7.
62. Ison MG, Nalesnik MA. An Update on Donor-derived Disease Transmission in Organ Transplantation. American Journal of Transplantation: Official Journal of the American Society of Transplantation and the American Society of Transplant Surgeons. 2011;11(6):1123–30.
63. Green M, Covington S, Taranto S, Wolfe C, Bell W, Biggins SW, et al. Donor-derived Transmission Events in 2013: A Report of the Organ Procurement Transplant Network Ad Hoc Disease Transmission Advisory Committee. Transplantation. 2015;99(2):282–7.
64. Reich DJ, Mulligan DC, Abt PL, Pruett TL, Abecassis MM, D'Alessandro A, et al. ASTS Recommended Practice Guidelines for Controlled Donation after Cardiac Death Organ Procurement and Transplantation. Am J Transplant. 2009;9(9):2004–11.
65. Todo S, Demetris AJ, Makowka L, Teperman L, Podesta L, Shaver T, et al. Primary Nonfunction of Hepatic Allografts with Preexisting Fatty Infiltration. Transplantation. 1989;47(5):903–5.
66. Kakizoe S, Yanaga K, Starzl TE, Demetris AJ. Frozen Section of Liver Biopsy for the Evaluation of Liver Allografts. Transplant Proc. 1990;22(2):416–7.
67. Zamboni F, Franchello A, David E, Rocca G, Ricchiuti A, Lavezzo B, et al. Effect of Macrovesicular Steatosis and Other Donor and Recipient Characteristics on the Outcome of Liver Transplantation. Clin Transplant. 2001;15(1):53–7.
68. Spitzer AL, Lao OB, Dick AA, Bakthavatsalam R, Halldorson JB, Yeh MM, et al. The Biopsied Donor Liver: Incorporating Macrosteatosis into High-risk Donor Assessment. Liver Transpl. 2010;16(7):874–84.
69. Sharkey FE, Lytvak I, Prihoda TJ, Speeg KV, Washburn WK, Halff GA. High-grade Microsteatosis and Delay in Hepatic Function after Orthotopic Liver Transplantation. Human Pathology. 2011;42(9):1337–42.
70. Fiorini RN, Kirtz J, Periyasamy B, Evans Z, Haines JK, Cheng G, et al. Development of an Unbiased Method for the Estimation of Liver Steatosis. Clin Transplant. 2004;18(6):700–6.
71. D'Alessandro AM, Kalayoglu M, Sollinger HW, Hoffmann RM, Reed A, Knechtle SJ, et al. The Predictive Value of Donor Liver Biopsies for the Development of Primary Nonfunction after Orthotopic Liver Transplantation. Transplantation. 1991;51(1):157–63.
72. McCormack L, Petrowsky H, Jochum W, Mullhaupt B, Weber M, Clavien PA. Use of Severely Steatotic Grafts in Liver Transplantation: A Matched Case-control Study. Ann Surg. 2007;246(6):940–6; discussion 6–8.
73. Angele MK, Rentsch M, Hartl WH, Wittmann B, Graeb C, Jauch KW, et al. Effect of Graft Steatosis on Liver Function and Organ Survival after Liver Transplantation. Am J Surg. 2008;195(2):214–20.
74. D'Alessandro E, Calabrese F, Gringeri E, Valente M. Frozen-section Diagnosis in Donor Livers: Error Rate Estimation of Steatosis Degree. Transplantation Proceedings. 2010;42(6):2226–8.
75. Fiorentino M, Vasuri F, Ravaioli M, Ridolfi L, Grigioni WF, Pinna AD, et al. Predictive Value of Frozen-section Analysis in the Histological Assessment of Steatosis before Liver Transplantation. Liver Transpl. 2009;15(12):1821–5.
76. Chen CL, Cheng YF, Yu CY, Ou HY, Tsang LL, Huang TL, et al. Living Donor Liver Transplantation: The Asian Perspective. Transplantation. 2014;97 Suppl 8:S3.
77. Markin RS, Wisecarver JL, Radio SJ, Stratta RJ, Langnas AN, Hirst K, et al. Frozen Section Evaluation of Donor Livers before Transplantation. Transplantation. 1993;56(6):1403–9.
78. Patwardhan VR, Curry MP. Reappraisal of the Hepatitis C Virus-positive Donor in Solid Organ Transplantation. Curr Opin Organ Transplant. 2015;20(3):267–75.
79. Ballarin R, Cucchetti A, Spaggiari M, Montalti R, Di Benedetto F, Nadalin S, et al. Long-term Follow-up and Outcome of Liver Transplantation from Anti-hepatitis C virus-positive Donors: A European Multicentric Case-control Study. Transplantation. 2011;91(11):1265–72.
80. Dodson SF, Issa S, Araya V, Gayowski T, Pinna A, Eghtesad B, et al. Infectivity of Hepatic Allografts with Antibodies to Hepatitis B Virus. Transplantation. 1997;64(11):1582–4.
81. Avelino-Silva VI, D'Albuquerque LA, Bonazzi PR, Song AT, Miraglia JL, De Brito Neves A, et al. Liver Transplant from Anti-HBc-positive, HBsAg-negative Donor into HBsAg-negative Recipient: Is It Safe? A Systematic Review of the Literature. Clin Transplant. 2010;24(6):735–46.
82. Adams D, Lacroix C, Antonini T, Lozeron P, Denier C, Kreib AM, et al. Symptomatic and Proven de Novo Amyloid Polyneuropathy in Familial Amyloid Polyneuropathy Domino Liver Recipients. Amyloid. 2011;18 Suppl 1:169–72.
83. Aziz S, Callen PW, Vincenti F, Hirose R. Rapidly Developing Nephrocalcinosis in a Patient with End-stage Liver Disease Who Received a Domino Liver Transplant from a Patient with Known Congenital Oxalosis. J Ultrasound Med. 2005;24(10):1449–52.
84. Lee SM, Speeg KV, Pollack MS, Sharkey FE. Progression of Morphological Changes after Transplantation of a Liver with Heterozygous Alpha-1 Antitrypsin Deficiency. Human Pathology. 2011.
85. Tanaka K, Kiuchi T. Living-donor Liver Transplantation in the New Decade: Perspective from the Twentieth to the Twenty-first Century. J Hepatobiliary Pancreat Surg. 2002;9(2):218–22.
86. Song GW, Lee SG. Living Donor Liver Transplantation. Curr Opin Organ Transplant. 2014;19(3):217–22.
87. Cheah YL, Simpson MA, Pomposelli JJ, Pomfret EA. Incidence of Death and Potentially Life-threatening Near-miss Events in Living Donor Hepatic Lobectomy: A World-wide Survey. Liver Transpl. 2013;19(5):499–506.
88. Nadalin S, Malago M, Valentin-Gamazo C, Testa G, Baba HA, Liu C, et al. Preoperative Donor Liver Biopsy for Adult Living Donor Liver Transplantation: Risks and Benefits. Liver Transpl. 2005;11(8):980–6.

89. Tran TT, Changsri C, Shackleton CR, Poordad FF, Nissen NN, Colquhoun S, et al. Living Donor Liver Transplantation: Histological Abnormalities Found on Liver Biopsies of Apparently Healthy Potential Donors. J Gastroenterol Hepatol. 2006;21(2):381–3.

90. Ryan CK, Johnson LA, Germin BI, Marcos A. One Hundred Consecutive Hepatic Biopsies in the Workup of Living Donors for Right Lobe Liver Transplantation. Liver Transpl. 2002;8(12):1114–22.

91. Trotter JF, Wachs M, Everson GT, Kam I. Adult-to-Adult Transplantation of the Right Hepatic Lobe from a Living Donor. The New England Journal of Medicine. 2002;346(14):1074–82.

92. Simpson MA, Pomfret EA. Checking the Harness: Safety for Living Liver Donors. Liver Transpl. 2012;18 Suppl 2:S15–9.

93. Minervini MI, Ruppert K, Fontes P, Volpes R, Vizzini G, de Vera ME, et al. Liver Biopsy Findings from Healthy Potential Living Liver Donors: Reasons for Disqualification, Silent Diseases and Correlation with Liver Injury Tests. Journal of Hepatology. 2009;50(3):501–10.

94. Lee JY, Kim KM, Lee SG, Yu E, Lim YS, Lee HC, et al. Prevalence and Risk Factors of Non-alcoholic Fatty Liver Disease in Potential Living Liver Donors in Korea: A Review of 589 Consecutive Liver Biopsies in a Single Center. Journal of Hepatology. 2007;47(2):239–44.

95. Rinella ME, Alonso E, Rao S, Whitington P, Fryer J, Abecassis M, et al. Body Mass Index as a Predictor of Hepatic Steatosis in Living Liver Donors. Liver Transpl. 2001;7(5):409–14.

96. Fan ST, Lo CM, Liu CL, Yong BH, Chan JK, Ng IO. Safety of Donors in Live Donor Liver Transplantation Using Right Lobe Grafts. Archives of Surgery. 2000;135(3):336–40.

97. Dorwal P, Gautam D, Sharma D, Singh DR, Raina V. Donor Biopsy in Living Donor Liver Transplantation: Is It Still Relevant in a Developing Country? Malays J Pathol. 2015;37(1):39–43.

98. Starzl TE. History of Liver and Other Splanchnic Organ Transplantation. In: Busuttil R, Klintmalm G, editors. Transplantation of the Liver. Philadelphia: W.B. Saunders Company; 1996. p. 3–22.

99. Rockey DC, Caldwell SH, Goodman ZD, Nelson RC, Smith AD. Liver Biopsy. Hepatology. 2009;49(3):1017–44.

100. Pathology BWGoLA. Importance of Liver Biopsy Findings in Immunosuppression Management: Biopsy Monitoring and Working Criteria for Patients with Operational Tolerance. Liver Transpl. 2012;18(10):1154–70.

101. Bellizzi AM, LeGallo RD, Boyd JC, Iezzoni JC. Hepatocyte Cytokeratin 7 Expression in Chronic Allograft Rejection. Am J Clin Pathol. 2011;135(2):238–44.

102. Demetris AJ, Jaffe R, Starzl TE. A Review of Adult and Pediatric Post-transplant Liver Pathology. Pathol Annu. 1987;22(Pt 2):347–86.

103. Sieders E, Peeters PM, TenVergert EM, de Jong KP, Porte RJ, Zwaveling JH, et al. Graft Loss after Pediatric Liver Transplantation. Annals of Surgery. 2002;235(1):125–32.

104. Kashyap R, Jain A, Reyes J, Demetris AJ, Elmagd KA, Dodson SF, et al. Causes of Retransplantation after Primary Liver Transplantation in 4000 Consecutive Patients: 2 to 19 Years Follow-up. Transplantation Proceedings. 2001;33(1–2):1486–7.

105. Jain A, Reyes J, Kashyap R, Dodson SF, Demetris AJ, Ruppert K, et al. Long-term Survival after Liver Transplantation in 4,000 Consecutive Patients at a Single Center. Ann Surg. 2000;232(4):490–500.

106. Rabkin JM, de La Melena V, Orloff SL, Corless CL, Rosen HR, Olyaei AJ. Late Mortality after Orthotopic Liver Transplantation. Am J Surg. 2001;181(5):475–9.

107. Kitchens WH, Yeh H, Markmann JF. Hepatic Retransplant: What Have We Learned? Clin Liver Dis. 2014;18(3):731–51.

108. Jain A, Demetris AJ, Kashyap R, Blakomer K, Ruppert K, Khan A, et al. Does Tacrolimus Offer Virtual Freedom from Chronic Rejection after Primary Liver Transplantation? Risk and Prognostic Factors in 1,048 Liver Transplantations with a Mean Follow-up of 6 Years. Liver Transpl. 2001;7(7):623–30.

109. McCashland T, Watt K, Lyden E, Adams L, Charlton M, Smith AD, et al. Retransplantation for Hepatitis C: Results of a U.S. Multicenter Retransplant Study. Liver Transpl. 2007;13(9):1246–53.

110. Kim KR, Ko GY, Sung KB, Yoon HK, Shin JH, Song HY, et al. Transjugular Liver Biopsy in Patients with Living Donor Liver Transplantation: Comparison with Percutaneous Biopsy. Liver Transplantation: Official Publication of the American Association for the Study of Liver Diseases and the International Liver Transplantation Society. 2008;14(7):971–9.

111. Astarcioglu I, Cursio R, Reynes M, Gugenheim J. Increased Risk of Antibody-mediated Rejection of Reduced-size Liver Allografts. J Surg Res. 1999;87(2):258–62.

112. Demetris AJ, Kelly DM, Eghtesad B, Fontes P, Wallis Marsh J, Tom K, et al. Pathophysiologic Observations and Histopathologic Recognition of the Portal Hyperperfusion or Small-for-Size Syndrome. Am J Surg Pathol. 2006;30(8):986–93.

113. Peralta C, Jiménez-Castro MB, Gracia-Sancho J. Hepatic Ischemia and Reperfusion Injury: Effects on the Liver Sinusoidal Milieu. Journal of Hepatology. 2013;59(5):1094–106.

114. Zhai Y, Petrowsky H, Hong JC, Busuttil RW, Kupiec-Weglinski JW. Ischaemia-Reperfusion Injury in Liver Transplantation–From Bench to Bedside. Nat Rev Gastroenterol Hepatol. 2013;10(2):79–89.

115. Hong JC, Yersiz H, Kositamongkol P, Xia VW, Kaldas FM, Petrowsky H, et al. Liver Transplantation Using Organ Donation after Cardiac Death: A Clinical Predictive Index for Graft Failure-free Survival. Arch Surg. 2011;146(9):1017–23.

116. de Vera ME, Lopez-Solis R, Dvorchik I, Campos S, Morris W, Demetris AJ, et al. Liver Transplantation Using Donation after Cardiac Death Donors: Long-term Follow-up from a Single Center. Am J Transplant. 2009;9(4):773–81.

117. Taner CB, Bulatao IG, Willingham DL, Perry DK, Sibulesky L, Pungpapong S, et al. Events in Procurement as Risk Factors for Ischemic Cholangiopathy in Liver Transplantation Using Donation after Cardiac Death Donors. Liver Transpl. 2012;18(1):100–11.

118. Kakizoe S, Yanaga K, Starzl TE, Demetris AJ. Evaluation of Protocol before Transplantation and after Reperfusion Biopsies from Human Orthotopic Liver Allografts: Considerations of Preservation and Early Immunological Injury. Hepatology. 1990;11(6):932–41.

119. Ludwig J, Batts KP, MacCarty RL. Ischemic Cholangitis in Hepatic Allografts. Mayo Clinic Proceedings. 1992;67(6):519–26.

120. Cameron AM, Busuttil RW. Ischemic Cholangiopathy after Liver Transplantation. Hepatobiliary Pancreat Dis Int. 2005;4(4):495–501.

121. Kocbiyik A, Demirhan B, Sevmis S, Budakoglu I, Karakayali H, Haberal M. Role of Postreperfusion Subcapsular Wedge Biopsies in Predicting Initially Poor Graft Function after Liver Transplantation. Transplantation Proceedings. 2009;41(7):2747–8.

122. Ali JM, Davies SE, Brais RJ, Randle LV, Klinck JR, Allison ME, et al. Analysis of Ischemia/Reperfusion Injury in Time-zero Biopsies Predicts Liver Allograft Outcomes. Liver Transpl. 2015;21(4):487–99.

123. Shahbazi N, Haeri H, Nasiri Toosi M, Jafarian A, Shahsiah R, Talebian Moghadam M, et al. Correlation of Histopathologic Findings of Non-graft Threatening Preservation/Reperfusion Injury in Time-zero Liver Needle Biopsies With Short-term Post-transplantation Laboratory Alterations. Hepat Mon. 2015;15(6):e30008.

124. Kukan M, Haddad PS. Role of Hepatocytes and Bile Duct Cells in Preservation-Reperfusion Injury of Liver Grafts. Liver Transpl. 2001;7(5):381–400.

125. Lunz J, Ruppert KM, Cajaiba MM, Isse K, Bentlejewski CA, Minervini M, et al. Re-examination of the Lymphocytotoxic Crossmatch in Liver Transplantation: Can C4d Stains Help in Monitoring? American Journal of Transplantation: Official Journal of the American Society of Transplantation and the American Society of Transplant Surgeons. 2012;12(1):171–82.

126. Dahm F, Georgiev P, Clavien PA. Small-for-Size Syndrome after Partial Liver Transplantation: Definition, Mechanisms of Disease and Clinical Implications. American Journal of Transplantation: Official Journal of the American Society of Transplantation and the American Society of Transplant Surgeons. 2005;5(11):2605–10.

127. Chan SC, Lo CM, Fan ST. Simplifying Living Donor Liver Transplantation. Hepatobiliary & Pancreatic Diseases International: HBPD INT. 2010;9(1):9–14.

128. Chan SC, Lo CM, Ng KK, Ng IO, Yong BH, Fan ST. Portal Inflow and Pressure Changes in Right Liver Living Donor Liver Transplantation Including the Middle Hepatic Vein. Liver Transpl. 2011;17(2):115–21.

129. Man K, Fan ST, Lo CM, Liu CL, Fung PC, Liang TB, et al. Graft Injury in Relation to Graft Size in Right Lobe Live Donor Liver Transplantation: A Study of Hepatic Sinusoidal Injury in Correlation with Portal Hemodynamics and Intragraft Gene Expression. Ann Surg. 2003;237(2):256–64.

130. Lautt WW. Mechanism and Role of Intrinsic Regulation of Hepatic Arterial Blood Flow: Hepatic Arterial Buffer Response. Am J Physiol. 1985;249(5 Pt 1):G549–56.

131. Eipel C, Abshagen K, Vollmar B. Regulation of Hepatic Blood Flow: The Hepatic Arterial Buffer Response Revisited. World J Gastroenterol. 2010;16(48):6046–57.

132. Kelly DM, Zhu X, Shiba H, Irefin S, Trenti L, Cocieru A, et al. Adenosine Restores the Hepatic Artery Buffer Response and Improves Survival in a Porcine Model of Small-for-Size Syndrome. Liver Transpl. 2009;15(11):1448–57.

133. Botha JF, Langnas AN, Campos BD, Grant WJ, Freise CE, Ascher NL, et al. Left Lobe Adult-to-Adult Living Donor Liver Transplantation: Small Grafts and Hemiportocaval Shunts in the Prevention of Small-for-Size Syndrome. Liver Transpl. 2010;16(5):649–57.

134. Michalopoulos GK. Principles of Liver Regeneration and Growth Homeostasis. Compr Physiol. 2013;3(1):485–513.

135. Starzl TE, Fung JJ. Themes of Liver Transplantation. Hepatology. 2010;51(6):1869–84.

136. Hessheimer AJ, Fondevila C, Taura P, Munoz J, Sanchez O, Fuster J, et al. Decompression of the Portal Bed and Twice-baseline Portal Inflow are Necessary for the Functional Recovery of a "Small-for-Size" Graft. Annals of Surgery. 2011;253(6):1201–10.

137. Fondevila C, Hessheimer AJ, Taura P, Sanchez O, Calatayud D, de Riva N, et al. Portal Hyperperfusion: Mechanism of Injury and Stimulus for Regeneration in Porcine Small-for-Size Transplantation. Liver Transplantation: Official Publication of the American Association for the Study of Liver Diseases and the International Liver Transplantation Society. 2010;16(3):364–74.

138. Kelly DM, Demetris AJ, Fung JJ, Marcos A, Zhu Y, Subbotin V, et al. Porcine Partial Liver Transplantation: A Novel Model of the "Small-for-Size" Liver Graft. Liver Transpl. 2004;10(2):253–63.

139. Yagi Y, Gilbertson JR. Digital Imaging in Pathology: The Case for Standardization. Journal of Telemedicine and Telecare. 2005;11(3):109–16.

140. Fukuhara T, Umeda K, Toshima T, Takeishi K, Morita K, Nagata S, et al. Congestion of the Donor Remnant Right Liver after Extended Left Lobe Donation. Transplant International: Official Journal of the European Society for Organ Transplantation. 2009;22(8):837–44.

141. Man K, Lo CM, Ng IO, Wong YC, Qin LF, Fan ST, et al. Liver Transplantation in Rats Using Small-for-Size Grafts: A Study of Hemodynamic and Morphological Changes. Arch Surg. 2001;136(3):280–5.

142. Asakura T, Ohkohchi N, Orii T, Koyamada N, Tsukamoto S, Sato M, et al. Portal Vein Pressure Is the Key for Successful Liver Transplantation of an Extremely Small Graft in the Pig Model. Transpl Int. 2003;16(6):376–82.

143. Ayata G, Pomfret E, Pomposelli JJ, Gordon FD, Lewis WD, Jenkins RL, et al. Adult-to-Adult Live Donor Liver Transplantation: A Short-term Clinicopathologic Study. Hum Pathol. 2001;32(8):814–22.

144. Pantanowitz L, Pomfret EA, Pomposelli JJ, Lewis WD, Gordon FD, Jenkins RL, et al. Pathologic Analysis of Right-lobe Graft Failure in Adult-to-Adult Live Donor Liver Transplantation. Int J Surg Pathol. 2003;11(4):283–94.

145. Bekker J, Ploem S, de Jong KP. Early Hepatic Artery Thrombosis after Liver Transplantation: A Systematic Review of the Incidence, Outcome and Risk Factors. American Journal of Transplantation: Official Journal of the American Society of Transplantation and the American Society of Transplant Surgeons. 2009;9(4):746–57.

146. Gunsar F, Rolando N, Pastacaldi S, Patch D, Raimondo ML, Davidson B, et al. Late Hepatic Artery Thrombosis after Orthotopic Liver Transplantation. Liver Transplantation: Official Publication of the American Association for the Study of Liver Diseases and the International Liver Transplantation Society. 2003;9(6):605–11.

147. Backman L, Gibbs J, Levy M, McMillan R, Holman M, Husberg B, et al. Causes

148. Demetris AJ, Qian SG, Sun H, Fung JJ. Liver Allograft Rejection: An Overview of Morphologic Findings. The American Journal of Surgical Pathology. 1990;14(Suppl 1):49–63.

149. Demetris A, Kakizoe S, S. O. Pathology of Liver Transplantation. In: Williams JW, editor. Hepatic Transplantation. Philadelphia: WB Saunders; 1990. p. 61–111.

150. Liu TC, Nguyen TT, Torbenson MS. Concurrent Increase in Mitosis and Apoptosis: A Histological Pattern of Hepatic Arterial Flow Abnormalities in Post-transplant Liver Biopsies. Mod Pathol. 2012;25(12):1594–8.

151. Ponziani FR, Zocco MA, Campanale C, Rinninella E, Tortora A, Di Maurizio L, et al. Portal Vein Thrombosis: Insight into Physiopathology, Diagnosis, and Treatment. World Journal of Gastroenterology: WJG. 2010;16(2):143–55.

152. Alvarez F. Portal Vein Complications after Pediatric Liver Transplantation. Curr Gastroenterol Rep. 2012;14(3):270–4.

153. Kuang AA, Renz JF, Ferrell LD, Ring EJ, Rosenthal P, Lim RC, et al. Failure Patterns of Cryopreserved Vein Grafts in Liver Transplantation. Transplantation. 1996;62(6):742–7.

154. Zahmatkeshan M, Geramizadeh B, Eshraghian A, Nikeghbalian S, Bahador A, Salahi H, et al. De Novo Fatty Liver due to Vascular Complications after Liver Transplantation. Transplantation Proceedings. 2011;43(2):615–7.

155. Zhang S, Dong Z, Zhang M, Xia Q, Liu D, Zhang JJ. Right Lobe Living-donor Liver Transplantation with or without Middle Hepatic Vein: A Meta-analysis. Transplantation Proceedings. 2011;43(10):3773–9.

156. Klintmalm G, Busuttil R. Transplantation of the Liver. Second ed. Klintmalm G, Busuttil R, editors. Philadelphia: Elsevier Saunders; 2005. 1485 p.

157. Sebagh M, Debette M, Samuel D, Emile JF, Falissard B, Cailliez V, et al. "Silent" Presentation of Veno-occlusive Disease after Liver Transplantation as Part of the Process of Cellular Rejection with Endothelial Predilection. Hepatology. 1999;30(5):1144–50.

158. Pascher A, Neuhaus P. Bile Duct Complications after Liver Transplantation. Transpl Int. 2005;18(6):627–42.

159. Ghobrial RM, Busuttil RW. Challenges of Adult Living-donor Liver Transplantation. J Hepatobiliary Pancreat Surg. 2006;13(2):139–45.

160. Akamatsu N, Sugawara Y, Hashimoto D. Biliary Reconstruction, Its Complications and Management of Biliary Complications after Adult Liver Transplantation: A Systematic Review of the Incidence, Risk Factors and Outcome. Transplant International: Official Journal of the European Society for Organ Transplantation. 2011;24(4):379–92.

161. Kochhar G, Parungao JM, Hanouneh IA, Parsi MA. Biliary Complications Following Liver Transplantation. World J Gastroenterol. 2013;19(19):2841–6.

162. Demetris AJ, Murase N, Nakamura K, Iwaki Y, Yagihashi A, Valdivia L, et al. Immunopathology of Antibodies as Effectors of Orthotopic Liver Allograft Rejection. Seminars in Liver Disease. 1992;12(1):51–9.

163. Demetris AJ, Jaffe R, Tzakis A, Ramsey G, Todo S, Belle S, et al. Antibody-mediated Rejection of Human Orthotopic Liver Allografts. A Study of Liver Transplantation across ABO Blood Group Barriers. American Journal of Pathology. 1988;132(3):489–502.

164. Demetris AJ, Lunz JG, 3rd, Specht S, Nozaki I. Biliary Wound Healing, Ductular Reactions, and IL-6/gp130 Signaling in the Development of Liver Disease. World J Gastroenterol. 2006;12(22):3512–22.

165. Verdonk RC, Buis CI, Porte RJ, van der Jagt EJ, Limburg AJ, van den Berg AP, et al. Anastomotic Biliary Strictures after Liver Transplantation: Causes and Consequences. Liver Transpl. 2006;12(5):726–35.

166. Verdonk RC, Buis CI, Porte RJ, Haagsma EB. Biliary Complications after Liver Transplantation: A Review. Scand J Gastroenterol Suppl. 2006 (243):89–101.

167. Verdonk RC, Buis CI, van der Jagt EJ, Gouw AS, Limburg AJ, Slooff MJ, et al. Nonanastomotic Biliary Strictures after Liver Transplantation, Part 2: Management, Outcome, and Risk Factors for Disease Progression. Liver Transpl. 2007;13(5):725–32.

168. Buis CI, Verdonk RC, Van der Jagt EJ, van der Hilst CS, Slooff MJ, Haagsma EB, et al. Nonanastomotic Biliary Strictures after Liver Transplantation, Part 1: Radiological Features and Risk Factors for Early vs. Late Presentation. Liver Transpl. 2007;13(5):708–18.

169. Song GW, Lee SG, Hwang S, Kim KH, Ahn CS, Moon DB, et al. Biliary Stricture is the Only Concern in ABO-incompatible Adult Living Donor Liver Transplantation in the Rituximab Era. Journal of Hepatology. 2014;61(3):575–82.

170. Foley DP, Fernandez LA, Leverson G, Chin LT, Krieger N, Cooper JT, et al. Donation after Cardiac Death: The University of Wisconsin Experience with Liver Transplantation. Ann Surg. 2005;242(5):724–31.

171. Demetris A, Crawford J, Nalesnik M, Randhawa P, Wu T, Minervini M. Transplantation Pathology of the Liver. In: Odze R, Goldblum J, Crawford JM, editors. Surgical Pathology of the GI Tract, Liver, Biliary Tract, and Pancreas. Philadelphia: WB Saunders; 2004. p. 909–66.

172. Pirenne J, Aerts R, Yoong K, Gunson B, Koshiba T, Fourneau I, et al. Liver Transplantation for Polycystic Liver Disease. Liver Transpl. 2001;7(3):238–45.

173. Minor T, Hachenberg A, Tolba R, Pauleit D, Akbar S. Fibrinolytic Preflush upon Liver Retrieval from Non-Heart Beating Donors to Enhance Postpreservation Viability and Energetic Recovery upon Reperfusion. Transplantation. 2001;71(12):1792–6.

174. Demetris AJ, Fontes P, Lunz JG, 3rd, Specht S, Murase N, Marcos A. Wound Healing in the Biliary Tree of Liver Allografts. Cell Transplant. 2006;15 Suppl 1:S57–65.

175. Demetris AJ, Nakamura K, Yagihashi A, Iwaki Y, Takaya S, Hartman GG, et al. A Clinicopathological Study of Human Liver Allograft Recipients Harboring Preformed IgG Lymphocytotoxic Antibodies. Hepatology. 1992;16(3):671–81.

176. Sanchez-Urdazpal L, Batts KP, Gores GJ, Moore SB, Steriolf S, Wiesner RH, et al. Increased Bile Duct Complications in Liver Transplantation across the ABO Barrier. Ann Surg. 1993;218(2):152–8.

177. Jorgensen JE, Waljee AK, Volk ML, Sonnenday CJ, Elta GH, Al-Hawary MM, et al. Is MRCP Equivalent to ERCP for Diagnosing Biliary Obstruction in Orthotopic Liver Transplant Recipients? A Meta-analysis. Gastrointest Endosc. 2011;73(5):955–62.

178. Boraschi P, Donati F. Postoperative Biliary Adverse Events Following Orthotopic Liver Transplantation: Assessment with Magnetic Resonance Cholangiography. World J Gastroenterol. 2014;20(32):11080–94.

179. Girometti R, Como G, Bazzocchi M, Zuiani C. Post-operative Imaging in Liver Transplantation: State-of-the-Art and Future Perspectives. World J Gastroenterol. 2014;20(20):6180–200.

180. Hartshorne N, Hartman G, Markin RS, Demetris AJ, Ferrell L. Bile Duct Hemorrhage: A Biopsy Finding after Cholangiography or Biliary Tree Manipulation. Liver. 1992;12(3):137–9.

181. Nagral A, Ben-Ari Z, Dhillon AP, Burroughs AK. Eosinophils in Acute Cellular Rejection in Liver Allografts. Liver Transpl Surg. 1998;4(5):355–62.

182. O'Leary JG, Michelle Shiller S, Bellamy C, Nalesnik MA, Kaneku H, Jennings LW, et al. Acute Liver Allograft Antibody-mediated Rejection: An Inter-institutional Study of Significant Histopathological Features. Liver Transpl. 2014;20(10):1244–55.

183. Lunz JG, 3rd, Contrucci S, Ruppert K, Murase N, Fung JJ, Starzl TE, et al. Replicative Senescence of Biliary Epithelial Cells Precedes Bile Duct Loss in Chronic Liver Allograft Rejection: Increased Expression of p21(WAF1/Cip1) as a Disease Marker and the Influence of Immunosuppressive Drugs. Am J Pathol. 2001;158(4):1379–90.

184. Demetris AJ. Distinguishing between Recurrent Primary Sclerosing Cholangitis and Chronic Rejection. Liver Transpl. 2006;12(11 Suppl 2):S68–72.

185. Demetris AJ, Crawford JM, Isse K, Minervini MI, Nalesnik MA, Rubin E, et al. Pathology of Liver and Hematopoietic Stem Cell Transplantation. In: Odze RD, Goldblum JR, editors. Surgical Pathology of the GI Tract, Liver, Biliary Tract and Pancreas 3rd ed. Philadelphia, PA: Elsevier/Saunders; 2015. p. 1408–61.

186. Clendenon JN, Aranda-Michel J, Krishna M, Taner CB, Willingham DL. Recurrent Liver Failure Caused by IgG4 Associated Cholangitis. Ann Hepatol. 2011;10(4):562–4.

187. Demetris AJ, Eghtesad B, Marcos A, Ruppert K, Nalesnik MA, Randhawa P, et al. Recurrent Hepatitis C in Liver Allografts: Prospective Assessment of Diagnostic Accuracy, Identification of Pitfalls, and Observations about Pathogenesis. Am J Surg Pathol. 2004;28(5):658–69.

188. O'Leary JG, Kaneku H, Demetris AJ, Marr JD, Shiller SM, Susskind BM, et al. Antibody-mediated Rejection as a Contributor to Previously Unexplained Early Liver Allograft Loss. Liver Transpl. 2014;20(2):218–27.

189. Kozlowski T, Andreoni K, Schmitz J, Hayashi PH, Nickeleit V. Sinusoidal C4d Deposits in Liver Allografts Indicate an Antibody-mediated Response: Diagnostic Considerations in the Evaluation of Liver Allografts. Liver Transpl. 2012;18(6):641–58.

190. Gelson W, Hoare M, Dawwas MF, Vowler S, Gibbs P, Alexander G. The Pattern of Late Mortality in Liver Transplant Recipients in the United Kingdom. Transplantation. 2011;91(11):1240–4.

191. Duffy JP, Kao K, Ko CY, Farmer DG, McDiarmid SV, Hong JC, et al. Long-term Patient Outcome and Quality of Life after Liver Transplantation: Analysis of 20-year Survivors. Ann Surg. 2010;252(4):652–61.

192. O'Leary JG, Demetris AJ, Friedman LS, Gebel HM, Halloran PF, Kirk AD, et al. The Role of Donor-specific HLA Alloantibodies in Liver Transplantation. Am J Transplant. 2014;14(4):779–87.

193. Salah A, Fujimoto M, Yoshizawa A, Yurugi K, Miyagawa-Hayashino A, Sumiyoshi S, et al. Application of Complement Component 4d Immunohistochemistry to ABO-compatible and ABO-incompatible Liver Transplantation. Liver Transpl. 2014;20(2):200–9.

194. Rose ML, West LJ. Accommodation: Does It Apply to Human Leukocyte Antigens? Transplantation. 2012;93(3):244–6.

195. Raut V, Uemoto S. Management of ABO-incompatible Living-donor Liver Transplantation: Past and Present Trends. Surg Today. 2011;41(3):317–22.

196. Haga H, Egawa H, Shirase T, Miyagawa A, Sakurai T, Minamiguchi S, et al. Periportal Edema and Necrosis as Diagnostic Histological Features of Early Humoral Rejection in ABO-incompatible Liver Transplantation. Liver Transpl. 2004;10(1):16–27.

197. Ruiz R, Tomiyama K, Campsen J, Goldstein RM, Levy MF, McKenna GJ, et al. Implications of a Positive Crossmatch in Liver Transplantation: A 20-year Review. Liver Transplantation: Official Publication of the American Association for the Study of Liver Diseases and the International Liver Transplantation Society. 2011.

198. Al-Sibae MR, Koffron AJ, Raofi V. Does a Positive Pretransplant Crossmatch Affect Long-term Outcome in Liver Transplantation? Transplantation. 2011;91(3):261–2.

199. Chan KM, Lee CS, Wu TJ, Lee CF, Chen TC, Lee WC. Clinical Perspective of Acute Humoral Rejection after Blood Type-compatible Liver Transplantation. Transplantation. 2011;91(5):e29–30.

200. O'Leary J, Kaneku H, Banuelos N, Jennings L, Klintmalm G, Terasaki P. Impact of IgG3 Subclass and C1q-fixing Donor Specific Antibodies on Rejection and Survival in Liver Transplantation. American Journal of Transplantation. 2015;(in press).

201. O'Leary JG, Kaneku H, Jennings L, Susskind BM, Terasaki PI, Klintmalm GB. Donor-specific Slloantibodies Are Associated with Fibrosis Progression after Liver Transplantation in Hepatitis C Virus-infected Patients. Liver Transpl. 2014;20(6):655–63.

202. Castillo-Rama M, Castro MJ, Bernardo I, Meneu-Diaz JC, Elola-Olaso AM, Calleja-Antolin SM, et al. Preformed Antibodies Detected by Cytotoxic Assay or Multibead Array Decrease Liver Allograft Survival: Role of Human Leukocyte Antigen Compatibility. Liver Transpl. 2008;14(4):554–62.

203. O'Leary JG, Klintmalm GB. Impact of Donor-specific Antibodies on Results of Liver Transplantation. Curr Opin Organ Transplant. 2013;18(3):279–84.

204. Taner T, Gandhi MJ, Sanderson SO, Poterucha CR, De Goey SR, Stegall MD, et al. Prevalence, Course and Impact of HLA Donor-specific Antibodies in Liver Transplantation in the First Year. Am J Transplant. 2012;12(6):1504–10.

205. Manez R, Kelly RH, Kobayashi M, Takaya S, Bronsther O, Kramer D, et al. Immunoglobulin G Lymphocytotoxic Antibodies in Clinical Liver Transplantation: Studies Toward Further Defining Their Significance. Hepatology. 1995;21(5):1345–52.

206. Doyle HR, Marino IR, Morelli F, Doria C, Aldrighetti L, McMichael J, et al. Assessing Risk in Liver Transplantation. Special Reference

207. Kozlowski T, Rubinas T, Nickeleit V, Woosley J, Schmitz J, Collins D, et al. Liver Allograft Antibody-mediated Rejection with Demonstration of Sinusoidal C4d Staining and Circulating Donor-specific Antibodies. Liver Transplantation: Official Publication of the American Association for the Study of Liver Diseases and the International Liver Transplantation Society. 2011;17(4):357–68.

208. Hubscher SG. Antibody-mediated Rejection in the Liver Allograft. Curr Opin Organ Transplant. 2012;17(3):280–6.

209. Demetris AJ, Bellamy C, Hubscher SG, O'Leary J, Randhawa PS, Feng S, et al. 2016 Comprehensive Update of the BANFF Working Group on Liver Allograft Pathology: Introduction of Antibody-mediated Rejection. Am J Transplant. 2016.

210. Haga H, Egawa H, Fujimoto Y, Ueda M, Miyagawa-Hayashino A, Sakurai T, et al. Acute Humoral Rejection and C4d Immunostaining in ABO Blood Type-incompatible Liver Transplantation. Liver Transpl. 2006;12(3):457–64.

211. Egawa H, Uemoto S, Inomata Y, Shapiro AM, Asonuma K, Kiuchi T, et al. Biliary Complications in Pediatric Living Related Liver Transplantation. Surgery. 1998;124(5):901–10.

212. Sebagh M, Farges O, Kalil A, Samuel D, Bismuth H, Reynes M. Sclerosing Cholangitis Following Human Orthotopic Liver Transplantation. The American Journal of Surgical Pathology. 1995;19(1):81–90.

213. Iacob S, Cicinnati VR, Dechêne A, Lindemann M, Heinemann FM, Rebmann V, et al. Genetic, Immunological and Clinical Risk Factors for Biliary Strictures Following Liver Transplantation. Liver International: Official Journal of the International Association for the Study of the Liver. 2012;32(8):1253–61.

214. Manez R, Kobayashi M, Takaya S, Bronsther O, Kramer D, Bonet H, et al. Humoral Rejection Associated with Antidonor Lymphocytotoxic Antibodies Following Liver Transplantation. Transplantation Proceedings. 1993;25(1 Pt 2):888–90.

215. Musat AI, Agni RM, Wai PY, Pirsch JD, Lorentzen DF, Powell A, et al. The Significance of Donor-specific HLA Antibodies in Rejection and Ductopenia Development in ABO Compatible Liver Transplantation. American Journal of Transplantation: Official Journal of the American Society of Transplantation and the American Society of Transplant Surgeons. 2011;11(3):500–10.

216. Bellamy CO. Complement C4d Immunohistochemistry in the Assessment of Liver Allograft Biopsy Samples: Applications and Pitfalls. Liver Transplantation: Official Publication of the American Association for the Study of Liver Diseases and the International Liver Transplantation Society. 2011;17(7):747–50.

217. Grabhorn E, Binder TM, Obrecht D, Brinkert F, Lehnhardt A, Herden U, et al. Long-term Clinical Relevance of De Novo Donor-specific Antibodies after Pediatric Liver Transplantation. Transplantation. 2015.

218. Markiewicz-Kijewska M, Kaliciński P, Kluge P, Piątosa B, Jankowska I, Rękawek A, et al. Immunological Factors and Liver Fibrosis in Pediatric Liver Transplant Recipients. Ann Transplant. 2015;20:279–84.

219. Wozniak LJ, Hickey MJ, Venick RS, Vargas JH, Farmer DG, Busuttil RW, et al. Donor-specific HLA Antibodies Are Associated with Late Allograft Dysfunction after Pediatric Liver Transplantation. Transplantation. 2015.

220. Ohe H, Uchida Y, Yoshizawa A, Hirao H, Taniguchi M, Maruya E, et al. Association of Anti-human Leukocyte Antigen and Anti-angiotensin II Type 1 Receptor Antibodies with Liver Allograft Fibrosis after Immunosuppression Withdrawal. Transplantation. 2014;98(10):1105–11.

221. Kosola S, Lampela H, Jalanko H, Makisalo H, Lohi J, Arola J, et al. Low-dose Steroids Associated with Milder Histological Changes after Pediatric Liver Transplantation. Liver Transpl. 2013;19(2):145–54.

222. Miyagawa-Hayashino A, Yoshizawa A, Uchida Y, Egawa H, Yurugi K, Masuda S, et al. Progressive Graft Fibrosis and Donor-specific Human Leukocyte Antigen Antibodies in Pediatric Late Liver Allografts. Liver Transpl. 2012;18(11):1333–42.

223. Yamada H, Kondou H, Kimura T, Ikeda K, Tachibana M, Hasegawa Y, et al. Humoral Immunity Is Involved in the Development of Pericentral Fibrosis after Pediatric Live Donor Liver Transplantation. Pediatr Transplant. 2012;16(8):858–65.

224. Girnita A, Mazariegos GV, Castellaneta A, Reyes J, Bentlejewski C, Thomson AW, et al. Liver Transplant Recipients Weaned off Immunosuppression Lack Circulating Donor-specific Antibodies. Hum Immunol. 2010;71(3):274–6.

225. Kaneku H, O'Leary JG, Banuelos N, Jennings LW, Susskind BM, Klintmalm GB, et al. De Novo Donor-specific HLA Antibodies Decrease Patient and Graft Survival in Liver Transplant Recipients. Am J Transplant. 2013;13(6):1541–8.

226. O'Leary JG, Cai J, Freeman R, Banuelos N, Hart B, Johnson M, et al. Proposed Diagnostic Criteria for Chronic Antibody-mediated Rejection in Liver Allografts. Am J Transplant. 2015.

227. Yoshitomi M, Koshiba T, Haga H, Li Y, Zhao X, Cheng D, et al. Requirement of Protocol Biopsy before and after Complete Cessation of Immunosuppression after Liver Transplantation. Transplantation. 2009;87(4):606–14.

228. Egawa H, Miyagawa-Hayashino A, Haga H, Teramukai S, Yoshizawa A, Ogawa K, et al. Non-inflammatory Centrilobular Sinusoidal Fibrosis in Pediatric Liver Transplant Recipients under Tacrolimus Withdrawal. Hepatology Research: The Official Journal of the Japan Society of Hepatology. 2012;42(9):895–903.

229. Demetris AJ, Adeyi O, Bellamy CO, Clouston A, Charlotte F, Czaja A, et al. Liver Biopsy Interpretation for Causes of Late Liver Allograft Dysfunction. Hepatology. 2006;44(2):489–501.

230. Demetris AJ, Lunz JG, 3rd, Randhawa P, Wu T, Nalesnik M, Thomson AW. Monitoring of Human Liver and Kidney Allograft Tolerance: A Tissue/Histopathology Perspective. Transpl Int. 2009;22(1):120–41.

231. Benitez C, Londono MC, Miquel R, Manzia TM, Abraldes JG, Lozano JJ, et al. Prospective Multicenter Clinical Trial of Immunosuppressive Drug Withdrawal in Stable Adult Liver Transplant Recipients. Hepatology. 2013.

232. Feng S, Demetris AJ, Ekong U, Girnita A, Kanaparthi S, Soppe C, et al., editors. Serum and Tissue DSA Subclass, Stellate and Endothelial Phenotype Monitoring in ITN029ST Tolerance Pediatric Liver Transplant Recipients over 5+ Years of Follow-up. Joint International Conference of

ILTS, ELITA & LICAGE; 2014; London.

233 Hubscher SG. What Is the Long-term Outcome of the Liver Allograft? Journal of Hepatology. 2011;**55**(3):702-17.

234 Smith RN, Colvin RB. Chronic Alloantibody Mediated Rejection. Semin Immunol. 2012;**24**(2):115-21.

235 Bellamy CO, Herriot MM, Harrison DJ, Bathgate AJ. C4d Immunopositivity Is Uncommon in ABO-compatible Liver Allografts, but Correlates Partially with Lymphocytotoxic Antibody Status. Histopathology. 2007;**50**(6):739-49.

236 Iacob S, Cicinnati VR, Lindemann M, Heinemann FM, Radtke A, Kaiser GM, et al. Donor-Specific Anti-HLA Antibodies and Endothelial C4d Deposition-Association with Chronic Liver Allograft Failure. Transplantation. 2015;**99**(9):1869-75.

237 Seemayer CA, Gaspert A, Nickeleit V, Mihatsch MJ. C4d Staining of Renal Allograft Biopsies: A Comparative Analysis of Different Staining Techniques. Nephrol Dial Transplant. 2007;**22**(2):568-76.

238 Nadasdy GM, Bott C, Cowden D, Pelletier R, Ferguson R, Nadasdy T. Comparative Study for the Detection of Peritubular Capillary C4d Deposition in Human Renal Allografts Using Different Methodologies. Hum Pathol. 2005;**36**(11):1178-85.

239 Bu X, Zheng Z, Yu Y, Zeng L, Jiang Y. Significance of C4d Deposition in the Diagnosis of Rejection after Liver Transplantation. Transplant Proc. 2006;**38**(5):1418-21.

240 Dankof A, Schmeding M, Morawietz L, Gunther R, Krukemeyer MG, Rudolph B, et al. Portal Capillary C4d Deposits and Increased Infiltration by Macrophages Indicate Humorally Mediated Mechanisms in Acute Cellular Liver Allograft Rejection. Virchows Arch. 2005;**447**(1):87-93.

241 Jain A, Mohanka R, Orloff M, Abt P, Romano J, Bryan L, et al. Characterization of CD4, CD8, CD56 Positive Lymphocytes and C4d Deposits to Distinguish Acute Cellular Rejection from Recurrent Hepatitis C in Post-liver Transplant Biopsies. Clin Transplant. 2006;**20**(5):624-33.

242 Krukemeyer MG, Moeller J, Morawietz L, Rudolph B, Neumann U, Theruvath T, et al. Description of B Lymphocytes and Plasma Cells, Complement, and Chemokines/Receptors in Acute Liver Allograft Rejection. Transplantation. 2004;**78**(1):65-70.

243 Sakashita H, Haga H, Ashihara E, Wen MC, Tsuji H, Miyagawa-Hayashino A, et al. Significance of C4d Staining in ABO-identical/Compatible Liver Transplantation. Mod Pathol. 2007;**20**(6):676-84.

244 Sawada T, Shimizu A, Kubota K, Fuchinoue S, Teraoka S. Lobular Damage Caused by Cellular and Humoral Immunity in Liver Allograft Rejection. Clin Transplant. 2005;**19**(1):110-4.

245 Troxell ML, Higgins JP, Kambham N. Evaluation of C4d Staining in Liver and Small Intestine Allografts. Arch Pathol Lab Med. 2006;**130**(10):1489-96.

246 Bouron-Dal Soglio D, Rougemont AL, Herzog D, Soucy G, Alvarez F, Fournet JC. An Immunohistochemical Evaluation of C4d Deposition in Pediatric Inflammatory Liver Diseases. Human Pathology. 2008;**39**(7):1103-10.

247 Aguilera I, Sousa JM, Gavilan F, Gomez L, Alvarez-Marquez A, Nunez-Roldan A. Complement Component 4d Immunostaining in Liver Allografts of Patients with de Novo Immune Hepatitis. Liver Transplantation: Official Publication of the American Association for the Study of Liver Diseases and the International Liver Transplantation Society. 2011;**17**(7):779-88.

248 Schmeding M, Dankof A, Krenn V, Krukemeyer MG, Koch M, Spinelli A, et al. C4d in Acute Rejection after Liver Transplantation–A Valuable Tool in Differential Diagnosis to Hepatitis C Recurrence. Am J Transplant. 2006;**6**(3):523-30.

249 Silva MA, Mirza DF, Murphy N, Richards DA, Reynolds GM, Wigmore SJ, et al. Intrahepatic Complement Activation, Sinusoidal Endothelial Injury, and Lactic Acidosis Are Associated with Initial Poor Function of the Liver after Transplantation. Transplantation. 2008;**85**(5):718-25.

250 Martelius T, Halme L, Arola J, Hockerstedt K, Lautenschlager I. Vascular Deposition of Complement C4d Is Increased in Liver Allografts with Chronic Rejection. Transpl Immunol. 2009;**21**(4):244-6.

251 Anonymous. Terminology for Hepatic Allograft Rejection. International Working Party. Hepatology. 1995;**22**(2):648-54.

252 Knechtle SJ, Kwun J. Unique Aspects of Rejection and Tolerance in Liver Transplantation. Seminars in Liver Disease. 2009;**29**(1):91-101.

253 Neuberger J. Incidence, Timing, and Risk Factors for Acute and Chronic Rejection. Liver Transpl Surg. 1999;**5**(4 Suppl 1):S30-6.

254 Demetris AJ, Ruppert K, Dvorchik I, Jain A, Minervini M, Nalesnik MA, et al. Real-time Monitoring of Acute Liver-allograft Rejection Using the BANFF Schema. Transplantation. 2002;**74**(9):1290-6.

255 Germani G, Rodriguez-Castro K, Russo FP, Senzolo M, Zanetto A, Ferrarese A, et al. Markers of Acute Rejection and Graft Acceptance in Liver Transplantation. World J Gastroenterol. 2015;**21**(4):1061-8.

256 Neil DA, Hubscher SG. Current Views on Rejection Pathology in Liver Transplantation. Transplant International: Official Journal of the European Society for Organ Transplantation. 2010;**23**(10):971-83.

257 Uemura T, Ikegami T, Sanchez EQ, Jennings LW, Narasimhan G, McKenna GJ, et al. Late Acute Rejection after Liver Transplantation Impacts Patient Survival. Clin Transplant. 2008;**22**(3):316-23.

258 Neil DA, Hubscher SG. Are Parenchymal Changes in Early Post-transplant Biopsies Related to Preservation-Reperfusion Injury or Rejection? Transplantation. 2001;**71**(11):1566-72.

259 Anonymous. BANFF Schema for Grading Liver Allograft Rejection: An International Consensus Document. Hepatology. 1997;**25**(3):658-63.

260 Yeh MM, Larson AM, Tung BY, Swanson PE, Upton MP. Endotheliitis in Chronic Viral Hepatitis: A Comparison with Acute Cellular Rejection and Non-alcoholic Steatohepatitis. The American Journal of Surgical Pathology. 2006;**30**(6):727-33.

261 Demetris AJ, Lasky S, Van Thiel DH, Starzl TE, Dekker A. Pathology of Hepatic Transplantation: A Review of 62 Adult Allograft Recipients Immunosuppressed with a Cyclosporine/Steroid Regimen. Am J Pathol. 1985;**118**(1):151-61.

262 McCaughan GW, Davies JS, Waugh JA, Bishop GA, Hall BM, Gallagher ND, et al. A Quantitative Analysis of T Lymphocyte Populations in Human Liver Allografts Undergoing Rejection: The Use of Monoclonal Antibodies

263. Steinhoff G, Behrend M, Wonigeit K. Expression of Adhesion Molecules on Lymphocytes/Monocytes and Hepatocytes in Human Liver Grafts. Hum Immunol. 1990;28(2):123–7.

264. Demetris AJ, Belle SH, Hart J, Lewin K, Ludwig J, Snover DC, et al. Intraobserver and Interobserver Variation in the Histopathological Assessment of Liver Allograft Rejection. The Liver Transplantation Database (LTD) Investigators. Hepatology. 1991;14(5):751–5.

265. Cong WM, Zhang SY, Wang ZL, Xue L, Liu YS, Zhang SH. [Pathologic Diagnosis of 1123 Post-transplant Liver Biopsies from 665 Liver Transplant Patients]. Zhonghua Bing Li Xue Za Zhi. 2005;34(11):716–9.

266. Netto GJ, Watkins DL, Williams JW, Colby TV, dePetris G, Sharkey FE, et al. Interobserver Agreement in Hepatitis C Grading and Staging and in the BANFF Grading Schema for Acute Cellular Rejection: The "Hepatitis C 3" Multi-institutional Trial Experience. Arch Pathol Lab Med. 2006;130(8):1157–62.

267. Demirhan B, Bilezikci B, Haberal AN, Sevmis S, Arat Z, Haberal M. Hepatic Parenchymal Changes and Histologic Eosinophilia as Predictors of Subsequent Acute Liver Allograft Rejection. Liver Transpl. 2008;14(2):214–9.

268. Hubscher S. Diagnosis and Grading of Liver Allograft Rejection: A European Perspective. Transplant Proc. 1996;28(1):504–7.

269. Ishak K, Baptista A, Bianchi L, Callea F, De Groote J, Gudat F, et al. Histological Grading and Staging of Chronic Hepatitis. Journal of Hepatology. 1995;22(6):696–9.

270. Tsamandas AC, Jain AB, Felekouras ES, Fung JJ, Demetris AJ, Lee RG. Central Venulitis in the Allograft Liver: A Clinicopathologic Study. Transplantation. 1997;64(2):252–7.

271. Krasinskas AM, Ruchelli ED, Rand EB, Chittams JL, Furth EE. Central Venulitis in Pediatric Liver Allografts. Hepatology. 2001;33(5):1141–7.

272. Krasinskas AM, Demetris AJ, Poterucha JJ, Abraham SC. The Prevalence and Natural History of Untreated Isolated Central Perivenulitis in Adult Allograft Livers. Liver Transpl. 2008;14(5):625–32.

273. Sanei MH, Schiano TD, Sempoux C, Fan C, Fiel MI. Acute Cellular Rejection Resulting in Sinusoidal Obstruction Syndrome and Ascites Postliver Transplantation. Transplantation. 2011;92(10):1152–8.

274. Demetris AJ, Duquesnoy RJ, Fung JJ, Murase N, Nalesnik M, Randhawa P, et al. Pathophysiology of Chronic Allograft Rejection [Internet]. Medscape Transplantation. 2000. Available from: www.transplantation.medscape.com/Medscape/transplantation/ClinicalMgmt/CM.v02/public/index.CM.v02.html.

275. Walter T, Dumortier J, Guillaud O, Hervieu V, Paliard P, Scoazec JY, et al. Rejection under Alpha Interferon Therapy in Liver Transplant Recipients. Am J Transplant. 2007;7(1):177–84.

276. Stanca CM, Fiel MI, Kontorinis N, Agarwal K, Emre S, Schiano TD. Chronic Ductopenic Rejection in Patients with Recurrent Hepatitis C Virus Treated with Pegylated Interferon Alfa-2a and Ribavirin. Transplantation. 2007;84(2):180–6.

277. Blakolmer K, Gaulard P, Mannhalter C, Swerdlow S, Fassati LR, Rossi G, et al. Unusual Peripheral T Cell Lymphoma Presenting as Acute Liver Failure and Reappearing in the Liver Allograft. Transplantation. 2000;70(12):1802–5.

278. Blakolmer K, Jain A, Ruppert K, Gray E, Duquesnoy R, Murase N, et al. Chronic Liver Allograft Rejection in a Population Treated Primarily with Tacrolimus as Baseline Immunosuppression: Long-term Follow-up and Evaluation of Features for Histopathological Staging. Transplantation. 2000;69(11):2330–6.

279. Demetris AJ. Spectrum of Chronic Hepatic Allograft Rejection and Arteriopathy and the Controversy of Centrilobular Necrosis. Liver Transpl. 2000;6(1):102–3.

280. Evans PC, Smith S, Hirschfield G, Rigopoulou E, Wreghitt TG, Wight DG, et al. Recipient HLA-DR3, Tumour Necrosis Factor-alpha Promoter Allele-2 (Tumour Necrosis Factor-2) and Cytomegalovirus Infection are Interrelated Risk Factors for Chronic Rejection of Liver Grafts. Journal of Hepatology. 2001;34(5):711–5.

281. O'Leary JG, Kaneku H, Susskind BM, Jennings LW, Neri MA, Davis GL, et al. High Mean Fluorescence Intensity Donor-specific Anti-HLA Antibodies Associated with Chronic Rejection Postliver Transplant. Am J Transplant. 2011;11(9):1868–76.

282. Pappo O, Ramos H, Starzl TE, Fung JJ, Demetris AJ. Structural Integrity and Identification of Causes of Liver Allograft Dysfunction Occurring More Than 5 Years after Transplantation. American Journal of Surgical Pathology. 1995;19(2):192–206.

283. Demetris AJ, Murase N, Starzl TE, Fung JJ. Pathology of Chronic Rejection: An Overview of Common Findings and Observations about Pathogenic Mechanisms and Possible Prevention. Graft. 1998;1:52–9.

284. Blakolmer K, Seaberg EC, Batts K, Ferrell L, Markin R, Wiesner R, et al. Analysis of the Reversibility of Chronic Liver Allograft Rejection Implications for a Staging Schema. Am J Surg Pathol. 1999;23(11):1328–39.

285. Demetris AJ, Fung JJ, Todo S, McCauley J, Jain A, Takaya S, et al. Conversion of Liver Allograft Recipients from Cyclosporine to FK506 Immunosuppressive Therapy–A Clinicopathologic Study of 96 Patients. Transplantation. 1992;53(5):1056–62.

286. White RM, Zajko AB, Demetris AJ, Bron KM, Dekker A, Starzl TE. Liver Transplant Rejection: Angiographic Findings in 35 Patients. AJR Am J Roentgenol. 1987;148(6):1095–8.

287. Freese DK, Snover DC, Sharp HL, Gross CR, Savick SK, Payne WD. Chronic Rejection after Liver Transplantation: A Study of Clinical, Histopathological and Immunological Features. Hepatology. 1991;13(5):882–91.

288. Hubscher SG, Buckels JA, Elias E, McMaster P, Neuberger JM. Reversible Vanishing Bile Duct Syndrome after Liver Transplantation: Report of 6 Cases. Transplantation Proceedings. 1991;23(1 Pt 2):1415–6.

289. Hubscher SG, Buckels JA, Elias E, McMaster P, Neuberger J. Vanishing Bile-duct Syndrome Following Liver Transplantation–Is It Reversible? Transplantation. 1991;51(5):1004–10.

290. van den Heuvel MC, de Jong KP, Boot M, Slooff MJ, Poppema S, Gouw AS. Preservation of Bile Ductules Mitigates Bile Duct Loss. Am J Transplant. 2006;6(11):2660–71.

291. Demetris A, Adams D, Bellamy C, Blakolmer K, Clouston A, Dhillon AP, et al. Update of the International BANFF Schema for Liver Allograft Rejection: Working Recommendations for the Histopathologic Staging and Reporting of Chronic Rejection. An International Panel. Hepatology. 2000;31(3):792–9.

292. O'Keeffe C, Baird AW, Nolan N, McCormick PA. Mast Cell Hyperplasia in Chronic Rejection after Liver Transplantation. Liver Transpl. 2002;8(1):50–7.

293. Sasaki M, Ikeda H, Haga H, Manabe T, Nakanuma Y. Frequent Cellular Senescence in Small Bile Ducts in Primary Biliary Cirrhosis: A Possible Role in Bile Duct Loss. The Journal of Pathology. 2005;205(4):451–9.

294. Rygiel KA, Robertson H, Willet JD, Brain JG, Burt AD, Jones DE, et al. T Cell-mediated Biliary Epithelial-to-Mesenchymal Transition in Liver Allograft Rejection. Liver Transplantation: Official Publication of the American Association for the Study of Liver Diseases and the International Liver Transplantation Society. 2010;16(5):567–76.

295. Crawford AR, Lin XZ, Crawford JM. The Normal Adult Human Liver Biopsy: A Quantitative Reference Standard. Hepatology. 1998;28(2):323–31.

296. Oguma S, Belle S, Starzl TE, Demetris AJ. A Histometric Analysis of Chronically Rejected Human Liver Allografts: Insights into the Mechanisms of Bile Duct Loss: Direct Immunologic and Ischemic Factors. Hepatology. 1989;9(2):204–9.

297. Moreira RK, Chopp W, Washington MK. The Concept of Hepatic Artery-bile Duct Parallelism in the Diagnosis of Ductopenia in Liver Biopsy Samples. The American Journal of Surgical Pathology. 2011;35(3):392–403.

298. Matsumoto Y, McCaughan GW, Painter DM, Bishop GA. Evidence that Portal Tract Microvascular Destruction Precedes Bile Duct Loss in Human Liver Allograft Rejection. Transplantation. 1993;56(1):69–75.

299. Neil DA, Hubscher SG. Histologic and Biochemical Changes during the Evolution of Chronic Rejection of Liver Allografts. Hepatology. 2002;35(3):639–51.

300. Nakazawa Y, Jonsson JR, Walker NI, Kerlin P, Steadman C, Lynch SV, et al. Fibrous Obliterative Lesions of Veins Contribute to Progressive Fibrosis in Chronic Liver Allograft Rejection. Hepatology. 2000;32(6):1240–7.

301. Rubin RH, Tolkoff-Rubin NE. Opportunistic Infections in Renal Allograft Recipients. Transplantation Proceedings. 1988;20(6 Suppl 8):12–8.

302. Kalil AC, Opal SM. Sepsis in the Severely Immunocompromised Patient. Current Infectious Disease Reports. 2015;17(6):487.

303. Fishman JA. Infections in Immunocompromised Hosts and Organ Transplant Recipients: Essentials. Liver Transpl. 2011;17 Suppl 3:S34–7.

304. Helfrich M, Ison MG. Opportunistic Infections Complicating Solid Organ Transplantation with Alemtuzumab Induction. Transpl Infect Dis. 2015.

305. Pedersen M, Seetharam A. Infections after Orthotopic Liver Transplantation. J Clin Exp Hepatol. 2014;4(4):347–60.

306. Bruminhent J, Razonable RR. Management of Cytomegalovirus Infection and Disease in Liver Transplant Recipients. World J Hepatol. 2014;6(6):370–83.

307. Fehr T, Cippa PE, Mueller NJ. Cytomegalovirus Post Kidney Transplantation: Prophylaxis versus Pre-emptive Therapy? Transpl Int. 2015.

308. Bai X, Rogers BB, Harkins PC, Sommerauer J, Squires R, Rotondo K, et al. Predictive Value of Quantitative PCR-based Viral Burden Analysis for Eight Human Herpesviruses in Pediatric Solid Organ Transplant Patients. J Mol Diagn. 2000;2(4):191–201.

309. Neoh CF, Snell G, Levvey B, Morrissey CO, Stewart K, Kong DC. Antifungal Prophylaxis in Lung Transplantation. International Journal of Antimicrobial Agents. 2014;44(3):194–202.

310. Razonable RR, Emery VC. Management of CMV Infection and Disease in Transplant Patients. 27–29 February 2004. Herpes: The Journal of the IHMF. 2004;11(3):77–86.

311. Lautenschlager I. CMV Infection, Diagnosis and Antiviral Strategies after Liver Transplantation. Transplant International: Official Journal of the European Society for Organ Transplantation. 2009;22(11):1031–40.

312. Razonable RR. Cytomegalovirus Infection after Liver Transplantation: Current Concepts and Challenges. World Journal of Gastroenterology: WJG. 2008;14(31):4849–60.

313. Eid AJ, Bakri SJ, Kijpittayarit S, Razonable RR. Clinical Features and Outcomes of Cytomegalovirus Retinitis after Transplantation. Transpl Infect Dis. 2008;10(1):13–8.

314. Demetris AJ, Nalesnik M, Randhawa P, Wu T, Minervini M, Lai C, et al. Histologic Patterns of Rejection and Other Causes of Liver Dysfunction. In: Busuttil RW, Klintmalm GB, editors. Transplantation of the Liver. Philadelphia: Elsevier Saunders; 2005. p. 1057–128.

315. Barkholt LM, Ehrnst A, Veress B. Clinical Use of Immunohistopathologic Methods for the Diagnosis of Cytomegalovirus Hepatitis in Human Liver Allograft Biopsy Specimens. Scand J Gastroenterol. 1994;29(6):553–60.

316. Mabruk MJ. In Situ Hybridization: Detecting Viral Nucleic Acid in Formalin-fixed, Paraffin-embedded Tissue Samples. Expert Review of Molecular Diagnostics. 2004;4(5):653–61.

317. O'Grady JG, Alexander GJ, Sutherland S, Donaldson PT, Harvey F, Portmann B, et al. Cytomegalovirus Infection and Donor/Recipient HLA Antigens: Interdependent Co-factors in Pathogenesis of Vanishing Bile-duct Syndrome after Liver Transplantation. Lancet. 1988;2(8606):302–5.

318. Lautenschlager I, Hockerstedt K, Jalanko H, Loginov R, Salmela K, Taskinen E, et al. Persistent Cytomegalovirus in Liver Allografts with Chronic Rejection. Hepatology. 1997;25(1):190–4.

319. Paya CV, Wiesner RH, Hermans PE, Larson-Keller JJ, Ilstrup DM, Krom RA, et al. Lack of Association between Cytomegalovirus Infection, HLA Matching and the Vanishing Bile Duct Syndrome after Liver Transplantation. Hepatology. 1992;16(1):66–70.

320. Nourse JP, Jones K, Gandhi MK. Epstein-Barr Virus-related Post-transplant Lymphoproliferative Disorders: Pathogenetic Insights for Targeted Therapy. American Journal of Transplantation: Official Journal of the American Society of Transplantation and the American Society of Transplant Surgeons. 2011;11(5):888–95.

321. Cesarman E. Gammaherpesvirus and Lymphoproliferative Disorders in Immunocompromised Patients. Cancer Lett. 2011;305(2):163–74.

322. Nalesnik MA. Clinicopathologic Characteristics of Post-transplant Lymphoproliferative Disorders. Recent Results Cancer Res. 2002;159:9–18.

323. Allen U, Preiksaitis J. Epstein-barr Virus and Posttransplant Lymphoproliferative Disorder in Solid Organ Transplant Recipients. Am J Transplant. 2009;9 Suppl 4:S87–96.

324. Verghese PS, Schmeling DO, Knight JA, Matas AJ, Balfour HH, Jr. The Impact of Donor Viral Replication at Transplant on Recipient Infections Posttransplant: A Prospective Study. Transplantation. 2015;99(3):602–8.

325. Jain A, Nalesnik M, Reyes J, Pokharna R, Mazariegos G, Green M, et al. Posttransplant Lymphoproliferative Disorders in Liver Transplantation: A 20-year experience. Ann Surg. 2002;236(4):429–36.

326. Hartmann C, Schuchmann M, Zimmermann T. Posttransplant Lymphoproliferative Disease in Liver Transplant Patients. Current Infectious Disease Reports. 2011;13(1):53–9.

327. Narkewicz MR, Green M, Dunn S, Millis M, McDiarmid S, Mazariegos G, et al. Decreasing Incidence of Symptomatic Epstein-Barr Virus Disease and Posttransplant Lymphoproliferative Disorder in Pediatric Liver Transplant Recipients: Report of the Studies of Pediatric Liver Transplantation Experience. Liver Transpl. 2013;19(7):730–40.

328. Koch DG, Christiansen L, Lazarchick J, Stuart R, Willner IR, Reuben A. Posttransplantation Lymphoproliferative Disorder–The Great Mimic in Liver Transplantation: Appraisal of the Clinicopathologic Spectrum and the Role of Epstein-Barr Virus. Liver Transpl. 2007;13(6):904–12.

329. Niller HH, Wolf H, Minarovits J. Regulation and Dysregulation of Epstein-Barr Virus Latency: Implications for the Development of Autoimmune Diseases. Autoimmunity. 2008;41(4):298–328.

330. Randhawa PS, Markin RS, Starzl TE, Demetris AJ. Epstein-Barr Virus-associated Syndromes in Immunosuppressed Liver Transplant Recipients. Clinical Profile and Recognition on Routine Allograft Biopsy. Am J Surg Pathol. 1990;14(6):538–47.

331. Randhawa PS, Jaffe R, Demetris AJ, Nalesnik M, Starzl TE, Chen YY, et al. The Systemic Distribution of Epstein-Barr Virus Genomes in Fatal Post-Transplantation Lymphoproliferative Disorders. An in Situ Hybridization Study. Am J Pathol. 1991;138(4):1027–33.

332. Randhawa PS, Jaffe R, Demetris AJ, Nalesnik M, Starzl TE, Chen YY, et al. Expression of Epstein-Barr Virus-encoded Small RNA (by the EBER-1 Gene) in Liver Specimens from Transplant Recipients with Post-transplantation Lymphoproliferative Disease. N Engl J Med. 1992;327(24):1710–4.

333. Jha B, Gajendra S, Sachdev R, Goel S, Sahni T, Raina V. Prompt Diagnosis and Management of Epstein-Barr Virus-associated Post-transplant Lymphoproliferative Disorder and Hemophagocytosis: A Dreaded Complication in a Post-liver Transplant Child. Pediatr Transplant. 2015.

334. Cockfield SM. Identifying the Patient at Risk for Post-transplant Lymphoproliferative Disorder. Transpl Infect Dis. 2001;3(2):70–8.

335. Bakker NA, van Imhoff GW, Verschuuren EA, van Son WJ. Presentation and Early Detection of Post-transplant Lymphoproliferative Disorder after Solid Organ Transplantation. Transpl Int. 2007;20(3):207–18.

336. Jamalidoust M, Geramizadeh B, Pouladfar G, Namayandeh M, Asaie S, Aliabadi N, et al. Epstein-Barr Virus DNAemia in Iranian Liver Transplant Recipients and Assessment of Its Variation in Posttransplant Lymphproliferative Disorder Patients by Quantitative Polymerase Chain Reaction Assay. Exp Clin Transplant. 2015;13 Suppl 1:306–11.

337. Randhawa P, Blakolmer K, Kashyap R, Raikow R, Nalesnik M, Demetris AJ, et al. Allograft Liver Biopsy in Patients with Epstein-Barr Virus-associated Posttransplant Lymphoproliferative Disease. Am J Surg Pathol. 2001;25(3):324–30.

338. Loginov R, Halme L, Arola J, Hockerstedt K, Lautenschlager I. Intragraft Immunological Events Associated with EBV DNAemia in Liver Transplant Patients. APMIS: acta pathologica, microbiologica, et immunologica Scandinavica. 2010;118(11):888–94.

339. Petrova M, Kamburov V. Epstein-Barr Virus: Silent Companion or Causative Agent of Chronic Liver Disease? World Journal of Gastroenterology: WJG. 2010;16(33):4130–4.

340. Harris N, Swerdlow S, Frizzera G, Knowles D, editors. Post-transplant Lymphoproliferative Disorders. Lyon: IARC Press; 2001.

341. Singavi AK, Harrington AM, Fenske TS. Post-transplant Lymphoproliferative Disorders. Cancer Treatment and Research. 2015;165:305–27.

342. Hubscher SG, Williams A, Davison SM, Young LS, Niedobitek G. Epstein-Barr Virus in Inflammatory Diseases of the Liver and Liver Allografts: An in Situ Hybridization Study. Hepatology. 1994;20(4 Pt 1):899–907.

343. Kobayashi M, Asano N, Fukushima M, Honda T. Three Different Histological Subtypes of Epstein-Barr Virus-negative Post-transplant Lymphoproliferative Disorder in a Patient with Hepatitis C Infection. International Journal of Hematology. 2014;100(3):307–11.

344. Morscio J, Dierickx D, Ferreiro JF, Herreman A, Van Loo P, Bittoun E, et al. Gene Expression Profiling Reveals Clear Differences between EBV-positive and EBV-Negative Posttransplant Lymphoproliferative Disorders. Am J Transplant. 2013;13(5):1305–16.

345. Montalbano M, Slapak-Green GI, Neff GW. Fulminant Hepatic Failure from Herpes Simplex Virus: Post Liver Transplantation Acyclovir Therapy and Literature Review. Transplantation Proceedings. 2005;37(10):4393–6.

346. Kusne S, Schwartz M, Breinig MK, Dummer JS, Lee RE, Selby R, et al. Herpes Simplex Virus Hepatitis after Solid Organ Transplantation in Adults. J Infect Dis. 1991;163(5):1001–7.

347. Javed S, Javed SA, Tyring SK. Varicella Vaccines. Current Opinion in Infectious Diseases. 2011.

348. Lucey MR, Terrault N, Ojo L, Hay JE, Neuberger J, Blumberg E, et al. Long-term Management of the Successful Adult Liver Transplant: 2012 Practice Guideline by the American Association for the Study of Liver Diseases and the American Society of Transplantation. Liver Transpl. 2013;19(1):3–26.

349. Basse G, Mengelle C, Kamar N, Ribes D, Selves J, Cointault O, et al. Disseminated Herpes Simplex Type-2 (HSV-2) Infection after Solid-organ Transplantation. Infection. 2008;36(1):62–4.

350. Riediger C, Sauer P, Matevossian E, Muller MW, Buchler P, Friess H. Herpes Simplex Virus Sepsis and Acute Liver Failure. Clinical Transplantation. 2009;23 Suppl 21:37–41.

351. Kusne S, Martin M, Shapiro R, Jordan M, Fung J, Alessiani M, et al. Early Infections in Kidney Transplant Recipients under FK 506. Transplantation Proceedings. 1991;23(1 Pt 2):956–7.

352. Abdel Massih RC, Razonable RR. Human Herpesvirus 6 Infections after Liver Transplantation. World J Gastroenterol. 2009;15(21):2561-9.

353. Razonable RR, Rivero A, Brown RA, Hart GD, Espy MJ, van Cruijsen H, et al. Detection of Simultaneous Beta-herpesvirus Infections in Clinical Syndromes due to Defined Cytomegalovirus Infection. Clin Transplant. 2003;17(2):114-20.

354. Lautenschlager I, Razonable RR. Human Herpesvirus-6 Infections in Kidney, Liver, Lung, and Heart Transplantation: Review. Transpl Int. 2012;25(5):493-502.

355. Lautenschlager I, Hockerstedt K, Linnavuori K, Taskinen E. Human Herpesvirus-6 Infection after Liver Transplantation. Clin Infect Dis. 1998;26(3):702-7.

356. Lautenschlager I, Harma M, Hockerstedt K, Linnavuori K, Loginov R, Taskinen E. Human Herpesvirus-6 Infection Is Associated with Adhesion Molecule Induction and Lymphocyte Infiltration in Liver Allografts. Journal of Hepatology. 2002;37(5):648-54.

357. Potenza L, Luppi M, Barozzi P, Rossi G, Cocchi S, Codeluppi M, et al. HHV-6A in Syncytial Giant-cell Hepatitis. The New England Journal of Medicine. 2008;359(6):593-602.

358. Andreoni M, Goletti D, Pezzotti P, Pozzetto A, Monini P, Sarmati L, et al. Prevalence, Incidence and Correlates of HHV-8/KSHV Infection and Kaposi's Sarcoma in Renal and Liver Transplant Recipients. J Infect. 2001;43(3):195-9.

359. Pietrosi G, Vizzini G, Pipitone L, Di Martino G, Minervini MI, Lo Iacono G, et al. Primary and Reactivated HHV8 Infection and Disease after Liver Transplantation: A Prospective Study. American Journal of Transplantation: Official Journal of the American Society of Transplantation and the American Society of Transplant Surgeons. 2011;11(12):2715-23.

360. Aseni P, Vertemati M, Minola E, Arcieri K, Bonacina E, Camozzi M, et al. Kaposi's Sarcoma in Liver Transplant Recipients: Morphological and Clinical Description. Liver Transplantation: Official Publication of the American Association for the Study of Liver Diseases and the International Liver Transplantation Society. 2001;7(9):816-23.

361. Benhammane H, Mentha G, Tschanz E, El Mesbahi O, Dietrich PY. Visceral Kaposi's Sarcoma Related to Human Herpesvirus-8 in Liver Transplant Recipient: Case Report and Literature Review. Case Reports in Oncological Medicine. 2012;2012:137291.

362. Lebbe C, Porcher R, Marcelin AG, Agbalika F, Dussaix E, Samuel D, et al. Human Herpesvirus 8 (HHV8) Transmission and Related Morbidity in Organ Recipients. Am J Transplant. 2013;13(1):207-13.

363. Pozo F, Tenorio A, de la Mata M, de Ory F, Torre-Cisneros J. Persistent Human Herpesvirus 8 Viremia before Kaposi's Sarcoma Development in a Liver Transplant Recipient. Transplantation. 2000;70(2):395-7.

364. Koneru B, Jaffe R, Esquivel CO, Kunz R, Todo S, Iwatsuki S, et al. Adenoviral Infections in Pediatric Liver Transplant Recipients. Jama. 1987;258(4):489-92.

365. Michaels MG, Green M, Wald ER, Starzl TE. Adenovirus Infection in Pediatric Liver Transplant Recipients. J Infect Dis. 1992;165(1):170-4.

366. Saad RS, Demetris AJ, Lee RG, Kusne S, Randhawa PS. Adenovirus Hepatitis in the Adult Allograft Liver. Transplantation. 1997;64(10):1483-5.

367. Perez D, McCormack L, Petrowsky H, Jochum W, Mullhaupt B, Clavien PA. Successful Outcome of Severe Adenovirus Hepatitis of the Allograft Following Liver Transplantation. Transplant Infectious Disease: An Official Journal of the Transplantation Society. 2007;9(4):318-22.

368. Hoffman JA. Adenoviral Disease in Pediatric Solid Organ Transplant Recipients. Pediatric Transplantation. 2006;10(1):17-25.

369. Kerensky T, Hasan A, Schain D, Trikha G, Liu C, Rand K, et al. Histopathologic Resolution of Adult Liver Transplantation Adenovirus Hepatitis with Cidofovir and Intravenous Immunoglobulin: A Case Report. Transplantation Proceedings. 2013;45(1):293-6.

370. Ronan BA, Agrwal N, Carey EJ, De Petris G, Kusne S, Seville MT, et al. Fulminant Hepatitis due to Human Adenovirus. Infection. 2014;42(1):105-11.

371. Cimsit B, Tichy EM, Patel SB, Rosencrantz R, Emre S. Treatment of Adenovirus Hepatitis with Cidofovir in a Pediatric Liver Transplant Recipient. Pediatr Transplant. 2012;16(3):E90-3.

372. McGrath D, Falagas ME, Freeman R, Rohrer R, Fairchild R, Colbach C, et al. Adenovirus Infection in Adult Orthotopic Liver Transplant Recipients: Incidence and Clinical Significance. J Infect Dis. 1998;177(2):459-62.

373. Ohori NP, Michaels MG, Jaffe R, Williams P, Yousem SA. Adenovirus Pneumonia in Lung Transplant Recipients. Hum Pathol. 1995;26(10):1073-9.

374. Zarrinpar A, Kaldas F, Busuttil RW. Liver Transplantation for Hepatocellular Carcinoma: An Update. Hepatobiliary & Pancreatic Diseases International: HBPD INT. 2011;10(3):234-42.

375. Washburn K, Halff G. Hepatocellular Carcinoma and Liver Transplantation. Curr Opin Organ Transplant. 2011;16(3):297-300.

376. Chok K. Management of Recurrent Hepatocellular Carcinoma after Liver Transplant. World J Hepatol. 2015;7(8):1142-8.

377. Schmeding M, Neumann UP. Liver Transplant for Cholangiocarcinoma: A Comeback? Exp Clin Transplant. 2015;13(4):301-8.

378. Grossman EJ, Millis JM. Liver Transplantation for Non-hepatocellular Carcinoma Malignancy: Indications, Limitations, and Analysis of the Current Literature. Liver Transplantation: Official Publication of the American Association for the Study of Liver Diseases and the International Liver Transplantation Society. 2010;16(8):930-42.

379. Hunt J, Gordon FD, Jenkins RL, Lewis WD, Khettry U. Sarcoidosis with Selective Involvement of a Second Liver Allograft: Report of a Case and Review of the Literature. Mod Pathol. 1999;12(3):325-8.

380. Vanatta JM, Modanlou KA, Dean AG, Nezakatgoo N, Campos L, Nair S, et al. Outcomes of Orthotopic Liver Transplantation for Hepatic Sarcoidosis: An Analysis of the United Network for Organ Sharing/Organ Procurement and Transplantation Network Data Files for a Comparative Study with Cholestatic Liver Diseases. Liver Transplantation: Official Publication of the American Association for the Study of Liver Diseases and the International Liver Transplantation Society. 2011;17(9):1027-34.

381. Pappo O, Yunis E, Jordan JA, Jaffe R, Mateo R, Fung J, et al. Recurrent and de Novo Giant Cell Hepatitis after Orthotopic Liver Transplantation. Am J Surg Pathol. 1994;18(8):804-13.

382 Starzl TE, Demetris AJ. Liver Transplantation: A 31-year Perspective. Part I. Curr Probl Surg. 1990;27(2):55–116.

383 Starzl TE, Demetris AJ. Liver Transplantation: A 31-year Perspective. Part II. Curr Probl Surg. 1990;27(3):123–78.

384 Starzl TE, Demetris AJ. Liver Transplantation: A 31-year Perspective. Part III. Curr Probl Surg. 1990;27(4):187–240.

385 Huang J. Ethical and Legislative Perspectives on Liver Transplantation in the People's Republic of China. Liver Transpl. 2007;13(2):193–6.

386 Saab S, Greenberg A, Li E, Bau SN, Durazo F, El-Kabany M, et al. Sofosbuvir and Simeprevir Is Effective for Recurrent Hepatitis C in Liver Transplant Recipients. Liver International: Official Journal of the International Association for the Study of the Liver. 2015.

387 Coilly A, Roche B, Duclos-Vallee JC, Samuel D. Optimal Therapy in Hepatitis C Virus Liver Transplant Patients with Direct Acting Antivirals. Liver International: Official Journal of the International Association for the Study of the Liver. 2015;35 Suppl 1:44–50.

388 Cavallari A, De Raffele E, Bellusci R, Miniero R, Vivarelli M, Galli S, et al. De Novo Hepatitis B and C Viral Infection after Liver Transplantation. World J Surg. 1997;21(1):78–84.

389 Jimenez-Perez M, Gonzalez-Grande R, Rando-Munoz FJ. Management of Recurrent Hepatitis C Virus after Liver Transplantation. World J Gastroenterol. 2014;20(44):16409–17.

390 Laverdure N, Scholtes-Brunel C, Rivet C, Heissat S, Restier L, Bacchetta J, et al. Paediatric Liver Transplanted Patients and Prevalence of Hepatitis E Virus. Journal of Clinical Virology: The Official Publication of the Pan American Society for Clinical Virology. 2015;69:22–6.

391 Eisenbach C, Longerich T, Fickenscher H, Schalasta G, Stremmel W, Encke J. Recurrence of Clinically Significant Hepatitis A Following Liver Transplantation for Fulminant Hepatitis A. Journal of Clinical Virology: The Official Publication of the Pan American Society for Clinical Virology. 2006;35(1):109–12.

392 Park GC, Hwang S, Yu YD, Park PJ, Choi YI, Song GW, et al. Intractable Recurrent Hepatitis A Virus Infection Requiring Repeated Liver Transplantation: A Case Report. Transplantation Proceedings. 2010;42(10):4658–60.

393 Gane E, Sallie R, Saleh M, Portmann B, Williams R. Clinical Recurrence of Hepatitis A Following Liver Transplantation for Acute Liver Failure. J Med Virol. 1995;45(1):35–9.

394 Fagan E, Yousef G, Brahm J, Garelick H, Mann G, Wolstenholme A, et al. Persistence of Hepatitis A Virus in Fulminant Hepatitis and after Liver Transplantation. J Med Virol. 1990;30(2):131–6.

395 Liu J, Zhang S, Wang Q, Shen H, Zhang M, Zhang Y, et al. Seroepidemiology of Hepatitis B Virus Infection in 2 Million Men Aged 21–49 Years in Rural China: A Population-based, Cross-sectional Study. The Lancet Infectious Diseases. 2015.

396 Zhang W, Ji Z, Wang L, Xiao D, Yan Y. A Meta-analysis of HBsAg-positive Rate among General Chinese Populations Aged 1–59 Years. Infectious Diseases (London, England). 2015:1–11.

397 Samuel D, Muller R, Alexander G, Fassati L, Ducot B, Benhamou JP, et al. Liver Transplantation in European Patients with the Hepatitis B Surface Antigen. The New England Journal of Medicine. 1993;329(25):1842–7.

398 Jiang L, Yan LN. Current Therapeutic Strategies for Recurrent Hepatitis B Virus Infection after Liver Transplantation. World Journal of Gastroenterology: WJG. 2010;16(20):2468–75.

399 Chen J, Yi L, Jia JD, Ma H, You H. Hepatitis B Immunoglobulins and/or Lamivudine for Preventing Hepatitis B Recurrence after Liver Transplantation: A Systematic Review. J Gastroenterol Hepatol. 2010;25(5):872–9.

400 Fung J, Lo R, Chan SC, Chok K, Wong T, Sharr W, et al. Outcomes Including Liver Histology after Liver Transplantation for Chronic Hepatitis B Using Oral Antiviral Therapy Alone. Liver Transpl. 2015.

401 Wesdorp DJ, Knoester M, Braat AE, Coenraad MJ, Vossen AC, Claas EC, et al. Nucleoside Plus Nucleotide Analogs and Cessation of Hepatitis B Immunoglobulin after Liver Transplantation in Chronic Hepatitis B Is Safe and Effective. Journal of Clinical Virology: The Official Publication of the Pan American Society for Clinical Virology. 2013;58(1):67–73.

402 Yurdaydin C, Idilman R. Therapy of Delta Hepatitis. Cold Spring Harbor Perspectives in Medicine. 2015.

403 Pascarella S, Negro F. Hepatitis D Virus: An Update. Liver International: Official Journal of the International Association for the Study of the Liver. 2011;31(1):7–21.

404 Govindarajan S, De Cock KM, Redeker AG. Natural Course of Delta Superinfection in Chronic Hepatitis B Virus-infected Patients: Histopathologic Study with Multiple Liver Biopsies. Hepatology. 1986;6(4):640–4.

405 Roche B, Samuel D. Liver Transplantation in Delta Virus Infection. Seminars in Liver Disease. 2012;32(3):245–55.

406 Demetris AJ, Jaffe R, Sheahan DG, Burnham J, Spero J, Iwatsuki S, et al. Recurrent Hepatitis B in Liver Allograft Recipients. Differentiation between Viral Hepatitis B and Rejection. Am J Pathol. 1986;125(1):161–72.

407 Demetris AJ, Todo S, Van Thiel DH, Fung JJ, Iwaki Y, Sysyn G, et al. Evolution of Hepatitis B Virus Liver Disease after Hepatic Replacement. Practical and Theoretical Considerations. Am J Pathol. 1990;137(3):667–76.

408 Zhang X, Xiang C, Zhou YH, Jiang A, Qin YY, He J. Effect of Statins on Cardiovascular Events in Patients with Mild to Moderate Chronic Kidney Disease: A Systematic Review and Meta-analysis of Randomized Clinical Trials. BMC Cardiovasc Disord. 2014;14:19.

409 Roche B, Samuel D. The Difficulties of Managing Severe Hepatitis B Virus Reactivation. Liver International: Official Journal of the International Association for the Study of the Liver. 2011;31 Suppl 1:104–10.

410 Harrison RF, Davies MH, Goldin RD, Hubscher SG. Recurrent Hepatitis B in Liver Allografts: A Distinctive Form of Rapidly Developing Cirrhosis. Histopathology. 1993;23(1):21–8.

411 Thung SN. Histologic Findings in Recurrent HBV. Liver Transpl. 2006;12(11 Suppl 2):S50–3.

412 Davies SE, Portmann BC, O'Grady JG, Aldis PM, Chaggar K, Alexander GJ, et al. Hepatic Histological Findings after Transplantation for Chronic Hepatitis B Virus Infection, Including a Unique Pattern of Fibrosing Cholestatic Hepatitis. Hepatology. 1991;13(1):150–7.

413 O'Grady JG, Smith HM, Davies SE, Daniels HM, Donaldson PT, Tan KC, et al. Hepatitis B Virus Reinfection after Orthotopic Liver Transplantation. Serological and Clinical Implications. Journal of Hepatology. 1992;14(1):104–11.

414 Yurdaydin C, Idilman R, Bozkaya H, Bozdayi AM. Natural History and Treatment of Chronic Delta Hepatitis. J Viral Hepat. 2010;17(11):749–56.

415 Salomao M, Verna EC, Lefkowitch JH, Moreira RK. Histopathologic Distinction between Fibrosing Cholestatic Hepatitis C and Biliary Obstruction. The American Journal of Surgical Pathology. 2013;37(12):1837–44.

416 Verna EC. Hepatitis Viruses and Liver Transplantation: Evolving Trends in Antiviral Management. Clin Liver Dis. 2014;18(3):575–601.

417 Verna EC, O'Leary JG. Hepatitis C Treatment in Patients on the Liver Transplant Waiting List. Curr Opin Organ Transplant. 2015;20(3):242–50.

418 Gane EJ. The Natural History of Recurrent Hepatitis C and What Influences This. Liver Transpl. 2008;14 Suppl 2:S36–44.

419 Ramirez S, Perez-Del-Pulgar S, Forns X. Virology and Pathogenesis of Hepatitis C Virus Recurrence. Liver Transpl. 2008;14 Suppl 2:S27–35.

420 McCaughan GW, Shackel NA, Bertolino P, Bowen DG. Molecular and Cellular Aspects of Hepatitis C Virus Reinfection after Liver Transplantation: How the Early Phase Impacts on Outcomes. Transplantation. 2009;87(8):1105–11.

421 Verna EC, Abdelmessih R, Salomao MA, Lefkowitch J, Moreira RK, Brown RS, Jr. Cholestatic Hepatitis C Following Liver Transplantation: An Outcome-based Histological Definition, Clinical Predictors, and Prognosis. Liver Transpl. 2013;19(1):78–88.

422 Berenguer M, Aguilera V, Prieto M, San Juan F, Rayon JM, Benlloch S, et al. Significant Improvement in the Outcome of HCV-infected Transplant Recipients by Avoiding Rapid Steroid Tapering and Potent Induction Immunosuppression. Journal of Hepatology. 2006;44(4):717–22.

423 Marcos A, Eghtesad B, Fung JJ, Fontes P, Patel K, Devera M, et al. Use of Alemtuzumab and Tacrolimus Monotherapy for Cadaveric Liver Transplantation: With Particular Reference to Hepatitis C Virus. Transplantation. 2004;78(7):966–71.

424 Eghtesad B, Fung JJ, Demetris AJ, Murase N, Ness R, Bass DC, et al. Immunosuppression for Liver Transplantation in HCV-infected Patients: Mechanism-based Principles. Liver Transpl. 2005;11(11):1343–52.

425 Thursz M, Yee L, Khakoo S. Understanding the Host Genetics of Chronic Hepatitis B and C. Seminars in Liver Disease. 2011;31(2):115–27.

426 Charlton MR, Thompson A, Veldt BJ, Watt K, Tillmann H, Poterucha JJ, et al. Interleukin-28B Polymorphisms Are Associated with Histological Recurrence and Treatment Response Following Liver Transplantation in Patients with Hepatitis C Virus Infection. Hepatology. 2011;53(1):317–24.

427 Fukuhara T, Taketomi A, Motomura T, Okano S, Ninomiya A, Abe T, et al. Variants in IL28B in Liver Recipients and Donors Correlate with Response to Peg-Interferon and Ribavirin Therapy for Recurrent Hepatitis C. Gastroenterology. 2010;139(5):1577–85, 85 e1–3.

428 Demetris AJ. Evolution of Hepatitis C Virus in Liver Allografts. Liver Transpl. 2009;15 Suppl 2:S35–41.

429 Chhatwal J, Kanwal F, Roberts MS, Dunn MA. Cost-effectiveness and Budget Impact of Hepatitis C Virus Treatment with Sofosbuvir and Ledipasvir in the United States. Ann Intern Med. 2015;162(6):397–406.

430 Berenguer M. Natural History of Recurrent Hepatitis C. Liver Transpl. 2002;8(10 Suppl 1):S14–8.

431 Berenguer M, Aguilera V, Prieto M, Carrasco D, Rayon M, San Juan F, et al. Delayed Onset of Severe Hepatitis C-related Liver Damage Following Liver Transplantation: A Matter of Concern? Liver Transpl. 2003;9(11):1152–8.

432 Dhanasekaran R, Sanchez W, Mounajjed T, Wiesner RH, Watt KD, Charlton MR. Impact of Fibrosis Progression on Clinical Outcome in Patients Treated for Post-transplant Hepatitis C Recurrence. Liver International: Official Journal of the International Association for the Study of the Liver. 2015.

433 Burton JR, Jr., Rosen HR. Acute Rejection in HCV-infected Liver Transplant Recipients: The Great Conundrum. Liver Transpl. 2006;12(11 Suppl 2):S38–47.

434 Moreira RK. Recurrent Hepatitis C and Acute Allograft Rejection: Clinicopathologic Features with Emphasis on the Differential Diagnosis between These Entities. Advances in Anatomic Pathology. 2011;18(5):393–405.

435 Asanza CG, Garcia-Monzon C, Clemente G, Salcedo M, Garcia-Buey L, Garcia-Iglesias C, et al. Immunohistochemical Evidence of Immunopathogenetic Mechanisms in Chronic Hepatitis C Recurrence after Liver Transplantation. Hepatology. 1997;26(3):755–63.

436 Rosen HR, Martin P. Hepatitis C Infection in Patients Undergoing Liver Retransplantation. Transplantation. 1998;66(12):1612–6.

437 Rosen HR, Martin P, Goss J, Donovan J, Melinek J, Rudich S, et al. Significance of Early Aminotransferase Elevation after Liver Transplantation. Transplantation. 1998;65(1):68–72.

438 Ferrell LD, Wright TL, Roberts J, Ascher N, Lake J. Hepatitis C Viral Infection in Liver Transplant Recipients. Hepatology. 1992;16(4):865–76.

439 Demetris AJ, Sebagh M. Plasma Cell Hepatitis in Liver Allografts: Variant of Rejection or Autoimmune Hepatitis? Liver Transpl. 2008;14(6):750–5.

440 Guido M, Burra P. De Novo Autoimmune Hepatitis after Liver Transplantation. Seminars in Liver Disease. 2011;31(1):71–81.

441 Castillo-Rama M, Sebagh M, Sasatomi E, Randhawa P, Isse K, Salgarkar AD, et al. "Plasma Cell Hepatitis" in Liver Allografts: Identification and Characterization of an IgG4-Rich Cohort. Am J Transplant. 2013;13(11):2966–77.

442 Fiel MI, Agarwal K, Stanca C, Elhajj N, Kontorinis N, Thung SN, et al. Posttransplant Plasma Cell Hepatitis (de Novo Autoimmune Hepatitis) Is a Variant of Rejection and May Lead to a Negative Outcome in Patients with Hepatitis C Virus. Liver Transpl. 2008;14(6):861–71.

443 Berardi S, Lodato F, Gramenzi A, D'Errico A, Lenzi M, Bontadini A, et al. High Incidence of Allograft Dysfunction in Liver Transplanted Patients Treated with Pegylated-interferon Alpha-2b and Ribavirin for Hepatitis C Recurrence: Possible de Novo Autoimmune Hepatitis? Gut. 2007;56(2):237–42.

444 Alvarez F, Berg PA, Bianchi FB, Bianchi L, Burroughs AK, Cancado EL,

et al. International Autoimmune Hepatitis Group Report: Review of Criteria for Diagnosis of Autoimmune Hepatitis. Journal of Hepatology. 1999;**31**(5):929–38.

445. Czaja AJ, Carpenter HA. Sensitivity, Specificity, and Predictability of Biopsy Interpretations in Chronic Hepatitis. Gastroenterology. 1993;**105**(6):1824–32.

446. Czaja AJ, Carpenter HA. Histological Findings in Chronic Hepatitis C with Autoimmune Features. Hepatology. 1997;**26**(2):459–66.

447. Khettry U, Huang WY, Simpson MA, Pomfret EA, Pomposelli JJ, Lewis WD, et al. Patterns of Recurrent Hepatitis C after Liver Transplantation in a Recent Cohort of Patients. Hum Pathol. 2007;**38**(3):443–52.

448. Kessel A, Toubi E. Chronic HCV-related Autoimmunity: A Consequence of Viral Persistence and Lymphotropism. Current Medicinal Chemistry. 2007;**14**(5):547–54.

449. Schiano TD, Te HS, Thomas RM, Hussain H, Bond K, Black M. Results of Steroid-based Therapy for the Hepatitis C-autoimmune Hepatitis Overlap Syndrome. The American Journal of Gastroenterology. 2001;**96**(10):2984–91.

450. Zekry A, Bishop GA, Bowen DG, Gleeson MM, Guney S, Painter DM, et al. Intrahepatic Cytokine Profiles Associated with Posttransplantation Hepatitis C Virus-related Liver Injury. Liver Transpl. 2002;**8**(3):292–301.

451. Narang TK, Ahrens W, Russo MW. Post-liver Transplant Cholestatic Hepatitis C: A Systematic Review of Clinical and Pathological Findings and Application of Consensus Criteria. Liver Transpl. 2010;**16**(11):1228–35.

452. Leroy V, Dumortier J, Coilly A, Sebagh M, Fougerou-Leurent C, Radenne S, et al. Efficacy of Sofosbuvir and Daclatasvir in Patients with Fibrosing Cholestatic Hepatitis C after Liver Transplantation. Clin Gastroenterol Hepatol. 2015.

453. Selzner N, Guindi M, Renner EL, Berenguer M. Immune-mediated Complications of the Graft in Interferon-treated Hepatitis C Positive Liver Transplant Recipients. Journal of Hepatology. 2011;**55**(1):207–17.

454. Wiesner RH, Demetris AJ, Belle SH, Seaberg EC, Lake JR, Zetterman RK, et al. Acute Hepatic Allograft Rejection: Incidence, Risk Factors, and Impact on Outcome. Hepatology. 1998;**28**(3):638–45.

455. Pischke S, Suneetha PV, Baechlein C, Barg-Hock H, Heim A, Kamar N, et al. Hepatitis E Virus Infection as a Cause of Graft Hepatitis in Liver Transplant Recipients. Liver Transpl. 2010;**16**(1):74–82.

456. Pischke S, Wedemeyer H. Chronic Hepatitis E in Liver Transplant Recipients: A Significant Clinical Problem? Minerva Gastroenterol Dietol. 2010;**56**(2):121–8.

457. Kamar N, Garrouste C, Haagsma EB, Garrigue V, Pischke S, Chauvet C, et al. Factors Associated with Chronic Hepatitis in Patients with Hepatitis E Virus Infection Who Have Received Solid Organ Transplants. Gastroenterology. 2011;**140**(5):1481–9.

458. Haagsma EB, Riezebos-Brilman A, van den Berg AP, Porte RJ, Niesters HG. Treatment of Chronic Hepatitis E in Liver Transplant Recipients with Pegylated Interferon Alpha-2b. Liver Transpl. 2010;**16**(4):474–7.

459. Kamar N, Abravanel F, Selves J, Garrouste C, Esposito L, Lavayssiere L, et al. Influence of Immunosuppressive Therapy on the Natural History of Genotype 3 Hepatitis-E Virus Infection after Organ Transplantation. Transplantation. 2010;**89**(3):353–60.

460. Haagsma EB, Niesters HG, van den Berg AP, Riezebos-Brilman A, Porte RJ, Vennema H, et al. Prevalence of Hepatitis E Virus Infection in Liver Transplant Recipients. Liver Transpl. 2009;**15**(10):1225–8.

461. Kamar N, Selves J, Mansuy JM, Ouezzani L, Peron JM, Guitard J, et al. Hepatitis E Virus and Chronic Hepatitis in Organ-transplant Recipients. N Engl J Med. 2008;**358**(8):811–7.

462. Aggarwal R, Jameel S. Hepatitis E. Hepatology. 2011;**54**(6):2218–26.

463. Behrendt P, Steinmann E, Manns MP, Wedemeyer H. The Impact of Hepatitis E in the Liver Transplant Setting. Journal of Hepatology. 2014;**61**(6):1418–29.

464. Halac U, Beland K, Lapierre P, Patey N, Ward P, Brassard J, et al. Chronic Hepatitis E Infection in Children with Liver Transplantation. Gut. 2011.

465. Peters van Ton AM, Gevers TJ, Drenth JP. Antiviral Therapy in Chronic Hepatitis E: A Systematic Review. J Viral Hepat. 2015.

466. Abravanel F, Lhomme S, Chapuy-Regaud S, Peron JM, Alric L, Rostaing L, et al. Performance of a New Rapid Test for Detecting Anti-hepatitis E Virus Immunoglobulin M in Immunocompetent and Immunocompromised Patients. Journal of Clinical Virology: The Official Publication of the Pan American Society for Clinical Virology. 2015;**70**:101–4.

467. Raczyńska J, Habior A, Pączek L, Foroncewicz B, Pawełas A, Mucha K. Primary Biliary Cirrhosis in the Era of Liver Transplantation. Ann Transplant. 2014;**19**:488–93.

468. Gautam M, Cheruvattath R, Balan V. Recurrence of Autoimmune Liver Disease after Liver Transplantation: A Systematic Review. Liver Transpl. 2006;**12**(12):1813–24.

469. Liaskou E, Henriksen EK, Holm K, Kaveh F, Hamm D, Fear J, et al. High-throughput T-cell Receptor Sequencing across Chronic Liver Diseases Reveals Distinct Disease-associated Repertoires. Hepatology. 2015.

470. Mendes F, Couto CA, Levy C. Recurrent and de Novo Autoimmune Liver Diseases. Clinics in Liver Disease. 2011;**15**(4):859–78.

471. Czaja AJ, Manns MP. Advances in the Diagnosis, Pathogenesis, and Management of Autoimmune Hepatitis. Gastroenterology. 2010;**139**(1):58–72 e4.

472. Venick RS, McDiarmid SV, Farmer DG, Gornbein J, Martin MG, Vargas JH, et al. Rejection and Steroid Dependence: Unique Risk Factors in the Development of Pediatric Posttransplant de Novo Autoimmune Hepatitis. Am J Transplant. 2007;**7**(4):955–63.

473. Inui A, Sogo T, Komatsu H, Miyakawa H, Fujisawa T. Antibodies against Cytokeratin 8/18 in a Patient with de Novo Autoimmune Hepatitis after Living-donor Liver Transplantation. Liver Transplantation: Official Publication of the American Association for the Study of Liver Diseases and the International Liver Transplantation Society. 2005;**11**(5):504–7.

474. Huguet S, Vinh J, Johanet C, Samuel D, Gigou M, Zamfir O, et al. Identification by Proteomic Tool of Atypical Anti-liver/Kidney Microsome Autoantibodies Targets in de Novo Autoimmune Hepatitis after Liver Transplantation. Ann N Y Acad Sci. 2007;**1109**:345–57.

475. Yamagiwa S, Kamimura H, Takamura M, Genda T, Ichida T, Nomoto M, et al. Presence of Antibodies against

Self Human Leukocyte Antigen Class II Molecules in Autoimmune Hepatitis. International Journal of Medical Sciences. 2014;11(9):850–6.

476 Maggiore G, Gonzales E, Sciveres M, Redon MJ, Grosse B, Stieger B, et al. Relapsing Features of Bile Salt Export Pump Deficiency after Liver Transplantation in Two Patients with Progressive Familial Intrahepatic Cholestasis Type 2. Journal of Hepatology. 2010;53(5):981–6.

477 Jara P, Hierro L, Martinez-Fernandez P, Alvarez-Doforno R, Yanez F, Diaz MC, et al. Recurrence of Bile Salt Export Pump Deficiency after Liver Transplantation. The New England Journal of Medicine. 2009;361(14):1359–67.

478 Siebold L, Dick AA, Thompson R, Maggiore G, Jacquemin E, Jaffe R, et al. Recurrent Low Gamma-glutamyl Transpeptidase Cholestasis Following Liver Transplantation for Bile Salt Export Pump (BSEP) Disease (Posttransplant Recurrent BSEP Disease). Liver Transplantation: Official Publication of the American Association for the Study of Liver Diseases and the International Liver Transplantation Society. 2010;16(7):856–63.

479 Sebagh M, Castillo-Rama M, Azoulay D, Coilly A, Delvart V, Allard MA, et al. Histologic Findings Predictive of a Diagnosis of de Novo Autoimmune Hepatitis after Liver Transplantation in Adults. Transplantation. 2013;96(7):670–8.

480 Abraham SC, Freese DK, Ishitani MB, Krasinskas AM, Wu TT. Significance of Central Perivenulitis in Pediatric Liver Transplantation. The American Journal of Surgical Pathology. 2008;32(10):1479–88.

481 Poupon R. Primary Biliary Cirrhosis: A 2010 Update. Journal of Hepatology. 2010;52(5):745–58.

482 Silveira MG, Talwalkar JA, Lindor KD, Wiesner RH. Recurrent Primary Biliary Cirrhosis after Liver Transplantation. Am J Transplant. 2010;10(4):720–6.

483 Bosch A, Dumortier J, Maucort-Boulch D, Scoazec JY, Wendum D, Conti F, et al. Preventive Administration of UDCA after Liver Transplantation for Primary Biliary Cirrhosis Is Associated with a Lower Risk of Disease Recurrence. Journal of Hepatology. 2015.

484 Sebagh M, Farges O, Dubel L, Samuel D, Bismuth H, Reynes M. Histological Features Predictive of Recurrence of Primary Biliary Cirrhosis after Liver Transplantation. Transplantation. 1998;65(10):1328–33.

485 Hubscher SG, Elias E, Buckels JA, Mayer AD, McMaster P, Neuberger JM. Primary Biliary Cirrhosis. Histological Evidence of Disease Recurrence after Liver Transplantation. Journal of Hepatology. 1993;18(2):173–84.

486 Jones DE, James OF, Portmann B, Burt AD, Williams R, Hudson M. Development of Autoimmune Hepatitis Following Liver Transplantation for Primary Biliary Cirrhosis. Hepatology. 1999;30(1):53–7.

487 Graziadei IW. Recurrence of Nonviral Liver Diseases after Liver Transplantation. Clin Liver Dis. 2014;18(3):675–85.

488 Demetris AJ, Markus BH, Esquivel C, Van Thiel DH, Saidman S, Gordon R, et al. Pathologic Analysis of Liver Transplantation for Primary Biliary Cirrhosis. Hepatology. 1988;8(4):939–47.

489 Kang YZ, Sun XY, Liu YH, Shen ZY. Autoimmune Hepatitis-primary Biliary Cirrhosis Concurrent with Biliary Stricture after Liver Transplantation. World J Gastroenterol. 2015;21(7):2236–41.

490 Bhanji RA, Mason AL, Girgis S, Montano-Loza AJ. Liver Transplantation for Overlap Syndromes of Autoimmune Liver Diseases. Liver International: Official Journal of the International Association for the Study of the Liver. 2013;33(2):210–9.

491 Li Y, Ayata G, Baker SP, Banner BF. Cholangitis: A Histologic Classification Based on Patterns of Injury in Liver Biopsies. Pathol Res Pract. 2005;201(8–9):565–72.

492 Vakiani E, Hunt KK, Mazziotta RM, Emond JC, Brown RS, Lefkowitch JH, et al. Hepatitis C-associated Granulomas after Liver Transplantation: Morphologic Spectrum and Clinical Implications. American Journal of Clinical Pathology. 2007;127(1):128–34.

493 Fosby B, Karlsen TH, Melum E. Recurrence and Rejection in Liver Transplantation for Primary Sclerosing Cholangitis. World Journal of Gastroenterology: WJG. 2012;18(1):1–15.

494 Ravikumar R, Tsochatzis E, Jose S, Allison M, Athale A, Creamer F, et al. Risk Factors for Recurrent Primary Sclerosing Cholangitis after Liver Transplantation. Journal of Hepatology. 2015.

495 Gelley F, Zadori G, Gorog D, Kobori L, Fehervari I, Gaman G, et al. Recurrence of Primary Sclerosing Cholangitis after Liver Transplantation – The Hungarian Experience. Interventional Medicine & Applied Science. 2014;6(1):16–8.

496 Sheng R, Campbell WL, Zajko AB, Baron RL. Cholangiographic Features of Biliary Strictures after Liver Transplantation for Primary Sclerosing Cholangitis: Evidence of Recurrent Disease. AJR Am J Roentgenol. 1996;166(5):1109–13.

497 Rai RM, Boitnott J, Klein AS, Thuluvath PJ. Features of Recurrent Primary Sclerosing Cholangitis in Two Consecutive Liver Allografts after Liver Transplantation. Journal of Clinical Gastroenterology. 2001;32(2):151–4.

498 Jeyarajah DR, Netto GJ, Lee SP, Testa G, Abbasoglu O, Husberg BS, et al. Recurrent Primary Sclerosing Cholangitis after Orthotopic Liver Transplantation: Is Chronic Rejection Part of the Disease Process? Transplantation. 1998;66(10):1300–6.

499 Carrasco-Avino G, Schiano TD, Ward SC, Thung SN, Fiel MI. Primary Sclerosing Cholangitis: Detailed Histologic Assessment and Integration Using Bioinformatics Highlights Arterial Fibrointimal Hyperplasia as a Novel Feature. Am J Clin Pathol. 2015;143(4):505–13.

500 Jaffe R. Liver Transplant Pathology in Pediatric Metabolic Disorders. Pediatr Dev Pathol. 1998;1(2):102–17.

501 Hansen K, Horslen S. Metabolic Liver Disease in Children. Liver Transplantation: Official Publication of the American Association for the Study of Liver Diseases and the International Liver Transplantation Society. 2008;14(5):713–33.

502 Zezos P, Renner EL. Liver Transplantation and Non-alcoholic Fatty Liver Disease. World J Gastroenterol. 2014;20(42):15532–8.

503 Merola J, Liapakis A, Mulligan DC, Yoo PS. Non-alcoholic Fatty Liver Disease Following Liver Transplantation: A Clinical Review. Clin Transplant. 2015;29(9):728–37.

504 Charlton MR, Burns JM, Pedersen RA, Watt KD, Heimbach JK, Dierkhising RA. Frequency and Outcomes of

505. Ong J, Younossi ZM, Reddy V, Price LL, Gramlich T, Mayes J, et al. Cryptogenic Cirrhosis and Posttransplantation Nonalcoholic Fatty Liver Disease. Liver Transpl. 2001;7(9):797-801.

506. Patil DT, Yerian LM. Evolution of Nonalcoholic Fatty Liver Disease Recurrence after Liver Transplantation. Liver Transpl. 2012;18(10):1147-53.

507. Hanouneh IA, Macaron C, Lopez R, Feldstein AE, Yerian L, Eghtesad B, et al. Recurrence of Disease Following Liver Transplantation: Nonalcoholic Steatohepatitis vs Hepatitis C Virus Infection. International Journal of Organ Transplantation Medicine. 2011;2(2):57-65.

508. Tevar AD, Clarke C, Wang J, Rudich SM, Woodle ES, Lentsch AB, et al. Clinical Review of Nonalcoholic Steatohepatitis in Liver Surgery and Transplantation. Journal of the American College of Surgeons. 2010;210(4):515-26.

509. Contos MJ, Cales W, Sterling RK, Luketic VA, Shiffman ML, Mills AS, et al. Development of Nonalcoholic Fatty Liver Disease after Orthotopic Liver Transplantation for Cryptogenic Cirrhosis. Liver Transpl. 2001;7(4):363-73.

510. Dumortier J, Giostra E, Belbouab S, Morard I, Guillaud O, Spahr L, et al. Non-alcoholic Fatty Liver Disease in Liver Transplant Recipients: Another Story of "Seed and Soil." The American Journal of Gastroenterology. 2010;105(3):613-20.

511. Malik SM, Ahmad J. Outcomes of Liver Transplantation in Patients with Cirrhosis due to Nonalcoholic Steatohepatitis versus Patients with Cirrhosis due to Alcoholic Liver Disease. Liver Transpl. 2010;16(4):533.

512. Malik SM, Devera ME, Fontes P, Shaikh O, Sasatomi E, Ahmad J. Recurrent Disease Following Liver Transplantation for Nonalcoholic Steatohepatitis Cirrhosis. Liver Transpl. 2009;15(12):1843-51.

513. Malik SM, deVera ME, Fontes P, Shaikh O, Ahmad J. Outcome after Liver Transplantation for NASH Cirrhosis. Am J Transplant. 2009;9(4):782-93.

514. Ayata G, Gordon FD, Lewis WD, Pomfret E, Pomposelli JJ, Jenkins RL, et al. Cryptogenic Cirrhosis: Clinicopathologic Findings at and after Liver Transplantation. Hum Pathol. 2002;33(11):1098-104.

515. Kim WR, Poterucha JJ, Porayko MK, Dickson ER, Steers JL, Wiesner RH. Recurrence of Nonalcoholic Steatohepatitis Following Liver Transplantation. Transplantation. 1996;62(12):1802-5.

516. Takata MC, Campos GM, Ciovica R, Rabl C, Rogers SJ, Cello JP, et al. Laparoscopic Bariatric Surgery Improves Candidacy in Morbidly Obese Patients Awaiting Transplantation. Surgery for Obesity and Related Diseases: Official Journal of the American Society for Bariatric Surgery. 2008;4(2):159-64; discussion 64-5.

517. Marszalek R, Ziemianski P, Lagiewska B, Pacholczyk M, Domienik-Karlowicz J, Trzebicki J, et al. The First Polish Liver Transplantation after Roux-en-Y Gastric Bypass Surgery for Morbid Obesity: A Case Report and Literature Review. Ann Transplant. 2015;20:112-5.

518. Brunt EM, Tiniakos DG. Histopathology of Nonalcoholic Fatty Liver Disease. World J Gastroenterol. 2010;16(42):5286-96.

519. Lucey MR. Liver Transplantation in Patients with Alcoholic Liver Disease. Liver Transplantation: Official Publication of the American Association for the Study of Liver Diseases and the International Liver Transplantation Society. 2011;17(7):751-9.

520. Bellamy CO, DiMartini AM, Ruppert K, Jain A, Dodson F, Torbenson M, et al. Liver Transplantation for Alcoholic Cirrhosis: Long Term Follow-up and Impact of Disease Recurrence. Transplantation. 2001;72(4):619-26.

521. Jimenez-Romero C, Justo-Alonso I, Cambra-Molero F, Calvo-Pulido J, Garcia-Sesma A, Abradelo-Usera M, et al. Incidence, Risk Factors and Outcome of de Novo Tumors in Liver Transplant Recipients Focusing on Alcoholic Cirrhosis. World J Hepatol. 2015;7(7):942-53.

522. Abosh D, Rosser B, Kaita K, Bazylewski R, Minuk G. Outcomes Following Liver Transplantation for Patients with Alcohol- versus Nonalcohol-induced Liver Disease. Can J Gastroenterol. 2000;14(10):851-5.

523. Conjeevaram HS, Hart J, Lissoos TW, Schiano TD, Dasgupta K, Befeler AS, et al. Rapidly Progressive Liver Injury and Fatal Alcoholic Hepatitis Occurring after Liver Transplantation in Alcoholic Patients. Transplantation. 1999;67(12):1562-8.

524. Molloy RM, Komorowski R, Varma RR. Recurrent Nonalcoholic Steatohepatitis and Cirrhosis after Liver Transplantation. Liver Transpl Surg. 1997;3(2):177-8.

525. Tang H, Boulton R, Gunson B, Hubscher S, Neuberger J. Patterns of Alcohol Consumption after Liver Transplantation. Gut. 1998;43(1):140-5.

526. Schieber K, Lindner M, Sowa JP, Gerken G, Scherbaum N, Kahraman A, et al. Self-reports on Symptoms of Alcohol Abuse: Liver Transplant Patients versus Rehabilitation Therapy Patients. Progress in Transplantation (Aliso Viejo, Calif). 2015;25(3):203-9.

527. Rice JP, Eickhoff J, Agni R, Ghufran A, Brahmbhatt R, Lucey MR. Abusive Drinking after Liver Transplantation Is Associated with Allograft Loss and Advanced Allograft Fibrosis. Liver Transpl. 2013;19(12):1377-86.

528. MacSween RN, Burt AD. Histologic Spectrum of Alcoholic Liver Disease. Seminars in Liver Disease. 1986;6(3):221-32.

529. Saragoca A, Moreira ML, Novais L, Vilar D, Silva HS, Baptista AS. Liver Injury in Chronic Alcoholism: Clinical, Laboratorial and Histological Correlation. Acta medica portuguesa. 1981(Suppl 2):65-74.

530. Pageaux GP, Bismuth M, Perney P, Costes V, Jaber S, Possoz P, et al. Alcohol Relapse after Liver Transplantation for Alcoholic Liver Disease: Does It Matter? Journal of Hepatology. 2003;38(5):629-34.

531. Hubscher SG. Recurrent Autoimmune Hepatitis after Liver Transplantation: Diagnostic Criteria, Risk Factors, and Outcome. Liver Transpl. 2001;7(4):285-91.

532. Kaneku H, O'Leary JG, Taniguchi M, Susskind BM, Terasaki PI, Klintmalm GB. Donor-specific Human Leukocyte Antigen Antibodies of the Immunoglobulin G3 Subclass Are Associated with Chronic Rejection and Graft Loss after Liver Transplantation. Liver Transpl. 2012;18(8):984-92.

533. Shaikh OS, Demetris AJ. Idiopathic Posttransplantation Hepatitis? Liver Transpl. 2007;13(7):943-6.

534. Aini W, Miyagawa-Hayashino A, Tsuruyama T, Hashimoto S, Sumiyoshi S, Ozeki M, et al. Telomere

535. Adeyi O, Fischer SE, Guindi M. Liver Allograft Pathology: Approach to Interpretation of Needle Biopsies with Clinicopathological Correlation. J Clin Pathol. 2010;**63**(1):47–74.

536. Gane E, Portmann B, Saxena R, Wong P, Ramage J, Williams R. Nodular Regenerative Hyperplasia of the Liver Graft after Liver Transplantation. Hepatology. 1994;**20**(1 Pt 1):88–94.

537. Devarbhavi H, Abraham S, Kamath PS. Significance of Nodular Regenerative Hyperplasia Occurring de Novo Following Liver Transplantation. Liver Transpl. 2007;**13**(11):1552–6.

538. Eguchi S, Takatsuki M, Hidaka M, Soyama A, Muraoka I, Tomonaga T, et al. Lack of Grafted Liver Rejuvenation in Adult-to-Pediatric Liver Transplantation. Digestive Diseases and Sciences. 2011;**56**(5):1542–7.

539. Espinasse G, Kamar N, Hurault C, Suc B, Fourtanier G, Montastruc JL, et al. Drug Exposure and Perceived Adverse Drug Events Reported by Liver-transplant Patients. Int J Clin Pharmacol Ther. 2009;**47**(3):159–64.

540. Sterneck M, Wiesner R, Ascher N, Roberts J, Ferrell L, Ludwig J, et al. Azathioprine Hepatotoxicity after Liver Transplantation. Hepatology. 1991;**14**(5):806–10.

541. Lefkowitch JH, Lobritto SJ, Brown RS, Jr., Emond JC, Schilsky ML, Rosenthal LA, et al. Ground-glass, Polyglucosan-like Hepatocellular Inclusions: A "New" Diagnostic Entity. Gastroenterology. 2006;**131**(3):713–8.

542. Mells G, Mann C, Hubscher S, Neuberger J. Late Protocol Liver Biopsies in the Liver Allograft: A Neglected Investigation? Liver Transpl. 2009;**15**(8):931–8.

543. Abraham SC, Poterucha JJ, Rosen CB, Demetris AJ, Krasinskas AM. Histologic Abnormalities Are Common in Protocol Liver Allograft Biopsies from Patients with Normal Liver Function Tests. The American Journal of Surgical Pathology. 2008;**32**(7):965–73.

544. Mells G, Neuberger J. Protocol Liver Allograft Biopsies. Transplantation. 2008;**85**(12):1686–92.

545. Ahmad W, Ijaz B, Gull S, Asad S, Khaliq S, Jahan S, et al. A Brief Review on Molecular, Genetic and Imaging Techniques for HCV Fibrosis Evaluation. Virology Journal. 2011;**8**(1):53.

546. T JSC, Jothimani D, Heneghan MA, Harrison PM. Non-invasive Assessment of Fibrosis in Liver Grafts due to Hepatitis C Virus Recurrence. Clinical Transplantation. 2011;**25**(3):345–51.

547. Demetris A, Crawford J, Minervini M, Nalesnik M, Ochoa E, Randhawa P, et al. Transplantation Pathology of the Liver. In: Odze R, Goldblum J, editors. Surgical Pathology of the GI Tract, Liver, Biliary Tract, and Pancreas. 2nd ed. Philadelphia: Saunders Elsevier; 2009. p. 1169–229.

548. Karimi MH, Geramizadeh B, Malek-Hosseini SA. Tolerance Induction in Liver. International Journal of Organ Transplantation Medicine. 2015;**6**(2):45–54.

549. Mastoridis S, Martinez-Llordella M, Sanchez-Fueyo A. Emergent Transcriptomic Technologies and Their Role in the Discovery of Biomarkers of Liver Transplant Tolerance. Front Immunol. 2015;**6**:304.

550. Bohne F, Londoño MC, Benítez C, Miquel R, Martínez-Llordella M, Russo C, et al. HCV-induced Immune Responses Influence the Development of Operational Tolerance after Liver Transplantation in Humans. Sci Transl Med. 2014;**6**(242):242ra81.

551. Kamada N. The Immunology of Experimental Liver Transplantation in the Rat. Immunology. 1985;**55**(3):369–89.

552. Feng S, Ekong UD, Lobritto SJ, Demetris AJ, Roberts JP, Rosenthal P, et al. Complete Immunosuppression Withdrawal and Subsequent Allograft Function among Pediatric Recipients of Parental Living Donor Liver Transplants. Jama. 2012;**307**(3):283–93.

553. Lerut J, Sanchez-Fueyo A. An Appraisal of Tolerance in Liver Transplantation. Am J Transplant. 2006;**6**(8):1774–80.

554. Murphy MS, Harrison R, Davies P, Buckels JA, Mayer AD, Hubscher S, et al. Risk Factors for Liver Rejection: Evidence to Suggest Enhanced Allograft Tolerance in Infancy. Arch Dis Child. 1996;**75**(6):502–6.

555. Talisetti A, Hurwitz M, Sarwal M, Berquist W, Castillo R, Bass D, et al. Analysis of Clinical Variables Associated with Tolerance in Pediatric Liver Transplant Recipients. Pediatric Transplantation. 2010;**14**(8):976–9.

556. Demetris AJ, Isse K. Tissue Biopsy Monitoring of Operational Tolerance in Liver Allograft Recipients. Curr Opin Organ Transplant. 2013;**18**(3):345–53.

557. Tisone G, Orlando G, Cardillo A, Palmieri G, Manzia TM, Baiocchi L, et al. Complete Weaning off Immunosuppression in HCV Liver Transplant Recipients Is Feasible and Favourably Impacts on the Progression of Disease Recurrence. Journal of Hepatology. 2006;**44**(4):702–9.

558. Wong T, Nouri-Aria KT, Devlin J, Portmann B, Williams R. Tolerance and Latent Cellular Rejection in Long-term Liver Transplant Recipients. Hepatology. 1998;**28**(2):443–9.

559. Takatsuki M, Uemoto S, Inomata Y, Egawa H, Kiuchi T, Fujita S, et al. Weaning of Immunosuppression in Living Donor Liver Transplant Recipients. Transplantation. 2001;**72**(3):449–54.

560. Ramos HC, Reyes J, Abu-Elmagd K, Zeevi A, Reinsmoen N, Tzakis A, et al. – Weaning of Immunosuppression in Long-term Liver Transplant Recipients. Transplantation. 1995;**59**(2):212–7.

561. Strehlau J, Pavlakis M, Lipman M, Shapiro M, Vasconcellos L, Harmon W, et al. Quantitative Detection of Immune Activation Transcripts as a Diagnostic Tool in Kidney Transplantation. Proc Natl Acad Sci U S A. 1997;**94**(2):695–700.

562. Sharma VK, Bologa RM, Li B, Xu GP, Lagman M, Hiscock W, et al. Molecular Executors of Cell Death–Differential Intrarenal Expression of Fas Ligand, Fas, Granzyme B, and Perforin during Acute and/or Chronic Rejection of Human Renal Allografts. Transplantation. 1996;**62**(12):1860–6.

563. Lipman ML, Stevens AC, Strom TB. Heightened Intragraft CTL Gene Expression in Acutely Rejecting Renal Allografts. J Immunol. 1994;**152**(10):5120–7.

564. Suthanthiran M. Molecular Analyses of Human Renal Allografts: Differential Intragraft Gene Expression during Rejection. Kidney Int Suppl. 1997;**58**:S15–21.

565. Suthanthiran M. Clinical Application of Molecular Biology: A Study of Allograft Rejection with Polymerase Chain Reaction. Am J Med Sci. 1997;**313**(5):264–7.

566. Strehlau J, Pavlakis M, Lipman M, Maslinski W, Shapiro M, Strom TB. The Intragraft Gene Activation of Markers Reflecting T-cell-activation and -Cytotoxicity Analyzed by Quantitative RT-PCR in Renal Transplantation. Clin Nephrol. 1996;46(1):30–3.

567. Adam B, Mengel M. Transplant Biopsy beyond Light Microscopy. BMC Nephrol. 2015;16:132.

568. Sis B, Mengel M, Haas M, Colvin RB, Halloran PF, Racusen LC, et al. BANFF '09 Meeting Report: Antibody Mediated Graft Deterioration and Implementation of BANFF Working Groups. American Journal of Transplantation: Official Journal of the American Society of Transplantation and the American Society of Transplant Surgeons. 2010;10(3):464–71.

569. Haas M, Sis B, Racusen LC, Solez K, Glotz D, Colvin RB, et al. BANFF 2013 Meeting Report: Inclusion of c4d-negative Antibody-mediated Rejection and Antibody-associated Arterial Lesions. Am J Transplant. 2014;14(2):272–83.

570. Shahzad K, Fatima A, Cadeiras M, Wisniewski N, Bondar G, Cheng R, et al. Challenges and Solutions in the Development of Genomic Biomarker Panels: A Systematic Phased Approach. Current Genomics. 2012;13(4):334–41.

571. Starling RC, Pham M, Valantine H, Miller L, Eisen H, Rodriguez ER, et al. Molecular Testing in the Management of Cardiac Transplant Recipients: Initial Clinical Experience. J Heart Lung Transplant. **25**. United States2006. p. 1389–95.

572. Deng MC, Eisen HJ, Mehra MR, Billingham M, Marboe CC, Berry G, et al. Noninvasive Discrimination of Rejection in Cardiac Allograft Recipients Using Gene Expression Profiling. Am J Transplant. 2006;6(1):150–60.

573. Deng MC, Eisen HJ, Mehra MR. Methodological Challenges of Genomic Research–The CARGO Study. Am J Transplant. **6**. Denmark2006. p. 1086–7.

574. Mehra MR, Parameshwar J. Gene Expression Profiling and Cardiac Allograft Rejection Monitoring: Is IMAGE Just a Mirage? J Heart Lung Transplant. **29**. United States: Copyright 2010 International Society for Heart and Lung Transplantation. Published by Elsevier Inc. All rights reserved. 2010. p. 599–602.

575. Pham MX, Deng MC, Kfoury AG, Teuteberg JJ, Starling RC, Valantine H. Molecular Testing for Long-term Rejection Surveillance in Heart Transplant Recipients: Design of the Invasive Monitoring Attenuation through Gene Expression (IMAGE) Trial. J Heart Lung Transplant. 2007;26(8):808–14.

576. Martinez-Llordella M, Lozano JJ, Puig-Pey I, Orlando G, Tisone G, Lerut J, et al. Using Transcriptional Profiling to Develop a Diagnostic Test of Operational Tolerance in Liver Transplant Recipients. J Clin Invest. 2008;118(8):2845–57.

577. Martinez-Llordella M, Puig-Pey I, Orlando G, Ramoni M, Tisone G, Rimola A, et al. Multiparameter Immune Profiling of Operational Tolerance in Liver Transplantation. Am J Transplant. 2007;7(2):309–19.

578. Kawasaki M, Iwasaki M, Koshiba T, Fujino M, Hara Y, Kitazawa Y, et al. Gene Expression Profile Analysis of the Peripheral Blood Mononuclear Cells from Tolerant Living-donor Liver Transplant Recipients. Int Surg. 2007;92(5):276–86.

579. Gehrau R, Maluf D, Archer K, Stravitz R, Suh J, Le N, et al. Molecular Pathways Differentiate Hepatitis C Virus (HCV) Recurrence from Acute Cellular Rejection in HCV Liver Recipients. Mol Med. 2011;17(7-8):824–33.

580. Gehrau R, Mas V, Archer KJ, Maluf D. Molecular Classification and Clonal Differentiation of Hepatocellular Carcinoma: The Step Forward for Patient Selection for Liver Transplantation. Expert rev. 2011;5(4):539–52.

581. von Ahlfen S, Missel A, Bendrat K, Schlumpberger M. Determinants of RNA Quality from FFPE Samples. PLoS One. 2007;2(12):e1261.

582. Kojima K, April C, Canasto-Chibuque C, Chen X, Deshmukh M, Venkatesh A, et al. Transcriptome Profiling of Archived Sectioned Formalin-fixed Paraffin-embedded (AS-FFPE) Tissue for Disease Classification. PLoS One. 2014;9(1):e86961.

583. Geiss GK, Bumgarner RE, Birditt B, Dahl T, Dowidar N, Dunaway DL, et al. Direct Multiplexed Measurement of Gene Expression with Color-coded Probe Pairs. Nature Biotechnology. 2008;26(3):317–25.

584. Tan PS, Nakagawa S, Goossens N, Venkatesh A, Huang T, Ward SC, et al. Clinicopathological Indices to Predict Hepatocellular Carcinoma Molecular Classification. Liver International: Official Journal of the International Association for the Study of the Liver. 2015.

585. Pfeffer LM, Li K, Fleckenstein JF, Marion TN, Diament J, Yang CH, et al. An Interferon Response Gene Signature Is Associated with the Therapeutic Response of Hepatitis C Patients. PLoS One. 2014;9(8):e104202.

586. Venkatesh A, Sun X, Hoshida Y. Prognostic Gene Signature Profiles of Hepatitis C-Related Early-stage Liver Cirrhosis. Genom Data. 2014;2:361–2.

587. Shannon CP, Balshaw R, Ng RT, Wilson-McManus JE, Keown P, McMaster R, et al. Two-stage, in Silico Deconvolution of the Lymphocyte Compartment of the Peripheral Whole Blood Transcriptome in the Context of Acute Kidney Allograft Rejection. PLoS One. 2014;9(4):e95224.

588. Oghumu S, Bracewell A, Nori U, Maclean KH, Balada-Lasat JM, Brodsky S, et al. Acute Pyelonephritis in Renal Allografts: A New Role for MicroRNAs? Transplantation. 2014;97(5):559–68.

589. Spivey TL, De Giorgi V, Zhao Y, Bedognetti D, Pos Z, Liu Q, et al. The Stable Traits of Melanoma Genetics: An Alternate Approach to Target Discovery. BMC genomics. 2012;13:156.

590. Khatri P, Roedder S, Kimura N, De Vusser K, Morgan AA, Gong Y, et al. A Common Rejection Module (CRM) for Acute Rejection across Multiple Organs Identifies Novel Therapeutics for Organ Transplantation. J Exp Med. 2013;210(11):2205–21.

591. Isse K, Lesniak A, Grama K, Roysam B, Minervini MI, Demetris AJ. Digital Transplantation Pathology: Combining Whole Slide Imaging, Multiplex Staining and Automated Image Analysis. American Journal of Transplantation: Official Journal of the American Society of Transplantation and the American Society of Transplant Surgeons. 2012;12(1):27–37.

592. Grant A, Neuberger J. Guidelines on the Use of Liver Biopsy in Clinical Practice. British Society of Gastroenterology. Gut. 1999;45 Suppl 4:Iv1–iv11.

593. Isse K, Grama K, Abbott IM, Lesniak A, Lunz JG, Lee WM, et al. Adding Value to Liver (and Allograft) Biopsy Evaluation Using a Combination of Multiplex Quantum Dot Immunostaining, High-resolution Whole-slide Digital Imaging, and Automated Image Analysis. Clin Liver Dis. 2010;14(4):669–85.

594. McGrath MA, Morton AM, Harnett MM. Laser Scanning Cytometry: Capturing the Immune System in Situ. Methods Cell Biol. 2011;102:231–60.

595. Harnett MM. Laser Scanning Cytometry: Understanding the Immune System in Situ. Nat Rev Immunol. 2007;7(11):897–904.

596. Takahashi H, Ruiz P, Ricordi C, Miki A, Mita A, Barker S, et al. In Situ Quantitative Immunoprofiling of Regulatory T Cells Using Laser Scanning Cytometry. Transplantation Proceedings. 2009;41(1):238–9.

597. Halasz T, Horvath G, Kiss A, Par G, Szombati A, Gelley F, et al. Evaluation of Histological and Non-invasive Methods for the Detection of Liver Fibrosis: The Values of Histological and Digital Morphometric Analysis, Liver Stiffness Measurement and APRI Score. Pathology Oncology Research: POR. 2015.

598. Manousou P, Burroughs AK, Tsochatzis E, Isgro G, Hall A, Green A, et al. Digital Image Analysis of Collagen Assessment of Progression of Fibrosis in Recurrent HCV after Liver Transplantation. Journal of Hepatology. 2013;58(5):962–8.

599. Isgro G, Calvaruso V, Andreana L, Luong TV, Garcovich M, Manousou P, et al. The Relationship between Transient Elastography and Histological Collagen Proportionate Area for Assessing Fibrosis in Chronic Viral Hepatitis. J Gastroenterol. 2013;48(8):921–9.

600. Calvaruso V, Dhillon AP, Tsochatzis E, Manousou P, Grillo F, Germani G, et al. Liver Collagen Proportionate Area Predicts Decompensation in Patients with Recurrent Hepatitis C Virus Cirrhosis after Liver Transplantation. J Gastroenterol Hepatol. 2012;27(7):1227–32.

601. Vanderbeck S, Bockhorst J, Kleiner D, Komorowski R, Chalasani N, Gawrieh S. Automatic Quantification of Lobular Inflammation and Hepatocyte Ballooning in Nonalcoholic Fatty Liver Disease Liver Biopsies. Human Pathology. 2015;46(5):767–75.

602. Neil DA, Roberts IS, Bellamy CO, Wigmore SJ, Neuberger JM. Improved Access to Histopathology Using a Digital System Could Increase the Organ Donor Pool and Improve Allocation. Transpl Int. 2014;27(8):759–64.

603. Mammas CS, Lazaris A, Kostopanagiotou G, Lemonidou C, Patsouris E. The Digital Microscopy in Organ Transplantation: Ergonomics of the Tele-pathological Evaluation of Renal and Liver Grafts. Studies in Health Technology and Informatics. 2015;213:287–90.

604. Jen KY, Olson JL, Brodsky S, Zhou XJ, Nadasdy T, Laszik ZG. Reliability of Whole Slide Images as a Diagnostic Modality for Renal Allograft Biopsies. Human Pathology. 2013;44(5):888–94.

605. Neil DA, Demetris AJ. Digital Pathology Services in Acute Surgical Situations. Br J Surg. 2014;101(10):1185–6.

606. Demetris AJ, Crawford JM, Minvervini MI, Nalesnik M, Ochoa E, Randhawa P, et al. Transplantation Pathology of the Liver. In: Odze R, Goldblum J, Crawford JM, editors. Surgical Pathology of the GI Tract, Liver, Biliary Tract, and Pancreas. (in press). Philadelphia: Saunders Elsever; 2008.

607. Quaglia AF, Del Vecchio Blanco G, Greaves R, Burroughs AK, Dhillon AP. Development of Ductopaenic Liver Allograft Rejection Includes a "Hepatitic" Phase Prior to Duct Loss. Journal of Hepatology. 2000;33(5):773–80.

608. Kemmer N, Kaiser T, Zacharias V, Neff GW. Alpha-1-Antitrypsin Deficiency: Outcomes after Liver Transplantation. Transplantation Proceedings. 2008;40(5):1492–4.

609. Wolff H, Otto G, Giest H. Liver Transplantation in Crigler-Najjar Syndrome. A Case Report. Transplantation. 1986;42(1):84.

610. Kaufman SS, Wood RP, Shaw BW, Jr., Markin RS, Rosenthal P, Gridelli B, et al. Orthotopic Liver Transplantation for Type I Crigler-Najjar Syndrome. Hepatology. 1986;6(6):1259–62.

611. Yamashita T, Ando Y, Okamoto S, Yohei M, Hitahara T, Ueda M, et al. Effect of Liver Transplantation on the Survival of Patients with Ordinary Onset Familial Amyloid Polyneuropathy in Japan. Amyloid. 2011;18 Suppl 1:180–1.

612. Seth AK, Badminton MN, Mirza D, Russell S, Elias E. Liver Transplantation for Porphyria: Who, When, and How? Liver Transplantation: Official Publication of the American Association for the Study of Liver Diseases and the International Liver Transplantation Society. 2007;13(9):1219–27.

613. Wahlin S, Stal P, Adam R, Karam V, Porte R, Seehofer D, et al. Liver Transplantation for Erythropoietic Protoporphyria in Europe. Liver Transplantation: Official Publication of the American Association for the Study of Liver Diseases and the International Liver Transplantation Society. 2011;17(9):1021–6.

614. Brandhagen DJ. Liver Transplantation for Hereditary Hemochromatosis. Liver Transpl. 2001;7(8):663–72.

615. Maheshwari A, Rankin R, Segev DL, Thuluvath PJ. Outcomes of Liver Transplantation for Glycogen Storage Disease: A Matched-control Study and a Review of Literature. Clinical Transplantation. 2011.

616. Matern D, Starzl TE, Arnaout W, Barnard J, Bynon JS, Dhawan A, et al. Liver Transplantation for Glycogen Storage Disease Types I, III, and IV. Eur J Pediatr. 1999;158 Suppl 2:S43–8.

617. Gartner JC, Jr., Bergman I, Malatack JJ, Zitelli BJ, Jaffe R, Watkins JB, et al. Progression of Neurovisceral Storage Disease with Supranuclear Ophthalmoplegia Following Orthotopic Liver Transplantation. Pediatrics. 1986;77(1):104–6.

618. Arnon R, Annunziato R, Miloh T, Wasserstein M, Sogawa H, Wilson M, et al. Liver Transplantation for Hereditary Tyrosinemia Type I: Analysis of the UNOS Database. Pediatric Transplantation. 2011;15(4):400–5.

619. Arnon R, Annunziato R, Schilsky M, Miloh T, Willis A, Sturdevant M, et al. Liver Transplantation for Children with Wilson Disease: Comparison of Outcomes between Children and Adults. Clinical Transplantation. 2011;25(1):E52–60.

Chapter 4

The Pathology of Heart Transplantation

E. Rene Rodriguez and Carmela D. Tan

Orthotopic heart transplantation is an effective therapy for end-stage heart disease of coronary and non-coronary etiology. Survival has continued to increase over time. The most common indications for cardiac transplantation in the adult have not changed in the last three decades: non-ischemic cardiomyopathies (54%) and ischemic disease (37%) [1]. In infancy, congenital heart disease is the most common indication for transplantation (56%) and cardiomyopathies account for 40% of heart transplants. In children older than ten years, the diagnosis of cardiomyopathy predominates (63%) [2]. The survival rate after cardiac transplantation currently is 81% at one year, 69% at five years, and better in high-volume centers [1].

The pathology of heart transplantation will be presented with emphasis on technical, morphologic, and interpretive aspects of the diagnosis. The working formulations of the International Society for Heart and Lung Transplantation (ISHLT) of 1990, 2005, 2011, and 2013 (ISHLT-WF-1990, ISHLT-WF-2005, ISHLT-WF-2011, and ISHLT-WF-2013) for the pathologic evaluation of transplant biopsies will be presented, including their evolution and current status. The pitfalls and caveats likely to be found in clinical practice, as well as controversial issues in the diagnosis of rejection in heart allografts, will be addressed.

The Endomyocardial Biopsy

The endomyocardial biopsy (EMB) remains as the gold standard diagnostic tool for the diagnosis of rejection in heart transplants. This diagnostic modality has a high sensitivity and specificity for the diagnosis of acute cellular rejection [3, 4]. No other current modality of cardiac imaging, serum markers, or molecular diagnostics has higher sensitivity and specificity than biopsies. In addition, the EMB has a very short turnaround of only a few hours, which directly impacts the decision-making process for the management of these patients [5]. Molecular testing has been developed for diagnosis of cellular rejection; however, to this date, the biopsy is far more informative for decision-making in real time because it can yield information about cellular rejection and antibody-mediated rejection.

Timing of the Biopsy: If possible, a baseline donor biopsy should be obtained at the time of the transplant to rule out myocarditis, ischemic injury, or other pathologic changes in the donor heart. In most heart transplant centers, surveillance protocol biopsies are done once a week for the first month, every two weeks for the second month, and every four to eight weeks from the 3rd to the 12th month.

Procurement of the Tissue: Bioptomes are used from either the jugular or femoral vein route to sample the right ventricular septal wall. Bioptomes (see Figure 4.1) are available in different sizes; therefore, the size of the pieces of tissue retrieved will differ slightly. The most common sizes in use are 7F (French) and 9F in adults and 3F, 5F, and 7F in pediatric age patients [6]. The cutting "jaws" procure adequate samples

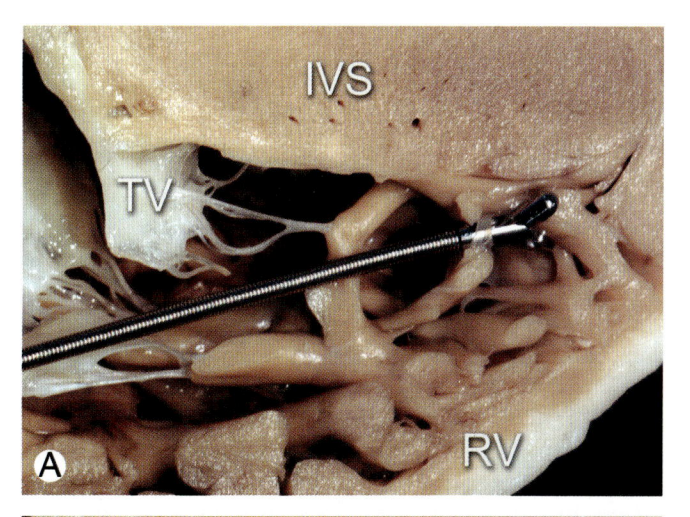

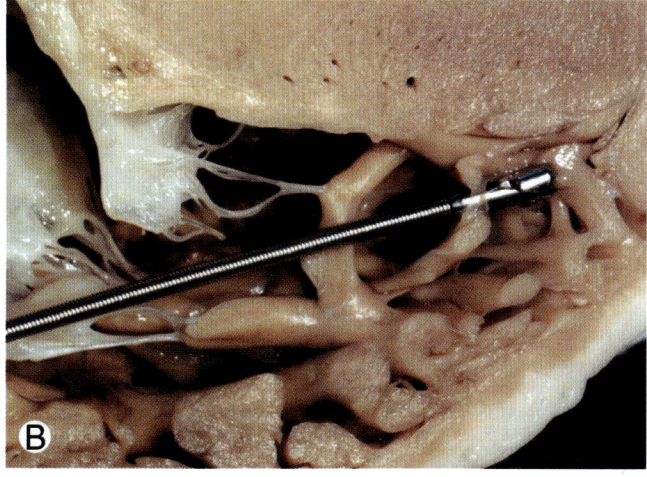

Figure 4.1 The bioptome is the instrument used to procure endomyocardial biopsies. In North America, most biopsies are procured from the right side of the heart via trans-jugular approach. The target is the interventricular septal myocardium. The two spoon-shaped cutters are opened (A) and placed against the interventricular septum. Closing the bioptome cutters (B) provides an adequate myocardial sample with minimal artifact.

of subendocardial myocardium, usually from the interventricular septum.

Minimum Number of Tissue Samples: Since acute cellular rejection is not uniformly distributed in the heart, it is important to take multiple samples during the biopsy procedure. Pomerance and Stovin [7] showed that if three biopsy pieces taken show no rejection, there is a 5% and 0% chance of missing a mild and moderate-to-severe rejection, respectively. However, if four pieces are examined, the false negative rate of mild rejection is further reduced to 2% [8]. Other investigators have emphasized that the extent of infiltration may also be important, given that if at least three of the four fragments are graded separately as mild rejection, with a calculated frequency of 13.57% of the time, the probability of missing moderate-severe rejection is as high as 25% [9].

The ISHLT-WF-1990 required four pieces of tissue examined and optional procurement of one piece of tissue for freezing and one for electron microscopy [10]. In comparison, the ISHLT-WF-2005 formulation calls for the examination of at least three pieces, and preferably four (or more) of myocardium, 50% of which must be evaluable myocardium and not biopsy site or scar [11]. Specimens that do not meet these criteria should be diagnosed as "inadequate biopsy" [10]. The revised working formulation does not require a separate piece of frozen tissue or tissue routinely fixed for electron microscopy [11].

Processing of the Endomyocardial Biopsy in the Pathology Laboratory: For optimal preservation, the tissue should be fixed immediately in the desired fixative that has been allowed to reach room temperature of 25°C. Cold fixative enhances contraction band artifact. The sample should not be allowed to sit on filter paper, gauze, or any other surface impregnated with saline for a long period of time. Saline is a very poor solution to preserve the morphology of myocardium and readily creates artifacts. Other fixatives or preservatives that maintain tissue antigens in a better state for immunohistochemistry or immunofluorescence studies can also be used. For research protocols, one or more pieces of tissue can be snap frozen for molecular studies.

The Gross Examination: The number of tissue pieces received should be documented on gross examination and always correlated with the number of pieces present in the glass slides for microscopic examination. Their average size and color should be described. Careful gross examination provides, in most instances, important information regarding the presence of myocardium, thickened endocardium, adipose tissue, chordae tendineae [12], blood clots, or small endocardial thrombi.

Handling of the Tissue: Fine microsurgery forceps may be used during gross exam in the pathology laboratory to avoid compression of the tissue. It can be safely transferred directly from the specimen container into a mesh-bag and then securely folded into the processing cassette. All the pieces obtained should be submitted without any triage, since they may have valuable information when examined with the microscope. White pieces,

Table 4.1 Acute Cellular Rejection

ISHLT-WF-1990	ISHLT-WF-2005
Grade 0 (No Acute Rejection)	Grade 0 R
Grade 1A (Focal, Mild Acute Rejection)	Grade 1 R Mild (interstitial and/or perivascular infiltrate with up to 1 focus of myocyte damage)
Grade 1B (Diffuse, Mild Acute Rejection)	
Grade 2 (Focal, Moderate Acute Rejection)	
Grade 3A (Multifocal Moderate Rejection)	Grade 2 R Moderate (two or more foci of infiltrate with associated myocyte damage)
Grade 3B (Diffuse, Borderline Severe Acute Rejection)	Grade 3 R Severe (diffuse infiltrate with multifocal myocyte damage ± edema ± hemorrhage ± vasculitis)
Grade 4 (Severe Acute Rejection)	

[10, 11]

which suggest that they are made up of thick endocardium, may actually be curled up, thus concealing some myocardium that will be visible on histologic sections. Likewise, pieces that look like blood clots may harbor a piece of myocardium in their core.

In our center, the entire biopsy (i.e., all four or more pieces) is processed as a frozen section specimen, and with proper technique, freezing artifact (such as ice crystals forming in the sarcoplasm of the myocytes) is avoided in almost all cases. This procedure allows us to evaluate the sample for both acute cellular rejection and antibody-mediated rejection in all the pieces, with a turnaround time of only a few hours.

Cardiac Allograft Rejection: Morphologic Aspects

The original ISHLT-WF-1990 working formulation [10] was revisited during the Heart Session of the BANFF Allograft Pathology group meeting in 2001. The meeting consensus was that while the working formulation had withstood the test of time, some areas for refinement in the cellular rejection grading approach and the lack of standard diagnostic criteria for antibody-mediated rejection needed to be addressed [13]. The formal revision was published in 2005 and included the refined diagnostic criteria for acute cellular rejection. In addition, criteria for antibody-mediated rejection were included for the first time [11, 14] (Table 4.1). A further revision of the working formulation for the diagnosis of antibody-mediated rejection was proposed in 2011 [15]. The current criteria from ISHLT [16] have been recently published. As with other solid organ allografts, cardiac allograft rejection can be divided into humoral and cellular rejection. Cellular rejection, in turn, can be sub-classified into hyperacute, acute, and chronic rejection on the basis of mechanism and duration of the process.

Hyperacute Rejection: This is a catastrophic, complement-mediated, immune attack to the graft that is triggered by preformed antibodies and occurs very quickly, usually within minutes to hours after the implantation of the graft. Predisposing factors that may play a role are preformed antibodies to epitopes of the ABO and HLA systems, multiple pregnancies, multiple surgeries requiring use of blood products, and even previous cardiac transplantation. The activation of the complement cascade produces severe endothelial cell damage, as well as platelet activation, followed by the clotting cascade and thrombosis. The morphologic findings include swelling of the endothelial cells (not easily documented by light microscopy), microthrombi, extravasation of red blood cells, and even microscopic hemorrhages, interstitial edema, and subsequently polymorphonuclear inflammatory infiltrates, followed by tissue necrosis. Gross examination may barely show any changes, focal areas of hemorrhage, or a combination of pallor and hemorrhages in the myocardium. Immunohistochemical studies may show deposits of IgM, IgG, and complement in the vessel walls as well as interstitial fibrin. Unfortunately, the pathologic examination of this type of rejection is usually done during the autopsy [17].

Acute Cellular Rejection

Effector Cells: Morphologically, acute cellular rejection is a mononuclear inflammatory response, predominantly lymphocytic, directed against the cardiac allograft. Granulocytes are also present in cases of severe rejection. The variable degrees of infiltration of the graft are used in the grading of rejection. Thus the rejection grades proposed in the working formulation are based mainly on the amount of inflammatory infiltrate and the presence of myocyte damage; the pattern of inflammatory infiltration plays a minor role. The subtypes of lymphocytes in cardiac biopsy tissue have not shown a reliable correlation between the extent and composition (CD4:CD8 ratio) of T lymphocytes infiltrating the graft and the histologic grading of rejection [18, 19]. However, other studies report a good correlation between the mean number of CD8+ T cells and the severity of rejection grade [20]. The discrepancy in these studies may be related to the fact that the immune response to the allograft is a continuous process in constant flux, while the biopsy provides, at best, "snap-shots" of the process for pathologic study. Some support to this notion is provided by the observation that if subsets of T lymphocytes are further classified on the basis of the presence of naïve cells (CD45RA) and memory or activated cells (CD45RO), naïve cells of the CD4 phenotype are more abundant in biopsy tissue during mild rejection. A shift toward activated CD8 phenotype is seen in moderate rejection [21]. An increase in the number of antigen-presenting cells (i.e., macrophages and dendritic cells) is also observed as a function of the severity of rejection [22, 23, 24, 25]. The role of regulatory cells in human cardiac allograft rejection is not well-defined. However, recent quantitative methods in biopsy material will allow better characterization of this subtype of T cells in cardiac allografts [26].

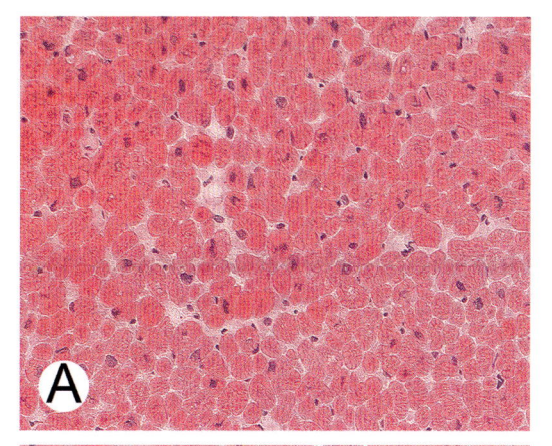

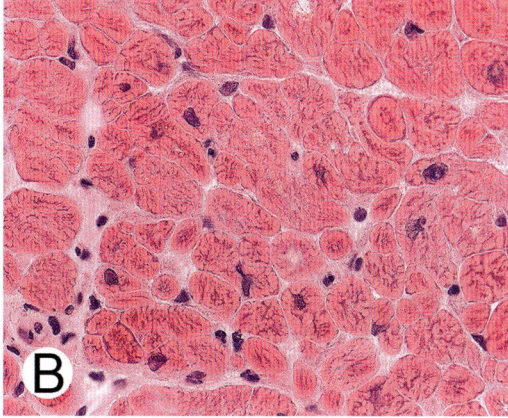

Figure 4.2 Endomyocardial biopsy of an allograft with rejection Grade 0 R. A. At low magnification, this frozen section of myocardium is shown without mononuclear cells infiltrates (H&E, X100) B. The myocytes show mild hypertrophy with enlarged hyperchromatic nuclei, but no evidence of any inflammatory infiltrates in the interstitium (H&E, X400).

B cell infiltrates are rarely present in mild rejection. However, a substantial increase in activated B lymphocytes and natural killer cells is seen in moderate rejection, suggesting their important role as promoters and effectors of cellular rejection [25].

Grading of Acute Cellular Rejection in Endomyocardial Biopsies: The rejection grades in the current ISHLT-WF-2005 have the added suffix R after the grade (Table 4.1), to indicate that these are the "revised" grades [11] as follows:

Grade 0 R (No Acute Cellular Rejection): In Grade 0 R, there is no evidence of mononuclear (lymphocytes/macrophages) inflammation or myocyte damage (see Figure 4.2).

Grade 1 R (Mild, Low-grade, Acute Cellular Rejection): Mild or low-grade rejection may manifest in one of two ways. First, perivascular and/or interstitial mononuclear cells (lymphocytes/macrophages) are present. In general, these cells respect myocyte borders, do not encroach on adjacent myocytes, and do not distort the normal architecture (see Figure 4.3). Second, one focus of mononuclear cells with associated myocyte damage may be present.

Grade 2 R (Moderate, Intermediate-grade, Acute Cellular Rejection): In Grade 2 R, two or more foci of mononuclear cells (lymphocytes/macrophages) with associated myocyte damage are present. Eosinophils may be present. The foci

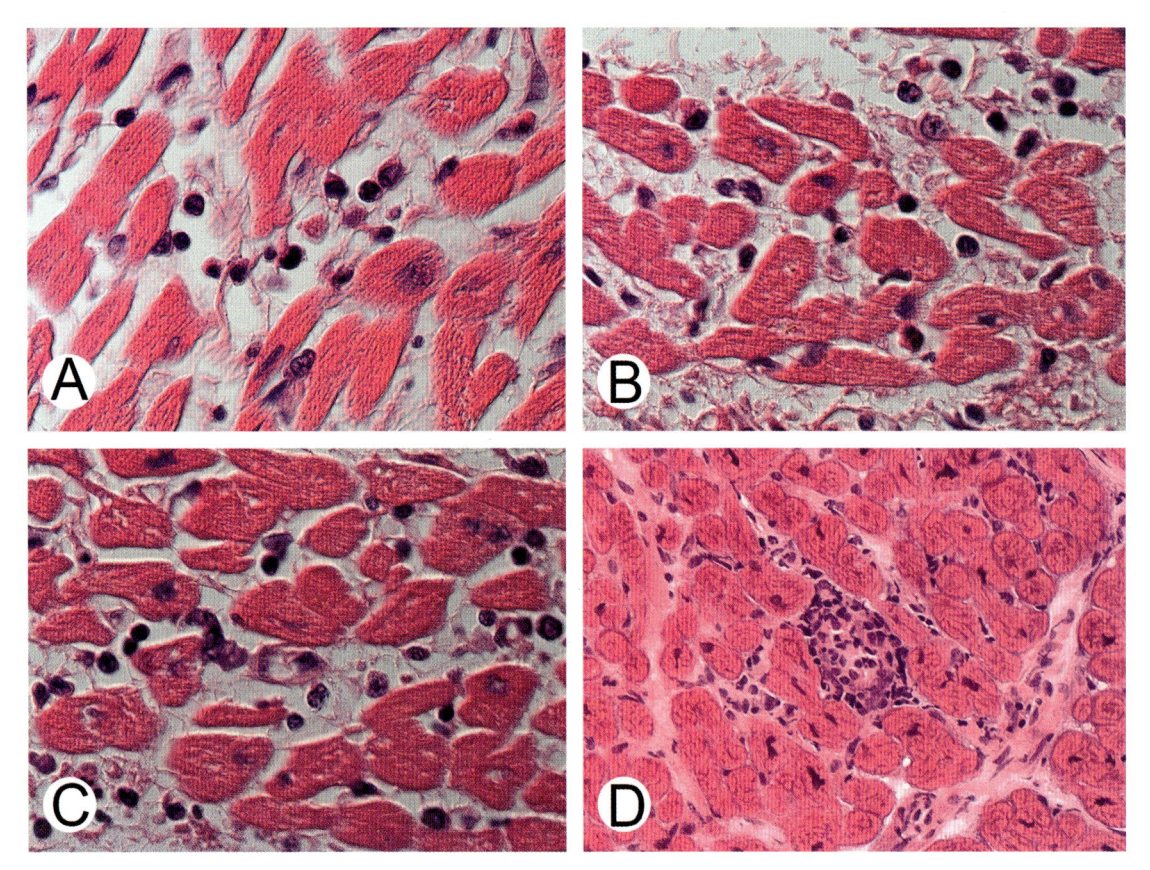

Figure 4.3 Rejection Grade 1 R. A. Light micrograph showing scant but conspicuous lymphocytes in the interstitium of the myocardium without evidence of necrosis, injury, or dropout of the myocytes (H&E, X 400). B. This micrograph shows a more abundant infiltration, with the lymphocytes distinctly surrounding individual myocytes in their perimysial spaces (H&E, X 400). C. A slightly different pattern of lymphocytic infiltrate is present in interstitial pattern (H&E, X400). D. A cluster of lymphocytes is present surrounding a small arteriole and also extending into the interstitial space. The infiltrate is discrete and clearly "vasculocentric" (H&E, X 300).

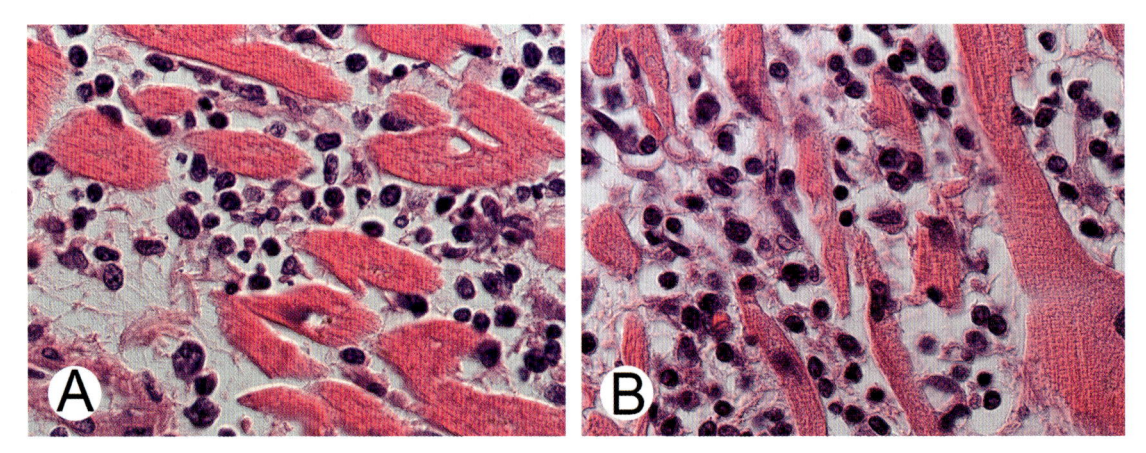

Figure 4.4 Rejection Grade 2 R. A. This biopsy shows multifocal lymphocytic infiltrates which expand the interstitial space (H&E, X 400). B. Myocyte dropout is clearly present, as well as distinct encroachment of the myocytes by the lymphocytic infiltrates (H&E, X 400).

may be distributed in one or more than one biopsy fragment. Intervening areas of uninvolved myocardium are present between the foci of rejection (see Figure 4.4). Low-grade rejection can be present in other biopsy pieces.

Grade 3 R (Severe, High-grade, Acute Cellular Rejection): A diffuse inflammatory process, either predominantly lymphocytes and macrophages or a polymorphous infiltrate, is present (see Figures 4.5 and 4.6). In most cases, the majority of biopsy fragments are involved, although the intensity of the infiltrate may vary between pieces. Multiple areas of associated myocyte damage are present. In the most severe forms of cellular (and humoral) rejection, edema, interstitial hemorrhage, and vasculitis may be present.

As described above, the predominant cellularity consists of T cells and macrophages (see Figure 4.7); however, for everyday diagnostic grading of rejection, it is not necessary to identify the subtypes of cells in these infiltrates.

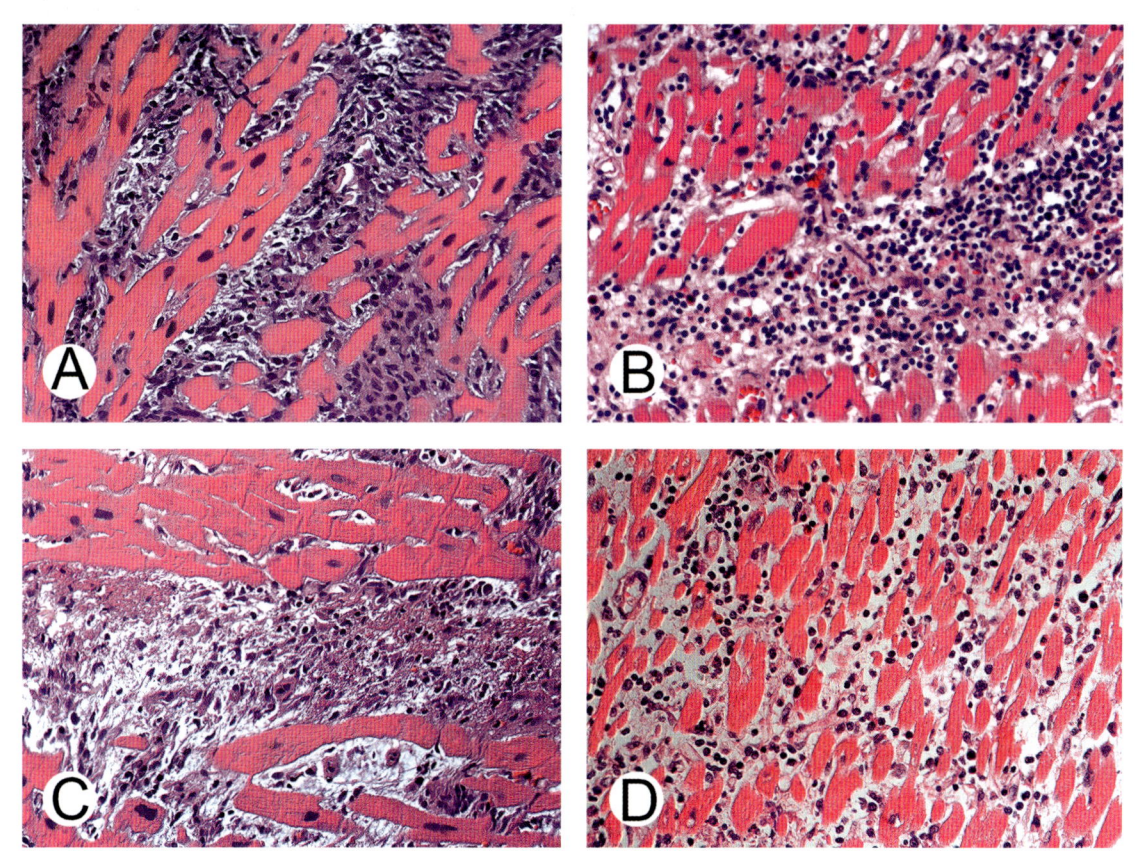

Figure 4.5 Rejection Grade 3 R. A. The myocardium is diffusely and extensively infiltrated by dense mononuclear inflammatory cells. These represent a Grade 3B in the ISHLTWF1990 (H&E, X100). B. The extensive inflammation can progress to the stage in which neutrophils and even vascular necrosis can be seen. C and D. In addition, marked interstitial edema accompanies the inflammatory infiltrate (H&E, X200).

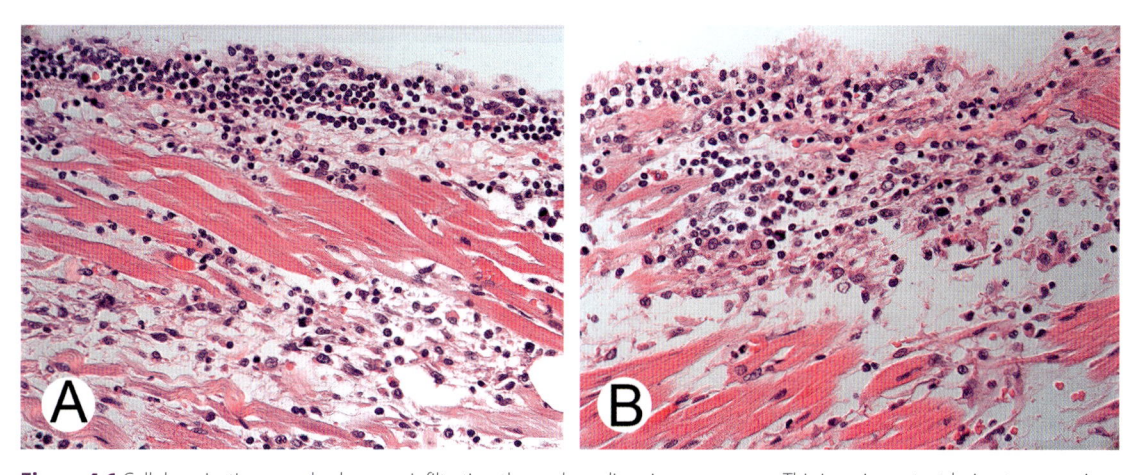

Figure 4.6 Cellular rejection can also be seen infiltrating the endocardium in severe cases. This is an important lesion to recognize as part of a cellular rejection episode and should not be confused with endocardial lymphocytic infiltrate (Quilty lesions, Figure 4.9). A and B. These micrographs show large and small lymphocytes and macrophages infiltrating the collagen fibers of the endocardium. There is also prominent edema. Occasional neutrophils and eosinophils are present. There is a distinct continuity of the infiltrate and the edema with the rejection infiltrate present in the myocardium (A and B. H&E, X400).

Non-rejection Biopsy Findings (Additional Information to Be Included in the Biopsy Report) (Table 4.2)

Adequacy of Biopsy. The term *inadequate biopsy* should be used when the specimen consists of less than three pieces [10, 11]. In addition, the term inadequate biopsy should also be used even when the number of pieces examined under the microscope is three, but the myocardium present in one or more of these pieces is less than 50% of the piece. The inadequate pieces usually consist of mostly or only endocardium, thrombus, granulation tissue from a previous biopsy site, or adipose tissue. It should be recognized however, that in some instances, valuable information such as rejection might be present in the other adequate biopsy pieces. Although a diagnosis of rejection cannot be rendered, the findings can be documented in the report as part of the histologic description or as a note.

Table 4.2 Non-rejection Findings

ISHLT-WF-1990	ISHLT-WF-2005
Ischemic Injury	*Ischemic injury*
A = up to three weeks post-transplant	Early – up to six weeks post-transplant
B = late ischemia	Late – related to allograft coronary disease
Quilty Effect	*Quilty Effect*
A = no myocyte encroachment	
B = with myocyte encroachment	
Infection	*Infection*
Lymphoproliferative disorder	*Lymphoproliferative disorder*

[10, 11]

Ischemic Injury (Perioperative): Early ischemic injury to the allograft may be related to prolonged ischemic time and histologically shows contraction band necrosis or coagulation necrosis (see Figure 4.8 A and B). Early perioperative necrosis may be due to events that affect the donor, such as catecholamine discharge, pressor therapy given during acute care, severe donor trauma, reimplantation damage, or early post-operative damage [27]. A biopsy of the septum taken at the time of implantation is informative, although the changes can be very subtle. During allograft monitoring, the working formulation makes a distinction between ischemia commonly seen up to the third week post-transplant representing perioperative injury and late ischemia that occurs after three or more months. Although this type of necrosis is usually clinically silent, these changes can compromise the function of the graft in various degrees if severe. Morphologically, there is clear evidence of myocyte necrosis, usually coagulative type, with hypereosinophilic myocytes, pyknotic nuclei, and even some karyorrhexis. Myocyte necrosis is usually out of proportion to the inflammatory infiltrate [11]. Healing may be delayed due to immunosuppression [27]. Necrotic areas are usually conspicuous, especially when stained with Masson trichrome. Calcification of myocytes sometimes occurs (see Figure 4.8 C). Myocyte vacuolization and fat necrosis may also be seen [27]. As healing ensues, the biopsy may show mixed inflammatory infiltrates, including lymphocytes,

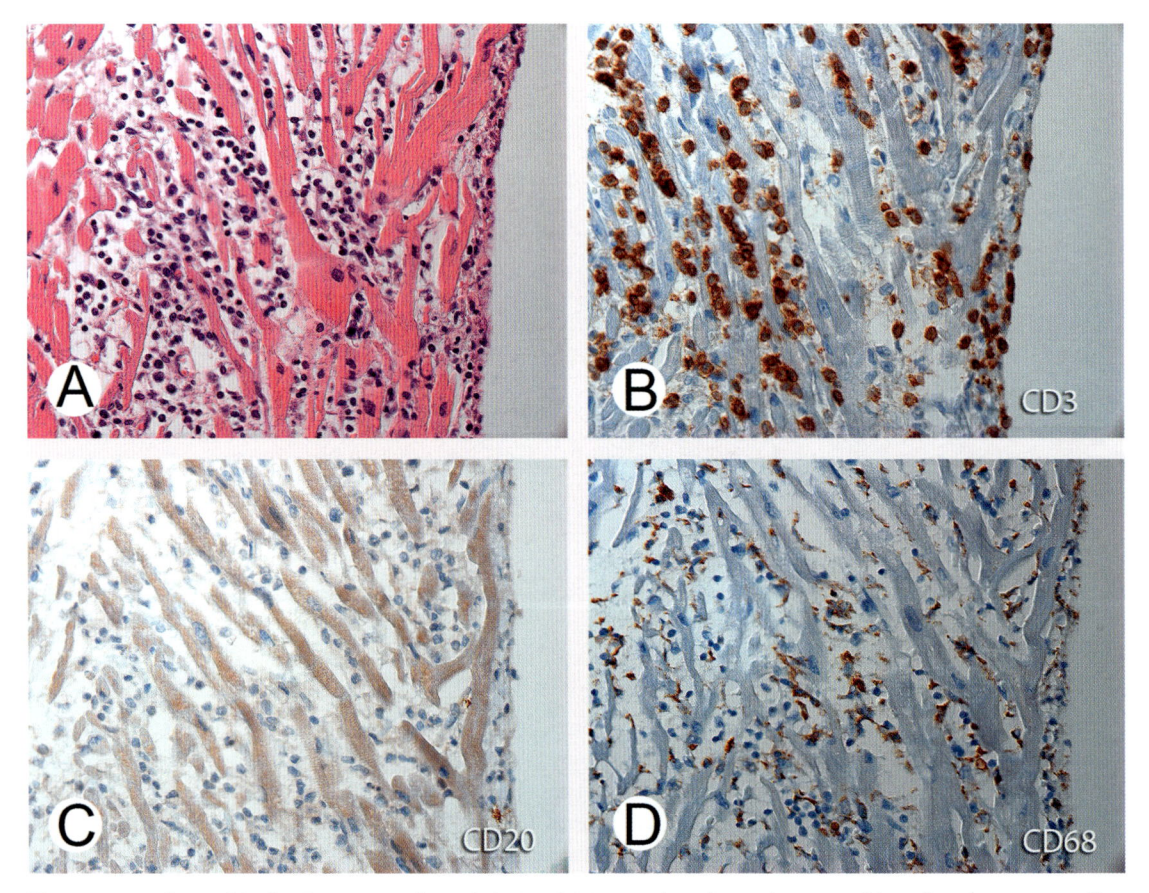

Figure 4.7 A. A focus of Grade 3 R rejection is shown (H&E, X200). B. Immunohistochemical staining of the cells in the rejection infiltrates shows predominance of T cells (CD3, X300). C. A much lesser amount of B cells is normally present (CD20, X300). D. Macrophages and dendritic cells are abundant in cell-mediated rejection (CD68, X300).

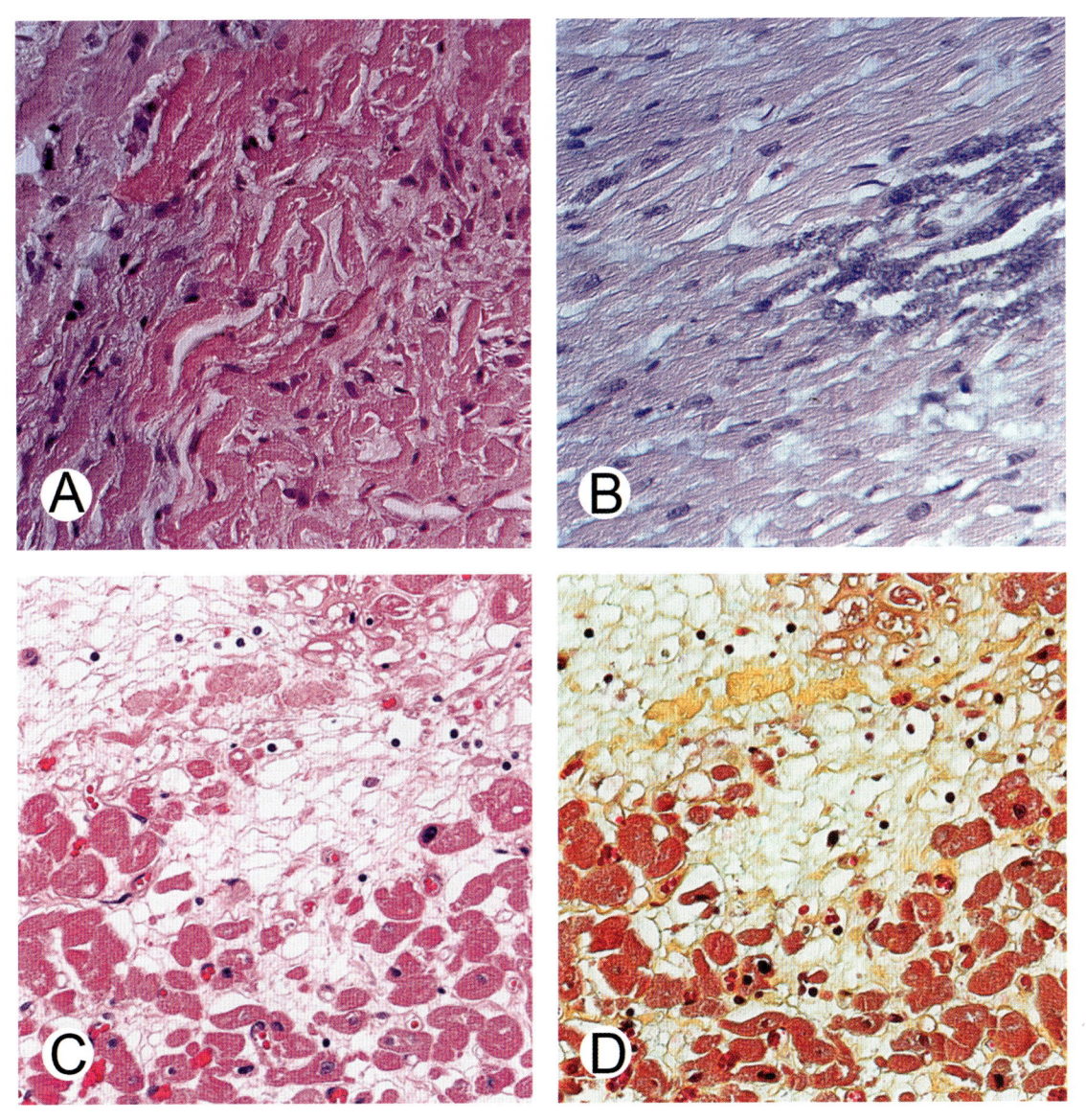

Figure 4.8 Ischemic injury. A. Hypereosinophilic, wavy, thinned myocytes with distinctly pyknotic nuclei and/or loss of nuclei which represent acute ischemic injury (H&E, X100). B. Focal calcification in the myocyte sarcoplasm starts within mitochondria in areas of ischemia. C and D. Healing ischemic focus with loose granulation tissue and early fibrosis (yellow in D) in an area of myocyte dropout is illustrated (C. H&E, X300, D. Movat pentachrome, X300).

macrophages, and eosinophils. This phenomenon may be seen in biopsies during the first six weeks. Further healing shows early interstitial fibrous tissue deposition and granulation tissue (see Figure 8 C and D) and eventually small replacement-type fibrous scars.

Ischemic Injury (Late): The assessment of the arterial changes of allograft vasculopathy in endomyocardial biopsies is usually precluded by the lack of vessels large enough to permit such an evaluation in the biopsy specimen. However, secondary myocardial changes, such as colliquative (liquefactive) myocytolysis and coagulation necrosis, can be easily identified. In the setting of cardiac allograft vasculopathy, ischemic foci are not associated with any significant mononuclear infiltrates. Thus, the diagnosis of late ischemic injury may be helpful in ruling out other potentially treatable etiologies that are part of the differential diagnoses for cardiac failure in transplant recipients, such as acute cellular rejection or antibody-mediated rejection [11].

Endocardial Lymphocytic Infiltrates (Quilty Effect): Endocardial lymphocytic infiltrates [28], also known as "Quilty effect" [29], are collections of T and B cells with histiocytes [30] seen in the endocardium of transplanted hearts (see Figure 4.9). Plasma cells are present in about half of these lesions. Occasional eosinophils and neutrophils may be seen [31]. Capillaries with red blood cells and sometimes prominent endothelial cells may be seen within the infiltrate. Several hypotheses have been proposed to explain the pathogenesis of these infiltrates, which include the use of cyclosporine A [32] to concomitant infection with Epstein-Barr virus [33], low local levels of cyclosporine A in the areas of endocardium where Quilty effect infiltrates develop [34], and idiosyncrasy to cyclosporine A [32], but

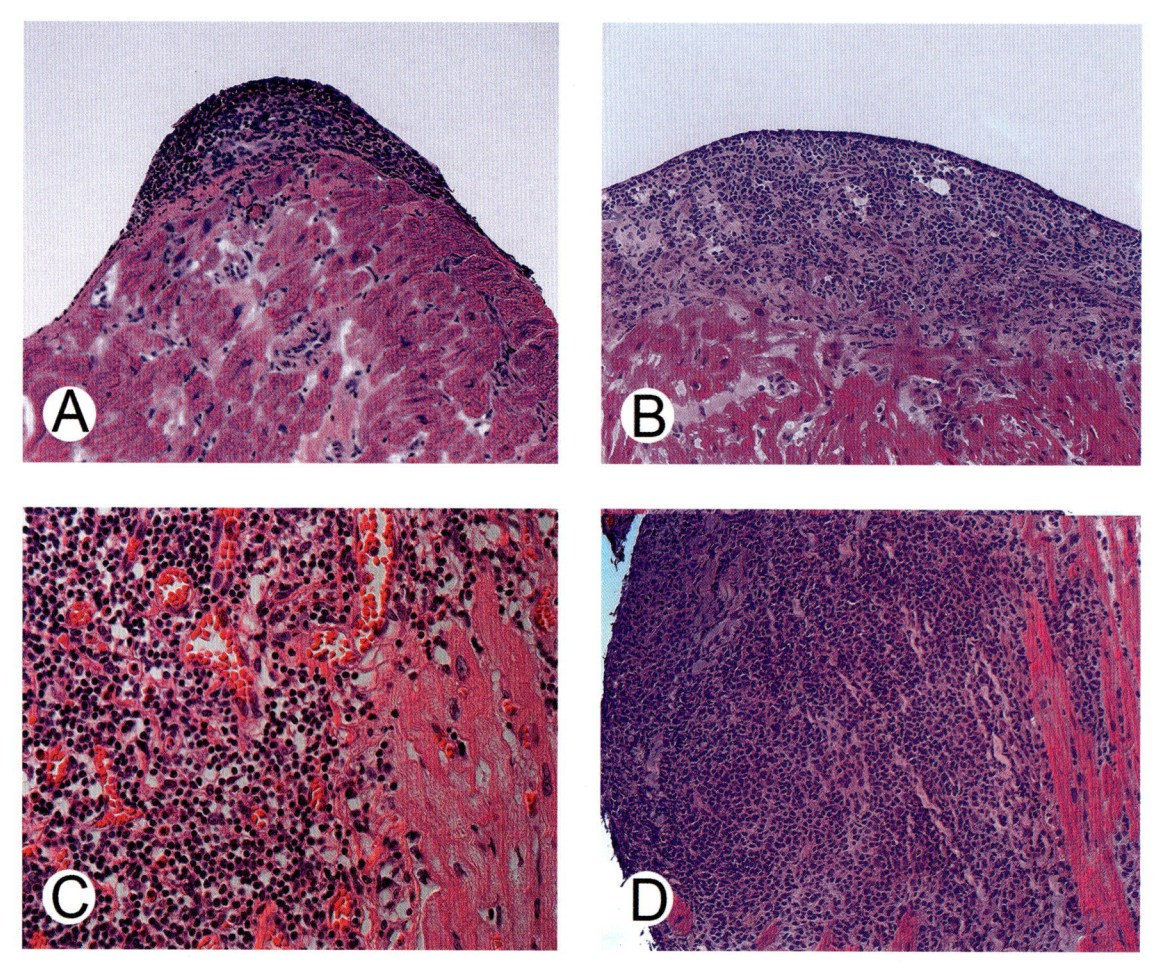

Figure 4.9 Endocardial lymphocytic infiltrates (Quilty lesions). A. Lymphocytic infiltrate contained within the endocardium and extending into the myocardium is shown in this biopsy. Such lesions used to be called Quilty type A in the ISHLT-WF-1990 (H&E, X 150). B. This frozen section shows a Quilty lesion distinctly contained within the endocardium and does not penetrate the subjacent myocardium. Small vessels are commonly present in Quilty lesions (but are more prominent in formalin-fixed paraffin-embedded tissue as shown in C) (H&E, X150). C. This endocardial infiltrate shows early infiltration of the myocardium. In addition, it shows conspicuous blood vessels filled with red blood cells. These are very characteristic and common in Quilty lesions (H&E, x 400). D. In this biopsy, the lymphocytic infiltrate clearly extends into the subjacent myocardium with finger-like projections. This used to be called Quilty B in the ISHLT-WF-1990 (H&E, X100).

none of these have been proven. However, one striking observation is that Quilty effect does not occur in the hearts of patients who are taking cyclosporine A, because they have received other organ transplants (i.e., liver, kidney) [35]. It seems to be a phenomenon that only occurs in the endocardium of cardiac allografts. It can be observed as early as the first post-transplant biopsy and tends to persist in subsequent biopsies of a given patient.

Quilty effect infiltrates may or may not be associated with rejection. The size of these infiltrates varies greatly, from a small cluster of mononuclear cells to grossly visible 2 mm lesions. Two morphologic patterns were recognized in the ISHLT-WF-1990, type A and type B. Type A was defined as confined to the endocardium and may be associated with areas that look like myocyte injury. Type B (invasive Quilty) extends into the subjacent myocardium [10] (see Figure 4.9 D). The ISHLT-WF-2005 removed the requirement to classify the Quilty lesions into A and B, since there is no clinical relevance to the distinction of these two patterns [11]. There is a rarely seen pattern in explanted allografts or in autopsy specimens in which lesions identical to Quilty effect are found deep in the myocardium besides the typical endocardial lymphocytic infiltrates.

Quilty Effect versus Moderate Rejection: The possible confusion of Quilty infiltrates with rejection [36] is still a problem for pathologists because of the obvious implications for therapy. One may imagine how a tangential section through the deeper myocardial end of a biopsy may show inflammatory infiltrates that look like rejection with myocyte damage if only a few levels of section are examined. However, if deeper sections are made, or better yet, if all the biopsy tissue is examined, it would soon become very obvious that in fact the inflammatory infiltrate in the myocardium is connected to a Quilty type lesion in the endocardium.

Quilty Effect versus Lymphoid Neoplasms: Exuberant Quilty lesions can be easily distinguished from lymphoid neoplasms by their cellular composition and location. See section on lymphoid neoplasms below.

In summary, endocardial lymphocytic infiltrates (Quilty effect) are lesions that are commonly seen in cardiac transplant biopsies, but until now lack any clinical relevance. In a study

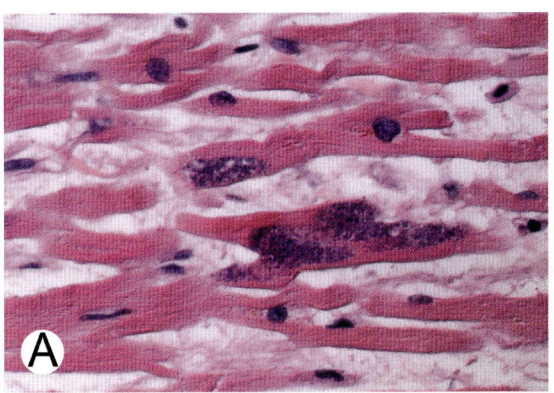

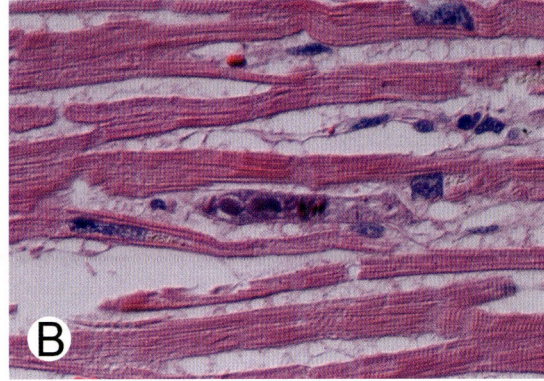

Figure 4.10 Infectious agents in endomyocardial biopsy. A. In this biopsy, there are two myocytes showing sarcoplasmic cysts filled with bradyzoites of Toxoplasma (H&E, X600). B. Cytomegalovirus inclusions are prominent in the nuclei of capillary endothelial cells (H&E X 600).

including 217 adults and 22 children observed during a period of ten years, the authors showed that 49% of adults and 68% of children show these infiltrates [29]. The important points in this study are that there seems to be no association between the endocardial infiltrates and: 1) grade of rejection; 2) subsequent development of vasculopathy (vascular chronic rejection); 3) development of lymphoma; and 4) viral infections (cytomegalovirus or Epstein-Barr virus).

Previous Biopsy Site: This is a common finding in transplant monitoring biopsies that can be seen in 53% [37] to 69% [38] of biopsies. This high frequency is due to the fact that, for a given patient, the anatomy of the inflow tract to the right ventricle is constant. During the biopsy procedure using the jugular approach, the ridges of the atrial anastomotic site, the right ventricular trabeculations, and the moderator band all contribute to guide the tip of the bioptome towards the same site in the interventricular septum. Gross examination at autopsy may show a patch of thickened endocardium measuring 1–2 cm in diameter in the mid-third of the right ventricular septum in patients who survived several months to years after the transplant. On light microscopy, the findings of this repetitive sampling of a small area of the septum vary with the interval between biopsies.

Pitfalls and Caveats in the Interpretation of Endomyocardial Biopsies for Surveillance

Although an enormous effort has been made to create a standard method for grading rejection [10, 11], there are several controversial points that are often identified by both pathologists and cardiologists in using the working formulation.

Myocyte Injury: A difficult issue in the interpretation of endomyocardial biopsies has been the inability to obtain consensus about the definition of myocyte damage and consequently in grading cellular rejection even among experienced pathologists trained in, and dedicated to, cardiovascular pathology [13]. The suggestion at the Banff 2001 conference was to focus on terminology that was more precise for pathologists, such as myocyte injury [13]. On light microscopic examination, this type of injury can encompass a spectrum of subtle to ominous changes. The subtle changes are more difficult to be noticed by the occasional observer. In a strict sense, simple changes in the myocytes such as vacuolization, hydropic change, or perinuclear halos [39] are at the somewhat milder side of the spectrum, whereas coagulation necrosis, myocytolysis, and nuclear pyknosis are at the very obvious worst end of the spectrum. Thus, the term "damage" is rather ambiguous. Unless there is clear coagulative necrosis or fragmentation of the sarcoplasm or typical nuclear changes such as pyknosis in the myocytes, the identification of "damaged" cells in hematoxylin-eosin stained paraffin sections is a subjective matter. Ultrastructural studies have clearly shown that subtle myocyte damage is present [40]. Myocyte degeneration is easily distinguished from necrosis. Damage to endothelial cells, basal lamina, or other components is also easily recognized [41]. Myocyte necrosis as defined by ultrastructural criteria is common in humoral rejection, whereas myocyte degeneration with the potential for recovery is more common in cellular rejection [42]. Ultrastructural studies have suggested that some of the myocyte damage seen during rejection may actually be a reversible process [40, 43]; however, by light microscopy, some of the myocyte changes that represent sub-lethal damage are indistinguishable from actual early necrosis.

Opportunistic Infections: It is well-known that the chronic therapy with immunosuppressive drugs to control rejection predisposes these patients to a large number of opportunistic infections, including viruses, bacteria, fungi, and protozoa. Bacterial infection is the most common type of infection, accounting for 67% of the cases in the last decade [44]. Viral infections are second in frequency (41%), with fungal and protozoal pathogens being responsible for the remaining 12% [45, 46]. The two most commonly reported opportunistic infections seen in EMB specimens are Toxoplasma and cytomegalovirus [47–49]. Other organisms reported to occur in heart transplant patients include: viruses-hepatitis B [50], hepatitis C [51], enteroviruses, parvovirus B19 [52], Epstein-Barr virus [52] and other herpes viruses, and adenovirus [52]; bacteria and mycobacteria [53–55]; fungi including Aspergillus [56, 57], Candida [57], Nocardia [44], and Mucor [58]; and protozoa including Pneumocystis [59], Toxoplasma [60] (see Figure 4.10 A), Leishmania [61], and reactivation of Chagas' disease [62]. In the

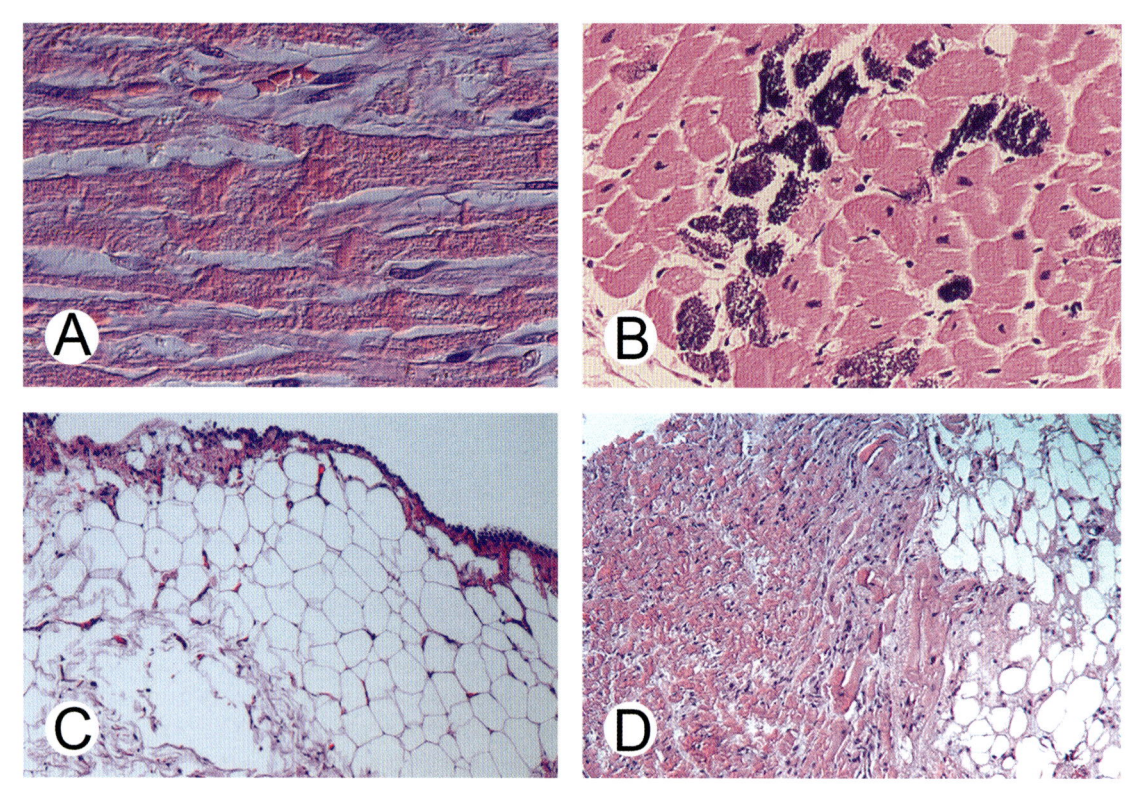

Figure 4.11 Other findings in post transplant endomyocardial biopsies. A. Contraction band artifact is relatively common in endomyocardial biopsies (H&E, X300). B. Dystrophic calcification of entire myocytes is also possible (H&E, X300). C. Cuboidal mesothelial cells are present (top), as well as adipose tissue in this biopsy. These findings distinctly indicate perforation of the myocardial wall (H&E, X400). D. This biopsy shows abundant adipose tissue, but in the absence of mesothelial cells or epicardial nerves, it cannot be diagnosed as a perforation (H&E, X 100).

pediatric heart transplant population, the pathogens reported include viruses (Cytomegalovirus, herpes simplex, Varicella-Zoster, respiratory viruses, and Epstein-Barr virus), bacteria (mycobacteria, Gram-positive, and Gram-negative), Toxoplasma, and Pneumocystis [57, 63, 64].

It should be noted that the identification of microorganisms in endomyocardial biopsy is difficult and should never be the only method to rule out infection. When examining a biopsy, hints of infection could include unusual inflammatory infiltrates such as the presence of granulocytes, plasma cells, and/or macrophages in a focus of inflammation without overt myocyte necrosis or dropout. Areas like these may harbor intracellular parasites (such as Toxoplasma) or fungal organisms which can be elusive on hematoxylin-eosin stain. Special stains for microorganisms should then be performed as needed. The pathologist should also look for viral inclusions in the nuclei of endothelial cells (see Figure 4.10 B), smooth muscle cells, or miscellaneous perivascular cells. Viral inclusions visible by light microscopy within the cardiac myocytes are quite rare.

Adipose Tissue: Perforation versus Infiltration: Adipocytes are normal cellular components of the heart mostly present in the epicardium. Microscopic foci of adipose tissue are usually present in the subendocardium and within the myocardium. These foci can be seen in all chambers, but are more commonly found in the right ventricular wall in obese patients and patients taking steroids. Thus, the pathologist should bear in mind that finding adipose tissue per se is not pathologic. An attempt should be made to define whether the adipose tissue seen in an endomyocardial biopsy is part of the ventricular wall, since it may also come from the epicardium (see Figure 4.11). Although the aim of a right ventricular biopsy procedure is to obtain samples from the right side of the interventricular septum, the bioptome may actually sample the right ventricular free wall. Therefore, when a focus of adipose tissue is found in an endomyocardial biopsy, the pathologist should make an effort to determine if this is subendocardial versus subepicardial adipose tissue. This can sometimes be easily determined by looking for the presence of mesothelial cell lining, which indicates the surface is actually epicardium (see Figure 4.11 C). The presence of ganglion cells or nerves is not indicative of perforation. However, due to the fibrinous and eventually fibrous pericarditis that usually develops after the transplant, it may be difficult to find mesothelial lining. In the latter case, the presence of nerves and ganglion cells may be suggestive of epicardial location, as these types of peripheral nerve tissue are common in the epicardium. However, a few weeks after the transplant, the organized pericarditis usually forms a dense protective layer around the myocardium that prevents the development of tamponade if there is perforation. The presence of adipose tissue in endomyocardial biopsies has been reported [65] and classified [66] in non-transplant patients. The presence of adipose tissue has been reported to occur in 4.62% of transplant biopsies in one study [66]. In transplant biopsies, there is also some tendency to see fat deposits in areas of previous biopsy site or perhaps foci of healing ischemic damage. Whether the use of steroids for the treatment of rejection increases the amount of adipose tissue in the endocardium is not known.

Lymphoid Neoplasms: Lymphoid neoplasms are reported to occur in 6% of all transplanted patients [67]. The role of Epstein-Barr virus in the pathogenesis of post-transplant lymphoproliferative disorders has been suggested [68, 69, 70, 71], but not clearly proven [72–73]. In most instances, these neoplasms are monoclonal B cell type [74] and their clinical presentation involves the lymph nodes, the central nervous system, systemic organs, or the transplanted organ itself [68]. Nevertheless, T cell lymphomas also occur [75]. Primary cardiac presentation of lymphoid neoplasms is not common [68]. Development of multiple myeloma is rare [76].

Biopsy-negative Allograft Dysfunction: The concept of biopsy-negative rejection or biopsy-negative allograft dysfunction has appeared in the heart transplant literature in recent years. It refers to cases in which there is nil or no cellular rejection in a biopsy to explain dysfunction of the allograft, thus suggesting that, in those instances, the dysfunction may be secondary to antibody-mediated rejection [77]. However, in centers that routinely evaluate biopsies for cellular and antibody-mediated rejection and rule out these two entities [78], this entity remains unexplained. Thus, the concept of true biopsy-negative allograft dysfunction, once antibody-mediated rejection has been ruled out, usually indicates that cardiac allograft vasculopathy may be the process responsible for the dysfunction and not cellular or antibody-mediated rejection.

Other Artifacts

Contraction Bands: This is a very common artifact seen in transplant and non-transplant heart biopsies. Several factors may influence the presence of contraction bands in the biopsy (see Figure 4.11 A). It may be the result of trauma to the myocardium induced when the bioptome cuts the tissue. It may also be induced by poor osmolarity of the medium in which the biopsy is placed before and during fixation, as well as the cold temperature of the medium of fixative (i.e. 4° C versus 22° C). Because of the high likelihood of finding contraction bands, they alone should never be the only criterion used to make a diagnosis of myocyte necrosis or ischemic injury.

Pinching or Forceps Artifact: This represents mechanical distortion of the tissue due to manipulation. The bioptome itself can induce this artifact, especially if its cutters are not very sharp (in the case of reusable bioptomes). It can also be induced during processing of the tissue in the pathology laboratory. An effort should be made to handle the tissue with care since this artifactual deformation may render the specimen uninterpretable.

Foreign Bodies: Occasional foreign bodies introduced at the time of the transplant can be seen such as gel-foam. It is also possible that the bioptome may actually sample fragments of indwelling catheters or the soft plastic cover of pacemaker leads. Giant cells containing birefringent material are most often seen in the subendocardium and should not be confused with a giant cell myocarditis.

Pseudohemorrhage: During the biopsy procedure, the spoon-shaped cutters of the bioptome can trap red blood cells and, at the time of biopsy, embed these cells into the myocardium by the pressure of the bioptome on the tissue. This produces artifactual pools that mimic hemorrhage. They are usually not accompanied by inflammatory cells or pathologic changes in the myocytes, thus making the distinction between artifact and rejection fairly easy.

"Telescoping" or Intussusception of Small Arteries: This occurs when a small muscular artery is sampled by the bioptome. Just before the bioptome cutters actually cut the tissue, the small artery is stretched and, as soon as it is cut, recoils into its own lumen. This can give the appearance of an occluded vessel or a small artery with vasculopathy. A coil of elastic lamina of these small arteries is usually determinant in showing that, in fact, there is an intussusception of the artery, thus making the distinction from vasculopathy rather obvious. It is uncommon to see this artifact occur in arterioles.

Dystrophic Calcification: There have been reports of various forms of calcification in the heart after transplantation (see Figure 4.11 B). In some patients, radiographic evidence of calcification has been shown in the native atria [79, 80] and in biopsy tissue [79]. In our experience, it is also uncommon to see dystrophic calcification of the ventricular myocardium in biopsies (see Figure 4.8). The myocytes and specifically the mitochondria show calcification. On light microscopy, the dystrophic calcification of the mitochondria is easily recognized as dark blue granular material within the myocytes. These granules are 1–2.5 micrometers in diameter. The granules may be seen in perinuclear location and also following the pattern of the sarcomeres. When abundant, they follow the contour of the whole myocyte. In some cases, a relationship between calcification of the mitochondria and cyclosporine therapy has been suggested [81]. Some conditions that have been associated with dystrophic calcification are sepsis, temporary uremia, hypomagnesemia, steroid therapy, alcoholism [79], and ischemic injury.

Chordae Tendineae and Valvular Tissue: Fragments of chordae tendineae are occasionally seen as part of the biopsy specimen [31]. They should be described and processed along with the biopsy. The clinical significance with regard to tricuspid dysfunction secondary to chordal rupture is varied [12, 82].

Antibody-mediated Rejection (The Humoral Arm of the Rejection Immune Response)

Antibody-mediated rejection (AMR) is an immunopathologic process in which donor-specific antibodies bind to antigen within the graft, leading to activation of the complement system and, in turn, result in injury to the graft. This type of rejection was first recognized as a distinct clinicopathologic entity in kidney transplant patients as an acute allograft rejection associated with the production of anti-donor reactive antibodies and poor prognosis [83]. AMR is poorly responsive to conventional immunosuppression which targets the cellular arm of the immune response. It has been postulated that the allorecognition and production of antibody may occur in any transplant and can span from subclinical to fully overt clinical AMR [84]. Old terminology in heart transplant literature such as vascular rejection, microvascular rejection, and humoral rejection should be avoided, since it has only led to confusion in the literature. The preferred terminology is AMR. For many years, it was said that AMR occurs early post-transplant (i.e. in the first three months) and the ISHLT-WF-1990 recommends AMR monitoring by immunofluorescence on all biopsies only up to six weeks post-transplant. This is clearly incorrect, as it is now known that AMR can and most commonly occurs months and even years after transplantation with formation of de novo antibodies [78, 85, 86].

Risk factors for developing AMR include pregnancy, previous transplantation, blood transfusions, sensitization by OKT3 induction therapy, use of ventricular assist devices, use of homografts in infants, presence of positive B cell flow cytometry crossmatch, and elevated panel-reactive antibodies [11, 87, 88]. The long-term outcome of AMR is not yet fully established in heart transplantation, but it has been suggested that an association exists with the development of cardiac allograft vasculopathy (CAV) and decreased survival [89, 90].

The ISHLT-WF-1990 did not provide a detailed pathologic classification of "humoral rejection" in biopsies (Table 4.3). Consequently, the true incidence of AMR was unknown and recognition of AMR as a real entity was not widely accepted. For more than a decade, there was no uniform set of diagnostic criteria provided to guide different transplant programs in the detection of this entity until the Banff Allograft Pathology group stressed the need for defined criteria for AMR [13]. In turn, the ISHLT-WF-2005 defined an initial set of standards to guide heart transplant centers around the world on how to evaluate endomyocardial biopsies for AMR (Table 4.3). This set included histologic and immunopathologic features. It suggested that the histologic features of AMR (see below under diagnostic criteria of AMR) should be identified in biopsies and this should prompt the use of immunopathologic examination [11, 14]. It is worth noting that evidence since has shown that the histologic criteria had rather low sensitivity and specificity for AMR [91]. Routine staining of all surveillance biopsies and biopsies for cause revealed that only approximately half of biopsies positive for complement deposition show histologic features of AMR, supporting the notion that complement activation precedes histologic changes in most instances [78]. The ISHLT-WF-2005 also required the presence of allograft dysfunction and circulating donor-specific antibodies in addition to pathologic evidence of AMR to make a definitive diagnosis of AMR.

The antibodies used in immunofluorescence evaluation for the diagnosis of AMR were varied and included antibodies to detect IgG, IgM, C3, C1q, fibrinogen, fibrin, and HLA-DR. But the presence of these antibodies did not always correlate with hemodynamic compromise or incidence of CAV, which resulted in decreased usefulness of staining for these antibodies [92]. Furthermore, a recent survey of North American centers regarding their diagnostic approach to AMR showed a chaotic situation with many more immunopathologic markers that have not been evaluated in large cohorts for sensitivity or specificity [93]. Evidence from large heart transplant centers in North America shows that while many markers such as immunoglobulins and some complement components (C3, C3c, C1q) may be detected in biopsies, the specificity and sensitivity of the immunoglobulins and some complement components are low as diagnostic [85] and prognostic markers of AMR [94, 95].

Diagnostic Criteria of AMR

Histopathologic Features: The histopathologic findings on light microscopy of endomyocardial biopsies as defined in the ISHLT-WF-2005 and its companion article on AMR [11, 14, 31] include capillary injury with endothelial cell swelling and intravascular macrophage accumulation (see Figure 4.12 A and B). On low magnification, the interstitium of the myocardium appears to be cellular and may superficially look similar to interstitial mononuclear cell infiltration of low-grade cellular rejection. The apparent cellularity of the biopsy on careful examination is due to either swollen capillary endothelial cells with enlarged vesicular nuclei or accumulation of macrophages within capillaries and venules. Macrophages appearing in Indian file pattern within capillaries in between longitudinally-oriented myocytes are also suggestive of intravascular accumulation. The difficulty of distinguishing endothelial cells from macrophages on hematoxylin-eosin stain only without the aid of immunostains prompted the recommendation to use "activated mononuclear cells" to include both cellular features.

Disruption of vascular integrity results in interstitial edema, and hemorrhage can be present together with neutrophils in and around capillaries. Intravascular thrombi and myocyte necrosis without cellular infiltration can also be identified [11, 14]. Edema or hemorrhage as an isolated finding may be an artifact of the biopsy procedure or processing and does not constitute as adequate histologic evidence of AMR. Hemorrhage, cellular necrosis with neutrophilic infiltrates, and vascular thrombosis represent the worst end of the morphologic spectrum of AMR. These constellations of histologic findings in severe AMR are rarely encountered in practice because of advances in the detection of pretransplantation HLA antibodies in heart transplant recipients.

As previously mentioned, the sensitivity of histopathologic findings alone (i.e., light microscopic features such as endothelial cell swelling and intravascular macrophages) is too low to serve as accurate screening parameters for AMR [91]. Consequently, it is strongly recommended to perform immunostaining to detect the presence of AMR. The histopathologic features of AMR, when present, often occur in a diffuse pattern and therefore are fairly easy to recognize. Changes involving only focal areas are sometimes encountered and its significance, in the absence of immunopathologic evidence of AMR, is unknown.

Immunostaining for Complement Split Products: Immunofluorescence methods for detection of AMR in tissues have evolved in the last decade. Some complement components, specifically C3d and C4d, are found to be more readily detected than antibodies and serve as very sensitive markers of

Table 4.3 Antibody-mediated Rejection

ISHLT-WF-1990	ISHLT-WF-2005	ISHLT-WF-2011 and 2013
Humoral rejection	Antibody-mediated rejection	Antibody-mediated rejection
Positive immunofluorescence, vasculitis, or severe edema in the absence of cellular infiltrate	AMR 0 = Negative for acute antibody-mediated rejection	pAMR 0 = Negative for pathologic AMR; both histological and immuno-pathological studies are negative
	AMR 1 = Positive for AMR	pAMR 1 (H+) = Histopathological AMR alone: histopathological findings present and immunopathological findings absent
	Histologic features of AMR	pAMR 1 (I+) = Immunopathologic AMR alone: Immunopathological findings present and histological findings absent
	Positive immunofluorescence or immunoperoxidase staining for AMR (positive CD68, C4d)	pAMR 2 = Pathologic AMR: both histological and immunopathological findings present
		pAMR 3 = Severe pathologic AMR: Rare cases of severe AMR with histopathological findings of interstitial hemorrhage, capillary fragmentation, mixed inflammation, endothelial cells pyknosis, karyorrhexis, marked edema

[10, 11, 15, 98]

rejection in endomyocardial biopsies for several reasons [96]. Antibodies bind to antigens with different avidity and either dissociate at varying rates, or are eliminated by shedding or internalization. In contrast, the process of complement activation yields split products of C4 and C3 that bind to the tissue where complement was activated. The longer half-lives of covalently-bounded complement split products C4d and C3d allow for increased sensitivity of complement detection. Among the components of the complement system, C3, followed by C4, are present in the highest concentration in serum; therefore, their split products are also deposited in tissues in the largest quantities [31]. Furthermore, the amplification steps in the complement cascade results in the generation of more C3 split products [97].

Immunostaining of Endomyocardial Biopsies Recommended in ISHLT-AMR-WF-2011 and 2013 [15, 98]

Immunofluorescence Staining: Immunofluorescence staining for the detection of complement activation is considered a more sensitive and specific method than immunohistochemical staining. A linear circumferential pattern of weak or strong staining in myocardial capillaries involving over half of the sampled capillaries is considered positive. The extent of capillary involvement is considered more important than the intensity of staining. The use of C4d and C3d immunofluorescence has shown excellent correlation with clinical AMR in medium size [85] and in large transplant centers [78] (see Figure 4.12 C through F). Therefore, the current recommendation includes both C4d and C3d staining. The use of other antibodies (HLA-DR, fibrin, and immunoglobulins) is rarely warranted.

Immunohistochemical Staining: For immunohistochemistry (IHC) on paraffin-embedded tissue, the latest working formulation recommends C4d and CD68 (or other appropriate macrophage marker). A positive C4d staining involves >50% of capillaries (multifocal or diffuse) with weak or strong intensity. On the other hand, the current threshold for a positive CD68 staining is set at >10% of the biopsy demonstrating intravascular macrophages. A concern is the lack of experience by pathologists in the interpretation of CD68 in the context of AMR. There is also poor correlation of CD68 staining pattern with intravascular macrophages observed on hematoxylin-eosin stain. The potential for misinterpretation is based on the fact that only intravascular macrophages should be interpreted as indicative of AMR. The interstitial macrophages should not be interpreted as indicative of AMR.

The interstitial macrophages, which can be increased in number in cellular rejection and ischemic injury, should not be interpreted as indicative of AMR.

The rationale for recommending IHC staining for both antibodies against C4d and CD68 is to gain experience in the evaluation of AMR in formalin-fixed paraffin-embedded tissue and to refine existing immunopathologic criteria through further validation studies. Limited experience using both stains indicated that there may be cases that are C4d-positive and CD68-negative and

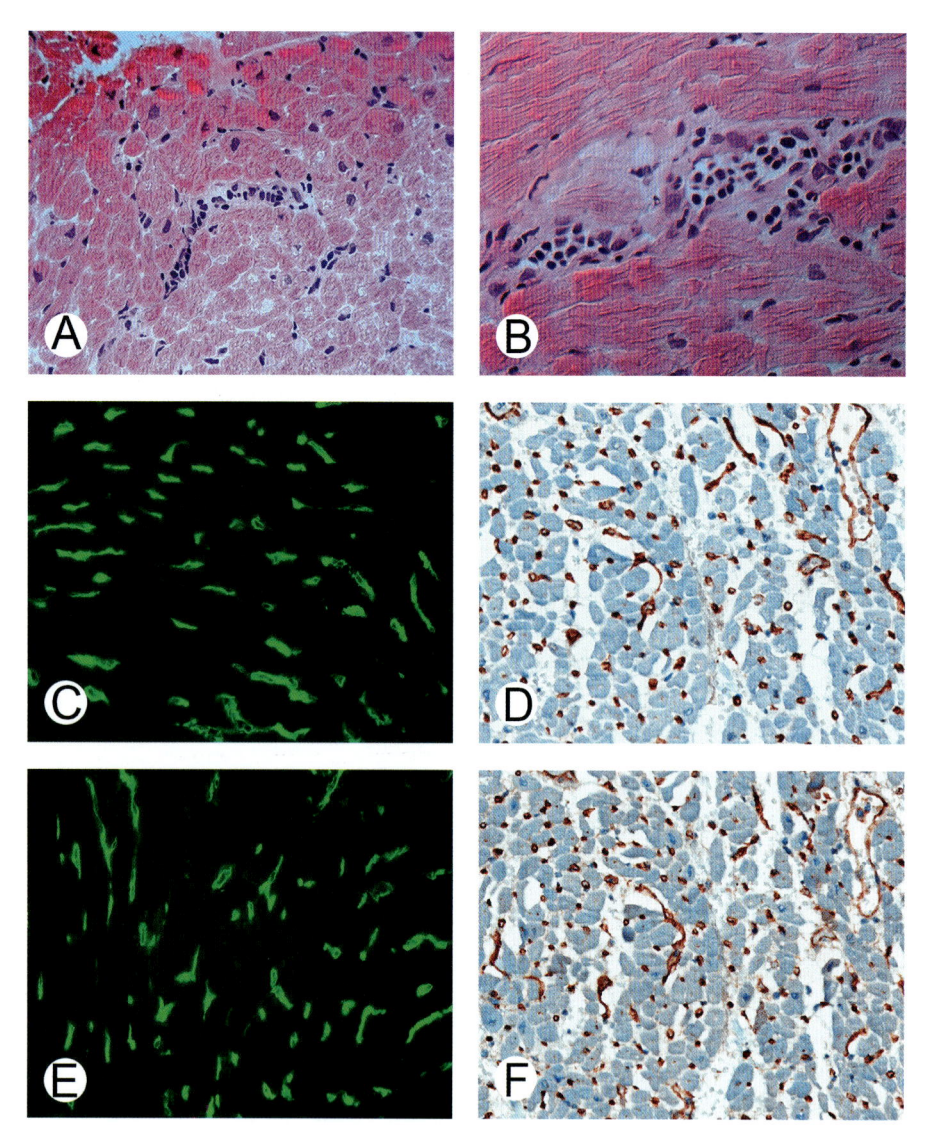

Figure 4.12 Antibody-mediated rejection. A. Low power view of an intramyocardial venule filled with mononuclear cells (H&E, 100X). B. In this field, a small arteriole distinctly shows intravascular macrophages (H&E, X 300). C. Immunofluorescence for C4d shows an intense capillary pattern deposition of this complement split product in this frozen endomyocardial biopsy tissue (C4d immunofluorescence (X300). D. The same complement split product C4d shown in a biopsy fixed in formalin. The pattern of positive deposition of C4d is identical (linear capillary staining) to the pattern seen on immunofluorescence (Immunohistochemistry for C4d. X 300). E and F. The same linear pattern of capillary staining is now demonstrating the presence of C3d in these two biopsies (E. Immunofluorescence for C3d. X 300. F. Immunohistochemistry for C3d. X300).

vice versa. The C4d-positive and CD68-negative cases may represent the same scenario as those C4d-positive cases without histopathologic features of AMR. However, the true incidence and significance of C4d-negative CD68-positive cases without histopathologic features is unknown. Likewise, the proportion of biopsies that are both C4d- and CD68-positive is not well established. While the recommendation calls for staining for both markers C4d and CD68, a positive result with either C4d or CD68 only is currently sufficient to fulfill the immunopathologic criteria for AMR.

Despite the availability of good reagents to detect C4d and C3d by immunohistochemistry, the ISHLT-WF-2011 stated that concomitant use of these two markers in immunohistochemistry had not been extensively evaluated in many high-volume centers [15]. However, recent study evidence [99] corroborated the findings that C4d and C3d used concomitantly show a strong correlation with clinical manifestations of AMR [78, 100]. There is, however, limited experience in the use of C3d in paraffin-embedded tissue due to commonly reported high background and nonspecific staining that interferes with accurate interpretation of C3d stains.

The 2013 ISHLT-working Formulation for Antibody-mediated Rejection Has the Following Grades:

pAMR 0: Negative for pathologic AMR: both histological and immunopathological studies are negative

pAMR 1 (H+): Histopathological AMR alone: histopathological findings present and immunopathological findings absent

pAMR 1 (I+): Immunopathologic AMR alone: immunopathological findings present and histological findings absent pAMR 2: Pathologic AMR: both histological and immunopathological findings present

pAMR 3: Severe pathologic AMR: rare cases of severe AMR with histopathological findings of interstitial hemorrhage, capillary fragmentation, mixed inflammation, endothelial cells pyknosis, karyorrhexis, and marked edema

While the ISHLT-WF-2005 recommended that these patients undergo assessment for circulating antibodies to HLA class I or II, as well as non-HLA donor antigens, the ISHLT-WF-AMR-2011 does not require correlation of the histologic or immunopathologic findings with the presence of donor-specific antibodies or allograft dysfunction. An EMB with no histologic or immunopathologic evidence of AMR is graded 0 (pAMR 0). If the immunofluorescence or immunohistochemical staining supports the histological features of AMR, the biopsy is considered positive (pAMR 2). The presence of either histologic or immunopathological findings only is considered pAMR 1 with a qualifier of H+ or I+. Note that occurrence of severe pathologic AMR or pAMR3 is very rare in current practice. The precise clinical correlation for each of these pathologic grades will continue to be established.

Indications for Immunostaining: The indications for immunostaining include the presence of histopathologic findings in the biopsy and allograft dysfunction, as well as monitoring highly sensitized patients and response to therapy in patients diagnosed with AMR. The ISHLT-AMR-WF-2011 states that initial immunostaining should be avoided in the first two weeks because of theoretical perioperative considerations such as ischemic injury [101] as potentially responsible for activating complement. However, the pattern of staining of capillaries in AMR is distinctly different than the sarcoplasmic staining of necrotic myocytes. This should not be a reason for not performing immunofluorescence during this period, particularly in highly sensitized patients.

Immunostaining, in addition to monitoring levels of donor-specific antibodies, can also be used to monitor response to therapy in patients with clinical AMR. Using immunofluorescence method, the staining intensity of C3d and C4d is observed to decrease as soon as one week after plasmapheresis is initiated, followed by disappearance of C3d and then C4d within one to two months in patients with clinical resolution of AMR.

It may also be prudent to continue to monitor patients with focal C4d or C3d staining, as well as those with diffuse staining for C4d only. Our personal experience with immunofluorescence staining indicates that some patients progress from focal to diffuse pattern and from C4d-positivity only to concomitant C4d and C3d-positivity within varying time intervals.

Mixed Acute Cellular and Antibody-mediated Rejection: Although most AMR episodes are associated with absent or at most mild acute cellular rejection, mixed rejections have also been reported to carry a significant risk of mortality [102, 103]. Mixed rejection may occur early or late [104] in the course of transplantation and is also associated with allograft dysfunction.

Diagnostic Consideration about Complement Split Products in the Diagnosis of AMR: While complement is activated through antibody in the classical pathway, one must remember that complement can also be activated during procedures such as extracorporeal circulation during surgery [105, 106], by ischemia/reperfusion injury and by induction therapy before transplant with anti-thymocyte globulin [101]. Thus, the mere presence of C4d or C3d alone in capillaries should not be equated with AMR.

In our experience, the use of C4d immunostaining alone is not a reliable tool. Instead, evaluation of endomyocardial biopsies for AMR should include staining for both C4d and C3d [85, 78] because the presence of both markers correlates highly with allograft dysfunction and the presence of elevated donor-specific antibodies.

Discrepancy between Immunopathology and Clinical Presentation: Activation of the complement cascade detected by immunostains for C4d and/or C3d is not always accompanied by dysfunction of the graft. Some authors have referred to this apparent lack of graft injury despite evidence of complement activation as "accommodation" in animal models [107] and in ABO-incompatible renal transplants [108]. One possible explanation is that complement activation is interrupted by a protective mechanism in the host. This suggests that unless the complement cascade proceeds to the formation of the membrane attack complex (MAC), there is no expected injury to the allograft. This complex is needed to form a "pore" that leads to loss of integrity of the cell membrane. In humans, it is well-known that there are regulators of complement activation (RCA) that can prevent the completion of the complement cascade at different stages of activation. The concept of subclinical AMR has also been proposed with the recognition of pathologic AMR diagnosed on routine surveillance biopsy of patients with stable hemodynamics. Patients with subclinical AMR appear to have worse survival than patients who never had positive biopsies for AMR. The appropriate management of these patients needs to be determined through large-scale prospective studies.

Regulators of Complement Activation: These regulators exert their effects at different points in the complement activation cascade, whether the activation occurs through the classic, alternate, or mannose binding lectin pathways. All these pathways converge at the point of generation of the enzymatic complexes known as the C3 convertases which, in turn, proceed to activate the remaining complement components required for the formation of the MAC. There are two main types of proteins that can regulate the activation of complement. These can be divided into the membrane-bound and soluble types. In humans, the membrane-bound regulators are CD35 or complement receptor 1 (CR1), CD46 or membrane cofactor protein (MCP), CD55 or decay-accelerating factor (DAF), CD59 or protectin, and C8-binding protein or homologous restriction factor (C8bp/HRF) [109, 110]. The soluble factors include the C1 inhibitor, C4 binding protein (C4bp),

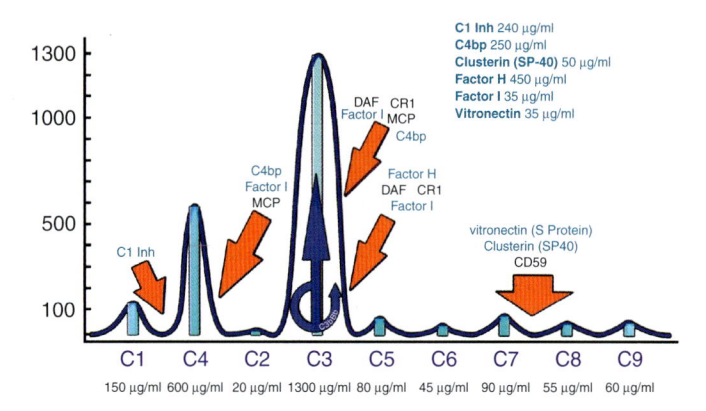

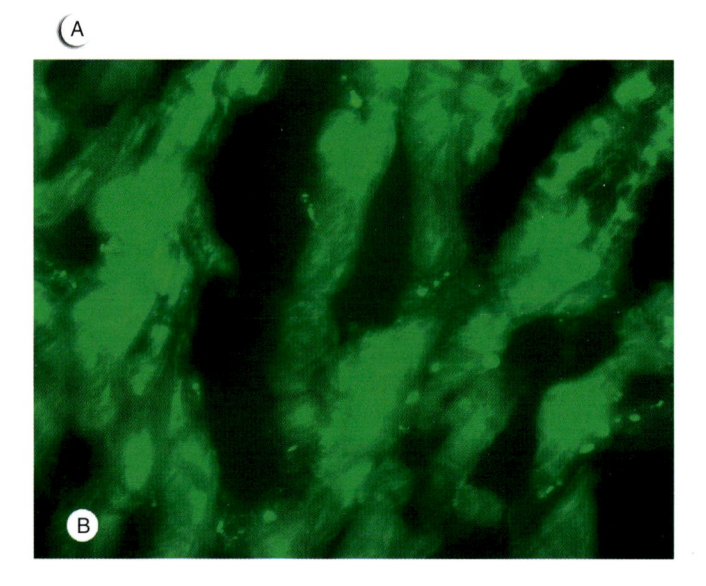

Figure 4.13 Serum concentration of complement components and regulators of complement activation. The serum concentration of the different complement factors in serum is shown in micrograms per milliliter. The activation of C3 is critical, as it augments both cellular and humoral immune response. C3 is enzymatically cleaved and activated by C4b2a of the classic pathway and C3bBb through an amplification loop of the alternative pathway. Its activation is an important amplification step because C3 is present in a larger molar amount and, once activated, it can further increase the activation of the rest of the cascade. Regulators of complement activation are composed of both plasma (blue letters) and membrane (black letters) proteins that inhibit the proteolytic subunits of classical and alternative pathways, thereby preventing the progression of the complement pathway to the membrane attack complex formation. MCP = membrane cofactor protein; DAF = decay accelerating factor; CR1 = complement receptor 1; C1 Inh = C1 inhibitor; C4bp = C4 binding protein. B. Decay accelerating factor (CD55) is demonstrated as granular pattern of fluorescence in the capillaries of this micrograph (Immunofluorescence for CD55, X600). The presence of CD55 is interpreted as the mechanism preventing progression of activation of the complement cascade from activation of C4 into activation of C3, and consequently no activation of the membrane attack complex.

factor I, factor H, clusterin, and S-Protein (vitronectin). Their points of action are shown in Figure 4.13 A [31].

There is little information about the expression of these RCA molecules in human heart transplantation. In heart transplants, DAF or CD55 is expressed locally in the myocardium [111]. In this study, a group of patients with complement deposition in endomyocardial biopsies was examined. The biopsies were stained by immunofluorescence for C4d, C3d, and DAF. There were two subgroups identified on the basis of allograft dysfunction present or absent. All patients had biopsy-proven C4d and C3d deposits. Patients with good response to therapy and resolution of the AMR episode showed intense tissue expression of CD55 in the endothelium of the allograft. Patients with poor outcomes had low or absent tissue expression of CD55. Thus, the local expression of DAF correlates with absence of allograft dysfunction in spite of C4d and C3d deposition in capillaries (see Figure 4.13 B).

Complement Staining Artifacts: Common artifactual staining seen in immunofluorescence microscopy of transplant biopsy includes autofluorescent lipofuscin deposits and nonspecific binding to collagen in the interstitium and to the internal elastic lamina of arteries. Necrotic myocytes likewise bind complement.

Platelets and Coagulation Factors in Rejection: The combination of antibodies and complement with inflammatory cells has great potential to injure the endothelial and smooth muscle cells of the vessels of the allograft [112]. It is known that stimulation through receptors for IgG or complement split products can activate macrophages, but stimulation through combinations of these receptors generates synergistic results. Thus, the effect of antibodies and complement efficiently integrate the activation of endothelial cells, platelets, and macrophages [112].

Alloantibodies can induce exocytosis of von Willebrand factor and P-selectin from endothelial cells and attachment of platelets within minutes. Consequently, platelets also adhere to and stimulate leukocytes, which are potentiated by complement activation. After attachment, platelets degranulate and release preformed mediators stored in their granules, such as platelet factor 4 and CXCL4 [113]. These effects may also play a role in the pathogenesis of CAV (see section on CAV below).

Thrombolytic and Coagulation Factors Have Also Been Implicated in Allograft Rejection and CAV: The notion that a hypercoagulable state may play a role in CAV has been supported by the finding that early elevation of tissue factor and fibrin and reduction of tissue plasminogen activator and antithrombin in human cardiac allografts are associated with both onset and severity of CAV and graft failure. As expected, impairment of fibrinolysis has also been correlated with CAV [114].

Cardiac Allograft Vasculopathy (CAV)

Allograft vasculopathy is the most difficult obstacle to long-term successful outcome in cardiac transplantation [31]. This problem is not unique to the heart and occurs in any solid organ graft in a similar manner [115]. Allograft vasculopathy (also called chronic rejection or accelerated graft arteriosclerosis, or transplant coronary artery disease) develops, over time, in practically all the transplanted hearts. In some patients, it develops in a few months, while in others, it develops after several years. The events leading to this vascular process are complex and include at least some of the following: native donor atherosclerosis [116], ischemic time of the graft [117], endothelial damage of diverse origins [118, 119], histocompatibility issues [120], arteritis [121], chronic humoral and cellular immune attack [122–125], fibrinolysis [126, 127], viral infections [128], serum lipids [129], and hormonal milieu [130]. The problem of vasculopathy is also seen in the pediatric population and follows a course similar to the one seen in adults [131, 132].

Vasculopathy involves both epicardial and intramural coronary arteries [31]. To understand the pathology, one should remember that the coronary vessels have three layers: the adventitia, the media, and the intima. In turn, each one of these anatomic layers is made of many different cellular and extracellular components. There is evidence that during the development of vasculopathy, a concerted series of events occurs that produce varying degrees of damage to each one of these structures (intima, media, adventitia, and vasa vasorum).

On gross examination, the epicardial coronary arteries may reveal a combination of focal eccentric lesions and, in other areas, uniform concentric thickening of the wall. However, in some instances, while there may be little or no gross evidence of vasculopathy in these epicardial coronary arteries, there is abundant pathology in the intramyocardial vessels. Careful exam of the cut surfaces of the ventricles often reveals thickened arteries (with a range diameter of 0.2 to 0.5 mm) with abundant perivascular fibrosis. These vessels are quite prominent on gross exam. Some allografts may show clear evidence of epicardial coronary atherosclerosis, which was present in the donor prior to the transplant [31, 116, 133]. In these cases, the allograft vasculopathy is superimposed over the atherosclerosis. If pre-existing atherosclerotic plaques are present, the morphology of the lesion may be eccentric, with more features of atheroma such as destruction of the internal elastic lamina, amorphous lipid-rich plaque, and cholesterol clefts. Long-term lesions of the epicardial coronaries may eventually look like conventional atherosclerosis and be indistinguishable from it.

The light microscopic morphology of the lesions seen as a result of vasculopathy is slightly different in epicardial than in medium or small arteries [31, 134]. If no atherosclerotic plaques are present, the typical vasculopathy lesions show concentric intimal proliferation (see Figure 4.14) composed of smooth muscle cells and less differentiated cells (myofibroblasts or "myointimal" cells). There is deposition of connective tissue components such as collagen and proteoglycans. The intramural coronary arteries usually show concentric uniform lesions consisting of intimal smooth muscle proliferation with or without lipoprotein deposition within the proliferating cells. The internal elastic lamina is usually intact or only focally disrupted, the media shows little to no lipoprotein deposition, and there usually is an adventitial cuff of fibrous tissue with or without mononuclear inflammatory infiltrates. The pathology of CAV in children is practically identical [135].

In some patients, frank vasculitis has been documented [122]. This usually affects the distal coronaries. Active vasculitis shows lymphocytes, plasma cells, and occasionally polymorphonuclear leukocytes. Fibrinoid necrosis may be seen in early stages. Thrombosed and recanalized vessels may represent healed vasculitis with thrombosis. Although small arteries or arterioles with vasculopathy may be seen in endomyocardial biopsies, there is no consistent correlation with the anatomic or functional status of epicardial coronary arteries [136]. Despite this lack of correlation, the presence of vasculopathy in the biopsy specimen, if any, should be recorded in the final report.

Recurrent Diseases in the Allograft and the Patient

A number of cardiac conditions have been shown to recur in the transplanted heart, including infections [62] and amyloidosis [137].

Depending on the cause of iron overload leading to heart transplantation [138], the iron overload may recur in the allograft [139]. Giant cell myocarditis [140, 141] can also rarely recur despite immunosuppression, [142] as does sarcoidosis [143, 144]. Administration of amiodarone pretransplant has been described to cause QT prolongation in the allograft [145]. Systemic disorders associated with genetic predisposition for recurrence have been reported, as in the case of recurrent thrombotic complications in a patient homozygous for prothrombin G20210A single nucleotide polymorphism [146] or recurrent aortic dissection after heart transplantation in a patient with Marfan's syndrome [147]. Vascular pathology complicated the postoperative course of a patient with Behcet's disease who developed a large pseudoaneurysm at the aortic anastomotic site [148]. Cardiac transplantation for unresectable primary cardiac sarcomas is controversial because of risks for local recurrence or metastatic disease. For instance, local recurrences of primary cardiac sarcomas have been described in both native right atrium [149] and the left pulmonary artery [150]. Recurrent EBV-related leiomyosarcoma has been described in young patients [151].

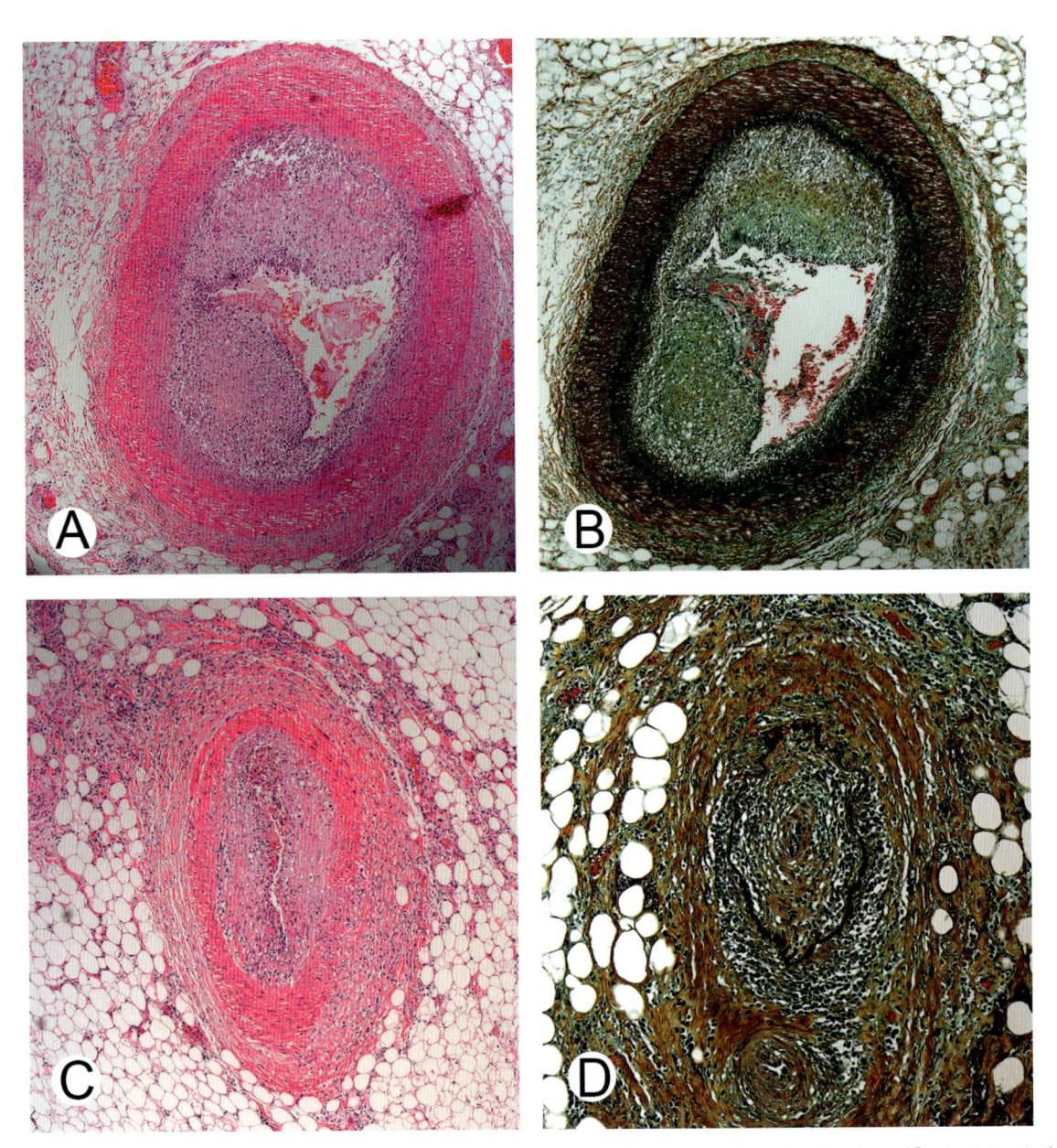

Figure 4.14 Cardiac allograft vasculopathy (CAV). A. Microscopic examination of an eccentric plaque showing the proliferative intima in the right half of an epicardial coronary artery (H&E, X10). B. The proliferative intima in this case is formed of mature extracellular matrix rich in glycosaminoglycans (green). The internal elastic lamina (black) is intact, and the media of the vessel is also intact (dark red) (Movat pentachrome, X10). C. This light micrograph shows an almost complete occlusion of the lumen by CAV in a small epicardial coronary artery branch (H&E, X10). D. The same artery stained with a Movat pentachrome shows the proliferative neointima of the CAV process as a glycosaminoglycan-rich extracellular matrix (green) (Movat pentachrome, X10).

References

1 Lund LH, Edwards LB, Kucheryavaya AY, Dipchand AI, Benden C, Christie JD, et al. The Registry of the International Society for Heart and Lung Transplantation: Thirtieth Official Adult Heart Transplant Report-2013; Focus Theme: Age. J Heart Lung Transplant. 2013;**32**(10):951–64.

2 Dipchand AI, Kirk R, Edwards LB, Kucheryavaya AY, Benden C, Christie JD, et al. The Registry of the International Society for Heart and Lung Transplantation: Sixteenth Official Pediatric Heart Transplantation Report-2013; Focus Theme: Age. J Heart Lung Transplant. 2013;**32**(10):979–88.

3 Zerbe TR, Arena V. Diagnostic Reliability of Endomyocardial Biopsy for Assessment of Cardiac Allograft Rejection. Hum Pathol. 1988;**19**(11):1307–14.

4 Wagner K, Oliver MC, Boyle GJ, Miller SA, Law YM, Pigula F, et al. Endomyocardial Biopsy in Pediatric Heart Transplant Recipients: A Useful Exercise? (Analysis of 1,169 Biopsies). Pediatr Transplant. 2000;**4**(3):186–92.

5 Mehra MR, Uber PA, Uber WE, Park MH, Scott RL. Anything but a Biopsy: Noninvasive Monitoring for Cardiac Allograft Rejection. Curr Opin Cardiol. 2002;**17**(2):131–6.

6 Balzer D, Moorhead S, Saffitz JE, Sekarski DR, Canter CE. Pediatric Endomyocardial Biopsy Performed Solely with Echocardiographic Guidance. J Am Soc Echocardiogr. 1993;**6**(5):510–5.

7 Pomerance A, Stovin PG. Heart Transplant Pathology: The British Experience. Journal of Clinical Pathology. 1985;**38**(2):146–59.

8. Spiegelhalter DJ, Stovin PG. An Analysis of Repeated Biopsies Following Cardiac Transplantation. Statistics in Medicine. 1983;2(1):33–40.

9. Sharples LD, Cary NR, Large SR, Wallwork J. Error Rates with which Endomyocardial Biopsy Specimens Are Graded for Rejection after Cardiac Transplantation. Am J Cardiol. 1992;70(4):527–30.

10. Billingham ME, Cary NR, Hammond ME, Kemnitz J, Marboe C, McCallister HA, et al. A Working Formulation for the Standardization of Nomenclature in the Diagnosis of Heart and Lung Rejection: Heart Rejection Study Group. The International Society for Heart Transplantation. J Heart Transplant. 1990;9(6):587–93.

11. Stewart S, Winters GL, Fishbein MC, Tazelaar HD, Kobashigawa J, Abrams J, et al. Revision of the 1990 Working Formulation for the Standardization of Nomenclature in the Diagnosis of Heart Rejection. J Heart Lung Transplant. 2005;24(11):1710–20.

12. Wiklund L, Suurkula MB, Kjellstrom C, Berglin E. Chordal Tissue in Endomyocardial Biopsies. Scandinavian Journal of Thoracic and Cardiovascular Surgery. 1994;28(1):13–8.

13. Rodriguez ER, International Society for H, Lung T. The Pathology of Heart Transplant Biopsy Specimens: Revisiting the 1990 ISHLT Working Formulation. J Heart Lung Transplant. 2003;22(1):3–15.

14. Reed EF, Demetris AJ, Hammond E, Itescu S, Kobashigawa JA, Reinsmoen NL, et al. Acute Antibody-mediated Rejection of Cardiac Transplants. J Heart Lung Transplant. 2006;25(2):153–9.

15. Berry GJ, Angelini A, Burke MM, Bruneval P, Fishbein MC, Hammond E, et al. The ISHLT Working Formulation for Pathologic Diagnosis of Antibody-mediated Rejection in Heart Transplantation: Evolution and Current Status (2005–2011). J Heart Lung Transplant. 2011;30(6):601–11.

16. Berry GJ, Burke MM, Andersen C, Bruneval P, Fedrigo M, Fishbein MC, et al. The 2013 International Society for Heart and Lung Transplantation Working Formulation for the Standardization of Nomenclature in the Pathologic Diagnosis of Antibody-mediated Rejection in Heart Transplantation. J Heart Lung Transplant. 2013;32(12):1147–62.

17. Rose AG, Cooper DK, Human PA, Reichenspurner H, Reichart B. Histopathology of Hyperacute Rejection of the Heart: Experimental and Clinical Observations in Allografts and Xenografts. J Heart Lung Transplant. 1991;10(2):223–34.

18. Schuurman HJ, Gmelig Meyling FH, Wijngaard PL, Van der Meulen A, Slootweg PJ, Jambroes G. Lymphocyte Status in Endomyocardial Biopsies and Blood after Heart Transplantation. J Pathol. 1989;159(3):197–203.

19. van Besouw NM, Balk AH, Mochtar B, Vaessen LM, Weimar W. Phenotypic Analysis of Lymphocytes Infiltrating Human Cardiac Allografts during Acute Rejection and the Development of Graft Vascular Disease. Transpl Int. 1996;9 Suppl 1:S234–6.

20. Higuchi ML, de Assis RV, Sambiase NV, Reis MM, Kalil J, Bocchi E, et al. Usefulness of T-cell Phenotype Characterization in Endomyocardial Biopsy Fragments from Human Cardiac Allografts. J Heart Lung Transplant. 1991;10(2):235–42.

21. Ibrahim S, Dawson DV, Van Trigt P, Sanfilippo F. Differential Infiltration by CD45RO and CD45RA Subsets of T Cells Associated with Human Heart Allograft Rejection. Am J Pathol. 1993;142(6):1794–803.

22. Mues B, Brisse B, Steinhoff G, Lynn T, Hewett T, Sorg C, et al. Diagnostic Assessment of Macrophage Phenotypes in Cardiac Transplant Biopsies. Eur Heart J. 1991;12 Suppl D:32–5.

23. Hoshinaga K, Mohanakumar T, Goldman MH, Wolfgang TC, Szentpetery S, Lee HM, et al. Clinical Significance of in Situ Detection of T Lymphocyte Subsets and Monocyte/Macrophage Lineages in Heart Allografts. Transplantation. 1984;38(6):634–7.

24. Gassel AM, Hansmann ML, Radzun HJ, Weyand M. Human Cardiac Allograft Rejection. Correlation of Grading with Expression of Different Monocyte/Macrophage Markers. Am J Clin Pathol. 1990;94(3):274–9.

25. Sorrentino C, Scarinci A, D'Antuono T, Piccirilli M, Di Nicola M, Pasquale M, et al. Endomyocardial Infiltration by B and NK Cells Foreshadows the Recurrence of Cardiac Allograft Rejection. The Journal of Pathology. 2006;209(3):400–10.

26. Takahashi H, Ruiz P, Ricordi C, Delacruz V, Miki A, Mita A, et al. Quantitative in Situ Analysis of FoxP3+ T Regulatory Cells on Transplant Tissue Using Laser Scanning Cytometry. Cell Transplant. 2012;21(1):113–25.

27. Fyfe B, Loh E, Winters GL, Couper GS, Kartashov AI, Schoen FJ. Heart Transplantation-associated Perioperative Ischemic Myocardial Injury. Morphological Features and Clinical Significance. Circulation. 1996;93(6):1133–40.

28. Kottke-Marchant K, Ratliff NB. Endomyocardial Lymphocytic Infiltrates in Cardiac Transplant Recipients. Incidence and Characterization. Arch Pathol Lab Med. 1989;113(6):690–8.

29. Joshi A, Masek MA, Brown BW, Jr., Weiss LM, Billingham ME. "Quilty" Revisited: A 10-year Perspective. Hum Pathol. 1995;26(5):547–57.

30. Luthringer DJ, Yamashita JT, Czer LS, Trento A, Fishbein MC. Nature and Significance of Epicardial Lymphoid Infiltrates in Cardiac Allografts. J Heart Lung Transplant. 1995;14(3):537–43.

31. Tan CD, Baldwin WM, 3rd, Rodriguez ER. Update on Cardiac Transplantation Pathology. Arch Pathol Lab Med. 2007;131(8):1169–91.

32. Suit PF, Kottke-Marchant K, Ratliff NB, Pippenger CE, Easely K. Comparison of Whole-blood Cyclosporine Levels and the Frequency of Endomyocardial Lymphocytic Infiltrates (the Quilty Lesion) in Cardiac Transplantation. Transplantation. 1989;48(4):618–21.

33. Nakhleh RE, Copenhaver CM, Werdin K, McDonald K, Kubo SH, Strickler JG. Lack of Evidence for Involvement of Epstein-Barr Virus in the Development of the "Quilty" Lesion of Transplanted Hearts: An in Situ Hybridization Study. J Heart Lung Transplant. 1991;10(4):504–7.

34. Freimark D, Czer LS, Aleksic I, Ruan XM, Admon D, Blanche C, et al. Pathogenesis of Quilty Lesion in Cardiac Allografts: Relationship to Reduced Endocardial Cyclosporine A. J Heart Lung Transplant. 1995;14(6 Pt 1):1197–203.

35. Barone JH, Fishbein MC, Czer LS, Blanche C, Trento A, Luthringer DJ. Absence of Endocardial Lymphoid Infiltrates (Quilty Lesions) in Nonheart Transplant Recipients Treated with Cyclosporine. J Heart Lung Transplant. 1997;16(6):600–3.

36. Marboe CC, Billingham M, Eisen H, Deng MC, Baron H, Mehra M, et al. Nodular Endocardial Infiltrates (Quilty Lesions) Cause Significant Variability in Diagnosis of ISHLT Grade 2 and 3A Rejection in Cardiac Allograft Recipients. J Heart Lung Transplant. 2005;24(7 Suppl):S219–26.

37. Foerster A, Simonsen S, Froysaker T. Heart Transplantation in Norway. Morphological Monitoring of Cardiac Allograft Rejection. A 3-year Follow-up. APMIS. 1988;96(1):14–24.

38. Sibley RK, Olivari MT, Ring WS, Bolman RM. Endomyocardial Biopsy in the Cardiac Allograft Recipient. A Review of 570 Biopsies. Ann Surg. 1986;203(2):177–87.

39. Kemnitz J, Cohnert T, Schafers HJ, Helmke M, Wahlers T, Herrmann G, et al. A Classification of Cardiac Allograft Rejection. A Modification of the Classification by Billingham. Am J Surg Pathol. 1987;11(7):503–15.

40. Myles JL, Ratliff NB, McMahon JT, Golding LR, Hobbs RE, Rincon G, et al. Reversibility of Myocyte Injury in Moderate and Severe Acute Rejection in Cyclosporine-treated Cardiac Transplant Patients. Arch Pathol Lab Med. 1987;111(10):947–52.

41. Hammond EH, Yowell RL. Ultrastructural Findings in Cardiac Transplant Recipients. Ultrastruct Pathol. 1994;18(1–2):213–20.

42. Hook S, Caple JF, McMahon JT, Myles JL, Ratliff NB. Comparison of Myocardial Cell Injury in Acute Cellular Rejection versus Acute Vascular Rejection in Cyclosporine-treated Heart Transplants. J Heart Lung Transplant. 1995;14(2):351–8.

43. McMahon JT, Ratliff NB. Regeneration of Adult Human Myocardium after Acute Heart Transplant Rejection. J Heart Transplant. 1990;9(5):554–67.

44. Haddad F, Deuse T, Pham M, Khazanie P, Rosso F, Luikart H, et al. Changing Trends in Infectious Disease in Heart Transplantation. J Heart Lung Transplant. 2010;29(3):306–15.

45. Miller LW, Naftel DC, Bourge RC, Kirklin JK, Brozena SC, Jarcho J, et al. Infection after Heart Transplantation: A Multiinstitutional Study. Cardiac Transplant Research Database Group. J Heart Lung Transplant. 1994;13(3):381–92; discussion 93.

46. Smart FW, Naftel DC, Costanzo MR, Levine TB, Pelletier GB, Yancy CW, Jr., et al. Risk Factors for Early, Cumulative, and Fatal Infections after Heart Transplantation: A Multiinstitutional Study. J Heart Lung Transplant. 1996;15(4):329–41.

47. Arbustini E, Grasso M, Diegoli M, Percivalle E, Grossi P, Bramerio M, et al. Histopathologic and Molecular Profile of Human Cytomegalovirus Infections in Patients with Heart Transplants. Am J Clin Pathol. 1992;98(2):205–13.

48. Holliman R, Johnson J, Savva D, Cary N, Wreghitt T. Diagnosis of Toxoplasma Infection in Cardiac Transplant Recipients Using the Polymerase Chain Reaction. Journal of Clinical Pathology. 1992;45(10):931–2.

49. Wagner FM, Reichenspurner H, Uberfuhr P, Weiss M, Fingerle V, Reichart B. Toxoplasmosis after Heart Transplantation: Diagnosis by Endomyocardial Biopsy. J Heart Lung Transplant. 1994;13(5):916–8.

50. Drescher J, Wagner D, Haverich A, Flik J, Stachan-Kunstyr R, Verhagen W, et al. Nosocomial Hepatitis B Virus Infections in Cardiac Transplant Recipients Transmitted during Transvenous Endomyocardial Biopsy. The Journal of Hospital Infection. 1994;26(2):81–92.

51. Fishman JA, Rubin RH, Koziel MJ, Periera BJ. Hepatitis C Virus and Organ Transplantation. Transplantation. 1996;62(2):147–54.

52. Breinholt JP, Moulik M, Dreyer WJ, Denfield SW, Kim JJ, Jefferies JL, et al. Viral Epidemiologic Shift in Inflammatory Heart Disease: The Increasing Involvement of Parvovirus B19 in the Myocardium of Pediatric Cardiac Transplant Patients. J Heart Lung Transplant. 2010;29(7):739–46.

53. Peters M, Schurmann D, Mayr AC, Heterzer R, Pohle HD, Ruf B. Immunosuppression and Mycobacteria Other than Mycobacterium Tuberculosis: Results from Patients with and without HIV Infection. Epidemiology and Infection. 1989;103(2):293–300.

54. Patel R, Roberts GD, Keating MR, Paya CV. Infections Due to Nontuberculous Mycobacteria in Kidney, Heart, and Liver Transplant Recipients. Clin Infect Dis. 1994;19(2):263–73.

55. LeMense GP, VanBakel AB, Crumbley AJ, 3rd, Judson MA. Mycobacterium Scrofulaceum Infection Presenting as Lung Nodules in a Heart Transplant Recipient. Chest. 1994;106(6):1918–20.

56. Morio F, Treilhaud M, Lepelletier D, Le Pape P, Rigal JC, Delile L, et al. Aspergillus Fumigatus Endocarditis of the Mitral Valve in a Heart Transplant Recipient: A Case Report. Diagn Microbiol Infect Dis. 2008;62(4):453–6.

57. Zaoutis TE, Webber S, Naftel DC, Chrisant MA, Kaufman B, Pearce FB, et al. Invasive Fungal Infections in Pediatric Heart Transplant Recipients: Incidence, Risk Factors, and Outcomes. Pediatr Transplant. 2011;15(5):465–9.

58. Almyroudis NG, Sutton DA, Linden P, Rinaldi MG, Fung J, Kusne S. Zygomycosis in Solid Organ Transplant Recipients in a Tertiary Transplant Center and Review of the Literature. Am J Transplant. 2006;6(10):2365–74.

59. Montoya JG, Giraldo LF, Efron B, Stinson EB, Gamberg P, Hunt S, et al. Infectious Complications among 620 Consecutive Heart Transplant Patients at Stanford University Medical Center. Clin Infect Dis. 2001;33(5):629–40.

60. Hermanns B, Brunn A, Schwarz ER, Sachweh JS, Seipelt I, Schroder JM, et al. Fulminant Toxoplasmosis in a Heart Transplant Recipient. Pathol Res Pract. 2001;197(3):211–5.

61. Golino A, Duncan JM, Zeluff B, DePriest J, McAllister HA, Radovancevic B, et al. Leishmaniasis in a Heart Transplant Patient. J Heart Lung Transplant. 1992;11(4 Pt 1):820–3.

62. Fiorelli AI, Santos RH, Oliveira JL, Jr., Lourenco-Filho DD, Dias RR, Oliveira AS, et al. Heart Transplantation in 107 Cases of Chagas' Disease. Transplant Proc. 2011;43(1):220–4.

63. Deen JL, Blumberg DA. Infectious Disease Considerations in Pediatric Organ Transplantation. Semin Pediatr Surg. 1993;2(4):218–34.

64. Braunlin EA, Canter CE, Olivari MT, Ring WS, Spray TL, Bolman RM, 3rd. Rejection and Infection after Pediatric Cardiac Transplantation. Ann Thorac Surg. 1990;49(3):385–90.

65. Cladellas M, Abadal ML, Ballester M, Obrador D, Crexells C, Matias-Guiu X, et al. Endomyocardial Diagnosis of Cardiac Lipomatosis. Catheterization and Cardiovascular Diagnosis. 1987;13(4):269–70.

66. Bonacina E, Recalcati F, Mangiavacchi M, Gronda E. Interstitial Myocardial Lipomatosis: A Morphological Study on Endomyocardial Biopsies and Diseased Hearts Surgically Removed for Heart Transplantation. Eur Heart J. 1989;10 Suppl D:100–2.

67. Gao SZ, Chaparro SV, Perlroth M, Montoya JG, Miller JL, DiMiceli S, et al. Post-transplantation Lymphoproliferative Disease in Heart and Heart-Lung Transplant Recipients: 30-year Experience at Stanford University. J Heart Lung Transplant. 2003;22(5):505–14.

68. Eisen HJ, Hicks D, Kant JA, Montone KT, Mull R, Pigott J, et al. Diagnosis of Posttransplantation Lymphoproliferative Disorder by Endomyocardial Biopsy in a Cardiac

Allograft Recipient. J Heart Lung Transplant. 1994;13(2):241–5.
69. Hanasono MM, Kamel OW, Chang PP, Rizeq MN, Billingham ME, van de Rijn M. Detection of Epstein-Barr Virus in Cardiac Biopsies of Heart Transplant Patients with Lymphoproliferative Disorders. Transplantation. 1995;60(5):471–3.
70. Schwend M, Tiemann M, Kreipe HH, Parwaresch MR, Kraatz EG, Herrmann G, et al. Rapidly Growing Epstein-Barr Virus-associated Pulmonary Lymphoma after Heart Transplantation. Eur Respir J. 1994;7(3):612–6.
71. Montone KT, Friedman H, Hodinka RL, Hicks DG, Kant JA, Tomaszewski JE. In Situ Hybridization for Epstein-Barr Virus NotI Repeats in Posttransplant Lymphoproliferative Disorder. Mod Pathol. 1992;5(3):292–302.
72. Lager DJ, Burgart LJ, Slagel DD. Epstein-Barr Virus Detection in Sequential Biopsies from Patients with a Posttransplant Lymphoproliferative Disorder. Mod Pathol. 1993;6(1):42–7.
73. Ohta H, Fukushima N, Ozono K. Pediatric Post-transplant Lymphoproliferative Disorder after Cardiac Transplantation. Int J Hematol. 2009;90(2):127–36.
74. Hanto DW, Birkenbach M, Frizzera G, Gajl-Peczalska KJ, Simmons RL, Schubach WH. Confirmation of the Heterogeneity of Posttransplant Epstein-Barr Virus-Associated B Cell Proliferations by Immunoglobulin Gene Rearrangement Analyses. Transplantation. 1989;47(3):458–64.
75. Kemnitz J, Cremer J, Gebel M, Uysal A, Haverich A, Georgii A. T-cell Lymphoma after Heart Transplantation. Am J Clin Pathol. 1990;94(1):95–101.
76. Chucrallah AE, Crow MK, Rice LE, Rajagopalan S, Hudnall SD. Multiple Myeloma after Cardiac Transplantation: An Unusual Form of Posttransplant Lymphoproliferative Disorder. Hum Pathol. 1994;25(5):541–5.
77. Fishbein MC, Kobashigawa J. Biopsy-negative Cardiac Transplant Rejection: Etiology, Diagnosis, and Therapy. Curr Opin Cardiol. 2004;19(2):166–9.
78. Tan CD, Sokos GG, Pidwell DJ, Smedira NG, Gonzalez-Stawinski GV, Taylor DO, et al. Correlation of Donor-specific Antibodies, Complement and Its Regulators with Graft Dysfunction in Cardiac Antibody-mediated Rejection. Am J Transplant. 2009;9(9):2075–84.
79. Cohnert TR, Kemnitz J, Haverich A, Dralle H. Myocardial Calcification after Orthotopic Heart Transplantation. J Heart Transplant. 1988;7(4):304–8.
80. Florence SH, Hutton LC, McKenzie FN, Kostuk WJ. Cardiac Transplantation: Postoperative Chest Radiographs. Canadian Association of Radiologists Journal = Journal l'Association canadienne des radiologistes. 1988;39(2):115–7.
81. Millane T, Wilson AJ, Patel MK, Jennison SH, Holt DW, Murday AJ, et al. Mitochondrial Calcium Deposition in Association with Cyclosporine Therapy and Myocardial Magnesium Depletion: A Serial Histologic Study in Heart Transplant Recipients. J Heart Lung Transplant. 1994;13(3):473–80.
82. Yankah AC, Musci M, Weng Y, Loebe M, Zurbruegg HR, Siniawski H, et al. Tricuspid Valve Dysfunction and Surgery after Orthotopic Cardiac Transplantation. Eur J Cardiothorac Surg. 2000;17(4):343–8.
83. Racusen LC, Colvin RB, Solez K, Mihatsch MJ, Halloran PF, Campbell PM, et al. Antibody-mediated Rejection Criteria – An Addition to the BANFF 97 Classification of Renal Allograft Rejection. Am J Transplant. 2003;3(6):708–14.
84. Takemoto SK, Zeevi A, Feng S, Colvin RB, Jordan S, Kobashigawa J, et al. National Conference to Assess Antibody-mediated Rejection in Solid Organ Transplantation. Am J Transplant. 2004;4(7):1033–41.
85. Rodriguez ER, Skojec DV, Tan CD, Zachary AA, Kasper EK, Conte JV, et al. Antibody-mediated Rejection in Human Cardiac Allografts: Evaluation of Immunoglobulins and Complement Activation Products C4d and C3d as Markers. Am J Transplant. 2005;5(11):2778–85.
86. Tan CD, Rodriguez ER. Diagnosis of Antibody-mediated Rejection in Cardiac Transplantation: A Call for Standardization. Current Opinion in Organ Transplantation. 2010.
87. Hammond EH, Wittwer CT, Greenwood J, Knape WA, Yowell RL, Menlove RL, et al. Relationship of OKT3 Sensitization and Vascular Rejection in Cardiac Transplant Patients Receiving OKT3 Rejection Prophylaxis. Transplantation. 1990;50(5):776–82.
88. Bishay ES, Cook DJ, Starling RC, Ratliff NB, Jr., White J, Blackstone EH, et al. The Clinical Significance of Flow Cytometry Crossmatching in Heart Transplantation. Eur J Cardiothorac Surg. 2000;17(4):362–9.
89. Michaels PJ, Espejo ML, Kobashigawa J, Alejos JC, Burch C, Takemoto S, et al. Humoral Rejection in Cardiac Transplantation: Risk Factors, Hemodynamic Consequences and Relationship to Transplant Coronary Artery Disease. J Heart Lung Transplant. 2003;22(1):58–69.
90. Taylor DO, Yowell RL, Kfoury AG, Hammond EH, Renlund DG. Allograft Coronary Artery Disease: Clinical Correlations with Circulating Anti-HLA Antibodies and the Immunohistopathologic Pattern of Vascular Rejection. J Heart Lung Transplant. 2000;19(6):518–21.
91. Hammond ME, Stehlik J, Snow G, Renlund DG, Seaman J, Dabbas B, et al. Utility of Histologic Parameters in Screening for Antibody-mediated Rejection of the Cardiac Allograft: A Study of 3,170 Biopsies. J Heart Lung Transplant. 2005;24(12):2015–21.
92. Bonnaud EN, Lewis NP, Masek MA, Billingham ME. Reliability and Usefulness of Immunofluorescence in Heart Transplantation. J Heart Lung Transplant. 1995;14(1 Pt 1):163–71.
93. Kucirka LM, Maleszewski JJ, Segev DL, Halushka MK. Survey of North American Pathologist Practices Regarding Antibody-mediated Rejection in Cardiac Transplant Biopsies. Cardiovasc Pathol. 2011;20(3):132–8.
94. Revelo MP, Stehlik J, Miller D, Snow GL, Everitt MD, Budge D, et al. Antibody Testing for Cardiac Antibody-mediated Rejection: Which Panel Correlates Best with Cardiovascular Death? J Heart Lung Transplant. 2011;30(2):144–50.
95. Rodriguez ER, Tan CD. Pathologic Evaluation for Antibody-mediated Rejection: Prognostic vs Diagnostic Markers? The Journal of Heart and Lung Transplantation: The Official Publication of the International Society for Heart Transplantation. 2011;30(2):136–8.
96. Baldwin WM, Ota H, Rodriguez ER. Complement in Transplant Rejection: Diagnostic and Mechanistic Considerations. Springer Semin Immunopathol. 2003;25(2):181–97.
97. Baldwin WM, 3rd, Kasper EK, Zachary AA, Wasowska BA, Rodriguez ER. Beyond C4d: Other Complement-related Diagnostic Approaches to Antibody-mediated Rejection. Am J Transplant. 2004;4(3):311–8.

98. Berry GJ, Burke MM, Anderson C, Bruneval P, Fedrigo M, Fishbein MC, et al. Isht Consensus Statement: International Society for Heart and Lung Transplantation 2013 Working Formulation for the Standardization of Nomenclature in the Pathologic Diagnosis of Antibody-mediated Rejection in Heart Transplantation. J Heart Lung Transplant. 2013;in press.

99. Miller DV, Everitt MD, Molina KM, Alharethi R, Budge D, Wachter B, et al. Clinical and Prognostic Significance of C3d and C4d Positive Immunopathology Pattern Versus C4d Positive Alone. Journal of Heart and Lung Transplantation. 2013;32(4):S20–S.

100. Rodriguez R, Moses JE, Adlington RM, Baldwin JE. A New and Efficient Method for O-quinone Methide Intermediate Generation: Application to the Biomimetic Synthesis of the Benzopyran Derived Natural Products (+/-)-Lucidene and (+/-)-Alboatrin. Organic & Biomolecular Chemistry. 2005;3(19):3488–95.

101. Baldwin WM, 3rd, Samaniego-Picota M, Kasper EK, Clark AM, Czader M, Rohde C, et al. Complement Deposition in Early Cardiac Transplant Biopsies Is Associated with Ischemic Injury and Subsequent Rejection Episodes. Transplantation. 1999;68(6):894–900.

102. Hammond EH, Yowell RL, Nunoda S, Menlove RL, Renlund DG, Bristow MR, et al. Vascular (Humoral) Rejection in Heart Transplantation: Pathologic Observations and Clinical Implications. J Heart Transplant. 1989;8(6):430–43.

103. Lones MA, Czer LS, Trento A, Harasty D, Miller JM, Fishbein MC. Clinical-pathologic Features of Humoral Rejection in Cardiac Allografts: A Study in 81 Consecutive Patients. J Heart Lung Transplant. 1995;14(1 Pt 1):151–62.

104. Loupy A, Cazes A, Guillemain R, Amrein C, Hedjoudje A, Tible M, et al. Very Late Heart Transplant Rejection Is Associated with Microvascular Injury, Complement Deposition and Progression to Cardiac Allograft Vasculopathy. Am J Transplant. 2011;11(7):1478–87.

105. Mollnes TE. Complement and Biocompatibility. Vox Sang. 1998;74 Suppl 2:303–7.

106. Mollnes TE. Biocompatibility: Complement as Mediator of Tissue Damage and as Indicator of Incompatibility. Experimental and Clinical Immunogenetics. 1997;14(1):24–9.

107. Williams JM, Holzknecht ZE, Plummer TB, Lin SS, Brunn GJ, Platt JL. Acute Vascular Rejection and Accommodation: Divergent Outcomes of the Humoral Response to Organ Transplantation. Transplantation. 2004;78(10):1471–8.

108. Haas M, Rahman MH, Racusen LC, Kraus ES, Bagnasco SM, Segev DL, et al. C4d and C3d Staining in Biopsies of ABO- and HLA-incompatible Renal Allografts: Correlation with Histologic Findings. Am J Transplant. 2006;6(8):1829–40.

109. Kirschfink M. Targeting Complement in Therapy. Immunol Rev. 2001;180:177–89.

110. Kim DD, Song WC. Membrane Complement Regulatory Proteins. Clinical Immunology (Orlando, Fla). 2006;118(2–3):127–36.

111. Gonzalez-Stawinski GV, Tan CD, Smedira NG, Starling RC, Rodriguez ER. Decay-accelerating Factor Expression May Provide Immunoprotection against Antibody-mediated Cardiac Allograft Rejection. J Heart Lung Transplant. 2008;27(4):357–61.

112. Wehner J, Morrell CN, Reynolds T, Rodriguez ER, Baldwin WM, 3rd. Antibody and Complement in Transplant Vasculopathy. Circ Res. 2007;100(2):191–203.

113. Kuo HH, Morrell CN, Baldwin WM, 3rd. Alloantibody Induced Platelet Responses in Transplants: Potent Mediators in Small Packages. Hum Immunol. 2012.

114. Labarrere CA, Woods JR, Hardin JW, Campana GL, Ortiz MA, Jaeger BR, et al. Early Prediction of Cardiac Allograft Vasculopathy and Heart Transplant Failure. Am J Transplant. 2011;11(3):528–35.

115. Libby P, Pober JS. Chronic Rejection. Immunity. 2001;14(4):387–97.

116. Tuzcu EM, Hobbs RE, Rincon G, Bott-Silverman C, De Franco AC, Robinson K, et al. Occult and Frequent Transmission of Atherosclerotic Coronary Disease with Cardiac Transplantation. Insights from Intravascular Ultrasound. Circulation. 1995;91(6):1706–13.

117. Gaudin PB, Rayburn BK, Hutchins GM, Kasper EK, Baughman KL, Goodman SN, et al. Peritransplant Injury to the Myocardium Associated with the Development of Accelerated Arteriosclerosis in Heart Transplant Recipients. Am J Surg Pathol. 1994;18(4):338–46.

118. Koskinen P, Lemstrom K, Bruggeman C, Lautenschlager I, Hayry P. Acute Cytomegalovirus Infection Induces a Subendothelial Inflammation (Endothelialitis) in the Allograft Vascular Wall. A Possible Linkage with Enhanced Allograft Arteriosclerosis. Am J Pathol. 1994;144(1):41–50.

119. Hosenpud JD, Morris TE, Shipley GD, Mauck KA, Wagner CR. Cardiac Allograft Vasculopathy. Preferential Regulation of Endothelial Cell-derived Mesenchymal Growth Factors in Response to a Donor-specific Cell-mediated Allogeneic Response. Transplantation. 1996;61(6):939–48.

120. Petrossian GA, Nichols AB, Marboe CC, Sciacca R, Rose EA, Smith CR, et al. Relation between Survival and Development of Coronary Artery Disease and Anti-HLA Antibodies after Cardiac Transplantation. Circulation. 1989;80(5 Pt 2):III122–5.

121. Smith SH, Kirklin JK, Geer JC, Caulfield JB, McGiffin DC. Arteritis in Cardiac Rejection after Transplantation. Am J Cardiol. 1987;59(12):1171–3.

122. Foerster A. Vascular Rejection in Cardiac Transplantation. A Morphological Study of 25 Human Cardiac Allografts. APMIS. 1992;100(4):367–76.

123. Hengstenberg C, Hufnagel G, Haverich A, Olsen EG, Maisch B. De Novo Expression of MHC Class I and Class II Antigens on Endomyocardial Biopsies from Patients with Inflammatory Heart Disease and Rejection Following Heart Transplantation. Eur Heart J. 1993;14(6):758–63.

124. Hosenpud JD, Everett JP, Morris TE, Mauck KA, Shipley GD, Wagner CR. Cardiac Allograft Vasculopathy. Association with Cell-mediated but Not Humoral Alloimmunity to Donor-specific Vascular Endothelium. Circulation. 1995;92(2):205–11.

125. Duquesnoy RJ, Kaufman C, Zerbe TR, Woan MC, Zeevi A. Presence of CD4, CD8 Double-negative and T-cell Receptor-Gamma-Delta-positive T

Cells in Lymphocyte Cultures Propagated from Coronary Arteries from Heart Transplant Patients with Graft Coronary Disease. J Heart Lung Transplant. 1992;11(3 Pt 2):S83–6.

126 Faulk WP, Labarrere CA, Nelson DR, Pitts D. Coronary Artery Disease in Cardiac Allografts: Association with Arterial Antithrombin. Transplant Proc. 1995;27(3):1944–6.

127 Labarrere CA, Pitts D, Nelson DR, Faulk WP. Coronary Artery Disease in Cardiac Allografts: Association with Depleted Arteriolar Tissue Plasminogen Activator. Transplant Proc. 1995;27(3):1941–3.

128 Koskinen PK. The Association of the Induction of Vascular Cell Adhesion Molecule-1 with Cytomegalovirus Antigenemia in Human Heart Allografts. Transplantation. 1993;56(5):1103–8.

129 Dong C, Redenbach D, Wood S, Battistini B, Wilson JE, McManus BM. The Pathogenesis of Cardiac Allograft Vasculopathy. Curr Opin Cardiol. 1996;11(2):183–90.

130 Herrington DM, Nanjee N, Achuff SC, Cameron DE, Dobbs B, Baughman KL. Dehydroepiandrosterone and Cardiac Allograft Vasculopathy. J Heart Lung Transplant. 1996;15(1 Pt 1):88–93.

131 Denfield SW. Cardiac Transplant Coronary Allograft Vasculopathy in Children: Achilles' Heel. Congenital Heart Disease. 2012;7(4):301.

132 Jeewa A, Dreyer WJ, Kearney DL, Denfield SW. The Presentation and Diagnosis of Coronary Allograft Vasculopathy in Pediatric Heart Transplant Recipients. Congenital heart disease. 2012;7(4):302–11.

133 Billingham ME. Histopathology of Graft Coronary Disease. J Heart Lung Transplant. 1992;11(3 Pt 2):S38–44.

134 Pucci AM, Forbes RD, Billingham ME. Pathologic Features in Long-term Cardiac Allografts. J Heart Transplant. 1990;9(4):339–45.

135 Berry GJ, Rizeq MN, Weiss LM, Billingham ME. Graft Coronary Disease in Pediatric Heart and Combined Heart-Lung Transplant Recipients: A Study of Fifteen Cases. J Heart Lung Transplant. 1993;12(6 Pt 2):S309–19.

136 Clausell N, Butany J, Molossi S, Lonn E, Gladstone P, Rabinovitch M, et al. Abnormalities in Intramyocardial Arteries Detected in Cardiac Transplant Biopsy Specimens and Lack of Correlation with Abnormal Intracoronary Ultrasound or Endothelial Dysfunction in Large Epicardial Coronary Arteries. J Am Coll Cardiol. 1995;26(1):110–9.

137 Luk A, Ahn E, Lee A, Ross HJ, Butany J. Recurrent Cardiac Amyloidosis Following Previous Heart Transplantation. Cardiovasc Pathol. 2010;19(4):e129–33.

138 Caines AE, Kpodonu J, Massad MG, Chaer R, Evans A, Lee JC, et al. Cardiac Transplantation in Patients with Iron Overload Cardiomyopathy. J Heart Lung Transplant. 2005;24(4):486–8.

139 Kuppahally SS, Hunt SA, Valantine HA, Berry GJ. Recurrence of Iron Deposition in the Cardiac Allograft in a Patient with Non-HFE Hemochromatosis. J Heart Lung Transplant. 2006;25(1):144–7.

140 Scott RL, Ratliff NB, Starling RC, Young JB. Recurrence of Giant Cell Myocarditis in Cardiac Allograft. J Heart Lung Transplant. 2001;20(3):375–80.

141 Chung L, Berry GJ, Chakravarty EF. Giant Cell Myocarditis: A Rare Cardiovascular Manifestation in a Patient with Systemic Lupus Erythematosus. Lupus. 2005;14(2):166–9.

142 Kong G, Madden B, Spyrou N, Pomerance A, Mitchell A, Yacoub M. Response of Recurrent Giant Cell Myocarditis in a Transplanted Heart to Intensive Immunosuppression. Eur Heart J. 1991;12(4):554–7.

143 Strecker T, Zimmermann I, Wiest GH. [Pulmonary and Cardiac Recurrence of Sarcoidosis in a Heart Transplant Recipient]. Dtsch Med Wochenschr. 2007;132(21):1159–62.

144 Luk A, Lee A, Ahn E, Soor GS, Ross HJ, Butany J. Cardiac Sarcoidosis: Recurrent Disease in a Heart Transplant Patient Following Pulmonary Tuberculosis Infection. Can J Cardiol. 2010;26(7):e273–5.

145 Schwarz ER, Czer LS, Simsir SA, Kass RM, Trento A. Amiodarone-induced QT Prolongation in a Newly Transplanted Heart Associated with Recurrent Ventricular Fibrillation. Cardiovascular Journal of Africa. 2010;21(2):109–12.

146 Miriuka SG, Langman LJ, Evrovski J, Miner SE, Kozuszko S, D'Mello N, et al. Thromboembolism in Heart Transplantation: Role of Prothrombin G20210A and Factor V Leiden. Transplantation. 2005;80(5):590–4.

147 Mullen JC, Lemermeyer G, Bentley MJ. Recurrent Aortic Dissection after Orthotopic Heart Transplantation. Ann Thorac Surg. 1996;62(6):1830–1.

148 Hollander SA, Yasnovsky JR, Reinhartz O, Chan F, Sandborg C, Hunt S, et al. Behcet's Disease and Heart Transplantation: A Word of Caution. J Heart Lung Transplant. 2010;29(11):1306–8.

149 Akhter SA, McGinty J, Konys JJ, Giesting RM, Merrill WH, Wagoner LE. Recurrent Primary Cardiac Malignant Fibrous Histiocytoma Following Orthotopic Heart Transplantation. J Heart Lung Transplant. 2004;23(12):1447–50.

150 Myruski KS, Manecke GR, Jr., Kotzur A, Wahrenbrock EA, Jamieson SW. Late Recurrence of Cardiac Sarcoma Presenting as Giant Pulmonary Artery Aneurysm. J Heart Lung Transplant. 2004;23(12):1445–6.

151 Bonatti H, Hoefer D, Rogatsch H, Margreiter R, Larcher C, Antretter H. Successful Management of Recurrent Epstein-Barr Virus-associated Multilocular Leiomyosarcoma after Cardiac Transplantation. Transplant Proc. 2005;37(4):1839–44.

Chapter 5: The Pathology of Lung Transplantation

Carol Farver and W. Dean Wallace

Introduction and Current State

The history of lung transplantation is relatively new with significant success occurring only in the past 20 years. The first human lung transplant was done by Hardy et al. in 1963 [1], but surgical complications, most commonly bronchial dehiscence and infection, precluded any significant long-term survival [2]. With improved surgical techniques and the advent of more effective immunosuppressant therapies such as cyclosporine, the 1980s saw considerable improvement in the long-term survival of these patients [3, 4].

Most transplants during this decade were performed in the setting of combined heart-lung transplantation [5, 6]. The first isolated lung transplantation series was published in 1990 by Cooper et al. and revealed 24 single- or bilateral-lung transplants with no hospital deaths. Since that time, the number of lung transplants has gradually increased to the current levels. Over the past 20 years, lung transplantation has emerged as a reasonable therapy for those patients with end-stage lung diseases. Over 39,000 lung transplants and 3,600 heart-lung transplants have been performed worldwide in adults [7] and 1,770 pediatric lung and heart-lung transplants [8] through June 2011. There are 178 centers worldwide that perform this procedure, with 50% of the transplants performed at the 30 busiest centers [7].

Most current lung transplants are bilateral lungs (20,831) with the remainder (13,271) being single-lung transplants [7]. Overall median survival for the most recent reporting year worldwide (2012) is 5.5 years and for those that survive at least one year, the median survival is 7.7 years with 53% of the lung transplants alive at five years [7]. The survival by disease is best in patients with cystic fibrosis (CF) at 7.1 years and worst in patients with idiopathic pulmonary fibrosis (IPF) at 4.3 years. Survival is usually related to disease-associated comorbidities and the age of the patient population referred for transplantation [9]. The better survival in the past decade can be best attributed to improved early survival with three-month survival improving from 81% to 90% and one-year survival improving from 70% to 81% [7, 10]. These improved outcomes are grounded in multiple changes in lung transplantation from better pre-screening and improved surgical procedures, to improved clinical care in the immediate postoperative time period, including intensive care management [10]. The predominant causes of death in the past 20 years have been over the long term due to non-cytomegalovirus (CMV) infections and graft failure for the first year and bronchiolitis obliterans syndrome (BOS) and non-CMV infections for the remainder [7].

Indications

The patients that are referred for lung transplantation are those with end-stage lung diseases where no effective medical therapeutic options are available. The most common pulmonary diseases to be transplanted are chronic obstructive pulmonary disease (COPD), usual interstitial pneumonia (UIP)/idiopathic pulmonary fibrosis (IPF), cystic fibrosis, pulmonary hypertension, and other interstitial lung diseases (Table 5.1). In each disease, the indications regarding referral for assessment for transplantation and timing of surgery varies with the availability of effective therapeutic options. For COPD, medical therapies for stabilizing the disease, including smoking cessation, decreasing environmental risk factors, and improved treatment of acute exacerbations due to infections [11], as well as surgical therapies such as lung volume resection surgery (LVRS), have improved survival in these patients without need for transplantation [12]. For IPF, similarly effective therapies have not been found; thus, lung transplantation has been increasing in these patients relative to COPD in the last few years and is now the most common cause for lung transplantation in the United States [9].

Allocation

In the first years of lung transplantation, the Organ Procurement and Transplantation Network (OPTN) allocated lungs for transplantation only to heart-lung transplant candidates. However, in 1990, OPTN amended these policies to include provisions for the allocation of donor lungs to isolated lung transplant candidates. The requirements for a patient to qualify for a donor lung included ABO match, the amount of time that candidates had accumulated on the waiting list, and location of the donor with local organ procurement organization (OPO) receiving first priority, then expanding to include a 500-nautical-mile concentric zone around the donor hospital [13].

In 2005, as increasing demand for lung transplantation overwhelmed the supply of donor lungs, the wait-time on lung transplant lists increased. With this, the federal government mandated the introduction of a new lung allocation system. The Organ Procurement and Transplantation Network (OPTN) changed the policy for lung allocation for transplantation from a system that allocated donor lungs based on waiting time to a system that allocated lungs based on lung allocation score (LAS). This model used medical urgency (risk for death without transplantation) and "net transplant benefit"

Table 5.1 Indication for Adult Lung Transplants Performed January 1995–June 2011

Diagnosis	Single Lung (n = 13,271) No. (%)	Bilateral/double (n = 20,831) No. (%)	Total (N = 34,102) No. (%)
COPD/emphysema	6,048 (45.6)	5,539 (26.6)	11,587 (34.0)
Pulmonary fibrosis			
Idiopathic	4,430 (33.4)	3,495 (16.8)	7,525 (23.2)
Other	498 (3.8)	659 (3.2)	1,157 (3.4)
Cystic fibrosis	219 (1.7)	5,469 (26.3)	5.688 (16.7)
a_1-Antitrypsin deficiency	741 (5.6)	1,332 (6.4)	2,073 (6.1)
Pulmonary arterial hypertension	82 (0.6)	982 (4.7)	1,064 (3.1)
Bronchiectasis	54 (0.4)	891 (4.3)	945 (2.8)
Sarcoidosis	251 (1.9)	614 (2.9)	865 (2.5)
Obliterative bronchiolitis	91 (0.7)	260 (1,2)	351 (1.0)
Retransplant			
Obliterative bronchiolitis	259 (2.0)	254 (1.2)	513 (1.5)
Not obliterative bronchiolitis	166 (1.3)	191 (0.9)	357 (1.0)
Connective tissue disease	140 (1.1)	281 (1.3)	421 (1.2)
Lymphangioleiomyomatosis	122 (0.9)	241 (1.2)	353 (1.1)
Congenital heart disease	45 (0.3)	248 (1.2)	293 (0.9)
Cancer	6 (0.0)	28 (0.1)	34 (0.1)
Other	119 (0.9)	347 (1.7)	466 (1.4)

COPD, chronic obstructive pulmonary disease.
(from Christie JC, et al., JHLT 2012; 10:1073–1086)

among approximately a dozen other factors to generate predictions of one year of survival with and without lung transplantation [14]. The LAS is calculated on the basis of survival of these predictions and each patient is given a score normalized to a 0–100 scale. Since the introduction of this new system in 2005, the number of actively listed patients has decreased to one-half of the pre-LAS level and wait time to transplantation has decreased from two to three years prior to this system to a current wait time of 35–200 days [14].

Donor Lungs

The donor pool of lungs available for transplantation has increased over the past decade as the selection criteria for donor lungs has been expanded. Prior to 1993, inclusion criteria for lung donation included an ABO blood group matched, and bilateral and single lungs from cadaveric donation after brain death (DBD) [15]. The "ideal" donor lung selection criteria included lungs from donors <55 years of age, of appropriate size, clear chest radiographs, <20 pack-year smoking history, absence of chest trauma, no evidence of aspiration or sepsis, absence of purulent secretions at bronchoscopy, absence of organisms on sputum Gram stain, and no history of primary pulmonary disease or active pulmonary infection [16, 17]. These criteria were based mostly on the belief that only the best lung would do without significant data to support this practice [18].

Since then, a variety of series have established that previously defined "marginal" or "extended criteria" lungs can be successfully transplanted without compromising long-term survival of the graft [18, 15]. Current suggestions for revision of the guidelines for donor lung selection have included lungs from the following: 1) Age <70 years, 2) ABO blood group compatible, 3) donation after brain death or donation after cardiac death donor, 4) approximate size match with minor surgical trimming or lobectomy as needed, minor diffuse, and moderate focal chest radiographic changes if stable/improving function, 5) tobacco history <40 pack-years, 6) chest trauma not relevant if good function 7) aspiration or minor sepsis acceptable if good, stable/improving function, 8) organism on Gram stain and ventilation time not relevant, and 9) primary donor pulmonary disease not acceptable, unless asthma [15].

In the future, expansion of the donor lung pool may also come from two other sources: 1) lobar donors, both cadaveric and living-related donors, especially for use in urgent lifesaving pediatric lung transplantation, and 2) lungs resuscitated for use using *ex vivo* lung perfusion (EVLP) methods [19, 20]. Though there is only early data that supports the use of EVLP-resuscitated lungs, some large studies have suggested at least equivalent outcomes for patients given EVLP-resuscitated donor lungs [20].

Explant Lung Evaluation

The role of the pathologist in the immediate post-operative time period is to pathologically evaluate the explanted lung with two major objectives in mind. First, the pathologist should confirm the pre-operative clinicopathologic diagnosis of the explanted lung. Most patients will have had either transbronchial or surgical biopsies prior to transplantation that may have been evaluated by both the referring pathologist in and the pathologist at the transplant referral center. These pre-operative pathologic evaluations are important to assure that the patient receives the appropriate therapy and accurate prognostications regarding the likely timeline for the clinical course of the patient in the pre-transplant time period. These pre-operative pathologic evaluations, though limited by the amount of tissue, are, nonetheless, usually quite accurate. In the author's (CF) experience of evaluating over 740 transplanted lungs, there were major discrepancies between pre- and post-transplant pathologic diagnosis in less than 4% of the cases. Nonetheless, careful and methodical evaluation of the explant is important. Most pathologists will inflate the explants with formalin and fix overnight in a large volume of formalin to assure optimal gross and microscopic evaluation. Photographs are essential to have on record, given the importance of gross pathology in establishing many of the fibroinflammatory diseases of the lung. The number of microscopic sections needed is determined at the time of the gross evaluation of the explant and hematoxylin and eosin stains as well as connective tissue stains are most useful.

The second objective in the evaluation of the explanted lung is to define other diseases in the explanted lung that might affect the post-operative clinical course. These include histologic evidence of active infections (granulomas, viral inclusions, or acute pneumonia patterns), as well as unexpected malignancies that may have been obscured by the advanced parenchymal disease on pre-operative imaging studies. For malignancies, the literature reports a rate of 3%–4% in explanted lungs, the overwhelming majority of which are carcinomas [21, 22] (also see following section: Recurrent Disease in the Lung Allograft).

For either infections or malignancies, post-operative clinical management may be affected. For infections, antibiotic therapies may be needed given the patient's new immunocompromised state, or, in the case of malignancies, either further staging work-up for lung primary neoplasms or further clinical work-up for those thought to be metastases to the lung may be needed. Given these possibilities, careful examination of the lung parenchyma for masses and evaluation of the surgical bronchial and vascular margins should be routine for each explanted lung, regardless of history.

Early Complications of Lung Transplantation

Primary Graft Dysfunction (Ischemic-Reperfusion Injury)

Primary graft dysfunction (PGD) is a form of severe ischemia/reperfusion injury in the newly transplanted lung and is a leading cause of immediate post-transplantation morbidity and mortality [23, 24]. Clinically, patients develop increasing hypoxemia and progressive radiographic pulmonary infiltrates with a known etiology [25]. PGD, also referred to by a variety of names including ischemia-reperfusion edema, noncardiogenic pulmonary edema, and post-transplantation acute respiratory distress (ARDS), is defined by a decreasing Pa_{O2}/F_{iO2} ratio in the presence of chest infiltrates at varying time points post-surgery [25, 24]. The extent of this decrease has been shown to predict long-term morbidity and mortality of the lung allograft. Thus, in an effort to standardize this definition and to more accurately define these outcomes, the ISHLT has defined a protocol for when these measurements are done in an effort to establish outcome definitions in clinical studies [26].

PGD manifests pathologically as diffuse alveolar damage (DAD) and pulmonary edema. Studies examining the pathogenesis suggest that in the early phase of the disease, donor macrophages and lymphocytes cause a release of free radicals that result in endothelial injury and pro-inflammatory agents, which, in turn, recruit circulating recipient neutrophils and lymphocytes that escalate the pathologic process [27]. Efforts going forward are focusing on finding specific molecular or biomarkers in either the bronchoalveolar lavage fluid (BALF) or in the tissue samples of the donor lung that will predict those patients that may be at risk for developing PGD. The most significant short and long-term morbidity in those patients that survive PGD is the development of bronchiolitis obliterans syndrome (BOS) [7].

Hyperacute Rejection

Hyperacute rejection (HAR) is a rare event in lung transplantation with six cases reported in the literature [28, 29, 30, 31, 32]. Clinically, the patients have done very poorly, with five of the six reported patients dying within two weeks of transplant [30]. The mechanism of injury is a result of high levels of donor-specific antibodies (DSAs) in the recipient that attack the donor lung in the minutes and hours post-transplantation. This causes antibody-antigen complexes binding to the endothelium, activation of complement, and massive vascular injury to the new lung (see Antibody-mediated Rejection section below). The reported pathologic pattern of injury in these patients is thought to be similar to that seen in AMR, i.e., diffuse alveolar damage with neutrophilic infiltrates and endothelial injury as manifested by thrombi formation [28, 29, 33]. Immunoglobulin deposition in the alveolar septae, vessels, and alveolar macrophages has been reported [28].

With improved pre-transplant crossmatch screening guidelines and increasingly sophisticated immunologic methodology [34], it is likely that this complication will remain very rare in the future.

Airway Complications

In the early years of lung transplantation, airway complications, predominantly anastomotic necrosis, and dehiscence were major complications in the post-operative period [35]. With the advances in surgical procedures and post-operative care, the incidence of anastomotic complications in the transplanted lung airway has diminished. Currently, the incidence of airway complications in lung transplantation is 7–18% [35, 36] with no difference in survival of those patients with and without airway complications [36, 35]. These complications are the result of a number of insults that the donor bronchus receives before, during, and after the transplant surgery. Graft preservation, donor bronchus ischemia, the surgical anastomotic technique, infection, and immunosuppression may all contribute [35]. The most common complication from these myriad of insults is airway stenosis [37, 38], which can occur either at, or in rare instances, distal to the anastomosis. When distal complications occur, they are most commonly in the bronchus intermedius due to its susceptibility to ischemia during the transplant surgery [36, 37]. Infections may involve either the entire airway or only the anastomotic site. These include bacterial infections that may be the result of organisms present in the donor airway prior to transplantation [36] and fungal infections, commonly *Aspergillus sp*, that are especially destructive and may require aggressive therapy including debridement [38, 39]. Finally, though immunosuppression has long been thought to increase airway complications, based on large retrospective studies, most now agree that though sirolimus, a rapamycin derivate, has been shown to have a high rate of severe airway complications in new lung transplants, steroids are not a risk factor in airway complications [40, 36].

Pathologic biopsies from these proximal airways may be done to assess the site for necrosis secondary to ischemia and for infections. This tissue commonly contains abundant granulation tissue in the early post-operative period, and, as healing occurs, this is replaced by a reparative mucosa with squamous metaplasia (see Figure 5.1). *Aspergillus* hyphae can be found (see Infections) and tissue organismal stains such as Grocott's methanimine silver (GMS) or Periodic acid Schiff (PAS) for fungal organisms are recommended.

Rejection in Lung Transplant Patients

Acute Cellular Rejection

Acute cellular rejection (ACR) in the lung is a result of the immune reaction of recipient lymphocytes recognizing as non-self the donor antigens on the surface of the lung allograft. These antigens are called major histocompatibility proteins (MHC) and are highly variable surface antigens. In humans, these antigens are referred to as human leucocyte antigens (HLA) and this recipient-donor mismatch can cause an immune response and tissue injury that manifests as lymphocyte aggregates within epithelial (airway) and endothelial (vessels) structures in the transplanted lung [41]. Solid organ transplantation became possible after the discovery of immunosuppression therapy that could suppress this response. However, solid organs, in general, and the lung, in particular, are not entirely protected from this immune injury.

The lung, compared to other organs, has a high incidence of acute cellular rejection, with the reported incidence in the first year post-transplantation ranging from 36%–55% [42, 43, 44] compared to the heart with 40% [45], the liver with <20% [46], and the kidney with 11% [47]. However, episodes of acute cellular rejection are rarely fatal in lung transplant patients, though their long-term effects on the lung may be associated with chronic rejection of the airways and vessels and could contribute to graft failure [48, 49]. Thus, close evaluation of the lung allograft for acute cellular rejection is required to assure adequate immune therapy and optimizing of the life of the allograft.

The clinical presentation of ACR has a wide range of symptoms from a relative asymptomatic presentation, to one with cough, which may be productive, dyspnea and fever, and, in the most severe cases, the patient may suffer acute respiratory distress [50]. Radiologic imaging of lung transplant patients with ACR by biopsy may reveal a variety of findings including ground-glass opacities, pleural effusions, and septal thickening [51]. However, overall, both clinical and radiologic imaging findings are not helpful in discriminating ACR from other processes [52].

Because of this potential for graft injury and the nonspecific clinical findings for ACR, lung transplant patients undergo routine monitoring of the lung for pathologic signs of acute rejection. Bronchoscopic biopsy is the main diagnostic tool used to evaluate the allograft for acute rejection and its sensitivity to detect rejection if present is greater than 80% [53]. Through this procedure, routine histologic samples are obtained and, when needed, cytological specimens can also

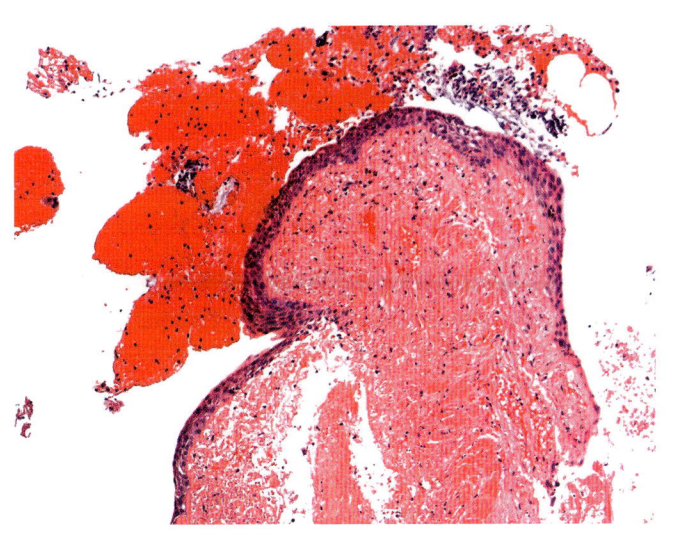

Figure 5.1 Subacute anastomotic site. The surface epithelium is squamous consistent with a metaplasia from previous injury and repair to the site. Also present is evidence of ongoing acute inflammation (Hematoxylin and eosin stain; original magnification 100x).

be acquired. These are then evaluated primarily for evidence of rejection and infection.

Appropriate technical handling of the transplant biopsies is important to obtain optimal information from the tissue and recommendations for this have been standardized in the ISHLT classification system [54]. The biopsies should be fixed in buffered formalin and undergo paraffin embedding. Paraffin tissue sections are cut and placed on microscopic glass slides (two to three sections/slides; three total slides) and stained with routine hematoxylin and eosin stains. Two additional slides are cut to be used, if needed, for a silver stain to evaluate for fungal organism, including *Pneumocystic jiroveci*, and the other for elastic fibers to highlight evidence of fibrosis, a marker of chronic rejection, especially in the airways. Additional studies for other infectious organisms, including immunohistochemical studies for cytomegalovirus (CMV) or Epstein-Barr virus (EBV), can be performed if clinically needed. Finally, most institutions may use either immunohistochemical or immunofluorescence staining for C4d in cases where morphology is suspicious for antibody-mediated rejection (AMR).

The number of tissue fragments needed in the biopsy for an adequate evaluation for the presence of rejection is not defined by the current working formulation (Revision of the Lung Rejection Study Group (LRSG) Working Formulation, 2007). However, the original 1990 Working Formulation and its successor in 1997 recommended that five pieces of alveolated lung or at least 100 alveoli are needed to adequately evaluate for the presence of rejection and that standard is continued by most centers today [55]. For those biopsies that have insufficient tissue for evaluation, a definitive diagnosis on the presence of absence of rejection is usually not given (see below).

Surgical Biopsy

Surgical biopsies are a less common diagnostic procedure than a transbronchial biopsy in lung transplant patients, despite their improved diagnostic yield. Large transplant centers report the incidence of surgical biopsies in this patient population as relatively low at 10%–41% [56], yet studies have shown that valuable treatment information is gained from invasive biopsies (open or video-assisted). Burdett et al. report in a retrospective study of 442 recipients that 51 invasive biopsies were performed in 45 patients and provided new, unsuspected diagnoses in 37% of the patients and confirmed the suspected clinical diagnosis in 47%. Further, in 57% of the cases, the information provided was clinically useful and led to a change in therapy [57]. Others have found less convincing results. Chaparro et al. found a benefit only beyond the 45-day post-transplant period [56] and Weill et al. found it helpful only when patients were undergoing a significant deterioration [51]. Useful information was found most often in patients with discrete lesions on imaging studies such as post-transplant lymphoproliferative disorders (PTLD) [57] and reported complications were minor and relatively uncommon, ranging from 11%–21%. No patient deaths directly related to the procedures were reported in any of the studies. Overall, invasive biopsies may provide clinically useful information in this patient population and should be handled similarly to TBBs,

including routine stains (hematoxylin and eosin), elastic stains, and tissue organismal stains when pathologically indicated. In addition, if mass lesions are present, additional tissue may be triaged for flow cytometric immunophenotypic analysis if PTLD is in the differential diagnosis.

Pathologic Grading of ACR

The classification system used to grade histologic rejection in these biopsies was defined initially by the Lung Rejection Study Group of the ISHLT in 1990 and is now in its third version [54]. The original working formulation, developed by pathologists in active lung transplantation centers, allows for the comparison of outcomes data among these institutions and is simple, reproducible, and an easily taught system. This original schema, which used a grading system of A and C for vascular rejection and B and D for airway rejection, was adopted by most of the centers and used for the subsequent five years with considerable success. In 1995, the grading schema was expanded to respond to new developments in the field. This second working formulation, published in 1996, emphasized the commonly held belief by pathologists at many large transplant centers based on their accumulated experience that the pathologic data needed to be interpreted within a broad clinical context to provide the optimum patient care. More specifically, infection and other sources of inflammation in the biopsy tissue needed to be excluded clinically for more accurate and reproducible grading [54].

The most recent revision of this grading system occurred in 2007 and continues to be used today (Table 5.2). The major

Table 5.2 Revised Working Formulation for Classification and Grading of Pulmonary Allograft Rejection

A: Acute rejection
Grade 0—none
Grade 1—minimal
Grade 2—mild
Grade 3—moderate
Grade 4—severe
B: Airway inflammation
Grade 0—none
Grade 1R—low-grade
Grade 2R—high-grade
Grade X—ungradeable
C: Chronic airway rejection—obliterative bronchiolitis
0—absent
1—present
D: Chronic vascular rejection—accelerated graft vascular sclerosis

"R" denotes revised grade to avoid confusion with 1996 scheme.
(From Stewart S, et al., JHLT 2007; 26:1229–1242.)

The Pathology of Lung Transplantation

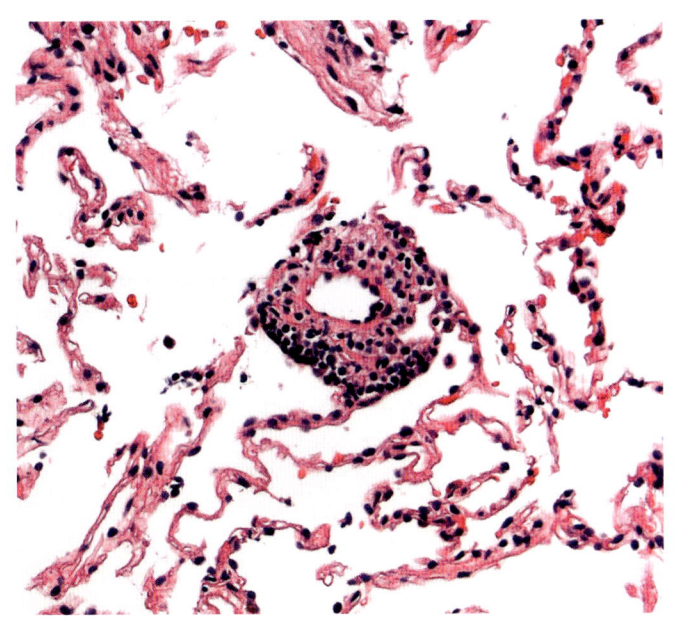

Figure 5.2 Minimal acute cellular rejection – Grade A1. Benign lymphocytes are in two to three layers encircling a small vessel (Hematoxylin and eosin stain; original magnification 200x).

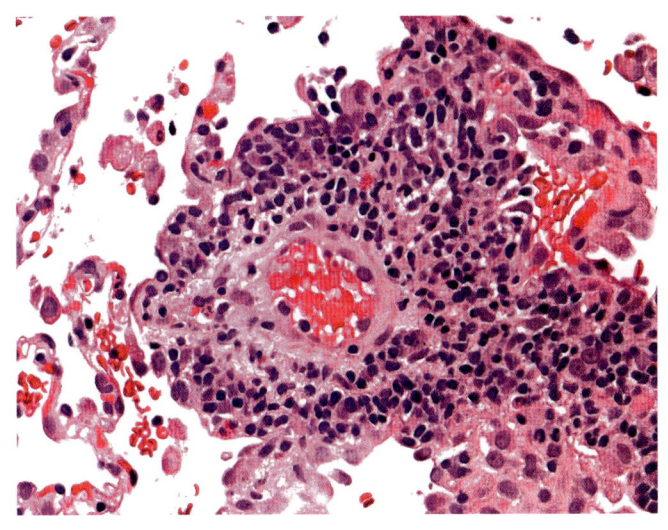

Figure 5.3 Mild acute cellular rejection – Grade A2. Benign lymphocytes with scattered activated and more plasmacytoid variants are present in multiple layers around a vessel. Eosinophils are part of the perivascular infiltrate and reactive endothelial cells consistent with endothelialitis are seen in the cross-section of the vessel (Hematoxylin and eosin stain; original magnification 400x).

changes in this document were the revision of the acute airway rejection grading system from a four-tier system (B1–B4) to a two-tier system with low-grade and high-grade and the grading of chronic airway rejection (C) without reference to the presence of inflammation. Finally, though recommendations were made for the pathologic evaluation of AMR, there was no consensus as to its role or diagnostic criteria in lung allograft rejection [54].

Acute cellular rejection in the lung is graded using two scales, A for acute cellular rejection, referring to acute cellular vascular rejection, and B for airway inflammation, referring to acute cellular airway rejection. A change from the previous working formulation is that the latter, grade B, is not labelled definitely as rejection in the latest working formulation, since some argue that given the overlap of morphologic features of acute cellular airway rejection with other etiologic influences such as infection, a more broad term of "airway inflammation" should be used [54]. However, in the absence of definitive infectious etiologies, this B grade refers to acute cellular airway rejection. Acute cellular rejection in the perivascular area is usually accompanied by rejection in the airways, especially in cases of moderate and severe cellular rejection [58], but ACR is the clinical trigger that prompts therapy even in the absence of airway rejection.

Acute Cellular Vascular Rejection

Acute cellular vascular rejection is graded on an A0–A4 scale, each increment representing an increasing amount of inflammation, first surrounding the vessels and then infiltrating out into the alveolar walls. The infiltrate is composed of lymphocytes, some with reactive faintly eosinophilic or "transformed" nuclei, macrophages, eosinophils, and neutrophils, the latter two acute inflammatory cell populations usually seen only in grade A2 and above. A diagnosis of ACR has no minimal number of vessels involved, requiring only a single vessel to show histologic evidence of rejection. Veins and venules are more commonly involved than arteries and arterioles. Finally, though the ACR may include a spectrum of grades, the grade given to the biopsy represents the highest grade present in the tissue.

Grade A0 (No Acute Rejection) is the grade given to the biopsy when no acute rejection is seen and adequate tissue is available for grading. Grade A1 (Minimal Acute Rejection) indicates the presence of lymphocytes encircling the vessels in layers two to three cells thick in the adventitia (see Figure 5.2). Though previous working formulations have accepted incomplete vascular cuffing consistent with rejection, the most recent working formulation states that the infiltrate must completely surround the vessel [54]. Unlike higher grades of acute rejection, no eosinophils or neutrophils are seen in this grade. Though subtle, this pathology can usually be seen even at low magnification if the tissue is free of artifacts.

Grade A2 (Mild Acute Rejection) also has a mononuclear infiltrate around vessels containing lymphocytes, many activated and plasmacytoid variants, as well as eosinophils. The infiltrate is more prominent than in Grade A1 with cell layers of three to five cells thick and easily visible at low magnification (see Figure 5.3). There may be sub-endothelial involvement of these mononuclear cells (endothelialitis). In addition, though airway inflammation is not commonly see in Grade A1, it is commonly found coexisting with Grade A2 [59]. No extension of this mononuclear infiltrate into the alveoli is seen in this grade, which distinguishes it from Grade A3 and Grade A4.

Grade A3 (Moderate Acute Rejection) consists of a dense, mononuclear infiltrate cuffing the vessels with frequent eosinophils and neutrophils and a prominent endothelialitis. The infiltrate, by definition, must extend into the adjacent alveolar walls, involving airspaces and septa and, in some cases, can

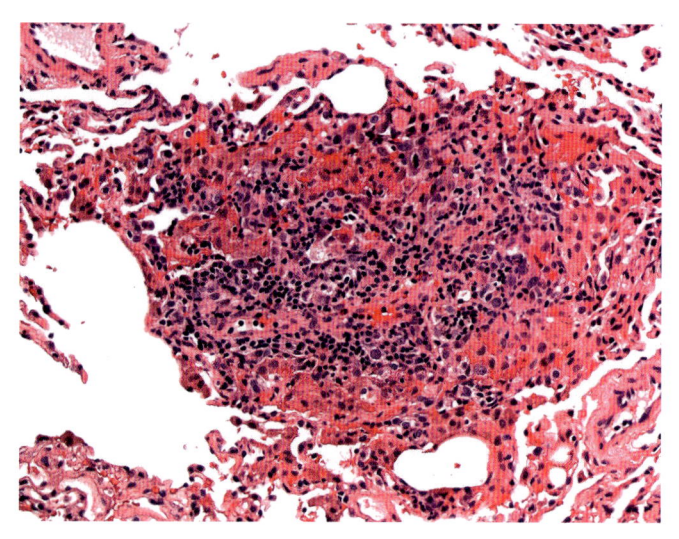

Figure 5.4 Moderate acute cellular rejection – Grade A3. The chronic inflammatory infiltrate in moderate acute rejection contains frequent eosinophils, and neutrophils may be present. In addition, this infiltrate spreads into the adjacent alveolar walls and causes some acute lung injury (Hematoxylin and eosin stain; original magnification 200x).

cause features of early acute lung injury, including reactive Type 2 pneumocyte hyperplasia and intra-alveolar fibrin. This infiltrate commonly extends into the alveolar space, resulting in clusters of alveolar macrophages, lymphocytes, and occasionally focal fibrin deposition, giving the lung parenchyma a more inflamed and atelectatic appearance (see Figure 5.4).

Grade A4 (Severe Acute Rejection), a grade seldom seen in transbronchial biopsies, is defined as diffuse involvement of the lung vessels and alveoli with mononuclear cell infiltrates and severe acute lung injury. The histologic features are those of diffuse interstitial pneumonia with intra-alveolar macrophages, fibrin, and perivascular inflammation with areas of both necrosis of the parenchyma and fibrinoid necrosis of the vessels (see Figure 5.5). The alveolar space may be filled with macrophages, fibrin, hemorrhage, and hyaline membranes and the abundance of neutrophils is characteristic of Grade A4 rejection. The vasculitis and perivascular prominence of the inflammation may be helpful in distinguishing Grade A4 acute rejection from diffuse alveolar damage. The latter has multiple etiologies, including infection or re-perfusion injury in the immediate post-transplantation period [60]. Both the reactive Type 2 pneumocyte hyperplasia and the endothelialitis are more prominent than that seen in Grade A3. With Grade A4 acute rejection, the inflammation commonly spills over into the adjacent large and small airways, resulting in infiltration of the epithelium with these inflammatory cells and ulceration [61]. Because of the abundance of acute inflammation including neutrophils, the primary differential diagnostic consideration to Grade A4 rejection is usually an infectious process. Organism stains and clinical information are often necessary to support the correct diagnosis.

For biopsies that have less than five pieces of tissue and are insufficient to adequately evaluate for rejection, a Grade of AX is given.

Airway Inflammation/Acute Cellular Airway Inflammation

Grading of the small airways for acute cellular airway rejection is based on the extent of a lymphocytic infiltrate of the airway and epithelium injury and is applicable to small airways only [54]. In the original 1990 Working Formulation, acute airway rejection was simply listed as present or absent, at the discretion of each institution [61]. In the 1996 revision, the grading of airway inflammation expanded to include B0 (no inflammation) to B4 (severe airway inflammation) [61]. However, not all members of the LRSG were convinced that the inflammation could be used solely to grade rejection, since it was also found in other settings (most notably infection); thus, the consensus was that this schema would need ongoing study. In the 2007 revision, the difficulty in discriminating the causes for the inflammation (predominantly rejection or infection) was officially acknowledged with the introduction of the generic term "airway inflammation" into the grading schema. In addition, because a consensus could not be reached regarding the criteria needed to reproducibly separate the airway inflammation into four separate grades, it was decided to collapse the grading schema down to a two-tier system, B1 R and B2 R (R for revised grade), retaining B0 for the absence of inflammation and BX for those biopsies in which the inflammation could not be adequately assessed for a number of reasons. These included cases in which no airways were present for evaluation, other inflammatory processes capable of producing the inflammation were present (such as infection), or tangential cuts of the tissue or crush artifact obscured the small airway present [54].

In airways with Grade B1 R, there are mononuclear cells forming patches or, in more prominent cases, a band within the submucosa of the small airways. The infiltrate may extend into the muscular wall of the bronchiole, but does not tend to involve the overlying bronchiolar epithelium and no significant epithelial injury is present (see Figure 5.6). Grade B2 R has a much more exuberant infiltrate and forms a dense band of more activated lymphocytes with plasmacytoid variants and significant numbers of eosinophils and neutrophils. This inflammation infiltrates the overlying bronchiolar epithelium, causing significant epithelial injury, taking the form of both apoptotic cells and areas of frank ulceration with cellular debris (see Figure 5.7). The acute inflammatory cells make it difficult to distinguish high-grade rejection from infection; however, a more prominent presence of neutrophils within the epithelium and lumen of the airway may be evidence of infection versus rejection. Viral bronchiolitis may induce a similar degree of airway-centered inflammation and epithelial injury. In these cases, careful review of the injured epithelial cells may reveal viral inclusions and immunohistochemistry studies, especially cytomegalovirus and herpes simplex virus, may demonstrate the viral inclusions.

Given the importance of the transbronchial biopsy in assessing rejection and dictating treatment, several studies have looked at the validity and reproducibility of the current classification system by assessing the interobserver variability. In general, these studies show that agreement between expert lung pathologists for acute rejection is variable from poor

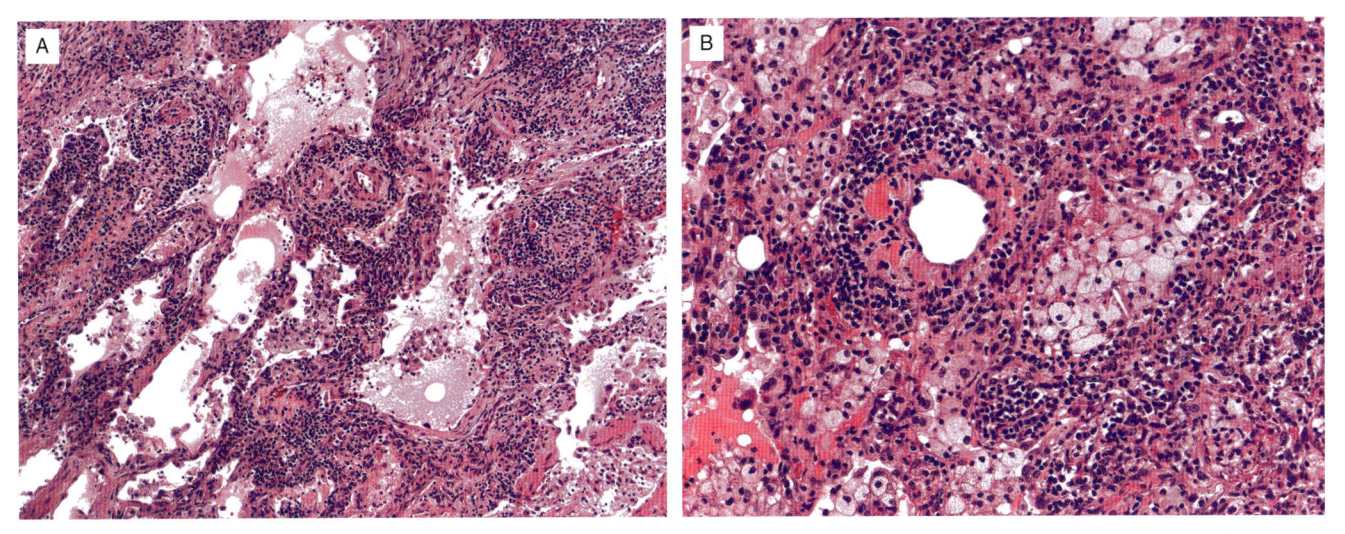

Figure 5.5 Severe acute cellular rejection. A: The lung shows diffuse involvement by an interstitial pneumonia with multiple vessels with a perivascular mononuclear cell infiltrate (Hematoxylin and eosin stain; original magnification 100x). B: Note the alveolar space filled with macrophages, fibrin and areas of neutrophilic infiltrate (Hematoxylin and eosin stain; original magnification 200x).

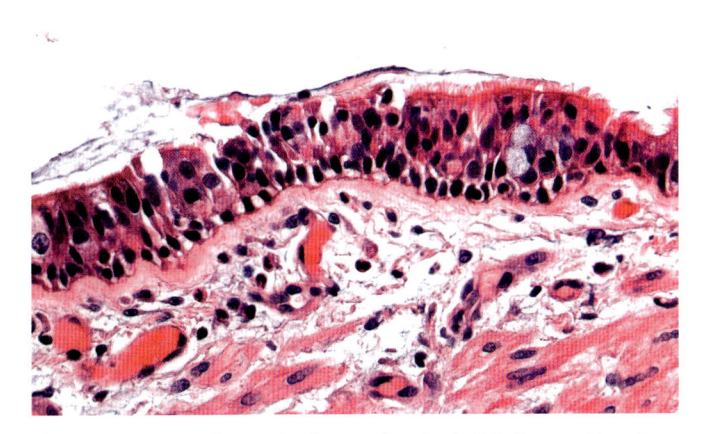

Figure 5.6 Airway inflammation, low-grade – Grade B1R. Scattered lymphocytes are present within the bronchiolar epithelium, but no significant epithelial injury is seen (Hematoxylin and eosin stain; original magnification 400x).

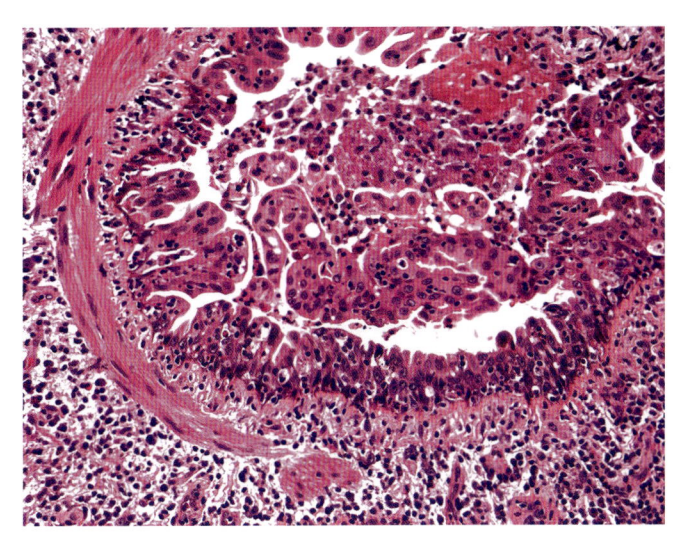

Figure 5.7 Airway inflammation, high-grade – Grade B2R. The chronic inflammation is quite exuberant with bands of activated lymphocytes and significant epithelial injury (Hematoxylin and eosin stain; original magnification 200x).

(kappa 0.183) [62] to moderate (kappa 0.47–0.79)[63, 64, 65] with most disagreement occurring for Grade A1 (minimal acute rejection) and most concurrence for Grade A2 (mild acute rejection). For airway inflammation, there was predominantly poor interobserver variability (kappa 0.035–0.46) [63, 65, 66] with significant concurrence occurring for Grade B0, no airway inflammation. These data argue for continued education to optimize and increase uniformity of the pathologic grading of acute rejection and for ongoing refinement of the current classification system to improve concordance among pathologists [62, 65].

BALF and ACR

The use of bronchoalveolar lavage (BAL) fluid analysis in monitoring rejection in the lung allograft remains an area of controversy. The evaluation of the various inflammatory cell populations in the lung, including those populating the alveoli and the interstitial compartment and the small and large airways becomes possible with bronchoscopy and bronchoalveolar lavage through the counting and immunophenotyping of inflammatory cells within the BALF. Through lavaging the lung allograft, it is estimated that over one million alveoli may be sampled [67], a considerably larger area of the lung than TBB can access. This would seem to give BAL a considerable advantage over TBB, given the patchy nature of rejection. However, though BAL is a primary tool used in assessment of the lung for infection [68] and is a common tool used when infection is suspected in lung transplantation patients [69], the promise of BAL as a more sensitive tool for diagnosing rejection has not been borne out for a number of reasons. First, the cellular composition of the BALF changes during the post-transplantation period. In the immediate aftermath of surgery, the total cell count is elevated, especially the neutrophils, probably due to a number of inflammatory insults including reperfusion injury [69, 70]. This cell count may remain elevated for years, making it difficult to establish a firm baseline with which to compare subsequent samples. Second, though acute rejection in the lung allograft is characterized by an increase in mononuclear inflammatory cells within the interstitium and the airspaces that increase with the grade of both acute vascular and airway rejection [54], granulocytes (eosinophils and neutrophils) also increase, [71] making it difficult to separate infection from rejection. Studies that compared the inflammatory cell findings in TBB specimens with those in BALF found the inflammatory cells in TBB are highly specific for rejection. However, the cellular changes in the BALF from lungs with rejection had increased proportions of lymphocytes in early rejection and neutrophils in later-occurring rejection, but were not specific for rejection [72, 73].

Finally, given the importance of T cells in rejection [74], studies that focused on subtypes of T cells in the BALF did show some correlation with CD4+ and CD8+ ratios with the presence of acute cellular rejection in the lung allograft [75] and with the development of chronic airway rejection [76, 43]. However, further studies to confirm these findings are needed before BALF is useful clinically in diagnosing rejection.

Antibody-mediated Rejection

Antibody-mediated rejection (AMR) results from injury to the allograft post-transplantation from anti-donor antibodies [77]. These donor-specific antibodies (DSAs) may be pre-formed and present pre-transplantation, arising from previous blood transfusions, pregnancy, or retransplant, or they may form *de novo* as new DSAs post-transplantation. In either case, these antibodies bind to the lung HLA class I or II, ABO blood group antigens (if ABO-incompatible transplantation has taken place), or, occasionally, non-HLA self-antigens [78, 79], usually on the endothelium of the microcirculation, the interface between the transplanted donor organ and the recipient blood, and activate the complement case that leads to the pathologic injury of the vessels of the organ [80]. In general, this injury is morphologically characterized by recruitment of leukocytes, endothelial cell lysis and death, and vascular thrombosis. Complement split products such as C4d can be markers of this injury, though the role of C4d in the lung remains unknown. Ultimately, the amount and type of DSAs present will determine the severity and duration of this injury and affect the prognosis of the transplanted organ [81, 82].

This form of allograft rejection has been shown to be clinically important in other solid organ transplants such as kidney and heart [83] and recent studies have reported that anti-HLA antibodies among lung transplant recipients decreases lung allograft survival [84, 85]. However, currently, there remains no consensus definition for AMR in the lung. In the 1996 working formulation, AMR was not in the classification or grading for lung rejection [61] and though the current 2007 working formulation includes a discussion of AMR, it concludes that the pathologic features for AMR in the lung are not yet definitive. Further, it introduces the term "capillary injury" (in place of capillaritis), stating that this may be the pattern of injury for AMR, but may also include a wider etiologic spectrum including infection and high grades of cellular rejection [54] adding further ambiguity to the definition.

The difficulty in defining AMR in the lung may be, in part, due to incomplete early studies. The working group from the National Conference to Assess Antibody-mediated Rejection in Solid Organ Transplantation has proposed a general classification system for humoral rejection that requires four necessary features for humoral rejection. These include detection of circulating HLA or donor-specific antibodies, C4d deposition in the allograft tissue, the presence of tissue pathology, and graft dysfunction [83] and most of the early studies did not study all four of these features. In those that reported tissue pathology, most reported an acute lung injury (ALI) pattern with neutrophils (see Figure 5.8 A) within alveolar septal capillaries or even definitive necrosis with evidence of pulmonary hemorrhage, all features at least suggestive of pulmonary capillaritis (see Figure 5.8 B) [86]. When C4d staining was performed, some found C4d deposition in lung allografts (see Figure 5.8 C) with this vascular pattern of injury [87, 88, 89], while others did not see C4d deposition when this vascular injury pattern was present [90]. These discrepancies may be a result of differing methodologies, difference in interpretation of the staining pattern, nonspecific staining of elastic tissue and fibrin, or the extremely low incidence of capillary-specific C4d-positivity in lung allograft biopsies.

More recently, the focus of study on AMR in the lung has been to follow the recommendations and construct a multi-disciplinary definition that includes clinical, immunologic, and pathologic criteria. With this, a clearer definition of AMR has begun to emerge. Most suggest that the tissue pathology of AMR in the lung is an ALI pattern with neutrophils in the septal capillaries [89, 90, 91, 92, 93, 94, 95, 96, 97]. Some have found the majority of biopsies reveal C4d + staining [91, 92, 93, 94, 97, 95, 98] and others found minimal or no staining for C4d [99]. Further, some report a lack of correlation of the presence of C4d staining and the presence of DSAs [96][93] and a lack of pathology in biopsies that may show either C4d or DSAs or both [100]. Finally, Yousem et al. compared the pathology of lung biopsies from lung transplant patients with ACR only and the pathology of lung biopsies from lung transplant patients with AMR (clinical graft dysfunction, DSAs, and C4d) and similar grades of ACR. He found that 3/23 AMR biopsies had capillaritis, but no ACR-only biopsies had capillaritis. Further, there was C4d staining in 74% of the biopsies from the AMR patients and C4d staining in 24% of the patient with ACR only with similar patterns of C4d staining (diffuse, multi-focal linear capillary pattern). These findings suggest that capillaritis may be a specific, but not sensitive, marker for AMR, while C4d staining may occur in lung biopsies, both in AMR as well as in high-grade ACR, and may not be specific for AMR in lung transplant biopsies [95].

In an effort to focus the future research efforts on AMR with the hope of bringing clarity to its multi-disciplinary definition, the Pathology Council of the International Society for Heart and Lung Transplantation (ISHLT) issued a summary statement with consensus points for pathologic diagnosis of pulmonary

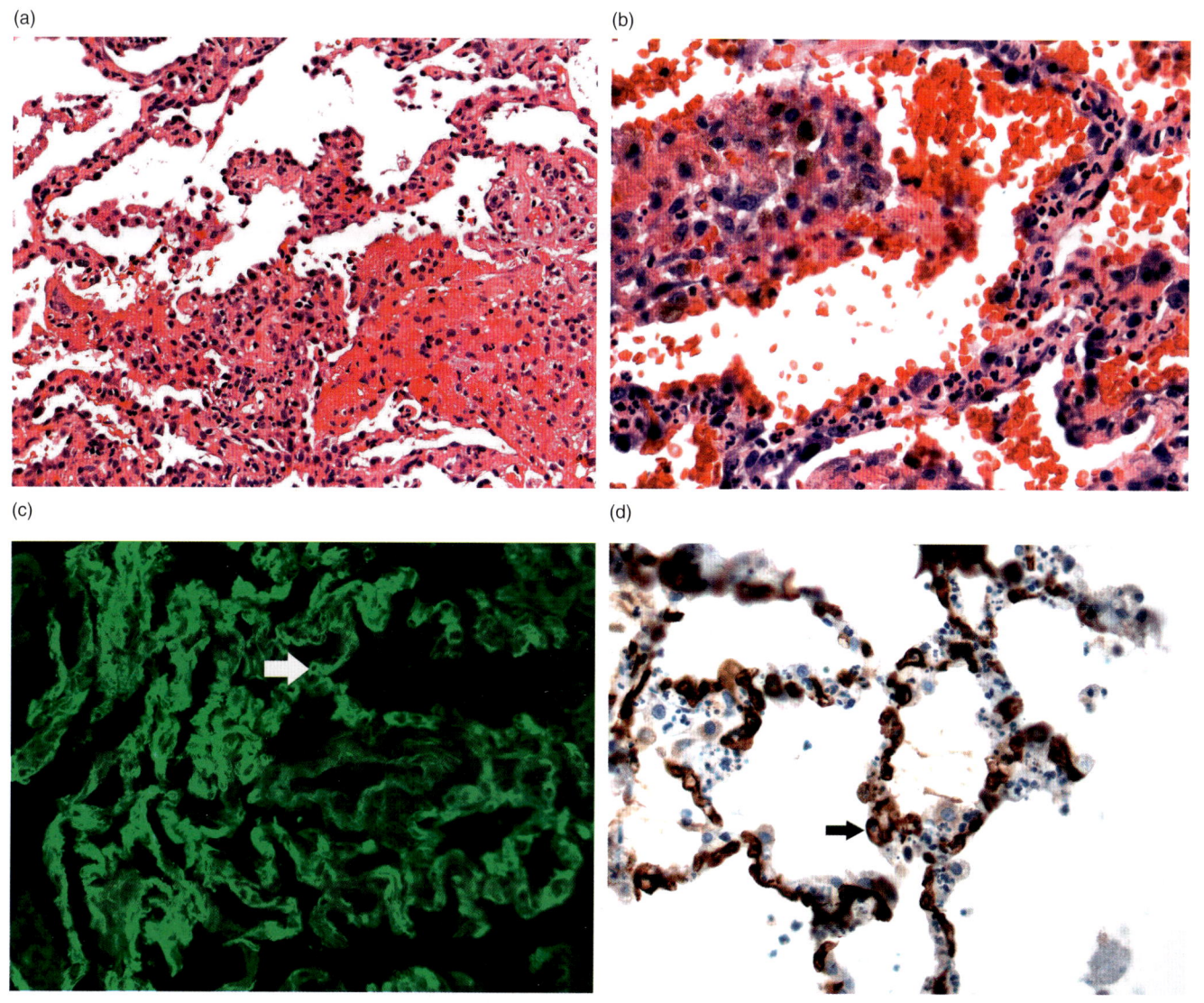

Figure 5.8 Antibody-mediated rejection. A. Acute lung injury with neutrophils. Alveolated lung shows acute lung injury with reactive Type 2 pneumocytes, intra-alveolar fibrin, and neutrophils within the septal capillaries (Hematoxylin and eosin stain; original magnification 200x). B. Capillaritis. The septal capillaries contain a marked neutrophilic infiltrate with necrosis of the capillary and hemosiderosis present in the adjacent alveolar space consistent with pulmonary hemorrhage (Hematoxylin and eosin stain; original magnification 400x). C. C4d Immunofluorescence. The fluorescent staining pattern is one of diffuse endothelial staining and "donut" type foci of capillary cross-sections (white arrow) (Original magnification 400x). D. C4d Immunohistochemistry. An antibody to C4d reveals diffuse capillary staining and cross-sectional staining (black arrow) of the capillary (Original magnification 400x).

antibody-mediated rejection [101]. In general, these six points recommend a multidisciplinary approach to the diagnosis that includes 1) clinical allograft dysfunction, circulation DSAs, pathologic findings; 2) histopathologic findings in AMR may be found in other settings including ACR, infection, graft preservation injury and drug reactions; 3) C4d staining should be done when certain histopathologic features are present, but the results of the staining need interpretation within a broad clinical context; 4) the presence of C4d staining must not connote a definitive diagnosis of AMR, i.e. "suggestive of"; 5) DSA studies should be drawn at the time of the biopsy or as close to that procedure as possible in order for meaningful correlation of the pathologic findings; and 6) centers should develop protocols to ensure future multi-center studies are possible[101]. Currently underway are large-scale multi-institutional studies with standardized protocols for tissue biopsy, DSA measurement, and C4d tissue staining with the hope of more conclusive data and a more definitive definition of AMR in the lung [102].

BALF and AMR

Only two studies have examined the role of BALF in the diagnosis of AMR. Girnita et al. evaluated soluble C4d with C4d fragment enzyme immunoassay and correlated the findings with tissue C4d deposition and anti-HLA donor-specific antibodies. They found positive correlation of soluble C4d with tissue C4d deposition and donor-specific antibodies, but the findings were not specific and a high false-positive result was found in the setting of CMV infection [99]. Miller et al. report a study of 26 lung transplant patients where analysis of BALF by enzyme immunoassay revealed elevated C4d in BALF correlated with anti-HLA antibodies. However, C4d elevations were also found in lung

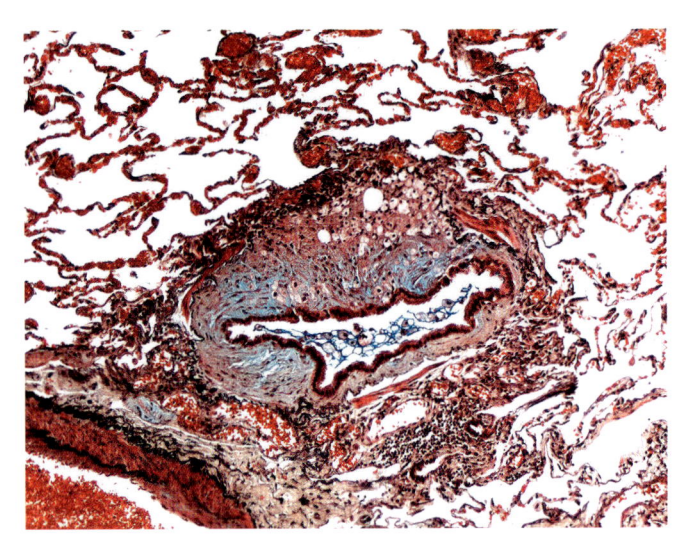

Figure 5.9 Chronic airway rejection, subtotal – Grade C1. There is significant narrowing of the small vessel by hyalinizing collagen in the subepithelial area with intact epithelium present (Movat stain; original magnification 100x).

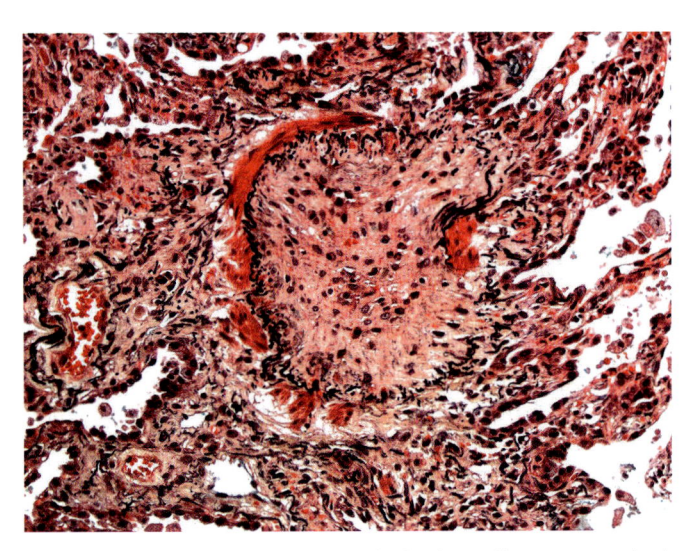

Figure 5.10 Chronic airway rejection, total – C1. The small airway is completely obliterated by collagen with loss of the bronchiolar epithelium (Movat stain; original magnification 100x).

transplantation with infection and in asymptomatic patients, suggesting that this may not be a unique finding in AMR [103].

Chronic Rejection

Airway

Chronic lung allograft dysfunction (CLAD) is a recently established term for all of the entities that give rise to the long-term dysfunction of the lung allograft that affects approximately 50% of lung transplant patients five years post-transplant [104]. These entities include restrictive allograft syndrome (RAS) and neutrophilic reversible allograft dysfunction (NRAD), characterized by a restrictive spirometric defect, and bronchiolitis obliterans syndrome (BOS), the most common form of CLAD, with obstructive pulmonary function pattern and air trapping on high resolution computed tomography [104]. The pathologic features of RAS and NRAD are not currently well-studied. The pathologic features of the BOS are known as constrictive or obliterative bronchiolitis (OB) and are the major limitation to long-term survival in the lung transplant patient [48]. Chronic airway rejection is a process by which collagenous type fibrosis occurs in the small airways as a sequela of the lymphocytic bronchiolitis. The lymphocytic infiltrate, which may be due to the airway inflammation of acute rejection [48, 49], results in cellular injury and death of the airway epithelium, leading to ulceration of the mucosa [105]. The subsequent fibrotic response is a result of the recruitment of fibroblasts into the airways and may be mediated via transforming growth factor–beta (TGF-β) overexpression in these fibroblasts [105]. This airway fibrosis may appear anywhere from a few months to several years after transplantation. The median time to presentation is 16–20 months [106]. This pathology is also quite patchy in the allograft and, therefore, the sensitivity of transbronchial biopsy (TBB) for the detection of chronic airway rejection at most centers ranges from 15%–40% [107] [44]. This sensitivity may increase with the number of tissue fragments and the experience of the bronchoscopist and the pathologist, but it remains a less sensitive measure than pulmonary function testing and it is more expensive and invasive. Therefore, surveillance TBBs for OB is no longer performed in most clinical transplant centers. Instead, a standardized formulation for the clinical diagnosis of OB or bronchiolitis obliterans syndrome (BOS), developed by the ISHLT and based on pulmonary function test results, is used to dictate therapy [2].

The pathology for chronic airway rejection is hyalinizing fibrosis comprised of type 3 collagen in the subepithelial area of the bronchiolar mucosa. This may be either concentric or eccentric and it gradually narrows (see Figure 5.9) and eventually obliterates the small airways (see Figure 5.10). As the fibrosis increases, the bronchiolar epithelium is lost and identification of the obliterated airway may be difficult. Connective tissue stains such as trichrome, elastic, or pentachrome stains are helpful in highlighting the elastica of the obliterated airway, as well as identifying evidence of early fibrosis. Mucostasis and/or foamy macrophages in or around these small airways may be evidence of early injury; however, dense fibrosis within the airway is needed for a definitive diagnosis [105]. Though previous Working Formulations considered the amount of chronic inflammation in the schema, the most recent grading system does not include this and consists of just two grades: Grade C0 if absent and Grade C1 if present.

Chronic inflammation, fibrosis, and eventually bronchiectasis may be present in large airways in lung allografts with both acute and chronic small airway rejection. These histologic findings may represent chronic injury from a number of insults that the allograft has suffered, including infection and aspiration, as well as rejection. Because these pathologic findings are not specific for rejection, they are not included in the 2006 Working Formulation, and are not graded as chronic airway rejection.

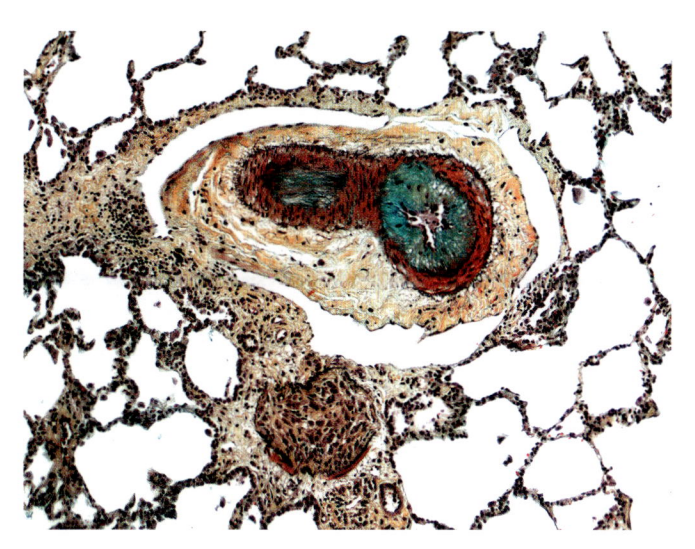

Figure 5.11 Chronic vascular rejection. An artery displays significant intimal fibrosis with early (blue) collagen deposition (Movat stain; original magnification 100x).

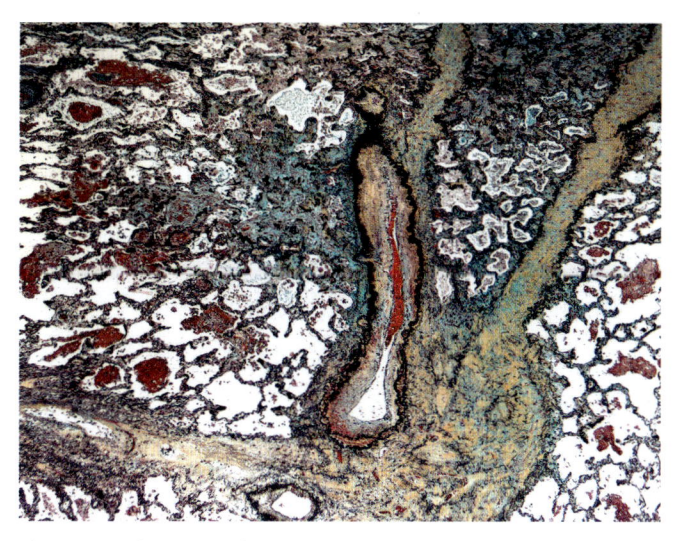

Figure 5.12 Chronic vascular rejection. A vein, outlined by black elastic fibers, is present within the interlobular septa and shows intimal fibrosis and luminal narrowing (Movat stain; original magnification 20x).

Vascular

The pathologic features of chronic vascular rejection have not received significant attention because the transbronchial biopsy does not reliably sample these lesions and the clinical significance of this pathology is not yet clear. However, a transplant-associated vasculopathy (TAV) in the arteries (see Figure 5.11) and veins (see Figure 5.12) of the lung has been described and is similar to those in other organs, including intimal fibrosis and variable transmural chronic inflammatory infiltrates. One report states that the intimal proliferation could be non-laminar eccentric and concentric and that the media of vessels can demonstrate mild extracellular matrix deposition with smooth muscle atrophy [108]. Grading chronic vascular rejection is similar to chronic airway rejection in that only its absence (Grade D0) or presence (Grade D1) is noted. The presence of intimal sclerosis in veins or venules is commonly seen in transplant transbronchial biopsies. These findings may form etiologies other than chronic rejection and should not be interpreted as chronic vascular rejection without evidence of pathology in the arteries or arterioles.

The concurrence of chronic airway and chronic vascular rejection is well-documented, leading to speculation regarding a causal link [109]. Recent research suggests that intimal fibrosis of the small vessels that supply the airways may correlate with the presence of OB. [110, 111] Because the high pressure bronchial circulation that supplies the oxygen to the lung is not reconnected during the transplantation procedure, the lung tissue, including the small airways, is more susceptible to hypoxic injury [112]. Further, there is some evidence that the loss of the bronchial circulation may lead to the destruction of the microvasculature, further compromising oxygenation in the lung allograft small airways, leading to epithelium injury, fibrosis, and eventually OB [113]. To support this hypothesis, some studies have documented reduction in small airway vasculature with the development of OB [114] and, further, in lungs where the bronchial circulation has been reconnected, there is a decreased incidence of OB [115].

Infections in Lung Transplant Recipients

Lung transplant patients are at significantly increased risk of pulmonary infections for a variety of reasons. As with all transplant organ recipients, lung transplant patients are immunocompromised by anti-rejection medications and as lung transplant recipients, they have specific mechanical problems including diminished mucociliary clearance and loss or reduction of the normal cough reflex from disruption of the normal neural connections to and from the lungs. These factors all lead to increased susceptibility to all forms of infections [54, 116, 117, 118].

The type of infection that occurs in the lung transplant patient is in part determined by the time frame in which it occurs relative to the time of transplantation [116]. Lung transplant candidates are often debilitated with limited respiratory function and ambulatory ability and may be immunocompromised by medication. Immediately post-transplant, the stress of major surgery and hospitalization predisposes to infection, the vast majority of which is bacterial in this setting.

As a major surgical procedure, lung transplantation predisposes patients to typical hospital-acquired (nosocomial) infections. In the first post-transplant month, patients are susceptible to typical nosocomial infections and the most common organisms are bacterial. From the end of the first month until the end of the sixth month, patients are generally under high levels of immunosuppression to prevent early-onset allograft rejection, and this is the period in which most fungal and viral infections occur. However, throughout the entire life of the transplant patient, the risk for fungal, viral, and other infections remains elevated above the normal population [54, 117, 119, 118].

After six months, immunosuppression is often reduced and infections tend to be community-acquired, but may be

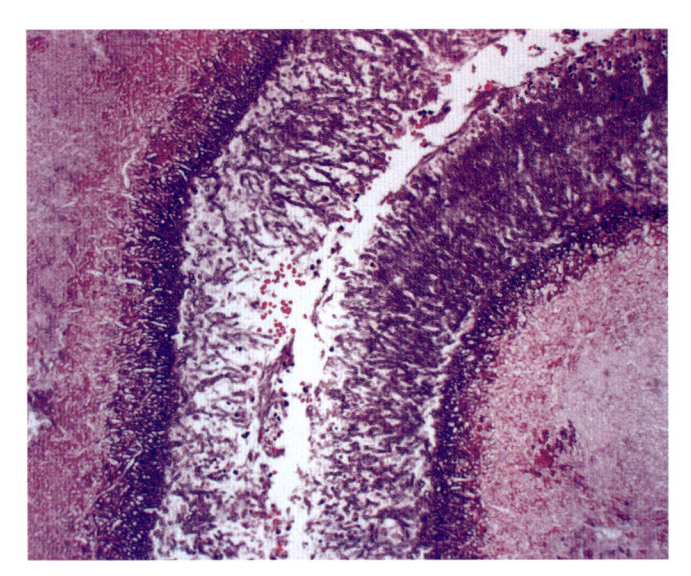

Figure 5.13 Area of clefting in mycetoma. Note the orderly and layered architecture of the fungal hyphae in the outer rim and disorderly clumping of organisms in the core (Periodic-acid Schiff stain; original magnification 200x).

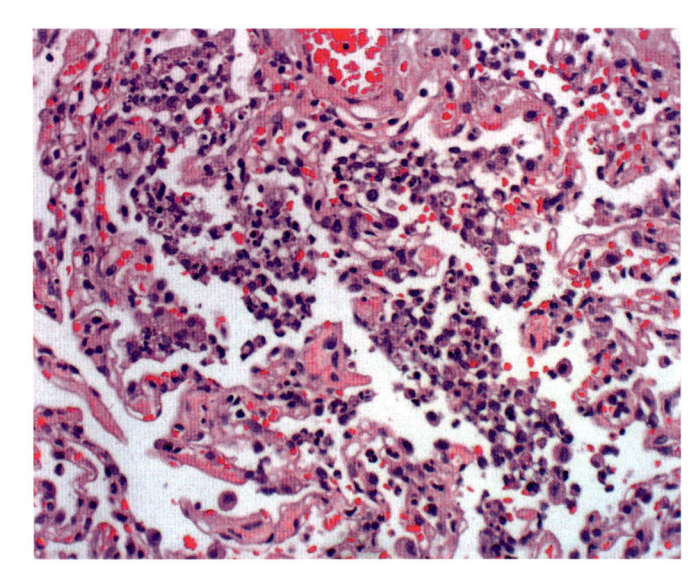

Figure 5.14 Acute bronchopneumonia. The alveolar air sacs are filled neutrophilic inflammation, but the alveolar walls are generally unremarkable (Hematoxylin and eosin stain; original magnification 400x).

inadvertently induced following treatment for late rejection. As an ironic corollary, acute and/or chronic rejection may be induced by CMV infection that appears to trigger the immune system [120, 121, 115]. It is a delicate clinical balance to offset the dangers of organ rejection while trying not to induce infection and vice versa.

Along with the time from transplant, the exposure history and geographic region the patient lives in may put the patient at risk for, and give diagnostic clues to, specific organisms.

Peri-operative Infections

Patients with significant architectural abnormalities of the lung parenchyma often have underlying organism colonization or infection at the time of transplantation. Cystic anomalies, especially in the setting of poor airflow, predispose to bacterial and fungal colonization. Common bacterial colonizers include *Pseudomonas*, *Burkholderia* and nontuberculous mycobacteria; fungal colonization often takes the form of a non-invasive fungus ball or mycetoma [122, 123, 117]. A mycetoma is composed of fungal hyphae within a cavity lined by bronchial epithelium and/or granulation tissue with acute and chronic inflammation (see Figure 5.13). Mycetomas and other noninvasive colonizing organisms may occur in any disease associated with cavitations such as cystic fibrosis, severe emphysema, primary ciliary dyskinesia, and lymphangioleiomyomatosis.

Thorough pathologic evaluation of the explanted lungs may uncover underlying colonization or low-grade infections that were previously undetected. One study found fungal infections in 5% of explanted lungs [124]. This is an important discovery as organisms in a latent stage, which may still be present in mediastinal lymph nodes, larger airways, or within the contralateral lung if the procedure was a unilateral transplant, may become active or more virulent as the patient becomes immunocompromised following the stress of major surgery and immunosuppression medications [123, 125]. Eradication of certain infections, such as *Staphylococcus aureus* and *Mycobacterium abscessus*, may reduce the risk of subsequent infectious complications in lung transplant recipients [126, 127].

First Month

In the first month after transplantation, the vast majority of infections are bacterial [128, 118]. Patients are evaluated for infectious complications by usual clinical parameters and infectious studies. Pathologic evaluation by transbronchial biopsy may reveal typical features of acute pneumonia if present (see Figure 5.14). The specific organism type can be classified by Gram stain if the bacteria are present; however, special stains to evaluate for organisms are generally not helpful for bacterial infections on the transbronchial biopsy unless the biopsy happened to sample the nidus of the infection. One helpful feature is the presence of sulfur granules which would indicate infection by *Actinomycetes* (see Figure 5.15). Otherwise, culture results may be necessary to prove the infection and determine organism type. It is important to remember antibiotics administered during the immediate post-transplant period may result in false negative culture results and clinicians may rely on the pathologist for diagnostic guidance [119, 118].

Histologic features of ischemia-reperfusion injury include acute lung injury with or without hyaline membranes and may overlap with acute pneumonia. If the biopsy is small or inadequate, it might not be possible for the pathologist to reliably determine if the acute injury process is infectious or not. The distinction can usually be made based on the degree of cellular inflammation and pattern of injury. Ischemia-reperfusion injury is generally diffuse, pauci-cellular, and neutrophils are only scattered throughout the alveolar walls and not concentrated in alveolar sacs [129, 130].

One to Six Months

After the initial post-transplant period, the incidence of bacterial infections declines and the incidence of opportunistic infections increases for at least the first six months. If there is

The Pathology of Lung Transplantation

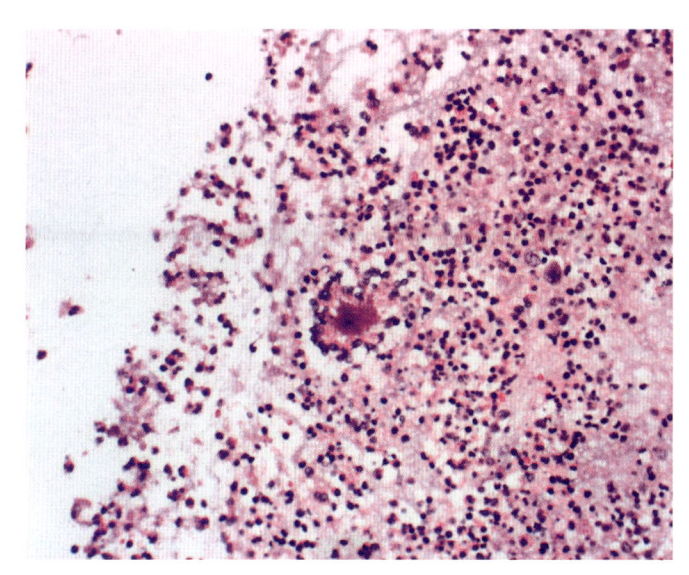

Figure 5.15 Splendore-Hoeppli effect (granular eosinophilic material with radiating neutrophils), consistent with *Actinomycetes*-associated sulfur granule in background of acute inflammation (Hematoxylin and eosin stain; original magnification 400x).

Table 5.3 Infections and Patterns of Injury in Transplanted Lungs

Infections	Patterns of Injury
Aspergillus	Mycetoma Airway colonization Colonization of anastomotic site Chronic necrotizing tracheobronchitis Granulomatous pneumonitis Invasive fungal pneumonia Diffuse alveolar damage
Candida	Airway colonization Colonization of anastomotic site Granulomatous pneumonitis Diffuse alveolar damage
Pneumocystis	Acute lung injury with frothy alveolar exudate Interstitial pneumonia Granulomatous pneumonitis Diffuse alveolar damage
Mycobacteria	Granulomatous pneumonitis
Virus	Diffuse alveolar damage Interstitial pneumonia Necrotizing tracheobronchitis (especially HSV) Necrotizing pneumonia (especially CMV, HSV, adenovirus) Giant cell pneumonia (RSV, parainfluenza, measles) Obliterative bronchiolitis (CMV, adenovirus)

clinical concern for infection, a history of infection, or histologic features suggestive of infection, infectious stains at the time of initial tissue processing should be performed. Even without these concerns, it may be prudent to prepare multiple unstained slides at the time of initial processing of the biopsy to better conserve tissue if special stains are needed and to reduce turn-around time if organism stains are needed. It should be noted that typical clinical features of infection may be masked in lung transplant recipients by anti-pyretic and immunosuppressive medications and pathologic evaluation may be the first indication of an infection.

Aspergillus

Aspergillus is a ubiquitous organism found all over the world. Aspergillus-associated lung disease manifests in many ways, from non-invasive colonization to diffusely angio-invasive infection (Table 5.3). The underlying health status of the patient generally determines the type of infection involved [122].

The endobronchial or transbronchial biopsy is often adequate to determine the presence of the organism, but the exact type of infection may require clinical-radiologic correlation or even larger surgical resection. The presence of intravascular fungal hyphae is pathognomonic for angio-invasive disease and should prompt an immediate notification to the managing clinical team. Determination of organism type is not reliable by light microscopic features alone and requires microbiologic correlation (see Figure 5.16). Other organisms with similar histology to *Aspergillus* include *Fusarium* and *Scedosporium* (previously *Pseudoallescheria*); however, if only rare and small fungal hyphae fragments are present on the biopsy, distinction from other hyphal organisms, such as *Zygomycetes* or even *Candida*, may be difficult and culture results may be necessary to determine species (see Figure 5.17) [54, 119, 118].

Ischemic airway disease at the tracheobronchial anastomotic site may lead to necrosis and become fertile ground for fungal colonization. Fungal organisms may be seen on organism stains in this necrotic tissue, including in necrotic cartilage (see Figure 5.18). These fungal organisms at the dehiscence site do not necessarily indicate an invasive fungal infection and should not be equated with angio-invasive fungal disease. One small study evaluating *Aspergillus* colonization at wound dehiscence sites showed universal response to antifungal treatment and/or surgical debridement (six out of six patients), in contrast to 50% mortality in patients with invasive fungal pneumonia or disseminated disease [122, 131, 132].

Other Fungal Organisms

Candida is another ubiquitous organism that more frequently colonizes the upper respiratory tract than results in pulmonary

The Pathology of Lung Transplantation

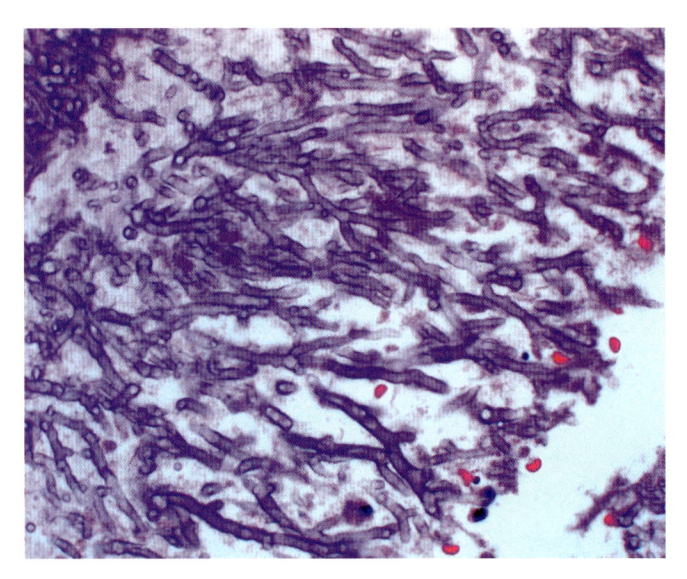

Figure 5.16 Septate fungal hyphae with 45 degree angle branching, consistent with, but not specific for, *Aspergillus* (Periodic-acid Schiff stain; original magnification 400x).

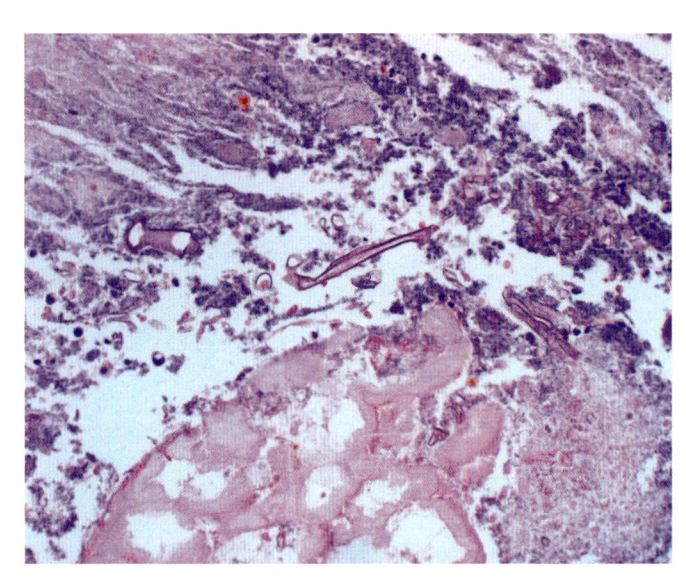

Figure 5.17 Irregular, ribbon-like fungal hyphae with inconspicuous septa in necrotic bronchial submucosa, consistent with invasive *Zygomycetes* (Periodic-Acid Schiff stain; original magnification 400x).

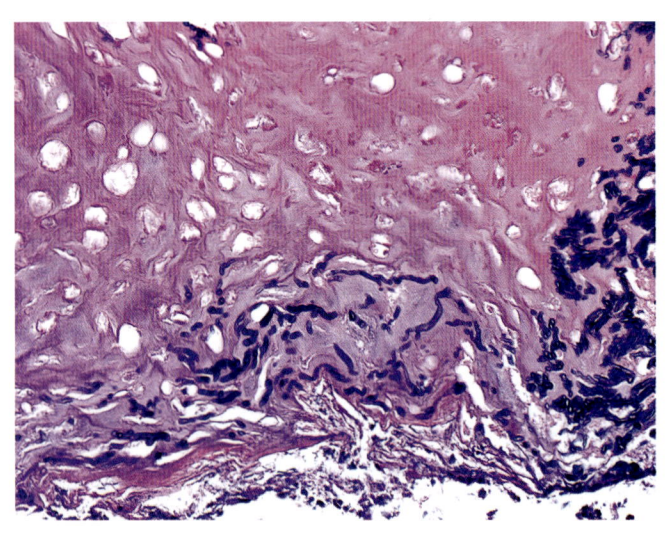

Figure 5.18 Fungal hyphae in necrotic cartilage at anastomosis site. The fungal hyphae have degenerating features and cannot be reliably classified by histologic morphology; microbiology cultures confirmed *Aspergillus* (Hematoxylin and eosin stain; original magnification 200x).

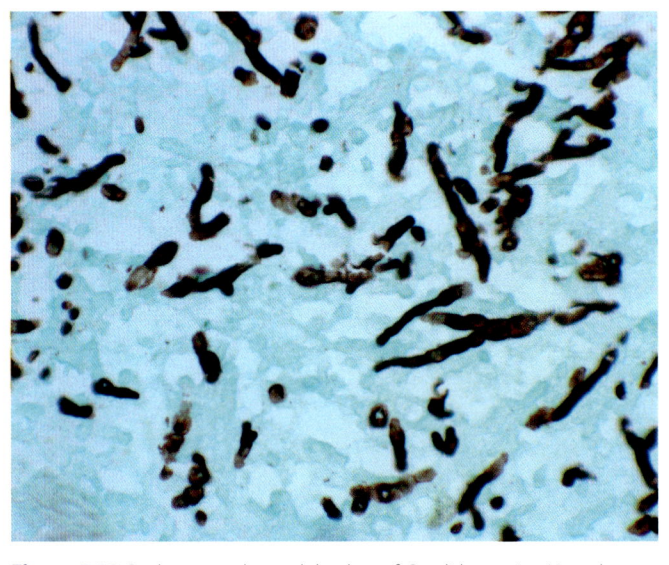

Figure 5.19 Oval yeast and pseudohyphae of *Candida* species. Note the pinching where the cells attach to one another (Grocott's methenamine silver stain; original magnification 400x).

disease. However, in the lung transplant setting, the various factors predisposing to infection can coalesce to tilt the organism-host interaction towards invasive infection. Patterns of infection include superficial airway invasion, especially at the anastomotic site, and bronchopneumonia with development of diffuse alveolar damage. *Candida* is characterized by non-branching pseudohyphae mixed with blastoconidial spores. True septate hyphae may sometimes be seen (see Figure 5.19). Histologic features of infection include: granulomatous reaction, giant cells, and evidence of tissue injury such as diffuse alveolar damage with hyaline membranes. *Candida* is often isolated from colonization of the upper airways culture contaminant and pathologic evaluation may be crucial to confirm pulmonary disease and inform clinical evaluation [131, 133, 132].

Pneumocystis jiroveci pneumonia is an uncommon pathogen in lung transplant patients due to the effectiveness of prophylactic antibiotics. However, in poorly compliant patients, infections may occur and are pathologically characterized by pauci-cellular frothy exudates in alveolar spaces. *Pneumocystis* cysts are three to five microns, non-budding, often appear to be collapsed and tend to be found in small clusters (see Figure 5.20). Other patterns of injury that have been reported include DAD, granulomatous pneumonitis, and sparse cellular infiltrates that may mimic acute rejection. Identification of the organism confirms the diagnosis. The cysts are not effectively stained with periodic acid-

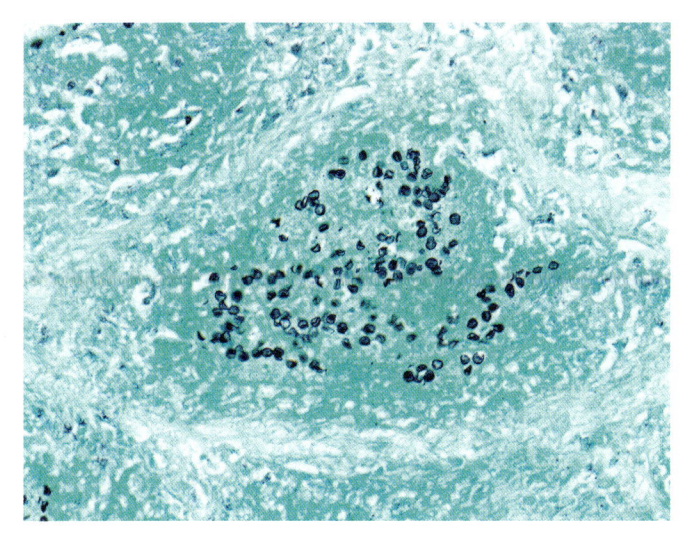

Figure 5.20 Non-budding cysts of *Pneumocystis*, approximately seven to eight microns in size, resembling dented ping-pong balls; some with a central black dot (Grocott's methenamine silver stain; original magnification 400x).

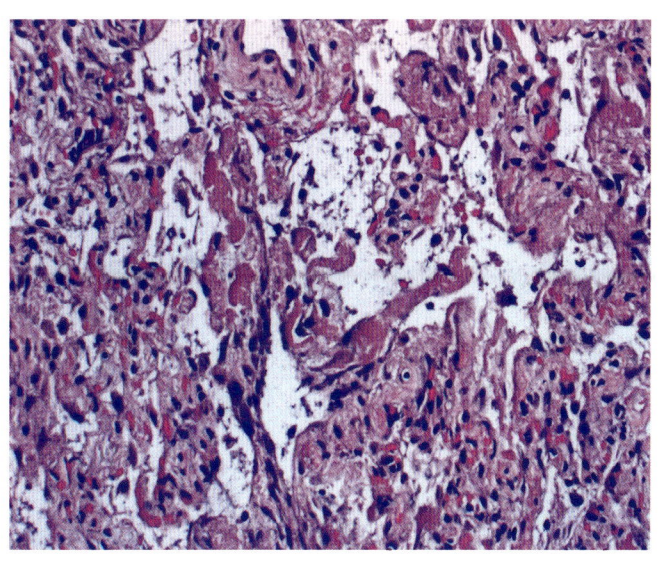

Figure 5.21 Diffuse alveolar damage with numerous hyaline membranes lining the alveolar sacs and alveolar walls expanded by edema and paucicellular inflammation. In some areas, cells have nuclear atypia with smudgy chromatin (Hematoxylin and eosin stain; original magnification 400x).

Schiff (PAS) and Grocott's methenamine silver (GMS) stain is recommended [134].

Viral Infection

As with fungal organisms, viral infections are a special concern for lung transplant recipients. Greater than 50% of pediatric lung transplant recipients develop respiratory viral infections [135]. The most common viral agent is CMV and infection usually occurs within the first six months. CMV infection may occur by viral transmission from the community or reactivation of a latent virus. CMV sero-negative recipients receiving lungs from CMV sero-positive donors are at greatest risk for CMV infection [136, 137]. The use of anti-viral prophylactic medication has reduced the rates of CMV disease, but has led to the development of "late-onset CMV disease" or drug resistance in up to 15% of patients [138]. As with the causes of many other atypical pulmonary infections, CMV can manifest a range of pathologic processes from rare non-pathologic viral inclusions to florid severe acute lung injury with diffuse alveolar damage (see Figure 5.21). The disease manifestation is usually determined by the underlying health status of the patient. Nevertheless, up to 15% of lung transplant patients with CMV infection are asymptomatic [54]. CMV infection is defined as evidence of viral replication with or without symptoms or tissue injury. In this setting, the presence of viral inclusions may not, of itself, indicate disease. Nevertheless, this finding needs to be clarified in the pathology report allowing the treating clinicians to carefully monitor the patient and adjust immunosuppressive medication as needed. CMV can be detected by a variety of methods, including evaluation of BAL lavage or blood by PCR, pp65 antigen assay, or rapid shell viral culture. Generally, if there are no clinical or histologic features to suggest viral disease, it is not cost-effective to perform immunohistochemistry stains on all biopsies [138, 139, 140].

The presence of tissue injury with demonstrable CMV inclusions is diagnostic of CMV pneumonitis. The tissue injury may range from mild interstitial pneumonia to severe acute lung injury with hyaline membranes. CMV most often infects pneumocytes and histiocytes, but may involve almost any cell type. The nuclear inclusions characteristically are large, amphophilic (or dark purple), and surrounded by a clear halo, giving a classic "owl-eye" appearance. Inclusions or viral particles may also be in the cell cytoplasm, but these are usually smaller and inconspicuous. Immunohistochemistry staining is necessary to confirm the diagnosis of CMV in the tissue and may help to identify the viral inclusions that may not be easily seen on the H&E stain (see Figure 5.22). In some cases, CMV pneumonitis may result in perivascular inflammation very similar to acute rejection. The identification of viral inclusions will help distinguish the two entities, but if viral inclusions are not seen and there is still some concern for CMV infection, the immunohistochemistry stain can assist in making the correct diagnosis. It may be difficult to determine if both CMV disease and acute rejection are occurring simultaneously [141, 120].

Recognition of CMV infection in lung transplants is particularly important due to the documented positive association between CMV infection and the development of BOS. Several studies have shown reduced freedom from BOS in CMV patients or benefit if treated prophylactically with anti-virals in patients who have serologic evidence of CMV infection [121, 142, 139].

Other opportunistic viruses that may be detected on transbronchial biopsy are adenovirus and herpes simplex virus (HSV). These are much less common than CMV, but need to be considered if viral inclusions are discovered but diagnostic studies do not confirm CMV. Adenovirus can cause a hemorrhagic and necrotizing pneumonia. Viral inclusions are limited to the nuclei and are smudgy. HSV infections begin in airway epithelium and result in necrotizing or ulcerating tracheobronchitis. Multinucleated giant cells with refractile or glassy-

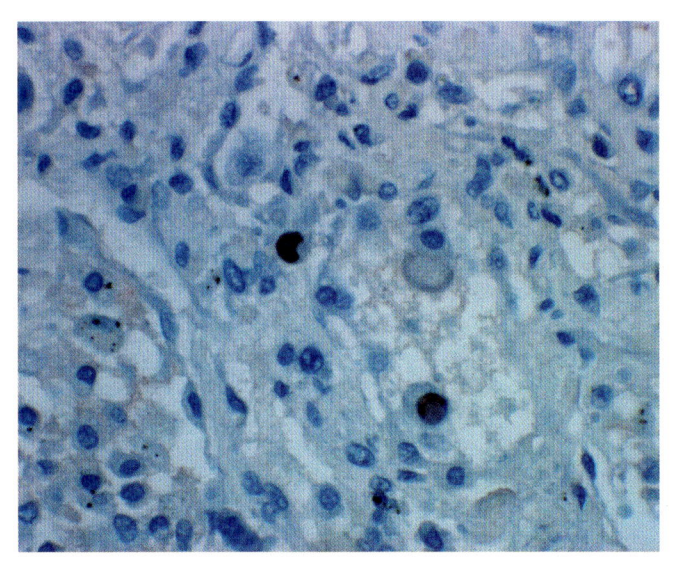

Figure 5.22 CMV immunohistochemistry stain highlighting two cells (Original magnification 600x).

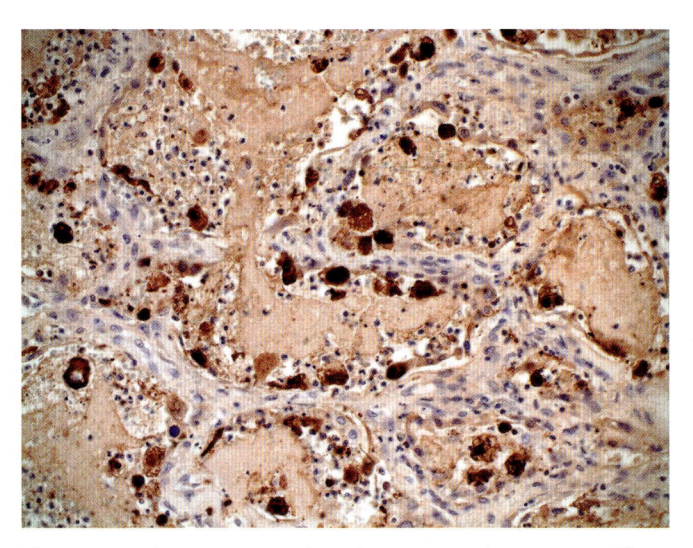

Figure 5.23 Adenovirus immunohistochemistry stain demonstrating diffuse infection of pneumocytes (Original magnification 400x).

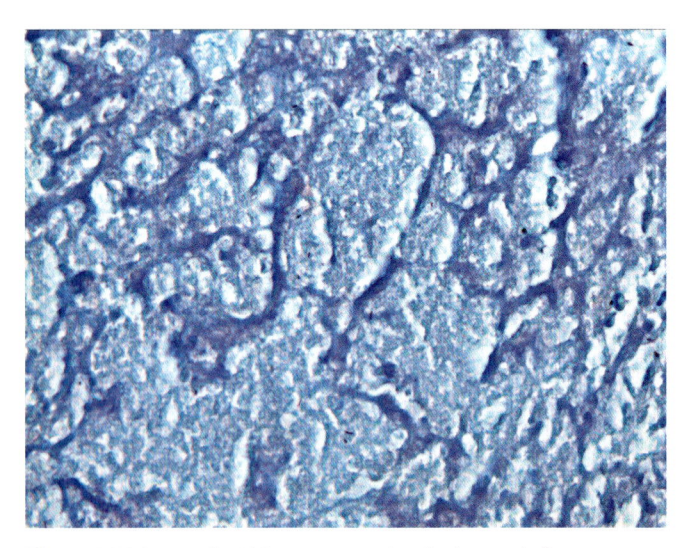

Figure 5.24 Scattered acid-fast positive rods in background of necrosis, consistent with *Mycobacterial* infection (Acid-fast bacillus stain; original magnification 600x).

appearing eosinophilic inclusions (Cowdry type A) may be seen in the area of necrosis. Both adenovirus and HSV may be identified by immunohistochemistry studies (see Figure 5.23) [138, 141].

Greater than Six Months

After six months, the immunosuppression can be reduced in many patients if there are no features of acute rejection on biopsy or evidence of graft dysfunction. In trying to optimize a given patient's maintenance immunosuppression regimen, it becomes a balancing act between managing the risk of infection versus managing the risk of chronic rejection. As immunosuppression is lowered, the risk of atypical infections is also reduced, but always remains above the general healthy population. Furthermore, other non-infectious complications of lung transplantation can slowly exacerbate, including chronic aspiration and chronic rejection through the development of obstructive small airway disease, BOS. In both settings, infections can develop.

Community acquired viral pneumonias are more common and tend to be more severe than in the general population. Influenza A/B, parainfluenza, respiratory syncytial virus, adenovirus, coronavirus, human metapneumovirus, and rhinovirus all may cause significant pulmonary complications in lung transplant patients [143]. As mentioned previously, adenovirus can cause severe necrotizing pneumonia, but influenza, parainfluenza, and RSV can also cause DAD and may induce acute rejection, which can lead to the development of OB [144]. Viral pneumonias may further be complicated by bacterial pneumonias leading to much more severe and life-threatening disease. Other than adenovirus, the histologic findings of most community acquired viral pneumonias are nonspecific and the diagnosis is determined by viral culture, antibody probes, or PCR studies [139].

Nontuberculous mycobacterial infections, especially *M. abscessus*, are being recognized more often in lung transplant patients (see Figure 5.24). *M. abscessus* has been associated with clinically significant pleuropulmonary and disseminated disease. The incidence is particularly high in cystic fibrosis patients and was found in 19.7% of pre-transplant patients in one study [123]. Pathologic evaluation of the explanted organs is especially important in these cases to ensure appropriate antibiotic coverage [145, 123, 146, 118]. One large study found mycobacterial infections, including extrapulmonary sites, occurring in 9% of lung transplant patients with a median time to diagnosis after transplant of 677 days. In this study, most pulmonary infections were due to *M. avium* complex, but this included three cases of "transient colonization" that were not treated [145].

Post-transplant Lymphoproliferative Disorders

Immunosuppression not only predisposes to infection, but also may induce post-transplant lymphoproliferative disorder

Table 5.4 Post-transplant Lymphoproliferative Disorders

1. Early lesions *plasmacytic hyperplasia/infectious mononucleosis-like PTLD*
2. Polymorphic PTLD
3. Monomorphic PTLD *(classified according to lymphoma it resembles)*
4. Classical Hodgkin lymphoma-type PTLD

from Swerdlow SH. Posttransplant Lymphoproliferative Disorders. In Classification of Tumors of Hematopoietic and Lymphoid Tissues. 4th ed. Lyon:IARC, 2008. pp. 343–349.

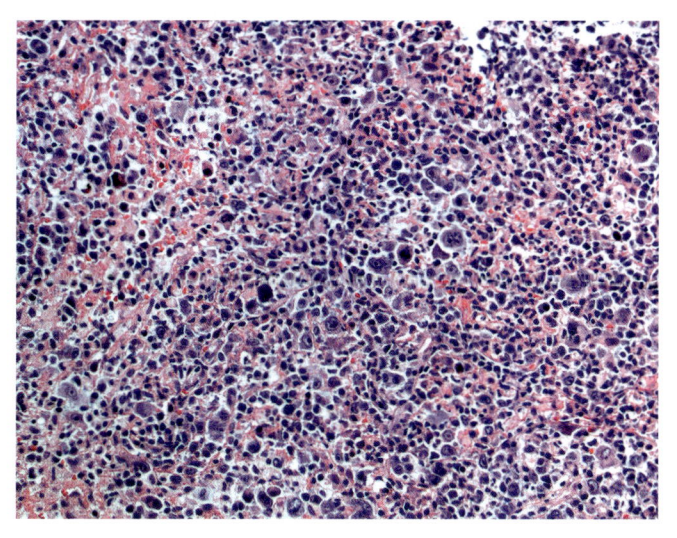

Figure 5.25 Post-transplant lymphoproliferative disorder (PTLD) – monomorphic large B cell type, EBV+. Lymphoplasmacytic infiltrate of monomorphic large B cells consistent with monomorphic PTLD (Hematoxylin and eosin stain; original magnificantion100x).

(PTLD), a potential complication and significant cause of morbidity in all transplant patients. Of solid organ transplants, lung transplant patients are among the highest at risk of developing PTLD and can occur in up to 6% of patients. The greatest risk of occurrence is during the first year post-transplant, but may occur any time [147]. Overall, 2%–3% of lung transplant deaths are due to PTLD [148]. PTLD is generally a disease of B lymphocytes and is most often due to dysregulation of cell cycle control induced by infection from Epstein-Barr virus (EBV) [149].

PTLD usually arises in the transplanted lung, but may also occur in other sites, especially the gastrointestinal tract and lymph nodes. Patients with EBV-negative serologies who receive organs from EBV-positive donors are at highest risk for the development of PTLD. This has led to the use of antiviral prophylactics in EBV-negative recipients and lower rates of PTLD [151]. PCR testing for EBV in the blood or BAL fluid may be a useful screening tool for PTLD in the first two years after transplantation, but pathologic analysis of tissue is required to confirm the diagnosis of PTLD [152, 153]. It is important to recognize that PTLD is often angiocentric in distribution and can mimic acute-cellular rejection. If histologic or clinical suspicions prompt the pathologist, immunohistochemistry, and EBV, EBER1 studies should be able to confirm the diagnosis. However, in patients more than two years out from transplantation, the incidence of EBV in cases of PTLD drops to less than 50% and EBV studies should not be used to screen for PTLD. Later onset of PTLD is more likely to be disseminated than early PTLD and has poorer prognosis [154].

The pathologic categories of PTLD have been revised by the WHO and are classified as: early, polymorphic, monomorphic, and classical Hodgkin lymphoma-type (Table 5.4) [155, 149].

Early Lesions

Early lesions are defined as lymphoid hyperplasia in the transplant patient with preservation of the normal lymphoid architecture. The two main categories of early lesions are plasmacytic hyperplasia (PH) and infectious mononucleosis (IM)-like PTLD and are more common in children and EBV-naïve adults. PH is characterized by a polyclonal proliferation of plasma cells and lymphocytes and IM-like PTLD resembles mononucleosis in the non-transplant setting. Most cases have demonstrable EBV by EBER1 or LMP1 studies. In the absence of EBV, it is difficult to distinguish early lesions of PTLD from a reactive process due to another cause.

Polymorphic PTLD (see Figure 5.25)

Polymorphic PTLD is composed of a combination of B and T lymphocytes, larger immunoblasts, and plasma cells. EBV studies may reveal the virus and facilitate the diagnosis. The recommended testing modality for EBV is EBER1 in situ hybridization, as it is more sensitive than EBV LMP1 immunohistochemistry staining, but a positive result with either study indicates EBV infection. If EBV and conventional immunohistochemistry studies are inconclusive for PTLD, T and B antigen receptor gene rearrangement studies will usually detect a clonal gene rearrangement and confirm the diagnosis. Suspicion for PTLD should be aroused if clusters of plasma cells or large immunoblast-like lymphocytes are seen on the biopsy or if there is clinical concern for PTLD. Generally, the B lymphocytes in PTLD will express CD19, CD20, CD43, CD79a, and CD45.

Monomorphic PTLD

Monomorphic PTLD has more typical features of lymphoma and is generally straightforward to diagnose if sufficiently sampled. The classification of the PTLD is based on the form of non-Hodgkin lymphoma it resembles. The most common type of monomorphic PTLD is diffuse large B cell lymphoma, but other types of NHL also occur. The association with EBV is more variable in the monomorphic form of PTLD than in other types. Monomorphic NK/T cell lymphomas have also been reported to arise as PTLD and include the full spectrum of tumor types, including extranodal nasal and cutaneous types. Most NK/T cell type monomorphic PTLD are EBV-negative [156].

Table 5.5 Recurrent Disease in Lung Transplant

Sarcoidosis

Bronchioloalveolar carcinoma (lepidic adenocarcinoma)

Hard metal pneumoconiosis

Pulmonary alveolar proteinosis

Lymphangioleiomyomatosis

Idiopathic pulmonary hemosiderosis

Pulmonary veno-occlusive disease

Pulmonary Langerhans cell histiocytosis

Diffuse panbronchiolitis

Strollo, D. C., et al. (2013). "Malignancies Incidentally Detected at Lung Transplantation: Radiologic and Pathologic Features." AJR Am J Roentgenol 201(1): 108–116.

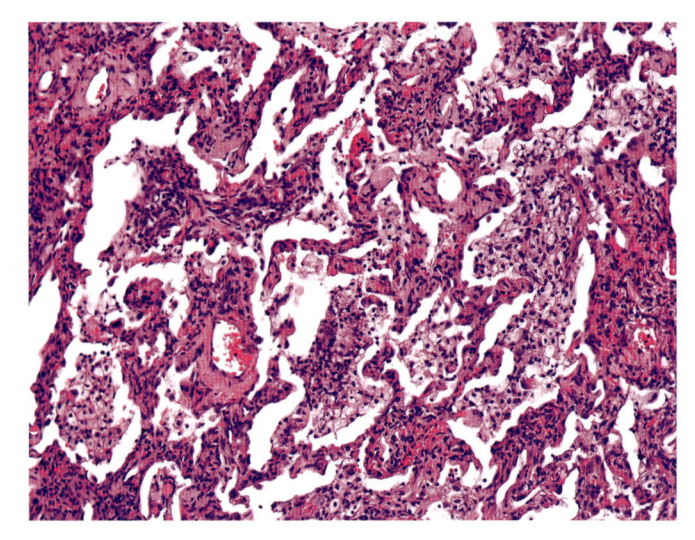

Figure 5.26 Clusters and sheets of alveolar foam cells with early interstitial fibrosis, characteristic of amiodarone toxicity (Hematoxylin and eosin stain; original magnification 200x).

Classical Hodgkin Lymphoma-type PTLD

Classical Hodgkin lymphomas (CHL) that develop in the post-transplant setting have the same histologic and immunophenotypic features as in the non-transplant setting and almost always are EBV-positive. CHL-PTLD is the least common type of PTLD and has been reported most frequently following bone marrow transplantation. The tumor is composed of a polymorphous mixture of inflammatory cells including: lymphocytes, histiocytes, plasma cells, and eosinophils. The classic Reed-Sternberg tumor cells are scattered throughout the infiltrate and are characteristically large with bilobed nuclei and large inclusion-like nucleoli. The Reed-Sternberg cells should express CD15 and CD30 [157]. In cases that are CD15-negative and CD20/CD79a-positive, the diagnosis of Hodgkin lymphoma-like PTLD should be considered [158, 155].

Drug-associated Effects in the Lungs

An unfortunate consequence of the immunomodulating medications that lung transplant recipients receive is the substantial risk for the development of infections and PTLD, which can markedly complicate medical management and compel clinicians to alter immunosuppression regimens to minimize these dangers while trying to stave off allograft rejection. A further potential consequence is injury to the allograft or another organ due to side effects of the medications that are utilized with the purpose of protecting the allograft.

Sirolimus is a common anti-rejection medication used in many organ transplants for its inhibitory effects on the activation of T and B lymphocytes. It is often favored over the calcineurin inhibitor class of immunosuppressives (tacrolimus and cyclosporin) because of its lack of renal toxicity. As a non-steroid, it also has the advantage of allowing patients to enroll in steroid-free immunosuppression protocols. The main disadvantage of sirolimus is lung toxicity, which seems to be exacerbated in lung transplant recipients. The range of reported patterns of lung injury attributable to sirolimus includes: airway dehiscence, subacute organizing pneumonia, alveolar hemorrhage, granulomatous pneumonitis, lymphoid interstitial pneumonia, vasculitis, and diffuse alveolar damage [159, 160]. The risk of airway dehiscence only occurs early after transplant and resolves after wound recovery and organ stabilization [161]. All other patterns of injury are nonspecific and a high degree of suspicion, coupled with close communication between pathologist and clinician, is needed to determine the probable diagnosis. Sirolimus-induced pulmonary toxicity can develop at any time, but is at highest risk during the first year after transplant [162]. The primary treatment is removal of the drug, but clinical and radiographic resolution may take two to three months [159].

As with the non-transplant setting, all pulmonary toxic medications can result in lung disease. Pathologic patterns of injury are usually nonspecific, but a detailed report of the histologic findings may allow the clinician to determine if a drug may be causing the injury. Amiodarone is a well-known cause of drug-induced pulmonary toxicity that is still sometimes used in the lung transplant setting for patients with atrial fibrillation. The pulmonary toxicity of amiodarone is well-documented and the classic pathologic feature is accumulation of foamy macrophages and pneumocytes (see Figure 5.26). However, these features are nonspecific and require careful clinical correlation to confirm the diagnosis. Amiodarone toxicity is dose-dependent and treatment is primarily withdrawal of the drug [163, 164]. Unfortunately, amiodarone may accumulate in the tissue and take several months to clear, so early diagnosis of toxicity is essential.

Recurrent Disease in the Lung Allograft

Recurrence of disease in the lung allograft is unusual and dependent on the original disease. Sarcoidosis is the most common of the various entities that have been reported to recur (Table 5.5). Features of the recurrent disease may be difficult to distinguish from allograft changes due to acute lung injury or rejection and may require clinical and radiologic correlation. The transbronchial biopsy has only a limited role

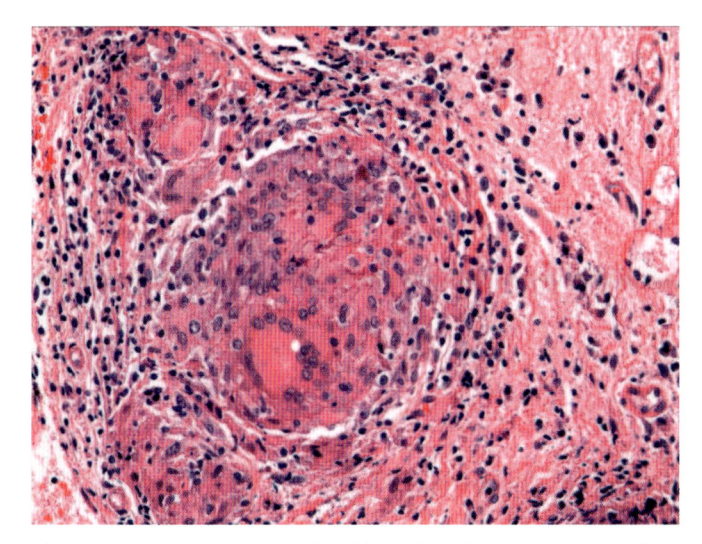

Figure 5.27 Non-necrotizing and well-formed (epithelioid) granuloma. This pattern of granulomatous inflammation is characteristic, but not specific for, sarcoidosis (Hematoxylin and eosin stain; original magnification 400x).

Figure 5.28 Granular and dense acellular proteinaceous material within alveolar sacs, consistent with pulmonary alveolar proteinosis (Hematoxylin and eosin stain; original magnification 100x).

in the diagnosis of the recurrent disease, and the pathologist may make the diagnosis at autopsy or upon evaluation of an explanted allograft lung.

In contrast to most other recurrent diseases, sarcoidosis is amenable to transbronchial biopsy due to the presence of the granulomas in the bronchovascular bundle. Sarcoidosis recurs in 10% of lung transplant recipients. Pathologic evaluation demonstrates non-necrotizing granulomas in a lymphatic distribution, especially prominent in the bronchovascular bundle (see Figure 5.27). The granulomas might be somewhat poorly formed if the patient has been on a course of steroids. Clinically, patients are at greater risk of chronic rejection than sarcoidosis interstitial lung disease and the recurrent disease rarely results in allograft failure [165, 166, 167, 168].

Neoplasms also have a high risk of recurrence. Invasive malignancy is a contraindication to transplantation and current ISHLT guidelines require a five-year disease-free interval following treatment of cancer prior to being listed for transplantation [169]. Nevertheless, undetected adenocarcinoma in situ (or lepidic adenocarcinoma if greater than 3 cm), which has no demonstrable tissue invasion, may occur in a background of underlying lung disease, especially COPD or interstitial fibrosis, and despite appearing to be entirely excised with the lung, there are case reports of recurrent disease [170, 171]. One study found incidentally detected lung cancer in 22 of 759 (2.9%) lung transplant recipients. Seventeen cases were primary lung cancers of which 13 (76%) were stage I or II [22] (Strollo, Dacic et al., 2013). Other cellular proliferative processes, such as lymphangioleiomyomatosis (LAM) and pulmonary Langerhans cell histiocytosis (PLCH), have also been reported to recur. Pulmonary veno-occlusive disease/pulmonary capillary hemangiomatosis (PVOD/PCH) is not thought of as a neoplasm, but also has been reported to occur [172, 173, 174].

Diseases caused by environmental exposures also have the potential to recur whether the patient continues to be exposed to the exogenous irritant or not; hard metal pneumoconiosis and desquamative interstitial pneumonia (DIP) are two examples. Interestingly, in a case of single-lung transplantation for giant cell interstitial pneumonia (now termed hard metal pneumoconiosis), inorganic particles were discovered in the explanted lung with the giant cells, but not in the transplanted lung, which also demonstrated features of giant cell interstitial pneumonia. It was speculated the giant cell reaction resulted from an autoimmune mechanism originally initiated by the inorganic particles and recurred in the transplanted lung possibly stimulated by the continued presence of the inorganic particles in the contralateral native lung [175].

Other Pulmonary Complications

Pulmonary alveolar proteinosis is an infrequent complication of lung transplant patients and may manifest as a recurrent disease. It is sometimes seen in patients with a history of ischemia-reperfusion injury. Pathologically, it is characterized by accumulation of acellular granular eosinophilic material within alveolar spaces, which is positive staining by the PAS stain (see Figure 5.28). The histologic features may be very similar to *Pneumocystis* pneumonia and other infections; appropriate histologic stains are necessary to exclude infection [176].

Pulmonary emboli are a relatively frequent occurrence in lung transplant patients, occurring in 36.4% of patients who died within 30 days of the lung transplantation. Overall, the incidence of pulmonary emboli has been estimated at up to 29% [177, 178]. The incidence of thromboembolism is higher in the lung transplant setting due to the numerous risk factors in this patient population including: immobility, older age, recent surgery, and increased rates of pneumonia [179]. It should be noted that thromboemboli are rarely sampled in transbronchial biopsies. If a small artery in a biopsy has a thrombus, it could be an in situ lesion and does not necessarily indicate embolic disease. The diagnosis of pulmonary embolism is determined by clinical and radiographic findings.

The immunosuppression of lung transplant patients also predisposes the patients to malignant disease other than PTLD. Up to 25% of ten-year survivors have at least one malignancy. After

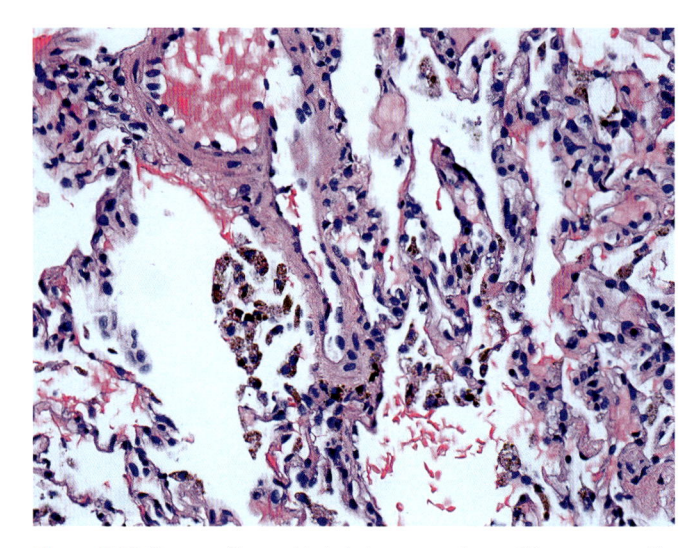

Figure 5.29 Clusters of hemosiderin-laden macrophages. When present diffusely throughout the biopsy, this is consistent with alveolar hemosiderosis (Hematoxylin and eosin stain; original magnification 400x).

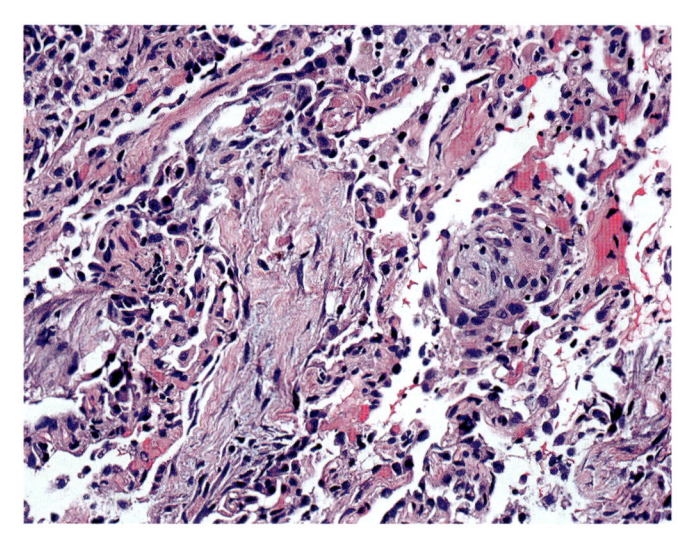

Figure 5.30 Polyps of early fibrosis. The collagen is pale staining and edematous with scattered fibroblasts, in contrast to more established hyalinized fibrosis that develops later on (Hematoxylin and eosin stain; original magnification 400x).

PTLD, the most common malignancies are squamous and basal cell carcinomas of the skin. After two years out from transplantation, skin cancer becomes more prevalent than PTLD. Primary lung carcinoma may develop in 3%–7% of native lungs of patients with contralateral transplants, especially in patients whose underlying disease is idiopathic pulmonary fibrosis or chronic obstructive pulmonary disease (COPD), as these are both associated within increased risk of lung carcinoma [170, 180, 181].

Another rare complication of lung transplantation is graft transmission of donor malignancy. An evaluation of the United Kingdom Transplant Registry database between January 1, 2001, and December 31, 2010, revealed 18 cases of donor-origin cancer (15 cases transmitted with the organ, three cases developed subsequently in the graph) from 30,756 transplants at a rate of 0.06%. The most common cancer types were renal cell carcinoma (six cases) and lung cancer (five cases). Earlier detection resulted in better survival (no deaths in 11 cases diagnosed ≤6 weeks of transplantation) [182]. The finding of potentially donor-origin cancer in the recipient patient should be reported promptly to the originating donor registry to prompt evaluation of other organ recipients from the original donor to be screened for malignancy.

Additional Findings in Lung Allograft Samples

Alveolar hemosiderosis is a common finding in the lung transplant transbronchial biopsy. These hemosiderin-laden macrophages are residue from alveolar hemorrhage and may be seen following most injuries to the lungs, including ischemia-reperfusion, infection, and rejection. In the absence of hemoptysis and/or diffuse ground-glass infiltrates, the significance of few hemosiderin-laden macrophages is usually negligible (see Figure 5.29) [54].

Likewise, organizing pneumonia (OP), consisting of plugs of fresh fibrous tissue in airspaces, is a very nonspecific finding and can be seen during the reparative process of almost any injury to the lungs (see Figure 5.30). OP is somewhat more significant than alveolar hemosiderosis and often indicates a pathologic process has occurred or is ongoing. The managing clinician may choose to treat the pathologic finding of OP as residual disease if the patient is still symptomatic or has radiographic evidence of a diffuse infiltrate.

Due to the loss or diminishment of the cough reflex in lung transplant patients, aspiration, and subsequent aspiration pneumonia can be a serious complication leading to infections and bronchiolitis obliterans [183]. The finding of foreign material, often with accompanying giant cells, is diagnostic of aspiration. *Actinomycetes* infection with sulfur granules is virtually pathognomonic for aspiration. Lipoid pneumonia with lipid-laden macrophages is also suspicious for aspiration, but may also be seen in post-obstructive changes, especially if the patient is suffering from bronchiolitis obliterans syndrome.

References

1. Hardy JD, Webb WR, Dalton ML, Jr., Walker GR, Jr. Lung Homotransplantation in Man: Report of the Initial Case. JAMA. 1963 Dec 21;**186**(12):1065–74.

2. Cooper JD, Billingham M, Egan T, Hertz MI, Higenbottam T, Lynch J, et al. A Working Formulation for the Standardization of Nomenclature and for Clinical Staging of Chronic Dysfunction in Lung Allografts. International Society for Heart and Lung Transplantation. J Heart Lung Transplant Off Publ Int Soc Heart Transplant. 1993 Oct;**12**(5):713–6.

3. Veith FJ, Hagstrom JW. Alveolar Manifestations of Rejection: An Important Cause of the Poor Results

3. with Human Lung Transplantation. Ann Surg. 1972 Mar;**175**(3):336–48.
4. Veith FJ, Kamholz SL, Mollenkopf FP, Montefusco CM. Lung Transplantation 1983. Transplantation. 1983 Apr;**35**(4):271–8.
5. Reitz BA, Wallwork JL, Hunt SA, Pennock JL, Billingham ME, Oyer PE, et al. Heart-Lung Transplantation: Successful Therapy for Patients with Pulmonary Vascular Disease. N Engl J Med. 1982 Mar 11;**306**(10):557–64.
6. Mallidi HR. Lung Transplantation. Tex Heart Inst J. 2012;**39**(6):852–3.
7. Christie JD, Edwards LB, Kucheryavaya AY, Benden C, Dipchand AI, Dobbels F, et al. The Registry of the International Society for Heart and Lung Transplantation: 29th Adult Lung and Heart-Lung Transplant Report-2012. J Heart Lung Transplant Off Publ Int Soc Heart Transplant. 2012 Oct;**31**(10):1073–86.
8. Benden C, Edwards LB, Kucheryavaya AY, Christie JD, Dipchand AI, Dobbels F, et al. The Registry of the International Society for Heart and Lung Transplantation: Fifteenth Pediatric Lung and Heart-Lung Transplantation Report–2012. J Heart Lung Transplant Off Publ Int Soc Heart Transplant. 2012 Oct;**31**(10):1087–95.
9. Kotloff RM, Thabut G. Lung Transplantation. Am J Respir Crit Care Med. 2011 Jul 15;**184**(2):159–71.
10. Kotsimbos T, Williams TJ, Anderson GP. Update on Lung Transplantation: Programmes, Patients and Prospects. Eur Respir Rev Off J Eur Respir Soc. 2012 Dec 1;**21**(126):271–305.
11. Decramer M, Janssens W, Miravitlles M. Chronic Obstructive Pulmonary Disease. Lancet. 2012 Apr 7;**379**(9823):1341–51.
12. Singer JP, Yusen RD. Defining Patient-reported Outcomes in Chronic Obstructive Pulmonary Disease: The Patient-centered Experience. Med Clin North Am. 2012 Jul;**96**(4):767–87.
13. Egan TM, Murray S, Bustami RT, Shearon TH, McCullough KP, Edwards LB, et al. Development of the New Lung Allocation System in the United States. Am J Transplant Off J Am Soc Transplant Am Soc Transpl Surg. 2006;**6**(5 Pt 2):1212–27.
14. Kotloff RM. Risk Stratification of Lung Transplant Candidates: Implications for Organ Allocation. Ann Intern Med. 2013 May 7;**158**(9):699–700.
15. Snell GI, Paraskeva M, Westall GP. Donor Selection and Management. Semin Respir Crit Care Med. 2013 Jun;**34**(3):361–70.
16. Snell GI, Westall GP. Selection and Management of the Lung Donor. Clin Chest Med. 2011 Jun;**32**(2):223–32.
17. Griffin SM, Robertson AGN, Bredenoord AJ, Brownlee IA, Stovold R, Brodlie M, et al. Aspiration and Allograft Injury Secondary to Gastroesophageal Reflux Occur in the Immediate Post-lung Transplantation Period (Prospective Clinical Trial). Ann Surg. 2013 Nov;**258**(5):705–12.
18. Reyes KG, Mason DP, Thuita L, Nowicki ER, Murthy SC, Pettersson GB, et al. Guidelines for Donor Lung Selection: Time for Revision? Ann Thorac Surg. 2010 Jun;**89**(6):1756–1764; discussion 1764–1765.
19. Medeiros IL, Pêgo-Fernandes PM, Mariani AW, Fernandes FG, do Vale Unterpertinger F, Canzian M, et al. Histologic and Functional Evaluation of Lungs Reconditioned by ex Vivo Lung Perfusion. J Heart Lung Transplant Off Publ Int Soc Heart Transplant. 2012 Mar;**31**(3):305–9.
20. Ingemansson R, Eyjolfsson A, Mared L, Pierre L, Algotsson L, Ekmehag B, et al. Clinical Transplantation of Initially Rejected Donor Lungs after Reconditioning ex Vivo. Ann Thorac Surg. 2009 Jan;**87**(1):255–60.
21. Belli EV, Landolfo K, Keller C, Thomas M, Odell J. Lung Cancer Following Lung Transplant: Single Institution 10 Year Experience. Lung Cancer Amst Neth. 2013 Sep;**81**(3):451–4.
22. Strollo DC, Dacic S, Ocak I, Pilewski J, Bermudez C, Crespo MM. Malignancies Incidentally Detected at Lung Transplantation: Radiologic and Pathologic Features. AJR Am J Roentgenol. 2013 Jul;**201**(1):108–16.
23. Lee JC, Christie JD. Primary Graft Dysfunction. Clin Chest Med. 2011 Jun;**32**(2):279–93.
24. Lee JC, Christie JD. Primary Graft Dysfunction. Proc Am Thorac Soc. 2009 Jan 15;**6**(1):39–46.
25. Suzuki Y, Cantu E, Christie JD. Primary Graft Dysfunction. Semin Respir Crit Care Med. 2013 Jun;**34**(3):305–19.
26. Barr ML, Schenkel FA, Bowdish ME, Starnes VA. Living Donor Lobar Lung Transplantation: Current Status and Future Directions. Transplant Proc. 2005 Nov;**37**(9):3983–6.
27. Fiser SM, Tribble CG, Long SM, Kaza AK, Cope JT, Laubach VE, et al. Lung Transplant Reperfusion Injury Involves Pulmonary Macrophages and Circulating Leukocytes in a Biphasic Response. J Thorac Cardiovasc Surg. 2001 Jun;**121**(6):1069–75.
28. Frost AE, Jammal CT, Cagle PT. Hyperacute Rejection Following Lung Transplantation. CHEST J. 1996 Aug 1;**110**(2):559–62.
29. Choi JK, Kearns J, Palevsky HI, Montone KT, Kaiser LR, Zmijewski CM, et al. Hyperacute Rejection of a Pulmonary Allograft. Immediate Clinical and Pathologic Findings. Am J Respir Crit Care Med. 1999 Sep;**160**(3):1015–8.
30. De Jesus Peixoto Camargo J, Marcantonio Camargo S, Marcelo Schio S, Noguchi Machuca T, Adélia Perin F. Hyperacute Rejection after Single Lung Transplantation: A Case Report. Transplant Proc. 2008 Apr;**40**(3):867–9.
31. Bittner HB, Dunitz J, Hertz M, Bolman MR 3rd, Park SJ. Hyperacute Rejection in Single Lung Transplantation–Case Report of Successful Management by Means of Plasmapheresis and Antithymocyte Globulin Treatment. Transplantation. 2001 Mar 15;**71**(5):649–51.
32. Scornik JC, Zander DS, Baz MA, Donnelly WH, Staples ED. Susceptibility of Lung Transplants to Preformed Donor-specific HLA Antibodies as Detected by Flow Cytometry. Transplantation. 1999 Nov 27;**68**(10):1542–6.
33. Nguyen BH, Zwets E, Schroeder C, Pierson RN, Azimzadeh AM. Beyond Antibody-mediated Rejection: Hyperacute Lung Rejection as a Paradigm for Dysregulated Inflammation. Curr Drug Targets Cardiovasc Haematol Disord. 2005 Jun;**5**(3):255–69.
34. Tait BD, Süsal C, Gebel HM, Nickerson PW, Zachary AA, Claas FHJ, et al. Consensus Guidelines on the Testing and Clinical Management Issues Associated with HLA and Non-HLA Antibodies in Transplantation. Transplantation. 2013 Jan 15;**95**(1):19–47.
35. Porhownik NR. Airway Complications Post Lung Transplantation. Curr Opin Pulm Med. 2013 Mar;**19**(2):174–80.
36. Santacruz JF, Mehta AC. Airway Complications and Management after Lung Transplantation: Ischemia, Dehiscence, and Stenosis. Proc Am Thorac Soc. 2009 Jan 15;**6**(1):79–93.

37. Hasegawa T, Iacono AT, Yousem SA. The Anatomic Distribution of Acute Cellular Rejection in the Allograft Lung. Ann Thorac Surg. 2000 May;**69**(5):1529–31.

38. Krishnam MS, Suh RD, Tomasian A, Goldin JG, Lai C, Brown K, et al. Postoperative Complications of Lung Transplantation: Radiologic Findings along a Time Continuum. Radiogr Rev Publ Radiol Soc N Am Inc. 2007 Aug;**27**(4):957–74.

39. Herrera JM, McNeil KD, Higgins RS, Coulden RA, Flower CD, Nashef SA, et al. Airway Complications after Lung Transplantation: Treatment and Long-term Outcome. Ann Thorac Surg. 2001 Mar;**71**(3):989–993; discussion 993–994.

40. Mulligan MS. Endoscopic Management of Airway Complications after Lung Transplantation. Chest Surg Clin N Am. 2001 Nov;**11**(4):907–15.

41. McManigle W, Pavlisko EN, Martinu T. Acute Cellular and Antibody-mediated Allograft Rejection. Semin Respir Crit Care Med. 2013 Jun;**34**(3):320–35.

42. Hopkins PM, Aboyoun CL, Chhajed PN, Malouf MA, Plit ML, Rainer SP, et al. Prospective Analysis of 1,235 Transbronchial Lung Biopsies in Lung Transplant Recipients. J Heart Lung Transplant Off Publ Int Soc Heart Transplant. 2002 Oct;**21**(10):1062–7.

43. Christie JD, Edwards LB, Kucheryavaya AY, Benden C, Dobbels F, Kirk R, et al. The Registry of the International Society for Heart and Lung Transplantation: Twenty-eighth Adult Lung and Heart-Lung Transplant Report—2011. J Heart Lung Transplant. 2011;**30**(10):1104–22.

44. Trulock EP, Christie JD, Edwards LB, Boucek MM, Aurora P, Taylor DO, et al. Registry of the International Society for Heart and Lung Transplantation: Twenty-fourth Official Adult Lung and Heart–Lung Transplantation Report—2007. J Heart Lung Transplant. 2007;**26**(8):782–95.

45. Patel JK, Kittleson M, Kobashigawa JA. Cardiac Allograft Rejection. The Surgeon. 2011;**9**(3):160–7.

46. Shetty S, Adams DH, Hubscher SG. Post-transplant Liver Biopsy and the Immune Response: Lessons for the Clinician. Expert Rev Clin Immunol. 2012 Sep;**8**(7):645+.

47. Perkins D, Verma M, Park KJ. Advances of Genomic Science and Systems Biology in Renal Transplantation: A Review. Semin Immunopathol. 2011;**33**(2):211–218.

48. Sharples LD, McNeil K, Stewart S, Wallwork J. Risk Factors for Bronchiolitis Obliterans: A Systematic Review of Recent Publications. J Heart Lung Transplant Off Publ Int Soc Heart Transplant. 2002 Feb;**21**(2):271–81.

49. Husain AN, Siddiqui MT, Holmes EW, Chandrasekhar AJ, McCabe M, Radvany R, et al. Analysis of Risk Factors for the Development of Bronchiolitis Obliterans Syndrome. Am J Respir Crit Care Med. 1999 Mar;**159**(3):829–33.

50. Whelan TPM, Hertz MI. Allograft Rejection after Lung Transplantation. Clin Chest Med. 2005 Dec;**26**(4):599–612, vi.

51. Shitrit D, Izbicki G, Fink G, Bendayan D, Aravot D, Saute M, et al. Late Postoperative Pleural Effusion Following Lung Transplantation: Characteristics and Clinical Implications. Eur J Cardio-Thorac Surg Off J Eur Assoc Cardio-Thorac Surg. 2003 Apr;**23**(4):494–6.

52. Martinu T, Chen D-F, Palmer SM. Acute Rejection and Humoral Sensitization in Lung Transplant Recipients. Proc Am Thorac Soc. 2009 Jan 15;**6**(1):54–65.

53. Hopkins PM, Aboyoun CL, Chhajed PN, Malouf MA, Plit ML, Rainer SP, et al. Association of Minimal Rejection in Lung Transplant Recipients with Obliterative Bronchiolitis. Am J Respir Crit Care Med. 2004 Nov 1;**170**(9):1022–6.

54. Stewart S, Fishbein MC, Snell GI, Berry GJ, Boehler A, Burke MM, et al. Revision of the 1996 Working Formulation for the Standardization of Nomenclature in the Diagnosis of Lung Rejection. J Heart Lung Transplant Off Publ Int Soc Heart Transplant. 2007 Dec;**26**(12):1229–42.

55. Chakinala MM, Ritter J, Gage BF, Lynch JP, Aloush A, Patterson GA, et al. Yield of Surveillance Bronchoscopy for Acute Rejection and Lymphocytic Bronchitis/Bronchiolitis after Lung Transplantation. J Heart Lung Transplant Off Publ Int Soc Heart Transplant. 2004 Dec;**23**(12):1396–404.

56. Chaparro C, Maurer JR, Chamberlain DW, Todd TR. Role of Open Lung Biopsy for Diagnosis in Lung Transplant Recipients: Ten-year Experience. Ann Thorac Surg. 1995 Apr;**59**(4):928–32.

57. Burdett CL, Critchley RJ, Black F, Barnard S, Clark SC, Corris PA, et al. Invasive Biopsy Is Effective and Useful after Lung Transplant. J Heart Lung Transplant Off Publ Int Soc Heart Transplant. 2010 Jul;**29**(7):759–63.

58. Husain AN, Siddiqui MT, Montoya A, Chandrasekhar AJ, Garrity ER. Post-lung Transplant Biopsies: An 8-year Loyola Experience. Mod Pathol Off J U S Can Acad Pathol Inc. 1996 Feb;**9**(2):126–32.

59. Marboe CC. Pathology of Lung Transplantation. Semin Diagn Pathol. 2007 Aug;**24**(3):188–98.

60. Sato M, Hwang DM, Ohmori-Matsuda K, Chaparro C, Waddell TK, Singer LG, et al. Revisiting the Pathologic Finding of Diffuse Alveolar Damage after Lung Transplantation. J Heart Lung Transplant Off Publ Int Soc Heart Transplant [Internet]. 2012 Feb 11 [cited 2012 Feb 25]; available from: www.ncbi.nlm.nih.gov/pubmed/22330935.

61. Yousem SA, Berry GJ, Cagle PT, Chamberlain D, Husain AN, Hruban RH, et al. Revision of the 1990 Working Formulation for the Classification of Pulmonary Allograft Rejection: Lung Rejection Study Group. J Heart Lung Transplant Off Publ Int Soc Heart Transplant. 1996 Jan;**15**(1 Pt 1):1–15.

62. Arcasoy SM, Berry G, Marboe CC, Tazelaar HD, Zamora MR, Wolters HJ, et al. Pathologic Interpretation of Transbronchial Biopsy for Acute Rejection of Lung Allograft Is Highly Variable. Am J Transplant Off J Am Soc Transplant Am Soc Transpl Surg. 2011 Feb;**11**(2):320–8.

63. Stephenson A, Flint J, English J, Vedal S, Fradet G, Chittock D, et al. Interpretation of Transbronchial Lung Biopsies from Lung Transplant Recipients: Inter- and Intraobserver Agreement. Can Respir J J Can Thorac Soc. 2005 Mar;**12**(2):75–7.

64. Colombat M, Groussard O, Lautrette A, Thabut G, Marrash-Chahla R, Brugière O, et al. Analysis of the Different Histologic Lesions Observed in Transbronchial Biopsy for the Diagnosis of Acute Rejection. Clinicopathologic Correlations during the First 6 Months after Lung Transplantation. Hum Pathol. 2005 Apr;**36**(4):387–94.

65. Bhorade SM, Husain AN, Liao C, Li LC, Ahya VN, Baz MA, et al. Interobserver Variability in Grading Transbronchial Lung Biopsy Specimens after Lung Transplantation. Chest. 2013 Jun;**143**(6):1717–24.

66. Chakinala MM, Ritter J, Gage BF, Aloush AA, Hachem RH, Lynch JP, et al. Reliability for Grading Acute Rejection

and Airway Inflammation after Lung Transplantation. J Heart Lung Transplant Off Publ Int Soc Heart Transplant. 2005 Jun;24(6):652–7.

67. Hunninghake GW, Gadek JE, Kawanami O, Ferrans VJ, Crystal RG. Inflammatory and Immune Processes in the Human Lung in Health and Disease: Evaluation by Bronchoalveolar Lavage. Am J Pathol. 1979 Oct;97(1):149–206.

68. Meyer KC. Bronchoalveolar Lavage as a Diagnostic Tool. Semin Respir Crit Care Med. 2007 Oct;28(5):546–60.

69. Tiroke AH, Bewig B, Haverich A. Bronchoalveolar Lavage in Lung Transplantation. State of the Art. Clin Transplant. 1999 Apr;13(2):131–57.

70. Zheng L, Orsida B, Whitford H, Levvey B, Ward C, Walters EH, et al. Longitudinal Comparisons of Lymphocytes and Subtypes between Airway Wall and Bronchoalveolar Lavage after Human Lung Transplantation. Transplantation. 2005 Jul 27;80(2):185–92.

71. Vos R, Vanaudenaerde BM, Verleden SE, De Vleeschauwer SI, Willems-Widyastuti A, Van Raemdonck DE, et al. Bronchoalveolar Lavage Neutrophilia in Acute Lung Allograft Rejection and Lymphocytic Bronchiolitis. J Heart Lung Transplant Off Publ Int Soc Heart Transplant. 2010 Nov;29(11):1259–69.

72. Clelland C, Higenbottam T, Stewart S, Otulana B, Wreghitt T, Gray J, et al. Bronchoalveolar Lavage and Transbronchial Lung Biopsy during Acute Rejection and Infection in Heart-Lung Transplant Patients. Studies of Cell Counts, Lymphocyte Phenotypes, and Expression of HLA-DR and Interleukin-2 Receptor. Am Rev Respir Dis. 1993 Jun;147(6 Pt 1):1386–92.

73. Tikkanen J, Lemström K, Halme M, Pakkala S, Taskinen E, Koskinen P. Cytological Monitoring of Peripheral Blood, Bronchoalveolar Lavage Fluid, and Transbronchial Biopsy Specimens during Acute Rejection and Cytomegalovirus Infection in Lung and Heart–Lung Allograft Recipients. Clin Transplant. 2001 Apr;15(2):77–88.

74. Wood KJ. Regulatory T Cells in Transplantation. Transplant Proc. 2011;43(6):2135–6.

75. Gregson AL, Hoji A, Saggar R, Ross DJ, Kubak BM, Jamieson BD, et al. Bronchoalveolar Immunologic Profile of Acute Human Lung Transplant Allograft Rejection. Transplantation. 2008 Apr;85(7):1056–9.

76. Slebos D-J, Postma DS, Koëter GH, Van Der Bij W, Boezen M, Kauffman HF. Bronchoalveolar Lavage Fluid Characteristics in Acute and Chronic Lung Transplant Rejection. J Heart Lung Transplant Off Publ Int Soc Heart Transplant. 2004 May;23(5):532–40.

77. Montgomery RA, Cozzi E, West LJ, Warren DS. Humoral Immunity and Antibody-mediated Rejection in Solid Organ Transplantation. Semin Immunol. 2011;23(4):224–34.

78. Dragun D, Catar R, Philippe A. Non-HLA Antibodies in Solid Organ Transplantation: Recent Concepts and Clinical Relevance. Curr Opin Organ Transplant. 2013 Aug;18(4):430–5.

79. Tiriveedhi V, Gautam B, Sarma NJ, Askar M, Budev M, Aloush A, et al. Pre-transplant Antibodies to Kα1 Tubulin and Collagen-V in Lung Transplantation: Clinical Correlations. J Heart Lung Transplant Off Publ Int Soc Heart Transplant. 2013 Aug;32(8):807–14.

80. Joudeh A, Saliba KA, Topping KA, Sis B. Pathologic Basis of Antibody-mediated Organ Transplant Rejection: From Pathogenesis to Diagnosis. Curr Opin Organ Transplant. 2013 Aug;18(4):478–85.

81. Colvin RB. Dimensions of Antibody-mediated Rejection. Am J Transplant Off J Am Soc Transplant Am Soc Transpl Surg. 2010 Jul;10(7):1509–10.

82. Snyder LD, Wang Z, Chen D-F, Reinsmoen NL, Finlen-Copeland CA, Davis WA, et al. Implications for Human Leukocyte Antigen Antibodies after Lung Transplantation: A 10-year Experience in 441 Patients. Chest. 2013 Jul;144(1):226–33.

83. Takemoto SK, Zeevi A, Feng S, Colvin RB, Jordan S, Kobashigawa J, et al. National Conference to Assess Antibody-mediated Rejection in Solid Organ Transplantation. Am J Transplant Off J Am Soc Transplant Am Soc Transpl Surg. 2004 Jul;4(7):1033–41.

84. Girnita AL, Duquesnoy R, Yousem SA, Iacono AT, Corcoran TE, Buzoianu M, et al. HLA-specific Antibodies are Risk Factors for Lymphocytic Bronchiolitis and Chronic Lung Allograft Dysfunction. Am J Transplant Off J Am Soc Transplant Am Soc Transpl Surg. 2005 Jan;5(1):131–8.

85. Girnita AL, McCurry KR, Zeevi A. Increased Lung Allograft Failure in Patients with HLA-specific Antibody. Clin Transpl. 2007;231–9.

86. Astor TL, Weill D, Cool C, Teitelbaum I, Schwarz MI, Zamora MR. Pulmonary Capillaritis in Lung Transplant Recipients: Treatment and Effect on Allograft Function. J Heart Lung Transplant Off Publ Int Soc Heart Transplant. 2005 Dec;24(12):2091–7.

87. Magro CM, Deng A, Pope-Harman A, Waldman WJ, Bernard Collins A, Adams PW, et al. Humorally Mediated Posttransplantation Septal Capillary Injury Syndrome as a Common Form of Pulmonary Allograft Rejection: A Hypothesis. Transplantation. 2002 Nov 15;74(9):1273–80.

88. Magro CM, Pope Harman A, Klinger D, Orosz C, Adams P, Waldman J, et al. Use of C4d as a Diagnostic Adjunct in Lung Allograft Biopsies. Am J Transplant Off J Am Soc Transplant Am Soc Transpl Surg. 2003 Sep;3(9):1143–54.

89. Ionescu DN, Girnita AL, Zeevi A, Duquesnoy R, Pilewski J, Johnson B, et al. C4d Deposition in Lung Allografts Is Associated with Circulating Anti-HLA Alloantibody. Transpl Immunol. 2005 Oct;15(1):63–8.

90. Wallace WD, Reed EF, Ross D, Lassman CR, Fishbein MC. C4d Staining of Pulmonary Allograft Biopsies: An Immunoperoxidase Study. J Heart Lung Transplant Off Publ Int Soc Heart Transplant. 2005 Oct;24(10):1565–70.

91. Girnita AL, McCurry KR, Yousem SA, Pilewski J, Zeevi A. Antibody-mediated Rejection in Lung Transplantation: Case Reports. Clin Transpl. 2006;508–10.

92. Westall GP, Snell GI, McLean C, Kotsimbos T, Williams T, Magro C. C3d and C4d Deposition Early after Lung Transplantation. J Heart Lung Transplant Off Publ Int Soc Heart Transplant. 2008 Jul;27(7):722–8.

93. Astor TL, Galantowicz M, Phillips A, Palafox J, Baker P. Pulmonary Capillaritis as a Manifestation of Acute Humoral Allograft Rejection Following Infant Lung Transplantation. Am J Transplant Off J Am Soc Transplant Am Soc Transpl Surg. 2009 Feb;9(2):409–12.

94. Morrell MR, Patterson GA, Trulock EP, Hachem RR. Acute Antibody-mediated Rejection after Lung Transplantation. J Heart Lung Transplant Off Publ Int Soc Heart Transplant. 2009 Jan;28(1):96–100.

95. Yousem SA, Zeevi A. The Histopathology of Lung Allograft Dysfunction Associated with the Development of Donor-specific HLA Alloantibodies. Am J Surg Pathol. 2012 Jul;36(7):987–92.

96. DeNicola MM, Weigt SS, Belperio JA, Reed EF, Ross DJ, Wallace WD. Pathologic Findings in Lung Allografts

97. Jacob EK, De Goey SR, Gandhi MJ. Positive Virtual Crossmatch with Negative Flow Crossmatch Results in Two Cases. Transpl Immunol. 2011 Jul;25(1):77–81.

98. Witt CA, Gaut JP, Yusen RD, Byers DE, Iuppa JA, Bennett Bain K, et al. Acute Antibody-mediated Rejection after Lung Transplantation. J Heart Lung Transplant Off Publ Int Soc Heart Transplant. 2013 Oct;32(10):1034–40.

99. Girnita AL, Lee TM, McCurry KR, Baldwin WM, Yousem SA, Detrick B, et al. Anti-human Leukocyte Antigen Antibodies, Vascular C4d Deposition and Increased Soluble C4d in Broncho-Alveolar Lavage of Lung Allografts. Transplantation. 2008 Jul;86(2):342–7.

100. Roberts JA, Barrios R, Cagle PT, Ge Y, Takei H, Haque AK, et al. The Presence of Anti-HLA Donor-specific Antibodies in Lung Allograft Recipients Does Not Correlate with C4d Immunofluorescence in Transbronchial Biopsy Specimens. Arch Pathol Lab Med. 2013 Oct 28;

101. Berry G, Burke M, Andersen C, Angelini A, Bruneval P, Calabrese F, et al. Pathology of Pulmonary Antibody-mediated Rejection: 2012 Update from the Pathology Council of the ISHLT. J Heart Lung Transplant Off Publ Int Soc Heart Transplant. 2013 Jan;32(1):14–21.

102. Mengel M, Sis B, Haas M, Colvin RB, Halloran PF, Racusen LC, et al. BANFF 2011 Meeting Report: New Concepts in Antibody-mediated Rejection. Am J Transplant Off J Am Soc Transplant Am Soc Transpl Surg [Internet]. 2012 Feb 2 [cited 2012 Feb 23]; available from: www.ncbi.nlm.nih.gov/pubmed/22300494.

103. Miller GG, Destarac L, Zeevi A, Girnita A, McCurry K, Iacono A, et al. Acute Humoral Rejection of Human Lung Allografts and Elevation of C4d in Bronchoalveolar Lavage Fluid. Am J Transplant Off J Am Soc Transplant Am Soc Transpl Surg. 2004 Aug;4(8):1323–30.

104. Verleden SE, Ruttens D, Vandermeulen E, van Raemdonck DE, Vanaudenaerde BM, Verleden GM, et al. Elevated Bronchoalveolar Lavage Eosinophilia Correlates with Poor Outcome after Lung Transplantation. Transplantation. 2013 Oct 23.

105. Weigt SS, DerHovanessian A, Wallace WD, Lynch JP 3rd, Belperio JA. Bronchiolitis Obliterans Syndrome: The Achilles' Heel of Lung Transplantation. Semin Respir Crit Care Med. 2013 Jun;34(3):336–51.

106. Boehler A, Estenne M. Obliterative Bronchiolitis after Lung Transplantation. Curr Opin Pulm Med. 2000 Mar;6(2):133–9.

107. Woo MS. Overview of Lung Transplantation. Clin Rev Allergy Immunol. 2008 Dec;35(3):154–63.

108. Saggar R, Ross DJ, Saggar R, Zisman DA, Gregson A, Lynch JP 3rd, et al. Pulmonary Hypertension Associated with Lung Transplantation Obliterative Bronchiolitis and Vascular Remodeling of the Allograft. Am J Transplant Off J Am Soc Transplant Am Soc Transpl Surg. 2008 Sep;8(9):1921–30.

109. Jiang X, Khan MA, Tian W, Beilke J, Natarajan R, Kosek J, et al. Adenovirus-mediated HIF-1α Gene Transfer Promotes Repair of Mouse Airway Allograft Microvasculature and Attenuates Chronic Rejection. J Clin Invest. 2011 Jun;121(6):2336–49.

110. Langenbach SY, Zheng L, McWilliams T, Levvey B, Orsida B, Bailey M, et al. Airway Vascular Changes after Lung Transplant: Potential Contribution to the Pathophysiology of Bronchiolitis Obliterans Syndrome. J Heart Lung Transplant Off Publ Int Soc Heart Transplant. 2005 Oct;24(10):1550–6.

111. Dhillon GS, Zamora MR, Roos JE, Sheahan D, Sista RR, Van der Starre P, et al. Lung Transplant Airway Hypoxia: A Diathesis to Fibrosis? Am J Respir Crit Care Med. 2010 Jul 15;182(2):230–6.

112. Nicolls MR, Zamora MR. Bronchial Blood Supply after Lung Transplantation without Bronchial Artery Revascularization. Curr Opin Organ Transplant. 2010 Oct;15(5):563–7.

113. Khan MA, Nicolls MR. Complement-mediated Microvascular Injury Leads to Chronic Rejection. Adv Exp Med Biol. 2013;734a:233–46.

114. Luckraz H, Goddard M, McNeil K, Atkinson C, Sharples LD, Wallwork J. Is Obliterative Bronchiolitis in Lung Transplantation Associated with Microvascular Damage to Small Airways? Ann Thorac Surg. 2006 Oct;82(4):1212–8.

115. Pettersson GB, Karam K, Thuita L, Johnston DR, McCurry KR, Kapadia SR, et al. Comparative Study of Bronchial Artery Revascularization in Lung Transplantation. J Thorac Cardiovasc Surg. 2013 Oct;146(4):894–900.e3.

116. Fishman JA, Rubin RH. Infection in Organ-transplant Recipients. N Engl J Med. 1998 Jun 11;338(24):1741–51.

117. Hafkin J, Blumberg E. Infections in Lung Transplantation: New Insights. Curr Opin Organ Transplant. 2009 Oct;14(5):483–7.

118. Burguete SR, Maselli DJ, Fernandez JF, Levine SM. Lung Transplant Infection. Respirol Carlton Vic. 2013 Jan;18(1):22–38.

119. Witt CA, Meyers BF, Hachem RR. Pulmonary Infections Following Lung Transplantation. Thorac Surg Clin. 2012 Aug;22(3):403–12.

120. Roux A, Mourin G, Fastenackels S, Almeida JR, Iglesias MC, Boyd A, et al. CMV Driven CD8(+) T-cell Activation Is Associated with Acute Rejection in Lung Transplantation. Clin Immunol Orlando Fla. 2013 Jul;148(1):16–26.

121. Paraskeva M, Bailey M, Levvey BJ, Griffiths AP, Kotsimbos TC, Williams TP, et al. Cytomegalovirus Replication within the Lung Allograft Is Associated with Bronchiolitis Obliterans Syndrome. Am J Transplant Off J Am Soc Transplant Am Soc Transpl Surg. 2011 Oct;11(10):2190–6.

122. Mehrad B, Paciocco G, Martinez FJ, Ojo TC, Iannettoni MD, Lynch JP 3rd. Spectrum of Aspergillus Infection in Lung Transplant Recipients: Case Series and Review of the Literature. Chest. 2001 Jan;119(1):169–75.

123. Chalermskulrat W, Sood N, Neuringer IP, Hecker TM, Chang L, Rivera MP, et al. Non-tuberculous Mycobacteria in End Stage Cystic Fibrosis: Implications for Lung Transplantation. Thorax. 2006 Jun;61(6):507–13.

124. Vadnerkar A, Clancy CJ, Celik U, Yousem SA, Mitsani D, Toyoda Y, et al. Impact of Mold Infections in Explanted Lungs on Outcomes of Lung Transplantation. Transplantation. 2010 Jan 27;89(2):253–60.

125. King CS, Khandhar S, Burton N, Shlobin OA, Ahmad S, Lefrak E, et al. Native Lung Complications in Single-lung Transplant Recipients and the Role of Pneumonectomy. J Heart Lung Transplant Off Publ Int Soc Heart Transplant. 2009 Aug;28(8):851–6.

126. Luong M-L, Morrissey O, Husain S. Assessment of Infection Risks Prior to Lung Transplantation. Curr Opin Infect Dis. 2010 Dec;23(6):578–83.

127. Watkins RR, Lemonovich TL. Evaluation of Infections in the Lung

127. Transplant Patient. Curr Opin Infect Dis. 2012 Apr;25(2):193–8.
128. Avery RK. Infections after Lung Transplantation. Semin Respir Crit Care Med. 2006 Oct;27(5):544–51.
129. De Perrot M, Liu M, Waddell TK, Keshavjee S. Ischemia-Reperfusion-Induced Lung Injury. Am J Respir Crit Care Med. 2003 Feb 15;167(4):490–511.
130. Christie JD, Carby M, Bag R, Corris P, Hertz M, Weill D, et al. Report of the ISHLT Working Group on Primary Lung Graft Dysfunction part II: Definition. A Consensus Statement of the International Society for Heart and Lung Transplantation. J Heart Lung Transplant Off Publ Int Soc Heart Transplant. 2005 Oct;24(10):1454–9.
131. Hosseini-Moghaddam SM, Husain S. Fungi and Molds Following Lung Transplantation. Semin Respir Crit Care Med. 2010 Apr;31(2):222–33.
132. Bhaskaran A, Hosseini-Moghaddam SM, Rotstein C, Husain S. Mold Infections in Lung Transplant Recipients. Semin Respir Crit Care Med. 2013 Jun;34(3):371–9.
133. Lease ED, Zaas DW. Update on Infectious Complications Following Lung Transplantation. Curr Opin Pulm Med. 2011 May;17(3):206–9.
134. Wang EHZ, Partovi N, Levy RD, Shapiro RJ, Yoshida EM, Greanya ED. Pneumocystis Pneumonia in Solid Organ Transplant Recipients: Not Yet an Infection of the Past. Transpl Infect Dis Off J Transplant Soc. 2012 Oct;14(5):519–25.
135. Liu M, Mallory GB, Schecter MG, Worley S, Arrigain S, Robertson J, et al. Long-term Impact of Respiratory Viral Infection after Pediatric Lung Transplantation. Pediatr Transplant. 2010 May;14(3):431–6.
136. Christie JD, Edwards LB, Aurora P, Dobbels F, Kirk R, Rahmel AO, et al. Registry of the International Society for Heart and Lung Transplantation: Twenty-fifth Official Adult Lung and Heart/Lung Transplantation Report–2008. J Heart Lung Transplant Off Publ Int Soc Heart Transplant. 2008 Sep;27(9):957–69.
137. Mitsani D, Nguyen MH, Kwak EJ, Silveira FP, Vadnerkar A, Pilewski J, et al. Cytomegalovirus Disease among Donor-positive/Recipient-negative Lung Transplant Recipients in the Era of Valganciclovir Prophylaxis. J Heart Lung Transplant Off Publ Int Soc Heart Transplant. 2010 Sep;29(9):1014–20.
138. Shah PD, McDyer JF. Viral Infections in Lung Transplant Recipients. Semin Respir Crit Care Med. 2010 Apr;31(2):243–54.
139. Uhlin M, Mattsson J, Maeurer M. Update on Viral Infections in Lung Transplantation. Curr Opin Pulm Med. 2012 May;18(3):264–70.
140. Shalhoub S, Husain S. Community-acquired Respiratory Viral Infections in Lung Transplant Recipients. Curr Opin Infect Dis. 2013 Aug;26(4):302–8.
141. Clark NM, Lynch JP 3rd, Sayah D, Belperio JA, Fishbein MC, Weigt SS. DNA Viral Infections Complicating Lung Transplantation. Semin Respir Crit Care Med. 2013 Jun;34(3):380–404.
142. Patel N, Snyder LD, Finlen-Copeland A, Palmer SM. Is Prevention the Best Treatment? CMV after Lung Transplantation. Am J Transplant Off J Am Soc Transplant Am Soc Transpl Surg. 2012 Mar;12(3):539–44.
143. Gottlieb J, Schulz TF, Welte T, Fuehner T, Dierich M, Simon AR, et al. Community-acquired Respiratory Viral Infections in Lung Transplant Recipients: A Single Season Cohort Study. Transplantation. 2009 May 27;87(10):1530–7.
144. Garantziotis S, Howell DN, McAdams HP, Davis RD, Henshaw NG, Palmer SM. Influenza Pneumonia in Lung Transplant Recipients: Clinical Features and Association with Bronchiolitis Obliterans Syndrome. Chest. 2001 Apr;119(4):1277–80.
145. Malouf MA, Glanville AR. The Spectrum of Mycobacterial Infection after Lung Transplantation. Am J Respir Crit Care Med. 1999 Nov;160(5 Pt 1):1611–6.
146. Gilljam M, Scherstén H, Silverborn M, Jönsson B, Ericsson Hollsing A. Lung Transplantation in Patients with Cystic Fibrosis and Mycobacterium Abscessus Infection. J Cyst Fibros Off J Eur Cyst Fibros Soc. 2010 Jul;9(4):272–6.
147. Reams BD, McAdams HP, Howell DN, Steele MP, Davis RD, Palmer SM. Posttransplant Lymphoproliferative Disorder: Incidence, Presentation, and Response to Treatment in Lung Transplant Recipients. Chest. 2003 Oct;124(4):1242–9.
148. Trulock EP, Edwards LB, Taylor DO, Boucek MM, Keck BM, Hertz MI. Registry of the International Society for Heart and Lung Transplantation: Twenty-second Official Adult Lung and Heart-Lung Transplant Report–2005. J Heart Lung Transplant Off Publ Int Soc Heart Transplant. 2005 Aug;24(8):956–67.
149. Evens AM, Roy R, Sterrenberg D, Moll MZ, Chadburn A, Gordon LI. Post-Transplantation Lymphoproliferative Disorders: Diagnosis, Prognosis, and Current Approaches to Therapy. Curr Oncol Rep. 2010 Nov;12(6):383–94.
150. Shitrit D, Shitrit AB-G, Dickman R, Sahar G, Saute M, Kramer MR. Gastrointestinal Involvement of Posttransplant Lymphoproliferative Disorder in Lung Transplant Recipients: Report of a Case. Dis Colon Rectum. 2005 Nov;48(11):2144–7.
151. Malouf MA, Chhajed PN, Hopkins P, Plit M, Turner J, Glanville AR. Anti-viral Prophylaxis Reduces the Incidence of Lymphoproliferative Disease in Lung Transplant Recipients. J Heart Lung Transplant Off Publ Int Soc Heart Transplant. 2002 May;21(5):547–54.
152. Wheless SA, Gulley ML, Raab-Traub N, McNeillie P, Neuringer IP, Ford HJ, et al. Post-transplantation Lymphoproliferative Disease: Epstein-Barr Virus DNA Levels, HLA-A3, and Survival. Am J Respir Crit Care Med. 2008 Nov 15;178(10):1060–5.
153. Michelson P, Watkins B, Webber SA, Wadowsky R, Michaels MG. Screening for PTLD in Lung and Heart-Lung Transplant Recipients by Measuring EBV DNA Load in Bronchoalveolar Lavage Fluid using Real Time PCR. Pediatr Transplant. 2008 Jun;12(4):464–8.
154. Paranjothi S, Yusen RD, Kraus MD, Lynch JP, Patterson GA, Trulock EP. Lymphoproliferative Disease after Lung Transplantation: Comparison of Presentation and Outcome of Early and Late Cases. J Heart Lung Transplant Off Publ Int Soc Heart Transplant. 2001 Oct;20(10):1054–63.
155. Campo E, Swerdlow SH, Harris NL, Pileri S, Stein H, Jaffe ES. The 2008 WHO Classification of Lymphoid Neoplasms and Beyond: Evolving Concepts and Practical Applications. Blood. 2011 May 12;117(19):5019–32.
156. Tiede C, Maecker-Kolhoff B, Klein C, Kreipe H, Hussein K. Risk Factors and Prognosis in T-cell Posttransplantation Lymphoproliferative Diseases: Reevaluation of 163 Cases. Transplantation. 2013 Feb 15;95(3):479–88.
157. Rowlings PA, Curtis RE, Passweg JR, Deeg HJ, Socié G, Travis LB, et al.

157. Increased Incidence of Hodgkin's Disease after Allogeneic Bone Marrow Transplantation. J Clin Oncol Off J Am Soc Clin Oncol. 1999 Oct;17(10):3122–7.

158. Pitman SD, Huang Q, Zuppan CW, Rowsell EH, Cao JD, Berdeja JG, et al. Hodgkin Lymphoma-like Posttransplant Lymphoproliferative Disorder (HL-like PTLD) Simulates Monomorphic B-cell PTLD both Clinically and Pathologically. Am J Surg Pathol. 2006 Apr;30(4):470–6.

159. Haydar AA, Denton M, West A, Rees J, Goldsmith DJA. Sirolimus-induced Pneumonitis: Three Cases and a Review of the Literature. Am J Transplant Off J Am Soc Transplant Am Soc Transpl Surg. 2004 Jan;4(1):137–9.

160. Khalife WI, Kogoj P, Kar B. Sirolimus-induced Alveolar Hemorrhage. J Heart Lung Transplant Off Publ Int Soc Heart Transplant. 2007 Jun;26(6):652–7.

161. King-Biggs MB, Dunitz JM, Park SJ, Kay Savik S, Hertz MI. Airway Anastomotic Dehiscence Associated with Use of Sirolimus Immediately after Lung Transplantation. Transplantation. 2003 May 15;75(9):1437–43.

162. Zaas DW. Update on Medical Complications Involving the Lungs. Curr Opin Organ Transplant. 2009 Oct;14(5):488–93.

163. Camus P, Martin WJ 2nd, Rosenow EC 3rd. Amiodarone Pulmonary Toxicity. Clin Chest Med. 2004 Mar;25(1):65–75.

164. Diaz-Guzman E, Mireles-Cabodevila E, Arrossi A, Kanne JP, Budev M. Amiodarone Pulmonary Toxicity after Lung Transplantation. J Heart Lung Transplant Off Publ Int Soc Heart Transplant. 2008 Sep;27(9):1059–63.

165. Gilman MJ, Wang KP. Transbronchial Lung Biopsy in Sarcoidosis. An Approach to Determine the Optimal Number of Biopsies. Am Rev Respir Dis. 1980 Nov;122(5):721–4.

166. Martinez FJ, Orens JB, Deeb M, Brunsting LA, Flint A, Lynch JP 3rd. Recurrence of Sarcoidosis Following Bilateral Allogeneic Lung Transplantation. Chest. 1994 Nov;106(5):1597–9.

167. Shah L. Lung Transplantation in Sarcoidosis. Semin Respir Crit Care Med. 2007 Feb;28(1):134–40.

168. Israel-Biet D, Valeyre D. Diagnosis of Pulmonary Sarcoidosis. Curr Opin Pulm Med. 2013 Sep;19(5):510–5.

169. Orens JB, Estenne M, Arcasoy S, Conte JV, Corris P, Egan JJ, et al. International Guidelines for the Selection of Lung Transplant Candidates: 2006 Update–A Consensus Report from the Pulmonary Scientific Council of the International Society for Heart and Lung Transplantation. J Heart Lung Transplant Off Publ Int Soc Heart Transplant. 2006 Jul;25(7):745–55.

170. Arcasoy SM, Hersh C, Christie JD, Zisman D, Pochettino A, Rosengard BR, et al. Bronchogenic Carcinoma Complicating Lung Transplantation. J Heart Lung Transplant Off Publ Int Soc Heart Transplant. 2001 Oct;20(10):1044–53.

171. Machuca TN, Keshavjee S. Transplantation for Lung Cancer. Curr Opin Organ Transplant. 2012 Oct;17(5):479–84.

172. Nine JS, Yousem SA, Paradis IL, Keenan R, Griffith BP. Lymphangioleiomyomatosis: Recurrence after Lung Transplantation. J Heart Lung Transplant Off Publ Int Soc Heart Transplant. 1994 Aug;13(4):714–9.

173. Dauriat G, Mal H, Thabut G, Mornex J-F, Bertocchi M, Tronc F, et al. Lung Transplantation for Pulmonary Langerhans' Cell Histiocytosis: A Multicenter Analysis. Transplantation. 2006 Mar 15;81(5):746–50.

174. Lee C, Suh RD, Krishnam MS, Lai CK, Fishbein MC, Wallace WD, et al. Recurrent Pulmonary Capillary Hemangiomatosis after Bilateral Lung Transplantation. J Thorac Imaging. 2010 Aug;25(3):W89–92.

175. Frost AE, Keller CA, Brown RW, Noon GP, Short HD, Abraham JL, et al. Giant Cell Interstitial Pneumonitis. Disease Recurrence in the Transplanted Lung. Am Rev Respir Dis. 1993 Nov;148(5):1401–4.

176. Albores J, Seki A, Fishbein MC, Abtin F, Lynch JP 3rd, Wang T, et al. A Rare Occurrence of Pulmonary Alveolar Proteinosis after Lung Transplantation. Semin Respir Crit Care Med. 2013 Jun;34(3):431–8.

177. Izbicki G, Bairey O, Shitrit D, Lahav J, Kramer MR. Increased Thromboembolic Events after Lung Transplantation. Chest. 2006 Feb;129(2):412–6.

178. Kahan ES, Petersen G, Gaughan JP, Criner GJ. High Incidence of Venous Thromboembolic Events in Lung Transplant Recipients. J Heart Lung Transplant Off Publ Int Soc Heart Transplant. 2007 Apr;26(4):339–44.

179. Yegen HA, Lederer DJ, Barr RG, Wilt JS, Fang Y, Bagiella E, et al. Risk Factors for Venous Thromboembolism after Lung Transplantation. Chest. 2007 Aug;132(2):547–53.

180. Dickson RP, Davis RD, Rea JB, Palmer SM. High Frequency of Bronchogenic Carcinoma after Single-Lung Transplantation. J Heart Lung Transplant Off Publ Int Soc Heart Transplant. 2006 Nov;25(11):1297–301.

181. Parada MT, Sepúlveda C, Alba A, Salas A. Malignancy Development in Lung Transplant Patients. Transplant Proc. 2011 Aug;43(6):2316–7.

182. Desai R, Collett D, Watson CJ, Johnson P, Evans T, Neuberger J. Cancer Transmission from Organ Donors-Unavoidable but Low Risk. Transplantation. 2012 Dec 27;94(12):1200–7.

183. Fisichella PM, Davis CS, Kovacs EJ. A Review of the Role of GERD-induced Aspiration after Lung Transplantation. Surg Endosc. 2012 May;26(5):1201–4.

Chapter 6

The Pathology of Intestinal and Multivisceral Transplantation

Phillip Ruiz, Jennifer Garcia, Ji Fan, Seigo Nishida, Thiago Beduschi, Akin Tekin, and Rodrigo Vianna

I Introduction and Background

The application of intestinal (ITx) and multivisceral transplantation (MVTx) as therapy for Short Gut Syndrome (SGS) and substantial gastrointestinal failure has evolved over the last 25 years so that these procedures have become an adjunct and invaluable complement to first-line intestinal rehabilitation [1]. A variety of transplant centers have garnered extensive experience and this has been critical to the observed continual improvement in graft and patient survival with these challenging organ transplants [2-4, 5]. Intestinal rehabilitation and enteral feeding, though highly effective [6, 7], can still be associated with numerous and often life-threatening complications, elevated costs, and altered quality of life issues [8]. The origins of the significant gastrointestinal compromise necessary to consider intestinal or multivisceral transplantation typically include catastrophic abdominal compartment injury, medical disease, and certain tumors in both pediatric and adult patients (Table 6.1), although the disorders impeding gut function tend to be different according to the age group [9]. Ultimately, the central binding physiological failure of the patients necessitating ITx and MVTx is a compromise of the absorptive function of the alimentary tract, ultimately resulting in severe malnourishment. Although there are discrete considerations beforehand, pediatric and adult patients can both receive alimentary tract grafts. A majority of these patients are maintained by enteral feeding prior to transplantation [8].

The effective execution of an intestinal or multivisceral transplant provides the recipient with a functioning gastrointestinal tract devoid of or with minimal dietary restrictions, boosted growth and development, and the possibility of an independent lifestyle [10]. There are variations in the surgical procedure for intestinal transplantation, depending upon the underlying pathological conditions compromising gut function and the clinical presentation of the transplant candidate. There may be an isolated intestinal allograft (ITx) or the intestine can be a component of a multivisceral transplant (MVTx), the latter representing an abdominal organ bloc that can include stomach, small and large intestine, liver, pancreas, and spleen; the omission of a liver allograft is known as a modified multivisceral transplant [11, 12]. The utilization of MVTx has seen an increase, with graft and patient survival being comparable and in some studies better compared to isolated intestinal transplantation [12]. To date, the overwhelming majority of over 2000 ITx or MVTx performed procedures have been with using diseased donor allografts, although a small proportion of ITx have been performed with living donors [13]. Improved evaluation and selection of appropriate donors and recipients, improved and constantly evolving immunosuppression, greater information on gut physiology and mucosal immunology, and advances in post-transplant monitoring, the latter addressed in this chapter, have all contributed to an observed upgrading in graft and recipient survival.

Table 6.1 Primary Disease of Patients Receiving Intestinal or Multivisceral Transplants*

Pediatric Disease
Gastroschisis
Midgut volvulus
Necrotizing enterocolitis
Chronic intestinal pseudo-obstruction
Intestinal atresia
Aganglionosis/Hirschsprung's
Retransplant
Microvillous involution inclusion
Malabsorption
Massive resection due to tumor
Adult disease
Ischemia
Crohn's disease
Trauma
Volvulus
Motility disorders
Desmoids
Retransplant
Gardner's syndrome
Superior mesenteric artery thrombosis
Superior mesenteric vein thrombosis
Pseudo-obstruction

Table 6.2 List of Potential Complications after Intestinal Transplantation

Acute rejection
Chronic rejection
Infection
PTLD
GVHD
Renal dysfunction
Bowel perforation
Pancreatitis
Anastomotic leakage
Others

The presentation of an intestinal or multivisceral graft into a recipient represents a colossal lymphoid and non-lymphoid cellular load to the recipient that, for the most part, is histoincompatible and highly immunogenic. The consequence of this antigenic inoculum is that ITx and MVTx, often more than with most other solid organ allografts, require significant and unlimited use of powerful immunosuppression in order to maintain the viability of the grafts in the face of a sustained and vigorous immune-mediated attack from the host. As mentioned in previous chapters, the significant immunosuppressed state places the organ recipient at risk for the development of malignancies and infections, as well as the potential for direct toxicities on several organ systems by the drugs themselves [14]. While our increased understanding of the mechanisms involved in intestinal graft rejection has allowed the design of interventional protocols that often now protect the recipient and graft from immunologically-based injury, the frequency of alloimmune-based host-derived immune response [15] and sometimes the graft immune response to the host (i.e., Graft-versus-Host Disease or GVHD) [16] in ITx and MVTx remains very high. Aside from the level and type of immunosuppression, other variables such as the type of host innate genetic polymorphisms present that may influence the level of host responsiveness [17], the ratio of effector to regulatory cell populations [18] and the degree and type of genetic disparity between the host and donor affect the host alloimmune response. Aside from complications associable with immune system perturbation, peripheral factors such as pre- and post-transplant alimentation protocols, previous abdominal surgeries, and co-morbidities associated with the underlying disease(s) of the host are important variables to consider. Table 6.2 provides a list of some of the complications experienced in alimentary graft transplants.

The critically important monitoring of intestinal graft function and patient status in the post-transplant period has evolved over the past several decades and the transplant pathologist, whether by biopsy evaluation and/or coordination of laboratory analysis, occupies a central role in the clinical team's vigilance of potential complications [19]. As such, the field of transplant pathology as it pertains to gastrointestinal transplantation has evolved into a discipline that coordinates traditional histologic biopsy examination with general and specialized clinical laboratory analysis (e.g., histocompatibility lab), comprehension of pathophysiological mechanisms associated with allograft intestine or the other transplanted abdominal viscera, and knowledge of developing molecular techniques [20].

In the case of MVTx, the pathologist is also required to have an expanded knowledge of surgical allografts not characteristically encountered (i.e., stomach, colon) and a cognizance of the spectrum of pathological changes contingent upon which area of the gastrointestinal tract is sampled (e.g., duodenal versus ileal). For example, there may be contemporaneous obtaining of biopsies from native organs such as esophagus, rectum, and skin, as well as biopsies from transplanted stomach, small intestine, large intestine, and liver. A valuable tool in many circumstances is comparison of native versus allograft tissues when one is trying to discriminate whether changes are exclusive to alloimmune responses (i.e., rejection), generalized pathologies (e.g., infection, PTLD), or graft-derived changes (GVHD, preservation injury). Although these patients have an exteriorized ostomy through which endoscopy is often performed, biopsies attained from the ostomy site are discouraged since there may be ongoing inflammatory responses reflected by histological inflammatory processes, fibrosis, and distorted architecture [21].

II Histopathological Evaluations

A combination of histopathological evaluation of the transplants and medical laboratory support are critical to all stages of clinical intestinal and multivisceral transplantation. This clinicopathological support extends through the pretransplant phases and continuously through the evaluation and maintenance of long-term surviving grafts [19, 22]. A preponderance of tissue samples taken from selected regions of ITx and MVTx allografts are visualized by endoscopy and sampling of mucosal areas is the typical tissue that is procured. Biopsies from intestinal and gastric allografts are technically obtained in a fashion similar to biopsies from the native organ counterparts. It is important that the endoscopist (preferably experienced with GI transplants) and pathologist have an ongoing communication in order to determine which regions to biopsy, mucosal endoscopic changes, location, characteristics, and distribution of any lesion(s) and whether it was limited to the graft or also involving native tissue. Biopsies should be noted from which area they are in taken, such as lesional, perilesional, and non-involved areas, since there can be a gamut of different histological changes between adjacent regions. Submucosal areas of allografts tend to only be assessed when there is surgical revision of problematic areas or when grafts are explanted. As with biopsies obtained from any transplanted organ, it is imperative that the transplant pathologist has a reasonable clinical history of the recipient (e.g., date of transplant, native disease or problem that necessitated the transplantation, current clinical symptoms), what the previous biopsy results were (if any), and as mentioned above, an impression of the endoscopic appearance of the organ. Many of the complications affecting gastrointestinal transplants have high clinical urgency and could rapidly lead to allograft dysfunction and potential graft loss. Thus, processing and evaluation of allograft biopsies should be as expeditious as possible (e.g., our laboratory provides two-hour turnaround time for permanent sections) and available seven days a week. One or two fragments per area should be placed immediately in an appropriate fixative (typically buffered formalin) and paraffin sections are typically cut at 0.5cm with multiple levels, since processes such as rejection may be geographically limited and not diffusely distributed. Hematoxylin and Eosin (H&E) stains are used for the initial evaluation. The histology lab and pathology service providing transplant pathology support should also incorporate specialized immunohistochemical (IHC), immunofluorescence (IF) (e.g., to infectious agents such as CMV, adenovirus), and in situ hybridization (ISH) techniques (e.g., EBV); additionally, the transplant pathology lab should also serve as an initiation point for graft tissue-derived molecular assays such as quantitative infectious agent evaluations, antigen receptor rearrangement studies for T and B cells, and specific gene arrays.

III Donor Organs and Preservation Injury

As with other solid organ transplants, procurement of intestinal or multivisceral donor organs from deceased individuals depends upon on a complex yet coordinated system whereby potential donors are identified based on an algorithm that incorporates various factors, including size (e.g., size of the recipient abdominal cavity; pediatric age), donor clinical history fittingness, and an exclusion of most infectious risk factors [23]. In the case of intestine or other abdominal viscera, gross surgical inspection of the donor organs during retrieval suffices to assess any possible lesions; rarely, frozen section evaluation by a pathologist is needed for ITx or MVTx. Concurrently, the testing laboratory must rapidly provide a wide-ranging battery of tests for assessing potential infectious pathogens in the proposed donor, and the clinical team must try to identify the status of the donor organs insofar as issues such as ischemic injury, possible tumors, and ongoing medical conditions that could compromise gut function. Consequently, though it is not typical that the pathologist is asked to evaluate a donor bowel or stomach prior to being transplanted like other allografts such as kidney and liver, there is extensive dependence upon the clinical lab results. The pathological evaluation of residual donor tissue has typically not shown any significant pathological changes aside from ischemic injury, as would be expected from graft preservation.

The recovery of deceased donor organs necessitates that there be a preservation of the viscera in cold solutions followed by a warm reperfusion of the grafts upon vascular anastomosis with the recipient blood supply. There is typically minimal "cold ischemic" time associated with gastrointestinal grafts, although there is almost always some degree of preservation-associated or ischemia reperfusion (I/R) injury to the allograft following this revascularization of the donor organs [24]. Ischemia/reperfusion injury in the gut [25] results in a torrent of physiological changes and alterations of various genes that may ultimately influence function of the allograft. Although clinically silent as far as short-term function in a majority of the cases, these I/R changes may still have considerable consequence to the organ's long-term success. For example, there may be significant effects on the allograft organ's eventual susceptibility to immune-mediated injury and physiological function. I/R injury results in numerous gene shifts (mostly upregulated) [26], including many genes associated with inflammation [27, 28]. The implication of these transcriptional gene changes in donor bowel grafts remains unspecified and there can only be an assumption that these changes in the harvested organs impact long-term graft function. It can be speculated that the use of "marginal" donors [29] would predispose the recipient to I/R injury, primary non-function or delayed graft function, and complications such as acute rejection.

Morphology: Following transplantation, a preponderance of ITx and MVTx transplants are examined with "protocol" biopsies, particularly in the initial weeks post-transplant; during this period, it is not unusual for mucosal biopsies to demonstrate preservation injury changes [30]. Gastrointestinal grafts undergoing mild preservation injury tend to demonstrate diffuse edema and swelling of the villi without a significant increase in the inflammatory cell infiltrate, some vascular congestion, and a separation of the surface epithelial lining from the underlying lamina propria (see Figure 6.1). As I/R injury progresses and becomes more severe, there are additional changes such as epithelial cell necrosis that can extend from the surface of the mucosa to the deep submucosa (see Figure 6.2). In general, the more severe forms of I/R injury are clinically or pathologically evident. However, these latter changes have been well-portrayed in the coordinated environment of experimental models of I/R injury; for example, several murine models show gradable and progressive changes from the mucosa that eventually evolve to transmural necrosis of the intestine [31, 32]; as noted, these latter changes are not typically apparent microscopically in a clinical situation unless there is severe I/R injury along with prolonged vascular compromise, in which case, the allograft tissues show ischemic changes similar to bowel ischemia in native organs. Several controlled models may indeed allow visualization of all changes in the human intestine undergoing I/R injury [33]. Presently, the morphology of stomach allografts undergoing I/R injury is not well-described.

IV Acute Rejection

Alloimmune effector processes include the induction and promulgation of recipient alloimmune lymphoid cell populations (cell-mediated or T cell rejection) and host B cell-derived alloantibodies (humoral or antibody-mediated rejection) in combination with nonspecific innate immune mechanisms. When these processes remain uncontrolled by regulatory processes or immunosuppression, they can constitute an assault of anti-graft inflammatory responses that clinically and pathologically are defined as acute rejection [18]. This potent collection of immune-based cell populations and soluble immune molecules can be arranged in variable combinations; depending upon these groupings, there is a clinical and pathological manifestation of different forms of injury that have classically been delineated morphologically and sometimes behaviorally as distinct forms of acute rejection. Due to the immense potential for acute rejection to reduce graft function and lead to organ loss, the detection and effective

The Pathology of Intestinal and Multivisceral Transplantation

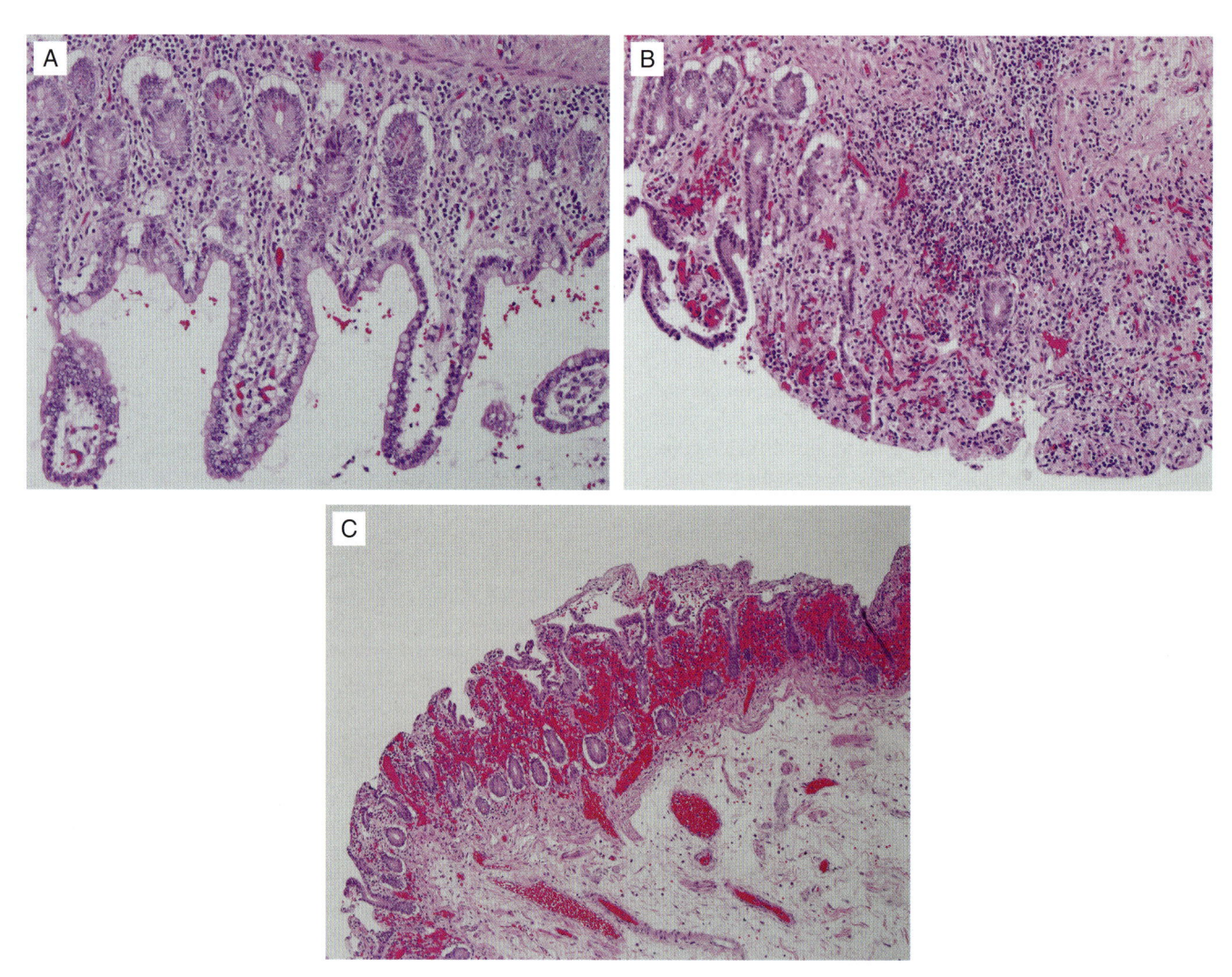

Figure 6.1 Preservation Injury (Original magnification x200, H&E). Small intestinal biopsies (a, b, c) several days after transplant shows swelling of the villi without a significant increase in the inflammatory cell infiltrate, some vascular congestion, and a separation of the surface epithelial lining from the underlying lamina propria.

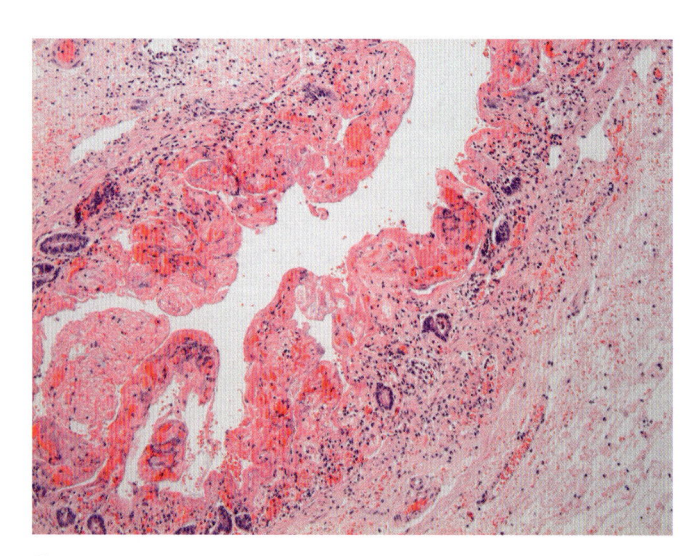

Figure 6.2 Preservation Injury (Original magnification x100, H&E). Example of more severe ischemia-reperfusion injury with prolonged vascular compromise showing mucosal hemorrhage and epithelial cell necrosis extending from the surface of the mucosa to the deep submucosa.

interruption of acute rejection in ITx and MVTx recipients, as with other solid organ transplants, remains an unceasing task and goal for transplant clinicians. However, in spite of the application of powerful immunosuppressive drugs, allograft acute rejection remains as an important and common complication in GI transplantation. The broad mechanisms involved in T cell-mediated and antibody-based forms of acute rejection are similar to other organ systems and beyond the scope of this chapter. Basically, recipient-derived B cells and T cells (the principal cells representing the adaptive immune response), in a complex interplay with innate immune populations including natural killer cells, dendritic cells, innate lymphoid cells (ILCs), and macrophages orchestrated through an assortment of immunomodulatory molecules [34], centrally participate in the genesis and culmination of immunological pathways that recognize the allogeneic GI tissue. There are multiple potential stimulatory targets in gastrointestinal tissue for immune effector cells and molecules, including parenchymal/epithelial cells (e.g., enterocytes, Paneth cells), vascular endothelial cells, and muscle, endocrine, and neural cells. Acute rejection-mediated injury or death of these various target cell populations in the bowel leads to clinical consequences such as fever, malabsorption, dysmotility, and ischemia [10, 23, 35]. Acute rejection of the bowel can progress rapidly due to the marked antigenicity and huge cellular mass of the bowel and, in some circumstances, can lead to exfoliation of the mucosa and submucosa [36, 37], transmural ischemia, and predisposition to translocation of luminal bacteria [38, 39], the latter scenario evolving to sepsis. It is therefore of vital importance that diagnosing acute rejection in small bowel and multivisceral transplantation be done promptly and precisely in order to avoid the menacing clinical consequences if rejection continues unabated in the host.

Clinical and endoscopic correlation is critical when considering the potential diagnosis of acute rejection. Bowel acute rejection can be associable with an assemblage of symptoms that can include increased fecal output (early on from their stoma), fever, and swelling [40]; these symptoms are not specific and other processes such as infection can also induce similar effects. In this regard, the endoscopically derived GI biopsy is often central to distinguishing these processes. Morphologically defined acute rejection in the absence of clinical symptoms is acknowledged as *subclinical rejection* (SCR) and this entity has been described in bowel allografts [41], comparable to several other solid organ transplants, including liver and kidney [42–44]. Typically, SCR is usually detected when biopsies are taken as part of protocol surveillance and the patients are clinically stable. SCR is potentially an important entity since patients with it may be at risk of a greater rate of eventual graft loss and some protocols treat SCR with additional immunosuppression. Adjunct non-invasive lab and biomarker assays, though currently lacking optimal specificity and sensitivity, are growing in use in order to further support a morphological diagnosis of acute rejection on the biopsy [45]. These tests include cytofluorographic analysis of peripheral immune cell populations [46], cytokine profiling, and the quantitation of distinct gene set changes [34]. Serial measurements of peripheral blood levels of the amino acid citrulline, though not specific for rejection, provide an assessment of viable intestinal mass, and this analyte is routinely measured at our institution in monitoring post-ITx and MVTx patients [47–49]. However, specificity in detecting acute (or chronic) rejection with citrulline alone does not appear possible; forthcoming algorithms with other markers of inflammation may yield more diagnostic specificity to the use of citrulline. In particular, an examination of molecules operative in GI acute rejection provide promise that limited gene sets, either from blood or from biopsies, will enhance the pathological diagnosis or refine the morphological impression seen in the biopsy [34]. Currently, however, histopathological examination of GI allograft biopsies remains as the most reliable and definitive method to diagnose rejection.

Morphology: The histopathology associated with acute rejection in biopsies after ITx or MVTx embodies a wide range of changes and fluctuates according to many variables with recipient, graft, and time post-transplant. The cataloging of acute rejection in small bowel and multivisceral transplantation, as with other solid organ allografts, utilizes terminology that derives from basic immunology (hyperacute rejection, accelerated acute rejection, acute vascular rejection, etc.) – with time, these terminologies have become more standardized. It is also now increasingly recognized that morphological changes associated with these subtypes of acute rejection also appear to be able to coexist (i.e., "mixed rejection"). Despite that, we will utilize a general classification, based on the general underlying etiology of the rejection, that being antibody-mediated or T cell-mediated but with the caveat being that all forms of rejection can coexist and that this is not an infrequent scenario.

a Antibody-mediated Rejection (AMR)

i Hyperacute and Accelerated Acute Rejection

Hyperacute and accelerated acute rejection are terms that outline the situation infrequently encountered in which an allograft organ is exposed to extremely high levels of alloantibodies that cross react with antigens on the organ (i.e., donor-specific antibodies) and is subsequently severely rejected within minutes to hours (*hyperacute rejection*) or a few days (*accelerated acute rejection*) following implantation [50, 51]. These potentially devastating forms of acute rejection tend to occur almost exclusively in the presensitized patient (i.e., pre-existing antibodies) and result in a severe antibody-mediated response in which the vasculature endothelium is the principal target, characterized histologically by vascular injury, thrombosis, and ischemic lesions. Experimental evidence of these forms of rejection in bowel allografts exists and documented clinical cases of hyperacute rejection in ITx or MVTx have been described [52], although this is a rare situation. The scarcity of hyperacute or accelerated acute rejection is a testament to the prognostic success of crossmatching of recipient sera by the histocompatibility lab with donor cells before GI transplantation; pre-transplant crossmatching was historically not the norm, although that has notably changed since the description of bowel hyperacute rejection episodes associated with the presence of pre-transplant donor-specific antibodies [53] [54, 55]. Grossly, the donor graft upon anastomosis immediately turns dusky in color and becomes hyperemic, resembling changes seen in other solid organ grafts experiencing hyperacute rejection.

The histopathological changes seen with hyperacute rejection of intestines include extensive mucosal congestion and necrosis with mixed acute inflammation and neutrophilic margination around vessels (see Figure 6.3). There is diffuse and severe vascular congestion with erythrocyte extravasation that extends from the mucosa through the entire thickness of the graft (transmural). Frank arteritis may be seen and native tissue tends to be unremarkable.

Curiously, these patients have the capacity to overcome this severe form of antibody-mediated acute rejection if there is aggressive intervention with plasmapheresis, treatment with anti-CD20 antibody (among other immunosuppression), and close monitoring [52, 54]. One patient we described with hyperacute rejection exhibited a full salvage of bowel graft function (normal graft morphology and asymptomatic) that coincided with reduction of titers of anti-donor antibodies and normal

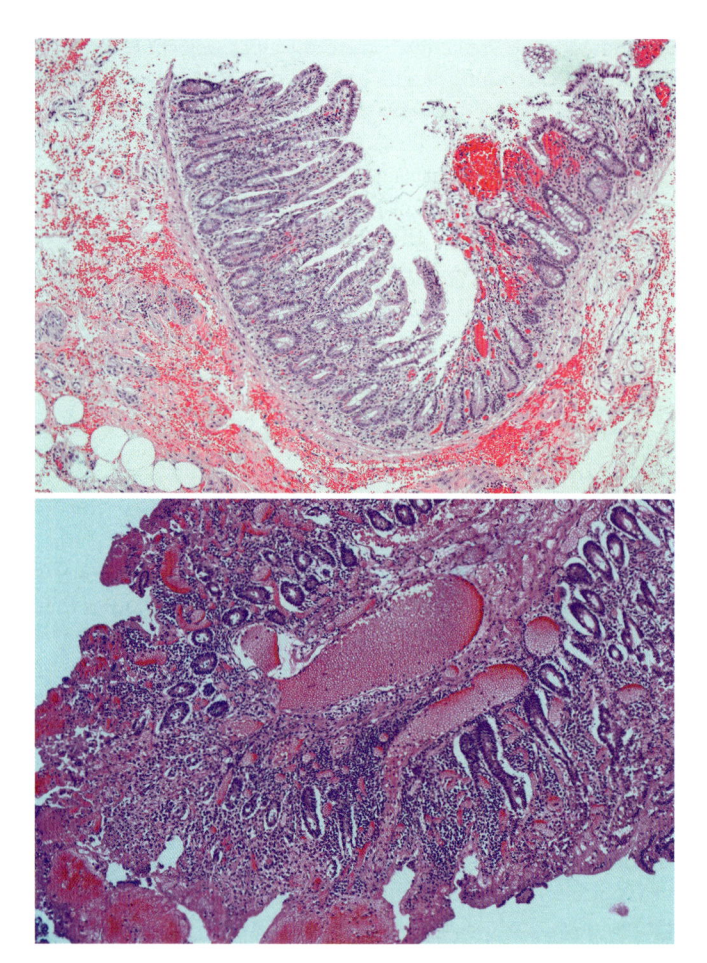

Figure 6.3 Hyperacute rejection (Original magnification 400x, H&E). Representative changes of bowel allograft on day two post-transplant undergoing hyperacute rejection due to high level of donor-specific alloantibodies. There is marked hemorrhage, vascular congestion, and mixed inflammatory cell infiltrate. Inflammatory cells were within several arteries.

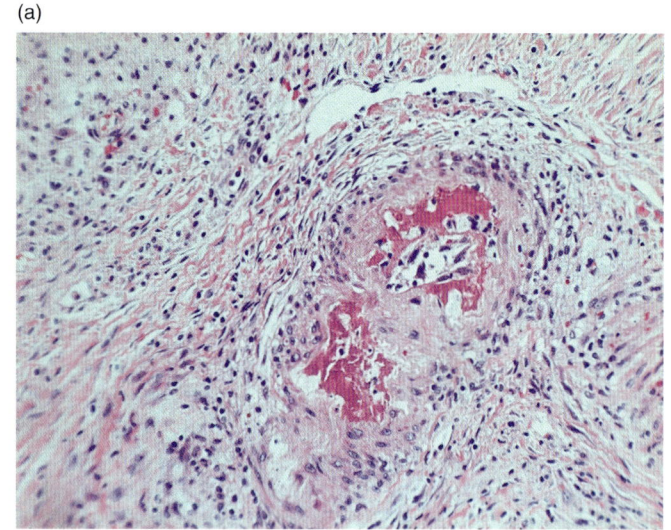

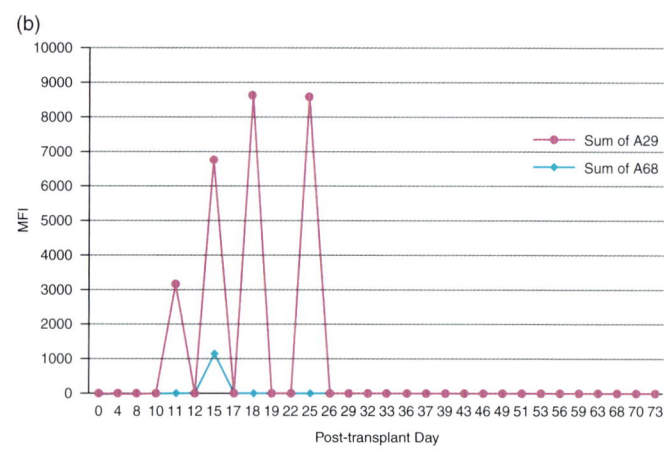

Figure 6.4 Acute antibody-mediated rejection – vasculitis (a) (Original magnification x400, H&E). Representative medium-sized artery in the submucosa of an intestinal allograft at day 25 post-transplant with high levels of donor-specific alloantibodies shown in (b), which is a chart showing the de novo post-transplant development of two class I alloantibodies. There was also simultaneous loss of crypts and focal fibrosis in lamina propria and submucosa.

endoscopic appearance [52]. Crossmatching is routinely performed at our center for all ITx and MVTx recipients.

On occasion, we have also found an accelerated AMR that occurred in the first several days following small bowel or multivisceral transplantation in which the recipients were sensitized with pre-existing alloantibodies and that morphologically demonstrated features of AMR described below, but not to the degree seen for hyperacute rejection.

ii Acute Antibody-mediated (Humoral) Rejection (AAMR)

As an entity, AAMR in human small bowel and multivisceral transplantation has become increasingly acknowledged over the past several years as an important cause of graft injury and dysfunction. The pathophysiology of AAMR originates with antibodies directed to alloantigens that then initiate a cascade of inflammation, coagulation, and other events that directly injure the transplant [53, 56, 57]. Consequently, identification of AAMR cannot be accomplished as a form of rejection without additional histochemical techniques and evidence of pre- and/or post-transplant alloantibody. Inflammation of arteries (vasculitis) can be one of the histological components of AAMR; however, this is not specific to antibodies since the cell-mediated arm of the immune response (T cell-mediated vasculitis) can also be an underlying cause of vasculitis in bowel allograft vessels. Severe forms of AAMR in small bowel transplants are often associated with alloantibody post-transplant sensitization of the recipient to donor antigens and subsequent rises in titers of pretransplant antibodies that were present at very low amounts before the transplant. The graft often demonstrates widespread inflammatory changes with a critical lesion being vasculitis of large-to-small arterial branches (see Figure 6.4). The vasculitis tends to show intimal edema and endothelial cell reactivity with an infiltration of acute and chronic inflammatory cells in the intimal layer of the artery. There are variable amounts of deposited complement components (e.g., C4d and C3d) and fibrinogen in lamina propria vasculature and larger vessels – monitoring and grading changes in the immunohistochemical expression of these molecules in sequential lesions can be an important adjunct pathological measurement. Left unchecked, the vasculitis can evolve to transmural inflammation with fibrin deposition and necrosis of the artery, causing severe ischemic injury to the graft. From time to time, selective arteries in the graft are affected more severely than others by the vasculitis. For example, mesenteric arteries can undergo AAMR and this can lead to sclerosing mesenteritis [58], a phenomenon that can be associated with increased alloantibodies. Severe vasculitis can also be evident in stomach and colon allografts with patterns as seen in the small bowel. When considering a differential diagnosis for this form of severe vasculitis only involving the transplant, other causes such as infectious agents (such as fungal or viral agents), neoplasia, drugs, and autoimmune processes should also be contemplated, although these are not common causes and characteristically would be distributed in native organs as well as the allograft. Larger vessel vasculitis is typically identified in explants or rejected organs or autopsies. Vasculitis tends to be relatively infrequent in mucosal biopsies; thus, the diagnosis of AAMR based upon severe vasculitis lesions in mucosal biopsies can be challenging in small bowel transplants.

AAMR also occurs in less severe forms in small bowel, stomach, and colon transplants and does so at a higher incidence than previously supposed. We have described alterations identifying early, mild, or evolving AAMR that can be isolated or occur in conjunction with T cell-mediated acute rejection [57]. These early and/or mild forms of AAMR appear associated in many cases with preexisting or post-transplant alloantibody formation with subtle, yet consistent mucosal morphological changes, often in the early period after transplantation. There is mild to diffuse, substantial vascular congestion with erythrocyte extravasation of the villous region and lamina propria microvasculature of the allograft mucosa (see Figure 6.5) and there may be no evidence of any significant vasculitis. There are various grades of congestion in the vasculature that can be graded (Table 6.3). Chronic inflammatory cells may or may not be increased and usually there is preservation of epithelial cells.

As stated above, supplementary tests can be very useful for assessment of humoral-based forms of acute rejection. For example, in suspected AAMR cases, an immunofluorescence or immunohistochemical panel for the presence of immunoglobulins (IgG, IgA, IgM) and complement components (C3, C4, C1q) fibrinogen, C3d, and C4d can be useful. In AAMR, there can be immunoglobulins deposited along vessels and within interstitium, along with complement components. We have also found C4d and C3d in small arteries and small capillaries in patients with milder or evolving forms of AAMR as in other transplanted organs and GI transplants undergoing severe antibody-mediated rejection (mentioned above) (see Figure 6.6). At this point, these subtle forms of AAMR do not demonstrate specific histopathological findings and some of these alterations can be found in ischemia, nonspecific enteritis, viral infections, and

Table 6.3 Scoring Grades for the Evaluation of Microvascular Changes during Acute Antibody-mediated Rejection in Gastrointestinal Allograft Mucosal Biopsies.

Grade	Histopathological Findings*
0	no significant congestion or extravasation
1	10%–40% of the tissue shows changes
2	40%–70% of the tissue shows changes
3	70% or greater portion of the tissues shows changes

* Capillaries, small venous and arterial branches in the lamina propria, and the submucosa are evaluated for the presence of dilatation and erythrocyte congestion. In addition, the surrounding interstitium is assessed for the presence of extravasated erythrocytes and edema. Scoring is calculated and based on the percentage of the overall biopsy.

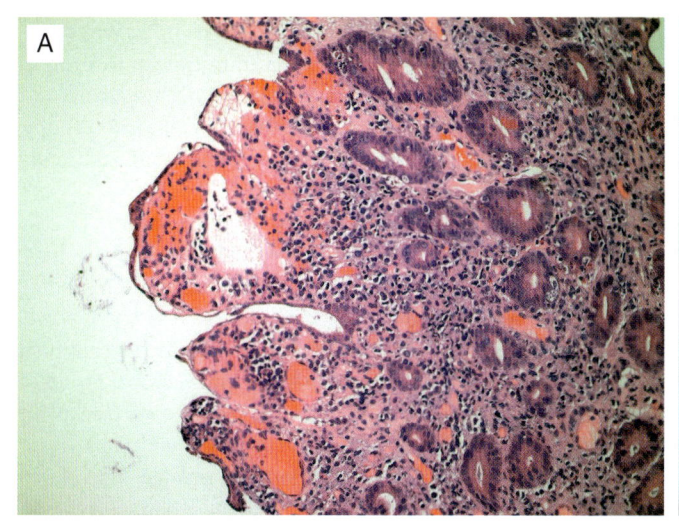

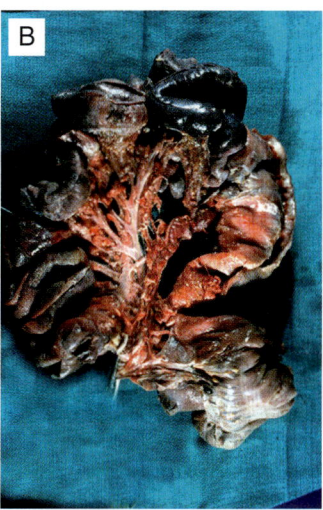

Figure 6.5 Acute antibody-mediated rejection (a) (Original magnification x400, H&E). Extensive vascular congestion of mucosal vasculature in patient with high levels of donor-specific alloantibodies. The interstitium also displays notable enteritis with epithelial apoptosis signifying concomitant acute cellular rejection. (b): Gross photomicrograph of the eventual bowel explant from the patient with segmental necrosis secondary to mesenteric artery thrombus, formed as a result of acute antibody-mediated rejection.

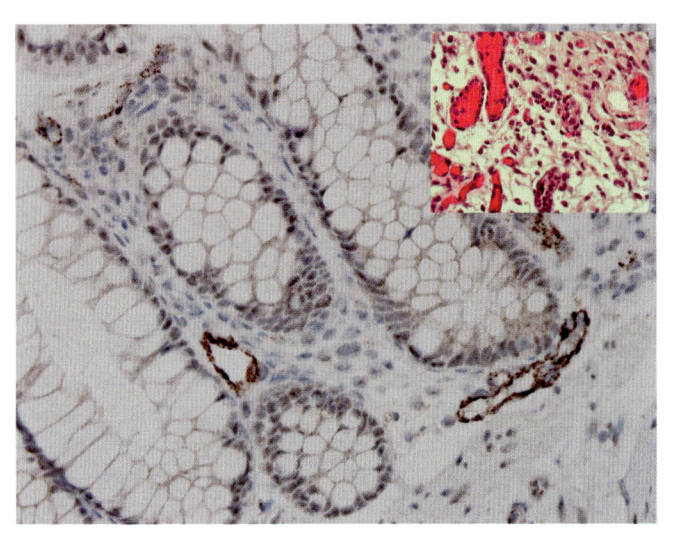

Figure 6.6 Acute antibody-mediated rejection (Original magnification x400). Graft undergoing antibody-mediated rejection with H&E showing significant vascular congestion and neutrophilic margination (Inset). Immunohistochemical staining for C4d in the same biopsy shows positive staining of the microvasculature of the mucosa.

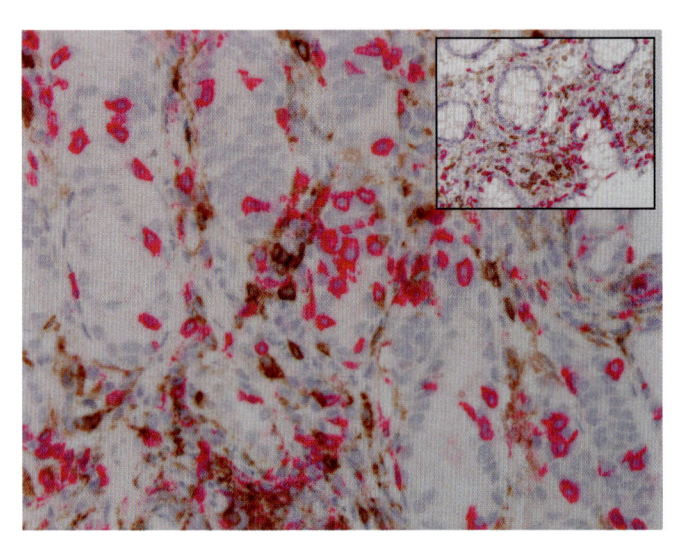

Figure 6.7 Acute T Cell-Mediated Acute Rejection (Original magnification 400x, two-color immunohistochemistry to CD4 and CD8). Two-color staining of gastrointestinal graft biopsy undergoing Acute T cell-mediated rejection, with CD4 (brown) and CD8 cells (red) within the interstitium and infiltrating glands. The CD4: CD8 ratio overall was estimated at 1:3.

mechanical vascular problems. Therefore, it is essential to incorporate the clinical history and lab values (e.g., alloantibody anti-donor titers), lesion distribution (allograft versus native tissue), other morphological findings (e.g., the presence of an acute inflammatory cell infiltrate or superficial epithelial changes with enteritis), and culture results. Furthermore, there should be a relationship of symptoms and histopathological resolution with supplemented immunosuppression concomitant with reduction of alloantibody concentrations.

b Acute T Cell-mediated (Cellular) Rejection

Acute T Cell-mediated Rejection (ACR) remains the most commonly recognized form of acute rejection in gastrointestinal (and other solid organ) transplants and can be present alongside other forms of rejection, as well as all other complications. Central among the pathophysiological processes functioning for this form of rejection is the recipient's T cell-mediated response to donor alloantigens. This is histologically characterized by a heterogeneous, lymphocyte-rich chronic inflammatory cell infiltrate that is primarily dispersed within the connective tissue/interstitial regions of organs with permeation and injuring of specific tissue parenchyma substructures [59]. Among the targeted gastrointestinal elements are cellular elements within crypts, glandular structures, as well as muscle, endothelial, and nerve cells. Functional and structural sequelae from this injury to the parenchyma can include metaplasia, apoptosis, and altered regulation of cell pathways.

Vascular compromise from the T cell-based alloimmune effector cell-based injury to the vessels can be particularly devastating (as with AAMR), since the vascular compromise subsequently leads to pervasive necrosis. The process of ACR in gastrointestinal allografts is involved and multifactorial, and one in which both CD4+ and CD8+ T cells are centrally involved (see Figure 6.7), analogous to other forms of allograft rejection. Crypt epithelial cell apoptosis is one of the foremost histological features associated with ACR in intestinal allografts [60] (see Figure 6.8), and appears principally due to CD8+ cytotoxic T cells induction of target cell apoptosis via the Granzyme B/Perforin-dependent granule-exocytosis pathway and Fas and Fas ligand–mediated cytotoxicity [34]. Non-CD8+ T cells also seem to potentially contribute to crypt epithelial cell apoptosis and acute allograft rejection in experimental animal models [61, 62].

There are regional differences in the gastrointestinal tracts insofar as susceptibility to ACR; for example, the ileum displays ACR more commonly, frequently, and more severely than duodenum or jejunum [63]. There may be severe infectious complications as a consequence of the heavy immunosuppression to treat ACR and alloimmune-mediated injury and impairment of mucosal barrier function (intestinal epithelial cells, intercellular tight junctions, and basement membranes) can result in bacterial translocation into the peritoneal space [39, 64].

Several classification schemes for grading acute T cell-mediated rejection (ACR) in small bowel/colon transplants have been described [59, 65], as well as a classification system for stomach [66]. A unified grading scheme for ACR in small bowel allografts was first developed in 2003 at the Eighth International Small Bowel Transplant Symposium by an international group of pathologists and clinicians experienced in small bowel transplant morphology [67] (Table 6.4). This scheme is now widely used and has been employed at our institution for greater than 4,000 biopsies [68]. To date, there appears to be good correlation between the morphological grading system and the clinical symptoms displayed by the recipient, as well as with inter-observer studies between different institutions (unpublished data).

The Pathology of Intestinal and Multivisceral Transplantation

Table 6.4 Characteristics of Acute Cellular rejection in Small Intestinal Allograft

Grade	Score	Description	Histopathological Findings
0	0	No evidence of acute rejection	Unremarkable histological changes that are essentially similar to normal native intestine.
IND	1	Indeterminate for acute rejection	A minor amount of epithelial cell injury or destruction; increase in crypt epithelial cell apoptosis, but with less than six apoptotic bodies per ten crypts; increased inflammatory infiltrate in lamina propria, mixed but primarily mononuclear inflammatory population; edema, blunting, vascular congestion can be present.
1	2	Acute cellular rejection, mild	Altered mucosal architecture (e.g. mild blunting of villi), edema, vascular congestion; increased crypt epithelial cell apoptosis (six or more apoptotic bodies per ten crypts); increased inflammatory infiltrate in lamina propria, mixed but primarily mononuclear inflammatory population with blastic and activated lymphocytes.
2	3	Acute cellular rejection, moderate	Features of Grade 1 as well as multiple; markedly increased crypt epithelial cell apoptosis (six or more apoptotic bodies per ten crypts), accompanied by foci of "confluent apoptosis"; whole gland necrosis, and/or crypt abscess; extensively increased inflammatory infiltrate in lamina propria, mixed but primarily mononuclear inflammatory population with blastic and activated lymphocytes; edema, vascular congestion, and blunting of villi of higher degree of Grade 1.
3	4	Acute cellular rejection, severe	Extensive morphological distortion and crypt damage with apoptosis, gland destruction, and associated mucosal ulceration; marked diffuse inflammatory infiltrate with blastic and activated lymphocytes, eosinophils, and neutrophils; granulation tissue and/or fibropurulent exudate with mucosal sloughing ("exfoliative rejection").

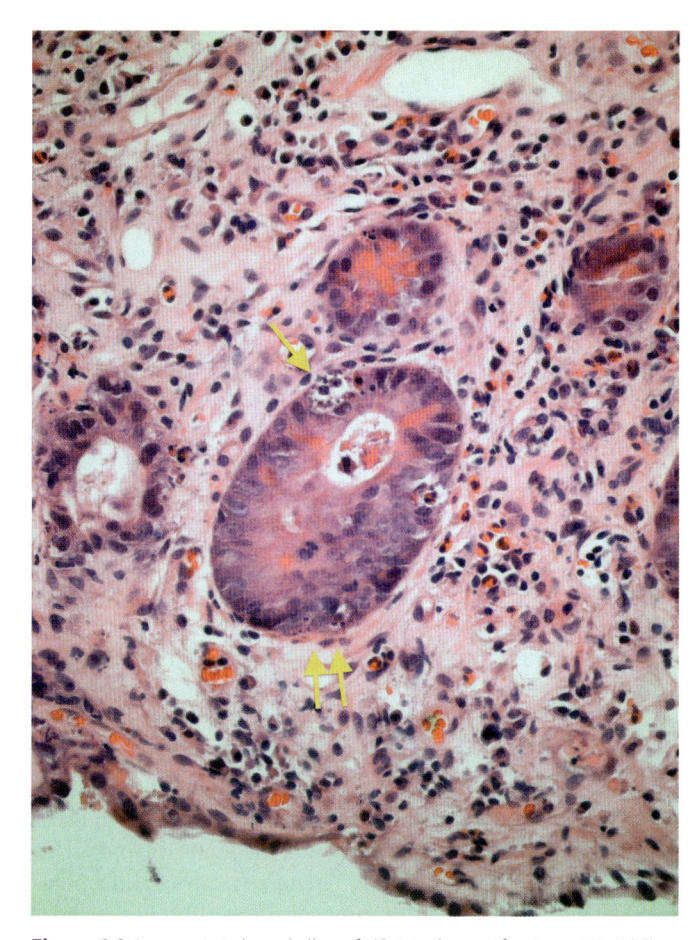

Figure 6.8 Apoptosis in bowel allograft (Original magnification x400, H&E). Bowel crypts demonstrating several forms of apoptosis of lining epithelial cells, including a larger "popcorn"-type of apoptosis (single arrow) and the more subtle forms of cellular degeneration (two arrows). Inflammatory cells are also infiltrating the gland.

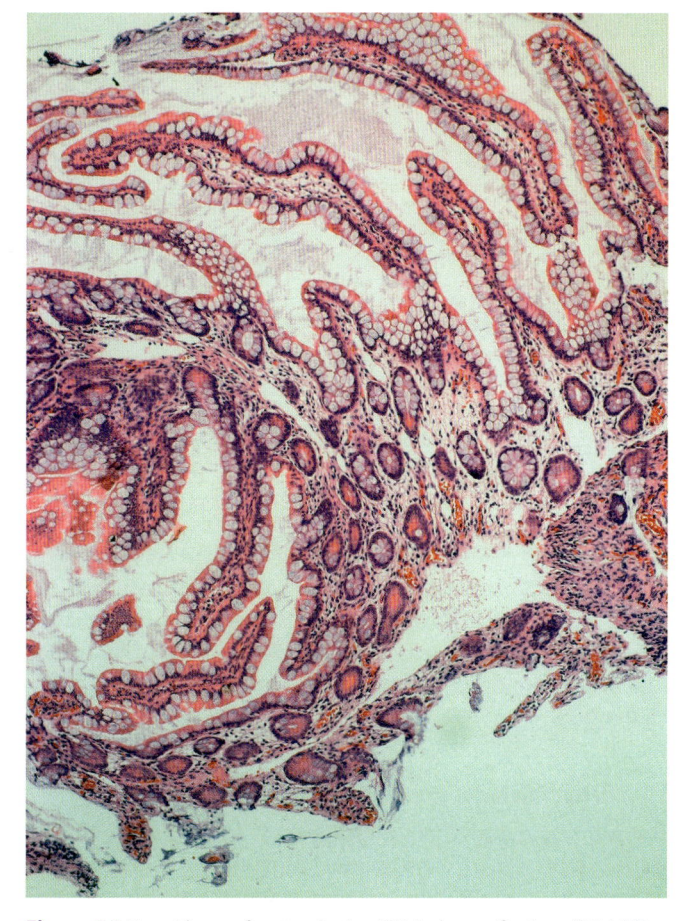

Figure 6.9 No evidence of acute rejection (Original magnification x200, H&E). Small bowel allograft seven days post-transplantation and showing no evidence of any significant alterations associated with acute rejection. Overall, the hematopoietic cell levels are less than seen with other immunosuppressive therapy.

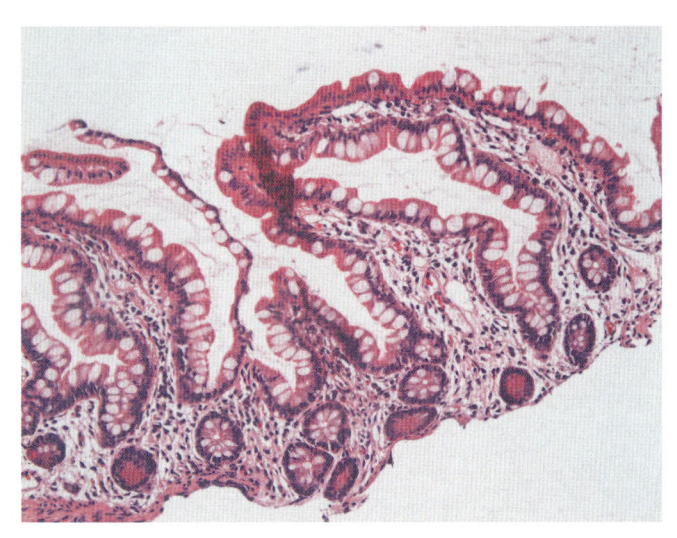

Figure 6.10 Indeterminate for acute rejection, Grade IND (Original magnification x100, H&E). Small bowel allograft with a subtle yet increased interstitial inflammatory infiltrate composed of lymphocytes, eosinophils, immunoblasts, some plasma cells, and occasional neutrophils along with mild blunting of villi.

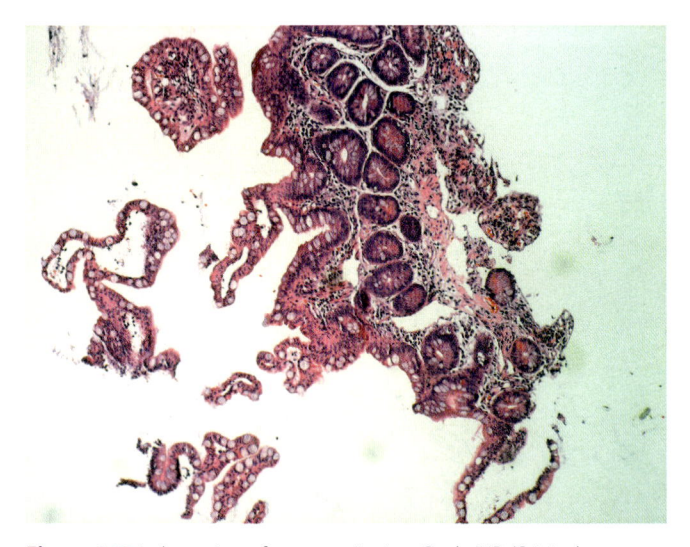

Figure 6.11 Indeterminate for acute rejection, Grade IND (Original magnification x100, H&E). Small bowel allograft with increased mixed interstitial inflammatory infiltrate, increased apoptosis, and architectural distortion.

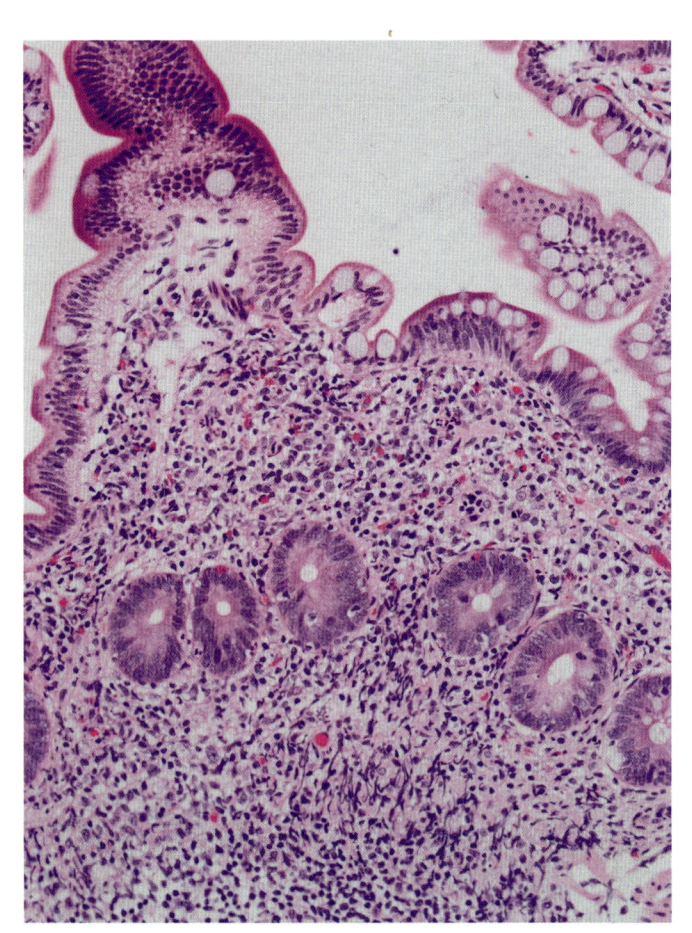

Figure 6.12 Acute cellular rejection, mild (Grade 1) (Original magnification x200, H&E). Mixed inflammatory infiltrate and several apoptotic bodies are seen in crypts (greater than six apoptotic bodies in ten crypts).

i No Evidence of Acute Rejection, Grade 0

The changes associated with this grade are essentially minimal or none (i.e., histomorphology is indistinguishable from normal bowel) in regards to acute rejection; however, other concurrent conditions (non-rejection) may be present (see Figure 6.9).

ii Indeterminate for Acute Rejection, Grade IND

The morphological alterations apparent in biopsies with this grade can be seen at any stage, including the early or resolving stages of ACR when there is a minor amount of epithelial cell injury or destruction, but nevertheless there is an added inflammatory infiltrate within the parenchyma. The inflammation tends to be composed of lymphocytes, eosinophils, immunoblasts, some plasma cells, and occasional neutrophils, with varying proportions and with the diffuse or focal intensity being visibly increased above normal (see Figures 6.10 and 6.11). Simultaneously, there is frequently also villous blunting, edema, and vascular congestion present, although these features are not obligatory for the diagnosis. Cryptitis with lymphocytes or eosinophils and epithelial apoptotic bodies are present. However, the number of apoptotic bodies does not reach the level designated for Grade 1 (mild) ACR.

iii Acute T Cell-mediated Acute Rejection (ACR), Mild, Grade 1

Mild ACR (Grade 1) demonstrates the crypt cell injury, inflammation, and all the other changes ascribed for the Indeterminate category (Grade IND), but at higher levels, including the level of apoptosis. In fact, classification of mild ACR necessitates six apoptotic bodies or above per ten crypts as the minimal cutoff, as designated in the International Grading Scheme [67]; other features typically include edema, congestion, and altered architecture such as villous blunting. The mixed chronic inflammatory cell infiltrate is mild-to-moderate intensity and inclines being diffusely distributed (see Figures 6.12, 6.13, 6.14, and 6.15), often with deeper extension to the submucosa and muscle. All of these morphological features, particularly the character and intensity of the infiltrate, can fluctuate according to the time

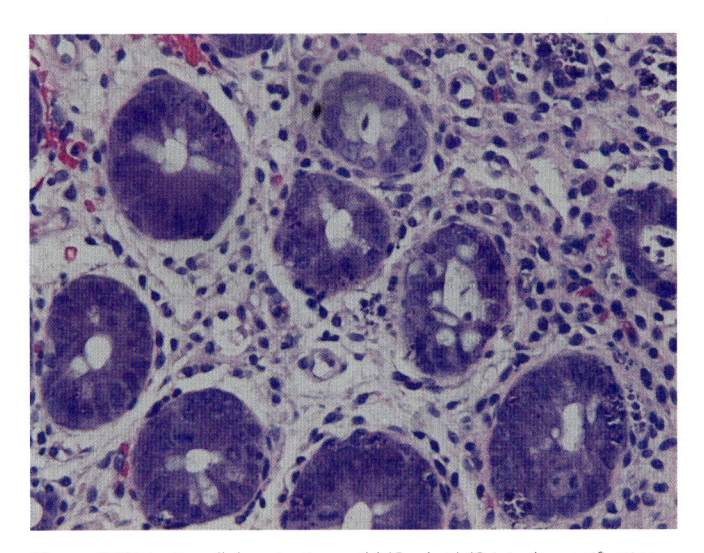

The Pathology of Intestinal and Multivisceral Transplantation

Figure 6.13 Acute cellular rejection, mild (Grade 1) (Original magnification x400, H&E). High magnification representation of inflammatory infiltrate and epithelial cells within crypts undergoing extensive apoptosis.

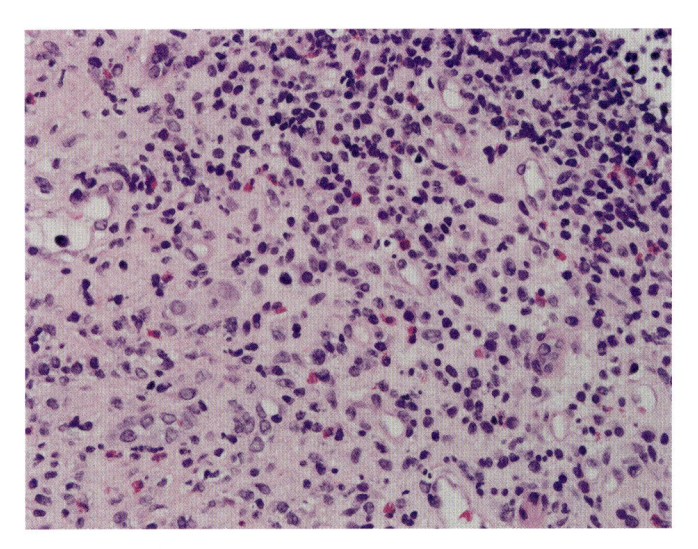

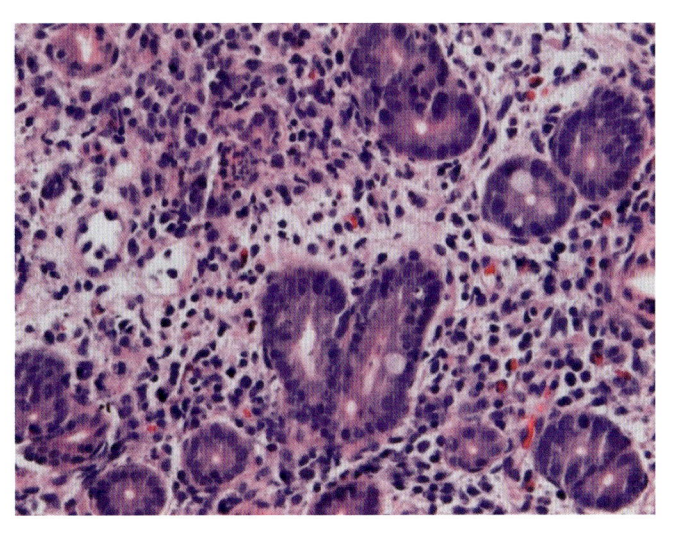

Figure 6.14 Acute cellular rejection, mild (Grade 1) (Original magnification x400, H&E). High magnification representation of inflammatory infiltrate with increased neutrophils and concomitant early antibody-mediated rejection; plasma cells and eosinophils.

Figure 6.15 Acute cellular rejection, mild (Grade 1) (Original magnification x400, H&E). High magnification representation of inflammatory infiltrate with increased eosinophils, plasma cells, and dilated microvasculature.

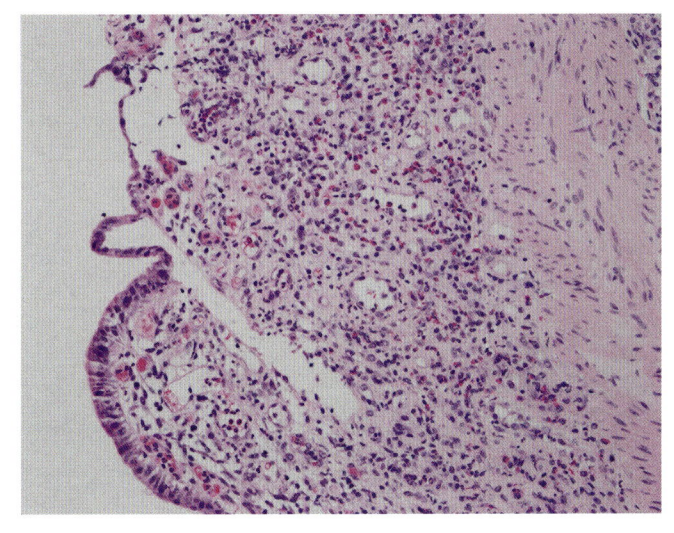

Figure 6.16 Acute cellular rejection, moderate (Grade 2) (Original magnification x200, H&E). Moderate- to severe-intensity, mixed inflammatory infiltrate with focal attenuation of surface epithelial lining, and dilated vasculature with PMN margination; apoptotic bodies were seen in crypts (greater than six apoptotic bodies in ten crypts).

after transplantation and which therapy is to be utilized for treatment of the ACR. Regenerative features such as mucin loss, epithelial cell nuclear enlargement, and hyperchromasia may also be present, contingent on the duration of the rejection. Vascular congestion and endothelialitis may be present with this and higher forms of ACR.

iv   Acute T Cell-mediated Acute Rejection (ACR), Moderate, Grade 2

ACR, moderate (Grade 2) shows the features of mild ACR, but with intensified crypt cell injury such that multiple and confluent apoptotic bodies are evident in single crypts. There may be whole gland necrosis and crypt abscesses. The inflammatory infiltrate in the lamina propria and submucosa is stereotypically more severe than with mild ACR and the nature of the infiltrate is mixed, but predominantly mononuclear inflammatory cell population, including blastic or activated lymphocytes, and mucosal architectural alteration tends to be significant. The moderate-to-severe intensity infiltrate is less affected by the time after transplantation, and villous blunting, edema, and vascular congestion are inclined to be more widespread with this higher degree than with Grade 1 rejection (see Figures 6.16, 6.17, 6.18, and 6.19).

v   Acute T Cell-mediated Acute Rejection (ACR), Severe, Grade 3

The development of severe (Grade 3) ACR can be catastrophic clinically and is a morphologically striking form of ACR. Although T cell-mediated rejection is central to this type of rejection, there is also often a humoral or alloantibody-mediated

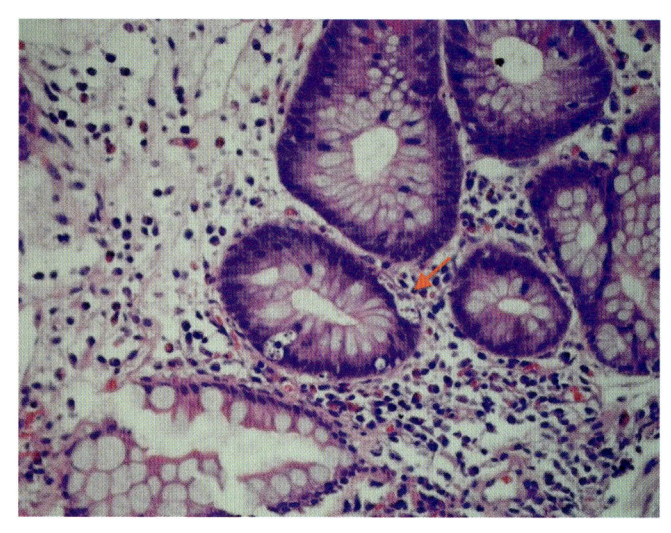

Figure 6.17 Acute cellular rejection, moderate (Grade 2) (Original magnification x400, H&E). Multiple apoptotic bodies in crypt (more than six apoptotic bodies per ten crypts) with some "confluent apoptosis" are seen (arrow).

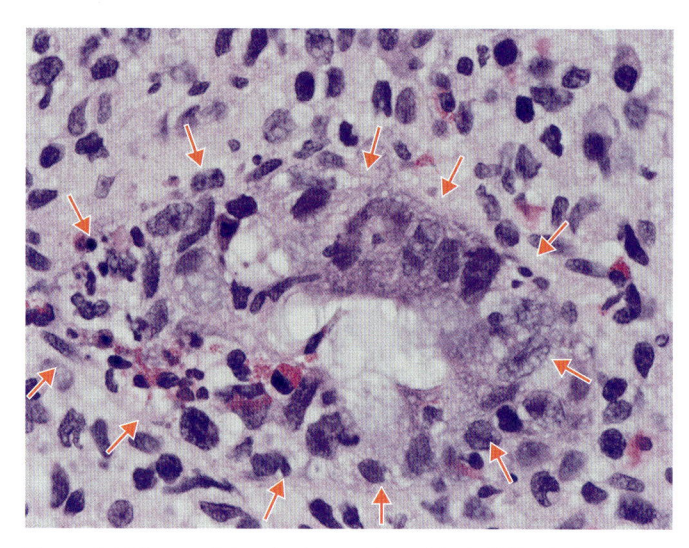

Figure 6.18 Acute cellular rejection, moderate (Grade 2) (Original magnification x1000, H&E). High magnification photomicrograph of crypt undergoing destruction with confluent apoptosis and inflammatory cells (including eosinophils) within the glandular basement membrane. The surrounding inflammatory cell infiltrate is intense in nature and mixed. Arrows delineate the edge of the crypt.

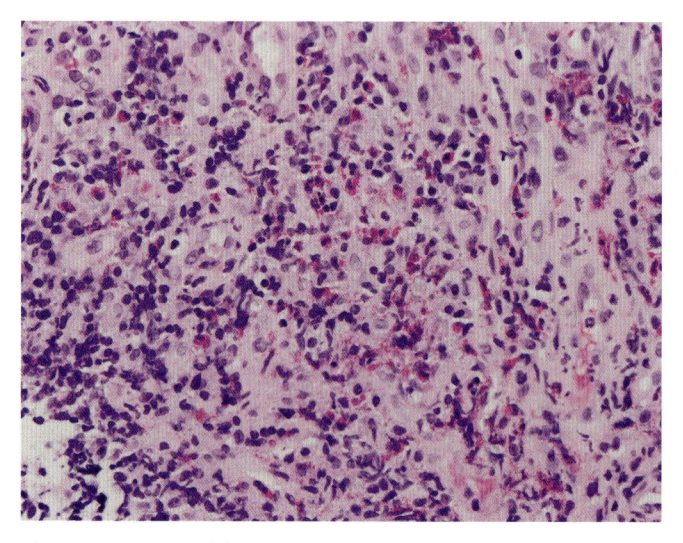

Figure 6.19 Acute cellular rejection, moderate (Grade 2) (Original magnification x400, H&E). High magnification representation of moderate-to-severe intensity inflammatory infiltrate with increased eosinophils, plasma cells, and neutrophils, often within epithelial lined structures.

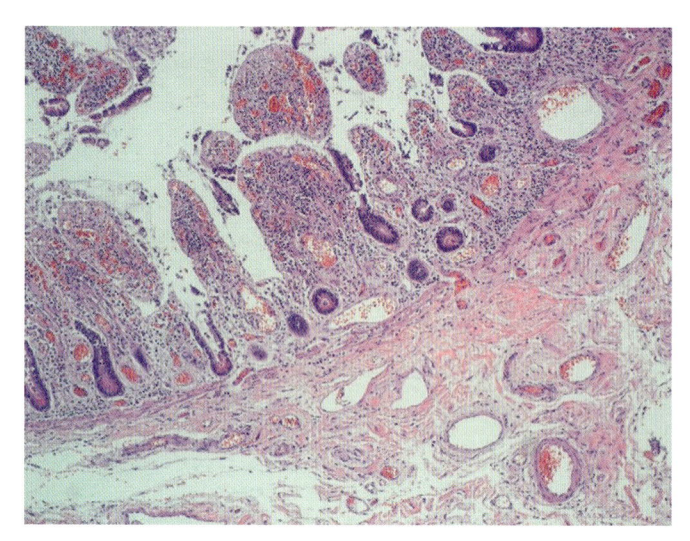

Figure 6.20 Acute cellular rejection, severe (Grade 3) (Original magnification x40, H&E). Extensive morphological distortions with marked diffuse inflammatory infiltrate are present. Severe denuding of villi with epithelial cell dropout is seen.

component and it can be considered a "mixed" acute rejection (ACR plus AAMR). Crypt cell injury and apoptosis, gland destruction, and related mucosal ulceration are pervasive features. The level of crypt epithelial apoptosis is variable; in fact, there may be a normal level of apoptosis among the surviving crypts, the latter that are often in a regenerative state. There is a marked diffuse inflammatory infiltrate with blastic or activated lymphocytes, eosinophils, and neutrophils. Since the tissue is often friable, it is not unusual to receive from the endoscopist only fragments of tissue with significant architectural alterations. Prolonged severe rejection can result in complete loss of the bowel histological architecture, and there may be predominantly granulation tissue and/or fibrinopurulent (pseudomembranous) exudate, with mucosal sloughing (see Figures 6.20, 6.21, and 6.22). Since mucosal ulceration can have different etiologies (e.g., ischemic and infectious processes), lesions not also having active crypt cell injury should not be classified as Grade 3 ACR, but rather "consistent with ACR, severe." The culmination of extensive severe rejection resulting in only sloughed, necrotic tissue has also been called "*exfoliative rejection*" [36, 37, 69]. Therefore, it is very useful to obtain tissue obtained from areas that grossly appear less involved. Left unabated, severe ACR can lead to intestinal graft loss.

c ACR in Colon and Stomach

With multivisceral transplantation, segments of the grafted alimentary tract aside from the small intestine can also be

The Pathology of Intestinal and Multivisceral Transplantation

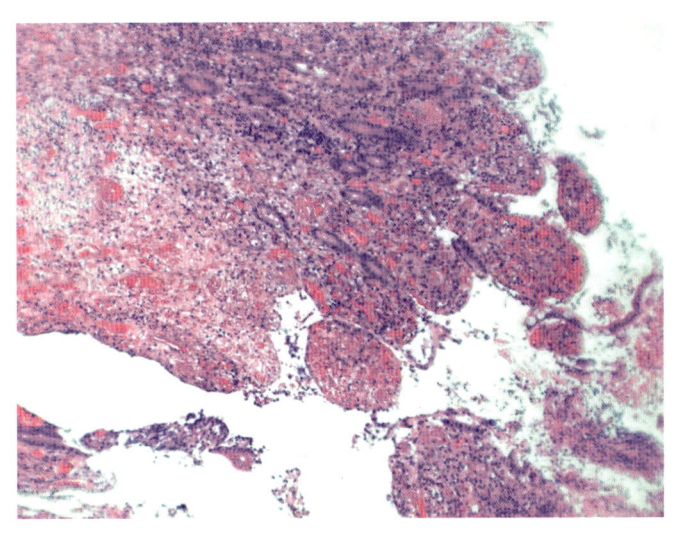

Figure 6.21 Acute cellular rejection, severe (Grade 3) (Original magnification x200, H&E). Mucosal architecture is extensively distorted with "ghosts" of villi, largely replaced by granulation tissue. The evaluation of crypt epithelial cell apoptosis is difficult because of complete loss of crypts. Dense inflammatory infiltrate is seen, which consists of mixed but predominantly mononuclear cell population with blastic and activated lymphocytes, eosinophils, and neutrophils. Marked vascular congestion is evident.

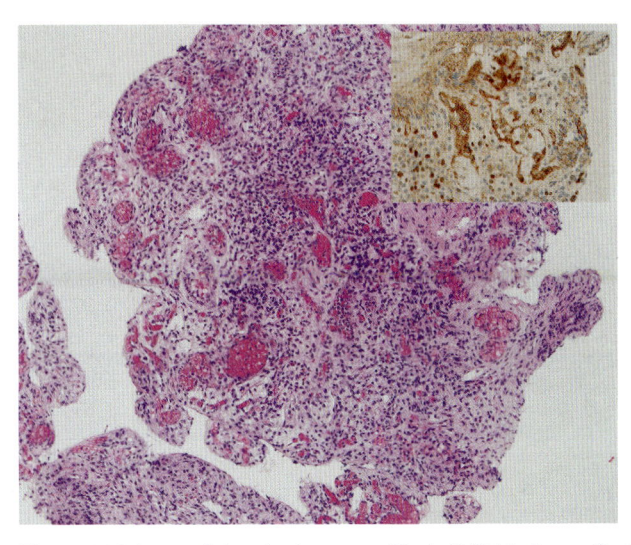

Figure 6.22 Acute cellular rejection, severe (Grade 3) (Original magnification x100, H&E). Hypervascular granulation tissue with complete loss of crypts and overall architecture. Dense inflammatory infiltrate is present in addition to neutrophilic margination. This case also had a component of antibody-mediated rejection (mixed rejection) and had abundant C4d deposition (see Figure 6.22a, 400x) by immunohistochemistry.

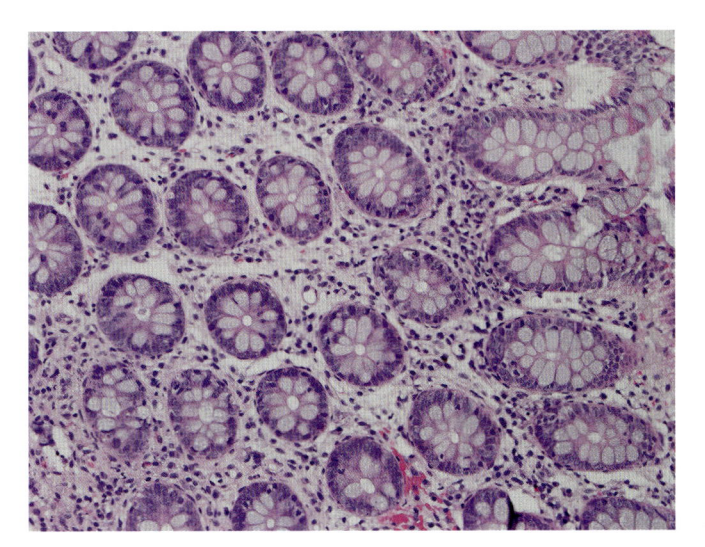

Figure 6.23 Acute cellular rejection, mild (Grade 1) of colon (Original magnification x200, H&E). Mixed inflammatory infiltrate and several apoptotic bodies are seen in crypts (greater than six apoptotic bodies in ten crypts).

complicated by the occurrence of acute and chronic rejection. The presence of ACR in colon allografts is manifested by comparable changes, as seen with the small intestine, and our experience with biopsies from this organ allograft is increasing as colon segments are included more often now with MVTx [70]. The arrangement and composition of the inflammatory cell infiltrate in colon ACR displays the same pattern as small bowel, as well as the epithelial cell injury in crypts (see Figure 6.23) and the same cell subpopulations appear involved (see Figure 6.24a–e). There can also be architectural distortion, goblet cell loss, and attenuation of the thickness of the surface epithelial cells. We apply the same criteria and grading system for the colon as we use in the small intestine [67, 68, 71]. There is often coexistent native colon in multivisceral transplant patients and obtaining tissue from native and allograft simultaneously can be useful to the pathologist in distinguishing alloreactive versus other inflammatory processes.

Stomach allografts can display ACR in all regions of this organ, exclusively or in combination with other inflammatory processes such as various forms of chronic gastritis and infectious processes. There is epithelial injury in the form of apoptosis and reactive changes, similar to small bowel and colon allografts. The degree of inflammation during acute rejection in the stomach is typically less compared to intestine such that corresponding grades of acute rejection in stomach do not demonstrate the same level of inflammation and epithelial injury as in small bowel or colon (see Figures 6.25, 6.26, 6.27, and 6.28). However, we have seen many situations where there is isolated gastric rejection or the grades of gastric rejection exceed other regions of the small bowel or colon. A grading scheme is useful (Table 6.5) to provide different levels of ACR and can be a worthwhile approach to appraising stomach allograft pathology to score individual morphological features [66].

V Chronic Rejection

Chronic allograft enteropathy (CAE) or chronic rejection of small bowel allografts is rising in incidence and recognition as graft survival progressively improves in ITx and MVTx [3, 72], and as such, it is becoming an important source of late graft loss in gastrointestinal transplantation. Chronic rejection of the bowel, as with other solid organ transplants, originates through a complex pathophysiological process, influenced by an interaction of several non-immune [73] and immune factors [74–77]. The nonspecific symptomology (e.g., protein losing enteropathy) for CAE tends to be progressive and unresponsive to therapy, and endoscopic information can include

The Pathology of Intestinal and Multivisceral Transplantation

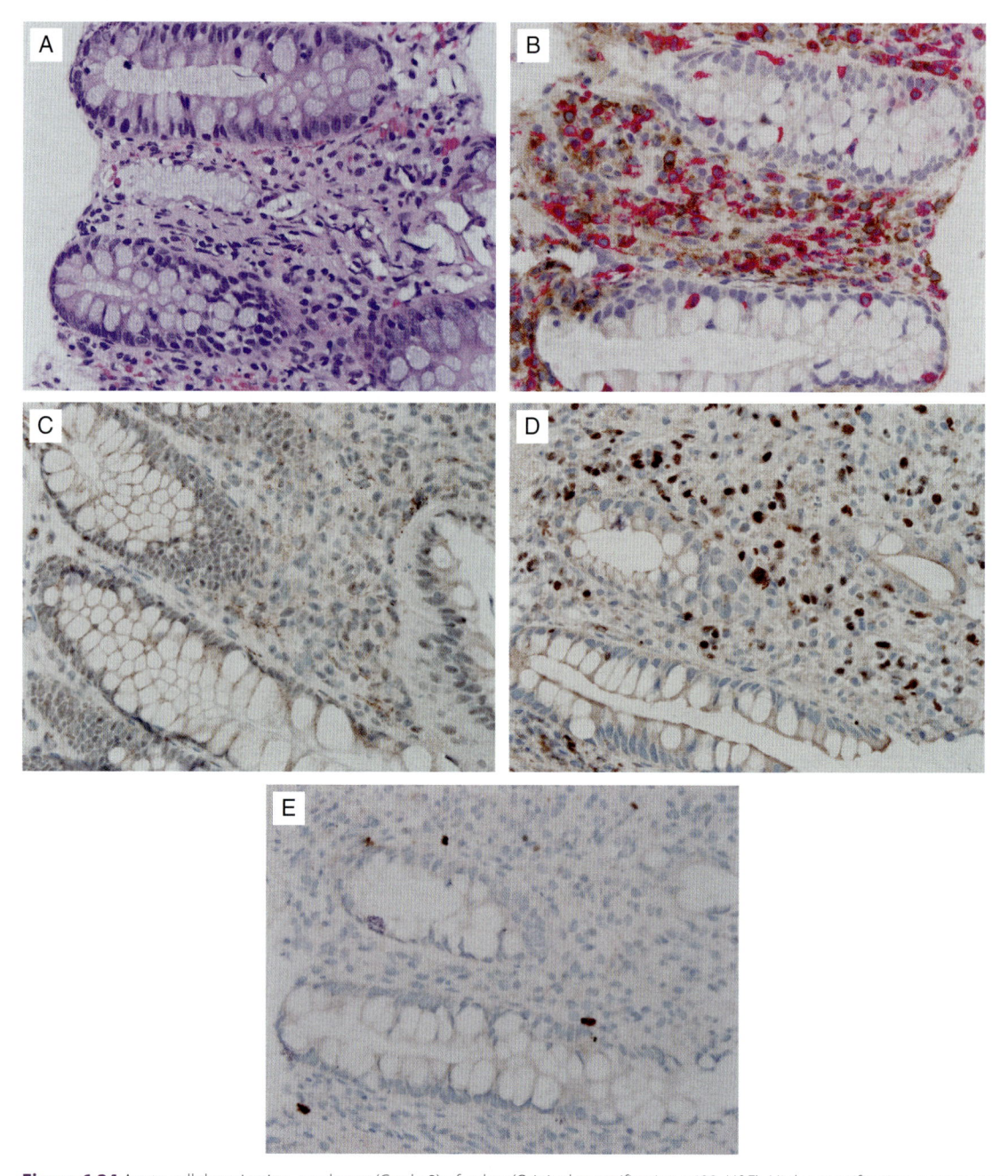

Figure 6.24 Acute cellular rejection, moderate (Grade 2) of colon (Original magnification x400, H&E). High magnification representation of moderate to severe intensity inflammatory infiltrate (see Figure 6.24a) with increased eosinophils, plasma cells, and neutrophils, and composed of CD4 (brown) and CD8 cells (red) within the interstitium and infiltrating glands. The CD4: CD8 ratio overall was estimated at 1:3 (see Figure 6.24b, two-color immunohistochemistry, 400x). There was no significant C4d deposition (see Figure 6.24 c, immunohistochemistry 400x), as this represented a T cell-mediated rejection. Tbet-positive cells were prominent (see Figure 6.24d, immunohistochemistry 400x) and related to T helper Type 1 cells; few FoxP3-positive cells (regulatory cells) were evident (see Figure 6.24e, immunohistochemistry 400x).

loss of villous structure with flattening; these findings are critical to correlate with the pathological findings of the mucosal biopsies (see Figures 6.29 and 6.30). Explanted bowels that are removed with severe chronic rejection grossly show a matted organ bloc due to abundant serosal adhesions, with transmural thickening, an irregular flattened mucosal surface, and intermittent ulcerations.

The pathognomonic microscopic lesion of bowel chronic rejection is concentric intimal thickening of small to large-sized arteries with fibrous changes, medial hypertrophy of smooth muscle cells interspersed with foam cells, and adventitial fibrosis [78] (see Figure 6.31). It is important to note that GI transplant mucosal biopsies are typically limited from being able to demonstrate the large vessel changes of chronic

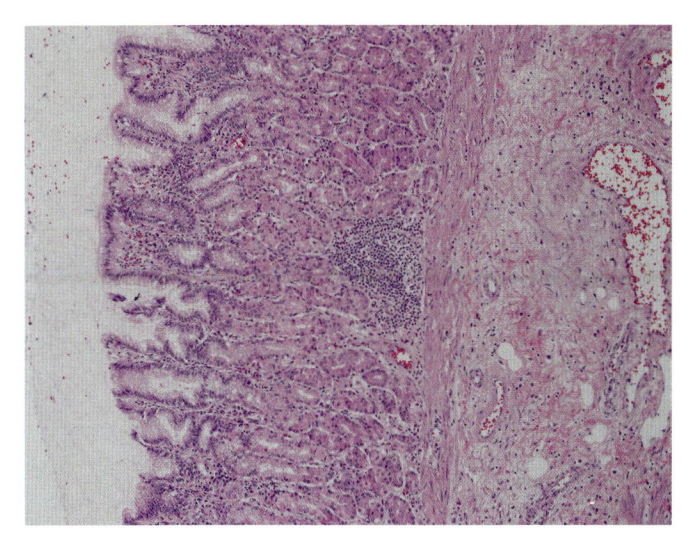

Figure 6.25 Indeterminate for acute rejection, Grade IND of stomach (Original magnification x100, H&E). Gastric allograft with increased mixed interstitial inflammatory infiltrate, focally increased apoptosis, and epithelial injury.

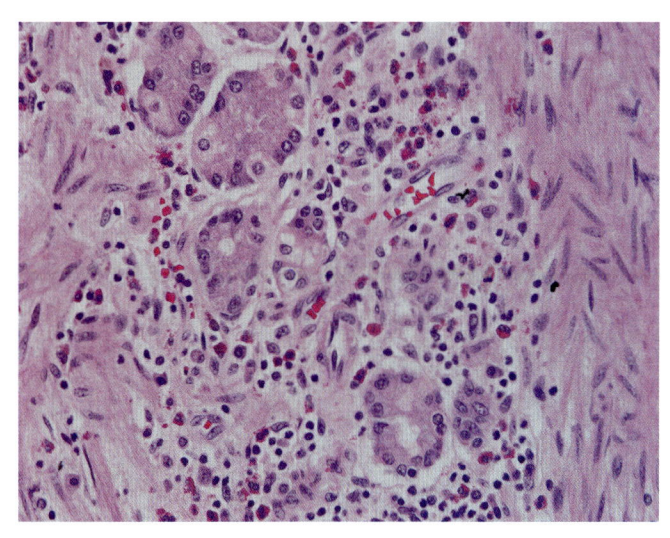

Figure 6.26 Indeterminate for acute rejection of stomach (Original magnification x400, H&E). Gastric allograft with increased mixed interstitial inflammatory infiltrate that includes lymphocytes, eosinophils, plasma cells, and epithelial injury.

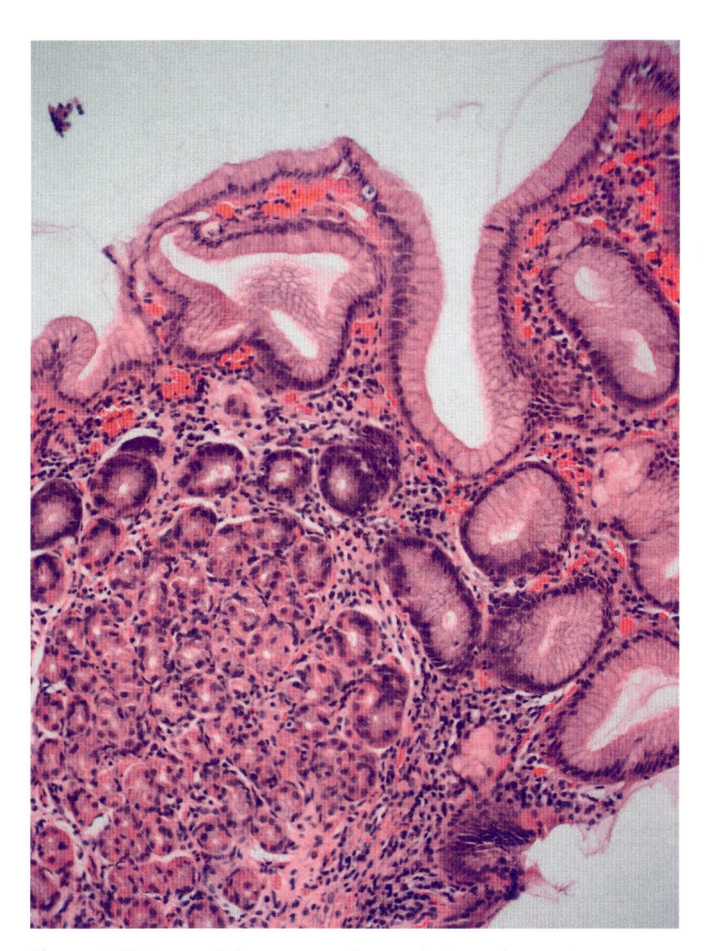

Figure 6.27 Acute cellular rejection of stomach (Original magnification x100, H&E). Gastric allograft displaying architectural disarray and significant increase of inflammatory infiltrate with epithelial apoptosis. Mild vascular congestion and extravasation are also seen.

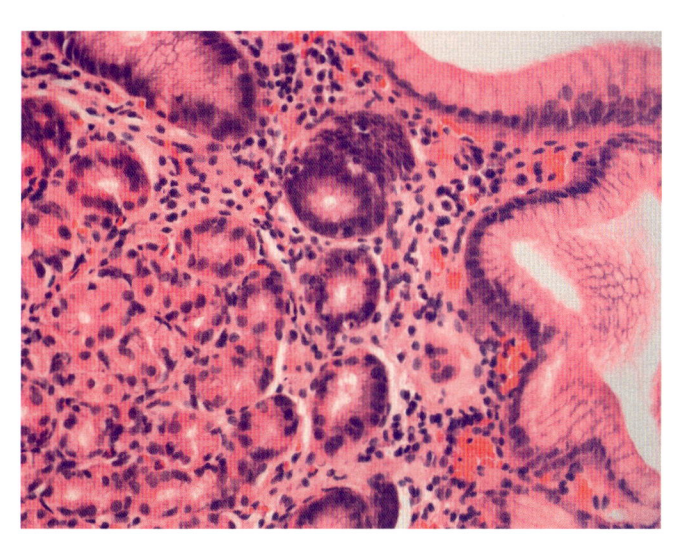

Figure 6.28 Acute cellular rejection of stomach (Original magnification x400, H&E). Several crypt epithelial cell apoptotic bodies and mixed inflammatory infiltrate with microvascular congestion is present.

rejection [79] [80] since these arteries are not usually present in these specimens. Occasional chronic inflammatory cells within the intimal space ("active" chronic allograft arteriopathy) or thrombi can be sometimes seen in arterial branches undergoing chronic rejection. Fibrosis can involve the mucosal, submucosal, and muscular layers, and there is associated crypt separation and disappearance, epithelial mucin loss, villous blunting, mucosal atrophy, and small arterial branches with evidence of transplant arteriopathy. Other microscopic changes can include ganglion cell destruction and hyperplasia, fibrinous serositis, and chronic inflammation; there may be ulceration and superimposed acute rejection.

In our experience, mucosal biopsies from GI allografts with CAE can be very useful in identifying the chronic injury (e.g., fibrosis, crypt loss and distortion, altered architecture) and, when incorporated with the clinical and endoscopic history, provide a practical suspicion for chronic rejection (see Figure 6.32). Appraisal and comparison of adjacent native tissue is very useful,

Table 6.5 Characteristics of Acute Cellular Rejection in Gastric Allograft

Grade	Description	Histopathological Findings
0	No evidence of acute rejection	Absent to very minimal inflammatory infiltrate; normal cytology and architecture (glandular structures arranged back-to-back).
IND	Indeterminate for acute rejection	Scattered mixed inflammatory infiltrate, edema, or focal congestion; normal architecture; normal cytology; no increased apoptotic bodies.
1	Acute cellular rejection, mild	Increased inflammation and apoptotic bodies, mild cytologic atypia, and mild architectural disarray.
2	Acute cellular rejection, moderate	Prominent mixed inflammatory infiltrate, increased cytologic atypia, vacuolization of parietal cells, erosion or ulceration of the surface epithelium, major architectural disarray, and increased or confluent apoptotic bodies.
3	Acute cellular rejection, severe	Significant distortion of the architecture with subtotal destruction of the gland and gastric pits, accompanied by ulceration.

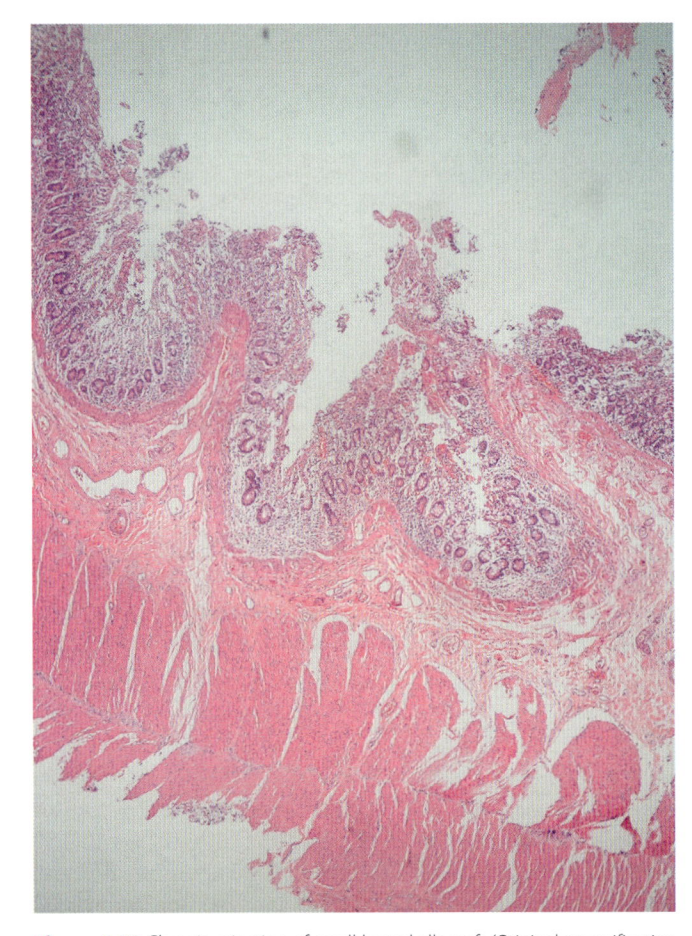

Figure 6.29 Chronic rejection of small bowel allograft (Original magnification x40, H&E). Explanted bowel undergoing chronic rejection. There is severe fibrosis in the lamina propria and submucosa with loss of crypts.

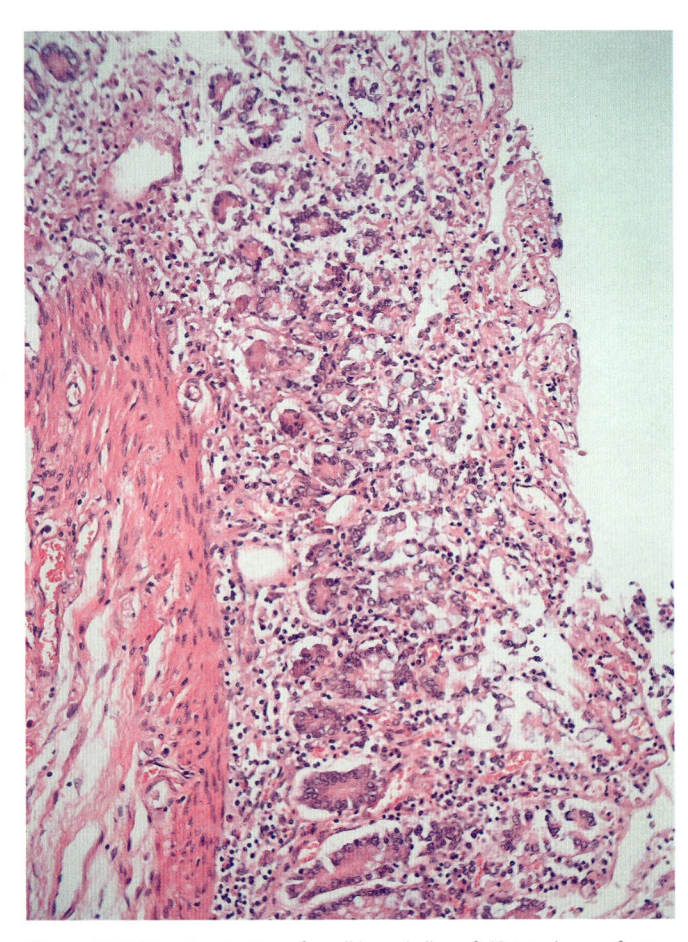

Figure 6.30 Chronic rejection of small bowel allograft (Original magnification x200, H&E). There is marked architectural distortion and glandular atrophy present.

since the latter can be unremarkable in CAE. A semiquantitative scoring template for the mucosal biopsy evaluation of chronic rejection (Table 6.6), along with immunohistochemical characterization of lymphoid and macrophage cell populations, is also useful in the identification and prognostication of GI chronic rejection [80]. To date, no consistently useful biomarkers or gene sets have been employed as auxiliary support of biopsies in diagnosing CAE.

VI Infections

The prolonged and high amount of immunosuppression with ITx and MVTx places these transplant patients at risk for several frequent complications, amongst the most important being the appearance of opportunistic infections [81–83]. These infections can manifest themselves systemically and/or

Table 6.6 Semiquantitative Grading Schema for Mucosal Fibrosis

Grade	Description	Histopathological findings
0	No fibrosis	No significant number of collagen fibers
1	Minimal fibrosis	Very few, although readily visible, collagen fibers
2	Mild fibrosis	Few collagen fibers arranged in bundle with preservation of the glandular architecture
3	Moderate fibrosis	Fibrous tissue in the lamina propria with decreased number of glands
4	Severe fibrosis	Areas devoid of glands and replaced by fibrous tissue

locally in the graft and adjacent native tissue (e.g., infectious gastritis, enteritis, or colitis); unfortunately, these infections can compromise graft function and place the host at risk of death in the absence of identification and therapy. Since GI graft infections with clinical symptoms can sometimes mimic acute rejection (e.g., diarrhea, fever) it must be distinguished by culture and/or biopsy appearance, since treatment often includes reduction in immunosuppression.

The gastrointestinal allograft can be involved by a number of viruses that can have distinguishing histopathological changes and be confirmed by immunohistochemical, culture, or molecular techniques. Among the most frequent viruses are rotavirus, adenovirus, calicivirus (human calicivirus: HuCV), herpes

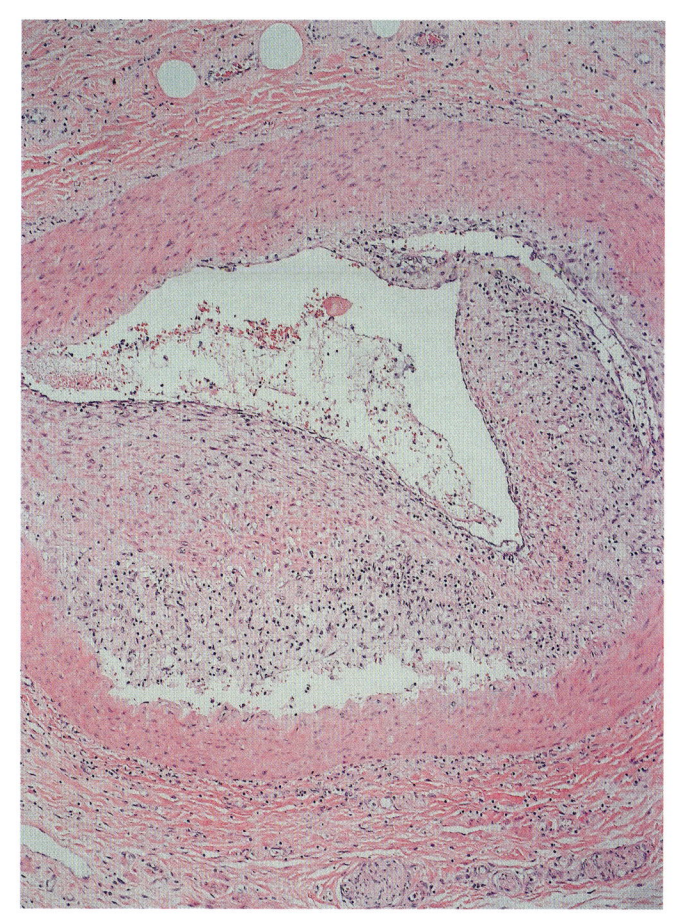

Figure 6.31 Chronic rejection of small bowel allograft (Original magnification x200, H&E). Marked myointimal hyperplasia and subendothelial accumulation of foamy macrophages and scattered lymphocytes (i.e., "active" allograft arteriopathy) are seen in obliterative arteriopathy in large-sized vessels in the deep submucosa.

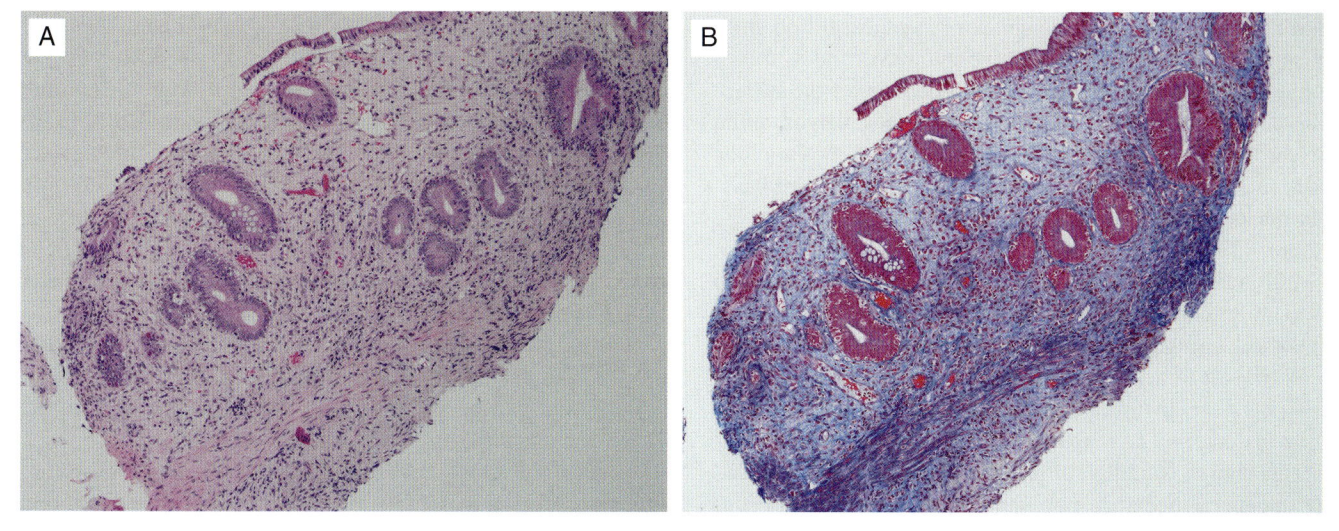

Figure 6.32 Chronic rejection of small bowel allograft (Original magnification x100, H&E, trichrome). Mucosal biopsy demonstrating chronic enteropathy with loss of glandular structures, architectural distortion (see Figure 6.32a), and extensive mucosal fibrosis (see Figure 6.32b, trichrome stain). This patient had longstanding acute cellular rejection, evident in this photomicrograph with a vigorous mixed inflammatory cell infiltrate and extensive epithelial injury and apoptosis.

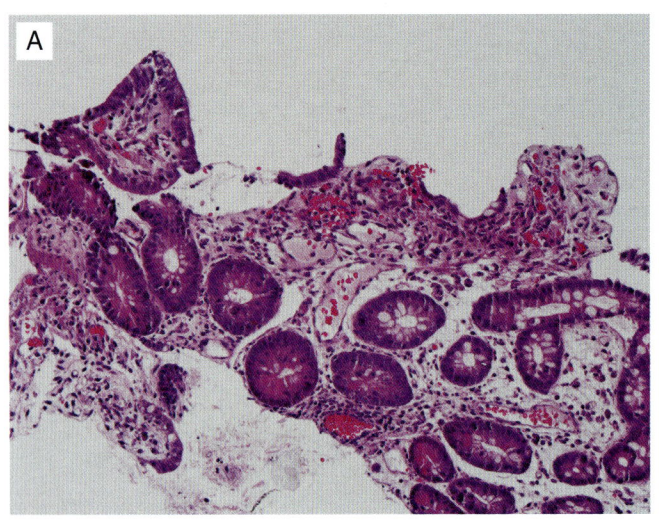

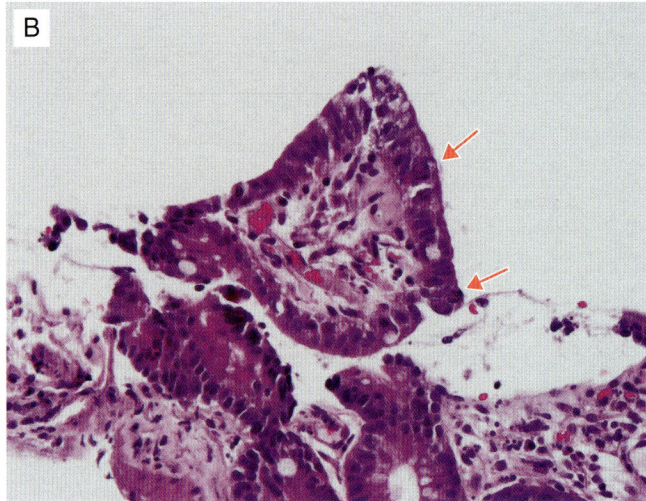

Figure 6.33 Adenovirus enteritis (Original magnification x200, x400). Mucosal biopsy showing mixed inflammatory cell infiltrate with disruption of the superficial lining epithelial cells, erosion, and increased vacuolization (see Figure 6.33a); higher magnification (see Figure 6.33b) demonstrates occasional subtle "smudge cells" (arrows) amidst the lining epithelium. These cells were positive for adenovirus by immunohistochemistry (not shown).

simplex virus (HSV), CMV, and EBV. In general, the presence of these viruses in GI tissue is complemented by an interstitial inflammation (e.g., gastritis, enteritis) that is composed of a varied acute and chronic inflammatory cell infiltrate with focal or diffuse epithelial damage, altered cell proliferation, and cytological changes [84]. Necrosis may be apparent, particularly in more severe cases. Unfortunately, the presence of a viral infection within the alimentary tract graft can commonly have concomitant acute rejection with one process often exacerbating the other. Thus, it remains important that the transplant pathologist consider the patient's clinical history and culture/molecular test results when evaluating the histology.

Adenovirus infections can be a baffling and perilous complication in GI transplantation, with sporadic reports of cases in ITx and MVTx [85, 86]. There can be subtle or prominent histopathology, sometimes with crypt cell have apoptosis and a mixed chronic inflammatory cell infiltrate, and disarray of the surface epithelial cells associated with the presence of enlarged, often hyperchromatic cells (see Figures 6.33 and 6.34). Eosinophilic nuclear inclusions, as well as "smudge cells" with enlarged basophilic nuclei and proliferation of surface enterocytes, may be apparent [87]. Immunohistochemistry, electron microscopy, and viral PCR assays (of tissue) for this virus are very useful to help identify the presence of this pathogen. Some of the histopathological changes associated with adenovirus infection can also be evident in acute rejection; therefore, it is critical to use all tools necessary to distinguish the processes. Rapid diagnosis of adenovirus enteritis is essential, because without proper treatment, the clinical condition of patients tends to rapidly worsen.

The general pediatric population commonly experiences Rotavirus and it can likewise complicate ITx and MVTx patients. The histopathological alterations associated with this virus are obscure and biopsies are not commonly procured to identify this pathogen. There may be superficial hyperplastic changes in the epithelium (see Figure 6.35), a mixed mucosal surface inflammatory infiltrate with occasional neutrophils, and cell debris. Deeper crypts tend not to be affected by the epithelial injury. There can be coexistence of acute rejection and rotaviral infections [88, 89].

Norwalk virus (Norovirus) is another gastrointestinal virus that has been described in intestinal transplant patients [90]. There are also a variety of relatively novel viruses that have been identified in human enteric tracts of persons with diarrhea, among them being Caliciviruses, which are non-enveloped, positive-stranded RNA viruses that can cause illness in animals and humans [91]. Calicivirus (HuCV) is a common cause of mild gastroenteritis and is composed of two pathogenic strains, Norwalk-like virus and Sapporo virus. HuCV results in protracted high-volume diarrhea in the general population and is usually uncovered by RT-PCR in fecal specimens. Histopathological alterations that have been reported include mixed lymphoplasmacytic infiltrate with a small number of neutrophils in lamina propria, blunting and flattening of villi, disarray, and reactive modifications of the superficial epithelium. Vacuolization of the surface epithelial cells can be prominent (see Figure 6.35) and there may be focal erosion [92]. There is also a loss of cellular polarity, increased apoptosis in the superficial epithelium and in the crypts, as well as in macrophages in the superficial portion of the lamina propria [93].

Cytomegalovirus (CMV) infection is among the most common infectious complications in GI transplant recipients [94] [95–97] and can be systemic or localized in its distribution. When causing enteritis, CMV can present as diarrhea, epigastric pain, and abdominal discomfort. Endoscopic examination can reveal mucosal erosions and ulcers in stomach and in small intestine. Histologically, there can be characteristic large CMV-infected cells with eosinophilic intranuclear inclusions surrounded by a clear halo and thickened nuclear membrane. Intranuclear inclusions can be identified in endothelial, stromal, smooth muscle, and epithelial cells often in the presence of a chronic inflammatory infiltrate,

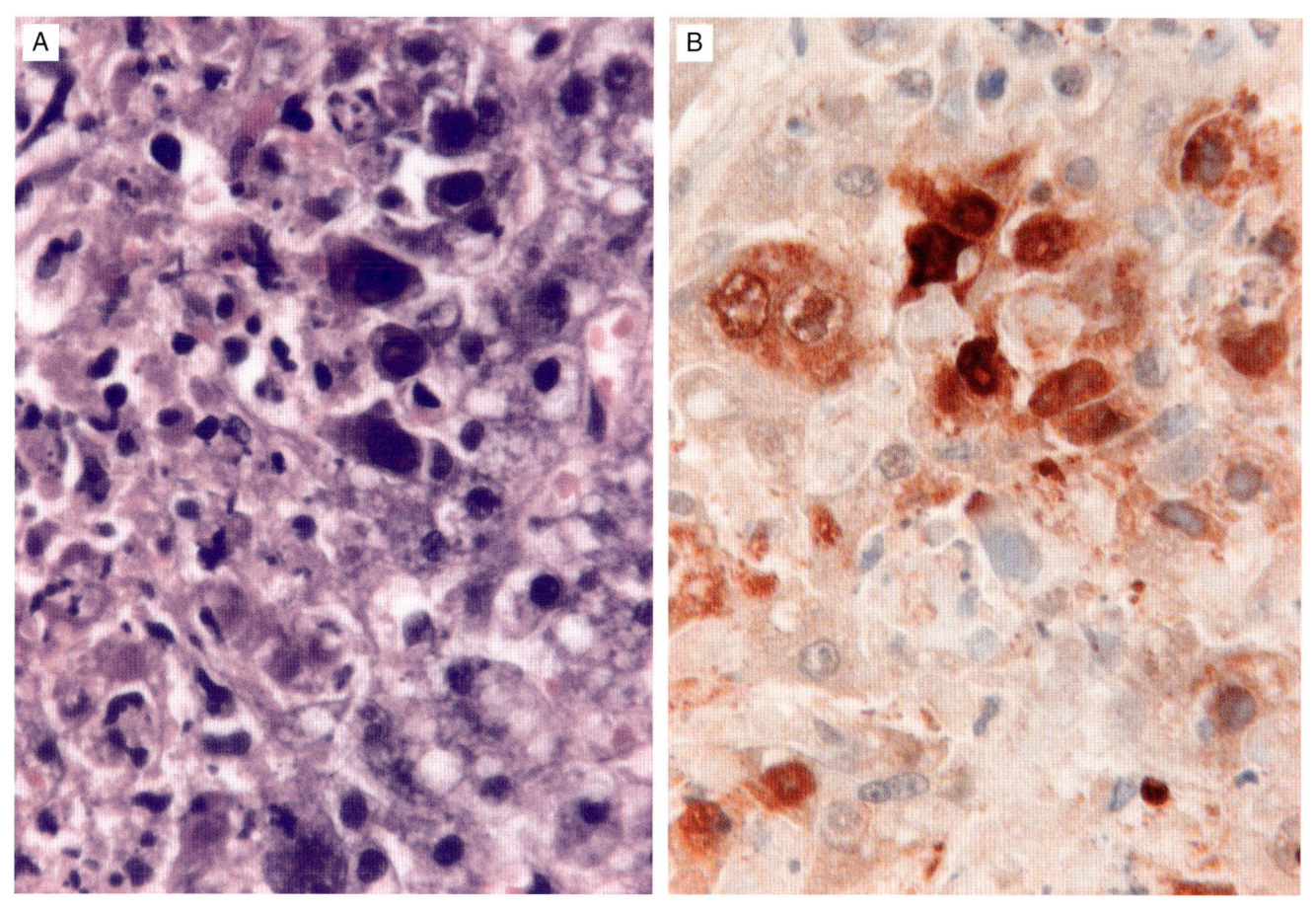

Figure 6.34 Adenovirus enteritis (Original magnification x400, H&E, Immunohistochemistry). Adenovirus inclusion bodies in small bowel allograft (see Figure 6.34a) and immunohistochemistry demonstrating adenovirus positive cells (see Figure 6.34b).

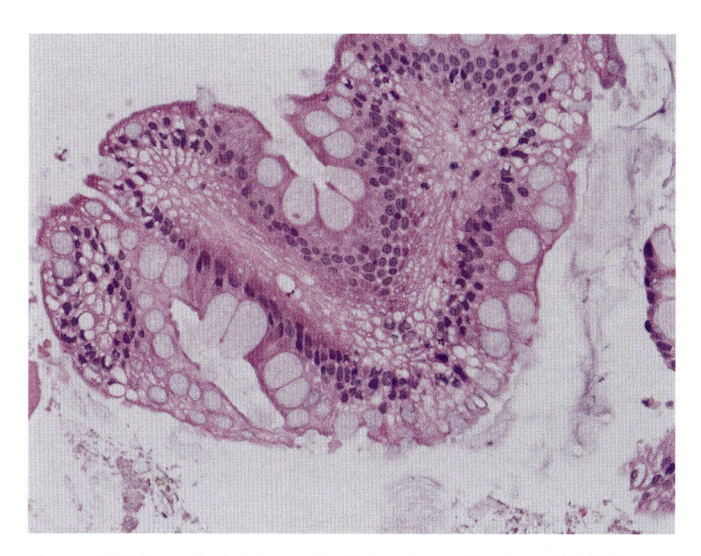

Figure 6.35 Suspected viral enteritis (Original magnification x400, H&E). Superficial epithelial cells with hyperplasia and vacuolization.

composed of lymphocytes and histiocytes, and with neutrophils at times observed in the lamina propria. Isolated intranuclear inclusions are sometimes hidden in dense chronic inflammatory infiltrates and hard to identify (see Figures 6.36–6.38). Immunohistochemical staining for CMV and PCR assay of tissues for CMV are helpful to confirm the diagnosis of CMV enteritis due to the obscuring at times of severe inflammatory cell infiltrates (see Figure 6.37).

In transplant patients, Herpes Simplex Virus (HSV) infection in the alimentary tract most commonly involves the oral cavity, esophagus, perianal area, and rectum, whereas HSV enteritis or colitis are relatively infrequent [98]. HSV enteritis can demonstrate aphthous and necrotic ulcers, mucosal erythema and friability, and inflammatory pseudopolypoid lesions by endoscopy. Microscopically, there is a mixed chronic inflammatory cell infiltrate with lymphoplasmacytic component and scattered eosinophils (see Figure 6.39). Virally infected cells can demonstrate eosinophilic intranuclear inclusions and multinucleation. Simultaneous culturing of the tissue and immunohistochemistry (Figure 6.40) is useful to confirm the diagnosis of HSV enteritis.

Epstein-Barr virus (EBV) acute infection is low in the ITx and MVTx population, but chronic infection is commonly associable with the development of PTLD.

Other herpesviruses that are latent, but which become reactivated subsequently bearing the capacity to infect and reoccur in intestinal and multivisceral transplant patients include HHV-6, HHV-7, and HHV-8 [99]. HHV-6 is closely related to CMV and

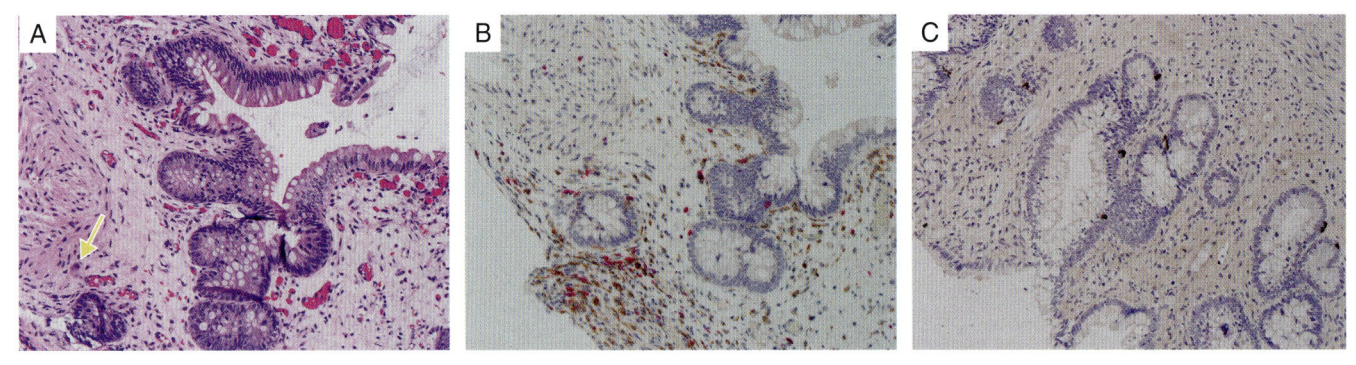

Figure 6.36 Cytomegalovirus enteritis (Original magnification x200, H&E; x200 immunohistochemistry for CD4/CD8; in situ hybridization for CMV, x200). Mucosal biopsy showing patchy mixed enteritis with occasional enlarged cells displaying hyperchromatic nuclei (arrow) (see Figure 6.36a). There is concomitant acute cellular rejection, mild (Grade 1) with focal erosion, increased vascularity, and focal loss of crypts. In addition, there were occasional EBV-positive cells present (not shown). Two-color immunohistochemistry to CD4/CD8 (see Figure 6.36b) shows a mild-to-moderate accumulation of both T cell subpopulations with a CD4: CD8 ratio of approximately 2:1. In situ hybridization to CMV shows positive cells present (see Figure 6.36 c). DNA was isolated from the biopsy and EBV and CMV levels were measured by PCR (EBV = 7,196,114 copies/100 ng DNA; CMV = 302,114 copies/100 ng DNA).

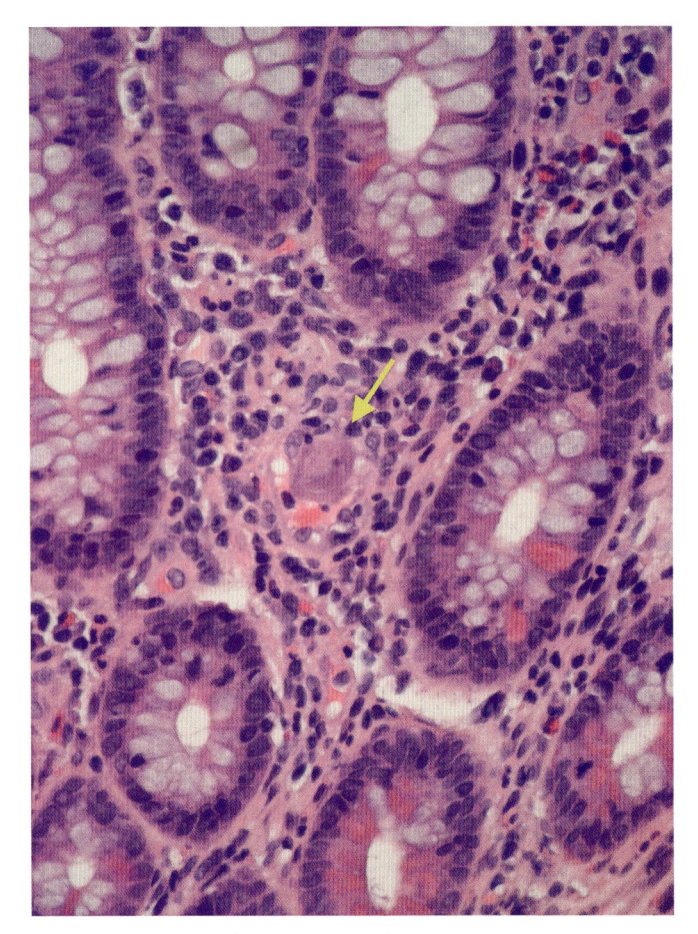

Figure 6.37 Cytomegalovirus enteritis (Original magnification x400, H&E). Amidst a prominent interstitial inflammatory cell infiltrate, Cytomegalovirus inclusion bodies (arrow) are present in small bowel allograft.

Figure 6.38 Cytomegalovirus enteritis (Original magnification x400, Immunohistochemistry). Immunohistochemistry demonstrating cytomegalovirus- (CMV) positive cells in bowel allograft.

can be classified into two classes, HHV-6A and HHV-6B. HHV-6 can be present in ileocolonic mucosa [100, 101] with immunohistochemical (see Figure 6.41) and molecular measurements are often very useful in determining the presence of the virus, which can cause symptoms of gastroenteritis. The histological findings are nonspecific and resemble changes present with a viral infection. Unlike the experience seen in liver transplant patients [102], we have not detected HHV-7 infection in the bowel and this apparently has a similar experience of bowel transplant centers [94], although in addition to skin infection and an acute febrile illness, diarrhea has been attributed to acute HHV-7 viremia and infection [103]. HHV-8 is also known

The Pathology of Intestinal and Multivisceral Transplantation

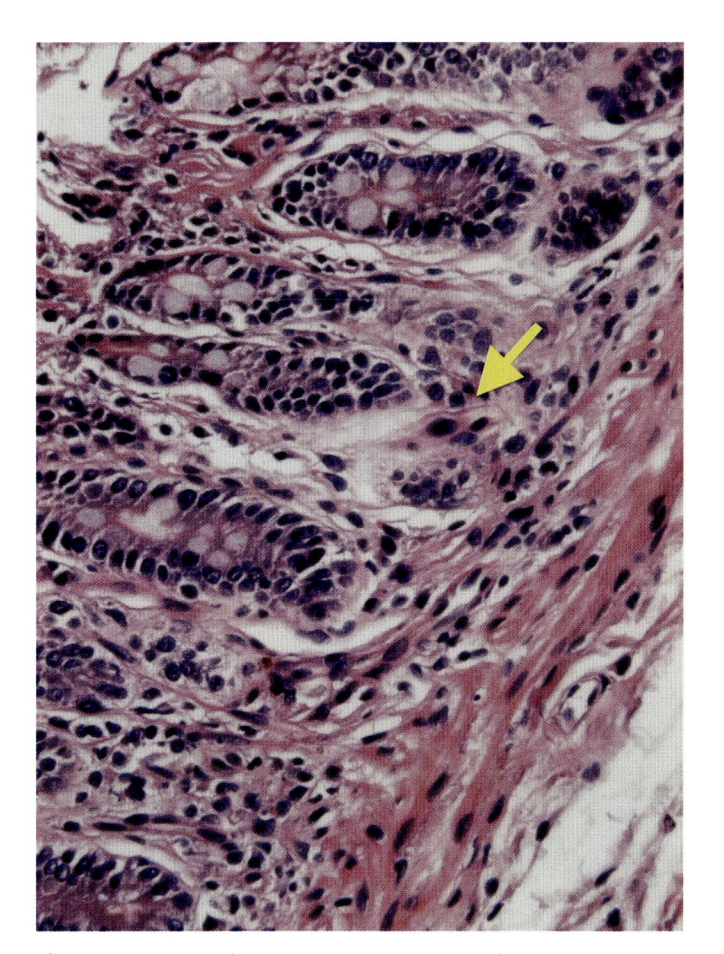

Figure 6.39 Section of colonic mucosa with Herpes infection, the arrow highlights the hyperchromatic changes in the enlarged infected cell within the interstitium, below the crypt (H&E, 400x).

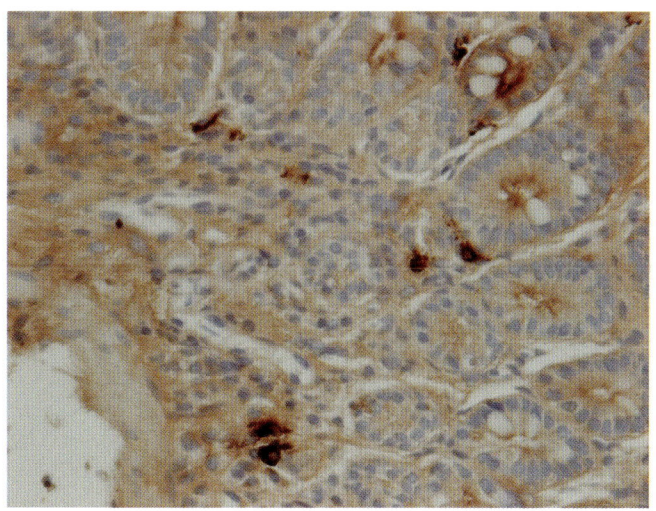

Figure 6.40 Immunohistochemistry to Herpes Simplex showing positive staining in a moderate number of cells within the interstitium. (400x).

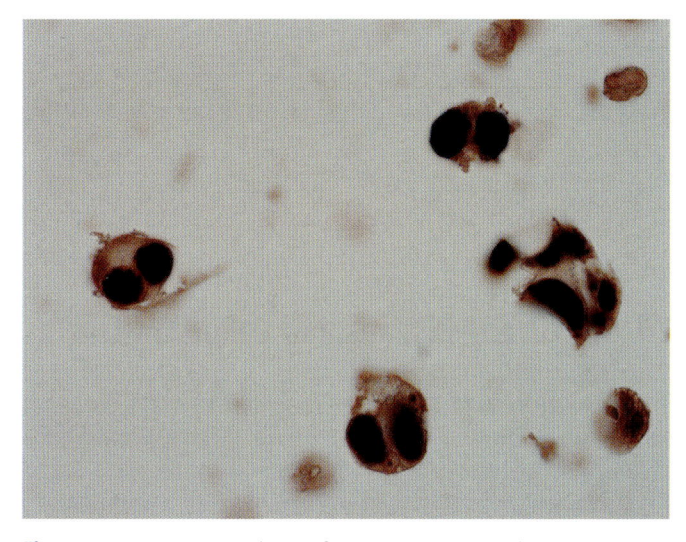

Figure 6.41 HHV-6 (Original magnification x1000, Immunohistochemistry). Immunohistochemistry demonstrating HHV-6-positive inflammatory cells.

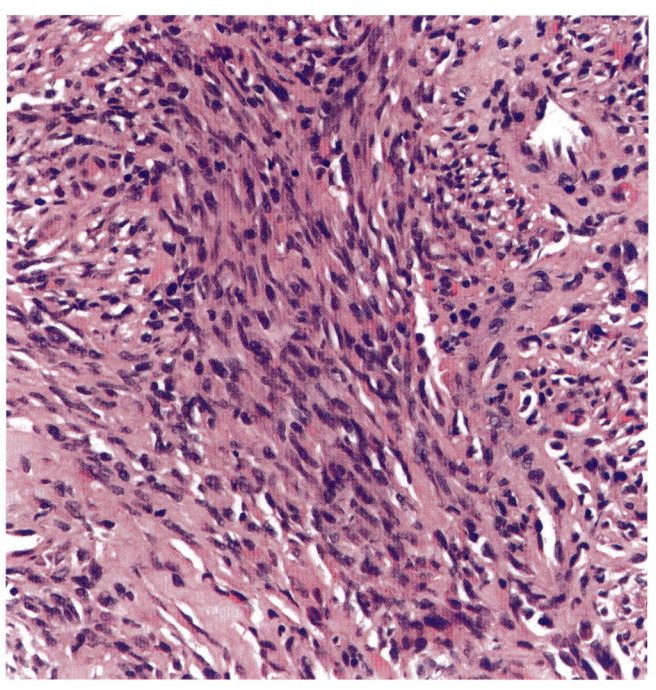

Figure 6.42 Kaposi's sarcoma in bowel (Original magnification x400). High magnification profile of classic Kaposi's sarcoma in bowel allograft and HHV-8-positive. The atypical tumor cells are spindle-shaped with vascular slits, inflammation, and total loss of normal bowel morphology.

as Kaposi's sarcoma-associated herpesvirus (KSHV) [104] and can typically involve solid organ transplant patients by the increased rate of occurrence of Kaposi's sarcoma (see Figure 6.42), primary effusion lymphoma, and Castleman's Disease [105]. The Kaposi's and lymphoma can primarily affect the bowel.

Bacterial overgrowth in bowel allografts (as compared to the density of the normal flora) can be seen and the pathologist should communicate this information. Among potentially important bacterial infections in bowel allografts are atypical mycobacteria that can cause significant graft dysfunction [106]. There are also several fungal and parasitic pathogens, including Candida (see Figure 6.43) and cryptosporidium [107] (see Figure 6.44), that are in the GI tract and which can involve the allograft.

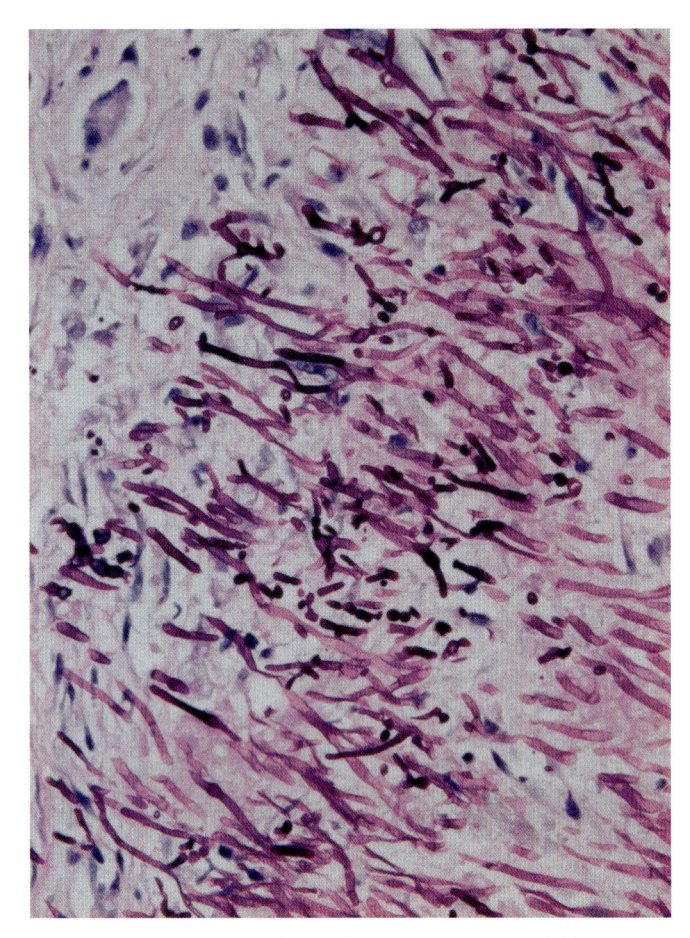

Figure 6.43 Candida (Original magnification x200, H&E). Candidal yeast forms in small bowel allograft.

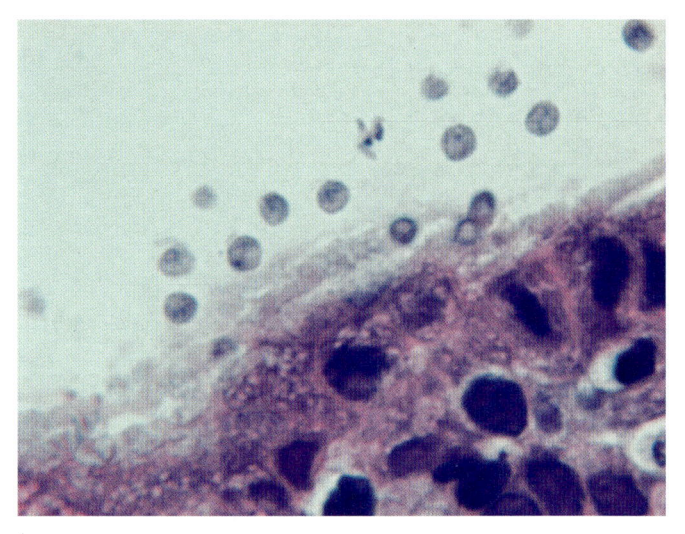

Figure 6.44 Cryptosporidium (Original magnification x400, H&E). Cryptosporidial organisms along mucosa of small bowel allograft.

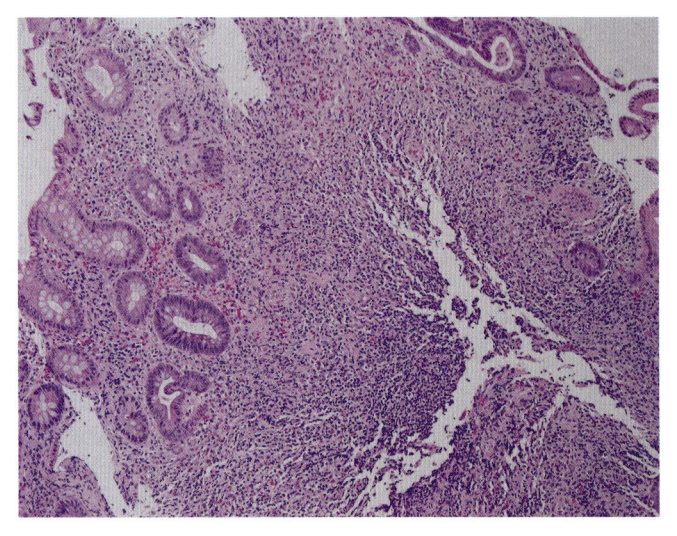

Figure 6.45 Inflammatory Bowel Disease (IBD) in allograft (Original magnification x100, H&E). Secondary IBD-like changes in long-term bowel allograft in patient that did not have IBD originally. There is extensive mixed chronic inflammatory infiltrate with glandular reactivity, occasional giant cells, superficial ulceration, and focal fibrosis.

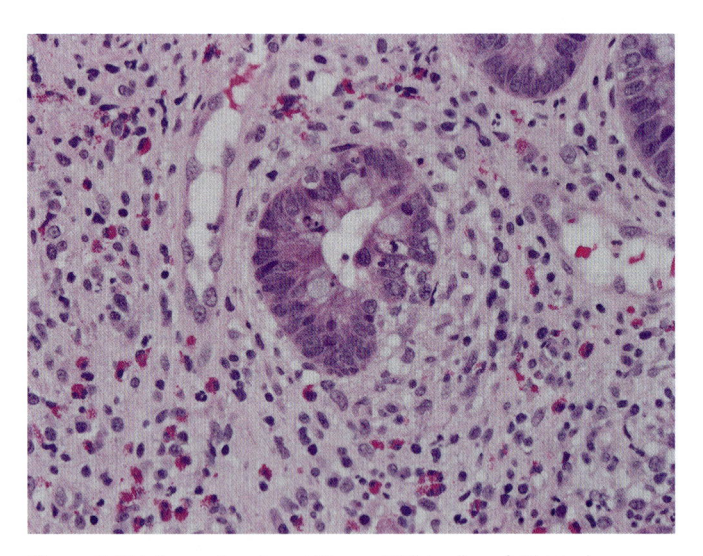

Figure 6.46 Inflammatory Bowel Disease (IBD) in allograft (Original magnification x400, H&E). Secondary IBD-like changes in long-term bowel allograft showing high magnification of acute colitis component, with neutrophils infiltrating crypt and surrounding mixed inflammatory cell infiltrate.

VII Recurrent Disease and Other Entities

The reappearance of original systemic or intestinal disease in the bowel allograft of ITx or MVTx patients is not a common occurrence. Generally, disease recurrence with GI transplants is not as frequent a complication as with other solid organ allografts (e.g., liver, kidney). Patients with inflammatory bowel disease (IBD) (e.g., Crohn's) [108, 109] receiving bowel allografts may show re-involvement in the transplant and this may be evident in the mucosal biopsies. There may also be secondary IBD involvement of GI allografts (see Figures 6.45 and 6.46) with certain systemic diseases such as Primary Sclerosing Cholangitis [110]. MVTx patients that originally

The Pathology of Intestinal and Multivisceral Transplantation

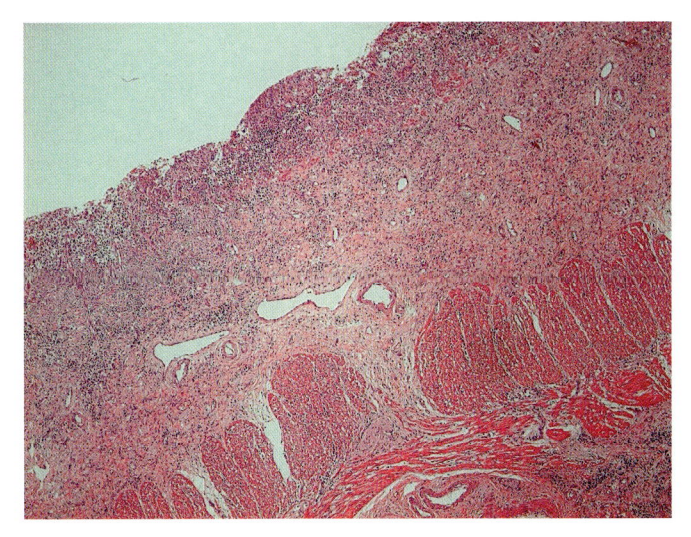

Figure 6.47 Intestinal ulcers (Original magnification x100 H&E). Persistent ulcer in small bowel allograft.

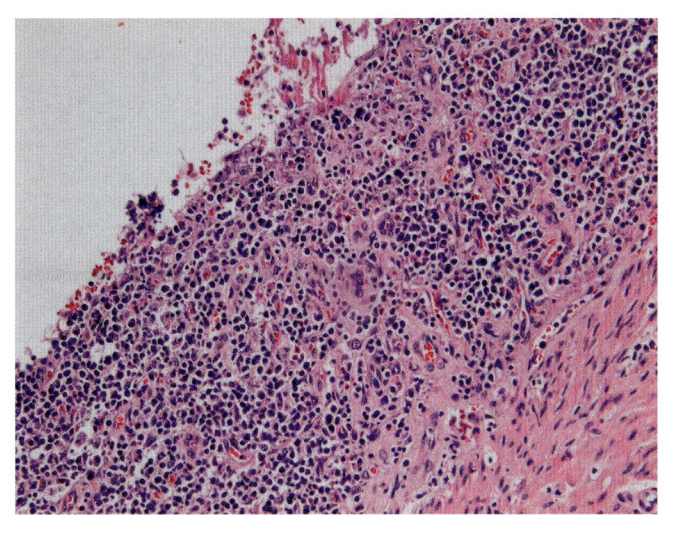

Figure 6.48 Intestinal ulcers (Original magnification x100 H&E). Persistent ulcer in small bowel allograft with prominent plasmacytic component. The lesion had a high EBV viral load from the paraffin block, but was negative for antigen receptor gene rearrangement studies.

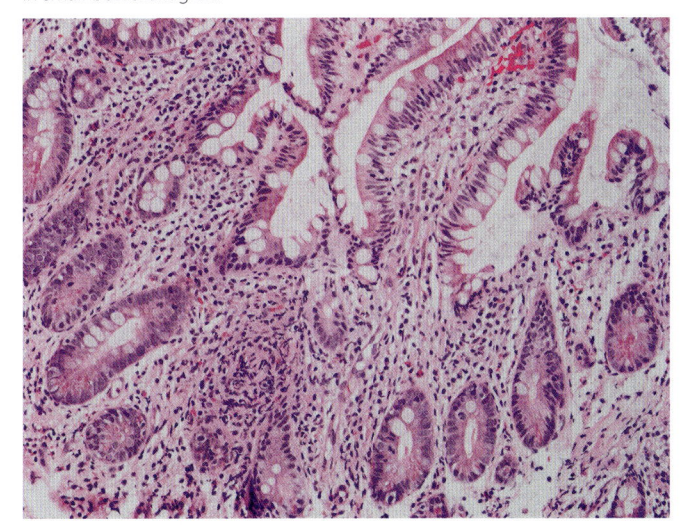

Figure 6.49 Chronic enteritis in intestinal allograft (Original magnification x200, H&E). Mixed chronic inflammatory cell infiltrate without notable epithelial apoptosis. Occasional eosinophils are present.

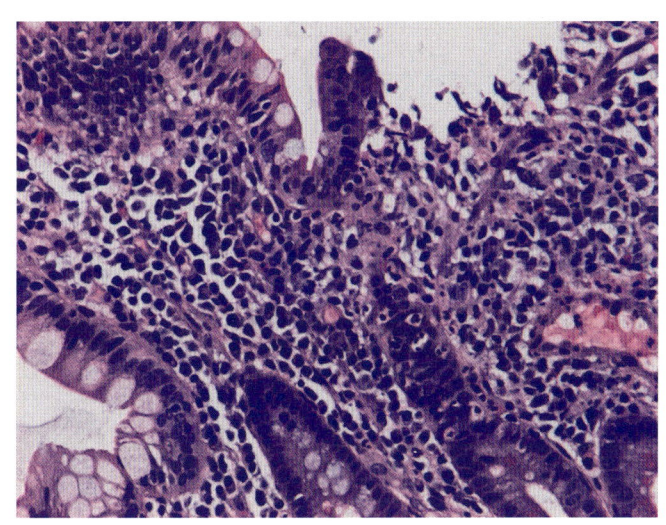

Figure 6.50 Acute and chronic enteritis in intestinal allograft (Original magnification x400, H&E). Higher magnification of patient with acute and chronic enteritis showing prominent plasma cell component and epithelial infiltration by neutrophils.

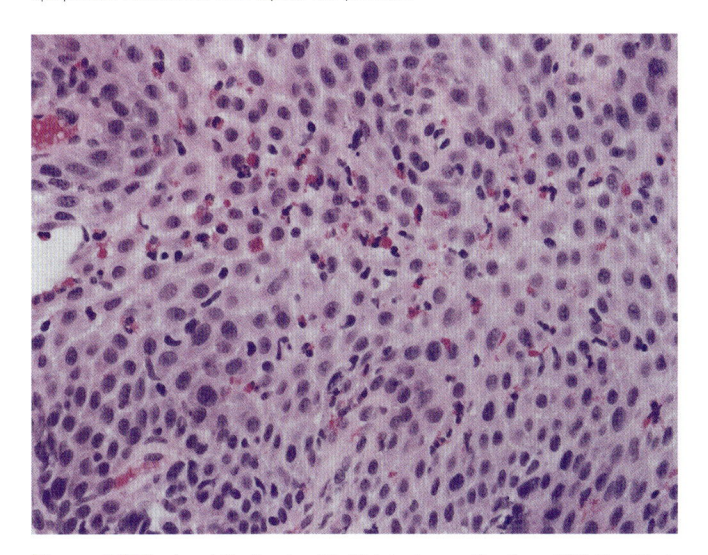

Figure 6.51 Eosinophilic Esophagitis (Original magnification x400). Stratified squamous epithelium of esophagus demonstrating numerous intraepithelial eosinophils. Patient was a multivisceral transplant recipient who also had increased eosinophilic infiltration throughout the GI tract.

had intra-abdominal neoplastic disorders (e.g., desmoid tumors) [111, 112] may display tumor recurrence after transplantation within intra-abdominal or extraperitoneal space.

A common complication in GI transplants is the manifestation of inflammatory lesions and processes that have an ambiguous or unexplained origin. For example, in some ITx and MVTx patients, there is the development later in the post-transplant course of persistent ulcers that can involve graft, native GI tissue, or both [113, 114]. These ulcers (see Figures 6.47 and 6.48) can originate from several causes, including EBV+ PTLD (the most common cause), smoldering acute rejection, infections, and some cases that remain of undetermined etiology.

Among other non-alloimmune miscellaneous inflammatory conditions that can affect the small intestinal allograft

205

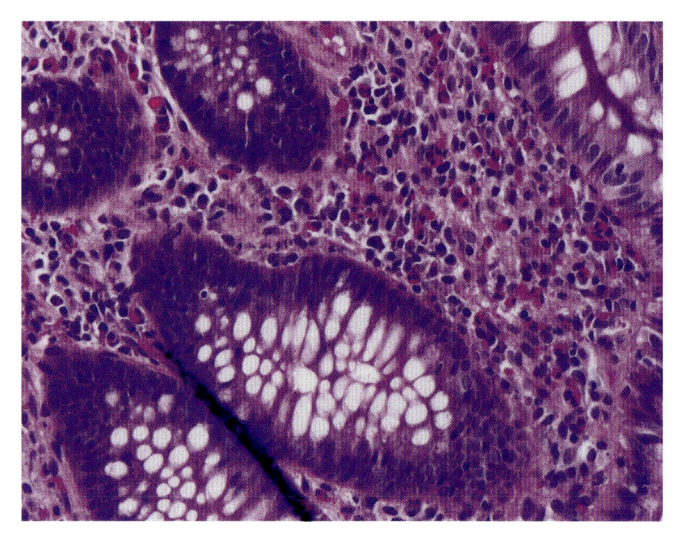

Figure 6.52 Eosinophilic colitis (Original magnification x400, H&E). Prominent and persistent chronic colitis (and enteritis) was present in the allografts of this multivisceral transplant patient with a very high proportion of eosinophils. The patient demonstrated increased allergic symptoms.

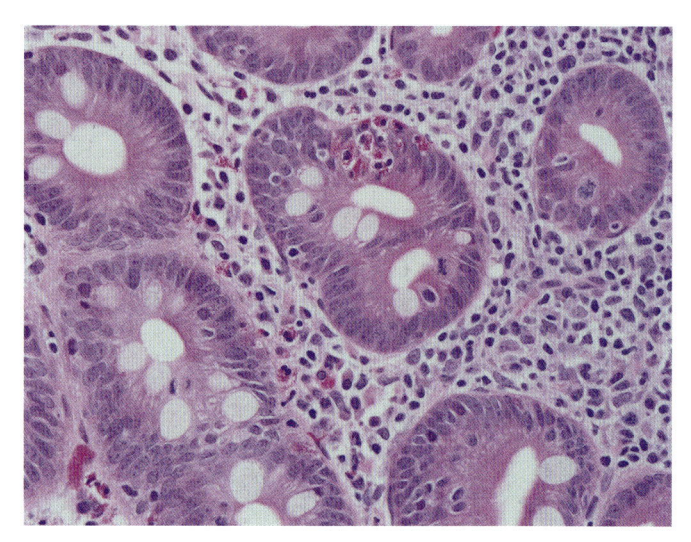

Figure 6.53 Eosinophilic colitis (Original magnification x400, H&E). Multivisceral transplant patient with an eosinophilic colitis showing epithelial infiltration by eosinophils.

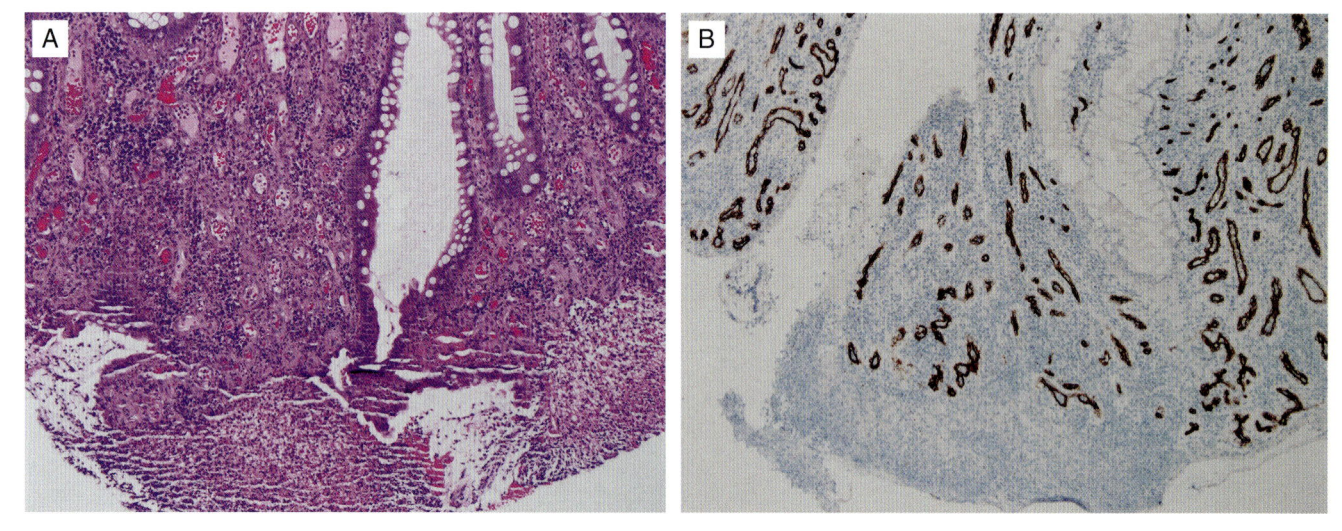

Figure 6.54 Hypervascular inflammatory lesion of bowel allograft (a. – original magnification x100, H&E). Severely inflamed area of mucosa with acute erosive component, hyperplasia of glands, and proliferation of vessels. Immunohistochemistry to CD34 (b. – original magnification x100, immunohistochemistry to CD34) highlights the large number of vessels, particularly near the surface of the lesion. Overall, this resembles a pyogenic granuloma.

and native small intestine [115, 116] is active enteritis of undetermined etiology. This entity is characterized by acute inflammation in lamina propria and/or surface epithelium with focal ulceration and crypt abscesses, occurring on a background of chronic inflammation (see Figures 6.49 and 6.50). Several potential pathogenic mechanisms of this entity are proposed, including stasis, altered bacterial flora, ischemia, prolapse, and mucolysis. Some NOD2 gene polymorphisms are associated with altered bacterial clearance and increased inflammatory infiltrate [17, 117–119].

It is not unusual for allograft and native gastrointestinal and colonic mucosa to demonstrate consistent infiltration with eosinophils [120]. Although there have been some associations with allergy, the particular pathophysiology remains unclear. There may also be an association with malabsorption, protein losing enteropathy, persistent acute rejection, and refractory ulcers. The eosinophilic infiltration can extend from the esophagus (e.g., eosinophilic esophagitis) (see Figure 6.51) throughout the entire GI tract (see Figures 6.52 and 6.53). On occasion, there may be hyperplastic polyps that form. Some inflammatory lesions have a high vascular component (e.g., hemangioma-like) with erosion and mucopurulent material, resembling a pyogenic granuloma of the skin [121] (see Figure 6.54).

Classical regenerative changes can transpire due to healing after acute rejection, infectious enteritis, or after ischemic injury.

Graft-versus-Host Disease (GVHD) can occur in skin, native alimentary tract, and other systems of ITx or MVTx patients

The Pathology of Intestinal and Multivisceral Transplantation

Table 6.7 Morphologic Categories of PTLD

1 "Early" lesions: Plasmacytic hyperplasia (PH) and Infectious Mononucleosis-like PTLD

Lymphoid proliferations that differ from typical reactive hyperplasia in having a diffuse proliferation of plasma cells and immunoblasts, but do not completely efface the architecture of the tissue.

2 Polymorphic PTLD

Destructive lesions composed of immunoblasts, plasma cells, and intermediate-sized lymphoid cells that efface the architecture of lymph nodes or form destructive extranodal masses.

3 Monomorphic PTLD

Monomorphic B cell PTLD

Sufficient architectural and cytologic atypia to be diagnosed as lymphoma on morphologic grounds, and expression of B cell antigens. Nodal architectural effacement and/or invasive tumoral growth in extranodal sites with confluent sheets of transformed cells.

Monomorphic T cell PTLD

Sufficient atypia and monomorphism to be recognized as neoplastic, and should be classified according to T cell neoplasms.

4 Hodgkin's Lymphoma and Hodgkin's Lymphoma-like PTLD

Since Reed-Sternberg-like cells may be seen in polymorphic PTLD, the diagnosis of Hodgkin's Lymphoma should be based on both classical morphologic and immunophenotypic features.

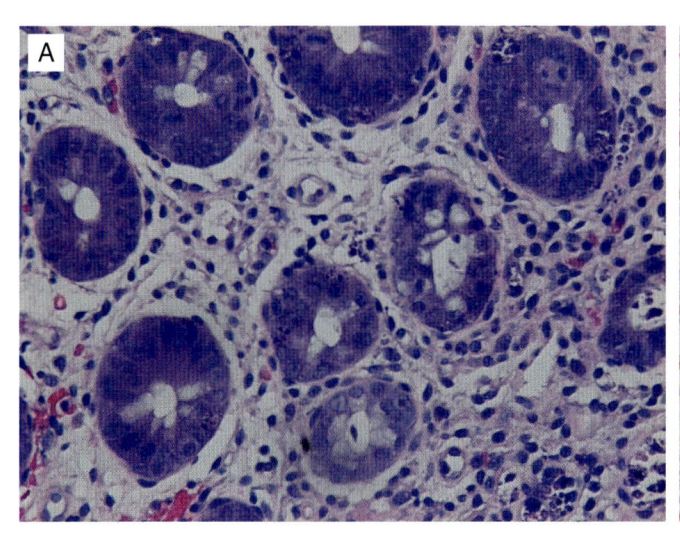

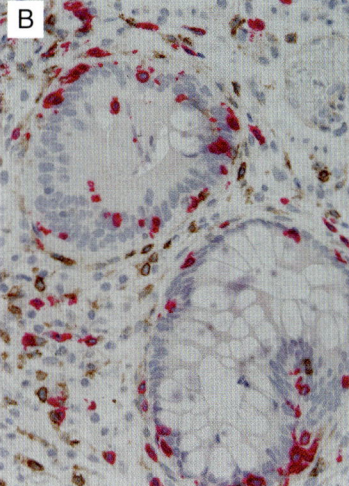

Figure 6.55 GVHD in native colon of patient with small intestinal allograft (Original magnification x400, 55a, H&E). High magnification of colonic epithelium showing significant apoptosis of the glandular lining cells in addition to a mixed colitis composed of CD4 (brown) and CD8 cells (red) within the interstitium and infiltrating glands. The CD4:CD8 ratio overall was estimated at 1:3 (see Figure 6.55b, two-color immunohistochemistry, 400x).

[122] [16, 123, 124]. The histopathological features of GVHD in native GI tissue can resemble acute cellular rejection with increased crypt epithelial cell apoptosis and inflammatory infiltrate (see Figure 6.55), thus the clinical history and origin of the tissue sample (whether from allograft or native) is critical to know in order to diagnose GVHD.

Compared to other solid organ allografts, there is a high incidence of Post-transplant Lymphoproliferative Disease (PTLD) in ITx and MVTx patients due to the prolonged immunosuppression [97, 125–127]. This common and serious complication escalates in frequency with extended duration of the time post-transplant and often does exhibit involvement of the allograft. While EBV infection is frequently associated with PTLD, EBV-negative PTLD can also transpire [128, 129]. The described histopathological progression of PTLD in the bowel includes an evolution from plasmacytic hyperplasia (an early lesion), polymorphic PTLD, monomorphic PTLD, and frank lymphoma (Table 6.7) [130]. The observation of lymphoplasmacytic infiltrates (i.e., plasmacytic hyperplasia), a suspected precursor lesion of PTLD, is common in bowel allograft biopsies as the time from transplant extends and epithelial structures may be effaced by the infiltrate (see Figures 6.56–6.60). EBV staining by EBER (see Figure 6.61) and immunostaining for the presence and relative composition of B and T cells within the infiltrate is useful in evaluating possible PTLD [131]. Antigen receptor gene rearrangement studies for T and B cell antigen receptors from the paraffin block can also be worthwhile for an assessment of potential monoclonality [128, 129]. Monomorphic

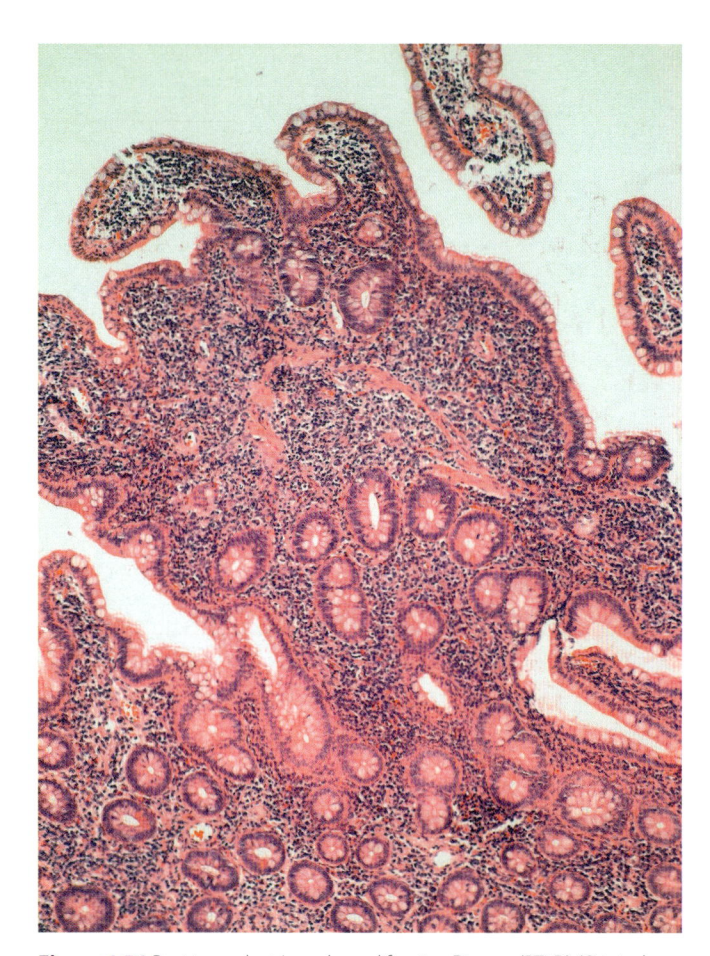

Figure 6.56 Post-transplant Lymphoproliferative Disease (PTLD) (Original magnification x100, H&E). Example of possible early PTLD. Moderate lymphoplasmacytic infiltrate with indeterminate for acute rejection is present. Gene rearrangement studies for T and B cell antigen receptors of this specimen suggested no B cell rearrangement.

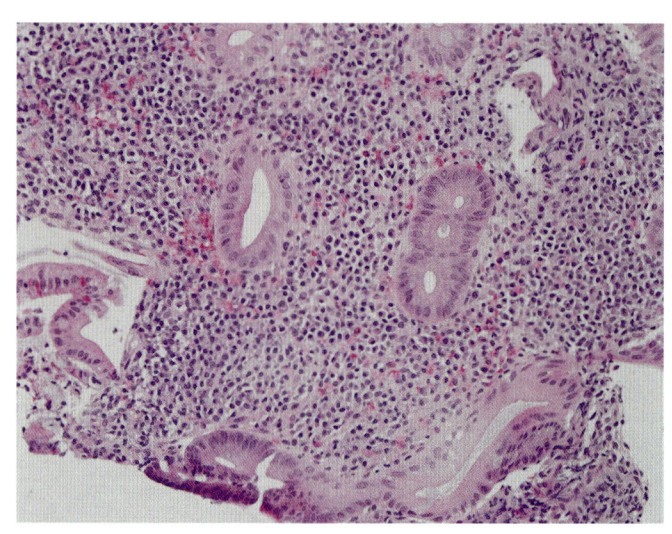

Figure 6.57 Post-transplant Lymphoproliferative Disease (PTLD) (Original magnification x200, H&E). Expansile mild lymphoplasmacytic infiltrate present with inflammatory infiltrate mainly consisting of lymphoplasmacytic population along with minor eosinophil component. There was minimal epithelial injury.

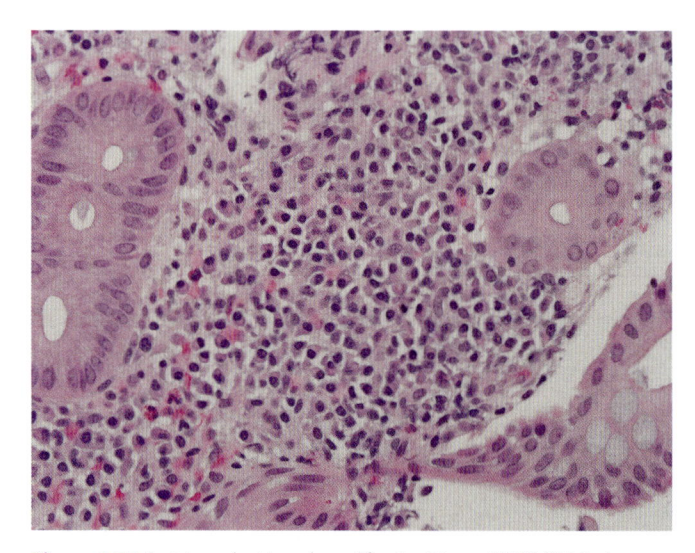

Figure 6.58 Post-transplant Lymphoproliferative Disease (PTLD) (Original magnification x400, H&E). Higher magnification of lymphoplasmacytic infiltrate. In situ hybridization for EBV was negative; however, gene rearrangement studies for T and B cell antigen receptors of this specimen suggested a B cell monoclonal population.

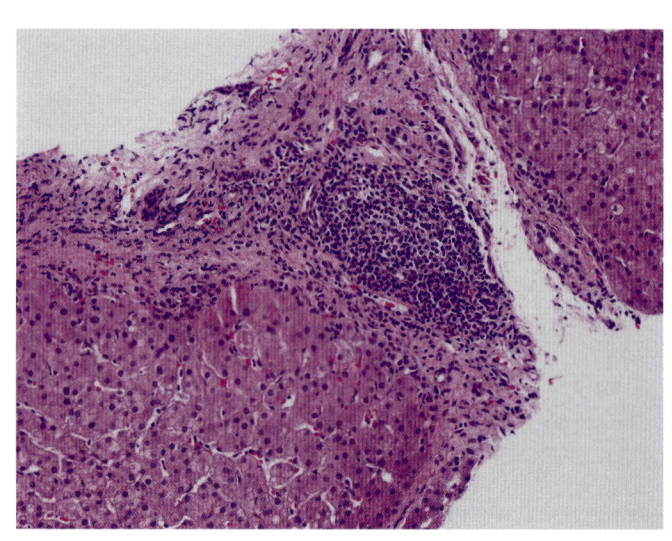

Figure 6.59 Post-transplant Lymphoproliferative Disease (PTLD) (Original magnification x200, H&E). Example of malignant lymphoma (PTLD), large B cell type involving liver allograft portal region in multivisceral transplant patient.

PTLDs can be of T or B cell origin [132, 133], and are recognized as neoplastic. PTLD lymphomas are classified according to their architectural and cytological features in a fashion identical to lymphomas occurring in native tissue [131].

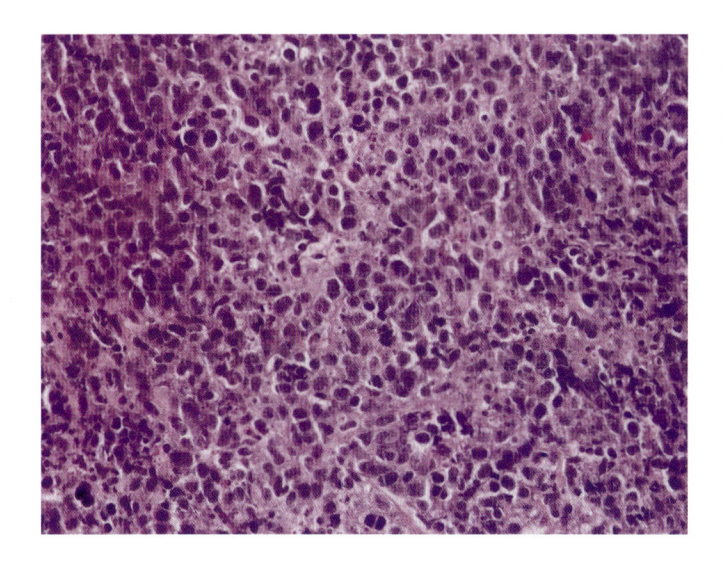

Figure 6.60 Post-transplant Lymphoproliferative Disease (PTLD) (Original magnification x400, H&E). Example of malignant lymphoma (PTLD), large B cell type within transplant colon with monomorphous, atypical lymphoid cells that were B cells by immunohistochemistry. Gene rearrangement studies for T and B cell antigen receptors of this specimen demonstrated a B cell monoclonal population.

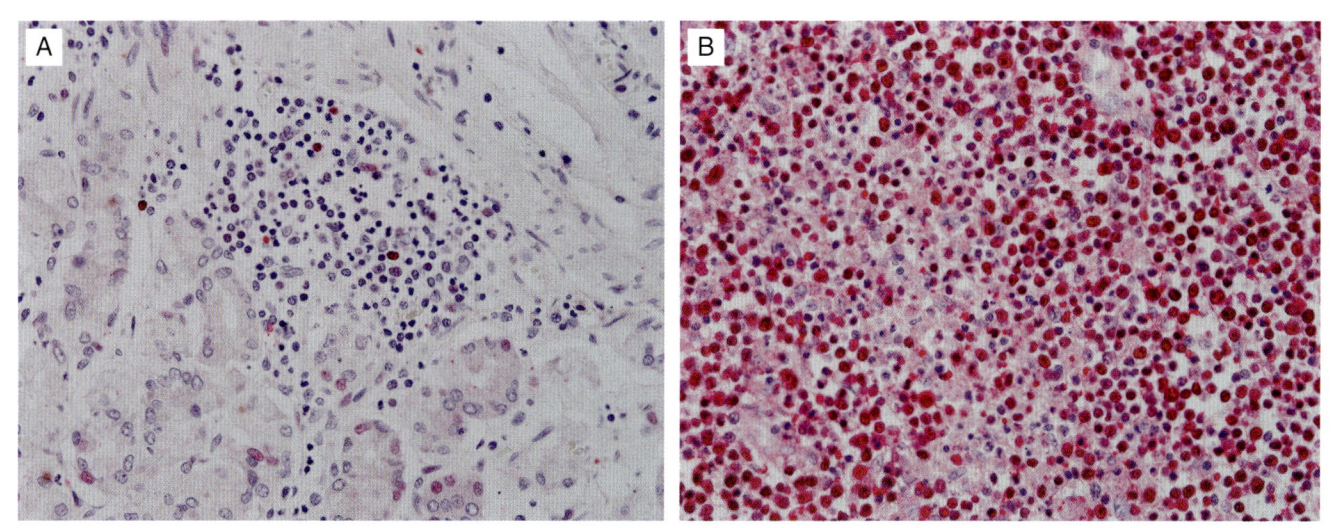

Figure 6.61 Post-transplant Lymphoproliferative Disease (PTLD) (a. – original magnification x200, EBV ISH). In situ hybridization for EBV shows mild number of positive cells. This patient had polymorphous PTLD. (b. – original magnification x200, EBV ISH). In situ hybridization for EBV shows extensive number of positive cells in B cell lymphoma that developed in intestinal transplant patient.

VIII Summary

Small intestinal transplantation has become a viable treatment option for patients with gastrointestinal failure and potential life-threatening complications due to parenteral nutrition. The surgical outcome, as well as short-term patient and graft survival, has improved dramatically over the past several decades. In part, this improvement is related to an advancement of surgical techniques, superior and more selective immunosuppressive agents, and a better conception of the causal nature of pathologic injury after transplantation. Regrettably, pathologic entities such as acute rejection, chronic rejection, infectious enteritis, and PTLD still endure as challenging impediments. Via histopathological evaluation of graft biopsies, transplant pathologists have been assigned with a critical role within the bowel transplant team. Pathologists are also obligated to understand and incorporate the clinical information of patients with the morphological changes of tissue samples in order to generate the most specific diagnosis to the treating physicians. Ultimately, the pathologist has the exciting charge of associating the pathological findings with the pathophysiologic mechanisms of graft injury in order to submit a realistic assessment of the probable clinical outcome.

References

1. Lacaille F. Intestinal Transplantation: Where Are We? Where Are We Going? Current Opinion in Organ Transplantation. 2012;17(3):248–9 10.1097/MOT.0b013e32835376e0.

2. LaRosa C, Baluarte HJ, Meyers KEC. Outcomes in Pediatric Solid-organ Transplantation. Pediatric Transplantation. 2011 Mar;15(2):128–41. PubMed PMID: 21309962. English.

3. Mazariegos GV. Intestinal Transplantation: Current Outcomes and Opportunities. Current Opinion in Organ Transplantation. 2009 Oct;14(5):515–21. PubMed PMID: 19623070. English.

4. Avitzur Y, Grant D. Intestine Transplantation in Children: Update 2010. Pediatric Clinics of North America. 2010 Apr;57(2):415–31. PubMed PMID: 20371045. English.

5. Fishbein TM. Intestinal Transplantation. New England Journal of Medicine. 2009 Sep 3;361(10):998–1008. PubMed PMID: 19726774. English.

6. Kocoshis SA. Medical Management of Pediatric Intestinal Failure. Semin Pediatr Surg. 2010 Feb;19(1):20–6. PubMed PMID: 20123270. Epub 2010/02/04. English.

7. Weimann A, Ebener C, Holland-Cunz S, Jauch KW, Hausser L, Kemen M, et al. Surgery and Transplantation – Guidelines on Parenteral Nutrition, Chapter 18. German Medical Science: GMS e-journal. 2009;7:Doc10. PubMed PMID: 20049072. PubMed Central PMCID: PMC2795372. Epub 2010/01/06. English.

8. Pironi L, Joly F, Forbes A, Colomb V, Lyszkowska M, Baxter J, et al. Long-term Follow-up of Patients on Home Parenteral Nutrition in Europe: Implications for Intestinal Transplantation. Gut. 2011 Jan;60(1):17–25. PubMed PMID: 21068130. Epub 2010/11/12. English.

9. Sauvat F, Fusaro F, Lacaille F, Dupic L, Bourdaud N, Colomb V, et al. Is Intestinal Transplantation the Future of Children with Definitive Intestinal Insufficiency? European Journal of Pediatric Surgery. 2008 Dec;18(6):368–71. PubMed PMID: 19023853. English.

10. Sudan D. Long-term Outcomes and Quality of Life after Intestine Transplantation. Current Opinion in Organ Transplantation. 2010 Jun;15(3):357–60. PubMed PMID: 20445450. English.

11. Ruiz P, Kato T, Tzakis A. Current Status of Transplantation of the Small Intestine. Transplantation. 2007 Jan 15;83(1):1–6. PubMed PMID: 17220781.

12. Tzakis AG, Kato T, Levi DM, Defaria W, Selvaggi G, Weppler D, et al. 100 Multivisceral Transplants at a Single Center. Annals of Surgery. 2005 Oct;242(4):480–90; discussion 91–3. PubMed PMID: 16192808.

13. Tzvetanov IG, Oberholzer J, Benedetti E. Current Status of Living Donor Small Bowel Transplantation. Curr Opin Organ Transplant. 2010 Jun;15(3):346–8. PubMed PMID: 20445448. Epub 2010/05/07. English.

14. Naesens M, Kuypers DRJ, Sarwal M. Calcineurin Inhibitor Nephrotoxicity. Clinical Journal of the American Society of Nephrology. 2009 February 2009;4(2):481–508.

15. Sirinek LP, O'Dorisio MS, Dunaway DJ. Accumulation of Donor-specific Cytotoxic T Cells in Intestinal Lymphoid Tissues Following Intestinal Transplantation. Journal of Clinical Immunology. 1995 Sep;15(5):258–65. PubMed PMID: 8537470. English.

16. Wu G, Selvaggi G, Nishida S, Moon J, Island E, Ruiz P, et al. Graft-versus-Host Disease after Intestinal and Multivisceral Transplantation. Transplantation. 2011 Jan 27;91(2):219–24. PubMed PMID: 21076376. Epub 2010/11/16. English.

17. Fishbein T, Novitskiy G, Mishra L, Matsumoto C, Kaufman S, Goyal S, et al. NOD2-expressing Bone Marrow-derived Cells Appear to Regulate Epithelial Innate Immunity of the Transplanted Human Small Intestine. Gut. 2008 Mar;57(3):323–30. PubMed PMID: 17965060.

18. Wood KJ, Goto R. Mechanisms of Rejection: Current Perspectives. Transplantation. 2012;93(1):1–10 .1097/TP.0b013e31823cab44.

19. Ruiz P. How Can Pathologists Help to Diagnose Late Complications in Small Bowel and Multivisceral Transplantation? Current Opinion in Organ Transplantation. 2012;17(3):273–9 10.1097/MOT.0b013e3283534eb0.

20. Ruiz P. Transplantation Pathology. 1st ed. Ruiz P, editor: Cambridge University Press; 2009.

21. Konigsrainer A, Ladurner R, Iannetti C, Steurer W, Ollinger R, Offner F, et al. The 'Blind Innsbruck Ostomy', a Cutaneous Enterostomy for Long-term Histologic Surveillance after Small Bowel Transplantation. Transplant International. 2007 Oct;20(10):867–74. PubMed PMID: 17711406. English.

22. Remotti H, Subramanian S, Martinez M, Kato T, Magid MS. Small-bowel Allograft Biopsies in the Management of Small-intestinal and Multivisceral Transplant Recipients: Histopathologic Review and Clinical Correlations. Arch Pathol Lab Med. 2012 Jul;136(7):761–71. PubMed PMID: 22742549. Epub 2012/06/30. English.

23. Ueno T, Fukuzawa M. Current Status of Intestinal Transplantation. Surgery Today. 2010 Dec;40(12):1112–22. PubMed PMID: 21110153. English.

24. Eltzschig HK, Eckle T. Ischemia and Reperfusion – From Mechanism to Translation. Nat Med. 2011;17(11):1391–401.

25. Mallick IH, Yang W, Winslet MC, Seifalian AM. Protective Effects of Ischemic Preconditioning on the Intestinal Mucosal Microcirculation Following Ischemia-Reperfusion of the Intestine. Microcirculation. 2005 Dec;12(8):615–25. PubMed PMID: 16284003. English.

26. Moore-Olufemi SD, Olufemi SE, Lott S, Sato N, Kozar RA, Moore FA, et al. Intestinal Ischemic Preconditioning after Ischemia/Reperfusion Injury in Rat Intestine: Profiling Global Gene Expression Patterns. Digestive Diseases and Sciences. 2010 Jul;55(7):1866–77. PubMed PMID: 19779973. Epub 2009/09/26. English.

27. Akalin E, O'Connell PJ. Genomics of Chronic Allograft Injury. Kidney International. 2010 Dec;78 Suppl 119: S33–7. PubMed PMID: 21116315. English.

28. Naito Y, Mizushima K, Yoshikawa T. Global Analysis of Gene Expression in Gastric Ischemia-Reperfusion: A Future Therapeutic Direction for Mucosal Protective Drugs. Digestive Diseases & Sciences. 2005 Oct;50 Suppl 1:S45–55. PubMed PMID: 16184421. English.

29. Stallone G, Infante B, Gesualdo L. Older Donors and Older Recipients in Kidney Transplantation. Journal of Nephrology. 2010 Sep–Oct;23 Suppl 15: S98–103. PubMed PMID: 20872377. English.

30. Quaedackers JS, Beuk RJ, Bennet L, Charlton A, oude Egbrink MG, Gunn AJ, et al. An Evaluation of Methods for Grading Histologic Injury Following Ischemia/Reperfusion of the Small

Bowel. Transplantation Proceedings. 2000 Sep;32(6):1307–10. PubMed PMID: 10995960. English.

31. Wasserberg N, Tzakis AG, Santiago SF, Ruiz P, Salgar SK. Anastomotic Healing in a Small Bowel Transplantation Model in the Rat. World Journal of Surgery. 2004 Jan;28(1):69–73. PubMed PMID: 14639489.

32. Beuk RJ, Tangelder GJ, Maassen RLJG, Quaedackers JSLT, Heineman E, Oude Egbrink MGA. Leucocyte and Platelet Adhesion in Different Layers of the Small Bowel during Experimental Total Warm Ischaemia and Reperfusion. British Journal of Surgery. 2008 Oct;95(10):1294–304. PubMed PMID: 18720462. English.

33. Grootjans J, Lenaerts K, Derikx JPM, Matthijsen RA, de Bruïne AP, van Bijnen AA, et al. Human Intestinal Ischemia-Reperfusion–Induced Inflammation Characterized: Experiences from a New Translational Model. The American Journal of Pathology. 2010 5//;176(5):2283–91.

34. Asaoka T, Island ER, Tryphonopoulos P, Selvaggi G, Moon J, Tekin A, et al. Characteristic Immune, Apoptosis and Inflammatory Gene Profiles Associated with Intestinal Acute Cellular Rejection in Formalin-fixed Paraffin-embedded Mucosal Biopsies. Transplant International. 2011;24(7):697–707.

35. Nayyar N, Mazariegos G, Ranganathan S, Soltys K, Bond G, Jaffe R, et al. Pediatric Small Bowel Transplantation. [Review] [26 refs]. Seminars in Pediatric Surgery. 2010;19(1):68–77. PubMed PMID: 20123276.

36. Kato T, Ruiz P, Tzakis A. Exfoliative Bowel Rejection–A Dangerous Loss of Integrity. Pediatric Transplantation. 2004 Oct;8(5):426–7. PubMed PMID: 15367275. English.

37. Park KT, Berquist WL, Pai R, Triadafilopoulos G. Exfoliative Rejection in Intestinal Transplantation. Digestive Diseases & Sciences. 2010 Dec;55(12):3336–8. PubMed PMID: 20683662. English.

38. Berney T, Kato T, Nishida S, Tector AJ, Mittal NK, Madariaga J, et al. Portal versus Systemic Drainage of Small Bowel Allografts: Comparative Assessment of Survival, Function, Rejection, and Bacterial Translocation. Journal of the American College of Surgeons. 2002 Dec;195(6):804–13. PubMed PMID: 12495313.

39. Cicalese L, Sileri P, Green M, Abu-Elmagd K, Kocoshis S, Reyes J. Bacterial Translocation in Clinical Intestinal Transplantation. Transplantation. 2001 May 27;71(10):1414–7. PubMed PMID: 11391228. English.

40. Tzakis AG, Kato T, Levi DM, Defaria W, Selvaggi G, Weppler D, et al. 100 Multivisceral Transplants at a Single Center. Annals of Surgery. 2005 Oct;242(4):480–90; discussion 91–3. PubMed PMID: 16192808. Pubmed Central PMCID: PMC1402343. English.

41. Takahashi H, Kato T, Selvaggi G, Nishida S, Gaynor JJ, Delacruz V, et al. Subclinical Rejection in the Initial Postoperative Period in Small Intestinal Transplantation: A Negative Influence on Graft Survival. Transplantation. 2007 Sep;84(6):689–96. PubMed PMID: ISI:000249841700006.

42. Mengel M. What Is the Significance of Subclinical Inflammation in Human Renal Allografts? It Depends! Transplantation. 2012;93(1):22–3.

43. Seron D, Moreso F. Protocol Biopsies in Renal Transplantation: Prognostic Value of Structural Monitoring. Kidney International. 2007 Sep;72(6):690–7. PubMed PMID: 17597702.

44. Choi BS, Shin MJ, Shin SJ, Kim YS, Choi YJ, Moon IS, et al. Clinical Significance of an Early Protocol Biopsy in Living-donor Renal Transplantation: Ten-year Experience at a Single Center. American Journal of Transplantation. 2005 Jun;5(6):1354–60. PubMed PMID: 15888041.

45. Mercer DF. Hot Topics in Postsmall Bowel Transplantation: Noninvasive Graft Monitoring Including Stool Calprotectin and Plasma Citrulline. Current Opinion in Organ Transplantation. 2011 Jun;16(3):316–22. PubMed PMID: 21505339. English.

46. Sageshima J, Ciancio G, Gaynor JJ, Chen L, Guerra G, Kupin W, et al. Addition of Anti-CD25 to Thymoglobulin for Induction Therapy: Delayed Return of Peripheral Blood CD25-positive Population. Clinical Transplantation. 2011 Mar-Apr;25(2):E132–5. PubMed PMID: 21083765. English.

47. Ruiz P, Tryphonopoulos P, Island E, Selvaggi G, Nishida S, Moon J, et al. Citrulline Evaluation in Bowel Transplantation. Transplantation Proceedings. 2010 Jan–Feb;42(1):54–6. PubMed PMID: 20172280. English.

48. David AI, Selvaggi G, Ruiz P, Gaynor JJ, Tryphonopoulos P, Kleiner GI, et al. Blood Citrulline Level Is an Exclusionary Marker for Significant Acute Rejection after Intestinal Transplantation. Transplantation. 2007 Nov 15;84(9):1077–81. PubMed PMID: 17998860.

49. Pappas PA, G Tzakis A, Gaynor JJ, Carreno MR, Ruiz P, Huijing F, et al. An Analysis of the Association between Serum Citrulline and Acute Rejection among 26 Recipients of Intestinal Transplant. American Journal of Transplantation. 2004 Jul;4(7):1124–32. PubMed PMID: 15196071.

50. Rose AG. Understanding the Pathogenesis and the Pathology of Hyperacute Cardiac Rejection. Cardiovascular Pathology. 2002 May–Jun;11(3):171–6. PubMed PMID: 12031770. English.

51. Terasaki PI, Cai J. Humoral Theory of Transplantation: Further Evidence. Current Opinion in Immunology. 2005 Oct;17(5):541–5. PubMed PMID: 16098722. English.

52. Ruiz P, Carreno M, Weppler D, Gomez C, Island E, Selvaggi G, et al. Immediate Antibody-mediated (Hyperacute) Rejection in Small-bowel Transplantation and Relationship to Cross-match Status and Donor-specific C4d-binding Antibodies: Case Report. Transplantation Proceedings. 2010 Jan–Feb;42(1):95–9. PubMed PMID: 20172288. English.

53. Tsai HL, Island ER, Chang JW, Gonzalez-Pinto I, Tryphonopoulos P, Nishida S, et al. Association between Donor-specific Antibodies and Acute Rejection and Resolution in Small Bowel and Multivisceral Transplantation. Transplantation. 2011 Jul 29. PubMed PMID: 21804443. Epub 2011/08/02. English.

54. Gerlach UA, Schoenemann C, Lachmann N, Koch M, Pascher A. Salvage Therapy for Refractory Rejection and Persistence of Donor-specific Antibodies after Intestinal Transplantation Using the Proteasome Inhibitor Bortezomib. Transplant International. 2011 May;24(5):e43–5. PubMed PMID: 21155900. English.

55. Kato T, Mizutani K, Terasaki P, Quintini C, Selvaggi G, Thompson J, et al. Association of Emergence of HLA Antibody and Acute Rejection in Intestinal Transplant Recipients: A Possible Evidence of Acute Humoral Sensitization. Transplantation

56. Dick AA, Horslen S. Antibody-mediated Rejection after Intestinal Transplantation. Curr Opin Organ Transplant. 2012 Jun;17(3):250–7. PubMed PMID: 22476220. Epub 2012/04/06. English.

57. Ruiz P, Garcia M, Pappas P, Berney T, Esquenazi V, Kato T, et al. Mucosal Vascular Alterations in Isolated Small-bowel Allografts: Relationship to Humoral Sensitization. American Journal of Transplantation. 2003 Jan;3(1):43–9. PubMed PMID: 12492709. English.

58. Ruiz P, Suarez M, Nishida S, de la Cruz V, Nicolas M, Weppler D, et al. Sclerosing Mesenteritis in Small Bowel Transplantation: Possible Manifestation of Acute Vascular Rejection. Transplantation Proceedings. 2003 Dec;35(8):3057–60. PubMed PMID: 14697979.

59. Lee RG, Nakamura K, Tsamandas AC, Abu-Elmagd K, Furukawa H, Hutson WR, et al. Pathology of Human Intestinal Transplantation. Gastroenterology. 1996 Jun;110(6):1820–34. PubMed PMID: 8964408.

60. Delacruz V, Garcia M, Mittal N, Nishida S, Levi D, Selvaggi G, et al. Immunoenzymatic and Morphological Detection of Epithelial Cell Apoptotic Stages in Gastrointestinal Allografts from Multivisceral Transplant Patients. Transplantation Proceedings. 2004 Mar;36(2):338–9. PubMed PMID: 15050151.

61. Krams SM, Hayashi M, Fox CK, Villanueva JC, Whitmer KJ, Burns W, et al. CD8+ cells Are Not Necessary for Allograft Rejection or the Induction of Apoptosis in an Experimental Model of Small Intestinal Transplantation. Journal of Immunology. 1998 Apr 15;160(8):3673–80. PubMed PMID: 9558067. English.

62. Ogura Y, Martinez OM, Villanueva JC, Tait JF, Strauss HW, Higgins JP, et al. Apoptosis and Allograft Rejection in the Absence of CD8+ T Cells. Transplantation. 2001 Jun 27;71(12):1827–34. PubMed PMID: 11455265. English.

63. Takahashi H, Selvaggi G, Nishida S, Weppler D, Levi D, Kato T, et al. Organ-specific Differences in Acute Rejection Intensity in a Multivisceral Transplant. Transplantation. 2006 Jan 27;81(2):297–9. PubMed PMID: 16436979.

64. Zou Y, Hernandez F, Burgos E, Martinez L, Gonzalez-Reyes S, Fernandez-Dumont V, et al. Bacterial Translocation in Acute Rejection after Small Bowel Transplantation in Rats. Pediatric Surgery International. 2005;21(3):208–11. PubMed PMID: 15756565.

65. Wu T, Abu-Elmagd K, Bond G, Nalesnik MA, Randhawa P, Demetris AJ. A Schema for Histologic Grading of Small Intestine Allograft Acute Rejection. Transplantation. 2003 Apr 27;75(8):1241–8. PubMed PMID: 12717210.

66. Garcia M, Delacruz V, Ortiz R, Bagni A, Weppler D, Kato T, et al. Acute Cellular Rejection Grading Scheme for Human Gastric Allografts. Human Pathology. 2004 Mar;35(3):343–9. PubMed PMID: 15017591.

67. Ruiz P, Bagni A, Brown R, Cortina G, Harpaz N, Magid MS, et al. Histological Criteria for the Identification of Acute Cellular Rejection in Human Small Bowel Allografts: Results of the Pathology Workshop at the VIII International Small Bowel Transplant Symposium. Transplantation Proceedings. 2004 Mar;36(2):335–7. PubMed PMID: 15050150.

68. Ruiz P, Takahashi H, Delacruz V, Island E, Selvaggi G, Nishida S, et al. International Grading Scheme for Acute Cellular Rejection in Small-bowel Transplantation: Single-center Experience. Transplantation Proceedings. 2010 Jan–Feb;42(1):47–53. PubMed PMID: 20172279. English.

69. Ishii T, Mazariegos GV, Bueno J, Ohwada S, Reyes J. Exfoliative Rejection after Intestinal Transplantation in Children. Pediatric Transplantation. 2003 Jun;7(3):185–91. PubMed PMID: 12756042. English.

70. Kato T, Selvaggi G, Gaynor JJ, Takahashi H, Nishida S, Moon J, et al. Inclusion of Donor Colon and Ileocecal Valve in Intestinal Transplantation. Transplantation. 2008 Jul;86(2):293–7. PubMed PMID: ISI:000257887500019.

71. Ruiz P, Weppler D, Nishida S, Kato T, Selvaggi G, Levi D, et al. International Grading Scheme for Acute Rejection in Small Bowel Transplantation: Implementation and Experience at the University of Miami. Transplantation Proceedings. 2006 Jul–Aug;38(6):1683–4. PubMed PMID: 16908246.

72. Nayyar N, Mazariegos G, Ranganathan S, Soltys K, Bond G, Jaffe R, et al. Pediatric Small Bowel Transplantation. Seminars in Pediatric Surgery. 2010 Feb;19(1):68–77. PubMed PMID: 20123276. English.

73. Murphy SP, Porrett PM, Turka LA. Innate Immunity in Transplant Tolerance and Rejection. Immunological Reviews. 2011 May;241(1):39–48. PubMed PMID: 21488888. English.

74. Baluja P, Haragsim L, Laszik Z. Chronic Allograft Nephropathy. Advances in Chronic Kidney Disease. 2006 Jan;13(1):56–61. PubMed PMID: 16412971.

75. Colvin RB, Hirohashi T, Farris AB, Minnei F, Collins AB, Smith RN. Emerging Role of B Cells in Chronic Allograft Dysfunction. Kidney International. 2010 Dec;78 Suppl 119:S13–7. PubMed PMID: 21116310. English.

76. Thaunat O, Patey N, Caligiuri G, Gautreau C, Mamani-Matsuda M, Mekki Y, et al. Chronic Rejection Triggers the Development of an Aggressive Intragraft Immune Response through Recapitulation of Lymphoid Organogenesis. J Immunol. 2010 July 1, 2010;185(1):717–28.

77. Takeda A, Horike K, Ohtsuka Y, Inaguma D, Goto N, Watarai Y, et al. Current Problems of Chronic Active Antibody-mediated Rejection. Clinical Transplantation. 2011 Jul;25 Suppl 23:2–5. PubMed PMID: 21623906. English.

78. Swanson BJ, Talmon GA, Wisecarver JW, Grant WJ, Radio SJ. Histologic Analysis of Chronic Rejection in Small Bowel Transplantation: Mucosal and Vascular Alterations. Transplantation. 2013;95(2):378–82 10.1097/TP.0b013e318270f370.

79. Tryphonopoulos P, Weppler D, Nishida S, Kato T, Levi D, Selvaggi G, et al. Mucosal Fibrosis in Intestinal Transplant Biopsies Correlates Positively with the Development of Chronic Rejection. Transplantation Proceedings. 2006 Jul–Aug;38(6):1685–6. PubMed PMID: 16908247.

80. Perez MT, Garcia M, Weppler D, Kato T, Delis S, Nishida S, et al. Temporal Relationships between Acute Cellular Rejection Features and Increased Mucosal Fibrosis in the Early Posttransplant Period of Human Small

81. Fryer JP. The Current Status of Intestinal Transplantation. Current Opinion in Organ Transplantation. 2008 Jun;13(3):266-72. PubMed PMID: 18685315. English.

82. Dijkstra G, Rings EHHM, van Dullemen HM, Bijleveld CMA, Meessen NEL, Karrenbeld A, et al. [Small Bowel Transplantation as a Treatment Option for Intestinal Failure in Children and Adults]. Nederlands Tijdschrift voor Geneeskunde. 2005 Feb 19;149(8):391-8. PubMed PMID: 15751317. Dunnedarmtransplantatie als behandeling van darmfalen bij kinderen en volwassenen. Dutch.

83. Abu-Elmagd K, Reyes J, Bond G, Mazariegos G, Wu T, Murase N, et al. Clinical Intestinal Transplantation: A Decade of Experience at a Single Center. Annals of Surgery. 2001 Sep;234(3):404-16; discussion 16-7. PubMed PMID: 11524593. PubMed Central PMCID: PMC1422031. English.

84. Ziring D, Tran R, Edelstein S, McDiarmid SV, Gajjar N, Cortina G, et al. Infectious Enteritis after Intestinal Transplantation: Incidence, Timing, and Outcome. Transplantation. 2005 Mar 27;79(6):702-9. PubMed PMID: 15785377. English.

85. McLaughlin GE, Delis S, Kashimawo L, Cantwell GP, Mittal N, Cirocco RE, et al. Adenovirus Infection in Pediatric Liver and Intestinal Transplant Recipients: Utility of DNA Detection by PCR. American Journal of Transplantation. 2003 Feb;3(2):224-8. PubMed PMID: 12603217.

86. Pinchoff RJ, Kaufman SS, Magid MS, Erdman DD, Gondolesi GE, Mendelson MH, et al. Adenovirus Infection in Pediatric Small Bowel Transplantation Recipients. Transplantation. 2003 Jul 15;76(1):183-9. PubMed PMID: 12865807. English.

87. Berho M, Torroella M, Viciana A, Weppler D, Thompson J, Nery J, et al. Adenovirus Enterocolitis in Human Small Bowel Transplants. Pediatric Transplantation. 1998 Nov;2(4):277-82. PubMed PMID: 10084729. English.

88. Giovanelli M, Gupte GL, Sharif K, Mayer DA, Mirza DF. Chronic Rejection after Combined Liver and Small Bowel Transplantation in a Child with Chronic Intestinal Pseudo-obstruction: A Case Report. Transplantation Proceedings. 2008 Jun;40(5):1763-7. PubMed PMID: 18589190. English.

89. Ziring D, Tran R, Edelstein S, McDiarmid SV, Vargas J, Cortina G, et al. Infectious Enteritis after Intestinal Transplantation: Incidence, Timing, and Outcome. Transplantation Proceedings. 2004 Mar;36(2):379-80. PubMed PMID: 15050165. English.

90. Florescu DF, Hill LA, McCartan MA, Grant W. Two Cases of Norwalk Virus Enteritis Following Small Bowel Transplantation Treated with Oral Human Serum Immunoglobulin. Pediatric Transplantation. 2008 05/;12(3):372-5.

91. Farkas T, Sestak K, Wei C, Jiang X. Characterization of a Rhesus Monkey Calicivirus Representing a New Genus of Caliciviridae. J Virol. 2008 Jun;82(11):5408-16. PubMed PMID: 18385231. PubMed Central PMCID: PMC2395209. Epub 2008/04/04. English.

92. Lynch M, Shieh W-J, Tatti K, Gentsch JR, Harris TF, Jiang B, et al. The Pathology of Rotavirus-associated Deaths, Using New Molecular Diagnostics. Clinical Infectious Diseases. 2003 November 15, 2003;37(10):1327-33.

93. Kaufman SS, Chatterjee NK, Fuschino ME, Magid MS, Gordon RE, Morse DL, et al. Calicivirus Enteritis in an Intestinal Transplant Recipient. American Journal of Transplantation. 2003 Jun;3(6):764-8. PubMed PMID: 12780570. English.

94. Pascher A, Klupp J, Schulz RJ, Dignass A, Neuhaus P. CMV, EBV, HHV6, and HHV7 Infections after Intestinal Transplantation without Specific Antiviral Prophylaxis. Transplantation Proceedings. 2004 Mar;36(2):381-2. PubMed PMID: 15050166. Epub 2004/03/31. English.

95. Bueno J, Green M, Kocoshis S, Furukawa H, Abu-Elmagd K, Yunis E, et al. Cytomegalovirus Infection after Intestinal Transplantation in Children. Clinical Infectious Diseases. 1997 Nov;25(5):1078-83. PubMed PMID: 9402361. PubMed Central PMCID: NIHMS239871 PMC2962562. English.

96. Furukawa H, Kusne S, Abu-Elmagd K, Green M, Reyes J, Starzl TE, et al. Effect of CMV Serology on Outcome after Clinical Intestinal Transplantation. Transplantation Proceedings. 1996 Oct;28(5):2780-1. PubMed PMID: 8908056. PubMed Central PMCID: NIHMS240402 PMC2956492. English.

97. Kocoshis SA. Small Bowel Transplantation in Infants and Children. Gastroenterology Clinics of North America. 1994 Dec;23(4):727-42. PubMed PMID: 7698829. English.

98. Gourishankar S MJ, Jhangri GS, Preiksaitis JK. Herpes Zoster Infection Following Solid Organ Transplantation: Incidence, Risk Factors and Outcomes in the Current Immunosuppressive Era. American Journal of Transplantation. 2004;4(1)(Jan):108-15.

99. Jenkins FJ, Rowe DT, Rinaldo CR. Herpesvirus Infections in Organ Transplant Recipients. Clinical and Diagnostic Laboratory Immunology. 2003 January 1, 2003;10(1):1-7.

100. Sipponen T, Turunen U, Lautenschlager I, Nieminen U, Arola J, Halme L. Human Herpesvirus 6 and Cytomegalovirus in Ileocolonic Mucosa in Inflammatory Bowel Disease. Scand J Gastroenterol. 2011 Nov;46(11):1324-33. PubMed PMID: 21879802. Epub 2011/09/02. English.

101. Halme L, Arola J, Höckerstedt K, Lautenschlager I. Human Herpesvirus 6 Infection of the Gastroduodenal Mucosa. Clinical Infectious Diseases. 2008 February 1, 2008;46(3):434-9.

102. Peigo MF, Thomasini RL, Puglia AL, Costa SC, Bonon SH, Boin IF, et al. Human Herpesvirus-7 in Brazilian Liver Transplant Recipients: A Follow-up Comparison between Molecular and Immunological Assays. Transpl Infect Dis. 2009 Dec;11(6):497-502. PubMed PMID: 19671120. Epub 2009/08/13. English.

103. Suga S, Yoshikawa T, Nagai T, Asano Y. Clinical Features and Virological Findings in Children with Primary Human Herpesvirus 7 Infection. Pediatrics. 1997 March 1, 1997;99(3):e4.

104. Cesarman E, Chang Y, Moore PS, Said JW, Knowles DM. Kaposi's Sarcoma-associated Herpesvirus-like DNA Sequences in AIDS-Related Body-Cavity-Based Lymphomas. New England Journal of Medicine. 1995;332(18):1186-91. PubMed PMID: 7700311.

105. Ariza-Heredia EJ, Razonable RR. Human Herpes Virus 8 in Solid Organ Transplantation. Transplantation. 2011 Oct 27;92(8):837-44. PubMed PMID: 21946171. Epub 2011/09/29. English.

106. Kato T, Dowdy L, Weppler D, Ruiz P, Thompson J, Raskin J, et al. Non-tuberculous Mycobacterial Associated Enterocolitis in Intestinal Transplantation. Transplantation Proceedings. 1998 Sep;30(6):2537–8. PubMed PMID: 9745476. English.

107. Delis SG, Tector J, Kato T, Mittal N, Weppler D, Levi D, et al. Diagnosis and Treatment of Cryptosporidium Infection in Intestinal Transplant Recipients. Transplantation Proceedings. 2002 May;34(3):951–2. PubMed PMID: 12034256.

108. Ningappa M, Higgs BW, Weeks DE, Ashokkumar C, Duerr RH, Sun Q, et al. NOD2 Gene Polymorphism rs2066844 Associates with Need for Combined Liver-Intestine Transplantation in Children with Short-gut Syndrome. American Journal of Gastroenterology. 2011 Jan;106(1):157–65. PubMed PMID: 20959815. English.

109. Sustento-Reodica N, Ruiz P, Rogers A, Viciana AL, Conn HO, Tzakis AG. Recurrent Crohn's Disease in Transplanted Bowel. [Erratum appears in Lancet 1997 Jul 26;350(9073):298]. Lancet. 1997 Mar 8;349(9053):688–91. PubMed PMID: 9078200. English.

110. Knight C, Murray KF. Hepatobiliary Associations with Inflammatory Bowel Disease. Expert rev. 2009 Dec;3(6):681–91. PubMed PMID: 19929587. English.

111. Chatzipetrou MA, Tzakis AG, Pinna AD, Kato T, Misiakos EP, Tsaroucha AK, et al. Intestinal Transplantation for the Treatment of Desmoid Tumors Associated with Familial Adenomatous Polyposis. Surgery. 2001 Mar;129(3):277–81. PubMed PMID: 11231455. English.

112. Moon JI, Selvaggi G, Nishida S, Levi DM, Kato T, Ruiz P, et al. Intestinal Transplantation for the Treatment of Neoplastic Disease. Journal of Surgical Oncology. 2005 Dec 15;92(4):284–91. PubMed PMID: 16299803. English.

113. Sarkar S, Selvaggi G, Mittal N, Cenk Acar B, Weppler D, Kato T, et al. Gastrointestinal Tract Ulcers in Pediatric Intestinal Transplantation Patients: Etiology and Management. Pediatric Transplantation. 2006 Mar;10(2):162–7. PubMed PMID: 16573601.

114. Turner D, Martin S, Ngan BY, Grant D, Sherman PM. Anastomotic Ulceration Following Small Bowel Transplantation. American Journal of Transplantation. 2006 Jan;6(1):236–40. PubMed PMID: 16433782. English.

115. Martland GT, Shepherd NA. Indeterminate Colitis: Definition, Diagnosis, Implications and a Plea for Nosological Sanity. Histopathology. 2007 Jan;50(1):83–96. PubMed PMID: 17204023. English.

116. Goldstein N, Dulai M. Contemporary Morphologic Definition of Backwash Ileitis in Ulcerative Colitis and Features that Distinguish It from Crohn Disease. American Journal of Clinical Pathology. 2006 Sep;126(3):365–76. PubMed PMID: 16880149. English.

117. Ningappa M, Higgs BW, Weeks DE, Ashokkumar C, Duerr RH, Sun Q, et al. NOD2 Gene Polymorphism rs2066844 Associates with Need for Combined Liver-Intestine Transplantation in Children with Short-gut Syndrome. The American Journal of Gastroenterology. 2010.

118. Fritz T, Niederreiter L, Adolph T, Blumberg RS, Kaser A. Crohn's Disease: NOD2, Autophagy and ER Stress Converge. Gut. 2011.

119. Janse M, Weersma RK, Sudan DL, Festen EAM, Wijmenga C, Dijkstra G, et al. Association of Crohn's Disease-associated NOD2 Variants with Intestinal Failure Requiring Small Bowel Transplantation and Clinical Outcomes. Gut. 2011 Jun;60(6):877–8; author reply 8–9. PubMed PMID: 20940282. English.

120. Rothenberg ME. Eosinophilic Gastrointestinal Disorders (EGID). The Journal of Allergy and Clinical Immunology. 2004 Jan;113(1):11–28; quiz 9. PubMed PMID: 14713902. Epub 2004/01/10. English.

121. Carmen Gonzalez-Vela M, Fernando Val-Bernal J, Francisca Garijo M, Garcia-Suarez C. Pyogenic Granuloma of the Sigmoid Colon. Ann Diagn Pathol. 2005 Apr;9(2):106–9. PubMed PMID: 15806519. Epub 2005/04/05. English.

122. Zhang Y, Ruiz P. Solid Organ Transplant-associated Acute Graft-versus-Host Disease. Arch Pathol Lab Med. 2010 Aug;134(8):1220–4. PubMed PMID: 20670147. Epub 2010/07/31. English.

123. Andres AM, Santamaria ML, Ramos E, Sarria J, Molina M, Hernandez F, et al. Graft-vs-Host Disease after Small Bowel Transplantation in Children. Journal of Pediatric Surgery. 2010;45(2):330–6. PubMed PMID: 20152346.

124. Triulzi DJ, Nalesnik MA. Microchimerism, GVHD, and Tolerance in Solid Organ Transplantation. Transfusion. 2001 Mar;41(3):419–26. PubMed PMID: 11274601.

125. Abu-Elmagd KM, Mazariegos G, Costa G, Soltys K, Bond G, Sindhi R, et al. Lymphoproliferative Disorders and de Novo Malignancies in Intestinal and Multivisceral Recipients: Improved Outcomes with New Outlooks. Transplantation. 2009 Oct 15;88(7):926–34. PubMed PMID: 19935465. English.

126. Pirenne J, Koshiba T, Geboes K, Emonds MP, Ferdinande P, Hiele M, et al. Complete Freedom from Rejection after Intestinal Transplantation Using a New Tolerogenic Protocol Combined with Low Immunosuppression. Transplantation. 2002 Mar 27;73(6):966–8. PubMed PMID: 11923701. English.

127. Ruiz P, Soares MF, Garcia M, Nicolas M, Kato T, Mittal N, et al. Lymphoplasmacytic Hyperplasia (Possibly Pre-PTLD) Has Varied Expression and Appearance in Intestinal Transplant Recipients Receiving Campath Immunosuppression. Transplantation Proceedings. 2004 Mar;36(2):386–7. PubMed PMID: 15050168.

128. Blaes AH, Morrison VA. Post-transplant Lymphoproliferative Disorders Following Solid-organ Transplantation. Expert Rev Hematol. 2010 Feb;3(1):35–44. PubMed PMID: 21082932. English.

129. Nourse JP, Jones K, Gandhi MK. Epstein-Barr Virus-related Post-transplant Lymphoproliferative Disorders: Pathogenetic Insights for Targeted Therapy. American Journal of Transplantation. 2011 May;11(5):888–95. PubMed PMID: 21521464. English.

130. Vardiman JW, Thiele J, Arber DA, Brunning RD, Borowitz MJ, Porwit A, et al. The 2008 Revision of the World Health Organization (WHO) Classification of Myeloid Neoplasms and Acute Leukemia: Rationale and Important Changes. Blood. 2009 July 30, 2009;114(5):937–51.

131. Parker A, Bowles K, Bradley JA, Emery V, Featherstone C, Gupte G,

et al. Diagnosis of Post-transplant Lymphoproliferative Disorder in Solid Organ Transplant Recipients – BCSH and BTS Guidelines. British Journal of Haematology. 2010 Jun;**149**(5):675–92. PubMed PMID: 20408847. English.

132 Berho M, Viciana A, Weppler D, Romero R, Tzakis A, Ruiz P. T Cell Lymphoma Involving the Graft of a Multivisceral Organ Recipient. Transplantation. 1999 Oct 27;**68**(8):1135–9. PubMed PMID: 10551642. English.

133 Sivaraman P, Lye WC. Epstein-Barr Virus-associated T-cell Lymphoma in Solid Organ Transplant Recipients. Biomedicine & Pharmacotherapy. 2001 Sep;**55**(7):366–8. PubMed PMID: 11669498. English.

Chapter 7

Pancreas and Islet Transplantation Pathology

Cinthia B. Drachenberg, and John C. Papadimitriou

List of Abbreviations
DM = diabetes mellitus, SPK = simultaneous kidney transplant, PTA = pancreas transplant alone, PAK = pancreas after kidney transplant, AMR = antibody-mediated allograft rejection, CMR = T cell-mediated allograft rejection, ACMR = acute T cell-mediated rejection, DSA = donor-specific antibody, IAC = interacinar capillaries, PTLD = post-transplant lymphoproliferative disorder, IAPP = islet amyloid polypeptide

I Introduction

Diabetes mellitus (DM), characterized by hyperglycemia, is the result of insufficient or defective insulin secretion and/or insulin activity. Although DM can result from multiple causes, the vast majority of patients can be classified in two types: DM type 1, typically resulting from immune-mediated destruction of the insulin-producing β cells, and DM type 2, which is more common and results from resistance to insulin action compounded with an inadequate compensatory insulin secretory response [1]. Over time, patients with DM develop extensive microvascular pathology leading to renal failure, retinopathy, systemic neuropathy, etc. These chronic complications are not only associated with a marked increase in morbidity and mortality, but also have significant impact on the patients' overall quality of life. In addition, patients with DM, particularly type 1, may have life-threatening acute complications such as diabetic ketoacidosis and severe hypoglycemia [1].

Treatment for DM type 1 consists of frequent, self-adjusted insulin administration (intensive insulin therapy). This type of treatment requires rigorous monitoring of blood glucose and interval testing of HbA1c. Despite significant improvement in glucose delivery systems, exogenous insulin therapy does not achieve complete normalization of HbA1c in many cases, and although the risk of secondary complications is decreased, it is not eliminated. In addition, insulin therapy carries a significant risk for hypoglycemia [2].

Given the limitations of intensive insulin therapy, there is a need for the development of other therapeutic options for DM, such as pancreas or islet transplantation. Although the slow advancement in the optimization of these treatments has precluded their widespread use, successful pancreas and islet transplantation are the only options that can currently provide complete normalization of the glucose metabolism [3–6]. As of 2010, more than 30,000 pancreas transplants were reported to the International Pancreas Transplant Registry and approximately 2,000 islet transplants have been performed worldwide [7, 8].

The majority of the topics covered in this chapter will refer to whole pancreas transplantation and only the last section will discuss the pathological aspects of islet transplantation.

Indications for Whole Pancreas Transplantation – Beta Cell Replacement Therapy

The surgical and immunosuppression-related risks of pancreas and islet transplantation are considered justified in insulin dependent diabetic patients with episodic hypoglycemic unawareness, or if there is rapid progression of the secondary diabetic complications. Marked improvement in the quality of life is reported by most patients with a functioning transplant [9].

The vast majority of whole pancreas transplants are done in patients with DM type 1, in whom a successful procedure results in normalization of the glucose metabolism and disappearance of the acute complications of the disease. Pancreas transplantation also results in prevention, stabilization, and in some cases, reversal of some of the long-term renal and neural complications of diabetes [3–6, 10, 11]. Pancreas transplantation is also indicated in a minority of patients with insulin-dependent DM type 2, this category representing only 5%–6% of patients undergoing pancreas transplantation [7, 12].

There are *three pancreas transplant types*, depending on the patient's kidney function. In patients with uremia/end-stage renal disease, a simultaneous pancreas-kidney (SPK) transplant is the treatment of choice, or alternatively the pancreas can be transplanted after a successful (previous) kidney transplant (pancreas after kidney, PAK). In contrast, a pancreas transplant alone (PTA) is used in non-uremic diabetic patients [13, 14]. A small fraction of pancreas transplants (approximately 4%) are not related to DM and are done in the context of multivisceral transplantation (i.e. with liver, intestine, and/or kidney transplants) [7].

In addition, pancreas transplantation is very rarely indicated in patients that have undergone surgical resection of the native pancreas (e.g. for a benign tumor) or if there is advanced chronic pancreatitis leading to exocrine as well as endocrine pancreas deficiency. In patients with pancreatectomy for benign disease, pancreas or islet autotransplantation should be considered before allotransplantation in order to avoid the need for immunosuppression [15].

Results of pancreas transplantation have continuously improved since the late '80s, with reported one-year graft survival rates of 85% for SPK, 78% for PAK, and 77% for PTA. Patient survival is excellent, in the order of 95%–96% at one year in all pancreas transplant types [16]. The improved graft outcomes are attributed to decreases in the technical and immunological failure rates, newer immunosuppressants, better diagnosis of rejection, and improved treatment of infections. In recent years, the risk of graft loss to acute rejection in technically successful transplants has decreased to 2%, 8%, and 10% at one year for SPK, PAK, and PTA cases, respectively. The most dramatic improvements have been achieved in the category of PTA. It is in this category where pancreas biopsies play the most decisive role for diagnosis of rejection [16–19].

The slower progress made with pancreas transplantation in comparison to other organ transplants is to a large extent related to the more challenging technical problems inherent to the organ itself. Difficulties related to high propensity to vascular thrombosis in the pancreas, issues with management of the pancreatic exocrine secretions, and manner of venous drainage have required constant technical improvements [20, 21].

Brief History of Pancreas Transplantation/Surgical Techniques

The first pancreas transplant was done in 1966 at the University of Minnesota, simultaneously with a kidney transplant (SPK) [22]. The pancreas exocrine secretions were managed by duct ligation, based on animal studies indicating that this would result in diffuse atrophy of the exocrine parenchyma allowing for the preservation of a vascularized endocrine component. The post-operative course, however, was complicated by a pancreatic fistula formation and pancreatitis. The patient was insulin-free for six days, but died a week later due to a pulmonary embolism [22]. After this initial experience, a dozen pancreas transplantations were done in the following years at the University of Minnesota with the exocrine secretions managed by cutaneous-graft duodenostomy (n=4) and enteric drainage (n=8) [23]. Venous drainage was most commonly directed through the iliac veins (systemic drainage). In the 1970s and 1980s, a variety of surgical techniques were tried by different centers, including enteric drainage, ureteral drainage, open duct drainage, and duct injection with synthetic polymers, but results were in general poor, resulting from both acute rejection and technical complications. Segmental pancreas transplantation was preferred over whole organ transplantation, initially [21].

By the early 1980s, only 105 pancreas transplants had been performed worldwide with equivalent proportions done in the United States and Europe. In 1983, a new technique was developed at the University of Wisconsin, based on the use of whole pancreas transplants and drainage of the exocrine secretions to the urinary bladder [24] (see Figure 7.1). Bladder drained pancreas transplants attained general acceptance in the 1990s and this technique was used in >80%–90% of cases. Significant complications such as hematuria, urine leaks, recurrent urinary tract infections, urethritis, and reflux pancreatitis were present in up to 25% of patients, eventually requiring conversion to enteric drainage. Although now used in a minority of centers, bladder drainage (pancreaticoduodenocystostomy

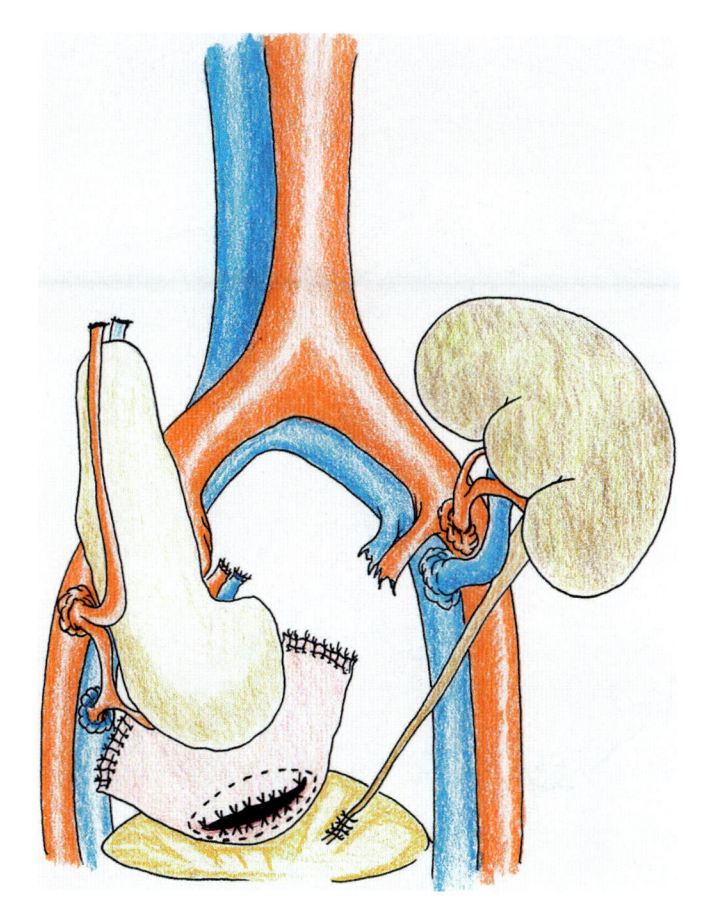

Figure 7.1 Schematic representation of pancreas and kidney transplants. The pancreatic exocrine secretions are drained in the urinary bladder and its venous drainage is systemic (iliac veins).

technique) has the advantage of allowing for the diagnostic use of the decrease in urinary amylase for the detection of acute rejection (see clinical diagnosis of rejection below). In the 1990s, marked decrease in the rates of immunologically-based graft losses were reported, related to the availability of more potent immunosuppressive drugs leading to further improvement in graft outcomes. Also, further refinements of the surgical techniques resulted in a return to enteric drainage as the preferred choice to avoid the common complications seen with bladder drainage (see Figure 7.2). Currently, enteric drainage is the most commonly used method to treat the exocrine secretions in SPK patients in whom elevations in creatinine is commonly used as a surrogate marker of pancreas rejection. Bladder drainage is still preferred by some for patients with solitary pancreas transplants, in order to take advantage of the diagnostic use of urinary amylase. In enteric drained transplants, venous drainage is preferably done into the portal vein (rather than in the iliac veins) to more closely resemble the physiological status [20] (see Figure 7.2).

II Diagnosis of Acute Allograft Rejection

Clinical Diagnosis of Acute Allograft Rejection

Symptoms are unusual in acute pancreas rejection; the clinical diagnosis, therefore, relies heavily on laboratory methods

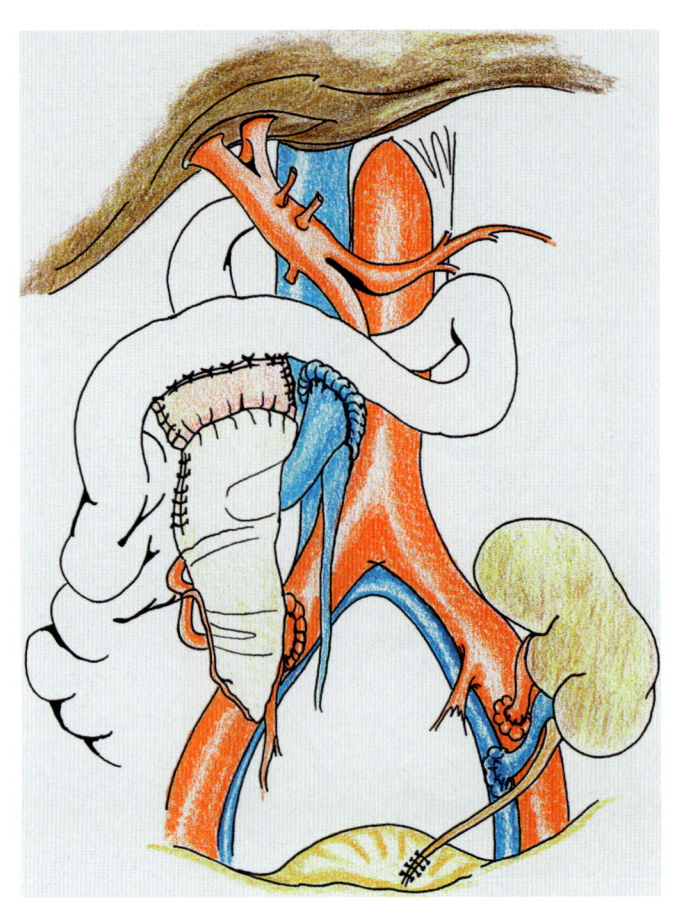

Figure 7.2 Schematic representation of pancreas and kidney transplants. The pancreatic exocrine secretions are drained into a loop of the small intestine (enteric drainage) and the venous drainage is to the portal system (portal venous drainage).

indicating abnormalities in the exocrine secretions (i.e. amylase, lipase) and/or the endocrine function (e.g., blood glucose). In pancreas transplants with exocrine drainage into the urinary bladder, serial measurements of amylasuria are useful for monitoring of acute rejection, if there is a decrease of >25% or >50% from the baseline [24–27]. Decrease in urine amylase, however, is not specific, and can be seen also in acute pancreatitis, graft thrombosis, duct obstruction, etc. When correlated with biopsy findings, decrease in urinary amylase had a specificity of 30% and a positive predictive value of 53% [28, 29].

Increase in amylase and lipase in serum are general markers of acinar cell injury and are useful for monitoring pancreas patients independently of the exocrine drainage technique [25–32]. Serum amylase and lipase typically increase in acute rejection, but also do so in acute pancreatitis and other inflammatory processes involving both the native and the transplanted pancreas. In acute rejection, a very pronounced increase in serum amylase and lipase is more characteristically associated with severe rejection; however, there is significant variability from patient to patient and the overall level of the pancreatic enzymes does not show good correlation with the lower rejection grades [32].

In contrast to abnormalities of the exocrine parameters (amylase and lipase) that are usually present in most forms of acute rejection, endocrine abnormalities such as hyperglycemia are relatively rare, occurring more often in severe or irreversible acute rejection typically associated with extensive parenchymal necrosis [32, 33]. In addition to severe rejection, hyperglycemia can be caused by other processes (i.e. recurrence of autoimmune disease, islet cell drug toxicity, and chronic rejection) [34, 35].

Development of chronic rejection/graft sclerosis leads to progressive impairment of glucose homeostasis that is usually accompanied by a gradual decrease in the levels of amylase and lipase in urine and/or serum [36, 37].

In patients with SPK transplants, monitoring of the renal function by serial serum creatinine levels is often used as a surrogate for rejection in both organs. Although this method is widely used in clinical practice, its absolute diagnostic value is questionable, since isolated rejection of one of these organs is not uncommon and may occur in up to 30% of cases [38].

Acute rejection presents earlier and is more common in PTA recipients [38, 39]. Similarly, graft loss from irreversible rejection occurred more frequently with PTA than with the other transplant types (9%, 15%, and 30% versus 2%, 3%, and 7% at one, two, and five years, respectively, in SPK) [17]. The availability of the percutaneous pancreas biopsy technique in these recipients, in whom the renal function is not available as a "sentinel," has significantly improved the outcomes in PTA [18, 38, 40]. Although overall outcomes continue to improve, *graft failure at five years* remains 40%–50% for PTA and PAK, in part due to difficulties in a timely diagnosis of rejection. The latter is of paramount importance to prevent subsequent development of graft sclerosis [41]. Repeated episodes of acute rejection, and particularly late acute rejection, significantly increase the risk for graft loss due to chronic rejection [37, 42–48]

Histological Diagnosis of Acute Rejection

Overall, the clinical markers of acute pancreas rejection have been shown to correlate with biopsy proven acute allograft rejection in approximately 80% of instances [40].

Due to the nonspecific nature of the laboratory tests, *needle core biopsies* are considered the gold standard for diagnosis of rejection [30–32, 38, 49–57].

III Pancreas Allograft Biopsies

The *percutaneous needle biopsy* technique was described by Allen et al. in the early 1990s [30]. Needle core biopsies are usually done under ultrasound or computer tomographic guidance, with 18 or 20 gauge needles [58–60]. Adequate tissue can be obtained in 85–90% of instances [40, 53, 56, 58, 60–63]. Significant complications have been reported in 2%–3% of cases (i.e. bleeding), none leading to graft loss [58, 60].

In patients with intestinal drainage, bowel loops are often interposed between the abdominal wall and the graft, interfering in the performance of percutaneous needle biopsies. This problem is circumvented with the use of the *laparoscopic biopsy* technique as an alternative to the percutaneous biopsy [64, 65].

Open (surgical wedge) biopsies are only done in selected cases when all the other methods fail to provide tissue adequate for diagnosis [55]. In patients with late development of hyperglycemia in whom the differential diagnosis includes recurrence of autoimmune Type 1 DM, performance of wedge biopsies is recommended [66–68].

In patients with bladder drainage, *cystoscopic transduodenal pancreas biopsies* can provide clinically useful information in the same manner as percutaneous core biopsies, but adequate pancreatic tissue is only obtained in 57%–80% of cases [69–75]. In comparison to the percutaneous biopsy technique, cystoscopic biopsies are considered more invasive and more costly [55]. Features of acute rejection can be recognized sometimes in samples containing only duodenal tissue, but in the absence of substantial comparative studies, it is unclear if a negative duodenal biopsy can rule out pancreas rejection [72, 73]. More recently, it has been proposed that duodenal samples obtained through upper gastrointestinal endoscopy from enteric drained pancreas allografts anastomosed to the proximal jejunum can be used to monitor the grafted pancreas. With this technique (*enteroscopic duodenal cuff biopsies*), Margreiter et al. [76] obtained diagnostic material in 75% of cases and identified pathological changes in a third of them. When the procedure was performed in patients with pancreas dysfunction, the duodenal sample demonstrated features consistent with rejection in 65% of cases [76].

Needle Core Biopsy Adequacy

Although the adequacy of any particular biopsy sample is ultimately determined by the examining pathologist, it is recommended that pancreas graft biopsies contain at least three lobular areas and their associated interlobular septa (see Figure 7.3). The latter typically contain veins and branches of the pancreatic duct. Arterial branches that follow separate courses, irregularly embedded in the parenchyma, are sampled with more difficulty. Due to the diagnostic importance ascribed to the arterial lesions, it is recommended that absence of arterial branches be specifically stated in the pathology report [77].

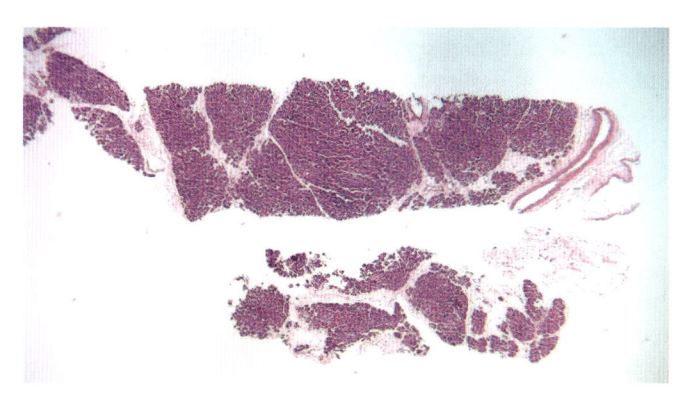

Figure 7.3 Low power view of a needle core biopsy of the pancreas. The lobular tissue is separated by fibrous septa containing vessels and ducts, but no inflammation. The acinar lobules are compact without evidence of acinar loss. The periphery of the lobules is more or less regular (i.e., there is no significant fragmentation of the lobules in the interface with the connective tissue).

Guidelines for Processing Pancreas Allograft Biopsies

For best diagnostic yield, it is recommended that at least two hematoxylin and eosin stained sections are examined from two different levels of the core. Five to ten adjacent/intervening unstained sections should be available in order to perform additional stains as needed (i.e., CMV stain).

It is recommended that C4d immunostain be performed in all biopsies. This stain is particularly indicated in the absence of other findings if the biopsy is performed for hyperglycemia, in patients with increased risk of humoral rejection (i.e., re-transplantation) and if there is margination of neutrophils or other inflammatory cells in the interacinar capillaries [78, 79].

Masson's trichrome stain can aid in the identification of specific structures or pathological changes (i.e., arterial walls, fibrinoid necrosis) and is also indicated in biopsies with suspected chronic rejection to demonstrate incipient interacinar fibrosis [77, 80].

In patients biopsied due to hyperglycemia, it is essential to perform stains for insulin and glucagon to identify selective loss of beta cells indicating recurrence of autoimmune disease [81].

Congo red stain should be performed to identify islet amyloid deposition if any amount of eosinophilic extracellular material is identified within the endocrine islets [82].

Correlation between Pancreas and Kidney Rejection in SPK

Animal studies have shown that acute rejections in kidney and pancreas grafts often occur together (synchronously) [83–86]. Interestingly, even in synchronous rejection, the histological grade or severity of rejection may be discordant between the two organs [83, 87].

In clinical practice, it is also assumed that SPK transplants are usually rejected synchronously, or at least in "tandem" with the kidney rejection preceding the pancreas rejection [85, 88]. Despite the general acceptance of this generalization, the occurrence of asynchronous rejection has been amply documented in SPK recipients [38, 89]. In a large study, based on concurrent biopsies of both organs, the pancreas and kidney showed synchronous rejection in 65% of episodes, with the pancreas and kidney being selectively involved in 22% and 13% of instances respectively. The possibility of isolated rejection in one of the organs in more than a third of cases underscores the need for considering selective renal or pancreatic biopsy evaluation even in patients with SPK [38, 40].

Protocol Biopsies

Few studies are available describing the histological findings in protocol biopsies. Protocol biopsies are defined as biopsies performed at specified time points, regardless of the graft function. In the prospective study of Stratta et al. [90] done in the cyclosporine era, mild rejection was identified in more than half of the patients (54%) in the first months post-transplantation. Despite treatment with steroids, 60% of these patients went on to develop recurrent biopsy-proven rejection within two months. The authors concluded that patients with rejection should have undergone standard treatment with antilymphocytic antibodies to prevent subsequent episodes of rejection and that protocol biopsies were essential for the identification of patients at risk of acute rejection [90].

In a recent study, Rogers et al. found acute rejection in 50% of protocol PTA biopsies done in the first and second months post-transplantation. Aggressive treatment of rejection in their cohort of PTA recipients significantly improved outcomes, comparable to results in the SPK transplants done at the same period [91].

A study of 30 patients with normal graft function biopsied at a mean of 15.4 months at the time of laparotomy for reasons unrelated to the pancreas graft showed that there was no evidence of rejection in most cases (83%). Of the five patients with histological – albeit subclinical – evidence of mild rejection, four subsequently developed accelerated chronic rejection and lost their grafts between 14 and 20 months post-transplantation [92].

A retrospective study evaluating protocol biopsies with BANFF grade indeterminate (old grade II, minimal rejection) concluded that these rarely progress to more severe degrees of inflammation [52].

IV Acute Allograft Rejection

Immunological Aspects

The mechanisms of acute allograft rejection in the pancreas are not different from those in other solid transplants, although the dual nature of the pancreas (i.e., exocrine and endocrine) justifies some special considerations. In the early post-transplantation period, most histopathological manifestations were related to the surgical trauma that invariably leads to some degree of pancreatitis (infiltration by neutrophils and macrophages with variable degrees of cell necrosis) [93–96]. Soon after implantation, the events related to antigen presentation are started, followed by T cell activation, generation of a large array of cytokines, and the capability for cell-mediated or humoral rejection.

Graft rejection depends highly on the degree of incompatibility between recipient and donor major histocompatibility complex (MHC) antigens [83]. MHC class I and II molecules are differentially expressed in exocrine and endocrine pancreatic tissues. Variations are also noted between a normal pancreas and a pancreas that is being rejected. In the normal pancreas, class I antigens are expressed weakly on islet cells and strongly on the ductal epithelium. In contrast, the normal acinar cells are negative for class I molecules [97]. Under normal circumstances, expression of class II antigens has not been demonstrated in any cell compartment [97]. In contrast, experimental studies have shown that in acute rejection the acinar cells overexpress class I and class II antigens. The latter are also expressed in ductal epithelium and endothelial cells, whereas class I antigens are expressed on the β cells [98, 99].

MHC disparities, specifically class II alloantibodies, have also been associated with an increased risk of humoral rejection and graft loss [100].

Although overlaps in the mechanisms of acute rejection do exist, the morphological findings are generally classified as "cell-mediated" or "antibody-mediated" [39, 101]. Morphologically, these categories are characterized by tissue infiltration by the effector inflammatory cells and by antibody/complement deposition in the vascular walls, respectively. In each of these pathways, the graft injury results from both antigen-specific immune damage and other nonspecific factors [39, 101].

The main effectors in cell-mediated rejection are T lymphocytes, monocytes, and eosinophils. Cytotoxic T lymphocytes (CTLs) lyse the target cell through specific antigen recognition pathways. CTLs release lytic molecules that cause among other effects, complement-like osmotic cell injury of the target cell (i.e., perforins, granzyme A and B, granulysin). Also, induction of apoptosis occurs through the former mechanism or when the CTL's Fas transmembrane glycoprotein binds to the Fas-ligand on the target cell. In contrast to CTLs, natural killer cells can lyse target cells independently of a specific antigen interaction. Well-developed, uncontrolled acute cell-mediated rejection is characterized by extensive inflammatory cell graft infiltration that invariably results in rapid or occasionally more protracted graft destruction [39, 102].

In antibody-mediated rejection, deposition of antibodies in the vascular walls is causative of direct injury by activation of the complement cascade and also through antibody dependent cell-mediated toxicity (ADCC) [100, 103]. Therefore, vascular injury and necrosis, development of thrombosis, and secondary ischemic parenchymal necrosis are characteristic of the more severe forms of antibody-mediated rejection (i.e., hyperacute rejection) [39, 101, 103]. Although initially thought to be only associated with immediate effects, more protracted forms of antibody-mediated rejection (acute versus hyperacute and chronic-active) are now being recognized [99, 104, 105]. Neutrophils are recruited in abundance in antibody-mediated rejection through the release of complement-derived chemokines. Neutrophils can be present also in the more severe forms of cell-mediated rejection, as well as in most forms of significant parenchymal injury [39, 101].

Different rejection patterns for the exocrine and endocrine components of the pancreas likely reflect variations of MHC expression, as well as other factors such as type and quality of the microvasculature, sensitivity to ischemia, etc. Experience with animal and clinical studies has shown that the acinar lobules are the primary target of T cell-mediated rejection, with less common involvement of the arterial walls. Acinar damage/drop-out and chronic vascular injury both lead to a fibrogenic reaction that represents the main feature of chronic rejection [106]. The islets are not directly affected in T cell-mediated acute rejection [31, 49, 83, 84, 86, 107–109]; however, the impact of AMR in pancreatic islets remains unclear. Whereas hyperglycemia was documented in early reports of AMR [79], this was a rare indication for biopsy in subsequent larger studies [110–113]. C4d staining in islet capillary endothelium was found in a fifth of samples from patients with DSA, but this did not correlate with hyperglycemia [113].

Morphological Features of Acute Allograft Rejection

Both in small and larger animal models, acute rejection is manifested with inflammatory infiltrates in the interstitium, consistent involvement of small veins, and variable more heterogeneous involvement of ducts [49, 106, 107, 114]. Acinar inflammation and acinar cell damage including apoptosis are also found to be characteristic of acute rejection [49, 84, 106, 115, 116]. The severe, more advanced forms of acute rejection display intimal arteritis, necrotizing vasculitis, thrombosis, and eventual parenchymal necrosis [106, 107]. Although islets are not the primary target in T cell-mediated rejection, extensive parenchymal necrosis is associated with secondary islet involvement and hyperglycemia [49, 84, 106, 107, 117].

With respect to clinical experience, examination of the first series of explanted pancreas allografts provided a glimpse of the spectrum of pathological changes that can be seen in these organs. Two weeks after implantation, the first pancreas allograft showed significant architectural disarray and fibrosis, likely secondary to the ligation of the pancreatic duct. In addition, there was a moderate amount of mononuclear cells in the interlobular septa and focally in the acini, consistent with acute T cell-mediated rejection. The islets were normal [22]. The dozens of cases done subsequently demonstrated that in contrast to cases with duct ligation, unrestricted drainage of the exocrine secretions allowed for maintenance of the exocrine pancreatic structure. From the experience with cases drained externally (cutaneous graft duodenostomy), it was concluded that inflammation of the exposed segment of the graft duodenum correlated with pancreas rejection [23].

In the following decades, seminal studies involving sequential and random samples consistently demonstrated similar histological findings as those seen in animal models [51, 118] (see Figures 7.4–7.10). The negative impact of intimal and transmural arteritis for the outcome of the graft was widely

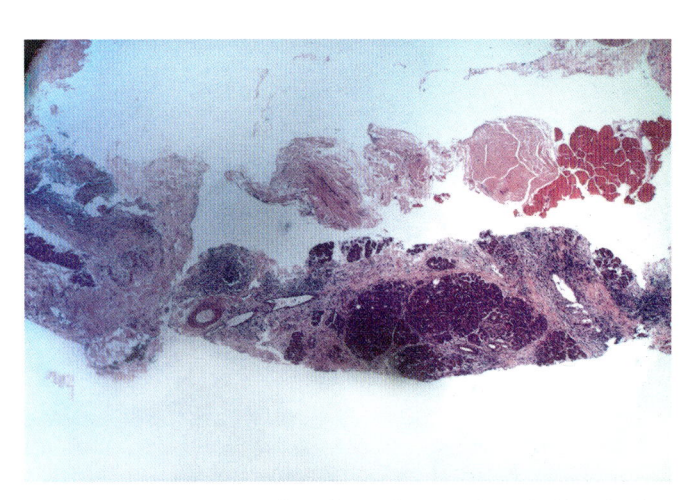

Figure 7.4 Low power view of needle core biopsy with marked lymphoid infiltrates in expanded septal areas. Severe episodes of acute rejection or undertreated T cell-mediated rejection results in progressive fibrosis. Note the fragmentation of the acinar contours that typically occurs in association with progression of the septal fibrosis.

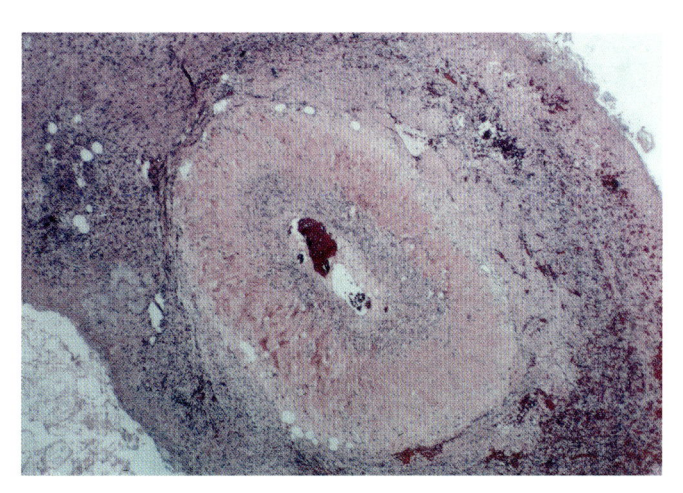

Figure 7.5A Cross section of thickened artery with active transplant arteriopathy characterized by intimal fibrosis with infiltrating mononuclear cells in the fibrotic area.

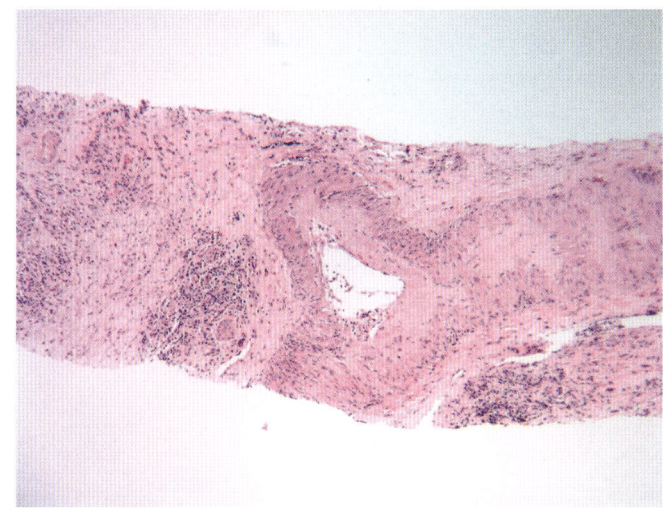

Figure 7.5B Focus of intimal arteritis and focal, sparse inflammation of subendothelial areas of fibrosis in an artery with significant fibrous narrowing. The septal areas are markedly expanded due to fibrosis with only rare remaining acini present (left of center).

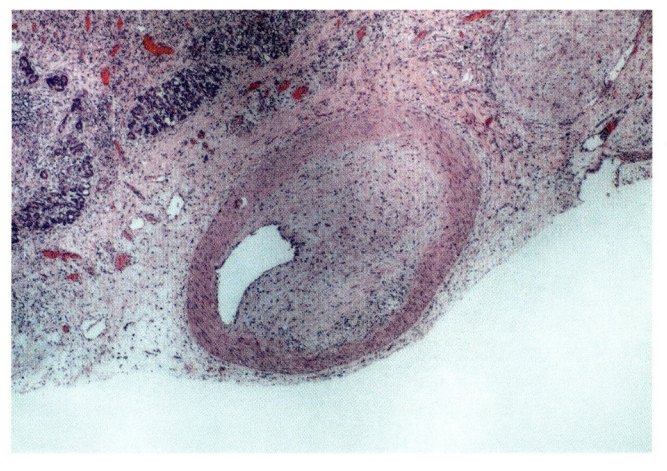

Figure 7.5C Asymmetric narrowing of artery with marked luminal narrowing and features of active transplant arteriopathy, characterized by infiltrating mononuclear cells in the fibrotic areas.

Pancreas and Islet Transplantation Pathology

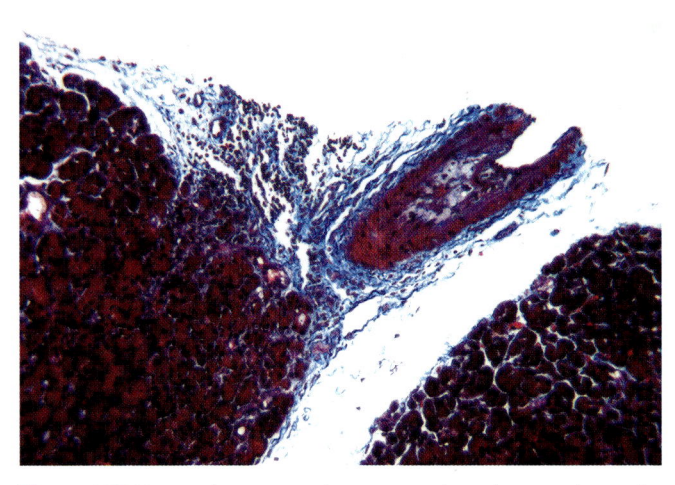

Figure 7.5D Variant of active transplant arteriopathy with accumulation of subendothelial foam cells and formation of neo-intima.

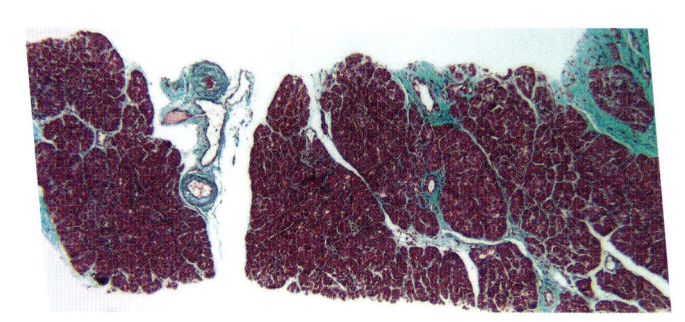

Figure 7.6A Medium power view of a needle core biopsy from a patient with a well-functioning graft 52 months post-transplantation. Note absence of inflammation or significant fibrosis, although two arterioles show circumferential hyalinosis likely related to calcineurin inhibitor toxicity.

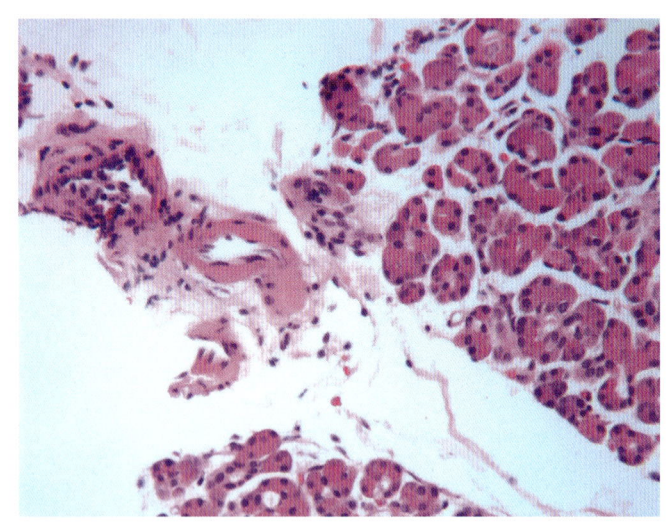

Figure 7.6B Well-functioning graft with arteriolar hyalinosis. There is no significant inflammation. Based on findings in adjacent sections, the structure to the left is a tangentially cut vessel without inflammation.

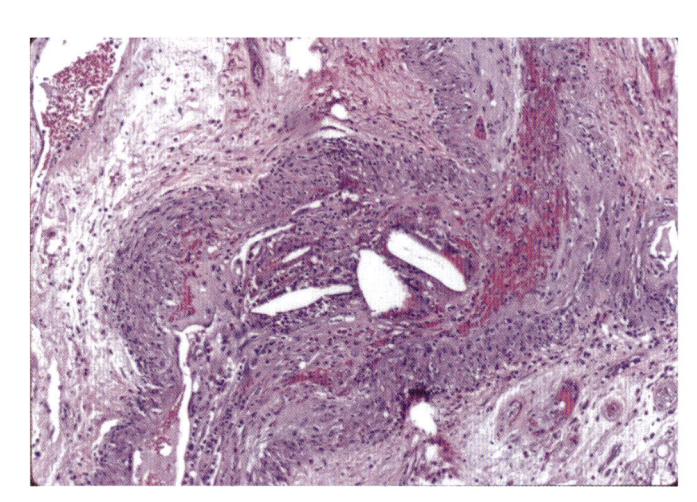

Figure 7.7 Artery occluded by atheroembolus found in pancreas biopsy from a patient with acute increase in serum amylase and lipase. There was no evidence of acute rejection.

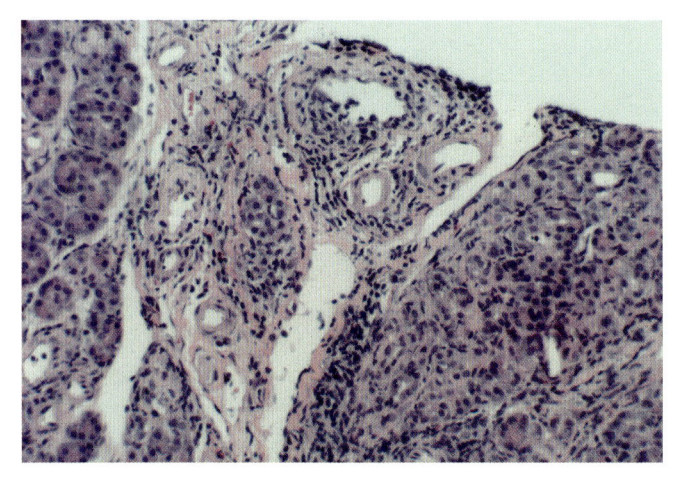

Figure 7.8A Acute T cell-mediated allograft rejection. This connective tissue septa contains active inflammation with involvement of a vein (venulitis) and a small duct. The inflammation extends to the adjacent lobule to the right.

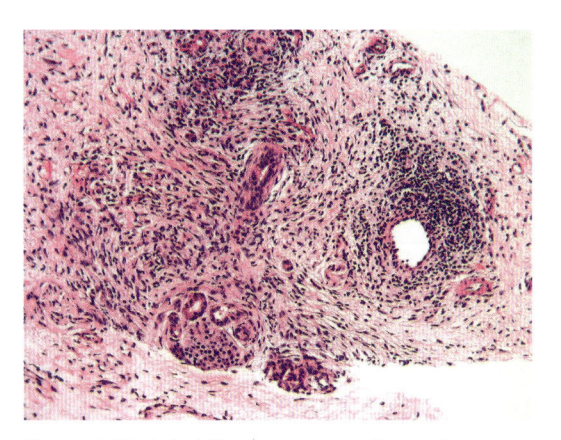

Figure 7.8B Marked fibrous expansion of a septal area in a patient with three previous episodes of biopsy proven and treated acute T cell-mediated rejection. There is marked mononuclear inflammation cuffing a vein, but without definite venulitis (right). On the top left, residual atrophic acinar tissue shows persistent lymphocytic inflammation suggesting ongoing T cell-mediated rejection. An islet in the bottom center is normal.

Pancreas and Islet Transplantation Pathology

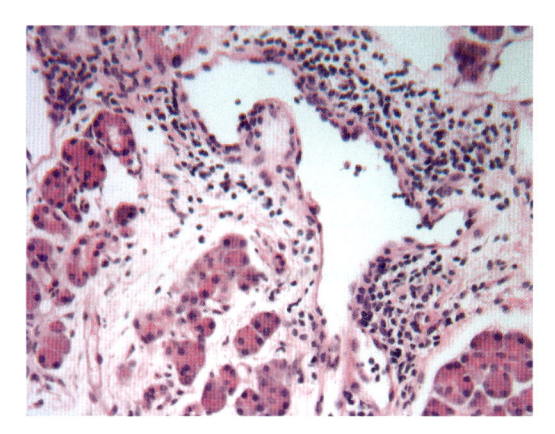

Figure 7.8C Mononuclear cuffing of a vein with questionable subendothelial lifting and endothelial cell damage. In the complete absence of any other findings, this biopsy could be classified as indetermined for acute rejection.

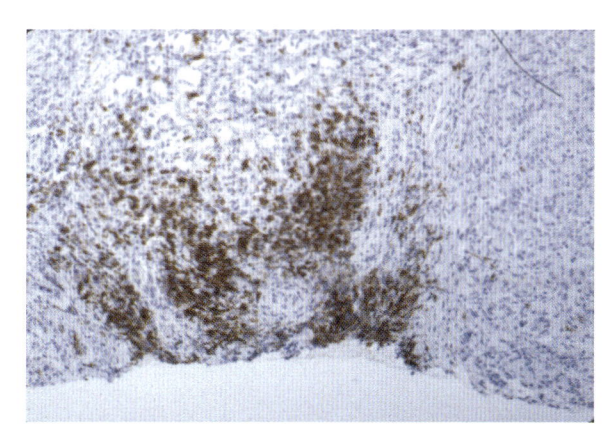

Figure 7.8D CD3 stain in a patient with acute cell-mediated allograft rejection demonstrates that the vast majority of the septal infiltrates consist of T lymphocytes. This is in contrast with cases of EBV-related PTLD.

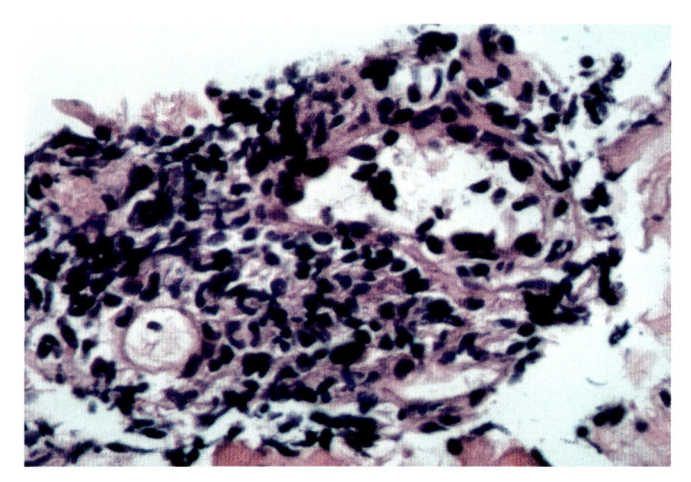

Figure 7.9A Venulitis. High power view of vein cuffed by activated (blastic) lymphocytes. Note endothelial cell damage: lifting of the endothelial lining and sloughing. Nuclear enlargement indicates endothelial cell activation.

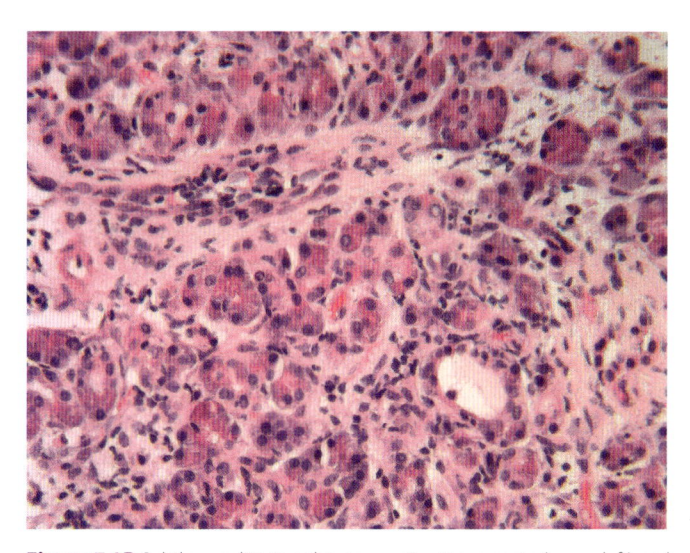

Figure 7.9B Subtle venulitis in a thin connective tissue septa (upper left) and incipient inflammation of a small duct (lower right). Note relatively sparse acinar inflammation in the slightly edematous connective tissue (left corner) and in the acini located above the small duct (right center).

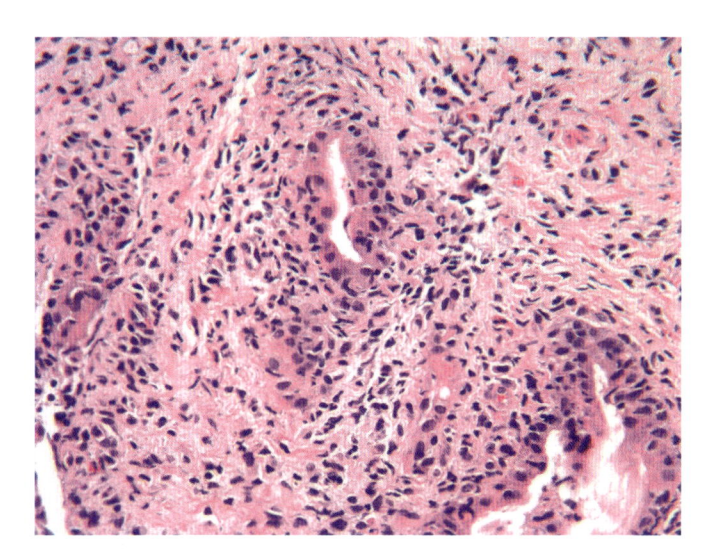

Figure 7.10 Inflamed septal area with pronounced ductitis, defined as permeation of the ductal epithelium by the inflammatory cells. There is also evidence of epithelial damage (loss of polarity, eosinophilic change in the cytoplasm, anisonucleosis).

recognized and accordingly, arterial involvement was used as a marker of severe rejection in the grading schema proposed by Nakhleh and Sutherland, based on a comparison of histological material from failed and functioning allografts [119]. In the 1990s, routine availability of needle core biopsies allowed for the recognition of the full spectrum of pathological changes in biopsies from well-functioning and rejecting allografts [30, 38, 44, 63, 72, 75, 90, 120, 121]. Based on the previous available studies and a systematic comparison of the histological changes in protocol and indication biopsies, a schema for grading acute rejection was developed at the University of Maryland which comprised six grades (0-V) [33]. The latter schema emphasized progressive changes ranging from lack of inflammation (Grade 0), to isolated involvement of fibrous septa (Grade I) and septal structures (Grade II), to acinar (Grade III) and arterial involvement (Grade IV). Parenchymal necrosis defined the most severe form of rejection (Grade V). The Maryland grading schema had overall a good correlation with ultimate graft outcomes and response to treatment [122], but long-term outcomes and response to antirejection treatment between Grades II and III were remarkably similar, likely reflecting grafts with milder forms of acute rejection in contrast to the higher grades (IV and V) [32]. In more recent years, a multidisciplinary group has worked in the development of a BANFF grading schema for pancreas allografts following the successful model used for other solid organ transplants (Table 7.1). This working grading schema will provide the framework for most histopathological considerations in this chapter [77, 99].

V Chronic Allograft Rejection/Graft Sclerosis

Pathogenetic Aspects

In the first months of post-transplantation, graft losses are more often related to surgical complications, idiopathic thrombosis, acute rejection, and peripancreatic infections [17, 36, 37, 123], but after the first year, chronic rejection – with or without superimposed acute rejection – accounts for the majority of graft losses [37]. Acute allograft rejection usually presents with sudden graft dysfunction that can be successfully treated in most instances, particularly in the case of T cell-mediated rejection. In contrast, chronic rejection is characterized by a slow, progressive decline in graft function and does not respond well to treatment [123].

Clear association has been found between acute rejection and chronic rejection in pancreas allografts recipients. Repeated, higher grade, and late (>1 year) episodes of acute rejection are all associated with an increased risk of chronic rejection and graft loss. In many cases, progressive fibrosis and acinar loss are observed over a prolonged period of time in serial biopsies [80, 124].

It is unclear if, in the pancreas, similar mechanisms operate for the propagation of tissue damage once a critical amount of parenchymal mass is lost, as is the case in the kidney. It is conceivable that in addition to the immune-mediated acinar cell and vascular injury, other factors play a role in the pathogenesis of graft sclerosis. The main histological findings in chronic rejection (septal fibrosis, acinar loss) are very similar to those of chronic pancreatitis in native organs. In native pancreas fibrosis, microcirculatory disturbances have been heavily implicated [96, 125]. These appear to play a very important role also in chronic allograft rejection/sclerosis [126]. Microvascular injury, inflammation, and obliteration are directly linked to progression to graft sclerosis in antibody-mediated allograft rejection (AMR) [113, 127].

As is the case with other organ transplants, pancreas allograft fibrosis most likely represents the end effect of cumulative injury (or injuries) of diverse immunological and non-immunological origins. Accordingly, the presence of graft sclerosis is not synonymous of chronic rejection, particularly in patients in whom a clear history of preceding episodes of acute rejection cannot be elicited. The use of the more encompassing term *chronic pancreas allograft rejection/graft sclerosis* is therefore recommended [37].

Clinical Diagnosis of Chronic Rejection/Graft Sclerosis

The clinical presentation of chronic rejection/graft sclerosis is nonspecific, with loss of glycemic control being the main clinical feature. Hyperglycemia may develop progressively or may be unmasked by infection or other physiologic stresses [123]. In addition, the exocrine tissue markers (e.g., blood or urinary amylase) progressively decrease and eventually disappear when extensive fibrosis develops in the graft [123]. In the context of chronic rejection, development of hyperglycemia indicates that the mass of functioning beta cells is significantly decreased and it heralds a short graft life [80, 123]. In general, there is no clinical marker for the monitoring of progressive loss of pancreas functional reserve, comparable to the serial measurements of serum creatinine or glomerular filtration rate in kidney transplantation, but progressive decline in C-peptide levels correlates with loss of functional beta cell mass [123].

Pancreas graft sclerosis can be suspected on imaging studies (ultrasound, MRI, CT), which typically show decrease in graft size, or there may be evidence of decreased parenchymal perfusion [128, 129].

In the early post-transplantation period, severe peripancreatic infections with abscess formation may lead to the observation of septal fibrosis resembling chronic rejection/graft sclerosis in biopsies obtained from the periphery of the graft. In those cases, the deeper parenchymal areas are not affected and resolution of the infection may allow for a normal graft life span [130].

Morphological Features of Chronic Rejection/Graft Sclerosis

Similar to animal models and to the experience with other organs, in the pancreas, chronic rejection is manifested histologically with progressive fibrosis arising from expansion of the fibrous septa leading to large areas of fibrosis intervening between atrophic acinar lobules (see Figure 7.4). With progression of graft sclerosis, the exocrine lobules appear fragmented by proliferating fibroblastic bundles randomly interspersed between the acini. All exocrine tissue is eventually lost, with some areas becoming unrecognizable except for occasional residual islets embedded in the dense scar tissue. Interestingly, although in most patients, disappearance of the acinar component forecasts progressive disappearance of islets as well, in a minority of patients, glycemic control has been maintained for some time even after extensive fibrosis had replaced the exocrine tissue [131].

Narrowing of the arterial branches due to proliferative intimal endarteritis/transplant arteriopathy is also characteristic of the process [37, 80, 106, 114, 129] (see Figure 7.5 a–d).

The role of chronic vascular injury in pancreas chronic rejection/graft sclerosis is unequivocal. Recent or organized thrombosis is routinely seen in pancreatectomies for chronic rejection. Late thrombosis leading to graft failure is typically superimposed on intimal arteritis or transplant arteriopathy

Table 7.1 BANFF Pancreas Allograft Rejection Grading Schema – 2011 Update Diagnostic Categories#

1 NORMAL Absent inflammation **or** inactive septal, mononuclear inflammation not involving ducts, veins, arteries, or acini. There is no graft sclerosis. The fibrous component is limited to normal septa and its amount is proportional to the size of the enclosed structures (ducts and vessels). The acinar parenchyma shows no signs of atrophy or injury.

2 INDETERMINATE Septal inflammation that appears active, but the overall features do not fulfill the criteria for mild cell-mediated acute rejection.

3 ACUTE T- CELL-MEDIATED REJECTION

– Grade I / Mild acute T cell-mediated rejection

Active septal inflammation (activated, blastic lymphocytes, ± eosinophils) involving septal structures, venulitis (subendothelial accumulation of inflammatory cells and endothelial damage in septal veins), and ductitis (epithelial inflammation and damage of ducts).

and/or

Focal acinar inflammation. No more than two inflammatory foci^ per lobule with absent or minimal acinar cell injury.

– Grade II / Moderate acute T cell-mediated rejection (requires differentiation from AMR)

Multifocal (but not confluent or diffuse) acinar inflammation (≥3 foci^ per lobule) with spotty (individual) acinar cell injury and drop-out.

and/or

Mild intimal arteritis (with minimal, <25% luminal compromise).

– Grade III / Severe acute T cell-mediated rejection (requires differentiation from AMR)

Diffuse, (widespread, extensive) acinar inflammation with focal or diffuse multicellular/confluent acinar cell necrosis.

and/or

Moderate or severe intimal arteritis, >25% luminal compromise.

and/or

Transmural inflammation – necrotizing arteritis.

4 ANTIBODY-MEDIATED REJECTION (AMR, See diagnostic components below*)

*Confirmed circulating donor-specific antibody (DSA)

*Morphological evidence of tissue injury (interacinar inflammation/capillaritis, acinar cell damage swelling/necrosis/apoptosis/drop-out, vasculitis, thrombosis)

*C4d positivity in interacinar capillaries (IAC, ≥5% of acinar lobular surface)

– **Acute AMR** three of three diagnostic components*

– **Consistent with acute AMR** two of three diagnostic components*

– **Requires exclusion of AMR** one of three diagnostic components*

See separate table for histological grading of acute AMR^

CHRONIC ACTIVE ANTIBODY-MEDIATED REJECTION Combined features of categories 4* and 6 in the absence of features of category 3.

5 CHRONIC ALLOGRAFT ARTERIOPATHY Arterial intimal fibrosis with mononuclear cell infiltration in fibrosis.

6 CHRONIC ALLOGRAFT REJECTION/GRAFT FIBROSIS

– Stage I (mild graft fibrosis)

Expansion of fibrous septa; the fibrosis occupies less than 30% of the core surface, but the acinar lobules have eroded, irregular contours. The central lobular areas are normal.

– Stage II (moderate graft fibrosis)

The fibrosis occupies 30%–60% of the core surface. The exocrine atrophy affects the majority of the lobules in their periphery (irregular contours) and in their central areas (thin fibrous strands criss-cross between individual acini).

– Stage III (severe graft fibrosis)

The fibrotic areas predominate and occupy more than 60% of the core surface with only isolated areas of residual acinar tissue and/or islets present.

Table 7.1 (cont.)

7 ISLET PATHOLOGY

- Recurrence of autoimmune DM
  - Insulitis
  - Selective ß cell loss
- Islet amyloid (amylin) deposition
- Islet cell drug toxicity

8 OTHER HISTOLOGICAL DIAGNOSIS Pathological changes not considered to be due to acute and/or chronic rejection. E.g., CMV pancreatitis, PTLD, etc.

\# Categories 2–8 may be diagnosed concurrently and should be listed in the diagnosis in the order of their clinicopathological significance.
^ Histological grading of acute AMR described in main text
Adapted from reference 99.

[37]. In patients with long-term grafts immunosuppressed with calcineurin inhibitors (cyclosporine, tacrolimus), there may be widespread arteriolar hyalinosis, but it is not clearly established if this contributes to the process of graft sclerosis [132] (see Figure 7.13). Furthermore, in patients with generalized atherosclerotic disease, atheroemboli have been demonstrated to lodge in the pancreas allograft, causing late pancreatitis and further ischemic compromise [133] (see Figure 7.7).

VI Pancreas Allograft Rejection BANFF Working Grading Schema

Diagnostic Categories; General Considerations

The diagnosis and grading of rejection are based on the global assessment of the biopsy.

The pancreas BANFF schema includes eight diagnostic categories that cover the range of histopathological changes in pancreas allografts. Similar to other transplanted organs, two main forms of allograft rejection are recognized: T cell-mediated (CMR) and antibody-mediated (AMR) [133]. For each of these rejection types, acute and chronic numerical scores, such as those used in the kidney BANFF grading schema or for the liver histology activity index, have not been defined for pancreas allograft biopsies.

Histological manifestations are identified and severity grades are defined [133, 134].

Specific Histological Features Utilized for the Diagnosis of Rejection

- *Septal inflammatory infiltrates*, predominantly mononuclear, including "blastic" (activated) lymphocytes and variable numbers of eosinophils. Eosinophils may be the predominant cell type in occasional cases (see Figure 7.8).
- *Venulitis*, defined as subendothelial accumulation of inflammatory cells and endothelial damage observed in septal veins (see Figure 7.9).
- *Ductitis*, defined as epithelial infiltration of branches of the pancreatic ducts by mononuclear or eosinophilic inflammation and evidence of ductal epithelial cell damage (see Fig 7.10).
- *Neural and perineural inflammation* of intrinsic parenchymal nerve branches.
- *Acinar inflammation*, defined by the presence of inflammatory infiltrates with similar characteristics as the septal infiltrates amidst the exocrine acini (see Figures 7.11–7.15).
- *Single cell and confluent acinar cell necrosis/apoptosis* in association to the acinar inflammation (see Figure 7.16).
- *Intimal arteritis*, defined as infiltration by mononuclear cells under the arterial endothelium (see Figures 7.17–7.19).
- *Necrotizing arteritis*, defined as transmural inflammation with focal or circumferential fibrinoid necrosis (see Figure 7.18).
- *Interacinar accumulation of neutrophils and/or macrophages* with or without capillary dilatation (capillaritis) (see Figures 7.20–7.22).
- *Microvascular injury* characterized by congestion of interacinar capillaries with small or confluent microhemorrhages that may be associated with foci of tissue necrosis (microvascular thrombi) (see Figure 7.23).
- *C4d-positive staining in interacinar capillaries* as a feature of antibody-mediated rejection, if in association with donor-specific antibodies in serum (see Figure 7.24).

Grading of Acute Allograft Rejection

Determination of the severity of acute T cell-mediated rejection is based on the evaluation of several components as described in Table 7.1. Specifically, *inflammation confined to the septa and septal structures* (veins, ducts) represents milder forms of rejection, more responsive to anti-rejection treatment and less likely to result in irreversible sclerosing sequelae [42]. By contrast, *intimal arteritis and necrotizing arteritis* define the more severe forms of acute pancreas rejection, because these arterial lesions are more refractory to anti-rejection treatment and are known to carry an increased risk for immediate and

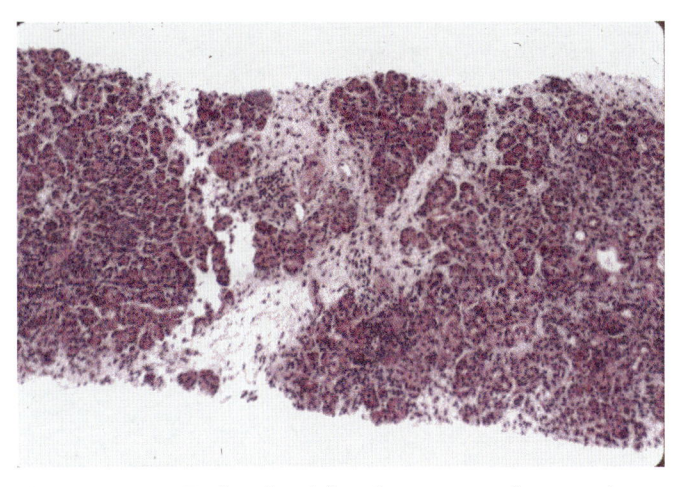

Figure 7.11 Acute T cell-mediated allograft rejection manifesting predominantly as acinar inflammation. The latter is patchy, involving clusters of acini (lower center and left).

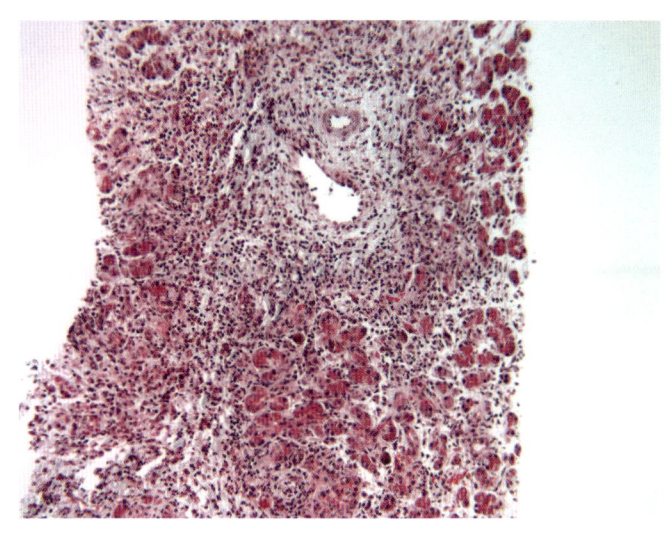

Figure 7.12 Representative field of a biopsy showing moderate acute T cell-mediated rejection. The inflammation involves the septal areas, as well as the acinar areas, in a diffuse manner. Only a few areas in the biopsy were free of inflammation.

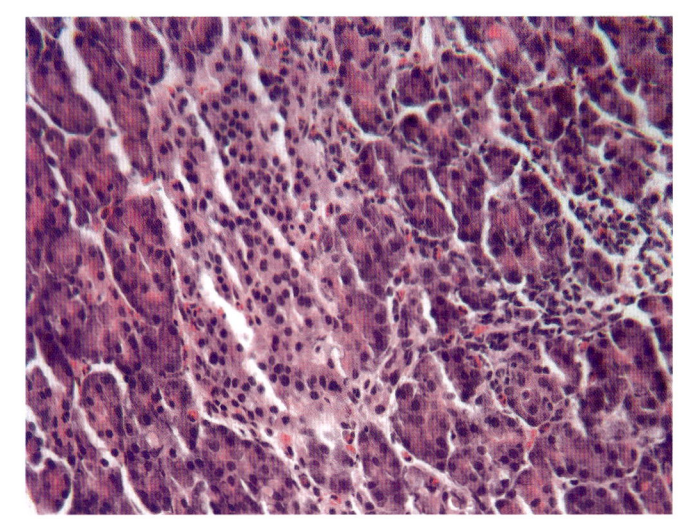

Figure 7.13A High power view of a focus of acinar inflammation, (right) composed of lymphocytes and eosinophils. Islets are not targeted in T cell-mediated rejection, although there are few eosinophils in the right upper part of the islet in continuity with the acinar inflammation.

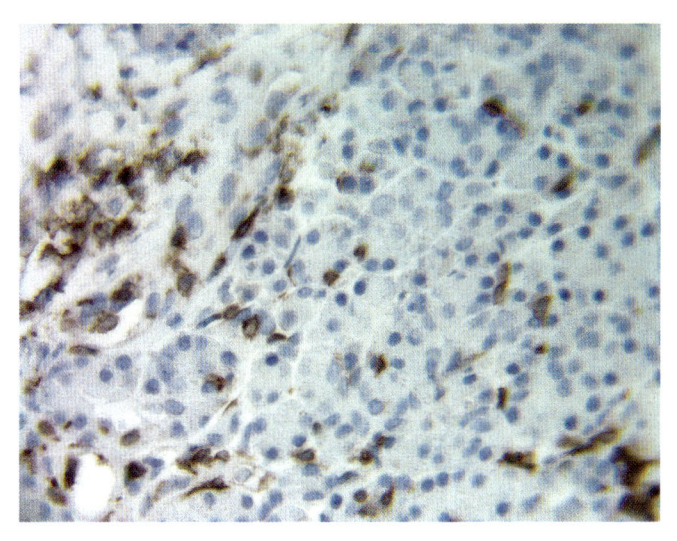

Figure 7.13B CD3 stain highlighting demonstrates tight association between T lymphocytes – main effectors in T cell-mediated rejection – and the acinar cells. The latter, together with ductal epithelium and endothelium of arteries and veins, are the main targets in acute T cell-mediated rejection.

subsequent graft thrombosis/loss and transplant arteriopathy [37]. The *extent of acinar inflammation* (focal versus multifocal-diffuse) and the *presence and extent of acinar cell injury* are also used to determine rejection severity based on evidence that extensive acinar injury and damage can lead to fibrosis and accelerated graft loss, if untreated or undertreated [42].

The severity of AMR is graded histologically as mild, moderate, or severe according to the extent of the interacinar infiltrates and the extent of microvascular injury and tissue damage as follows: Grade I/mild acute AMR: well-preserved architecture, mild monocytic-macrophagic or mixed (monocytic-macrophagic/neutrophilic) infiltrates with rare acinar cell damage, and *minimal or no evidence* of microvascular injury.

Grade II/moderate acute AMR: overall preservation of the architecture with significant interacinar monocytic-macrophagic or mixed (monocytic-macrophagic/neutrophilic) infiltrates with or without evidence of capillary dilatation (capillaritis) *associated with* significant microvascular injury manifested as congestion and extravasation of red blood cells (microhemorrhages) and multicellular acinar cell injury and drop-out.

Grade III/severe acute AMR: architectural disarray, scattered inflammatory infiltrates in a background of pronounced microvascular injury with interstitial hemorrhage, multifocal and confluent parenchymal necrosis. Arterial and venous wall necrosis and thrombosis may be present [99].

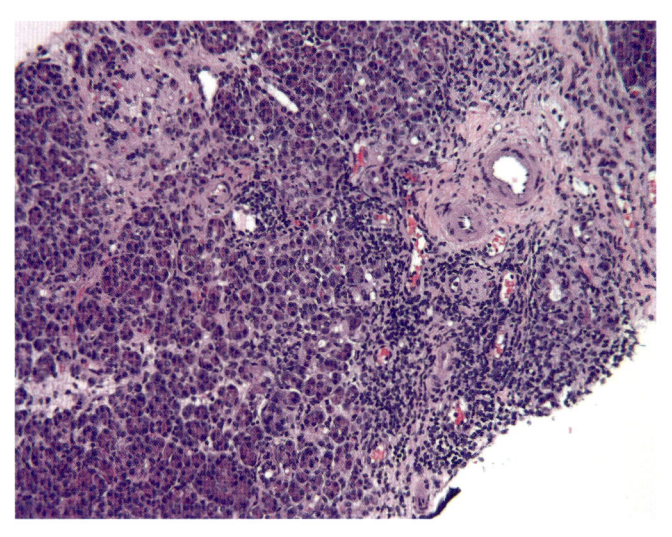

Figure 7.14A Acute T cell-mediated allograft rejection manifesting as septal inflammation with early acinar involvement (right low center).

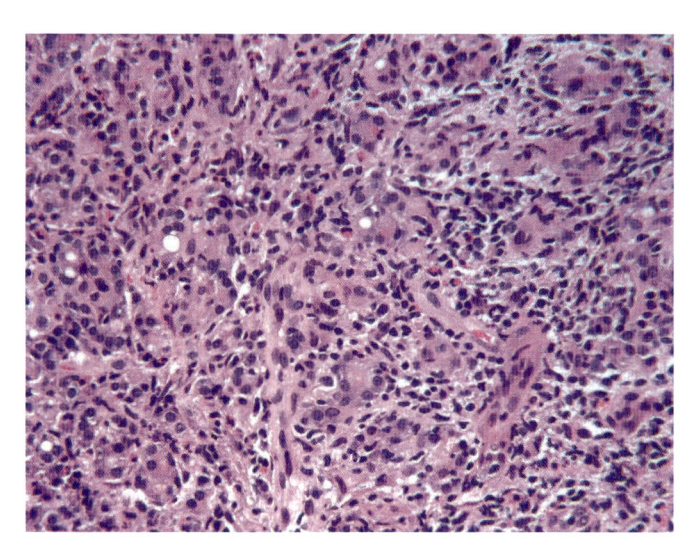

Figure 7.14B Significant inflammation in acute T cell-mediated allograft rejection. Numerous acinar cells show cytoplasmic vacuolization.

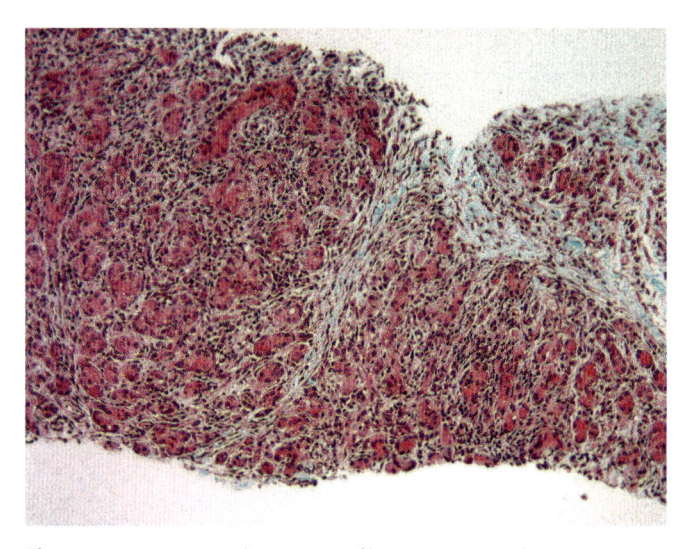

Figure 7.15 Masson's trichrome stain of biopsy represented in Figure 7.14 shows developing interacinar fibrosis.

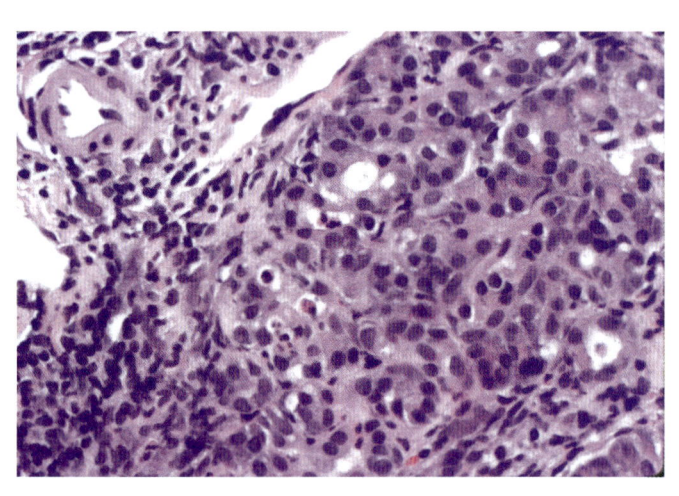

Figure 7.16A Moderate acute T cell-mediated allograft rejection defined by multifocal acinar inflammation and single cell (spotty) acinar cell damage. Only a small area of the biopsy is depicted here at high magnification in order to appreciate acinar cell vacuolization and occasional cell undergoing apoptosis (center left).

Diagnostic Categories: Specific Considerations

BANFF Category 1: Normal: Inflammatory infiltrates are absent, *or* very sparse, inactive, mononuclear (i.e., small lymphocytes, rare plasma cells). If there is slight inflammation, this is focal and confined to the septa with lack of involvement of any of the septal structures (vessels, ducts, nerves) (see Figures 7.24–7.26).

An adequate biopsy (see above) with these histological characteristics essentially rules out a diagnosis of cell-mediated acute rejection. Accordingly, these types of findings are more often encountered in protocol biopsies of well-functioning grafts [33, 92].

It should be emphasized, however, that "normal"-appearing biopsies may be also encountered under other clinical circumstances. Specifically, in patients biopsied for hyperglycemia, the differential diagnosis includes three main processes: A) Late phase of recurrent autoimmune disease, i.e., after resolution of isletitis [34, 135] (see below). This process can only be recognized by the evaluation of immunohistochemical stains for insulin and glucagon demonstrating selective loss of beta cells; B) Drug toxicity that is primarily characterized by vacuolization and damage of islet cells; [35] C) Grade 1 acute antibody-mediated rejection. It is noteworthy that an essentially normal biopsy was found in the first well-documented case of acute antibody-mediated rejection [79] (see Figure 7.24). It is therefore recommended that negative biopsies in patients with graft dysfunction are stained for C4d to rule out antibody-mediated rejection.

BANFF Category 2: Indeterminate For Rejection This category is defined by the presence of focal septal inflammation that displays features of activation (blastic changes, ± eosinophils), but the overall features do not fulfill the criteria for mild rejection (i.e., partial cuffing of a septal vein or duct but lacking any evidence of endothelial or epithelial involvement, etc.) (see Figures 7.27–7.29).

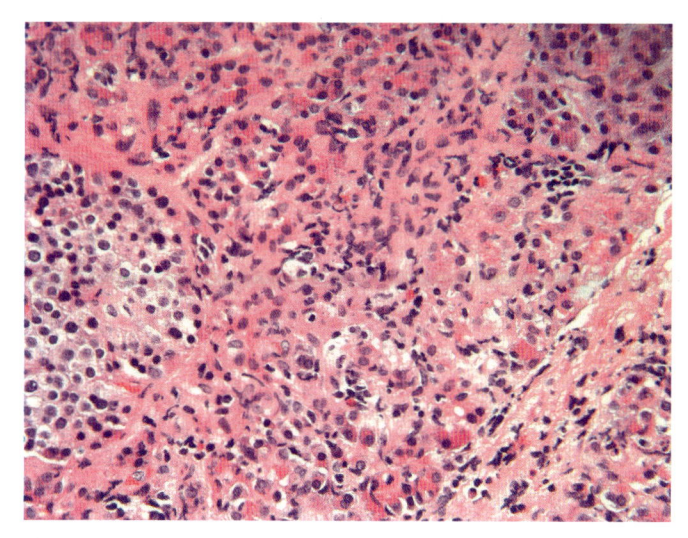

Figure 7.16B Medium power view of areas of multicellular acinar cell damage. Note marked acinar cell vacuolization and dissolution of the acinar architecture (lower center). An islet mostly free of inflammation is seen to the left.

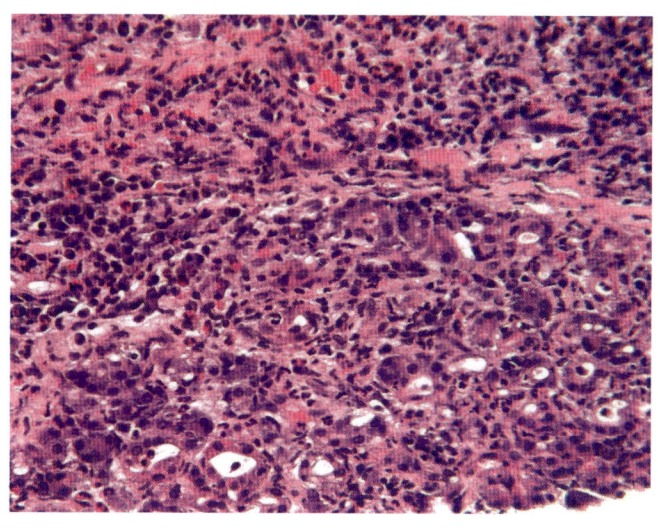

Figure 7.16C Representative area of biopsy with severe acute T cell-mediated rejection defined by extensive inflammation of septa and acini and evidence of acinar cell damage. Note dissolution of the acinar architecture in the lower right areas and secondary infiltration by neutrophils. C4d stain was negative.

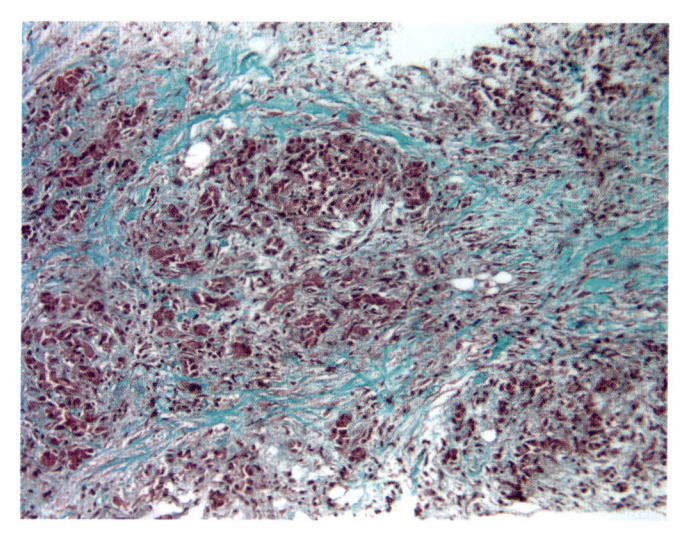

Figure 7.16D Diffuse acinar inflammation and multicellular acinar cell damage are precursors of acinar atrophy/fibrosis as observed in this biopsy obtained six weeks after the biopsy represented in Figure 7.16B.

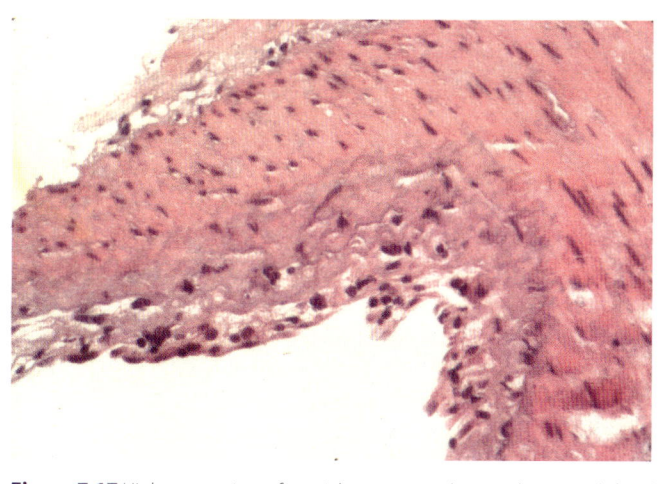

Figure 7.17 High power view of arterial segment with intimal arteritis defined as subendothelial accumulation of inflammatory cells with lifting and partial sloughing of the endothelial lining.

These histological features can be seen in protocol biopsies of well-functioning grafts, as well as in patients biopsied for graft dysfunction. Similarly to the "borderline" category in the kidney, these changes may represent early as well as treated acute rejection, or alternatively may be entirely nonspecific [32, 33, 92].

The treatment of patients with biopsies showing *"indeterminate"* features may vary depending on the indication for biopsy, and ultimately depends on clinical judgment. In accordance with the heterogeneous nature of the "indeterminate" histological changes, response to treatment varies significantly in comparison to biopsies with definite acute cell-mediated rejection that are usually responsive to treatment [32].

BANFF Category 3: Acute T Cell-mediated Rejection: Graded as mild, moderate, or severe (Grades I, II, and II, respectively), based on the identification of lesions that have been shown to prognosticate progressively worse outcomes [32, 33, 42, 51, 119].

Mild Acute T Cell-mediated Rejection (Grade I)

This grade is defined by the presence of septal inflammatory infiltrates that not only have features of activation ("blastic" lymphocytes, variable numbers of eosinophils), but also involve septal structures (veins, ducts) and ± focal acinar inflammation. These findings may vary from septal area to area; however, any degree of venulitis (subendothelial accumulation of inflammatory cells and endothelial damage in septal veins) or ductitis (epithelial inflammation and damage of pancreatic ducts) is sufficient for the diagnosis of mild-Grade I, cell-mediated rejection. Inflammation of peripheral nerve branches coursing through the parenchyma is also a feature of rejection, although this is a rare finding due to the scarcity of these structures in biopsy material.

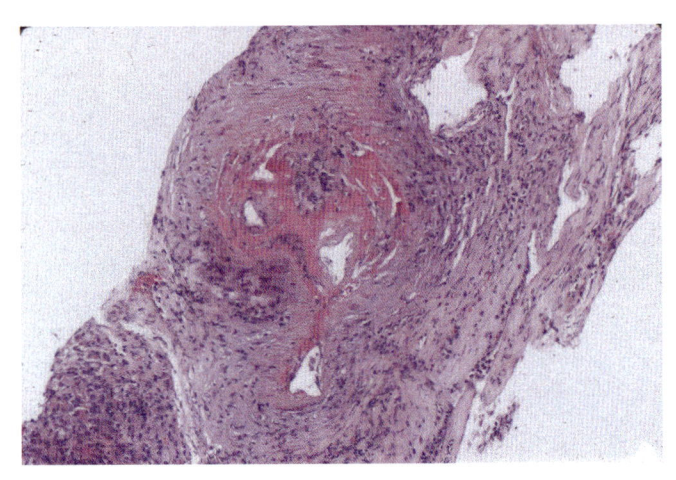

Figure 7.18 Necrotizing arteritis (in a patient whose rejection was refractory to anti-rejection treatment). The wall of a distorted artery is completely replaced by bright red amorphous material indicating fibrinoid necrosis. Note the presence of inflammation in the fibrotic connective tissue around the artery and in the adjacent acinar tissue (lower left), consistent with the history of ongoing rejection.

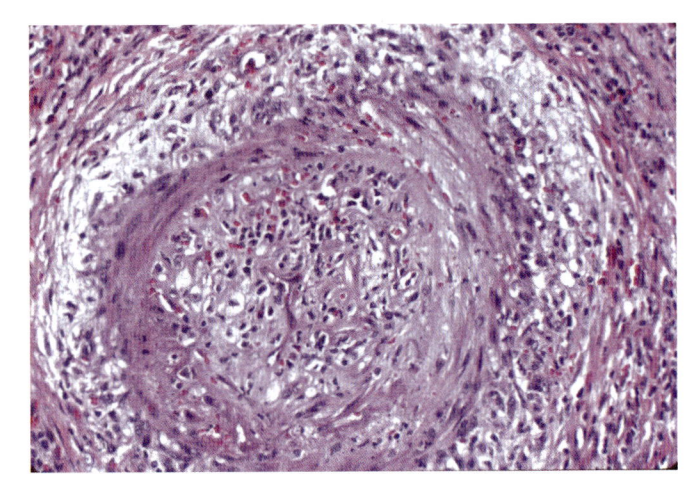

Figure 7.19 Arterial cross section with transmural inflammation and necrosis (arteritis) in the lower half of its circumference. Note slit-like lumen and neo-intima formation (left of center) resulting from severe expansion of the subendothelial areas due to accumulation of inflammatory cells and loose fibroblastic-myofibroblastic proliferation. The latter features indicate that in addition to the acute injury (arteritis), there is a subacute to chronic component.

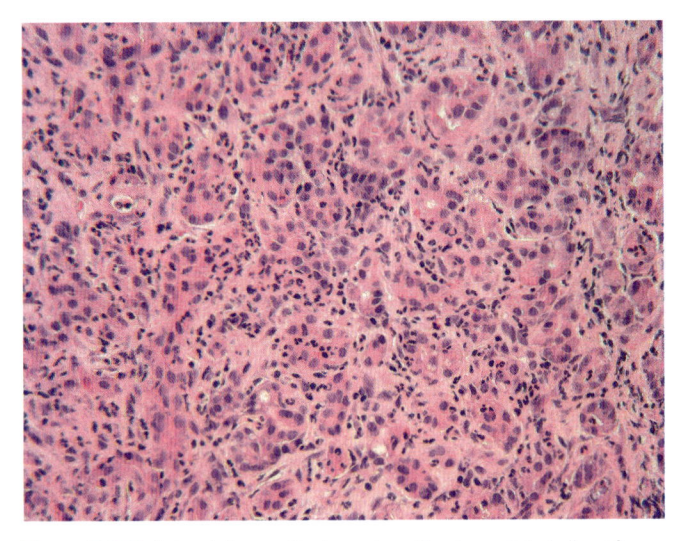

Figure 7.20A Acinar inflammation in acute antibody-mediated allograft rejection. In this case, the inflammation predominantly consists of neutrophils accumulating in capillaries and interstitium.

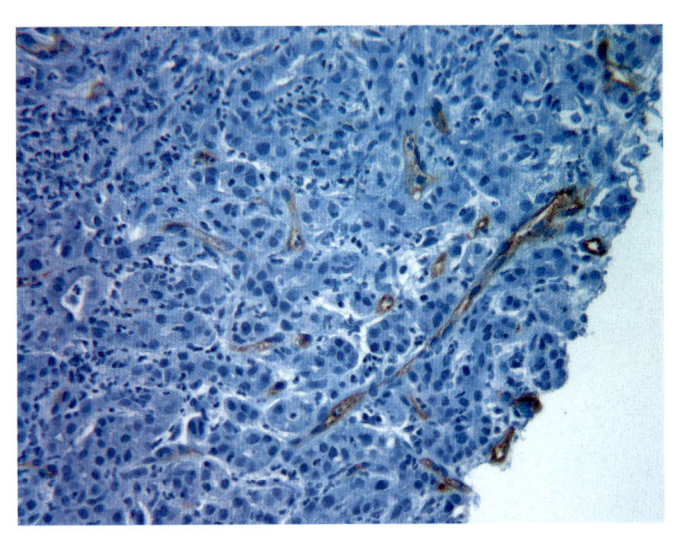

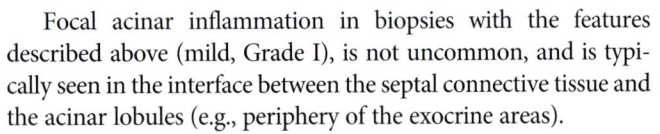

Figure 7.20B Acute antibody-mediated rejection (see Figure 7.20A). C4d stain demonstrates complement deposition in microvasculature.

Focal acinar inflammation in biopsies with the features described above (mild, Grade I), is not uncommon, and is typically seen in the interface between the septal connective tissue and the acinar lobules (e.g., periphery of the exocrine areas).

Due to sampling variations, in some cases, the foci of acinar inflammation appear to be completely separate from the septal inflammation within "deeper" areas of the lobules.

Mild cell-mediated rejection-Grade I also includes cases in which, due to sampling, septal involvement is not present and only focal acinar inflammation is appreciated.

In any case, in mild-Grade I rejection, the acinar inflammation should be clearly focal (i.e., no more than two inflammatory foci per lobule, as defined below) and should be lacking evidence of acinar cell injury (apoptosis, necrosis).

Recognition of an acinar inflammatory lesion/focus is not difficult at medium-to-high power; however, in order to avoid ambiguity, the grading schema provides a specific definition (collection of at least ten lymphocytes/eosinophils within an acinar area), particularly for cases in which the septal inflammation is mild or absent and the diagnosis of mild (Grade I) cell-mediated rejection will hinge on the acinar lesions only. The composition of the acinar inflammation is typically similar to that of the septal infiltrates (mixture of activated and small lymphocytes with variable numbers of eosinophils).

Biopsies with the features defining this rejection grade are occasionally found in patients with well-functioning grafts [32, 91, 92], but are more commonly seen in biopsies performed for graft dysfunction (typically increase in amylase/lipase in serum, or decrease in urinary amylase in bladder drained grafts). The main histological differential diagnosis in this category is CMV pancreatitis, which is often patchy in nature [136] (see Figures 7.34–7.38).

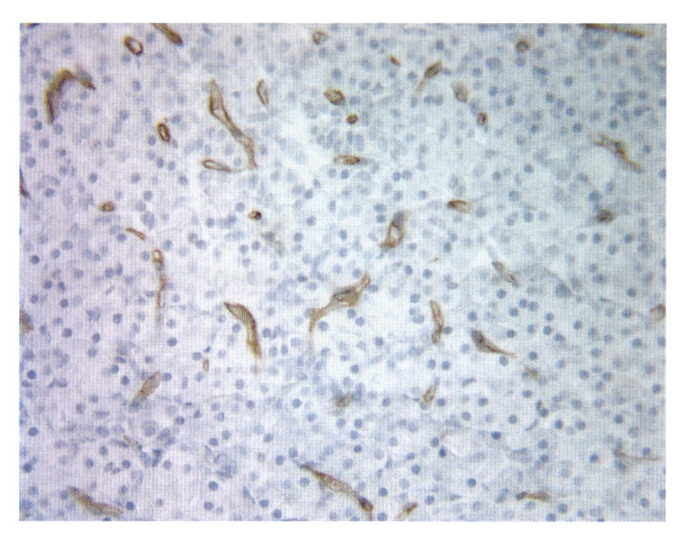

Figure 7.21 C4d stain in biopsy performed for increased serum amylase. A diagnosis of mild T cell-mediated rejection was made based on septal changes not depicted here. HLA type II donor-specific antibodies were identified concurrently. Interacinar inflammation was insignificant.

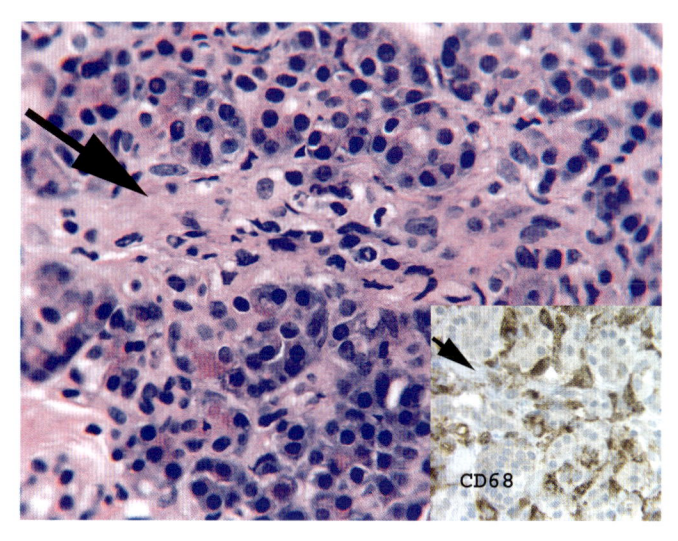

Figure 7.22 Early, mild, acute AMR. High power view of acinar and interstitial areas shows overall preservation of the architecture and very subtle inflammation. Insert: CD68 staining of the same area of the biopsy shows a large numbers of macrophages that are not clearly evident on the H&E. Arrows mark an interstitial area for orientation.

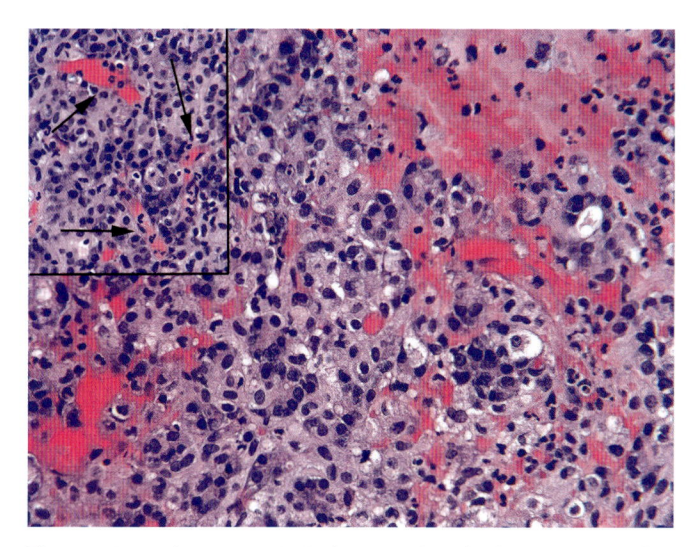

Figure 7.23 Moderate acute AMR. The parenchymal architecture is overall preserved; however, microvascular injury manifested as microhemorrhagic foci is significant. Capillaritis was identified only in rare fields (insert, arrows).

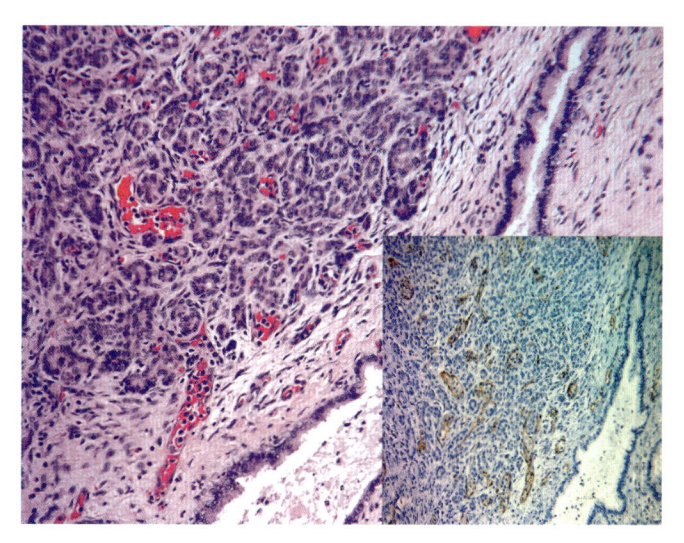

Figure 7.24A Ongoing AMR appears with microvascular congestion and inflammation, including prominent capillaritis. Note diffuse incipient acinar atrophy and increase in interacinar fibrous tissue. Diffuse C4d staining in the microvasculature.

Moderate Acute T Cell-mediated Rejection (Grade II)

This grade can be defined by two histological features that may be identified either in isolation or concurrently.

Multifocal Acinar Inflammation: The most common presentation of this grade consists of multiple foci (≥3 foci per lobule) of acinar inflammation and associated spotty (individual) acinar cell injury and drop-out. The acinar inflammatory involvement in this grade should be identified with ease at medium power; however, the involvement should not be confluent/diffuse. From a practical point of view, completely un-inflamed acinar/exocrine areas should be easily identified between the inflamed foci. Absence of confluent inflammation will differentiate this grade from the next-higher category (see below). Significant acinar inflammation is always associated with evidence of acinar cell injury [137, 138], but in this grade, the latter should be spotty (isolated). Specifically, acinar cell injury may appear as any of the following: cellular drop-out (empty spaces equaling the size of individual cells), cytoplasmic swelling and vacuolization, nuclear pyknosis, apoptotic bodies, and single cell lytic necrosis (see Figure 7.16).

Minimal Intimal Arteritis: Alternatively, depending on sampling variations, the category of moderate cell-mediated rejection-Grade II can be defined by the sole presence of mild, focal intimal arteritis defined by the presence of rare, occasional, but clearly defined, subendothelial (intimal) mononuclear cells. The latter changes may or may not be accompanied by the complete constellation of inflammatory changes described earlier in the septa and lobules (see Figures 7.39–7.42).

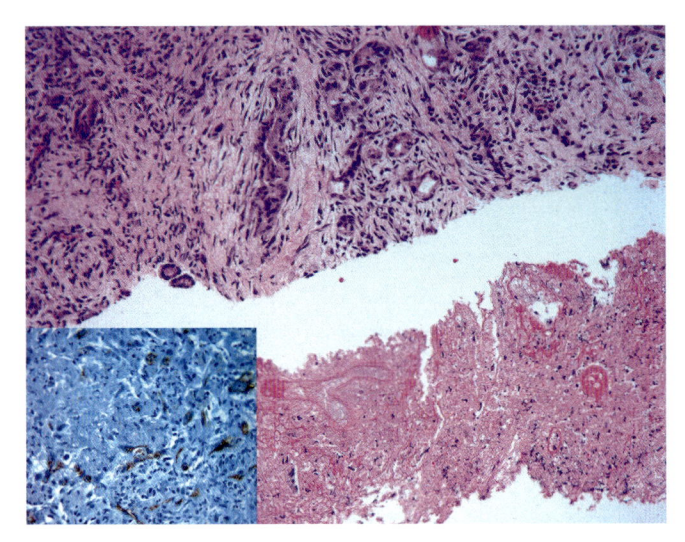

Figure 7.24B Severe acute and chronic AMR evolving for a period of three weeks. The core in the bottom shows necrosis; the outline of necrotic vessels can be discerned. The core in the top shows progression of fibrosis with pronounced loss of the acinar component. Microvascular inflammation subtle-to-absent; however, C4d stain remains positive in the viable areas. Severe acute antibody-mediated allograft rejection is characterized by areas of parenchymal necrosis, the extent of which is variable, mostly depending on the size and number of vessels affected by necrosis and thrombosis.

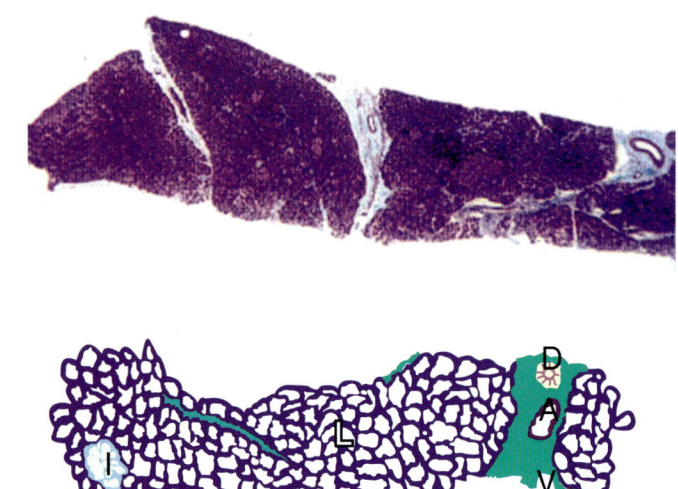

Figure 7.25A Microphotograph and diagram representing normal proportions between the connective and acinar tissues in a protocol biopsy of a well-functioning graft 12 months post-transplantation. The periphery of the acinar lobules is smooth and the acinar component is compact with total absence of interacinar connective tissue. An adequate biopsy should contain a minimum of three lobular areas and associated septa.

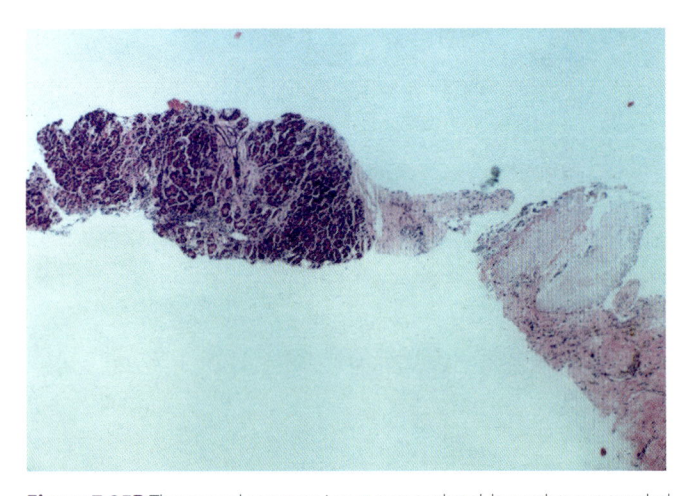

Figure 7.25B The normal pancreas is not encapsulated, but rather surrounded by poorly defined connective tissue that may become prominent after transplantation due to reactive and reparative mechanisms. Needle biopsies may demonstrate a variety of changes in the peripancreatic connective tissue, including fat necrosis (extreme right). The latter is more commonly seen early after transplantation.

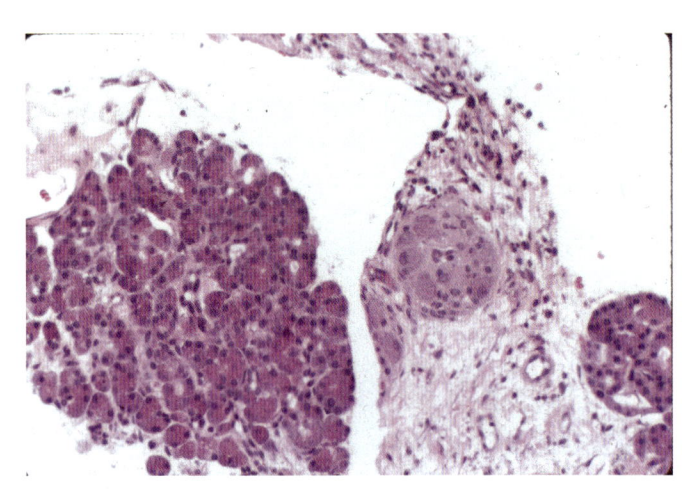

Figure 7.25C Ganglion cell clusters may be identified rarely in pancreas allograft biopsies. These should not be confused with cytomegalovirus cytopathic changes.

From a clinical point of view, biopsies with features of moderate cell-mediated rejection-Grade II are typically found in patients with graft dysfunction (usually increase in amylase/lipase in serum or decrease in urinary amylase in bladder drained grafts).

Severe Acute T Cell-mediated Rejection (Grade III)

This grade can be defined by three histological features that may be identified ether in isolation or concurrently.

Severe Acinar Inflammation and Acinar Cell Damage: This entity is characterized by confluent/diffuse (widespread, extensive) acinar inflammation with associated focal or diffuse multicellular/confluent acinar cell necrosis. The inflammation may be predominantly lymphoid or may contain abundant eosinophils or variable amounts of neutrophils. By definition, there should be none or only rare, focal areas of completely uninflamed acinar/exocrine parenchyma (see Figure 7.16).

Moderate or Severe Intimal Arteritis: Defined as easily identifiable (e.g., more than six to eight) lymphocytes within the intima of an involved muscular artery, and is by itself sufficient to justify a diagnosis of severe T cell-mediated rejection-Grade III (see Figure 7.40). Moderate or severe intimal arteritis is usually associated with some evidence of intimal injury (i.e., endothelial cell hypertrophy, fibrin leakage, coating neutrophils and/or macrophages, activation of intimal myofibroblasts).

Necrotizing Arteritis: Transmural arterial inflammation leading to complete or partial circumferential necrosis also

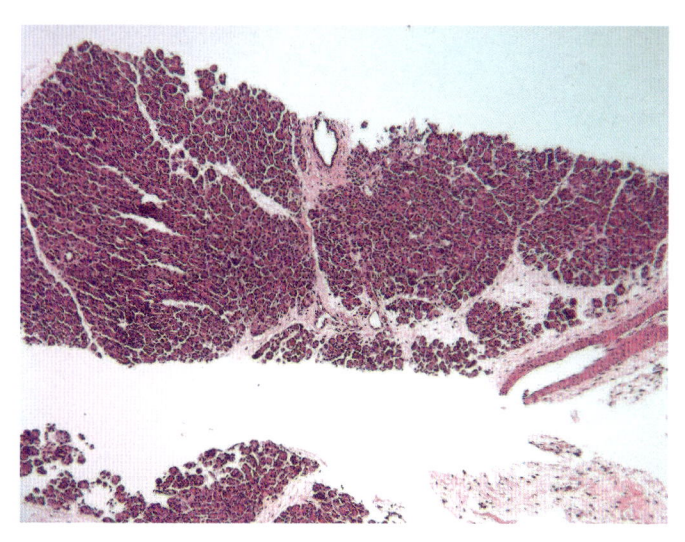

Figure 7.26 Representative area of a needle core biopsy in a patient with a well-functioning graft. There are very sparse inflammatory cells in the septa and mild interstitial edema. These findings are nonspecific; there is no evidence of acute cell-mediated rejection.

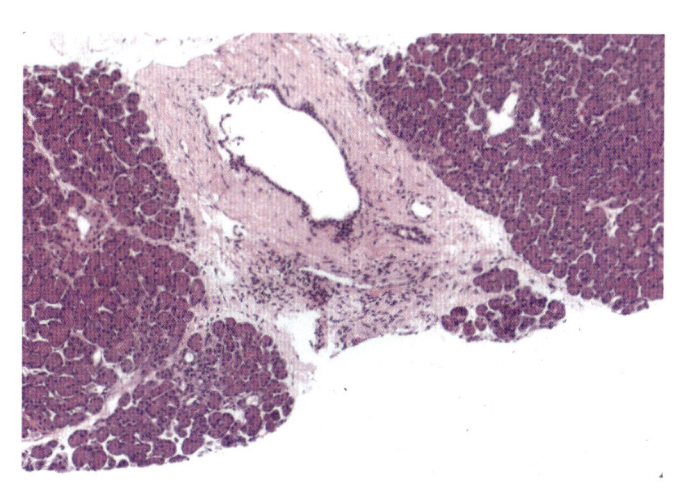

Figure 7.27 Single focus of septal inflammation sparing vein and duct found in a biopsy of a patient with fluctuating serum amylase and lipase. The inflammation appears inactive and is likely nonspecific. The patient was treated with bolus steroids with no clear response.

defines severe cell-mediated rejection. Transmural fibrinoid arterial necrosis is, however, more often associated with antibody-mediated rejection. C4d staining and search for donor-specific antibodies is therefore necessary to rule out humoral rejection if necrotizing arteritis is identified (see Figure 7.41).

Each of the three lesions used to define severe cell-mediated rejection portend poor outcome to the graft because they are associated with, or lead to, irreversible parenchymal damage. The short- and long-term impact to the organ will depend on the extent of acinar damage and the size and the number of the arteries affected by intimal arteritis or necrosis.

Confluent acinar inflammation and necrosis are invariably followed by some degree of secondary collagenization of the interacinar areas and eventual loss or disappearance of the exocrine component in the affected area. Changes of this nature markedly alter the microvascular environment of the graft on which the islets depend to maintain an adequate function [96, 125, 139, 140].

Similar to other solid organ transplants, intimal arteritis is associated with an increased risk of immediate or delayed thrombosis (see Figure 7.42). This lesion is also a precursor of transplant arteriopathy [37].

Transmural arteritis/vasculitis is associated with an immediate likelihood of thrombosis and secondary parenchymal infarction. Biopsies with histological findings corresponding to this category are characteristically associated with graft dysfunction/failure, often including hyperglycemia [32, 33].

BANFF Category 4: Antibody-mediated Rejection
Antibody-mediated rejection (AMR) in the pancreas is increasingly recognized as an important cause of graft failure due to its poor response to currently available treatments [78, 79, 110, 111, 113, 141–143]. AMR is caused by antibodies directed against donor-specific human leukocyte antigen (HLA) molecules or other cell surface antigens [144] and more often results from a strong anamnestic antibody response to previous antigenic exposure (i.e., previous islet transplantation, re-transplantation, pregnancy, etc.). Post-transplant development of *de novo* donor-specific antibody (DSA) may also occur, with or without association with known triggering factors such as vaccinations, viral infections, etc. [144–150].

DSA Studies

Diagnosis and treatment of AMR require laboratory measurements for circulating DSA at regular intervals after transplantation, at the time of biopsy, and whenever rejection is suspected. Specific clinical settings may require implementation of protocols tailored to individual patients (i.e., desensitization protocols, weaning of immunosuppression, etc.) [151–153]. The clinical relevance of anti-HLA antibody levels and specificities, as well as the significance of antibodies to non-HLA antigens (e.g., MHC class I-related chain A [MICA], auto antigens, etc.) continue to be debated [152, 153]. Although an earlier study found a strong association between DSA to MHC class II and chronic allograft rejection/graft loss, subsequent studies have not found significant clinicopathological differences between DSA to class I and class II antigens. Antibodies to MICA were associated with histopathological features of AMR in the pancreas in one series [99].

C4d Staining

Circulating DSA directed against endothelial cells leads to widespread activation of the complement and coagulation cascades in the vascular walls with consequent engagement of inflammatory mediators [105]. The complement fragment C4d is generated via the classical (antibody-induced) activation pathway and in contrast to other complement components, is resistant to shedding and degradation, remaining detectable in vessel walls for at least several days following the initial immunological event [154, 155]. C4d staining in renal biopsies performed for allograft dysfunction is predictive of poorer graft outcomes and helps identify patients with AMR. In pancreas allograft biopsies, C4d staining is typically absent in cases of

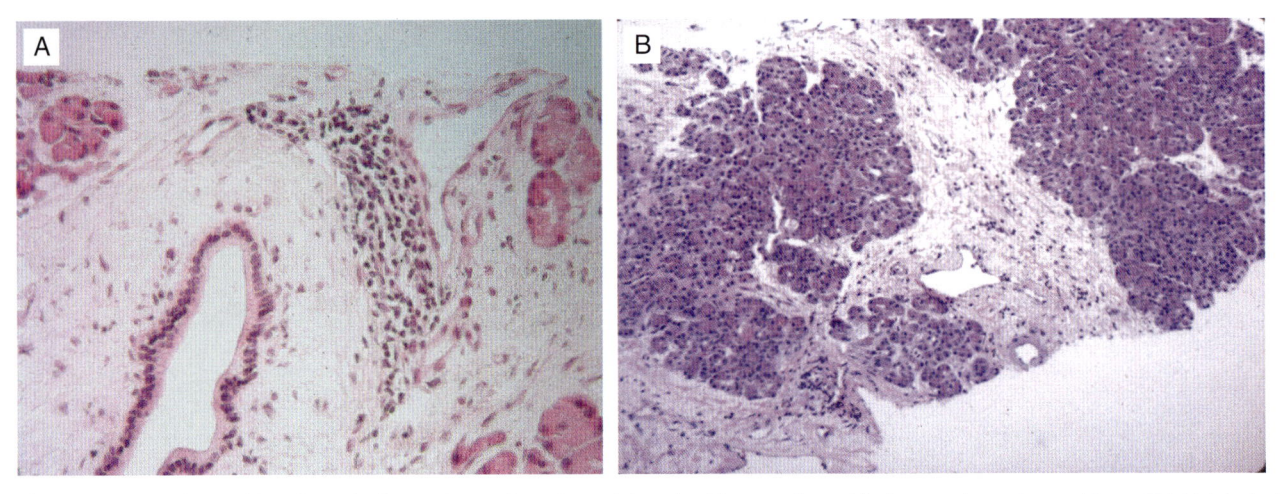

Figure 7.28 One of several foci of septal inflammation sparing veins and ducts in a biopsy performed for increase in amylase and lipase. This histological picture is compatible with a diagnosis of "indetermined" for acute rejection.

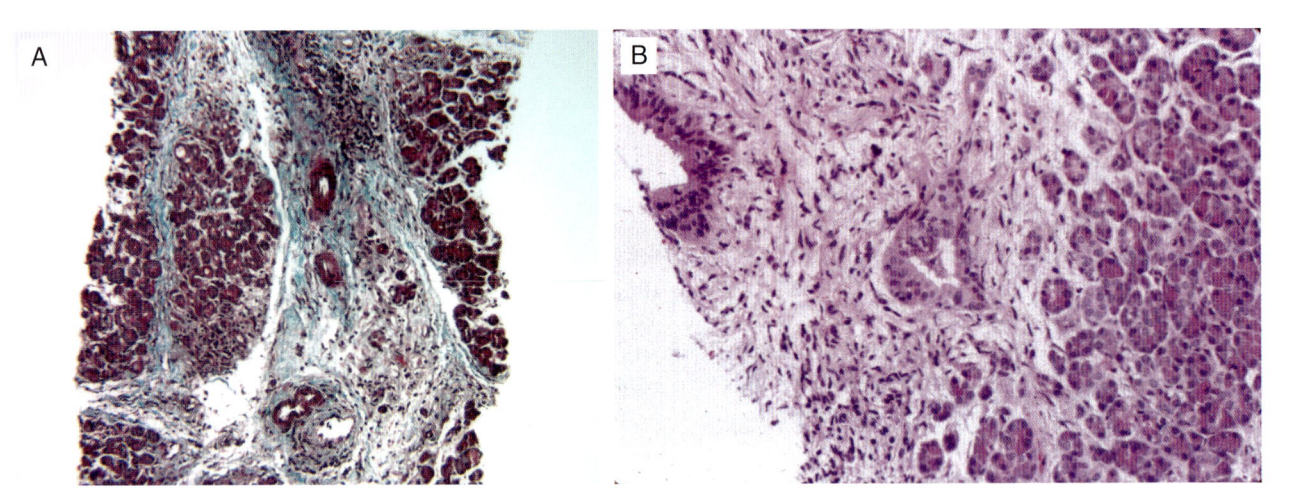

Figure 7.29A and B Biopsies performed two and three weeks after the biopsies represented in Figures 7.30A and B respectively show features found in "treated" acute rejection. The histological findings are more difficult to be classified and may fall in the categories of "indetermined" for rejection or mild rejection. Note incipient septal fibrosis with early fragmentation of the periphery of the exocrine lobules.

pure acute ACMR or in protocol biopsies from well-functioning grafts [110, 113].

Both immunohistochemical and immunofluorescence C4d stains are adequate for diagnosis and yield a similar staining pattern in interacinar capillaries (IAC; Figure). In renal and cardiac allograft biopsies, the immunofluorescence technique has been reported to yield stronger staining compared to the immunohistochemical method, but the difference was not considered significant for clinical purposes [104, 156]. Comparison of the two methods in pancreas allograft biopsies showed that, with the immunofluorescence technique, the estimated areas of lobular IAC staining were 10%–50% larger than with the immunohistochemical method. The threshold for C4d positivity in pancreas-allograft biopsies is set at ≥5% because most centers perform the staining on paraffin-embedded sections. A low threshold is preferable if immunohistochemical staining is used, considering that studies in the kidney and the pancreas have shown that both focal and diffuse C4d staining were associated with poorer graft outcomes [110, 113, 157]. C4d staining in parenchymal-IAC is to be reported semiquantitatively based on the extent of exocrine lobular biopsy surface staining, as follows: Negative <5%, Focal 5%–50% and Diffuse >50%. Only linear or granular staining along the IAC correlates with the presence of circulating DSA. In contrast, staining in other tissue components, such as the endothelium of larger vessels including veins and arteries, interstitial or septal connective tissue, and peripancreatic soft tissues, is considered nonspecific [113, 158].

Acute Antibody-mediated Rejection

The diagnosis of *acute pancreatic AMR* is based on the clinicopathological combination of: a) circulating donor-specific antibodies, b) morphological evidence of microvascular tissue injury (see below), and c) C4d staining in interacinar capillaries. A diagnosis of "*suspicious for AMR*" is reached if only two of the three elements are present, but the identification of only one

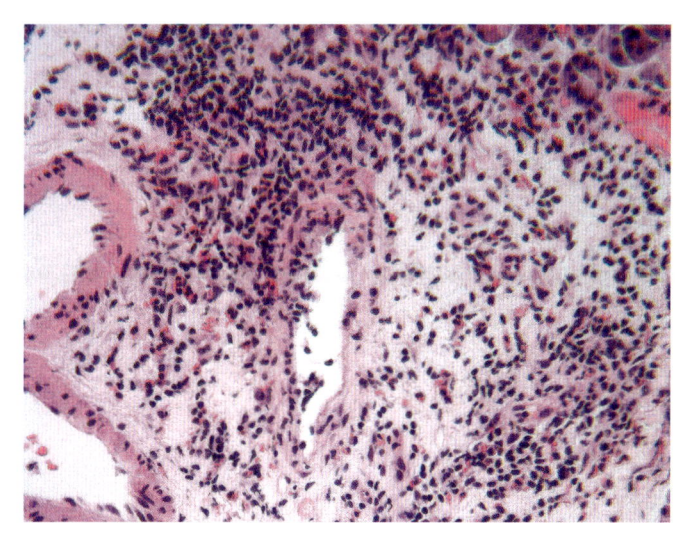

Figure 7.30A Active (blastic) lymphocytic and eosinophilic septal inflammation with early venulitis in acute T cell-mediated allograft rejection.

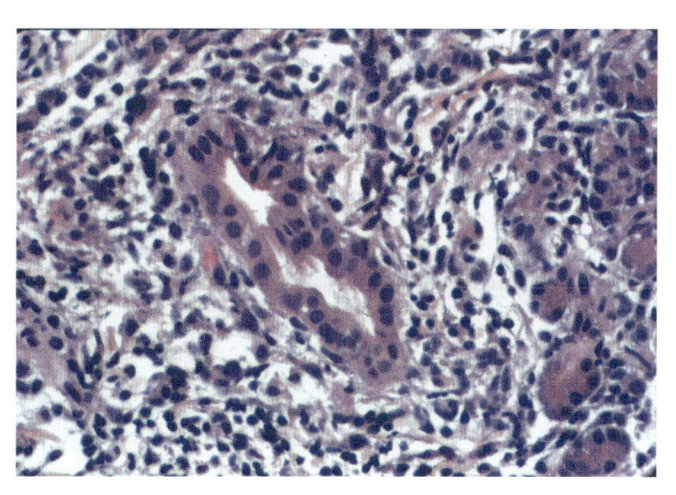

Figure 7.30B Pancreatic duct surrounded and focally permeated by prominent septal inflammation with features of activation (blastic transformation), including occasional markedly atypical nuclei (top left).

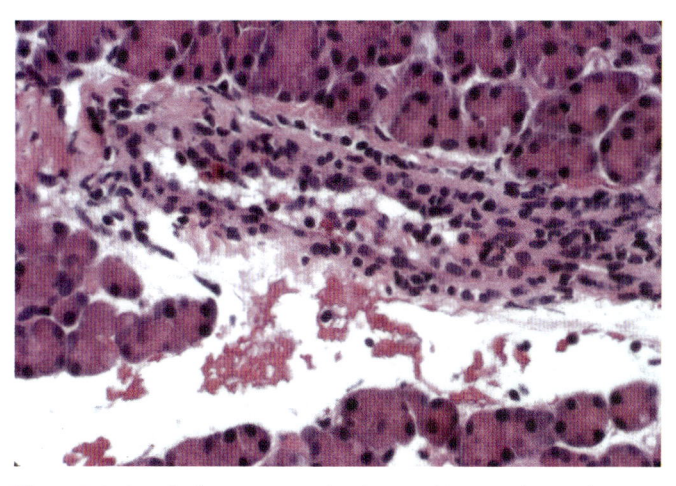

Figure 7.31 Septal inflammation confined to septal/perivenular area; however, diagnostic of acute rejection due to the presence of marked endothelial damage (lifting, vacuolization, and focal sloughing). The inflammation has features of activation (blastic changes), and there are eosinophils.

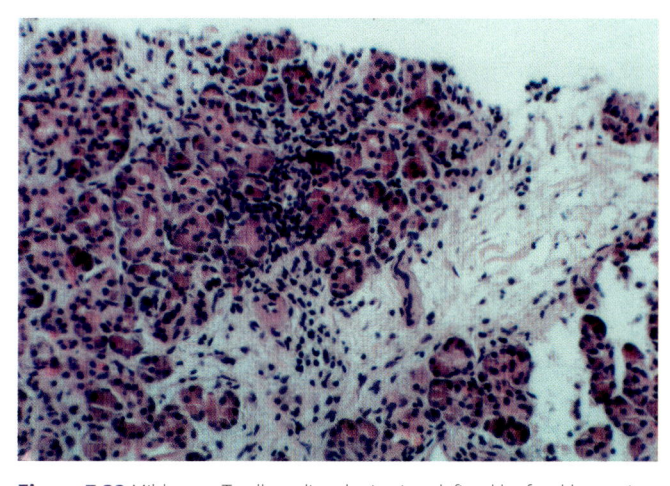

Figure 7.32 Mild acute T cell-mediated rejection defined by focal but active acinar inflammation in the interface with the septal connective tissue. The biopsy was from a patient with a bladder-drained pancreas allograft who presented with decrease in urine amylase. Amylase levels normalized after antirejection treatment.

diagnostic element is not sufficiently diagnostic or "suspicious" of AMR. Graft dysfunction is not required for the diagnosis of acute AMR [99]. The rationale behind the current guidelines for the diagnosis of AMR is based on the perceived strengths and limitations of the currently available tools (DSA, C4d, and histological findings), taking advantage of their complementary value. A diagnosis of "suspicious for AMR" increases the sensitivity of the schema by addressing clinical situations in which a complete constellation of elements is not identified (i.e., only two of the three elements are present). Specifically, cases of C4d-negative, as well as cases in which anti HLA DSA cannot be documented – albeit rare – can be encountered in clinical practice [99, 104, 159, 160]. Similar to the kidney, microvascular inflammation/injury found with concurrent detection of circulating DSA strongly suggests AMR independently of positive C4d staining [104, 113, 142, 161].

Treatment of acute AMR is indicated if all three or two elements are present, whereas rigorous clinical surveillance is recommended in the last setting (i.e., only one parameter is present) [77, 110, 111, 113, 160].

Spectrum of AMR in Pancreas Allografts

The clinicopathological manifestations of AMR range from immediate graft loss to ongoing microvascular inflammation leading to protracted graft sclerosis-fibrosis. A high degree of suspicion is required for the recognition of milder or more indolent forms of AMR that are potentially treatable. Biopsy evaluation remains the gold standard for the diagnosis of acute allograft rejection and is necessary to discriminate between ACMR and AMR, which require different treatments [111].

Hyperacute Rejection –– Significant levels of preformed circulating antidonor antibodies at the time of transplantation lead to

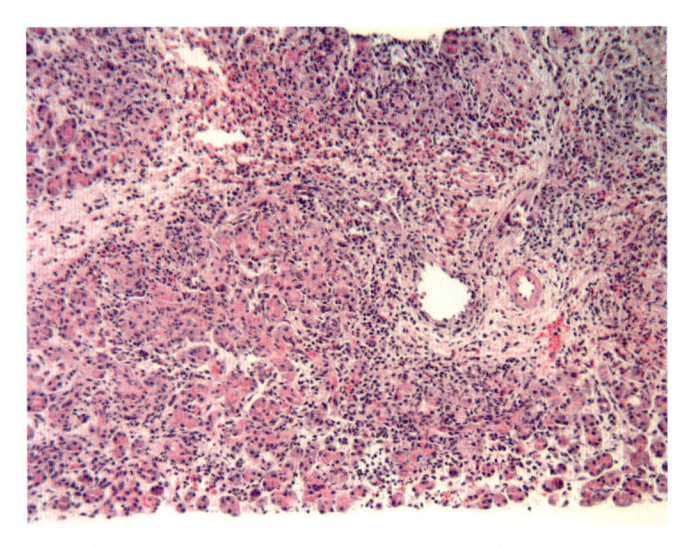

Figure 7.33 Moderate acute T cell-mediated allograft rejection. In contrast to the biopsy in Figure 7.36, the inflammation involves extensively the periphery of the acinar lobules, as well as areas more distant from the septa.

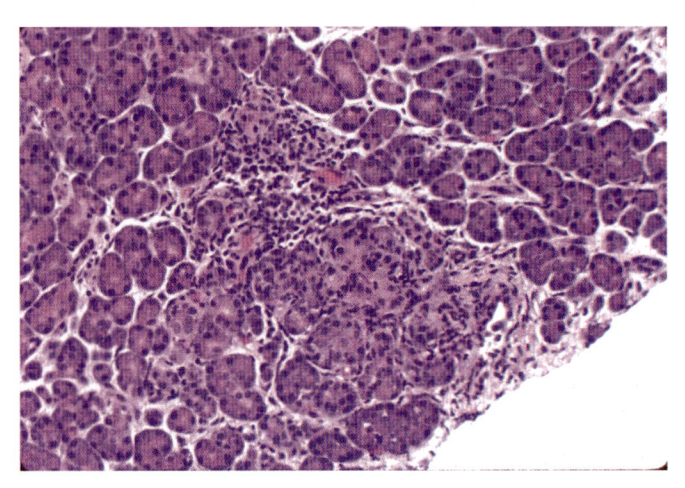

Figure 7.34A Medium power view of a focus of acinar inflammation in mild acute T cell-mediated rejection. Note that the inflammation is confined and the surrounding areas show normal acini. Acinar cell inflammation is not significant.

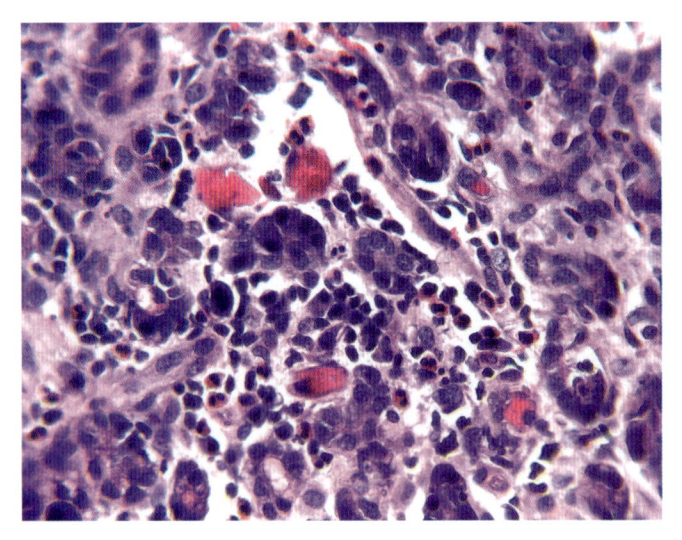

Figure 7.34B High power view of an inflammatory focus demonstrating the intimate association between the activated appearing inflammatory infiltrates and the acinar cells. The inflammation is mixed, composed of lymphocytes, eosinophils, and some plasma cells.

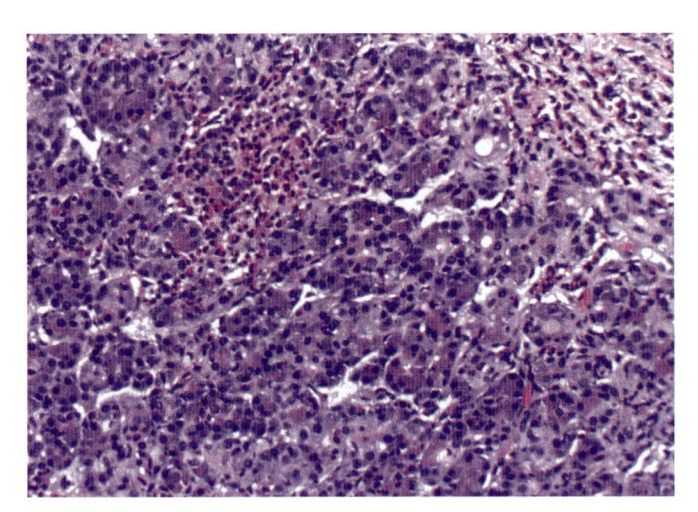

Figure 7.35 Septal and acinar inflammation in acute T cell-mediated allograft rejection with a predominance of eosinophils.

hyperacute rejection with immediate graft destruction through diffuse arterial and venous wall necrosis and associated thrombosis. Routine pre-transplant crossmatching has effectively eliminated this entity from clinical practice. In pancreas allografts, the recognition of *hyperacute rejection* has been obscured by the high propensity of this organ for early graft thrombosis that may or may not be related to rejection [37, 162]. Sibley [118] first described a case of hyperacute rejection in a patient with a negative pretransplant crossmatch, but high-level panel-reactive antibody (PRA) when retested after the removal of the thrombosed organ. Similar cases were described later, with graft loss occurring either immediately (*hyperacute rejection*) or within hours post-transplantation in which circulating DSA were also identified retrospectively in the setting of an initially negative cytotoxic crossmatches [37]. The features of severe, irreversible AMR have been studied in experimental models of hyperacute rejection. Edema, congestion, spotty acinar cell injury (i.e., vacuolization, degranulation, and necrosis), and capillary and venular neutrophilic margination occur within minutes of revascularization. Graft destruction occurs within a few hours and is characterized by confluent hemorrhagic necrosis in acini, islets and ducts, prominent neutrophilic infiltrates, and widespread fibrinoid vascular necrosis and thrombosis (see Figure 7.43) [103]. Immunoglobulin (IgG) and complement deposition including C4d staining can be found outlining necrotic arteries and veins [37].

Acute AMR – – Most cases of acute AMR are diagnosed in the first six months post-transplantation (75%), but late AMR is not unusual [78, 79, 110, 111, 113, 143, 158, 163–165]. Graft dysfunction, most commonly exocrine abnormalities (increase in serum amylase/lipase or decrease in urine amylase levels), is the

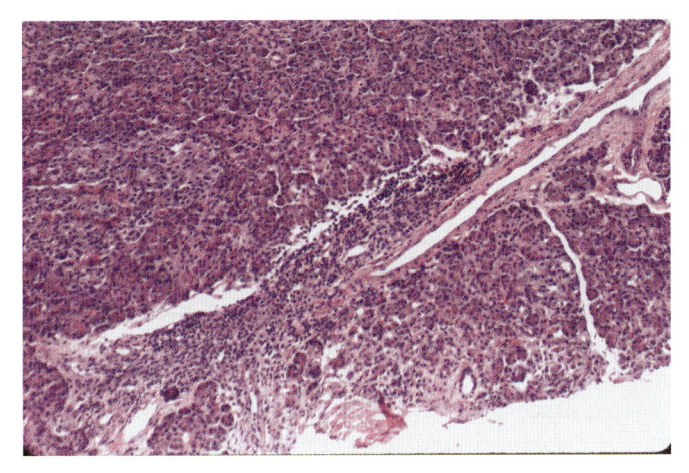

Figure 7.36 Early T cell-mediated acute allograft rejection with inflammation mostly confined to the connective tissue septa.

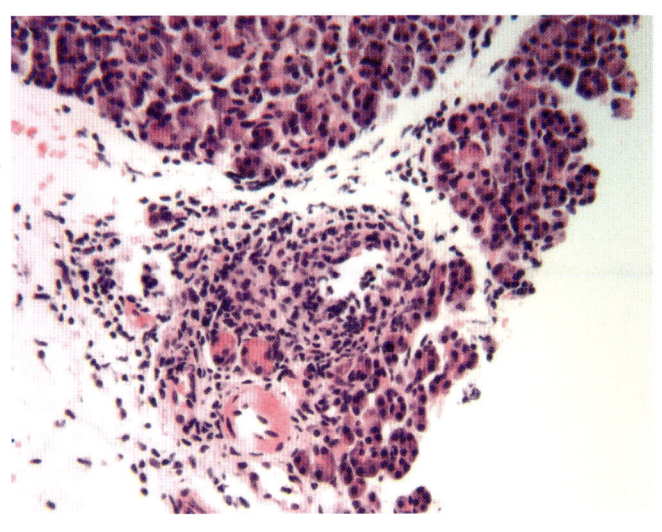

Figure 7.37 Typical example of venulitis, characterizing early cell-mediated acute allograft rejection.

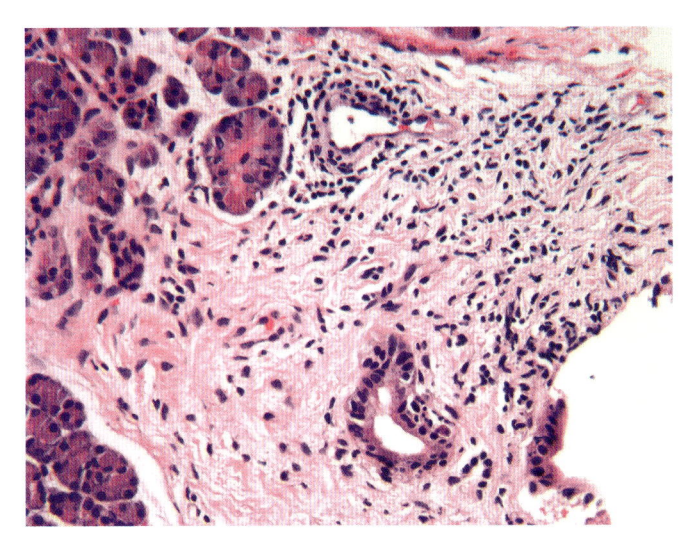

Figure 7.38A Mild cell-mediated acute allograft rejection. There is mild cuffing of the vein, but the predominant lesion is ductitis with prominent cell damage, including apoptosis (lower right of center) and epithelial sloughing in the larger duct.

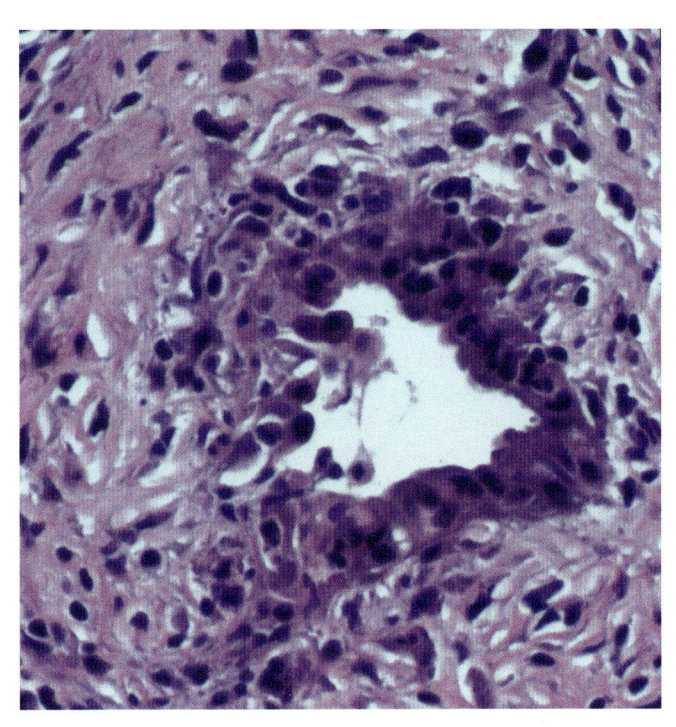

Figure 7.38B Ductitis in acute T cell-mediated rejection. Epithelial cell degeneration and reactive/regenerative atypia is noted in association with the intraepithelial inflammation.

indication for allograft biopsy in 55%–70% of cases followed by combined exocrine and endocrine abnormalities (15%–20%). Isolated endocrine dysfunction (hyperglycemia) appears to be a relatively rare indication for allograft biopsy (6%–8%) in the setting of acute AMR [110, 111, 113, 143, 158]. From the clinical point of view, ACMR and acute AMR cannot be distinguished from each other, hence the importance of DSA monitoring and biopsy evaluation. The unusual association between AMR and pancreatic panniculitis has been reported [165].

Chronic Active AMR –– Chronic exposure to circulating DSA was suspected in one of the first cases of documented pancreatic AMR [78] in which the predominant findings were graft fibrosis leading to graft failure. The diagnosis of *chronic active AMR* is based on the triad: (i) morphological features of acute AMR (two or three AMR diagnostic components, Table X), (ii) absence of features of ACMR, and (iii) underlying graft fibrosis (BANFF diagnostic category X). In the strict sense, use of this diagnostic category indicates that graft fibrosis or graft loss is attributed primarily to ongoing AMR, and therefore requires that other causes of graft fibrosis/sclerosis are ruled out, such as previous episodes of ACMR (acute T cell-mediated rejection). In clinical practice, a combination of chronic T cell-mediated rejection and chronic active AMR may occur together and a completely accurate determination of the main cause of graft fibrosis or loss may require evaluation of serial allograft biopsies.

Distortion of the lobular architecture with partial obliteration of the microvasculature secondary to interstitial fibrosis and

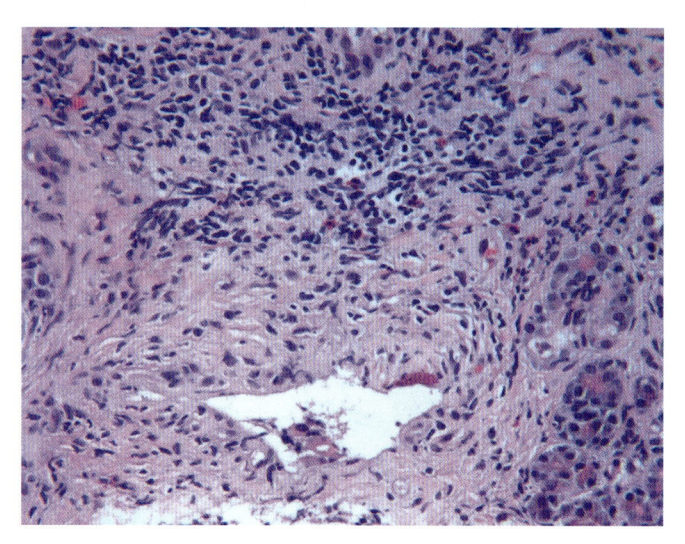

Figure 7.38C Marked epithelial damage secondary to acute T cell-mediated allograft rejection resulted in sloughing of the ductal epithelium. Only a few epithelial cells with reactive changes are noted in the lower segment of the ductal circumference.

acinar atrophy is characteristic of chronic active AMR. C4d stain positivity, however, is typically identified in residual IAC, often highlighting some recognizable underlying lobular architecture (see Figure 7.44). Vascular fibrinoid necroses, with recent or organized thrombosis, are findings supportive of ongoing antibody-mediated rejection. As with all situations where humoral rejection is suspected, correlation with the presence of donor-specific antibodies is required for diagnosis [78, 79, 101, 141].

Mixed ACMR and AMR — A significant proportion of biopsies with C4d positivity and documented DSA also show generalized increase in interstitial inflammation in septa and acini, as well as edema that strongly suggest a mixed rejection reaction (T cell-mediated and antibody-mediated [110]). In clinical practice, cases of stereotypical isolated AMR or ACMR can be classified by a systematic evaluation of the various features described in Table 7.1; however, it is not unusual for the two processes to coexist in the same biopsy (mixed rejection) and appear with overlapping features. In these situations, it is important that the pathology report clearly indicates the type of rejection present (AMR, ACMR, or mixed), estimates the degree of activity (mild, moderate, or severe) of each process, and indicates the extent of fibrosis (stage) [166].

BANFF Category 5: Chronic Allograft Arteriopathy
Except for necrotizing transmural arteritis, arterial inflammation was considered to be an expression of T cell-mediated rejection [104]. Recent studies, however, have shown that intimal arteritis and arterial lesions overall are often associated with DSA and AMR [167–170].

This category is defined by the presence of "active transplant arteriopathy" characterized by narrowing of the arterial lumen by a subendothelial proliferation of fibroblasts, myofibroblasts, and smooth muscle cells with superimposed evidence of ongoing inflammatory activity. The latter consists of infiltration of the subintimal fibrous proliferation by mononuclear cells, typically T cells and macrophages (see Figure 7.5). Although rarely seen in needle biopsies due to sampling issues, this lesion is consistently present in pancreatectomies from failed grafts due to chronic rejection [37, 171].

The entity of active transplant arteriopathy is included in the grading schema because according to clinical and experimental studies, this lesion is likely intermediate between intimal arteritis and inactive chronic transplant arteriopathy, both of which are associated with shortened graft survival in all solid organ transplants. The extent of the histological changes and the amount of inflammatory infiltrates appears to correlate with suboptimal immunosuppression [171]. The identification of this lesion has clinical impact potentially, as the process of ongoing vascular injury leading to further arterial narrowing may be halted with optimization of the immunosuppression treatment [101]. Chronic allograft arteriopathy increases the risk of late graft thrombosis and graft loss [37].

BANFF Category 6: Chronic Allograft Rejection/Graft Sclerosis
Histological grading of chronic rejection/graft sclerosis in the pancreas has been shown to correlate with graft survival; i.e., mild fibrosis is associated with lengthy graft survival, and severe fibrosis heralds a limited time of remaining graft function [80]. Furthermore, despite its notoriously patchy nature, the progression of pancreas allograft fibrosis can be reliably assessed in core biopsies through a semiquantitative grading schema that is both simple and reproducible. Grading is based on the semiquantitative determination of the proportion of sclerotic/fibrotic areas versus the remaining acinar/lobular tissue [80].

Three grades are recognized in this diagnostic category: mild graft sclerosis-Chronic Grade I; moderate graft sclerosis-Chronic Grade II; and severe graft sclerosis-Chronic Grade III, based on the identification of <30, 30–60, and >60% of fibrosis in the biopsy core, respectively (see Figures 7.45–7.46).

Transplant arteriopathy closely parallels the degree of fibrosis. Despite their major physiopathological importance, the vascular lesions are not used for grading of chronic rejection/graft sclerosis, because vascular disease that is fully appreciated in pancreatectomy specimens appears only sporadically in needle core biopsies [172]. Similarly, evaluation of endocrine islets is not used for grading because their disappearance does not follow a predictable course in relationship to that of graft fibrosis [131].

Inflammatory infiltrates associated with ongoing acinar cell injury, venulitis, and/or ductal inflammation indicate active T cell-mediated allograft rejection. Arterial inflammation (intimal arteritis, transmural arteritis, transplant arteriopathy) is also diagnostic of ongoing rejection and thought to be associated with both ACMR and AMR [167–169]. An attempt should be made to both grade acute rejection and stage chronic rejection/graft sclerosis based on the key histological features specified on each diagnostic category.

BANFF Category 7: Islet Pathology
Preservation of islet integrity and function is the main objective of pancreas transplantation. Unfortunately, a significant proportion of patients require insulin administration despite receiving a technically successful pancreas transplant. The main purpose of this category is the recognition of recurrent

Pancreas and Islet Transplantation Pathology

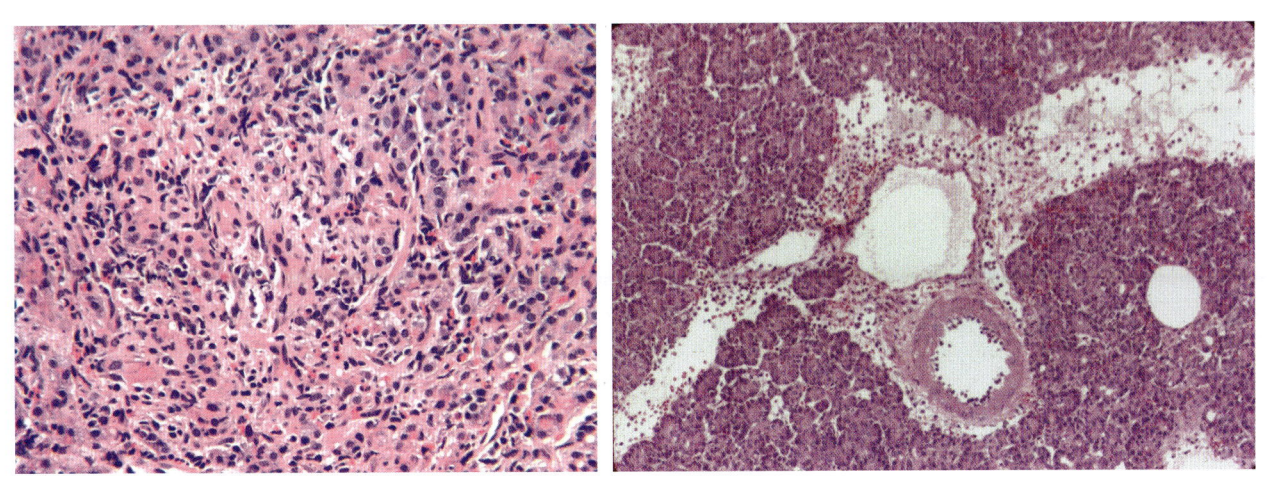

Figure 7.39 Moderate T cell-mediated allograft rejection defined by the presence of mild intimal arteritis. Marked septal edema and mild septal inflammation are also present.

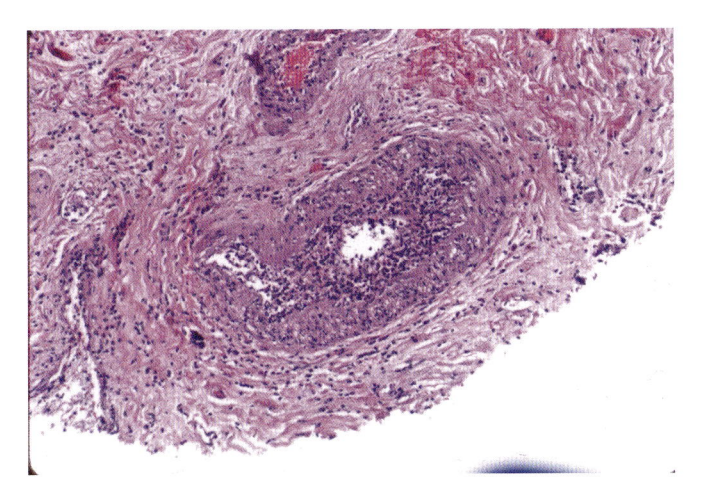

Figure 7.40 Severe intimal arteritis with marked narrowing of the lumen.

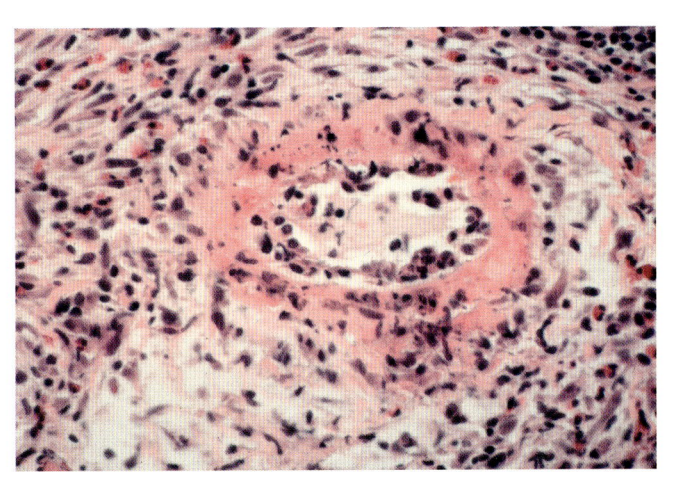

Figure 7.41 Severe acute T cell-mediated allograft rejection defined by arterial branch showing intimal arteritis, transmural inflammation, and fibrinoid necrosis. C4d stain was negative.

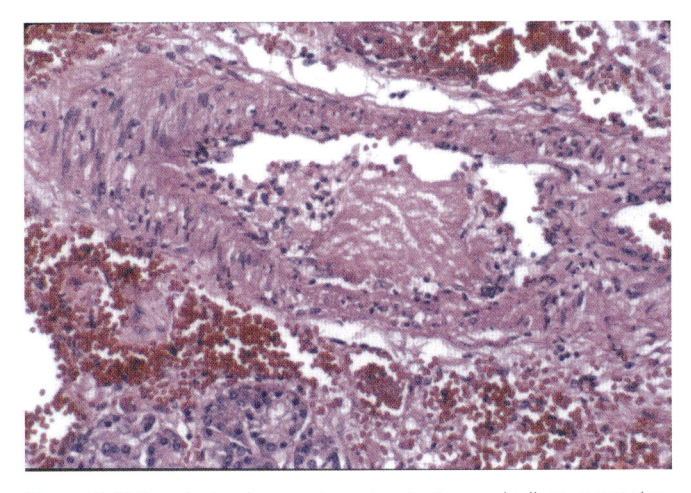

Figure 7.42 Vascular involvement in acute rejection markedly increases the risk of thrombosis as observed in this artery showing intimal arteritis (best appreciated in the extreme left of the vessel) and an associated recent thrombus.

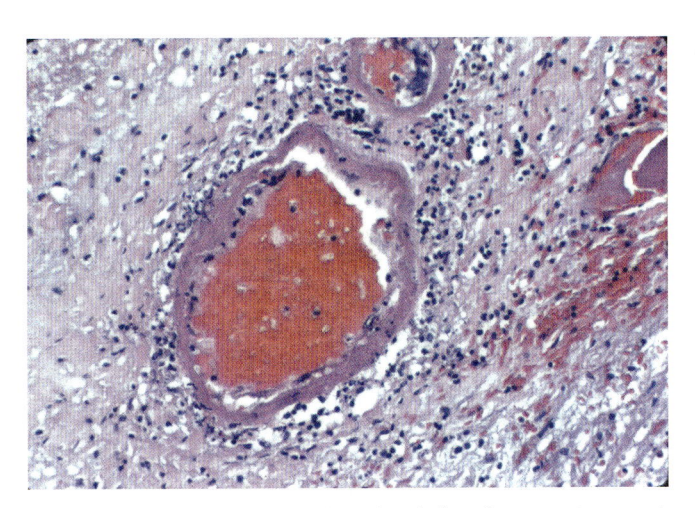

Figure 7.43A Severe acute antibody-mediated allograft rejection is rare and presents with acute graft failure within hours or days of transplantation. Histologically, there is diffuse fibrinoid necrosis of the vasculature and associated thrombosis as represented in the picture.

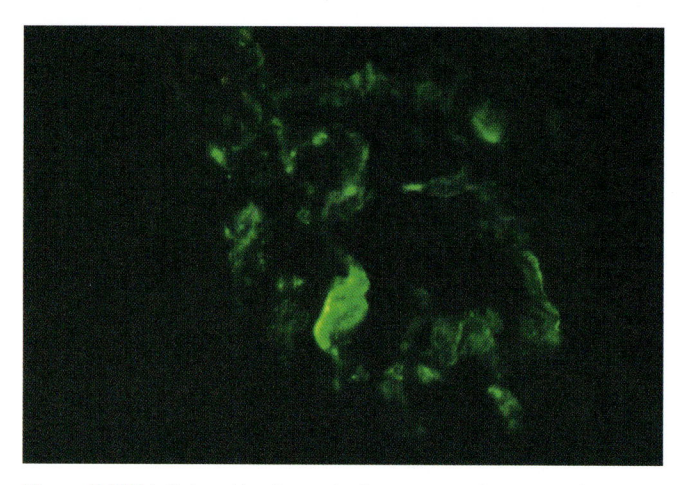

Figure 7.43B IgG deposition in arteries (same case as Figure 7.43A).

autoimmune diabetes mellitus (characterized by *insulitis (isletitis)* and/or *selective β cell loss*), deposition of *islet amyloid* (amylin), and islet cell *drug toxicity*. [166].

BANFF Category 8: Other Histological Diagnosis
A variety of other pathological processes affecting the pancreas allografts have histopathological manifestations. Identification of any of these processes may be achieved in isolation or concurrently with other diagnostic categories in the schema.

VII Other Forms of Pancreas Graft Pathology

Surgical Complications

Graft Thrombosis
Of the surgical complications that are grouped together under the category of technical failure (leaks, bleeding, thrombosis, infections, and pancreatitis), thrombosis continues to be the leading cause of non-immunological graft loss with higher rates seen in PAK and PTA cases with enteric drainage [17, 162].

Thrombosis in large- and medium-size vessels of the pancreas is routinely found in pancreatectomy specimens performed at any time post-transplantation [37]. Pancreas graft thrombosis occurs in different settings, including:

Thrombosis in Otherwise Normal Pancreas: This is the prime example of early graft thrombosis leading to graft loss for "technical failure." In these grafts, the only pathological changes consist of recent vascular thrombosis and bland ischemic parenchymal necrosis. There is no underlying vascular pathology or any other specific histological change [37] (see Figure 7.47). Lack of obvious histological changes does not rule out ultrastructural or subtle functional damage in these organs, since older donor age and longer cold ischemia times are associated with increased risk for early thrombosis. The pancreas has intrinsically a low blood flow compared to other solid organs. Perioperative inflammation and edema, as well as microvascular and endothelial damage relating to donor/procurement factors and organ preservation, all contribute to further compromise of the blood flow. Similarly, factors associated with ischemic pancreatitis (see below), such as longer cold ischemia times, have been associated with increased incidence of early graft thrombosis [17, 162].

- *Thrombosis in association with acute rejection* may occur at any time post-transplantation and is typically the result of vascular injury due to cell-mediated acute rejection (see Figures 7.42 and 7.43). Accordingly, the most common underlying lesion in this form of thrombosis is intimal arteritis. More unusual is the presence of underlying transmural inflammation and/or necrotizing arteritis. Thrombosis is also a characteristic feature of the different variants of humoral rejection, including the so-called accelerated rejection described above.

- *Late graft thrombosis* is a recognized cause of late graft loss. This process is also associated to underlying vascular pathology that may be immune-mediated (acute or chronic active cell-mediated vascular rejection) or may be non–immune-related (i.e., atherosclerosis) [37].

Post-transplantation (Ischemic) Pancreatitis
A significant number of patients with pancreas transplants require early re-laparotomy due to surgical complications. The most common reasons for re-laparotomy are intra-abdominal infections and graft pancreatitis, pancreas graft thrombosis, and anastomotic leak. The need for re-laparotomy is associated with a decrease in patient and graft survival [173].

Graft pancreatitis in the early post-transplantation period is secondary to ischemic injury, which causes dissolution of the cellular structures and spillage of pancreatic cell contents leading to acute inflammation. The incidence and severity of graft pancreatitis correlates with the length of cold ischemia time and is directly related to disturbances of the microcirculation in the reperfusion period [174–178]. Grafts from older donors appear to have a higher probability to develop graft pancreatitis presumably due to vascular quality issues. Less common causes of graft pancreatitis are impairment of drainage of exocrine secretions [174–176].

The morphology of post-transplant graft pancreatitis is similar to that of native pancreatitis. The main histological features being infiltration by neutrophils and macrophages, enzymatic necrosis of fat and parenchyma, and edema of the interlobular septa [179]. The more severe forms of graft pancreatitis appear with extensive hemorrhagic necrosis (see Figure 7.48).

Ischemia-reperfusion injury not only plays an important role in the development of graft pancreatitis, but also appears to be causally related to vascular thrombosis after pancreas transplantation (see above). Massive thrombosis of large blood vessels is associated with extensive coagulation necrosis of the graft and rapid loss of graft function. On the other hand, thrombosis in small blood vessels is associated with patchy coagulation necrosis of acinar tissue. These findings may be subtle and do overlap with those of acute pancreatitis [37].

Mild ischemia-reperfusion injury can be identified histologically in most samples obtained within the first week post-transplantation. This is characterized by spotty acinar cells drop-out, spotty apoptosis, flattening of the acinar cells, and otherwise minimal inflammation [94, 178]. Another manifestation of ischemia is the present of marked acinar and islet cell

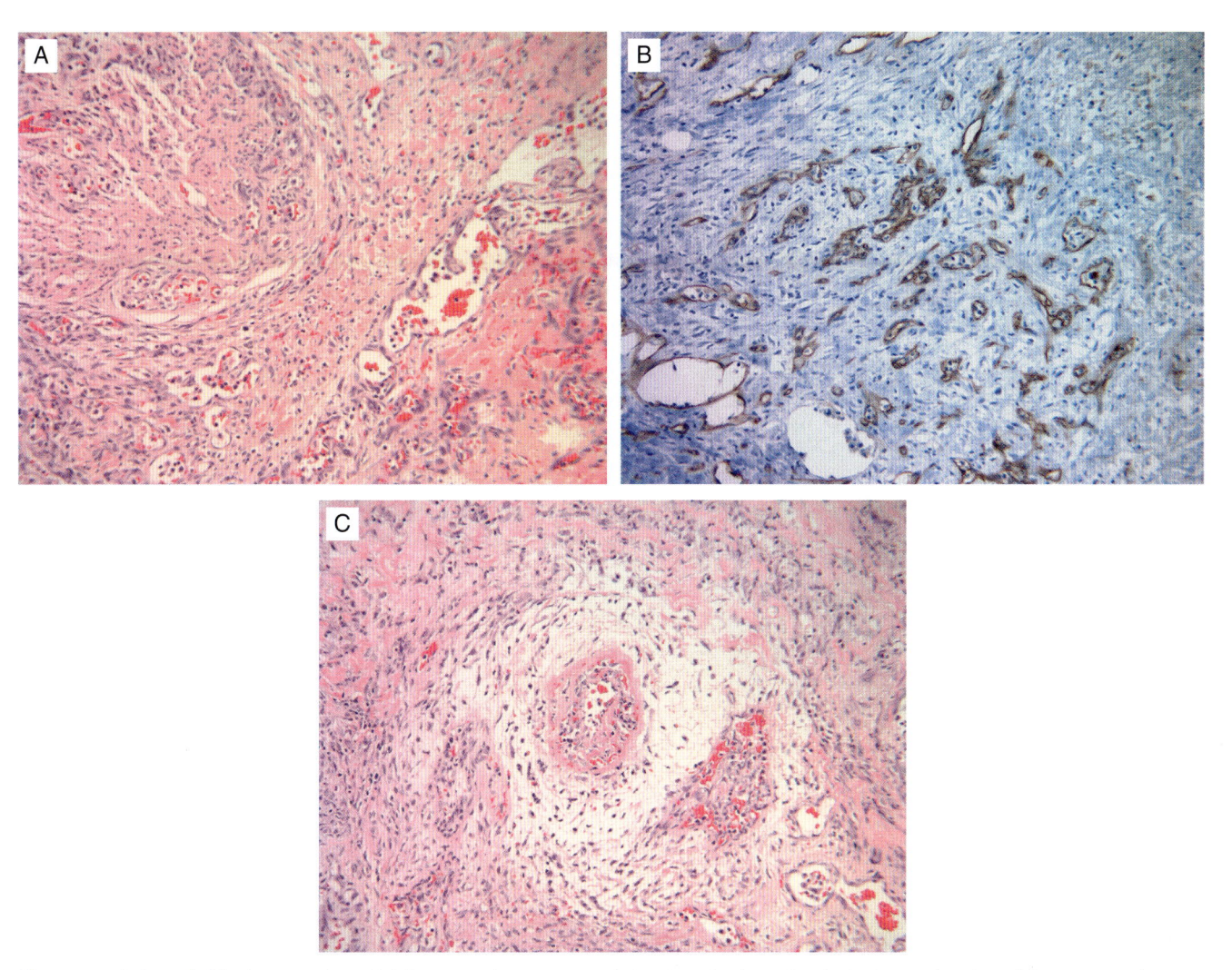

Figure 7.44A, B, and C Nephrectomy for graft failure secondary to acute and chronic antibody-mediated rejection resulting in graft loss two months post-transplantation. A: Complete loss of exocrine and endocrine structures with prominent residual vascular structures. B: C4d stains strongly the capillary-size vessels. C: Larger vessels showed fibrinoid necrosis and thrombosis with recanalization.

cytoplasmic swelling and vacuolization. In this setting, islet cell ballooning and spotty islet cell drop-out may occur that should be distinguished from islet drug toxicity [35].

Post-transplant Infectious Pancreatitis/Peripancreatitis/Fluid Collection/Peripancreatic Abscess

Infectious peripancreatitis is a relatively common early complication of pancreas transplantation, often secondary to ischemic graft pancreatitis [180–182] (see Figure 7.49).

Infected intra-abdominal fluid collections are treated conservatively with percutaneous drainage and antibiotics; however, abdominal exploration for drainage and debridement is often required [183, 184]. Needle biopsies obtained from the grafted pancreas during these surgical procedures show variable degrees of mixed inflammation, predominantly septally located. The inflammation is composed of lymphocytes, eosinophils, neutrophils, and less numerous plasma cells. A typical finding in these biopsies is the presence of dissecting bundles of active, tissue culture-like, connective tissue with abundant fibroblasts (see Figure 7.50). The fibrous bands run between the exocrine lobules, giving the biopsy a "cirrhotic" appearance. The fibrosis becomes more pronounced as time passes if the peripancreatic infected fluid collection persists [80]. The periphery of the acinar lobules usually shows some involvement by the inflammation. Typically, however, the acinar parenchyma per se shows proportionally little inflammation and acinar damage [130]. Correlation with microbiological studies is useful confirming the infectious nature of the process. It is important to remember that immunosuppression is often decreased in infected patients; therefore, concurrent acute rejection is not uncommon in biopsies from patients with intra-abdominal/peripancreatic abscesses. A high level of suspicion for concurrent acute rejection is warranted in this setting.

In the absence of acute rejection, septal fibrosis seen in biopsies from patients that require one or more re-laparotomies remains confined to the periphery (surface) of the graft and

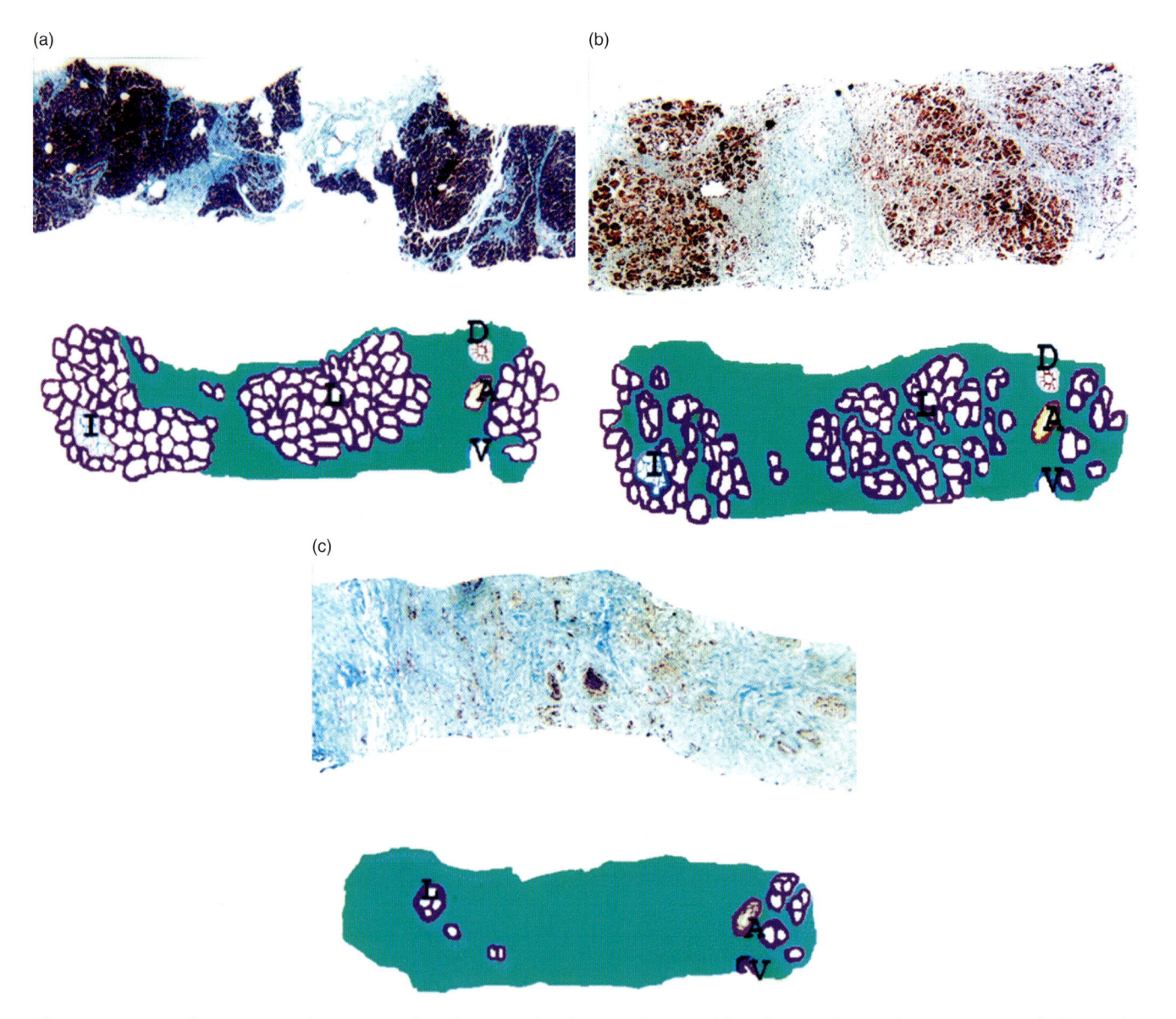

Figure 7.45 A, B, and C: Low power photomicrographs and corresponding diagrams showing mild, moderate, and severe chronic rejection/graft sclerosis (chronic Grades I, II, and III, respectively) characterized by progressive increase in fibrosis and acinar atrophy.

therefore superficial fibrotic biopsies may not represent the status of the whole organ.

Necrotizing infectious: Duodeno-pancreatitis with abscess formation can present at any time post-transplantation, but occurs often in the first months after transplantation. A variety of organisms can be cultured from these grafts, most commonly enterobacteria (Enterobacter cloacae, Proteus mirabilis) and Methicillin-resistant Staphylococcus aureus (MRSA). Fungal infections, more often from Candida sp. and mixed bacterial/fungal infection, are not uncommon [173, 184, 185]. Necrotizing pancreatitis can be rarely secondary to CMV infection [186].

Anastomotic Leak: Infection, ischemia, and poor surgical technique may lead to dehiscence of the anastomosis between the duodenal cuff and the urinary bladder or small intestine [173]. Pathological examination of grafts resected for this reason may show specific causes such as CMV-related perforation, or may only show nonspecific changes such as necrosis in the area around the anastomosis and acute inflammation. The adjacent peritoneal surfaces typically show acute fibrinous or purulent serositis.

Viral infections

Cytomegalovirus Infection

The use of newer more potent immunosuppressive drugs such as tacrolimus and mycophenolate mofetil are potentially associated with an increase in all types of infections (bacterial, fungal, and viral). Antiviral drugs are used prophylactically in many transplant centers to prevent CMV infection. There is evidence that prophylaxis for CMV delays the infection and reduces its severity [187–190].

Although the incidence of CMV disease in kidney-pancreas transplants may be up to 22% in donor positive-recipient negative cases, the actual diagnosis of CMV graft pancreatitis

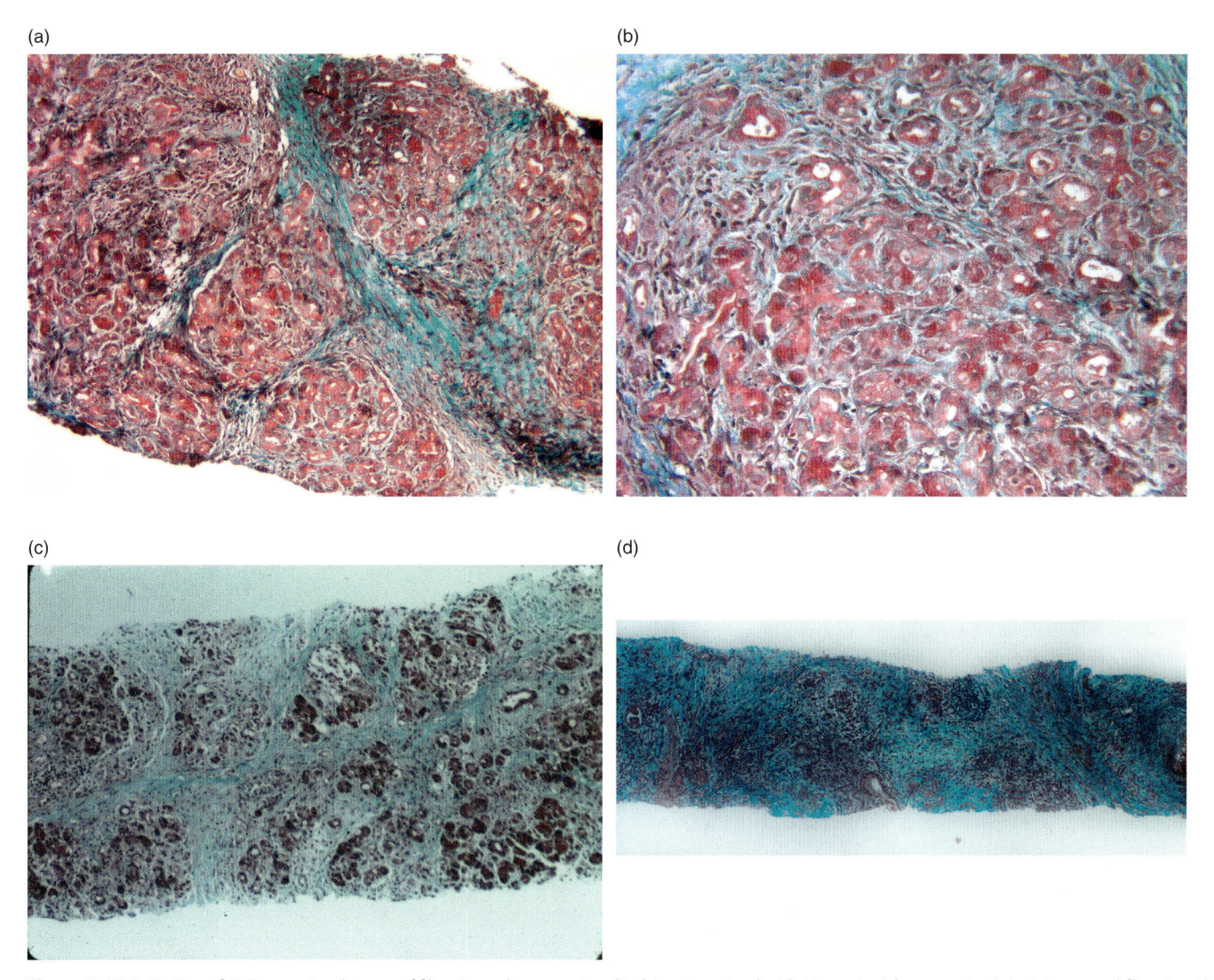

Figure 7.46 A, B, C, and D Progressive degrees of fibrosis can be appreciated in biopsies stained with Masson's trichrome stain. A: Incipient septal fibrosis with minimal extension to the acini. B: High power view of acinar area with incipient peri-acinar fibrosis. C: Moderate fibrosis with expansion of fibrous septa and "fragmentation" of the lobules due to periacinar and intraacinar fibrosis. D: Diffuse fibrosis with essential disappearance of the exocrine component and replacement by fibrous tissue and inflammatory infiltrates.

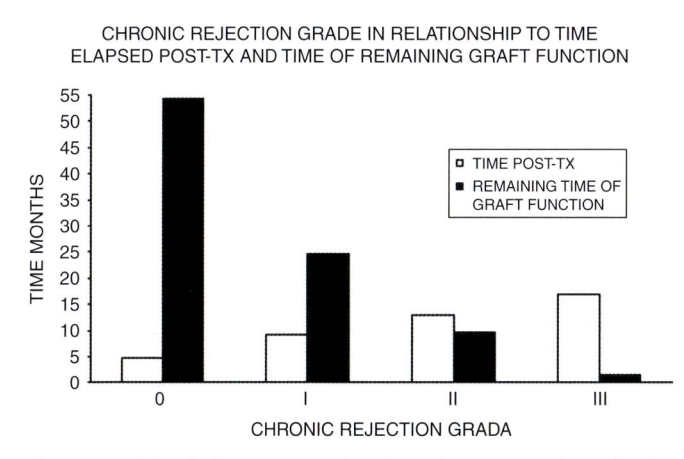

Figure 7.46E Graph demonstrating the relationship between the grade of chronic rejection/graft sclerosis and shortened graft survival.

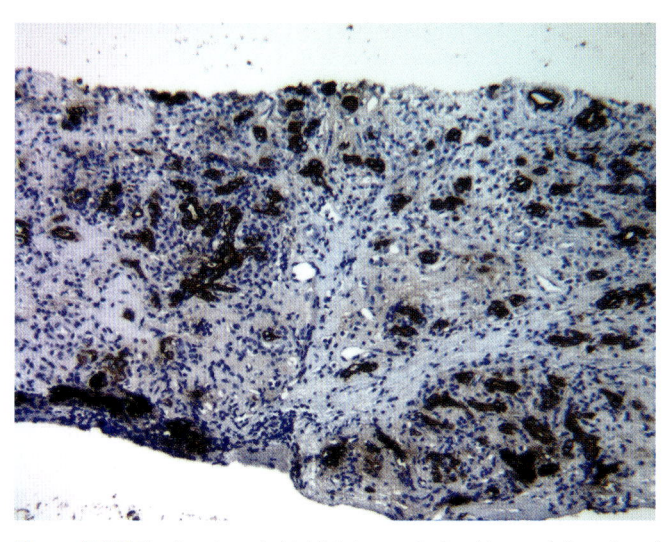

Figure 7.46F Cytokeratin stain highlighting marked architectural distortion of the exocrine parenchyma that mainly consists of residual ductules.

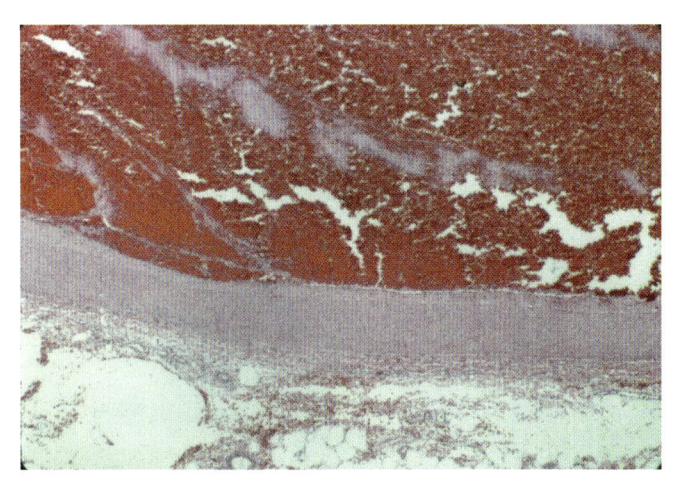

Figure 7.47 Thrombosed artery due to "technical failure." The arteries were normal except for the presence of recent thrombi. The patient underwent pancreatectomy 24 hours post-transplantation.

is rare. Klassen et al., reported biopsy proven CMV pancreatitis in four patients. The diagnosis was made 18 weeks to 44 months after transplantation. With prolonged ganciclovir treatment, clinical and histological resolution of the infection was achieved in all patients [136].

The clinical presentation of CMV graft pancreatitis is indistinguishable from acute rejection, e.g. increase in serum amylase and lipase. Similarly, on percutaneous needle biopsies, both acute allograft rejection and mild CMV pancreatitis may present with modest, predominantly lymphocytic acinar inflammation [136]. In addition, venous endothelial inflammation resembling venulitis may also occur in CMV infection. Eosinophils are more common in rejection, but may be present in small numbers in CMV infection as well. Neutrophils may be present in association with areas of necrosis or acinar cell damage in both rejection and CMV pancreatitis. Due to the morphological similarities between rejection and CMV infection, evidence of viral cytopathic changes should be sought systematically in all graft biopsies, independently of the clinical setting (see Figure 7.51). Multiple tissue sections and CMV stains should be performed if deemed necessary to rule out the viral infection [136].

Severe cases of CMV infection may present with intractable gastrointestinal hemorrhage and/or duodenal-cuff perforation [187–190]. Necrotizing CMV infection with abscess formation [191] and development of a CMV-related arterio-venous fistula [192] have been reported.

EBV-related Post-transplant Lymphoproliferative Disorder

PTLD occurs in 1%–3% of pancreas transplant recipients [193–197]. Most PTLD are EBV-related, and of B cell lineage. The time of occurrence after transplantation appears to depend on the intensity of immunosuppression and varies from few weeks to several years after transplantation. Very rare PTLD are of T cell lineage and these tend to occur later after transplantation [198].

EBV-related PTLD include a wide range of processes from benign hyperplastic, to overtly malignant lymphoid proliferations. On the most benign end of the spectrum (plasmacytic hyperplasia), the patients present with generalized types of symptoms and lymphadenopathy rather than with graft dysfunction, and therefore, graft biopsies usually play no role in the diagnostic work up. Graft involvement is not unusual in the other forms of PTLD (polymorphic B cell hyperplasia/lymphoma, immunoblastic lymphoma), as previously reported in the kidney. Graft involvement by monomorphic PTLD/lymphoma is recognized by the presence of monomorphic atypical immunoblasts of B cell lineage. Extensive parenchymal infiltration and geographic areas of necrosis are common in these cases [198] (see Figure 7.52).

Polymorphic PTLD, on the other hand, may be difficult to differentiate from acute cellular rejection. The differentiation between the two processes is very difficult in the earlier stages of polymorphic PTLD, particularly if there is a component of concurrent acute rejection [193]. Evaluation of T and B cell markers (e.g., CD3, CD20) can aid by the identification of the predominant cellular component in different areas of the biopsy. Acute rejection is characterized by a predominant population of T cells (typically more than 75%) and a minor population of B cells that form aggregates no larger than 200–300 microns. In contrast, the identification of large, confluent, nodular B cell aggregates are consistent with graft involvement by PTLD [193]. The presence of marked cytological atypia in infiltrates predominantly composed of immunoblastic and plasmacytoid cells also favors PTLD. Eosinophils are present in variable proportions both in acute rejection and in PTLD. Immunoglobulin light chain restriction can be demonstrated in patients with polymorphic B cell hyperplasia and is typically found in lymphoma.

EBV-related PTLD is confirmed with in-situ hybridization for EBV encoded RNAs (EBER) that mark a significant proportion of the atypical cells. Also, stains for LMP-1 (EBV latent membrane protein) are usually positive in a variable proportion of the cells (see Figure 7.52).

Other minor features of pancreas allograft involvement by EBV-related PTLD have been described. All sizes of veins are consistently infiltrated by the atypical B cells with associated lifting and damage of the endothelium similar to that seen in acute rejection. Also, nerves and adjacent soft tissues are usually extensively infiltrated by the lymphoproliferative process. With respect to the arteries, if concurrent T cell-mediated rejection is present in the form of intimal arteritis, the subendothelial infiltrates are predominantly composed of T cells, in contrast to the predominant population of B cells seen in the areas of PTLD. In the absence of vascular rejection, the arterial walls appear to be consistently resistant to permeation by the atypical B cell infiltrates.

Lastly, the random involvement seen in cases of PTLD with areas of parenchyma that may be completely free of infiltrates contrasts with the more diffuse involvement of the pancreas seen in the severe forms of T cell-mediated acute rejection [33, 193].

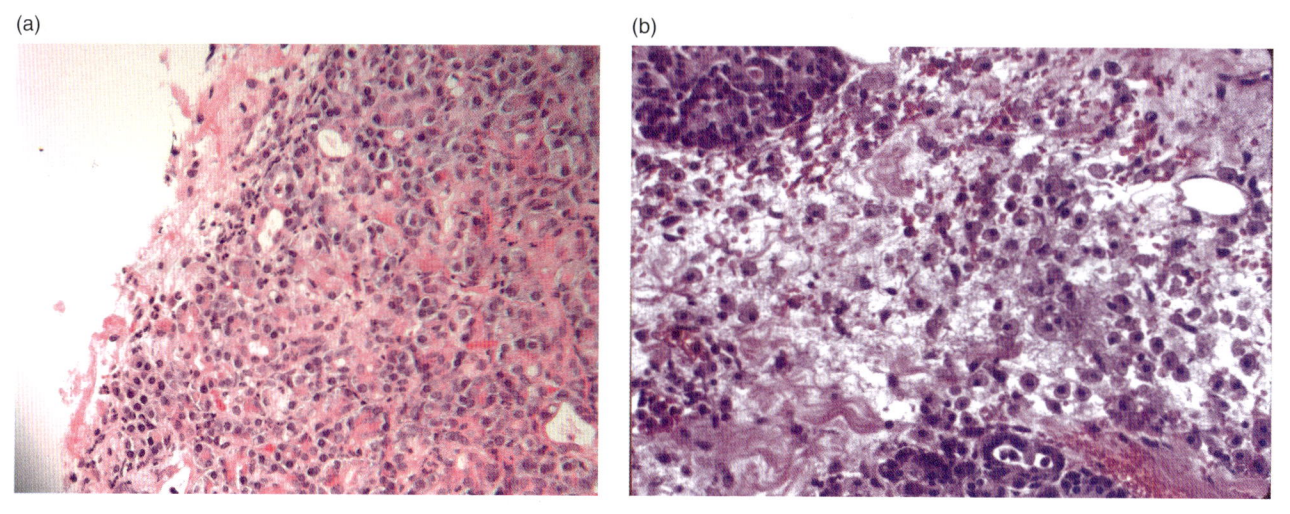

Figure 7.48A and B Ischemic pancreatitis A: Mild ischemic pancreatitis characterized by clusters of neutrophils in the connective tissue septa and nearby acini. B: More pronounced acute pancreatitis shows areas of fat necrosis with scattered lipid-laded macrophages, septal (interstitial) edema, and patchy hemorrhages.

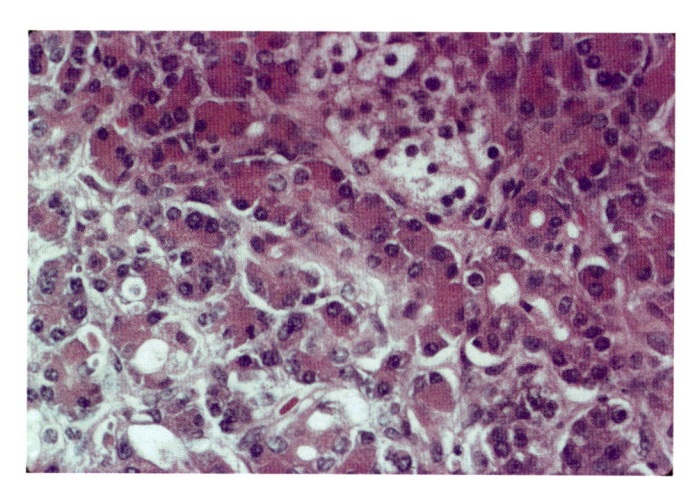

Figure 7.48C Ischemic injury is manifested as acinar and islet cell vacuolization with spotty cell drop-out. The acinar changes are better appreciated in the bottom half of the image.

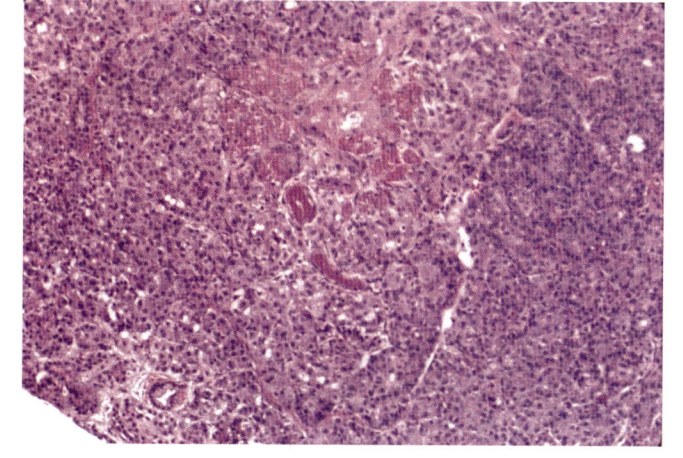

Figure 7.48D Ischemic injury and ischemic pancreatitis are associated with an increased risk of thombosis. Focal acinar necrosis with thrombosis of small associated vessels was found in this needle core biopsy performed 48 hours before pancreatectomy showing diffuse arterial and venous thrombosis, but no evidence of T cell-mediated or humoral rejection.

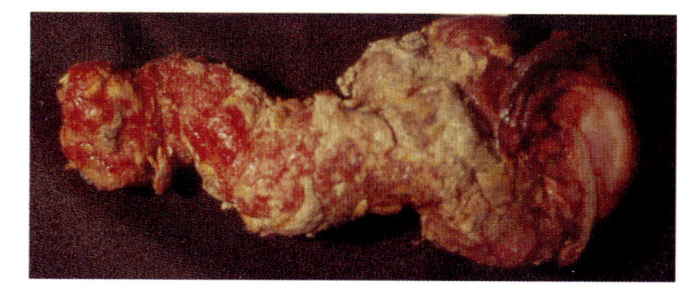

Figure 7.49 Graft pancreatectomy for severe bacterial peripancreatitis and extensive formation of peripancreatic abscesses.

Islet Graft Pathology

Nonspecific Islet Pathology

There is no experimental or clinical evidence that the endocrine islets are targeted in T cell-mediated alloimmune reactions. Islet pathology in acute and chronic allograft rejection is in essence nonspecific, secondary to the overall degree of acute parenchymal injury and ensuing fibrosis/sclerosis [80]. The pathological findings consist of islet inflammation and occasional necrosis, in a degree proportional to the severity of acute rejection. The inflammation is therefore random and the cells infiltrating the islets are similar to the surrounding inflammatory infiltrates, more or less representing a "spillover" phenomenon [108, 130].

In long-term pancreas allografts, islet distribution and morphology to a large extent reflect ongoing injury and repair. Extensive collagenization in chronic rejection leads to fragmentation of exocrine lobules as well as of islets that acquire irregular shapes and may consist of only few cell clusters with irregular distribution, nevertheless still containing a mixture of both insulin and glucagon producing cells. Conversely, in some grafts, aggregates of large but otherwise normal appearing islets

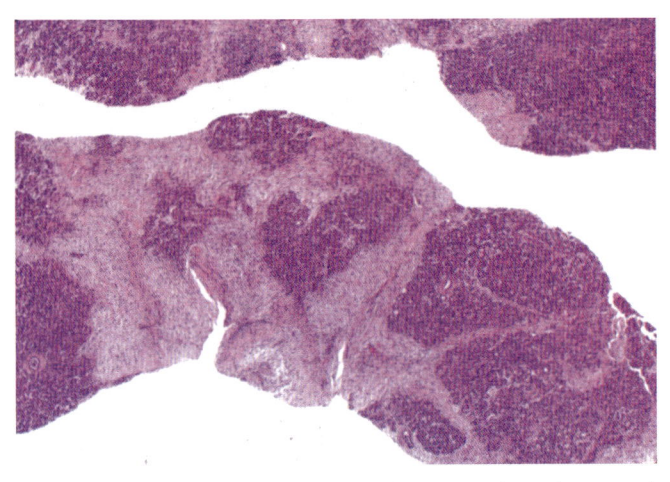

Figure 7.50 Biopsies obtained at the time of laparotomy for exploration and "wash-out" in patients with peripancreatic infections or fluid collections often show reactive changes in the pancreatic parenchyma. These consist of active fibroblastic proliferation of fibrous septa that may appear markedly expanded, separating adjacent exocrine lobules.

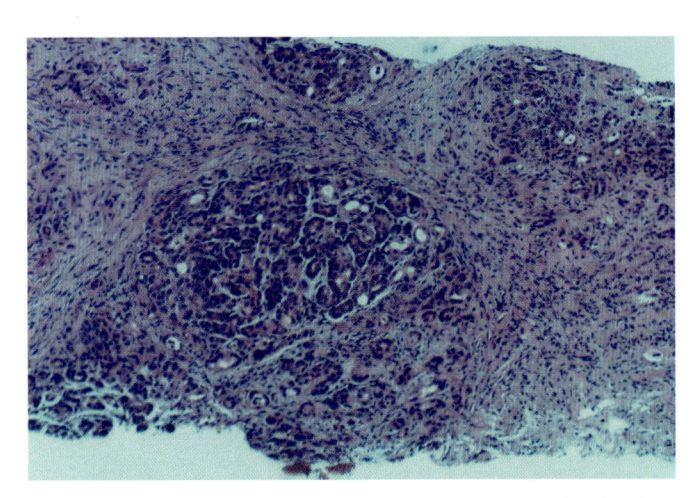

Figure 7.50B The areas of pancreas in the periphery of the graft and in direct continuity with the infection may become atrophic in a manner that may resemble chronic rejection/graft sclerosis. The most important distinguishing factor is the clinical history (i.e., recent transplantation and evidence of peripancreatic infection or fluid collection).

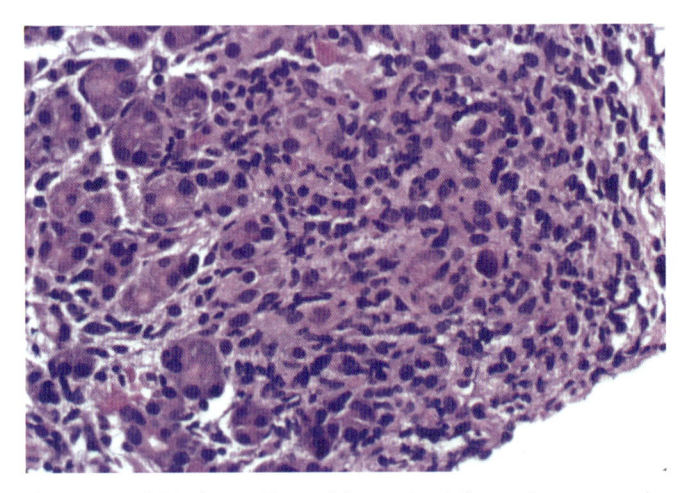

Figure 7.51 CMV infection. Focus of dense acinar inflammation composed predominantly of mononuclear cells (lymphocytes and macrophages). The viral cytopathic changes are subtle (note occasional atypical nuclei center right). Careful search for viral cytopathic changes is necessary in any transplant biopsy before a diagnosis of rejection is rendered.

may reflect compensatory hyperplasia [109]. Insulinomas or other islet cell tumors have not been described in pancreas allografts [199]. Islet cell atypia, hyperchromasia is seen in less than 5% of cases independently of the cause of the biopsy and is of unknown etiology or significance [108].

Recurrence of Type I Diabetes Mellitus

Type 1 diabetes is an autoimmune disease that can as such recur after pancreas transplantation. Recurrence of autoimmune disease is, however, a rare process that has been documented in approximately a dozen cases [135, 200, 201]. This process is characterized by selective autoimmune-mediated destruction of beta cells in an analogous manner as occurs in Type 1 diabetes in the native pancreas. The diagnosis of recurrent disease is made with the combination of sudden or progressive lack of glycemic control associated with selective loss of the insulin producing beta cells in the graft and persistence of the other types of islet cells, particularly the glucagon-producing alpha cells. In few cases, the active phase of beta cell destruction has been demonstrated, consisting of mononuclear cell infiltration (isletitis) [201]. Similarly to the disease in the native pancreas, the inflammation is centered in islets still containing beta cells and the isletitis resolves when beta cells disappear. An additional similarity between the native and graft disease is the occasional accumulation of amorphous eosinophilic deposits composed of amylin, within the diseased islets [201, 202] (see Figure 7.53).

The first reported cases of recurrent diabetes mellitus occurred in transplants from identical twins or HLA-identical siblings that were non-immunosuppressed or received minimal immunosuppression. In non-immunosuppressed patients, disease recurrence occurred within weeks after transplantation. In some cases, isletitis resolved after introduction or increase in immunosuppression [34, 135]. HLA-mismatched transplants from cadaveric donors are also susceptible to recurrence of the autoimmune diabetes with selective beta cell destruction but this occurs rarely. The rarity of recurrent Type I diabetes mellitus in whole pancreas transplantation has been attributed to the inclusion of donor lymphoid tissue with the transplanted pancreas. This would lead to modulatory effects from recipient chimerism for a donor T cell subset (RT6.2) [203].

In addition to the clinical and histological findings, the diagnosis of recurrent autoimmune disease is aided by the demonstration of islet cell auto-antibodies in serum (GAD 65 and IA-2); however, these may also be found in patients with no clinical evidence of autoimmune disease recurrence. In a study comparing patients with chronic graft failure versus patients with well-functioning grafts, islet cell auto-antibodies before transplantation and at the time of graft failure were significantly higher in the former group. Also, patients with failed grafts showed an increase in auto-antibodies at the time of loss of graft function [204].

From the pathological point of view, it is important to emphasize that the active destructive phase consisting of

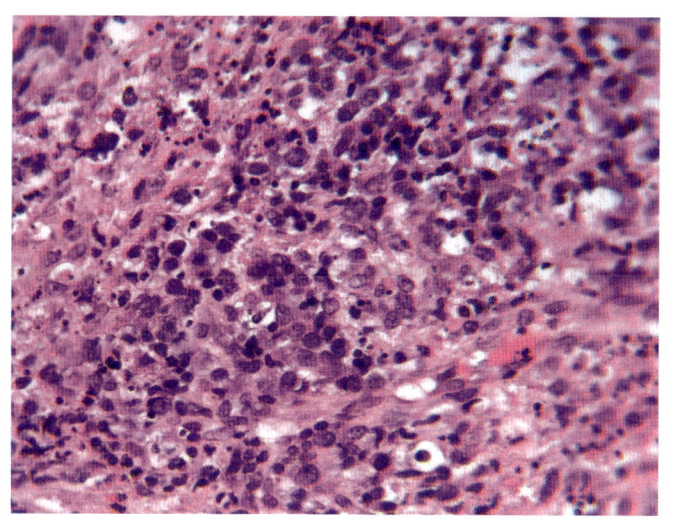

Pancreas and Islet Transplantation Pathology

Figure 7.52A EBV-related PTLD. Markedly atypical inflammation distending septal area. The presence of necrosis (abundant nuclear fragments) is helpful for the diagnosis of PTLD.

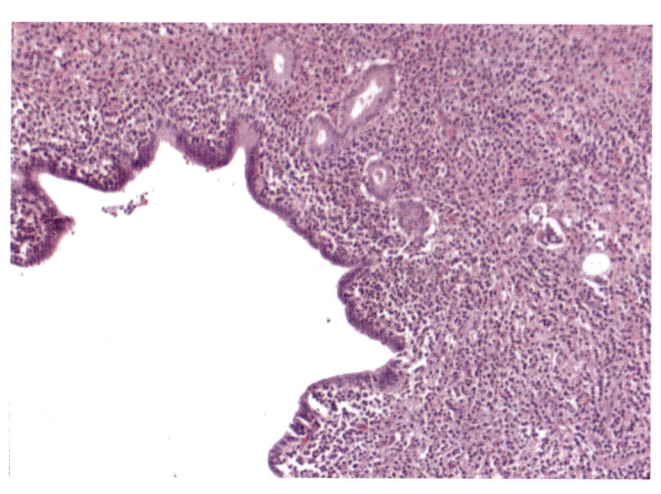

Figure 7.52B EBV-related PTLD. Pancreatic duct surrounded by dense inflammatory infiltrates.

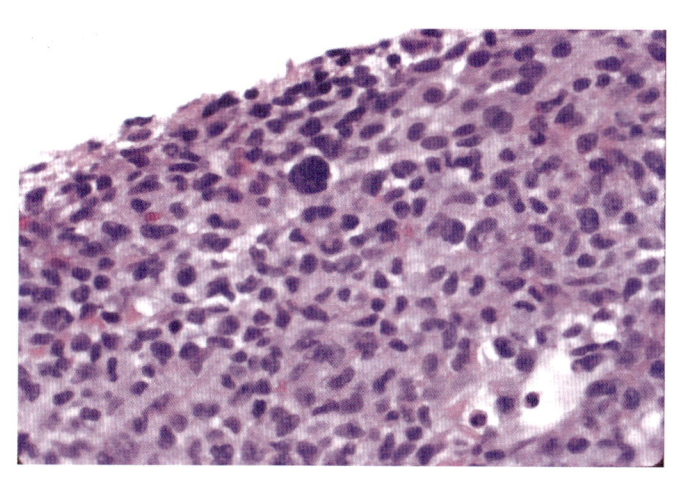

Figure 7.52C High magnification view of monomorphic EBV-related PTLD.

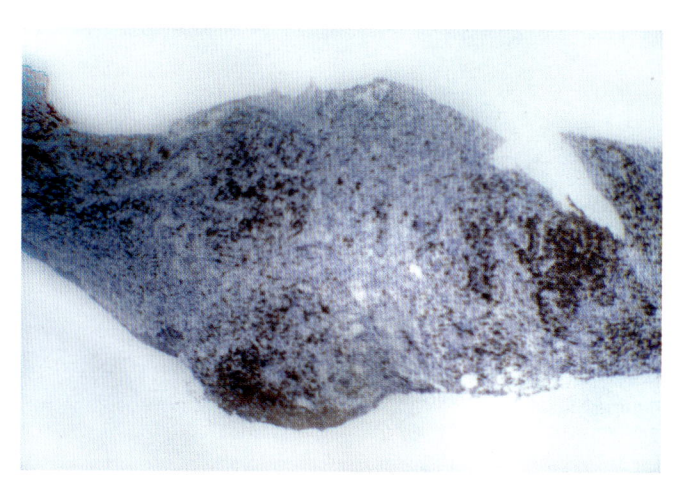

Figure 7.52D CD20 stain highlights large, nodular, and expansile B cell aggregates in a needle core biopsy from a patient with early graft involvement by EBV-related PTLD.

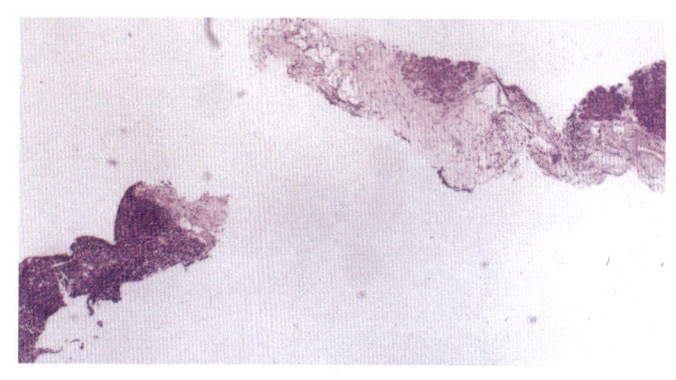

Figure 7.52E In rare occasions, pancreas transplant needle core biopsies may contain benign lymphoid tissue from the peripancreatic tissues (left lower corner) that should not be confused with a lymphoproliferative disorder.

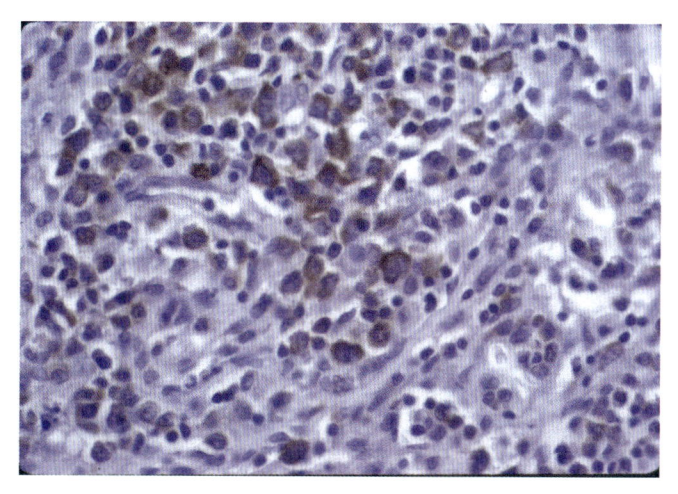

Figure 7.52F LMP-1 (EBV latent membrane protein-1) highlights numerous positive cells in a case of polymorphous EBV-related PTLD.

247

isletitis with progressive and selective loss of beta cells is transient and may be patchy. It is recommended that wedge biopsies be evaluated to avoid sampling errors. In the inactive phase (after the disappearance of beta cells and associated isletitis), the pancreas may look superficially normal or may show only minimal fibrosis. The diagnosis can only be made with the immunohistochemical demonstration of lack of insulin-insulin producing cells in islets [66–68, 205]. After a prolonged period of time, the islets as a whole can disappear [135, 206].

Islet Cell Drug Toxicity

In the pre-cyclosporine era, post-transplant diabetes mellitus occurred in almost half of renal transplant patients secondary to the use of large doses of corticosteroids. Older age, higher body weight, family history of abnormal glucose metabolism, and African-American or Hispanic descent are associated with higher incidence of post-transplant diabetes mellitus. The latter is believed to result from a combination of insulin resistance with a relative deficiency of insulin production. Insulin resistance results from decreased insulin receptor number and affinity, impaired glucose uptake, and probable inhibition on insulin secretion by beta cells [1].

The use of cyclosporine and tacrolimus has markedly improved the outcome in pancreas transplantation. In addition to nephrotoxicity, hirsutism/alopecia, neurological, and gastrointestinal side effects, both of these drugs can cause abnormalities in glucose metabolism. Hyperglycemia is more commonly seen in patients receiving tacrolimus.

In animal studies, cyclosporine administration has been associated with reduction in insulin secretion, diminished beta cell density, decreased insulin synthesis, and defective insulin secretion. Similar morphological findings have been seen also with tacrolimus [207]. The incidence of hyperglycemia in patients receiving cyclosporine and tacrolimus is reported to be 11%–19% and 15%–29% respectively. Most

Figure 7.52G In-situ hybridization for EBER (EBV encoded RNAs) is confirmatory of a diagnosis of EBV-related PTLD.

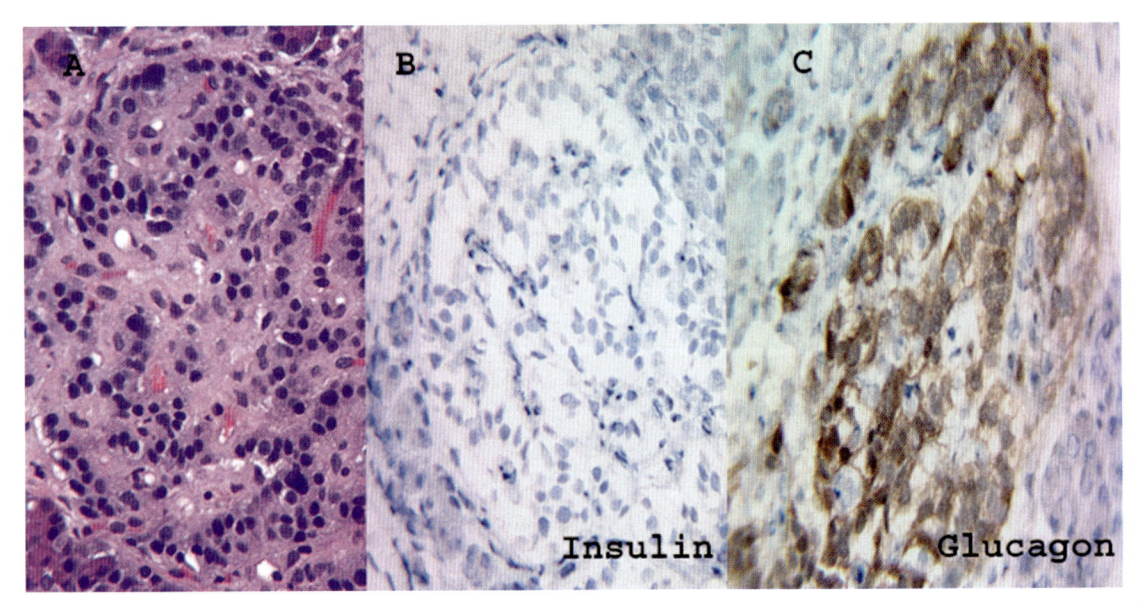

Figure 7.53A, B, and C Recurrence of diabetes mellitus in pancreas allograft. A: On Hematoxylin and Eosin stain, the islet is only remarkable for focal accumulation of amorphous eosinophilic material consistent with amylin as it occurs in diabetes mellitus in the native pancreas. The acinar tissue is normal. B: Negative insulin stain. The absence of isletitis is consistent with the complete loss of beta cells. C: Glucagon stain highlights remaining alpha cells that represent the vast majority of the islet cells.

Pancreas and Islet Transplantation Pathology

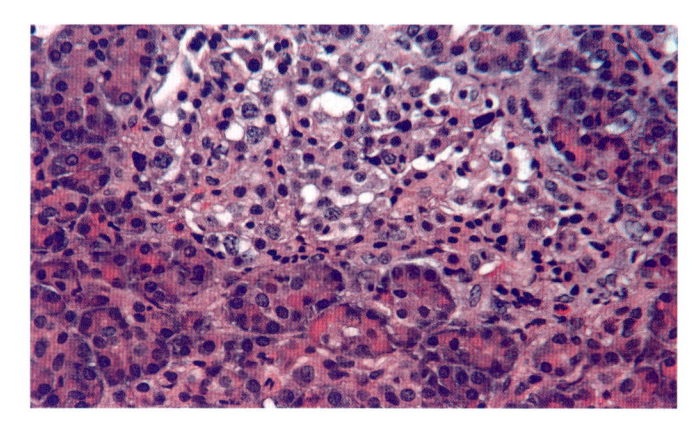

Figure 7.54A Calcineurin inhibitor islet cell toxicity is characterized by marked islet cell vacuolization and occasional islet cell apoptosis or drop-out. The biopsy was obtained in a patient presenting with hyperglycemia and high levels of FK506 (tacrolimus). Note lack of vacuolization of acinar cells and lack of inflammation.

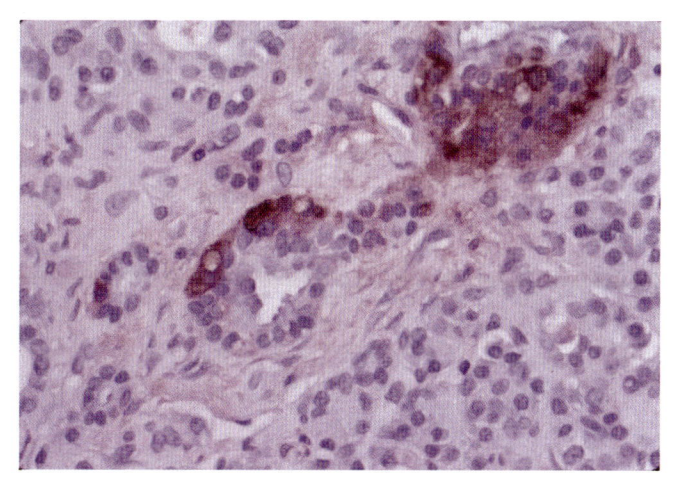

Figure 7.55 Nesidioblastosis. Insulin producing cells in pancreatic duct, appearing after severe ischemic injury. This likely represents a reactive/regenerative phenomenon.

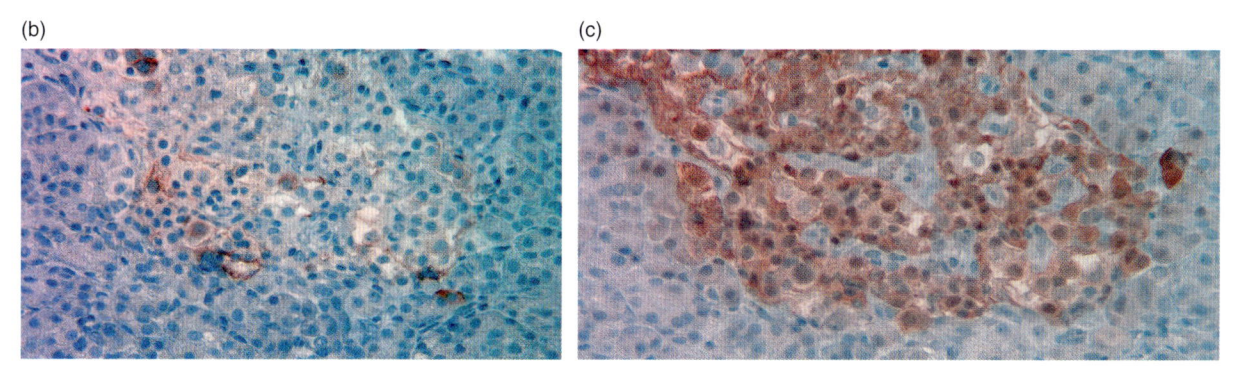

Figure 7.54B (Insulin stain) and C (Glucagon stain). A weak "washed-out" pattern of staining for insulin is seen in comparison to staining for glucagon.

patients had also received steroids and this represents a confounding factor [207].

The morphological findings in biopsies from patients with clinical evidence of drug toxicity consist of cytoplasmic swelling and vacuolization of islet cells. The islets appear optically clear and stand out from the more eosinophilic acinar parenchyma. In more severe cases, islet cell drop-out with formation of empty spaces (lacunae) can be seen if there is confluent islet cell drop-out. Rarely, intra-islet apoptotic cell fragments can be identified [35] (see Figure 7.54).

Immunoperoxidase stains for insulin and glucagon show diminished staining for insulin in beta cells in comparison to controls. This is the light microscopic counterpart of the marked loss of insulin dense core granules seen in beta cells by electron microscopy. The latter study shows preservation of the peripheral non-beta cells in the islets. The histological changes, as well as the clinical findings, are reversible with reduction or discontinuation of the drug. Hyperglycemia and the histological evidence of drug toxicity are worsened with the concurrent use of pulse steroids to treat acute rejection [35]. Islet toxicity should be less common under the current steroid sparing immunosuppression protocols.

Islet Amyloid

Islet deposition of Amylin (also known as islet amyloid polypeptide (IAPP)) can be demonstrated rarely in pancreas transplants with the Congo red stain. Amylin, a protein normally co-secreted with insulin by the beta cells, is present in the beta cell secretory granules together with C peptide [82]. In hyperglycemic states (i.e., Type 2 diabetes mellitus) with hyperinsulinemia, excessive secretion of IAPP leads to accumulation of insoluble aggregates in the form of amyloid. Deposition of amylin in otherwise normal pancreatic islets is usually associated with loss of glycemic control (hyperglycemia) [82, 208–210].

Nesidioblastosis

This is most likely a regenerative change leading to differentiation of adult pancreatic ductal epithelium into insulin-producing cells (see Figure 7.55). Nesidioblastosis was also demonstrated in one animal model of pancreas transplantation [211].

In systematic studies of pancreas graft biopsies, nesidioblastosis was found in approximately 4% of samples, with or without evidence of graft rejection. In most instances, the change was associated with documented previous injury (i.e., ischemic pancreatitis) and subsequent regenerative changes. The process had no discernible clinical significance [108, 109]. Nesidioblastosis has been associated with hypoglycemia in one report [212].

Duodenal Graft Pathology

In whole organ pancreas allografts, the exocrine drainage anastomosis is typically done through a segment of the graft duodenum. In patients with urinary bladder drainage, histological samples of the duodenal graft can be obtained by the cystoscopic biopsy technique. Duodenal tissue can be also obtained fortuitously through the percutaneous route.

Acute rejection in the duodenum most commonly occurs concurrently with pancreas rejection, but rejection can also occur independently in each of these organs [72]. Mild acute duodenal rejection is manifested by an increase in the inflammatory cells in the lamina propria with mild villous blunting and apoptosis of epithelial cells. Severe rejection has confluent epithelial necrosis with total loss of the epithelial lining. Necrosis can extend to all layers, including the muscularis propria. Arterial involvement (i.e., intimal arteritis, vasculitis) are diagnostic of rejection and may be seen also in the duodenum [72]. A case of perforation due to duodenal rejection has been reported [213].

Other forms of duodenal pathology amenable to be diagnosed with cystoscopic biopsies are ischemic and infectious duodenal ulcers (i.e., CMV, bacterial, fungal), Foley catheter trauma, and bladder tumors, etc. [214]. Recurrent urological complications may require conversion of a bladder-drained pancreas transplant to enteric drainage [17, 120].

VIII Gross and Microscopic Evaluation of Failed Allografts

Graft pancreatectomy specimens usually consist of the whole pancreas and attached portion of duodenum. The latter is present in continuity either with a loop of recipient's small intestine or a patch of urinary bladder wall (see Figures 7.1 and 7.2). Macroscopic evaluation of an explanted pancreas can be best accomplished if the pathologist understands the complexity of the technical issues in pancreas transplantation (see section on history of surgical techniques).

Systematic histological evaluation of failed grafts is necessary for accurate classification of the cause of graft loss. Minimum histological sampling should include cross sections of all large vessels and several sections from the parenchyma to include an adequate number of medium-sized and small vessels. The number of histological sections depends on each case, usually ranging from four to ten sections to allow for the most important structures to be sampled.

Specific Guidelines for Gross and Microscopic Evaluation

- Large arteries and veins: evaluate for thrombosis (recent and organized), intimal arteritis, transplant vasculopathy, donor atherosclerosis, etc.
- Random samples from parenchyma (viable and necrotic, usually three to five sections): evaluate for evidence of ischemia/pancreatitis, acute rejection, chronic rejection, presence of infectious organisms, etc.
- Area of anastomosis: evaluate for dehiscence (leak) and serositis.
- Samples from any other lesions: masses (i.e., PTLD), cysts, abscesses, lymph nodes, etc.

Ancillary Studies

- Immunoperoxidase stains for insulin and glucagon should be performed to evaluate for selective destruction of beta cells due to recurrence of autoimmune disease. These cases may show near normal parenchyma with no significant evidence of fibrosis/acinar loss, such as it is seen in chronic rejection.
- C4d stain is necessary to determine if there is a component of humoral rejection present (see above).
- Frozen tissue samples for immunofluorescence stains for immunoglobulins and complement in cases suspected to represent hyperacute/accelerated acute rejection.
- Electron microscopy may be used to demonstrate selective beta cell loss in recurrence of diabetes type 1 or beta cell degeneration in calcineurin inhibitor toxicity.

IX Other Complications of Pancreas Transplantation with Histopathological Manifestations

Thrombotic Microangiopathy: A well-known complication of transplantation and has been described in SPK patients. Clinicopathological evidence of pancreas involvement is however lacking, even in patients with systemic manifestations of the process [215].

Graft-versus-Host Disease: Secondary to pancreas transplantation, it has been well-documented, but is rare with an overall incidence of <.5% [216, 217]. The diagnosis is based on the characteristic clinical and pathological findings secondary to gastrointestinal, hepatic, and skin involvement. The presence of donor HLA or DNA material in the affected organs or in peripheral blood confirms the diagnosis.

Polyomavirus Infection: *Polyomavirus nephropathy* is considered one of the main causes of renal graft loss in SPK [218]. Since the infection is confined to the kidney allograft, the diagnosis relies on the demonstration of viral cytopathic changes in a renal biopsy. Urinary cytology and viral loads in blood are useful additional tools for diagnosis.

Gastrointestinal Drug Toxicity: Chronic diarrhea is one of the common side effects of Mycophenolate mofetil use. The most typical pathological changes in colonic biopsies performed in this context show strong similarities to those changes seen in other immunosuppressive states, namely, increased crypt cell apoptosis. Florid cases resemble intestinal acute Graft-versus-Host Disease. Dose reduction or discontinuation of the drug leads to clinical and histological improvement [219].

Adenovirus

Adenovirus has been associated with hemorrhagic cystitis in renal transplant patients, and in rare occasions, renal parenchyma involvement has been demonstrated (adenovirus pyelonephritis). There has been only one report of adenovirus infection in a combined kidney-pancreas transplant recipient. Adenovirus type 11 was demonstrated in some renal tubules, but the pancreas allograft continued to have normal function and apparently was not affected [220].

Neoplasia

A single case of pancreatic adenocarcinoma originating in a pancreas allograft has been reported [221].

X Histological Aspects of Islet Transplantation

For islet transplantation (IT), islet suspensions typically weighing 5–10 g in aggregate are injected in the portal vein to be distributed throughout the whole liver, which has an average weight of 1.5 kg. Hence, histological analysis of IT is not done routinely due to difficulties obtaining diagnostic graft samples. Toso et al. [222] described findings in islets and adjacent liver tissue in percutaneous liver core biopsies and autopsy samples from 16 and 2 patients, respectively. Islets were present in 31% of liver core biopsies, with the likelihood of their identification being in direct relationship to the size of the biopsy. Autopsy studies in IT recipients have shown multiple foci of grafted islets in liver tissue, with the liver parenchyma adjacent to the islet foci often showing localized steatosis [222]. Overall, the islets had similar cellular composition to native islets and only minimal inflammation (insulitis) was seen in few cases independently of the clinical presentation at the time of the tissue evaluation [222]. Lack of immunological damage (either allo- or autoimmune) was found in liver tissue obtained at the time of autopsy from one patient with two failed IT. Although both IT had failed six months after transplantation, insulin producing cells were clearly identified [223].

The limited histological studies of IT suggest that functional failure of the islets may result from a variety of factors including metabolic or microenvironmental stresses such as localized islet ischemia, toxic injuries, failure of islets to regenerate, etc. A concurrent low-grade immunologic rejection reaction is likely to be also present, but appears to be of less significance [222, 223].

C4d staining has been consistently negative in IT samples evaluated histologically, despite the fact that a significant proportion of recipients develop DSA [222–224].

Generalized deposition of islet amyloid (IAPP) was found in the islets of a patient who died of myocardial infarction five years after the first of three intraportal islet infusions [209]. Exhaustive studies of liver samples from the autopsies of patients that had previously received IT showed amyloid deposition in the islets of three out of four patients, further indicating the possibility that amyloid deposition plays a role in the long-term fate of transplanted islets [208].

References

1. Pirart J. Diabetes Mellitus and Its Degenerative Complications: A Prospective Study of 4,400 Patients Observed between 1947 and 1973 (Parts 1 & 2). Diabetes Care. 1978;**1**:168–88, 252–63.
2. Hirsch IB, Farkas-Hirsch R, Skyler JS. Intensive Insulin Therapy for Treatment of type I Diabetes. Diabetes Care. 1990 Dec;**13**(12):1265–83. PubMed PMID: 2276310.
3. Paty BW, Lanz K, Kendall DM, Sutherland DE, Robertson RP. Restored Hypoglycemic Counterregulation Is Stable in Successful Pancreas Transplant Recipients for up to 19 Years after Transplantation. Transplantation. 2001 Sep 27;**72**(6):1103–7. PubMed PMID: 11579308.
4. Secchi A, Di Carlo V, Martinenghi S, La Rocca E, Caldara R, Spotti D, et al. Effect of Pancreas Transplantation on Life Expectancy, Kidney Function and Quality of Life in Uraemic Type 1 (Insulin-dependent) Diabetic Patients. Diabetologia. 1991 Aug;34 Suppl 1:S141–4. PubMed PMID: 1936682.
5. Sudan D, Sudan R, Stratta R. Long-term Outcome of Simultaneous Kidney-Pancreas Transplantation: Analysis of 61 Patients with More Than 5 Years Follow-up. Transplantation. 2000 Feb 27;**69**(4):550–5. PubMed PMID: 10708110.
6. Robertson RP, Davis C, Larsen J, Stratta R, Sutherland DE. Pancreas and Islet Transplantation in Type 1 Diabetes. Diabetes Care. 2006 Apr;**29**(4):935. PubMed PMID: 16567844.
7. Gruessner AC, Sutherland DE, Gruessner RW. Pancreas Transplantation in the United States: A Review. Curr Opin Organ Transplant. 2010 Feb;**15**(1):93–101. PubMed PMID: 20009932.
8. Vrochides D, Paraskevas S, Papanikolaou V. Transplantation for Type 1 Diabetes Mellitus. Whole Organ or Islets? Hippokratia. 2009 Jan;**13**(1):6–8. PubMed PMID: 19240814. PubMed Central PMCID: 2633258. Epub 2009/02/26. English.
9. Voruganti L, Sells R. Quality of Life of Diabetic Patients after Combined Pancreatic-Renal Transplantation. Clin Transpl. 1989;**3**:78–82.
10. Fioretto P, Mauer M. Reversal of Diabetic Nephropathy: Lessons from Pancreas Transplantation. Journal of Nephrology. 2012 Jan–Feb;**25**(1):13–8. PubMed PMID: 22241641.
11. Khairoun M, de Koning EJ, van den Berg BM, Lievers E, de Boer HC, Schaapherder AF, et al. Microvascular Damage in Type 1 Diabetic Patients Is Reversed in the First Year after Simultaneous Pancreas-Kidney Transplantation. Am J Transplant. 2013 May;**13**(5):1272–81. PubMed PMID: 23433125.
12. Margreiter C, Resch T, Oberhuber R, Aigner F, Maier H, Sucher R, et al. Combined Pancreas-Kidney Transplantation for Patients with End-stage Nephropathy Caused by Type-2 Diabetes Mellitus. Transplantation. 2013 Apr 27;**95**(8):1030–6. PubMed PMID: 23407544.
13. Gruessner RW, Sutherland DE, Gruessner AC. Mortality Assessment for Pancreas Transplants. Am J Transplant. 2004 Dec;**4**(12):2018–26. PubMed PMID: 15575904.

14. Gruessner RW, Gruessner AC. Pancreas Transplant Alone: A Procedure Coming of Age. Diabetes Care. 2013 Aug;36(8):2440-7. PubMed PMID: 23881967. PubMed Central PMCID: 3714504.

15. Gruessner RW, Manivel C, Dunn DL, Sutherland DE. Pancreaticoduodenal Transplantation with Enteric Drainage Following Native Total Pancreatectomy for Chronic Pancreatitis: A Case Report. Pancreas. 1991 Jul;6(4):479-88. PubMed PMID: 1876604.

16. Andreoni KA, Brayman KL, Guidinger MK, Sommers CM, Sung RS. Kidney and Pancreas Transplantation in the United States, 1996–2005. Am J Transplant. 2007;7(5 Pt 2):1359-75. PubMed PMID: 17428285.

17. Gruessner AC, Sutherland DE. Pancreas Transplant Outcomes for United States (US) and Non-US Cases as Reported to the United Network for Organ Sharing (UNOS) and the International Pancreas Transplant Registry (IPTR) as of June 2004. Clin Transplant. 2005 Aug;19(4):433-55. PubMed PMID: 16008587.

18. Kuo PC, Johnson LB, Schweitzer EJ, Klassen DK, Hoehn-Saric EW, Weir MR, et al. Solitary Pancreas Allografts. The Role of Percutaneous Biopsy and Standardized Histologic Grading of Rejection. Arch Surg. 1997 Jan;132(1):52-7. PubMed PMID: 9006553.

19. Rogers J, Farney AC, Al-Geizawi S, Iskandar SS, Doares W, Gautreaux MD, et al. Pancreas Transplantation: Lessons Learned from a Decade of Experience at Wake Forest Baptist Medical Center. The Review of Diabetic Studies: RDS. 2011 Spring;8(1):17-27. PubMed PMID: 21720669. PubMed Central PMCID: 3143673.

20. Stratta RJ, Gaber AO, Shokouh-Amiri MH, Reddy KS, Egidi MF, Grewal HP, et al. A Prospective Comparison of Systemic-bladder versus Portal-enteric Drainage in Vascularized Pancreas Transplantation. Surgery. 2000 Feb;127(2):217-26. PubMed PMID: 10686988.

21. Gruessner R, Sutherland D. Transplantation of the Pancreas: History of Pancreas Transplantation. Springer; 1st edition (April 27, 2004) Chapter 11.

22. Kelly WD, Lillehei RC, Merkel FK, Idezuki Y, Goetz FC. Allotransplantation of the Pancreas and Duodenum along with the Kidney in Diabetic Nephropathy. Surgery. 1967 Jun;61(6):827-37. PubMed PMID: 5338113.

23. Lillehei RC, Simmons RL, Najarian JS, Weil R, Uchida H, Ruiz JO, et al. Pancreatico-Duodenal Allotransplantation: Experimental and Clinical Experience. Ann Surg. 1970 Sep;172(3):405-36. PubMed PMID: 4918002.

24. Sollinger HW, Odorico JS, Knechtle SJ, D'Alessandro AM, Kalayoglu M, Pirsch JD. Experience with 500 Simultaneous Pancreas-Kidney Transplants. Ann Surg. 1998 Sep;228(3):284-96. PubMed PMID: 9742912.

25. Prieto M, Sutherland DE, Fernandez-Cruz L, Heil J, Najarian JS. Urinary Amylase Monitoring for Early Diagnosis of Pancreas Allograft Rejection in Dogs. J Surg Res. 1986 Jun;40(6):597-604. PubMed PMID: 2427798.

26. Prieto M, Sutherland DE, Fernandez-Cruz L, Heil J, Najarian JS. Experimental and Clinical Experience with Urine Amylase Monitoring for Early Diagnosis of Rejection in Pancreas Transplantation. Transplantation. 1987 Jan;43(1):73-9. PubMed PMID: 2432705.

27. Nankivell BJ, Allen RD, Bell B, Wilson T, Chapman JR. Factors Affecting Urinary Amylase Excretion after Pancreas Transplantation. Transplant Proc. 1990 Oct;22(5):2156-7. PubMed PMID: 1699331.

28. Benedetti E, Najarian JS, Gruessner AC, Nakhleh RE, Troppmann C, Hakim NS, et al. Correlation between Cystoscopic Biopsy Results and Hypoamylasuria in Bladder-drained Pancreas Transplants. Surgery. 1995 Nov;118(5):864-72. PubMed PMID: 7482274.

29. Moukarzel M, Benoit G, Charpentier B, Bouchard P, Bensadoun H, Verdelli G, et al. Is Urinary Amylase a Reliable Index for Monitoring Whole Pancreas Endocrine Graft Function? Transplant Proc. 1992 Jun;24(3):925-6. PubMed PMID: 1376534.

30. Allen RD, Wilson TG, Grierson JM, Greenberg ML, Earl MJ, Nankivell BJ, et al. Percutaneous Biopsy of Bladder-drained Pancreas Transplants. Transplantation. 1991 Jun;51(6):1213-6. PubMed PMID: 1710842. Epub 1991/06/01. English.

31. Bartlett ST, Kuo PC, Johnson LB, Lim JW, Schweitzer EJ. Pancreas Transplantation at the University of Maryland. Clin Transpl. 1996:271-80. PubMed PMID: 9286577.

32. Papadimitriou JC, Drachenberg CB, Wiland A, Klassen DK, Fink J, Weir MR, et al. Histologic Grading of Acute Allograft Rejection in Pancreas Needle Biopsy: Correlation to Serum Enzymes, Glycemia, and Response to Immunosuppressive Treatment. Transplantation. 1998 Dec 27;66(12):1741-5. PubMed PMID: 9884270.

33. Drachenberg CB, Papadimitriou JC, Klassen DK, Racusen LC, Hoehn-Saric EW, Weir MR, et al. Evaluation of Pancreas Transplant Needle Biopsy: Reproducibility and Revision of Histologic Grading System. Transplantation. 1997 Jun 15;63(11):1579-86. PubMed PMID: 9197349.

34. Sutherland DE, Goetz FC, Sibley RK. Recurrence of Disease in Pancreas Transplants. Diabetes. 1989 Jan;38 Suppl 1:85-7. PubMed PMID: 2642862.

35. Drachenberg CB, Klassen DK, Weir MR, Wiland A, Fink JC, Bartlett ST, et al. Islet Cell Damage Associated with Tacrolimus and Cyclosporine: Morphological Features in Pancreas Allograft Biopsies and Clinical Correlation. Transplantation. 1999 Aug 15;68(3):396-402. PubMed PMID: 10459544.

36. Humar A, Khwaja K, Ramcharan T, Asolati M, Kandaswamy R, Gruessner RW, et al. Chronic Rejection: The Next Major Challenge for Pancreas Transplant Recipients. Transplantation. 2003 Sep 27;76(6):918-23. PubMed PMID: 14508354.

37. Drachenberg CB, Papadimitriou JC, Farney A, Wiland A, Blahut S, Fink JC, et al. Pancreas Transplantation: The Histologic Morphology of Graft Loss and Clinical Correlations. Transplantation. 2001 Jun 27;71(12):1784-91. PubMed PMID: 11455259.

38. Bartlett ST, Schweitzer EJ, Johnson LB, Kuo PC, Papadimitriou JC, Drachenberg CB, et al. Equivalent Success of Simultaneous Pancreas Kidney and Solitary Pancreas Transplantation. A Prospective Trial of Tacrolimus Immunosuppression with Percutaneous Biopsy. Ann Surg. 1996 Oct;224(4):440-9; discussion 9-52. PubMed PMID: 8857849.

39. Dallman M. Immunobiology of Graft Rejection. In: Ginns LC, Cosimi AB, Morris PJ, eds. Transplantation. 1988:23-42.

40. Klassen DK, Hoen-Saric EW, Weir MR, Papadimitriou JC, Drachenberg CB, Johnson L, et al. Isolated Pancreas Rejection in Combined Kidney Pancreas Transplantation.

41. Kandaswamy R, Stock PG, Skeans MA, Gustafson SK, Sleeman EF, Wainright JL, et al. OPTN/SRTR 2011 Annual Data Report: Pancreas. Am J Transplant. 2013 Jan;13 Suppl 1:47–72. PubMed PMID: 23237696.

42. Papadimitriou JC. Diffuse Acinar Inflammation is the Most Important Histological Predictor of Chronic Rejection in Pancreas Allografts. Transplantation. 2006;82(1 Suppl 2):223.

43. Tesi RJ, Henry ML, Elkhammas EA, Davies EA, Ferguson RM. The Frequency of Rejection Episodes after Combined Kidney-Pancreas Transplant–The Impact on Graft Survival. Transplantation. 1994 Aug 27;58(4):424–30. PubMed PMID: 8073510.

44. Stegall MD. Surveillance Biopsies in Solitary Pancreas Transplantation. Acta Chir Austriaca 2001;33:6.

45. Stratta RJ. Late Acute Rejection after Pancreas Transplantation. Transplant Proc. 1998 Mar;30(2):646. PubMed PMID: 9532215.

46. Stratta RJ. Graft Failure after Solitary Pancreas Transplantation. Transplant Proc. 1998 Mar;30(2):289. PubMed PMID: 9532043.

47. Stratta RJ. Patterns of Graft Loss Following Simultaneous Kidney-Pancreas Transplantation. Transplant Proc. 1998 Mar;30(2):288. PubMed PMID: 9532042.

48. Basadonna GP, Matas AJ, Gillingham KJ, Payne WD, Dunn DL, Sutherland DE, et al. Early versus Late Acute Renal Allograft Rejection: Impact on Chronic Rejection. Transplantation. 1993 May;55(5):993–5. PubMed PMID: 8497913.

49. Allen RD, Grierson JM, Ekberg H, Hawthorne WJ, Williamson P, Deane SA, et al. Longitudinal Histopathologic Assessment of Rejection after Bladder-drained Canine Pancreas Allograft Transplantation. Am J Pathol. 1991 Feb;138(2):303–12. PubMed PMID: 1992759.

50. Atwell TD, Gorman B, Larson TS, Charboneau JW, Ingalls Hanson BM, Stegall MD. Pancreas Transplants: Experience with 232 Percutaneous US-guided Biopsy Procedures in 88 Patients. Radiology. 2004 Jun;231(3):845–9. PubMed PMID: 15163821. Epub 2004/05/28. English.

51. Boonstra JG, van der Pijl JW, Smets YF, Lemkes HH, Ringers J, van Es LA, et al. Interstitial and Vascular Pancreas

Transplantation. 1996 Mar 27;61(6):974–7. PubMed PMID: 8623171.

Rejection in Relation to Graft Survival. Transpl Int. 1997;10(6):451–6. PubMed PMID: 9428119.

52. Casey ET, Smyrk TC, Burgart LJ, Stegall MD, Larson TS. Outcome of Untreated Grade II Rejection on Solitary Pancreas Allograft Biopsy Specimens. Transplantation. 2005 Jun 27;79(12):1717–22. PubMed PMID: 15973174.

53. Kuhr CS, Davis CL, Barr D, McVicar JP, Perkins JD, Bachi CE, et al. Use of Ultrasound and Cystoscopically Guided Pancreatic Allograft Biopsies and Transabdominal Renal Allograft Biopsies: Safety and Efficacy in Kidney-Pancreas Transplant Recipients. J Urol. 1995 Feb;153(2):316–21. PubMed PMID: 7815571.

54. Laftavi MR, Gruessner AC, Bland BJ, Aideyan OA, Walsh JW, Sutherland DE, et al. Significance of Pancreas Graft Biopsy in Detection of Rejection. Transplant Proc. 1998 Mar;30(2):642–4. PubMed PMID: 9532213.

55. Laftavi MR, Gruessner AC, Bland BJ, Foshager M, Walsh JW, Sutherland DE, et al. Diagnosis of Pancreas Rejection: Cystoscopic Transduodenal versus Percutaneous Computed Tomography Scan-guided Biopsy. Transplantation. 1998 Feb 27;65(4):528–32. PubMed PMID: 9500628.

56. Lee BC, McGahan JP, Perez RV, Boone JM. The Role of Percutaneous Biopsy in Detection of Pancreatic Transplant Rejection. Clin Transplant. 2000 Oct;14(5):493–8. PubMed PMID: 11048995.

57. Papadimitriou JC. Role of Histopathology Evaluation in Pancreas Transplantation. Current Opinion in Organ Transplantation. 2002;7:185–90.

58. Klassen DK, Weir MR, Cangro CB, Bartlett ST, Papadimitriou JC, Drachenberg CB. Pancreas Allograft Biopsy: Safety of Percutaneous Biopsy-results of a Large Experience. Transplantation. 2002 Feb 27;73(4):553–5. PubMed PMID: 11889428.

59. Klassen DK, Weir MR, Schweitzer EJ, Bartlett ST. Isolated Pancreas Rejection in Combined Kidney-Pancreas Transplantation: Results of Percutaneous Pancreas Biopsy. Transplant Proc. 1995 Feb;27(1):1333–4. PubMed PMID: 7533380.

60. Aideyan OA, Schmidt AJ, Trenkner SW, Hakim NS, Gruessner RW, Walsh JW. CT-guided Percutaneous Biopsy of Pancreas Transplants. Radiology. 1996 Dec;201(3):825–8. PubMed PMID: 8939238. Epub 1996/12/01. English.

61. Bernardino M, Fernandez M, Neylan J, Hertzler G, Whelchel J, Olson R. Pancreatic Transplants: CT-guided Biopsy. Radiology. 1990 Dec;177(3):709–11. PubMed PMID: 2243974.

62. Gaber AO, Gaber LW, Shokouh-Amiri MH, Hathaway D. Percutaneous Biopsy of Pancreas Transplants. Transplantation. 1992 Sep;54(3):548–50. PubMed PMID: 1384187.

63. Gaber LW, Stratta RJ, Lo A, Egidi MF, Shokouh-Amiri MH, Grewal HP, et al. Role of Surveillance Biopsies in Monitoring Recipients of Pancreas Alone Transplants. Transplant Proc. 2001 Feb–Mar;33(1–2):1673–4. PubMed PMID: 11267464.

64. Silver JM, Vitello JM, Benedetti E. Laparoscopic-guided Biopsy of Pancreatic Transplant Allograft. J Laparoendosc Adv Surg Tech A. 1997 Oct;7(5):319–22. PubMed PMID: 9453878.

65. Kayler LK, Merion RM, Rudich SM, Punch JD, Magee JC, Maraschio MA, et al. Evaluation of Pancreatic Allograft Dysfunction by Laparoscopic Biopsy. Transplantation. 2002 Nov 15;74(9):1287–9. PubMed PMID: 12451267. Epub 2002/11/27. English.

66. Burke GW, 3rd, Vendrame F, Pileggi A, Ciancio G, Reijonen H, Pugliese A. Recurrence of Autoimmunity Following Pancreas Transplantation. Current Diabetes Reports. 2011 Oct;11(5):413–9. PubMed PMID: 21660419.

67. Pugliese A, Reijonen HK, Nepom J, Burke GW, 3rd. Recurrence of Autoimmunity in Pancreas Transplant Patients: Research Update. Diabetes Management. 2011 Mar;1(2):229–38. PubMed PMID: 21927622. PubMed Central PMCID: 3171830.

68. Vendrame F, Pileggi A, Laughlin E, Allende G, Martin-Pagola A, Molano RD, et al. Recurrence of Type 1 Diabetes after Simultaneous Pancreas-Kidney Transplantation, Despite Immunosuppression, Is Associated with Autoantibodies and Pathogenic Autoreactive CD4 T-cells. Diabetes. 2010 Apr;59(4):947–57. PubMed PMID: 20086230. PubMed Central PMCID: 2844842.

69. Perkins JD, Munn SR, Marsh CL, Barr D, Engen DE, Carpenter HA. Safety and Efficacy of Cystoscopically Directed Biopsy in Pancreas Transplantation. Transplant Proc. 1990 Apr;22(2):665–6. PubMed PMID: 2327014.

70. Jones JW, Nakhleh RE, Casanova D, Sutherland DE, Gruessner RW.

Cystoscopic Transduodenal Pancreas Transplant Biopsy: A New Needle. Transplant Proc. 1994 Apr;26(2):527-8. PubMed PMID: 8171538.

71. Lowell JA, Bynon JS, Nelson N, Hapke MR, Morton JJ, Brennan DC, et al. Improved Technique for Transduodenal Pancreas Transplant Biopsy. Transplantation. 1994 Mar 15;57(5):752-3. PubMed PMID: 8140640.

72. Nakhleh RE, Benedetti E, Gruessner A, Troppmann C, Goswitz JJ, Sutherland DE, et al. Cystoscopic Biopsies in Pancreaticoduodenal Transplantation. Are Duodenal Biopsies Indicative of Pancreas Dysfunction? Transplantation. 1995 Sep 27;60(6):541-6. PubMed PMID: 7570948.

73. Nakhleh RE, Sutherland DE, Benedetti E, Goswitz JJ, Gruessner RW. Diagnostic Utility and Correlation of Duodenal and Pancreas Biopsy Tissue in Pancreaticoduodenal Transplants with Emphasis on Therapeutic Use. Transplant Proc. 1995 Feb;27(1):1327-8. PubMed PMID: 7878902.

74. Casanova D, Gruessner R, Brayman K, Jessurun J, Dunn D, Xenos E, et al. Retrospective Analysis of the Role of Pancreatic Biopsy (Open and Transcystoscopic Technique) in the Management of Solitary Pancreas Transplants. Transplant Proc. 1993 Feb;25(1 Pt 2):1192-3. PubMed PMID: 8442083.

75. Carpenter HA, Engen DE, Munn SR, Barr D, Marsh CL, Ludwig J, et al. Histologic Diagnosis of Rejection by using Cystoscopically Directed Needle Biopsy Specimens from Dysfunctional Pancreatoduodenal Allografts with Exocrine Drainage into the Bladder. Am J Surg Pathol. 1990 Sep;14(9):837-46. PubMed PMID: 2389814.

76. Margreiter C, Aigner F, Resch T, Berenji AK, Oberhuber R, Sucher R, et al. Enteroscopic Biopsies in the Management of Pancreas Transplants: A Proof of Concept Study for a Novel Monitoring Tool. Transplantation. 2012 Jan 27;93(2):207-13. PubMed PMID: 22134369.

77. Drachenberg CB, Odorico J, Demetris AJ, Arend L, Bajema IM, Bruijn JA, et al. BANFF Schema for Grading Pancreas Allograft Rejection: Working Proposal by a Multi-disciplinary International Consensus Panel. Am J Transplant. 2008 Jun;8(6):1237-49. PubMed PMID: 18444939.

78. Carbajal R, Karam G, Renaudin K, Maillet F, Cesbron A, Rostaing L, et al. Specific Humoral Rejection of a Pancreas Allograft in a Recipient of Pancreas after Kidney Transplantation. Nephrol Dial Transplant. 2007 Mar;22(3):942-4. PubMed PMID: 17210592.

79. Melcher ML, Olson JL, Baxter-Lowe LA, Stock PG, Posselt AM. Antibody-mediated Rejection of a Pancreas Allograft. Am J Transplant. 2006 Feb;6(2):423-8. PubMed PMID: 16426331.

80. Papadimitriou JC, Drachenberg CB, Klassen DK, Gaber L, Racusen LC, Voska L, et al. Histological Grading of Chronic Pancreas Allograft Rejection/Graft Sclerosis. Am J Transplant. 2003 May;3(5):599-605. PubMed PMID: 12752316.

81. Tyden G, Reinholt FP, Sundkvist G, Bolinder J. Recurrence of Autoimmune Diabetes Mellitus in Recipients of Cadaveric Pancreatic Grafts. N Engl J Med. 1996 Sep 19;335(12):860-3. PubMed PMID: 8778604.

82. Westermark P, Andersson A, Westermark GT. Islet Amyloid Polypeptide, Islet Amyloid, and Diabetes Mellitus. Physiol Rev. 2011 Jul;91(3):795-826. PubMed PMID: 21742788. Epub 2011/07/12. English.

83. Gruessner RW, Nakhleh R, Tzardis P, Schechner R, Platt JL, Gruessner A, et al. Differences in Rejection Grading after Simultaneous Pancreas and Kidney Transplantation in Pigs. Transplantation. 1994 Apr 15;57(7):1021-8. PubMed PMID: 7513096.

84. Nakhleh RE, Sutherland DE, Tzardis P, Schechner R, Gruessner RW. Correlation of Rejection of the Duodenum with Rejection of the Pancreas in a Pig Model of Pancreaticoduodenal Transplantation. Transplantation. 1993 Dec;56(6):1353-6. PubMed PMID: 8279003.

85. Severyn W, Olson L, Miller J, Kyriakides G, Rabinovitch A, Flaa C, et al. Studies on the Survival of Simultaneous Canine Renal and Segmental Pancreatic Allografts. Transplantation. 1982 Jun;33(6):606-12. PubMed PMID: 7048662.

86. Vogt P, Hiller WF, Steiniger B, Klempnauer J. Differential Response of Kidney and Pancreas Rejection to Cyclosporine Immunosuppression. Transplantation. 1992 Jun;53(6):1269-72. PubMed PMID: 1604483.

87. Gruessner RW, Sutherland DE, Troppmann C, Benedetti E, Hakim N, Dunn DL, et al. The Surgical Risk of Pancreas Transplantation in the Cyclosporine Era: An Overview. J Am Coll Surg. 1997 Aug;185(2):128-44. PubMed PMID: 9249080.

88. Hawthorne WJ, Allen RD, Greenberg ML, Grierson JM, Earl MJ, Yung T, et al. Simultaneous Pancreas and Kidney Transplant Rejection: Separate or Synchronous Events? Transplantation. 1997 Feb 15;63(3):352-8. PubMed PMID: 9039922.

89. Reinholt FP, Tyden G, Bohman SO, al. E. Pancreatic Juice Cytology in the Diagnosis of Pancreatic Graft Rejection. Clin Transpl. 1988;2:127-33.

90. Stratta RJ, Taylor RJ, Grune MT, Sindhi R, Sudan D, Castaldo P, et al. Experience with Protocol Biopsies after Solitary Pancreas Transplantation. Transplantation. 1995 Dec 27;60(12):1431-7. PubMed PMID: 8545870.

91. Rogers J, Iskandar S, Farney A, al. E. Surveillance Pancreas Biopsies in Solitary Pancreas Transplantation: A Shot in the Dark. Am J Transplant. 2007;7, Suppl 2:251.

92. Drachenberg CB, Papadimitriou JC, Schweitzer E, Philosophe B, Foster C, Bartlett ST. Histological Findings in "Incidental" Intraoperative Pancreas Allograft Biopsies. Transplant Proc. 2004 Apr;36(3):780-1. PubMed PMID: 15110661.

93. Benz S, Pfeffer F, Adam U, Schareck W, Hopt UT. Impairment of Pancreatic Microcirculation in the Early Reperfusion Period during Simultaneous Pancreas-Kidney Transplantation. Transpl Int. 1998;11 Suppl 1:S433-5. PubMed PMID: 9665033.

94. Benz S, Schnabel R, Morgenroth K, Weber H, Pfeffer F, Hopt UT. Ischemia/Reperfusion Injury of the Pancreas: A New Animal Model. J Surg Res. 1998 Mar;75(2):109-15. PubMed PMID: 9655083.

95. Troppmann C, Gruessner AC, Papalois BE, Sutherland DE, Matas AJ, Benedetti E, et al. Delayed Endocrine Pancreas Graft Function after Simultaneous Pancreas-Kidney Transplantation. Incidence, Risk Factors, and Impact on Long-term Outcome. Transplantation. 1996 May 15;61(9):1323-30. PubMed PMID: 8629291.

96. Uhlman D, Ludwig S, Geissler F, Tannapfel A, Hauss J, Witzigmann H. Importance of Microcirculatory Disturbances in the Pathogenesis of Pancreatitis. Zentralbl Chir. 2001;126:873-8.

97. Daar AS, Fuggle SV, Fabre JW, Ting A, Morris PJ. The Detailed Distribution of HLA-A, B, C Antigens in Normal Human Organs. Transplantation. 1984 Sep;38(3):287-92. PubMed PMID: 6591601.

98. Steiniger B, Klempnauer J, Wonigeit K. Altered Distribution of Class I and Class II MHC Antigens during Acute Pancreas Allograft Rejection in the Rat. Transplantation. 1985 Sep;40(3):234–9. PubMed PMID: 3898487.

99. Drachenberg CB, Torrealba JR, Nankivell BJ, Rangel EB, Bajema IM, Kim DU, et al. Guidelines for the Diagnosis of Antibody-mediated Rejection in Pancreas Allografts-Updated BANFF Grading Schema. Am J Transplant. 2011 Sep;11(9):1792–802. PubMed PMID: 21812920.

100. Pelletier RP, Hennessy PK, Adams PW, VanBuskirk AM, Ferguson RM, Orosz CG. Clinical Significance of MHC-reactive Alloantibodies that Develop after Kidney or Kidney-Pancreas Transplantation. Am J Transplant. 2002 Feb;2(2):134–41. PubMed PMID: 12099515.

101. Solez K, Colvin RB, Racusen LC, Sis B, Halloran PF, Birk PE, et al. BANFF '05 Meeting Report: Differential Diagnosis of Chronic Allograft Injury and Elimination of Chronic Allograft Nephropathy ('CAN'). Am J Transplant. 2007 Mar;7(3):518–26. PubMed PMID: 17352710.

102. Le Moine A, Goldman M, Abramowicz D. Multiple Pathways to Allograft Rejection. Transplantation. 2002 May 15;73(9):1373–81. PubMed PMID: 12023610.

103. Hawthorne WJ, Griffin AD, Lau H, Hibbins M, Grierson JM, Ekberg H, et al. Experimental Hyperacute Rejection in Pancreas Allotransplants. Transplantation. 1996 Aug 15;62(3):324–9. PubMed PMID: 8779677.

104. Solez K, Colvin RB, Racusen LC, Haas M, Sis B, Mengel M, et al. BANFF 07 Classification of Renal Allograft Pathology: Updates and Future Directions. Am J Transplant. 2008 Apr;8(4):753–60. PubMed PMID: 18294345.

105. Drachenberg CB, Papadimitriou JC. Endothelial Injury in Renal Antibody-mediated Allograft Rejection: A Schematic View Based on Pathogenesis. Transplantation. 2013 May 15;95(9):1073–83. PubMed PMID: 23370711.

106. Steiniger B, Klempnauer J. Distinct Histologic Patterns of Acute, Prolonged, and Chronic Rejection in Vascularized Rat Pancreas Allografts. Am J Pathol. 1986 Aug;124(2):253–62. PubMed PMID: 3526910.

107. Dietze O, Konigsrainer A, Habringer C, Krausler R, Klima G, Margreiter R. Histological Features of Acute Pancreatic Allograft Rejection after Pancreaticoduodenal Transplantation in the Rat. Transpl Int. 1991 Dec;4(4):221–6. PubMed PMID: 1786060.

108. Drachenberg CB, Papadimitriou JC, Klassen DK, Weir MR, Bartlett ST. Distribution of Alpha and Beta Cells in Pancreas Allograft Biopsies: Correlation with Rejection and Other Pathologic Processes. Transplant Proc. 1998 Mar;30(2):665–6. PubMed PMID: 9532226.

109. Drachenberg CB, Papadimitriou JC, Weir MR, Klassen DK, Hoehn-Saric E, Bartlett ST. Histologic Findings in Islets of Whole Pancreas Allografts: Lack of Evidence for Recurrent Cell-mediated Diabetes Mellitus. Transplantation. 1996 Dec 27;62(12):1770–2. PubMed PMID: 8990360.

110. de Kort H, Munivenkatappa RB, Berger SP, Eikmans M, van der Wal A, de Koning EJ, et al. Pancreas Allograft Biopsies with Positive c4d Staining and Anti-donor Antibodies Related to Worse Outcome for Patients. Am J Transplant. 2010 Jul;10(7):1660–7. PubMed PMID: 20455878.

111. Rangel EB, Malheiros DM, de Castro MC, Antunes I, Torres MA, Crescentini F, et al. Antibody-mediated Rejection (AMR) after Pancreas and Pancreas-Kidney Transplantation. Transpl Int. 2010 Jun;23(6):602–10. PubMed PMID: 20028489. English.

112. Torrealba JR, Odorico J. Antibody-mediated Rejection of the Pancreas Allograft. Transplantation. 2009 Jul 27;88(2):292–3. PubMed PMID: 19623030. Epub 2009/07/23. English.

113. Torrealba JR, Samaniego M, Pascual J, Becker Y, Pirsch J, Sollinger H, et al. C4d-positive Interacinar Capillaries Correlates with Donor-specific Antibody-mediated Rejection in Pancreas Allografts. Transplantation. 2008 Dec 27;86(12):1849–56. PubMed PMID: 19104433.

114. Carpenter HA, Engen DE, Munn SR, Barr DT, Marsh CL, Ludwig J, et al. Histologic Features of Rejection in Cystoscopically Directed Needle Biopsies of Pancreatoduodenal Allografts in Dogs and Humans. Transplant Proc. 1990 Apr;22(2):707–8. PubMed PMID: 2327023.

115. Knoop M, McMahon RF, Jones CJ, Hutchinson IV. Apoptosis in Pancreatic Allograft Rejection–Ultrastructural Observations. Exp Pathol. 1991;41(4):219–24. PubMed PMID: 2070844.

116. Dubernard JM, Traeger J, Touraine JL, Betuel H, Malik MC. Rejection of Human Pancreatic Allografts. Transplant Proc. 1980 Dec;12(4 Suppl 2):103–6. PubMed PMID: 7013184.

117. Oberhuber G, Schmid T, Thaler W, Klima G, Margreiter R. The Pattern of Rejection after Combined Stomach, Small Bowel, and Pancreas Transplantation in the Rat. Transpl Int. 1993;6(5):296–8. PubMed PMID: 8216709.

118. Sibley RK. Pancreas Transplantation. In: Sale GE ed. The Pathology of Organ Transplantation. Boston Butterworths. 1990;179.

119. Nakhleh RE, Sutherland DE. Pancreas Rejection. Significance of Histopathologic Findings with Implications for Classification of Rejection. Am J Surg Pathol. 1992 Nov;16(11):1098–107. PubMed PMID: 1471730.

120. Boudreaux JP, Nealon WH, Carson RC, Fish JC. Pancreatitis Necessitating Urinary Undiversion in a Bladder-drained Pancreas Transplant. Transplant Proc. 1990 Apr;22(2):641–2. PubMed PMID: 1691545.

121. Sutherland DE, Casanova D, Sibley RK. Role of Pancreas Graft Biopsies in the Diagnosis and Treatment of Rejection after Pancreas Transplantation. Transplant Proc. 1987 Feb;19(1 Pt 3):2329–31. PubMed PMID: 3274517.

122. Papadimitriou JC, Wiland A, Drachenberg CB, Klassen DK, Bartlett ST. Effectiveness of Immunosuppressive Treatment for Recurrent or Refractory Pancreas Allograft Rejection: Correlation with Histologic Grade. Transplant Proc. 1998 Dec;30(8):3945. PubMed PMID: 9865254.

123. Klassen D. Chronic Rejection in Pancreas Transplantation. Graft. 1998;(Suppl. II):74–6.

124. Brayman K, Morel P, Chau C, Stevens B, Goetz FC, Sutherland DE. Influence of Rejection Episodes on the Relationship between Exocrine and Endocrine Function in Bladder-drained Pancreas Transplants. Transplant Proc. 1992 Jun;24(3):921–3. PubMed PMID: 1376533.

125. Schilling MK, Redaelli C, Reber PU, Friess H, Signer C, Stoupis C, et al. Microcirculation in Chronic Alcoholic Pancreatitis: A Laser Doppler Flow

125. Study. Pancreas. 1999 Jul;19(1):21-5. PubMed PMID: 10416687.
126. Nakhleh RE, Gruessner RW. Ischemia due to Vascular Rejection Causes Islet Loss after Pancreas Transplantation. Transplant Proc. 1998 Mar;30(2):539-40. PubMed PMID: 9532169.
127. Munivenkatappa RP, J.C.; Drachenberg, C.B. Accelerated Pancreas Allograft Sclerosis due to Allograft Rejection Pathology Case Reviews. 2012;17(6):229-35.
128. Fattahi R, Modanlou KA, Bieneman BK, Soydan N, Balci NC, Burton FR. Magnetic Resonance Imaging in Pancreas Transplantation. Topics in Magnetic Resonance Imaging: TMRI. 2009 Feb;20(1):49-55. PubMed PMID: 19687726.
129. Vandermeer FQM, M.AA; Frazier, A.A.; Wong-You-Cheong, J.J. Imaging of Whole-organ Pancreas Transplants Radiographics. 2012;32(2):411-35.
130. Drachenberg CB, Papadimitriou JC. The Inflamed Pancreas Transplant: Histological Differential Diagnosis. Semin Diagn Pathol. 2004 Nov;21(4):255-9. PubMed PMID: 16273944.
131. Gruessner R. Immunobiology, Diagnosis, and Treatment of Pancreas Allograft Rejection. Pancreas Transplantation. 2004 2004; Gruessner RWG and Sutherland DER Ed. (Springer-Verlag):349-80.
132. Burke GW, Ciancio G, Cirocco R, Markou M, Olson L, Contreras N, et al. Microangiopathy in Kidney and Simultaneous Pancreas/Kidney Recipients Treated with Tacrolimus: Evidence of Endothelin and Cytokine Involvement. Transplantation. 1999 Nov 15;68(9):1336-42. PubMed PMID: 10573073.
133. Matsukuma S, Suda K, Abe H. Histopathological Study of Pancreatic Ischemic Lesions Induced by Cholesterol Emboli: Fresh and Subsequent Features of Pancreatic Ischemia. Hum Pathol. 1998 Jan;29(1):41-6. PubMed PMID: 9445132.
134. BANFF Schema for Grading Liver Allograft Rejection: An International Consensus Document. Hepatology. 1997 Mar;25(3):658-63. PubMed PMID: 9049215.
135. Sibley RK, Sutherland DE, Goetz F, Michael AF. Recurrent Diabetes Mellitus in the Pancreas Iso- and Allograft. A Light and Electron Microscopic and Immunohistochemical Analysis of Four Cases. Lab Invest. 1985 Aug;53(2):132-44. PubMed PMID: 3894793.
136. Klassen DK, Drachenberg CB, Papadimitriou JC, Cangro CB, Fink JC, Bartlett ST, et al. CMV Allograft Pancreatitis: Diagnosis, Treatment, and Histological Features. Transplantation. 2000 May 15;69(9):1968-71. PubMed PMID: 10830244.
137. Noronha IL, Oliveira SG, Tavares TS, Di Petta A, Dominguez WV, Perosa M, et al. Apoptosis in Kidney and Pancreas Allograft Biopsies. Transplantation. 2005 May 15;79(9):1231-5. PubMed PMID: 15880076.
138. Boonstra JG, Wever PC, Laterveer JC, Bruijn JA, van der Woude FJ, ten Berge IJ, et al. Apoptosis of Acinar Cells in Pancreas Allograft Rejection. Transplantation. 1997 Oct 27;64(8):1211-3. PubMed PMID: 9355845.
139. Henderson JR, Moss MC. A Morphometric Study of the Endocrine and Exocrine Capillaries of the Pancreas. Q J Exp Physiol. 1985 Jul;70(3):347-56. PubMed PMID: 3898188.
140. Olsson R, Carlsson PO. The Pancreatic Islet Endothelial Cell: Emerging Roles in Islet Function and Disease. Int J Biochem Cell Biol. 2006;38(4):492-7. PubMed PMID: 16162421.
141. Papadimitriou JC. Antibody Mediated Rejection in Pancreas Allografts. Ninth BANFF Conference on Allograft Pathology. 2007 June 23-29.
142. de Kort H, Roufosse C, Bajema IM, Drachenberg CB. Pancreas Transplantation, Antibodies and Rejection: Where Do We Stand? Curr Opin Organ Transplant. 2013 Jun;18(3):337-44. PubMed PMID: 23619511.
143. Troxell ML, Koslin DB, Norman D, Rayhill S, Mittalhenkle A. Pancreas Allograft Rejection: Analysis of Concurrent Renal Allograft Biopsies and Posttherapy Follow-up Biopsies. Transplantation. 2010 Jul 15;90(1):75-84. PubMed PMID: 20548259.
144. Einecke G, Sis B, Reeve J, Mengel M, Campbell PM, Hidalgo LG, et al. Antibody-mediated Microcirculation Injury Is the Major Cause of Late Kidney Transplant Failure. Am J Transplant. 2009 Nov;9(11):2520-31. PubMed PMID: 19843030.
145. Loupy A, Hill GS, Suberbielle C, Charron D, Anglicheau D, Zuber J, et al. Significance of C4d BANFF Scores in Early Protocol Biopsies of Kidney Transplant Recipients with Preformed Donor-specific Antibodies (DSA). Am J Transplant. 2011 Jan;11(1):56-65. PubMed PMID: 21199348. English.
146. Gaber LW. Pancreas Allograft Biopsies in the Management of Pancreas Transplant Recipients: Histopathologic Review and Clinical Correlations. Archives of Pathology & Laboratory Medicine. 2007 Aug;131(8):1192-9. PubMed PMID: 17683181. English.
147. Waki K, Terasaki PI, Kadowaki T. Long Term Pancreas Allograft Survival in Simultaneous Pancreas Kidney Transplantation by Era: UNOS Registry Analysis. Diabetes Care. 2010 May 11;33(8):1789-91. PubMed PMID: 20460444.
148. Fabio V, Daniele F, Monica DD, Simone G, Luciana MM, Margherita O, et al. Pancreas Rejection after Pandemic Influenzavirus A(H(1)N(1)) Vaccination or Infection: A Report of Two Cases. Transpl Int. 2010 Mar;24(3):e28-e9. PubMed PMID: 21121966. English.
149. Katerinis I, Hadaya K, Duquesnoy R, Ferrari-Lacraz S, Meier S, van Delden C, et al. De Novo Anti-HLA Antibody after Pandemic H1N1 and Seasonal Influenza Immunization in Kidney Transplant Recipients. American Journal of Transplantation: Official Journal of the American Society of Transplantation and the American Society of Transplant Surgeons. 2011 Aug;11(8):1727-33. PubMed PMID: 21672157. Epub 2011/06/16. English.
150. Zanone MM, Favaro E, Quadri R, Miceli I, Giaretta F, Romagnoli R, et al. Association of Cytomegalovirus Infections with Recurrence of Humoral and Cellular Autoimmunity to Islet Autoantigens and of Type 1 Diabetes in a Pancreas Transplanted Patient. Transplant International: Official Journal of the European Society for Organ Transplantation. 2010 Mar 1;23(3):333-7. PubMed PMID: 19906032. Epub 2009/11/13. English.
151. Howell WM, Harmer A, Briggs D, Dyer P, Fuggle SV, Martin S, et al. British Society for Histocompatibility & Immunogenetics and British Transplantation Society Guidelines for the Detection and Characterisation of Clinically Relevant Antibodies in Allotransplantation. Int J Immunogenet. 2010 Dec;37(6):435-7. PubMed PMID: 20670336.
152. Leffell MS, Zachary AA. Antiallograft Antibodies: Relevance, Detection, and Monitoring. Curr Opin Organ Transplant. 2010 Feb;15(1):2-7. PubMed PMID: 19898236.

153. Zeevi A, Lunz JG, 3rd, Shapiro R, Randhawa P, Mazariegos G, Webber S, et al. Emerging Role of Donor-specific Anti-human Leukocyte Antigen Antibody Determination for Clinical Management after Solid Organ Transplantation. Human Immunology. 2009 Aug;70(8):645–50. PubMed PMID: 19527760.

154. Feucht HE, Opelz G. The Humoral Immune Response towards HLA Class II Determinants in Renal Transplantation. Kidney Int. 1996 Nov;50(5):1464–75. PubMed PMID: 8914011.

155. Minami K, Murata K, Lee CY, Fox-Talbot K, Wasowska BA, Pescovitz MD, et al. C4d Deposition and Clearance in Cardiac Transplants Correlates with Alloantibody Levels and Rejection in Rats. Am J Transplant. 2006 May;6(5 Pt 1):923–32. PubMed PMID: 16611328. English.

156. Miller DV, Roden AC, Gamez JD, Tazelaar HD. Detection of C4d Deposition in Cardiac Allografts: A Comparative Study of Immunofluorescence and Immunoperoxidase Methods. Archives of Pathology & Laboratory Medicine. 2010 Nov;134(11):1679–84. PubMed PMID: 21043822.

157. Haririan A, Kiangkitiwan B, Kukuruga D, Cooper M, Hurley H, Drachenberg C, et al. The Impact of c4d Pattern and Donor-specific Antibody on Graft Survival in Recipients Requiring Indication Renal Allograft Biopsy. Am J Transplant. 2009 Dec;9(12):2758–67. PubMed PMID: 19845596. English.

158. Munivenkatappa RB, Philosophe B, Papadimitriou JC, Drachenberg CB. Interacinar c4d Staining in Pancreas Allografts. Transplantation. 2009 Jul 15;88(1):145–6. PubMed PMID: 19584698.

159. Sis B, Halloran PF. Endothelial Transcripts Uncover a Previously Unknown Phenotype: C4d-negative Antibody-mediated Rejection. Curr Opin Organ Transplant. 2010 Feb;15(1):42–8. PubMed PMID: 20009933.

160. Niederhaus SVL, G.E.; Lorentzen, D.F.; Robillard, D.J.; Sollinger, H.W.; Pirsch, J.D.; Torrealba, J.R.; Odorico, J.S. Acute Cellular and Antibody-mediated Rejection of the Pancreas Allograft: Incidence, Risk Factors and Outcomes. Am J of Transplant 2013;in press.

161. Papadimitriou JC, Drachenberg CB, Munivenkatappa R, Ramos E, Nogueira J, Sailey C, et al. Glomerular Inflammation in Renal Allografts Biopsies after the First Year: Cell Types and Relationship with Antibody-mediated Rejection and Graft Outcome. Transplantation. 2010 Dec 27;90(12):1478–85. PubMed PMID: 21042235. Epub 2010/11/03. English.

162. Troppmann C, Gruessner AC, Benedetti E, Papalois BE, Dunn DL, Najarian JS, et al. Vascular Graft Thrombosis after Pancreatic Transplantation: Univariate and Multivariate Operative and Nonoperative Risk Factor Analysis. J Am Coll Surg. 1996 Apr;182(4):285–316. PubMed PMID: 8605554.

163. Pascual J, Pirsch JD, Odorico JS, Torrealba JR, Djamali A, Becker YT, et al. Alemtuzumab Induction and Antibody-mediated Kidney Rejection after Simultaneous Pancreas-Kidney Transplantation. Transplantation. 2009 Jan 15;87(1):125–32. PubMed PMID: 19136902. Epub 2009/01/13. English.

164. Pascual J, Samaniego MD, Torrealba JR, Odorico JS, Djamali A, Becker YT, et al. Antibody-mediated Rejection of the Kidney after Simultaneous Pancreas-Kidney Transplantation. J Am Soc Nephrol. 2008 Apr;19(4):812–24. PubMed PMID: 18235091. PubMed Central PMCID: 2390970.

165. Prikis M, Norman D, Rayhill S, Olyaei A, Troxell M, Mittalhenkle A. Preserved Endocrine Function in a Pancreas Transplant Recipient with Pancreatic Panniculitis and Antibody-mediated Rejection. Am J Transplant. 2010 Dec;10(12):2717–22. PubMed PMID: 21114649.

166. Drachenberg CB, Torrealba JR, Nankivell BJ, Rangel EB, Bajema IM, Kim DU, et al. Guidelines for the Diagnosis of Antibody-mediated Rejection in Pancreas Allografts-Updated BANFF Grading Schema. American Journal of Transplantation: Official Journal of the American Society of Transplantation and the American Society of Transplant Surgeons. 2011 Sep;11(9):1792–802. PubMed PMID: 21812920. Epub 2011/08/05. English.

167. Hirohashi T, Uehara S, Chase CM, DellaPelle P, Madsen JC, Russell PS, et al. Complement Independent Antibody-mediated Endarteritis and Transplant Arteriopathy in Mice. Am J Transplant. 2010 Mar;10(3):510–7. PubMed PMID: 20055805. English.

168. Shimizu T, Ishida H, Shirakawa H, Omoto K, Tsunoyama K, Tokumoto T, et al. Clinicopathological Analysis of Acute Vascular Rejection Cases after Renal Transplantation. Clin Transplant. 2010 Jul;24 Suppl 22:22–6. PubMed PMID: 20590689. English.

169. Sis B, Einecke G, Chang J, Hidalgo LG, Mengel M, Kaplan B, et al. Cluster Analysis of Lesions in Nonselected Kidney Transplant Biopsies: Microcirculation Changes, Tubulointerstitial Inflammation and Scarring. American Journal of Transplantation: Official Journal of the American Society of Transplantation and the American Society of Transplant Surgeons. 2010 Feb;10(2):421–30. PubMed PMID: 20055794. Epub 2010/01/09. English.

170. Lefaucheur C, Loupy A, Vernerey D, Duong-Van-Huyen JP, Suberbielle C, Anglicheau D, et al. Antibody-mediated Vascular Rejection of Kidney Allografts: A Population-based Study. Lancet. 2013 Jan 26;381(9863):313–9. PubMed PMID: 23182298.

171. Wieczorek G, Bigaud M, Menninger K, Riesen S, Quesniaux V, Schuurman HJ, et al. Acute and Chronic Vascular Rejection in Nonhuman Primate Kidney Transplantation. Am J Transplant. 2006 Jun;6(6):1285–96. PubMed PMID: 16686753.

172. Sharma S, Green KB. The Pancreatic Duct and Its Arteriovenous Relationship: An Underutilized Aid in the Diagnosis and Distinction of Pancreatic Adenocarcinoma from Pancreatic Intraepithelial Neoplasia. A Study of 126 Pancreatectomy Specimens. Am J Surg Pathol. 2004 May;28(5):613–20. PubMed PMID: 15105649.

173. Troppmann C, Gruessner AC, Dunn DL, Sutherland DE, Gruessner RW. Surgical Complications Requiring Early Relaparotomy after Pancreas Transplantation: A Multivariate Risk Factor and Economic Impact Analysis of the Cyclosporine Era. Ann Surg. 1998 Feb;227(2):255–68. PubMed PMID: 9488525.

174. Grewal HP, Garland L, Novak K, Gaber L, Tolley EA, Gaber AO. Risk Factors for Postimplantation Pancreatitis and Pancreatic Thrombosis in Pancreas Transplant Recipients. Transplantation. 1993 Sep;56(3):609–12. PubMed PMID: 8212156.

175. Gruessner RW, Dunn DL, Gruessner AC, Matas AJ, Najarian JS, Sutherland DE. Recipient Risk Factors Have an Impact on Technical Failure and Patient and Graft Survival Rates in Bladder-drained Pancreas Transplants.

175 Transplantation. 1994 Jun 15;**57**(11):1598–606. PubMed PMID: 8009594.

176 Gruessner RW, Troppmann C, Barrou B, Dunn DL, Moudry-Munns KC, Najarian JS, et al. Assessment of Donor and Recipient Risk Factors on Pancreas Transplant Outcome. Transplant Proc. 1994 Apr;**26**(2):437–8. PubMed PMID: 8171491.

177 Obermaier R, Benz S, Kortmann B, Benthues A, Ansorge N, Hopt UT. Ischemia/Reperfusion-induced Pancreatitis in Rats: A New Model of Complete Normothermic in Situ Ischemia of a Pancreatic Tail-segment. Clin Exp Med. 2001 Mar;**1**(1):51–9. PubMed PMID: 11467402.

178 Schulak JA, Franklin WA, Stuart FP, Reckard CR. Effect of Warm Ischemia on Segmental Pancreas Transplantation in the Rat. Transplantation. 1983 Jan;**35**(1):7–11. PubMed PMID: 6337436.

179 Busing M, Hopt UT, Quacken M, Becker HD, Morgenroth K. Morphological Studies of Graft Pancreatitis Following Pancreas Transplantation. Br J Surg. 1993 Sep;**80**(9):1170–3. PubMed PMID: 8402124.

180 Hesse UJ, Sutherland DE, Simmons RL, Najarian JS. Intra-abdominal Infections in Pancreas Transplant Recipients. Ann Surg. 1986 Feb;**203**(2):153–62. PubMed PMID: 3511866.

181 Patel BK, Garvin PJ, Aridge DL, Chenoweth JL, Markivee CR. Fluid Collections Developing after Pancreatic Transplantation: Radiologic Evaluation and Intervention. Radiology. 1991 Oct;**181**(1):215–20. PubMed PMID: 1887034.

182 Knight RJ, Bodian C, Rodriguez-Laiz G, Guy SR, Fishbein TM. Risk Factors for Intra-abdominal Infection after Pancreas Transplantation. Am J Surg. 2000 Feb;**179**(2):99–102. PubMed PMID: 10773142.

183 Hiatt JR, Fink AS, King W, 3rd, Pitt HA. Percutaneous Aspiration of Peripancreatic Fluid Collections: A Safe Method to Detect Infection. Surgery. 1987 May;**101**(5):523–30. PubMed PMID: 3554575.

184 Letourneau JG, Hunter DW, Crass JR, Thompson WM, Sutherland DE. Percutaneous Aspiration and Drainage of Abdominal Fluid Collections after Pancreatic Transplantation. AJR Am J Roentgenol. 1988 Apr;**150**(4):805–9. PubMed PMID: 2450446.

185 Nobrega J, Halvorsen RA, Letourneau JG, Snover D, Sutherland D. Cystic Central Necrosis of Transplanted Pancreas. Gastrointest Radiol. 1990 Summer;**15**(3):202–4. PubMed PMID: 2340994.

186 Fernandez-Cruz L, Sabater L, Gilabert R, Ricart MJ, Saenz A, Astudillo E. Native and Graft Pancreatitis Following Combined Pancreas-Renal Transplantation. Br J Surg. 1993 Nov;**80**(11):1429–32. PubMed PMID: 7504566.

187 Humar A, Uknis M, Carlone-Jambor C, Gruessner RW, Dunn DL, Matas A. Cytomegalovirus Disease Recurrence after Ganciclovir Treatment in Kidney and Kidney-Pancreas Transplant Recipients. Transplantation. 1999 Jan 15;**67**(1):94–7. PubMed PMID: 9921803.

188 Ishibashi M, Bosshard S, Fukuuchi F, Lefrancois N, Martin X, Touraine L, et al. Incidence of CMV Infection in Simultaneous Pancreas and Kidney Transplantation: Comparative Study of Two Surgical Procedures of Segmental Pancreas versus Whole Bladder-drained Pancreas. Transplant Proc. 1996 Oct;**28**(5):2859–60. PubMed PMID: 8908101.

189 Keay S. CMV Infection and Disease in Kidney and Pancreas Transplant Recipients. Transpl Infect Dis. 1999;**1** Suppl 1:19–24. PubMed PMID: 11565582.

190 Lo A, Stratta RJ, Egidi MF, Shokouh-Amiri MH, Grewal HP, Kisilisik AT, et al. Patterns of Cytomegalovirus Infection in Simultaneous Kidney-Pancreas Transplant Recipients Receiving Tacrolimus, Mycophenolate Mofetil, and Prednisone with Ganciclovir Prophylaxis. Transpl Infect Dis. 2001 Mar;**3**(1):8–15. PubMed PMID: 11429034.

191 Backman L, Brattstrom C, Reinholt FP, Andersson J, Tyden G. Development of Intrapancreatic Abscess–A Consequence of CMV Pancreatitis? Transpl Int. 1991 Jun;**4**(2):116–21. PubMed PMID: 1654918.

192 Fernandez JA, Robles R, Ramirez P, Bueno FS, Rodriguez JM, Lujan JA, et al. Arterioenteric Fistula due to Cytomegalovirus Infection after Pancreas Transplantation. Transplantation. 2001 Sep 15;**72**(5):966–8. PubMed PMID: 11571472.

193 Drachenberg CB, Abruzzo LV, Klassen DK, Bartlett ST, Johnson LB, Kuo PC, et al. Epstein-Barr Virus-related Posttransplantation Lymphoproliferative Disorder Involving Pancreas Allografts: Histological Differential Diagnosis from Acute Allograft Rejection. Hum Pathol. 1998 Jun;**29**(6):569–77. PubMed PMID: 9635676.

194 Heyny-von Haussen R, Klingel K, Riegel W, Kandolf R, Mall G. Posttransplant Lymphoproliferative Disorder in a Kidney-Pancreas Transplanted Recipient: Simultaneous Development of Clonal Lymphoid B-cell Proliferation of Host and Donor Origin. Am J Surg Pathol. 2006 Jul;**30**(7):900–5. PubMed PMID: 16819335.

195 Keay S, Oldach D, Wiland A, Klassen D, Schweitzer E, Abruzzo LV, et al. Posttransplantation Lymphoproliferative Disorder Associated with OKT3 and Decreased Antiviral Prophylaxis in Pancreas Transplant Recipients. Clin Infect Dis. 1998 Mar;**26**(3):596–600. PubMed PMID: 9524829.

196 Rehbinder B, Wullstein C, Bechstein WO, Probst M, Engels K, Kriener S, et al. Epstein-Barr Virus-associated Posttransplant Lymphoproliferative Disorder of Donor Origin after Simultaneous Pancreas-Kidney Transplantation Limited to Pancreas Allograft: A Case Report. Am J Transplant. 2006 Oct;**6**(10):2506–11. PubMed PMID: 16869797.

197 Kroes AC, van der Pijl JW, van Tol MJ, van Krieken JH, Falk KI, Gratama JW, et al. Rapid Occurrence of Lymphoproliferative Disease after Pancreas-Kidney Transplantation Performed during Acute Primary Epstein-Barr Virus Infection. Clin Infect Dis. 1997 Mar;**24**(3):339–43. PubMed PMID: 9114182.

198 Paya CV, Fung JJ, Nalesnik MA, Kieff E, Green M, Gores G, et al. Epstein-Barr Virus-induced Posttransplant Lymphoproliferative Disorders. ASTS/ASTP EBV-PTLD Task Force and The Mayo Clinic Organized International Consensus Development Meeting. Transplantation. 1999 Nov 27;**68**(10):1517–25. PubMed PMID: 10589949.

199 Dombrowski F, Klingmuller D, Pfeifer U. Insulinomas Derived from Hyperplastic Intra-hepatic Islet Transplants. Am J Pathol. 1998 Apr;**152**(4):1025–38. PubMed PMID: 9546363.

200 Petruzzo P, Andreelli F, McGregor B, Lefrancois N, Dawahra M, Feitosa LC, et al. Evidence of Recurrent Type I Diabetes Following HLA-mismatched

200. Pancreas Transplantation. Diabetes Metab. 2000 May;26(3):215–8. PubMed PMID: 10880896.
201. Ruiz P. Recurrence of Type 1 Diabetes in Pancreas Transplantation. Ninth BANFF Conference on Allograft Pathology. 2007 June 23–29, 2007.
202. Gong W, Liu ZH, Zeng CH, Peng A, Chen HP, Zhou H, et al. Amylin Deposition in the Kidney of Patients with Diabetic Nephropathy. Kidney Int. 2007 Jul;72(2):213–8. PubMed PMID: 17495860.
203. Bartlett ST, Schweitzer EJ, Kuo PC, Johnson LB, Delatorre A, Hadley GA. Prevention of Autoimmune Islet Allograft Destruction by Engraftment of Donor T Cells. Transplantation. 1997 Jan 27;63(2):299–303. PubMed PMID: 9020334.
204. Braghi S, Bonifacio E, Secchi A, Di Carlo V, Pozza G, Bosi E. Modulation of Humoral Islet Autoimmunity by Pancreas Allotransplantation Influences Allograft Outcome in Patients with Type 1 Diabetes. Diabetes. 2000 Feb;49(2):218–24. PubMed PMID: 10868938.
205. Laughlin E, Burke G, Pugliese A, Falk B, Nepom G. Recurrence of Autoreactive Antigen-specific CD4+ T Cells in Autoimmune Diabetes after Pancreas Transplantation. Clinical Immunology. 2008 Jul;128(1):23–30. PubMed PMID: 18455963. PubMed Central PMCID: 2531116.
206. Sibley RK. Morphologic Features of Chronic Rejection in Kidney and Less Commonly Transplanted Organs. Clin Transplant. 1994 Jun;8(3 Pt 2):293–8. PubMed PMID: 8061371.
207. Hirano Y, Fujihira S, Ohara K, Katsuki S, Noguchi H. Morphological and Functional Changes of Islets of Langerhans in FK506-treated Rats. Transplantation. 1992 Apr;53(4):889–94. PubMed PMID: 1373536.
208. Westermark GT, Davalli AM, Secchi A, Folli F, Kin T, Toso C, et al. Further Evidence for Amyloid Deposition in Clinical Pancreatic Islet Grafts. Transplantation. 2012 Jan 27;93(2):219–23. PubMed PMID: 22193043. Epub 2011/12/24. English.
209. Westermark GT, Westermark P, Berne C, Korsgren O. Widespread Amyloid Deposition in Transplanted Human Pancreatic Islets. N Engl J Med. 2008 Aug 28;359(9):977–9. PubMed PMID: 18753660. Epub 2008/08/30. English.
210. Westermark P. Amyloid in the Islets of Langerhans: Thoughts and some Historical Aspects. Ups J Med Sci. 2011 May;116(2):81–9. PubMed PMID: 21486192. PubMed Central PMCID: 3078536. Epub 2011/04/14. English.
211. Dudek RW, Lawrence IE, Jr., Hill RS, Johnson RC. Induction of Islet Cytodifferentiation by Fetal Mesenchyme in Adult Pancreatic Ductal Epithelium. Diabetes. 1991 Aug;40(8):1041–8. PubMed PMID: 1860556.
212. Semakula C, Pambuccian S, Gruessner R, Kendall D, Pittenger G, Vinik A, et al. Clinical Case Seminar: Hypoglycemia after Pancreas Transplantation: Association with Allograft Nesidiodysplasia and Expression of Islet Neogenesis-associated Peptide. J Clin Endocrinol Metab. 2002 Aug;87(8):3548–54. PubMed PMID: 12161473.
213. Esterl RM, Stratta RJ, Taylor RJ, Radio SJ. Rejection with Duodenal Rupture after Solitary Pancreas Transplantation: An Unusual Cause of Severe Hematuria. Clin Transplant. 1995 Jun;9(3 Pt 1):155–9. PubMed PMID: 7549053.
214. Hakim NS, Gruessner AC, Papalois BE, Troppmann C, Dunn DL, Sutherland DE, et al. Duodenal Complications in Bladder-drained Pancreas Transplantation. Surgery. 1997 Jun;121(6):618–24. PubMed PMID: 9186461.
215. Rangel EB, Gonzalez AM, Linhares MM, Araujo SR, Franco MF, de Sa JR, et al. Thrombotic Microangiopathy after Simultaneous Pancreas-Kidney Transplantation. Clin Transplant. 2007 Mar–Apr;21(2):241–5. PubMed PMID: 17425752.
216. Weinstein A, Dexter D, KuKuruga DL, Philosophe B, Hess J, Klassen D. Acute Graft-versus-Host Disease in Pancreas Transplantation: A Comparison of Two Case Presentations and a Review of the Literature. Transplantation. 2006 Jul 15;82(1):127–31. PubMed PMID: 16861952.
217. Wijkstrom M, Sutherland D. Acta Chir Austriaca. 2001;33:5174–7.
218. Gaber LW, Egidi MF, Lo A, Gaber AO. Renal Pathology and Clinical Presentations of Polyomavirus Nephropathy in Simultaneous Kidney Pancreas Transplant Recipients Compared with Kidney Transplant Recipients. Transplant Proc. 2004 May;36(4):1095–6. PubMed PMID: 15194381.
219. Papadimitriou JC, Cangro CB, Lustberg A, Khaled A, Nogueira J, Wiland A, et al. Histologic Features of Mycophenolate Mofetil-related Colitis: A Graft-versus-Host Disease-like Pattern. Int J Surg Pathol. 2003 Oct;11(4):295–302. PubMed PMID: 14615824.
220. Mathur S, Squiers E, Tatum A, Szmalc F, Daucher J, Welker D, et al. Adenovirus Infection of the Renal Allograft with Sparing of Pancreas Graft Function in the Recipient of a Combined Kidney-Pancreas Transplant. Transplantation. 2000;65(1):138–41.
221. Roza AM, Johnson C, Juckett M, Eckels D, Adams M. Adenocarcinoma Arising in a Transplanted Pancreas. Transplantation. 2001 Sep 27;72(6):1156–7. PubMed PMID: 11579317.
222. Toso C, Isse K, Demetris AJ, Dinyari P, Koh A, Imes S, et al. Histologic Graft Assessment after Clinical Islet Transplantation. Transplantation. 2009 Dec 15;88(11):1286–93. PubMed PMID: 19996928.
223. Smith RN, Kent SC, Nagle J, Selig M, Iafrate AJ, Najafian N, et al. Pathology of an Islet Transplant 2 Years after Transplantation: Evidence for a Nonimmunological Loss. Transplantation. 2008 Jul 15;86(1):54–62. PubMed PMID: 18622278.
224. Campbell PM, Senior PA, Salam A, Labranche K, Bigam DL, Kneteman NM, et al. High Risk of Sensitization after Failed Islet Transplantation. Am J Transplant. 2007 Oct;7(10):2311–7. PubMed PMID: 17845564.

Chapter 8

Pathology of Hematopoietic Stem Cell Transplantation

Lazaros J. Lekakis and Krishna V. Komanduri

Overview

Hematopoietic stem cell transplantation (HCT) is a procedure aiming to regenerate bone marrow function either when it is purposely destroyed by high dose anti-neoplastic therapy, or when it is grossly dysfunctional (e.g., in cases of bone marrow failure syndromes, leukemia, enzymopathies, hemoglobinopathies, or immunodeficiencies). The donor of the stem cells can be the patient (autologous HCT) or someone else (allogeneic HCT, which can be performed using donors that are related or unrelated and derived from bone marrow, mobilized peripheral blood stem cells, or umbilical cord blood). Allogeneic HCT (allo-HCT) results in the development of a new immune system in the transplanted recipient. This can result in an attack of healthy recipient tissues by the donor immune system (graft-versus-host disease, GVHD), an undesired condition that is associated with significant morbidity and mortality. With a similar mechanism, however, the donor immune system can attack malignant cells (graft-versus-tumor effect, GVT; or graft-versus-leukemia effect, GVL) and cure certain malignancies.

Graft-versus-Leukemia Responses and Conditioning Intensity

The original rationale for allo-HCT in the treatment of hematologic malignancies relied on the use of high-dose, fully ablative conditioning (combining either cytotoxic chemotherapy and/or radiation) to induce greater proportional reduction of recipient cancer burden than possible with lower (and sub-ablative) doses of cytoreductive agents. The recognition of the GVL effect resulted from studies demonstrating that the depletion of T cells from allogeneic donor grafts was associated with higher rates of relapse following allo-HCT. Further studies then demonstrated that infusion of isolated donor lymphocytes (DLI) could induce relapses occurring after allo-HCT, even when unaccompanied by antineoplastic chemotherapy [1]. Indeed, the recognition of the importance of GVL responses after allo-HCT led to modern approaches wherein the doses of antineoplastic chemotherapy were significantly lowered to decrease the historically high morbidity of HCT (reduced-intensity conditioning, RIC), relying on GVL responses to fully eradicate malignant cells that may survive even fully ablative conditioning regimens.

Nonmyeloablative Conditioning

Occasionally, the pre-transplant chemotherapy is of so low intensity as to just prevent the rejection of the donor stem cells without the goal of eliminating recipient hematopoiesis (nonmyeloablative conditioning, NMA), letting the engrafted donor immune system be almost entirely responsible for the anti-neoplastic effect. Patients with post-HCT relapse of hematologic neoplasms can often be cured with infusion of more donor lymphocytes after dropping the immunosuppression (donor lymphocyte infusion, DLI) [1]. Although NK cells have been implicated, GVL is mainly a T cell-mediated process [2]. This is supported by the fact that the relapse rate is higher after allo-HCT using grafts that are either T cell depleted (TCD) or derived from an identical (syngeneic) donor. Similarly, chronic graft-versus-host disease (cGVHD) is associated with lower rates of relapse. The sensitivity of hematologic malignancies to GVL varies, with CML, follicular lymphoma (FL), and mantle cell lymphoma being the most sensitive and ALL, Burkitt's, and DLBCL being the most resistant entities [3]. Therefore, the intensity of conditioning utilized varies depending on the presumed sensitivity of the underlying malignancy to the GVL response, and on the ability of the recipient to tolerate intensive therapy.

Tumor-associated Antigens

In GVL, cytotoxic lymphocytes (CTL) recognize the neoplastic cells because of antigenic differences between recipient and donor. In such cases, usually we have both GVHD and GVL simultaneously. Frequently though, neoplastic cells can express unique antigens (tumor associated antigens, TAA) that can be recognized by CTL. Such antigens include rearranged immunoglobulin receptors or rearranged T cell receptor (TCR) or viral proteins or even specific antigens that are over-expressed by the tumors (cancer-testis antigens, Her-2 in breast cancer, PR1 and WT1 in leukemias, MAGE in melanomas, etc.) [1] [2]. Some tumor cells like CML cells and indolent lymphoma cells can be efficient antigen presenting cells (APCs) under certain conditions and facilitate their own demise [4]. This is one of the reasons that GVL is so strong in CML and FL. Primed CTL can kill their target cancer cells through secretion of perforin, granzymes, or through FasL that induce apoptosis on cancer cells [5]. NK-mediated killing may depend on mismatches of KIR ligands between donor NK cells and recipient tumor cells. In the absence of an inhibitory KIR ligand, donor NK cells do not receive tonic inhibition signals and are primed to attack. NK cells become more aggressive when they recognize specific antigens on the surface of cancer cells (for example, MICA/MICB molecules that can activate NK cells through the NKG2D receptor). NK cells kill their targets mainly with perforin and granzymes like CTLs. When CTL attack tumors because of recognition of TAA and when NK cells attack because of KIR ligand mismatch, GVL can happen without GVHD [6, 7].

Source of Hematopoietic Stem Cells (HSC)

The original source of HSC was exclusively the bone marrow (BM). Later studies demonstrated the ability to utilize peripheral blood which, after treatment with filgrastim or plerixafor (with or without chemotherapy), becomes enriched with HSC that migrate outside the BM (peripheral blood stem cells, PBSC) [8] [9]. The donor can be the patient himself (auto-HCT), an HLA-matched-related donor (MRD-allo), an HLA-matched unrelated person (MUD-allo), cord units (UCBT), or a haplo-identical relative (haplo-HCT). Although the collection of PBSC is easier for the donor, their use in the allo-HCT setting is associated with higher rates of cGVHD, which is likely due to the increased proportions of T cells, relative to marrow grafts [10]. Since there is a positive correlation between cGVHD and GVL, there is a theoretical justification for the use of PBSC in malignancies at high risk for relapse. When, however, the underlying disease is non-neoplastic or when the relapse risk of the malignancy is low, marrow is usually preferred, since the risk of GVHD is not associated with lower risk of relapse, as in the setting of HCT for malignancies. HCT can be curative for otherwise incurable diseases, but it is a toxic treatment with innumerable complications that can affect the quality of life or can even be lethal.

Indications for Autologous HCT

This section reviews major indications, by disease, for HCT and highlights important studies establishing modern indications for HCT in these respective settings.

Multiple Myeloma

Multiple studies have shown either an OS or a PFS benefit when high doses of melphalan are used (typically 200 mg/m^2) before auto-HCT [11]. Studies have also shown benefit from a second auto-HCT, especially for those without satisfactory response to the 1st auto-HCT or for patients with the t(11;14) translocation [12]. Most of the transplant centers, however, do only one transplant followed by lenalidomide and/or bortezomib maintenance [13, 14]. The role of allo-HCT in myeloma is still uncertain. Although an Italian study showed benefit from a NMA allo after an auto [15], an American trial did not verify the results and nowadays, allo-HCT for myeloma in USA is done only as part of a clinical trial. The role for auto-HCT in amyloidosis is questionable and may be harmful in patients with >2 organs involved and/or severe cardiac involvement [16].

Chemosensitive B Cell Non-Hodgkin Lymphoma (B-NHL) and Mantle Cell Lymphoma

Older European studies have shown survival benefits of auto-HCT in follicular lymphoma (FL) that relapsed and then responded to salvage chemotherapy [17]. Similarly, DLBCL patients who have a chemosensitive relapse get a survival benefit or even cure with auto-HCT [18]. Controversy still exists if auto-HCT is of any benefit in the rituximab era in high-risk patients (age-adjusted IPI score of 3) with DLBCL in CR1. A major cooperative group trial (SWOG S9704) was positive, but included some patients who did not receive rituximab as part of the initial chemotherapy (Proceedings of ASCO, 2011). In mantle cell lymphoma (MCL) the best PFS intervals have been obtained in patients who received poly-chemotherapy (usually incorporating cytarabine) combined with rituximab followed by auto-HCT in CR1 [19, 20]. It was shown recently that the use of post-transplant rituximab maintenance improved the survival of patients with Mantle cell Lymphoma who had an auto-HCT in CR1. Patients with relapsed MCL who did not have a previous auto-HCT usually do not get durable benefit with auto-HCT and allo-HCT may be more appropriate for them [19, 21].

The most commonly used conditioning regimens for lymphomas are: BEAM (carmustine, etoposide, cytarabine, and melphalan), BEAC (carmustine, etoposide, cytarabine, and cyclophosphamide), CBV (cyclophosphamide, carmustine, and etoposide), and Bu-Mel (busulfan and melphalan). For CD20+ NHL, rituximab is usually added. The enthusiasm of adding radio-immunotherapy to BEAM for CD20+ NHL has been tampered by a negative phase III trial that did not show benefit of adding Bexxar (anti-CD20 monoclonal antibody, mAb, labeled with I^{131}) to BEAM chemotherapy [22]. A new trial assessing Zevalin added to BEAM (anti-CD20 mAb attached to Y^{90}) is underway. Recently patients with Primary B-cell CNS lymphoma frequently have an auto-HCT in CR1 with Rituximab-Thiotepa-Busulfan and Cyclophosphamide (R-TBC regimen).

Hodgkin's Lymphoma

Patients with Hodgkin's lymphoma can also be cured (~50%) if they have relapsed and show chemosensitivity to a salvage regimen. Cures can sometimes (~30%) be achieved with auto-HCT in HL even in patients who do not have chemosensitive relapse [23] [24]. The use of brentuximab vedotin (anti-CD30 immunotoxin) maintenance has improved PFS after auto-HCT in patients with high-risk Hodgkin Lymphoma.

Peripheral T Cell Lymphomas

Peripheral T cell lymphoma, non-otherwise specified (PTCL-NOS), ALK-negative anaplastic large cell lymphomas (ALCL), and angio-immunoblastic T cell lymphomas (AITL), as well as high-risk subcutaneous panniculitis-like αβ lymphoma (especially if hemophagocytosis is evident), have a high relapse rate even if they respond completely to induction chemotherapy. Most authorities believe that patients with such lymphomas in CR1 get a benefit from auto-HCT, because relapses are usually not salvageable by an auto-HCT, but only by an allo-HCT [25] [26].

Germ Cell Tumors

Relapsed or resistant germ cell tumors can be salvaged even in the case of refractoriness to cisplatin with a tandem carboplatin-etoposide auto-HCT [27].

Neuroblastoma

Neuroblastoma patients with high-risk features (age>1 yr., N-Myc amplification, or metastatic disease) have an EFS benefit with auto-HCT, especially if this is performed with the combination of busulfan and Melphalan (Bu-Mel) [28].

The role of auto-HCT in Ewing sarcoma and in severe auto-immune diseases is controversial. A European study did not show benefit from auto-HCT in Ewing [29, 30]. Auto-HCT in auto-immune diseases is associated with higher morbidity and mortality and there is a plethora of new drugs that were approved in the last years for rheumatoid arthritis, multiple sclerosis, and systemic lupus. Auto-HCT for such diseases should be done only in the context of clinical trials.

Indications for Allogeneic HCT

Acute Myeloid Leukemia (AML)

Allo-HCT is the treatment of choice in relapsed AML and is the only treatment with a curative potential (although modest) in refractory AML. In 1st CR, allo-HCT is recommended for high-risk and intermediate-risk disease based on a meta-analysis of high quality phase III trials that showed survival benefit [31]. Good-risk AML should not be transplanted in CR1. The latter group of good-risk AML consists of a) acute promyelocytic leukemia (APL), b) t(8;21), inv 16, or t(16;16) AML if they do not harbor c-kit mutation (the so-called Core-Binding Factor Leukemias, CBF-AML), c) AML with NPM-1, or CEBPα mutations as long as they do not have a concurrent Flt-3 mutation.

The most commonly used conditioning regimens for AML (before allo-HCT) include total body irradiation with cyclophosphamide (TBI-Cy), busulfan with cyclophosphamide (Bu-Cy), and fludarabine and Busulfan (Flu-Bu). The latter is an ablative regimen with low toxicity and low 100-day mortality because of the introduction of intravenous busulfan and is currently preferred by many big centers [32]. Two recent retrospective studies have demonstrated the superiority of intravenous busulfan to TBI in combination with Cy, with the major improvement resulting from reduced non-relapse mortality. Clofarabine that has better anti-leukemic activity than fludarabine has also been used with busulfan (Clo-Bu), but it is still unclear if it leads to a superior survival rate, due to increases in morbidity [33]. For older patients, RIC with fludarabine and Melphalan (Flu-Mel) or even a truly NMA regimen of fludarabine and low-dosed (2 Gy) TBI are the most commonly used.

Acute Lymphoblastic Leukemia (ALL)

Although the outcomes of ALL in adults have improved with the introduction of the principles of pediatric protocols and the use of imatinib for ALL with the Philadelphia chromosome translocation (Ph+), there is evidence suggesting that adult patients benefit from allo-HCT in CR1 as long as they can tolerate the combination of total body irradiation and etoposide (TBI-VP16). The largest phase III trial showed a survival benefit for such patients if they had standard risk disease [34]. Although this trial used only sibling donors, most modern studies suggest that the outcomes after sibling or well-matched unrelated donor transplants are approximately equal [35]. For higher-risk adult patients, most institutions perform allo-HCT in CR1, since this is associated with much lower relapse risk, especially for certain subgroups like CD10-negative pro-B ALL that is usually associated with MLL translocations [36] and early precursor T-ALL that is commonly associated with Ikaros deletions [37, 38]. It is uncertain if monitoring of minimal residual disease (MRD) by multicolor flow cytometry and the incorporation of targeting agents (anti-CD22 immunotoxins like inotuzumab ozogamicin or the bi-specific antibody blinatumomab with anti-CD3 and anti-CD19 properties) will decrease the use of allo-HCT for ALL in the future [39]. Recently, investigators used chimeric antigen receptor T cells (CAR-T cells, usually against CD19, equipped with 1–2 co-stimulatory receptors) with encouraging results [40] [41]. The use of non-TBI regimens (e.g., Clofarabine with busulfan) has been successfully tried in older adults for ALL [42].

Chronic Myelogenous Leukemia (CML)

Historically, CML was one of the most frequent indications for allo-HCT. However, the development of targeted therapies based on tyrosine kinase inhibitors (TKI) has resulted in long-term disease-free survival with minimal toxicity for the vast majority of CML patients. In the TKI era, allo-HCT is usually reserved for patients who either have accelerated or blast-phase CML or have chronic-phase progressing through at least two TKI (e.g., imatinib, nilotinb, dasatinib, ponatinib). The most commonly used conditioning regimens in CML are Bu-Cy and TBI-Cy [43].

Chronic Lymphocytic Leukemia (CLL)

Allo-HCT is usually considered in CR1/PR1 in CLL patients with the adverse prognostic finding of deletion of chromosome 17p (17p-). It is usually done in CR2 or PR1 in patients' deletion of chromosome 11q (11q-). For patients without 11q- or 17p-, allo-HCT can be performed in CR2/PR2 for patients who progressed early after the first immunochemotherapy regimen (for example, less than three years after therapy using the combination of fludarabine, cyclophosphamide, and rituximab, FCR). Allo-HCT is usually not considered for patients who have an initially long remission after first-line therapy [44]. The conditioning is usually RIC (Fludarabine in combination with melphalan) or NMA (FCR or Flu-TBI 2Gy). Residual disease and incomplete donor chimerism after transplant can respond to DLI. The use of new and very powerful anti-leukemic drugs like Ibrutinib, Acalabrutinib (both Bruton Tyrosine Kinase Inhibitors) and Venetoclax (BH3 mimetic) have created a trend to postpone allo-HCT for CLL for later in the course after the patient has failed at least one of these drugs, even for high risk disease (17p- CLL).

Other Lymphoproliferative Disorders

FL and MCL patients can be cured by an allo-HCT even if they already had an auto-HCT because GVL is very strong in these diseases. Usually the option of allo-HCT in these diseases is considered only in cases of relapse after auto-HCT or if disease is relatively chemorefractory. On the other hand, GVL is not as strong in HL and DLBCL; therefore, allo-HCT is considered only after optimal cytoreduction with salvage therapy following auto-HCT failure. Relapsed PTCL NOS, ALK-negative ALCL, AITL, and subcutaneous panniculitis-like lymphoma are considered for allo-HCT in first relapse, because auto-HCT usually does not work well for such diseases in the relapsed setting. T cell prolymphocytic leukemia (T-PLL), adult T cell leukemia/lymphoma (ATLL) and extranodal T/NK lymphoma, nasal type (unless it is stage I and gets into a CR with chemoradiation), as well as γδ hepatosplenic lymphoma, are considered for allo-HCT in CR1. Enteropathy-associated T cell lymphoma (EATL) and Sezary syndrome may also be considered for allo-HCT, which can be curative [44].

Marrow Failure Syndromes

Aplastic anemia patients usually receive allo-HCT as first-line therapy if they are younger than 40 years old and have a matched-sibling donor. If they are older, immunosuppressive therapy with anti-thymocyte globulin and cyclosporine (ATG-CsA) is the preferred initial therapy and allo-HCT is used if immunosuppressive therapy is not successful, typically after waiting three to six months to assess the clinical response, which may be delayed. The conditioning regimen for aplastic anemia is typically ATG with cyclophosphamide (+/- low dose TBI for MUD allo-HCT), although many trials show encouraging results with incorporation of fludarabine in the conditioning regimen [45]. It is essential to rule out Fanconi anemia in young aplastic patients [46], because Fanconi patients are conditioned differently. Most of the other marrow failure syndromes are also treated with allo-HCT (Fanconi, dyskeratosis congenita, Shwachman-Diamond syndrome, and amegakaryocytic thrombocytopenia).

Myelodysplastic Syndromes (MDS)

Myelodysplastic syndromes are typically incurable and may progress either to bone marrow failure or to acute leukemia. Since the incidence of MDS increases with age, comorbidties are a major limiting factor that adversely influences survival following treatment of elderly patients. Unfortunately, few clinical therapies have been demonstrated to be helpful. DNA Methyltransferase inhibitors (DNMTI) like azacytidine and decitabine can prolong PFS or OS, but do not cure the disease. Allo-HCT is curative in the majority of patients who are transplanted with low marrow blast counts, but may not be possible in many patients with MDS, given the prevalence of limiting comorbidities and/or advanced age.

In most patients presenting with MDS, azacytidine or decitabine is typically administered as initial therapy unless the burden of leukemic blasts is high, in which cases, AML induction is used. The International Prognosis Scoring System (IPSS) can be a guide in terms of which patients may benefit most from early transplantation. A large meta-analysis showed that transplant is detrimental for low-risk patients, but is beneficial in Int-2 and high-risk patients [47]. The decision when to transplant IPSS-1 is more complex and depends on the presence of adverse cytogenetics, the percentage of marrow blasts, the frequency of infections and transfusions, and the response to DNMTI [48, 49]. Patients with monosomy 7 or requiring frequent transfusions without response to DNMTIs should be considered for early transplantation. Deferasirox or other iron chelation therapy should be used before transplant to avoid the complications of iron overload. Given the typical age and comorbidities present in most MDS patients, RIC conditioning (Flu-Mel, Flu-Bu with reduced busulfan dosing) is preferred because of reduced toxicity and similar overall survival, although decreased conditioning intensity does increase the likelihood of relapse[48, 49].

Myeloproliferative Neoplasms

Selected younger patients with myelofibrosis and with good performance status can be cured with allo-HCT [50, 51]. Atypical CML, chronic myelomonocytic leukemia (CMML), juvenile myelomonocytic leukemia (JMML), and MDS/MPN, NOS, as well as aggressive systemic mastocytosis, can be cured with allo-HCT.

Hemoglobinopathies

Both thalassemia and sickle cell disease (SCD) patients can be cured with allo-HCT. The optimal conditioning regimen for these diseases is under investigation. The risk of graft rejection in thalassemia is relatively higher and increases with the number of transfusions received before transplant. In thalassemia, the outcome can be predicted by the degree of iron overload. For thalassemic patients who have not had sufficient therapy with chelating agents and for those with hepatomegaly and liver fibrosis, the outcome is worse [52]. Bone marrow is usually preferred as the source of HSC to prevent chronic GVHD. For the same reason, ATG is used even for related transplants. For severe SCD, very early transplantation may be considered, since some of the complications of this disease are irreversible. Survival is better when transplant is done earlier for severe SCD. Interestingly, favorable outcomes of allogeneic transplantation in patients with hemoglobinopathies have been noted even when complete donor chimerism can't be achieved [53]. Stable mixed chimerism may be sufficient for satisfactory outcomes, when sufficient normal red cells are produced by the donor graft to reduce disease-related complications.

Immunodeficiencies

Examples include severe combined immunodeficiency (SCID), leukocyte adhesion defect (LAD), adenosine deaminase (ADA) deficiency, Chediak-Higashi syndrome, and chronic granulomatous disease. In all of these defects, diagnosis, as well as allo-HCT, should be performed early to avoid morbidity and mortality associated with opportunistic infections [54]. The conditioning regimen does not have to be intense, since rejection rate is usually low secondary to the underlying immunodeficiency. Because cord units are more readily available and usually do not carry EBV or CMV, they are frequently used to facilitate early transplantation in immunodeficient patients, particularly since outcomes in infants transplanted with cord blood are generally favorable. Recent studies have also considered the possibility of HIV eradication via the selection of allogeneic donors homozygous for the CCR5-δ32 mutation that decreases the permissiveness of HIV infection via co-receptor binding [55].

Inborn Errors of Metabolism

Some of these disorders (e.g., leukodystrophies and lysosomal storage diseases like Gaucher, fucosidosis, Hurler disease, and Hunter disease) can be cured with allo-HCT [56, 57]. Other diseases like Niemann-Pick disease cannot be cured with allo-HCT. It is imperative the transplant be performed early in these disorders before irreversible organ damage happens.

Hematopoietic Stem Cells (HSC), Homing, and Mobilization

HSC are remarkable for their properties of pluripotent differentiation, self-renewal, and unlimited replicative potential. One of the cardinal properties of HSC is their ability to reconstitute long-term hematopoiesis (more than few months) in a myeloablated severely immunodeficient mouse strain (e.g., NOD-SCID mice knocked out for the γ-subunit of the receptor for IL-2). They express multiple efflux pumps, including P-glycoprotein, that make them relatively resistant to chemotherapy. With these pumps, they are able to efflux some membrane dyes like Hoechst 33342, a property that is useful for their identification. Besides the efflux pumps, they possess properties that may confer chemoresistance; for example, they highly express aldehyde dehydrogenase that protects them from cyclophosphamide. Their immunophenotype is CD34+ /CD38-/CD90+/CD133+/VEGFR2+/CD150+/CD45RA$^{negative/dim}$/HLA-DR$^{negative/dim}$)/CD71-. Because of their efflux pumps, they are dimly stained with rhodamine-123 or Hoechst 33342. The CD34 marker is not specific for HSC since 2%–5% of bone marrow cells express the CD34 marker when only rare (<~1 in 10^5 cells) marrow cells are true HSC. Similarly, CD34-negative HSC have been described [58–61].

HSC reside in very delicate niches in the bone marrow, where support from surrounding cells and the extracellular matrix is essential for their function. These niches are either close to sinusoids (vascular niches) where HSC tend to proliferate, or close to the periosteum (endosteal niches) where HSC reside, mostly in a dormant state. Stem cell factor (SCF, kit ligand, steel factor) is essential for the maintenance of HSC in the perivascular niche and the sources of SCF in that microenvironment are endothelial cells and perivascular stromal cells expressing the leptin receptor. Thrombopoietin, Flt-3 ligand, and IL-3 also play significant roles in the maintenance of HSC. These cytokines transmit signals to the nucleus through pathways that activate mainly the transcription factors of the Homeobox family, including HoxA9 and HoxB4. Similarly, the stromal-derived factor-1 (SDF-1, CXCL12) via binding to CXCR4 not only helps to retain HSC in the bone marrow, but has an important role for HSC survival and proliferation. The Notch ligands of the Delta family are mainly expressed by osteoblasts and endothelial cells and transmit mitogenic signals to HSC [62]. Likewise, the Wnt/β-catenin pathway is essential not only for the maintenance of normal HSC, but also for the survival of leukemic stem cells through signals transmitted to the nucleus by the transcription factor TCF/LEF [63, 64]. In contrast, the TGFβ-Smad pathway inhibits the proliferation of HSC; similarly, the Angiopoetin-1/Tie-2 axis promotes quiescence of HSC in their niche [65]. Surprisingly, the EGF-EGFR axis protects and governs the regeneration of HSC after a myelosuppressive insult [66] through downregulation of the pro-apoptotic factor PUMA.

The HSC remain in their niches mainly through three interactions: CXCL12(SDF-1)-CXCR4, CD106(VCAM)-CD49d(VLA-4), and SCF-Kit (CD117). The CXCR4, CD49d, and Kit receptors are expressed in the HSC and interact with CXCL12, CD106, and SCF that are either expressed or secreted by niche cells of mesenchymal origin. Two important cellular producers of CXCL12 are the nestin+ mesenchymal stem cells (MSCs) and the CXCL12 abundant reticular cells (CARs) [59]. Adjacent CD68+ macrophages facilitate the production of CXCL12 by MSCs and CARs. Norepinephrine secreted by nerve fibers of the autonomous nervous system activates β3 receptors leading to a downregulation of CXCL12 production, mainly by nestin+ MSCs, and lets HSC escape the niche in a mechanism that follows a circadian rhythm [67, 68]. Parathyroid hormone increases HSC number by stimulating the proliferation of nestin+ MSCs [69].

Extracellular matrix plays a role in the retention of HSC to the niche. Fibronectin binds also to CD49d and hyaluronan to CD44 and to RHAMM (CD168). CD44d, CD44, and CD168 are expressed by HSC. The binding of fibronectin to VLA-4 mediates intracellular signals to the HSC mainly through the paxillin-FAK complex, which in turn activates the PI3 K and Ras pathways. Such signals regulate the cytoskeleton, but also can increase proliferation. Finally, the 67 KDa laminin receptor (which is known to be metastasis facilitator) is overexpressed in filgrastim mobilized HSC and probably plays a significant role in the HSC egress from the bone marrow [70].

HSC Mobilization

Filgrastim (filgrastim) is the most commonly used factor to mobilize HSC to escape from the BM and is usually given in a dose of 10 mcg/kg starting four days before the first apheresis day and is continued daily during apheresis. Filgrastim makes nestin+ MSCs dysfunctional and decreases the transcription of CXCL12 and expression of CD106 and SCF via two mechanisms: depletion of niche macrophages and stimulation of sympathetic nerve fibers [71]. The role of neutrophil-derived proteases like cathepsin, metalloproteinases, and elastase in filgrastim-induced HSC mobilization is not considered as important as initially believed.

Furthermore, due to the sympathetic innervations of the niche, administration of β2 agonists in mice increased HSC mobilization [67, 72]. Filgrastim alone is sufficient in most cases of mobilization of allogeneic donors. Mobilization of autologous HSC can be problematic, especially if the patients have received multiple lines of chemotherapy prior to attempted mobilization, in which case filgrastim alone may result in suboptimal collections.

It is known that chemotherapy itself mobilizes HSC. The most frequent chemotherapy used to mobilize HSC is cyclophosphamide, which kills osteoblasts and macrophages in the endosteal niche and induces HSC proliferation. Cyclophosphamide [73] can work synergistically with filgrastim, and when it is used, collection usually starts in the second week (day 11) after cyclophosphamide administration. Intermediate doses of cyclophosphamide (1500 mg/m^2) can be given in the outpatient setting and are probably safer than the older regimens of high-dose cyclophosphamide that were more likely to be complicated by infection, requiring hospitalization and presenting a greater risk of urothelial toxicity and profound myelosuppression. Many factors can decrease HSC mobilization, including advanced age, a history of prior marrow irradiation, heavy pre-treatment with chemotherapy, and especially the prior use of alkylating agents, purine analogs, and lenalidomide.

Plerixafor is a CXCR4 antagonist that works by disrupting the CXCR4-CXCL12 bond, thereby releasing HSC from the niche. It is administered the evening before the planned stem cell collection and usually given in combination with filgrastim, facilitating collections possible for patients who have failed filgrastim alone [74]. However, approximately one-third of patients who failed mobilization are not able to collect desired numbers of HSC, even with the use of plerixafor. Previously, marrow collection was considered in failed mobilizers, but is now rarely performed in this situation, since marrow yields are typically decreased commensurately. Sometimes such "poor mobilizers" are able to collect the safe threshold of two million CD34+ cells/kg with the combination of all three approaches (chemotherapy, filgrastim, and plerixafor), but obviously new approaches are needed [8]. Such an approach is to further weaken the HSC interaction with the niche that is integrin-mediated, as with CD49d inhibitors like BIO5192 [75] or natalizumab (a mAb inhibitor of α4 integrin already approved for multiple sclerosis) [76]. Additional CXCR4 inhibitors are in clinical trials (POL6326 and BTK140) [77] and use of PTH or β2 agonists has been proposed. Since HSC express sphingosine-1 phosphate receptors, experiments have shown that S1P mimetics like SEW2871 (but not fingolimod) increase plerixafor-induced HSC mobilization [78].

Allogeneic Donor Selection

In general, HLA-matched sibling donors (MSD) are preferred over matched unrelated donors (MUD), although the outcome differences in most experienced centers have diminished and are often considered to be minimal, especially with the best-matched MUD donors. Syngeneic transplants (e.g., from identical twins) are usually avoided because of the absence of significant GVL effects. If a living HLA-matched donor is not available and transplant is considered necessary, either an umbilical cord blood transplantation (UCBT) or a haplo-identical transplant (haplo-HCT) is pursued. UCBT in adults usually involve two cord units (double UCBT, dUCBT) and haplo-HCT requires *in vitro* or *in vivo* donor T cell depletion in order to avoid potentially lethal GVHD. The reason that UCBT and haplo-HCT are usually not performed more broadly is that the infectious complication rates are higher and the GVL effect is delayed and possibly weaker. The advantage is that in both cases, donor availability is more immediate in case an urgent transplant is required.

Donors should have good functional status, without significant co-morbidities and free of malignancies, HIV, and hepatitis viruses. Increasing donor age is associated with higher incidence of GVHD and for that reason, among similarly matched donors, the youngest one is usually preferred. Since allo-HCT is performed with increased frequency in older individuals, a relevant question is if the outcome will be better with older sibling donors or with younger MUDs. Recently, it was showed that in such situations, the sibling is preferred even when older, since mortality and GVHD rates were higher with MUDs [79]. In some cases, a sibling is mismatched in only one HLA antigen with the recipient, but there are completely matched MUDs available. In such cases, the completely matched MUD should be selected, according to a Japanese analysis [80]. Among similarly matched donors, if age is not an issue, CMV serostatus is often considered. If the recipient is CMV seronegative, there is a risk of CMV transmission if the donor is seropositive. Nevertheless, if the recipient is CMV seropositive, the likelihood of clinically significant CMV reactivation may be decreased due to the adoptive transfer of donor graft T cells to the recipient that are CMV-experienced [81, 82]. If age, HLA match, and CMV serostatus are similar between potential donors, ABO-matched donors are preferred. This is true, since recipient isohemagglutinins are expected to attack donor RBC, increasing the risk of hemolysis and transfusion requirements after transplant. When the source of stem cells is marrow rather than an apheresis product, and a major ABO mismatch is present, it is necessary for the donor product to be depleted of RBC before infusion to avoid major hemolytic reactions; this usually results in some HSC loss and a lower final HSC dose infused, potentially leading to delays in engraftment, depending on the resulting progenitor cell dose.

For non-malignant diseases, and for malignant diseases of lower risk for relapse, including those that are in remission before HCT, marrow may be the preferred HSC source, since it is associated with lower rates of cGVHD than with PBSC, due to lower donor graft T cell numbers. Various clinical studies have demonstrated that patients with CML in chronic phase, as well as patients with hemoglobinopathies and aplastic anemia, have better outcomes with BM-derived HSC than with PBSC.

In MUD HCT, the donor-recipient pair should not have more than one allelic mismatch at least in the GVHD direction (i.e., donor lymphocytes should not see more than one discordant HLA antigen in the recipient), to avoid a high-risk of GVHD. The relevant HLA antigens that are usually checked before transplants are the class I antigens HLA-A, -B, -C; and the class II antigens HLA-DR and -DQ, although many institutions do not count a mismatch in DQ since a NMDP large-scale analysis in 2007 showed no survival disadvantage with DP or DQ mismatches [83]. Most institutions believe that in the absence of any better donor, a 7/8 MUD (matched at HLA-A, B, C, and DR) is acceptable. Mismatches at HLA-C and HLA-B are better tolerated and preferred over HLA-DR or HLA-A mismatches. It should be emphasized that a perfect match at 12 loci (i.e., considering both DQ and DP, if available) may be desirable, since European reports have shown higher GVHD with DP-mismatches, which may be associated with recipient anti-HLA-DP antibodies (especially in multiparous women), potentially increasing the risk of graft rejection [84, 85].

A recent CIBMTR analysis showed that for transplants in adult AML patients, survival was similar between 8/8 MUD and MSD HCT; however, early mortality was higher with 7/8 MUD HCT (RR=1.4, compared to MSD HCT), although this survival difference lost its significance with longer follow-up [86]. Since GVHD rates are higher with MUD HCT, most centers apply some form of T cell depletion (TCD). The most widely used method is *in vivo* depletion with anti-thymocyte globulin (ATG) and although alemtuzumab is also frequently used instead of ATG, it has been associated with high rates of relapses and opportunistic infections. Lower than traditional doses of alemtuzumab are more acceptable and have been successfully tried [87]. A challenge on the dogma of using ATG for MUD allo-HCT came from Soiffer et al., who showed in a retrospective analysis that in vivo TCD with ATG impaired survival after reduced intensity conditioning MUD HCT [88]. Others have recently used post-transplant cyclophosphamide for in vivo TCD, which may lessen or eliminate the need for methotrexate and calcineurin inhibitors for GVHD prophylaxis in the MSD and MUD setting [89].

If an HLA-matched donor is not available, then a family member who is haplo-identical with the recipient may be used. In such cases, TCD is obligatory and usually this happens ex vivo in the stem cell product using antibodies directed against T cell antigens. Another method is the ex vivo positive selection of CD34+ cells. A third method is in vivo TCD with post-transplant use of cyclophosphamide. In an attempt to maximize the GVT effect given the absence of T cells in the graft, investigators have tried to use donors whose NK cells are predicted to be reactive against the recipient neoplastic cells based on killer cell immunoglobulin-like receptors (KIR) and mismatches with their ligands (KIR-L). KIR on NK cells can recognize HLA molecules that, upon engagement, can send inhibitory signals to the NK cells. Conversely, the absence of such ligands in the recipient can lower the activation threshold of donor NK cells. Such strategy of KIR/KIR-L mismatching has been shown to decrease relapse rates in the setting of haploidentical transplantation for myeloid leukemias [90]. This effect is not as pronounced outside of the haplo-HCT setting, and this difference is thought to be dependent on the greater importance of NK alloreactivity in the setting of T cell depletion. Very potent immunosuppressive recipient conditioning is necessary to avoid graft rejection in the haploidentical setting and this traditionally required the use of a strong ablative regimen; recently, reduced intensity conditioning regimens have been successfully used. More recently, it was shown that AML was less likely if the NK cells in the graft were positive for the activating receptor KIR2DS1, provided that the NK cells had at least one HLA-C1 allele [91]. Unfortunately, at this point, no routine screen for minor histocompatibility or KIR gene mismatches is done.

Less stringent matching is required for cord blood grafts. Most centers accept 4/6 matches (antigenic class I matching at HLA-A, B, and high resolution class II molecular matching at HLA-DRB1). The cell dose should be at least 30 million nucleated cells per kg (of recipient weight) and at least 200,000 CD34+ cells per kg. If these criteria are not fulfilled, then more than one cord units are typically used [92]. Recently, CIBMTR data showed that additional matching at HLA-C reduces treatment-related mortality (TRM) [93]. Screening of the recipient for anti-HLA antibodies is recommended in both the UCBT and haplo-HCT settings by many centers to find the graft with the lowest risk for rejection [94]. When this is not possible, depletion of the anti-HLA antibody may be attempted with plasma exchange and/or medications like steroids, intravenous immunoglobulin, and/or rituximab.

Expansion of cord units before infusion has been attempted in order to accelerate engraftment. De Lima et al. [95] described a technique where Stro-3+ MSCs were co-cultured with one of the two intended to infuse cord units in the presence of SCF, filgrastim, TPO, and Flt3. WBC engrafted on day +15, as opposed to day +24, for unmanipulated grafts. The acceleration of platelet engraftment was less pronounced. In a previous report, Delaney et al. reported on the engraftment of ten patients who received two cord blood units, one of which was expanded in the presence of immobilized Delta-1 (ligand for Notch), SCF, Flt3, TPO, IL-3, and IL-6. In this report, neutrophil engraftment occurred at a median of day +16, as compared to day +26 in historic controls [96]. Co-administration of haploidentical TCD grafts together with cord units has been performed in order to achieve faster neutrophil engraftment from the haplo-unit as a bridge to cord blood engraftment [97]. Expansion of CD34+ UCB cells in the presence of nicotinamide has also accelerated both neutrophil and platelet engraftment [98]. Multiple approaches are being pursued to facilitate UCB stem cell homing (e.g., *ex vivo* treatment of the cord units with dimethyl-PGE2, fucosylation of the cord unit, or *in vivo* administration of sitagliptin to the recipient) [99, 100] [101].

Graft Failure

Failure of initial engraftment (primary graft failure) and subsequent loss of engraftment or donor chimerism (secondary graft failure) is a serious complication and can be mediated by diverse immune mechanisms. Apart from specific anti-donor antibodies, T cells and NK cells can also reject the graft. One of the main aims of preparative regimens and post-transplant immunosuppression is to avoid rejection caused by residual host anti-donor immunity. Regulatory T cells in the mouse model have been shown to offer immune protection to the HSC niche [102–104] [105].

Once graft failure occurs, re-transplantation from the same or different donors may be attempted after intense immunosuppressive preparation. It is interesting that in such salvage attempts, the incidence of severe GVHD is high and may even be lethal [106]. In the case of incomplete (or mixed) donor chimerism, the infusion of donor T cells is frequently what is needed; however, this should be avoided if recipient chimerism predominates, because this can lead to lethal marrow aplasia. It is interesting that the higher the stem cell dose, the faster the engraftment kinetics and the lower the rejection rate. Two million CD34+ donor stem cells per kg is considered to be a safe dose, but higher stem cell doses are preferred. Even with "megadoses" of PBSC, the incidence of GVHD is not increased, perhaps because of the stable proportion of regulatory T cells in the graft.

Transfusion Support after HCT

After HCT, asymptomatic patients receive platelet transfusions to prevent spontaneous bleeding, usually above 10,000/μL, and also receive PRBCs (often to keep the hemoglobin concentration above 8 gm/dL) to minimize the risk of tissue hypoxia, activation of anaerobic metabolism, and also to prevent bleeding, as higher hemoglobin values are associated with improved vascular wall integrity and less bleeding. All blood products administered to immunocompromised transplant recipients should be irradiated to prevent transfusion-mediated GVHD, which can be lethal, mediated by transfused lymphocytes that attack the hematopoietic cells of immunosuppressed patients, potentially causing lethal marrow aplasia. Products should also be leukocyte reduced to avoid the transmission of viruses that are dormant inside white cells and to prevent infusion reactions (mainly fever) associated with cytokines produced by white cells. If the filtering of white cells is efficient, there is definitely less allo-immunization against HLA that sometimes causes problems with platelet transfusions (platelet transfusion refractoriness). If there is adequate filtration, the development of anti-HLA antibodies is about the same with both pooled platelet and apheresis platelet transfusion, which is more difficult to find. If the recipient and the donor are both CMV seronegative, it is safer to transfuse CMV-negative blood products to prevent primary CMV infection, which may be life-threatening in the immunocompromised host.

Frequently there is an ABO mismatch between stem cell donor and recipient. This is called major ABO mismatch when the recipient is the producer of isohemagglutinins (e.g., donor A, recipient O) and minor ABO mismatch when the donor has produced the isohemagglutinins (e.g., recipient A, donor O). When both the donor and the recipient have produced isohemagglutinins, then we call the ABO mismatch bidirectional (e.g., recipient A, donor B).

In the cases of major or bidirectional ABO mismatch, when an RBC-rich product is used (mainly marrow products), donor RBC are removed in order to prevent acute hemolytic reactions. After transplant, recipients of a major ABO-mismatched transplant receive transfusions of O group PRBCs until the titer of isohemagglutinins is undetectable and the recipient changes blood group (acquires the donor's blood group). The most serious complication after a major ABO-mismatched HCT is pure red cell aplasia that is the result of isohemagglutinin attack against RBC precursors in the bone marrow. The treatment is usually supportive with transfusions until the titer of isohemagglutinins is decreased and allows red cell production. Nevertheless, there have been cases where surviving memory B cells or plasma cells survived the conditioning and continued to produce antibodies. In such cases, withdrawal of immunosuppression may allow the donor T cells to attack the residual recipient antibody-producing cells. Rituximab and plasma exchange have been used successfully in this setting. In case of incomplete donor chimerism co-existing with post-HCT pure red cell aplasia, DLI can help.

In the case of minor ABO mismatch, there is a risk of recipient RBC hemolysis either by a high titer of isohemagglutinins already contained in the HCT product or by new isohemagglutinins produced by donor lymphocytes (which can lead to a delayed hemolytic reaction). In the case of a high titer of preformed isohemagglutinins against recipient RBC, some centers perform RBC exchange in the recipient to decrease the population of RBCs destined to be targeted by the donor isohemagglutinins. Others have proposed the removal of plasma from the stem cell product if the isohemagglutinin titer is high (1:128 or higher). In the setting of minor ABO mismatch, group O PRBCs are given post-HCT.

When plasma or platelets need to be transfused to a recipient of an ABO-mismatched HCT, every effort should be made to avoid products rich in isohemagglutinins against red cells circulating in the recipient. In the worst mismatch (bidirectional), AB plasma or platelets are preferred until establishment of a permanent post-HCT PRBC group. In cases of major ABO mismatch, platelets or plasma of the same ABO group with donor's blood group are transfused. In cases of minor mismatch, platelets and plasma of the same ABO group with the recipient are infused (until full donor erythropoiesis is established). In cases of Rh major mismatch and proof of presence of anti-Rh antibodies in the recipient, red cell depletion of the stem cell product is done when the graft contains high volumes of donor RBCs (e.g., bone marrow products) [107–109] [110, 111].

Frequently, platelet transfusions post-HCT are not associated with a satisfactory increase of the patient's platelet count. Checking platelet counts one hour after platelet transfusion is a very good predictor of effective platelet transfusion. If the corrected count increment (CCI) is <5000, the platelet transfusion was not effective in raising platelet count and the most common problem is an antibody. CCI is calculated as follows: CCI = (post-transfusion – pre-transfusion platelet count) × body surface area × 10^{11} / number of transfused platelets. One apheresis platelet unit usually contains three to four × 10^{11} platelets. In most cases, the antibody responsible for platelet transfusion refractoriness is an anti-HLA antibody. In such cases, HLA-matched platelets (partially matched at HLA-A and HLA-B) are transfused. In cases that this does not solve the problem, platelet crossmatching may be performed to identify a unit that does not react with the serum of the patient [112, 113] [114].

Hematopoietic and Immune Reconstitution after HCT

It is difficult to generalize the process of immune reconstitution post-transplant because this depends on many factors like the type of transplant, the source of stem cells, the use of ATG, the age of the patient, the nature of the underlying disease and of previous treatments, the intensity of the conditioning regimen, and the development of GVHD [115, 116].

Neutrophils engraft usually within 10–17 days post-transplant (slightly faster if filgrastim is used). While the recovery of an absolute neutrophil count above 500 cells/μl is associated with relative freedom from disease caused by endogenous pathogens, multiple reports have demonstrated the presence of qualitative neutrophil defects after HCT. Phagocytosis and respiratory burst may take up to two months to normalize, while chemotaxis is especially impaired in the context of GVHD. Trials of GM-CSF or filgrastim have improved some of the functional defects, but results have been inconsistent [117]. The use of steroids for GVHD is deleterious for phagocytes, since they compromise the respiratory burst and the killing of fungi [118]. Paradoxically, fungal exotoxins may increase ROS production, potentially increasing the inflammation associated with fungal infection and mediating tissue injury [119]. Immunosuppressive medications that are used to prevent GVHD can inhibit phagocyte chemotaxis (mTOR and calcineurin inhibitors), as well as superoxide production and release of antibacterial products like lysozyme, lactoferrin, and elastase. Infection with cytomegalovirus (CMV) may not only decrease neutrophil numbers (via direct myelosuppressive effects, and also due to the effects of antiviral agents, including ganciclovir), but can also impair neutrophil function and contribute to a more aggressive course of bacterial infections [120]. Since there is a delay in the post-transplant reconstitution of adaptive immunity (both T and B), impaired neutrophil function can be secondary due to attenuated cytokine production by T cells and to decreased opsonization resulting from reduced antibody production.

Polymorphisms of genes implicated in the innate immune response have been associated with higher incidence of infections. Mannose binding lectin 2 (MBL2) gene polymorphisms increase the rate of bacterial infections [121] and likewise polymorphisms of the Toll-Like Receptor 4 (TLR4) gene increases the risks of fungal infections, especially Aspergillus [122]. Defects in mucosal integrity and low levels of IgA and lysozyme contribute to a higher incidence of post-HCT skin, gastrointestinal, and respiratory infections.

The first subset of lymphocytes that recovers post-transplantation is the NK cells. It takes about a month for them to reach a plateau number and their function seems to be preserved even in the context of GVHD. Their immunophenotype initially is that of $CD16^{dim}$ $CD56^{bright}$ and they are able to kill micro-organisms, and postulated to also kill cancer cells [123, 124]. In the allo-HCT mouse setting, donor NK cells are able to kill recipient antigen presenting cells (APCs), and thus they decrease the GVHD rate. By killing recipient T cells, NK cells may facilitate donor engraftment; furthermore, NK-mediated killing of myeloid leukemic cells in the context of KIR/KIR-ligand mismatch may decrease relapse rates, at least in the setting of T cell depletion as in haploidentical HCT.

Although NK cells recover relatively soon after allo-HCT, the recovery of invariant NKT cells (iNKT) depends on the use of TCD. Without ATG or ex vivo TCD, iNKT cells recover as fast as NK cells, but in the T cell-depleted setting, it may take a year before they recover. They produce high quantities of IFNγ and they appear to be important for the control of mycobacterial infections. They are also able to produce IL-4 under different polarizing conditions, in which case they can protect against GVHD, based on murine modeling [125–127].

Donor dendritic cells may take up to six months to replace the relative radio- and chemo-resistant population of recipient tissue dendritic cells. They play a significant role in the antigen presentation of recipient antigens to donor T cells and thus to the initiation of acute GVHD [128]. The recovery of plasmacytoid dendritic cells (pDCs) is more delayed than that of myeloid dendritic cells (mDCs), and this may contribute to the increased incidence of viral infections post-HCT, since pDCs are sources of high quantities of IFNα.

The reconstitution of the adaptive immune system is slower, especially after allo-HCT. B cell numbers are very low in the first few months, though (like NK cells) may recover more quickly after CBT, presumably due to the relative T lymphopenia found in that setting[129]. GVHD can further delay B cell reconstitution. Recovery of relatively normal B cell numbers may take up to six months after auto-HCT and longer after allo-HCT. Naïve B cells (IgD+ CD27-) appear first, followed by memory B cells (CD27+). Antibody diversity and repertoire are diminished after HCT, which increases the frequency of infections. Somatic hypermutation of IgH genes may not be evident until almost a year after an allo-HCT [130–132]. Nevertheless, B cells may play a significant role in chronic GVHD. In chronic GVHD, autoreactive B cells are maintained through increased BAFF (B cell activating factor) levels, leading to the activation of Akt and ERK pathways and the inactivation of Bim (through ERK-induced Bim phosphorylation). Inactivation of Bim decreases the apoptotic rate of these B cells [133]. Immunosuppressive medications, used for GVHD prophylaxis and therapy, and intravenous immunoglobulin administration can further delay the recovery of humoral immunity. At least six months after HCT, recipients begin immunizations even if they or their donors had been vaccinated previously, to facilitate the recovery of lost recall responses against microbes.

T cell reconstitution after HCT follows a different course. The memory and the effector T cells derived from the donor are the ones that expand initially. This process is more efficient for CD8 cells than for CD4 cells. During the first year post-allo-HCT, the CD4/CD8 ratio is reversed. T cell depleted grafts and use of ATG or alemtuzumab delay T cell recovery further [134–138]. The immune reconstitution after UCBT is very slow. Although NK and B cells recover relatively fast, T cell recovery lags behind and takes a year or even longer to match the recovery seen after MSD or T cell replete MUD HCT. Because of the delayed T cell recovery after UCBT, the rate of opportunistic infections is higher and persists for long period of time [129, 139]. Nevertheless, the brisk recovery of NK cells after UCBT that usually have low levels of the inhibitory receptor NKG2A may contribute to lower than expected rates of relapse [6, 140].

Until the late 1990s, when two studies demonstrated conclusively that thymopoiesis persists throughout the life of most healthy adults, the thymus was thought to be largely vestigial beyond adolescence [141, 142]. Due to primary and secondary effects of cancer (and its therapy) on thymopoiesis, resulting in variable delays in recovery of T cell production after HCT, the development of naïve T cells with broad T cell receptor (TCR) repertoire is markedly slow (years). The thymus is also a target of GVHD [143], so patients with GVHD are severely immunocompromised and this worsens with the use of immunosuppressive medications that treat GVHD. Because recipient thymopoiesis theoretically generates T cells tolerant to self, but able to fight neoplasms and microbes, many efforts have been focused on enhancing the recovery recipient thymopoiesis. IL-7 is important for thymic regeneration [144-146] and has already been safely administered in adult recipients of TCD allo-HCT. Encouraging TCR diversity and T cell numerical recovery was observed. In the T cell-depleted HCT setting, however, there is a concern that administration of IL-7 may increase GVHD. Keratinocyte growth factor (KGF) [147], growth hormone, and the use of GnRH analogues (medical castration) have also been suggested to enhance thymopoiesis [148]; however, conclusive clinical data in the HCT setting are lacking.

Regulatory T cells (Treg, CD4+ CD25+ FoxP3+ CD127-) have been reported to decrease GVHD without inhibiting GvL. They probably play a role in reducing the severity or occurrence of GVHD after allo-HCT. Their presence and expansion may also contribute to the beneficial role of autologous transplant in auto-immune diseases like scleroderma and multiple sclerosis. Multiple groups are working on adoptive therapy of these cells in the HCT setting, as this has been demonstrated to be feasible, safe, and potentially effective in the setting of CBT [149]. Another study demonstrated Treg infusion in the haploidentical setting was able to facilitate the subsequent infusion of modest doses of conventional T cells without resulting in significant GVHD [150].

Due to the delayed recovery of T cells after allo-HCT, which can be more pronounced after haplo-HCT and after UCBT, infections with viruses are common. To overcome this problem, recently studies have examined the utility of the adoptive transfer of ex vivo manufactured T cells with specificity against EBV, CMV, and adenoviruses together, with the remarkable ability to prevent or treat multiple clinically significant infections without causing GVHD [151].

Infections after HCT

Infections are similar in the pre-engraftment period between allo-HCT and auto-HCT recipients. Mucositis increases the risk of febrile neutropenia. Bloodstream bacterial infections usually result from bacterial translocation from the GI tract or from infection of indwelling catheters. The most common gram-positive infections are caused by coagulase-negative *Staphylococci*, while more serious infections may be caused by *Staphylococcus aureus* and *Streptococcus viridans*, both of which can cause septic shock and endocarditis. Culture-negative neutropenic fever in the pre-engraftment period is usually caused by gram-positive bacteria, especially *Bacillus* species. The most dramatic infections are the gram-negative septicemias, many of which can be rapidly lethal if appropriate antibiotics are not instituted early. Gram-negative bacteria causing infections in the pre-engraftment syndrome include *Pseudomonas, E.coli, Klebsiella, Enterobacter, Acinetobacter, Citrobacter, Legionella pneumophila*, and *Stenotrophomonas maltophilia*. *Legionella* and *S. maltophilia* cause pneumonia, while the rest of the aforementioned bacteria are frequently associated with broad resistance to antibiotics (ESBL: extended-spectrum beta-lactamase producing bacteria, MDR: multi-drug resistant species, KPC: *Klebsiella pneumonia* carbapenemase-producing bacteria etc.). Neutropenic fever after transplant is usually treated with broad-spectrum anti-pseudomonal penicillins, cephalosporins, or carbapenems (e.g., cefepime, meropenem, or piperacillin/tazobactam) [152]. Vancomycin is often added [153], especially for patients known to be colonized with methicillin-resistant *Staphylococci* or when signs of catheter-related infection are present. Aminoglycosides (tobramycin or amikacin) are added either from the beginning or when the infection is associated with hypotension or hypoxemia, but may be associated with a greater risk of nephrotoxicity.

Diarrhea after HCT is frequent and because of antibiotic use in these patients, infections with *Clostridium difficile* are present in about 15% of patients with post-HCT diarrhea. Fidaxomicin, which is FDA-approved for the treatment of difficult cases of *C. difficile* diarrhea, is now being assessed for its safety and efficacy to prevent *C. difficile* diarrhea in post-HCT recipients [154-156]. Another cause of antibiotic-related hemorrhagic diarrhea has been recently identified to be the bacterium *Klebsiella oxytoca* [157] [158], which is also known to cause sepsis in transplanted patients. It has been reported that recipients of UCBT may experience an antibiotic-responsive colitis syndrome with histologic similarities with inflammatory bowel disease. Recently, the cause of this syndrome was identified [159] to be the bacterium *Bradyrhizobium enterica*. When the diarrhea is suspected to be infectious, stool specimens are assessed for *Salmonella, Shigella, E. coli* 0157:H7, and ova and parasites. *Entamoeba histolytica, Strongyloides*, and *Giardia* infections should be ruled out in certain populations.

Fungi now cause fewer infections than bacteria in the pre-engraftment period, probably as a result of the widespread use of azole prophylaxis and because prolonged neutropenia is no longer common after allo-HCT, except in the setting of CBT. Nevertheless, infections with fluconazole-resistant *Candida krusei* and *C. glabrata* may occur, as may infections caused by pathogenic molds. Among the latter, *Aspergillus* and *Fusarium* species are the most common. Zygomycosis, either with sinus or/and lung involvement, occurs usually in acute leukemia patients with prolonged periods of antecedent neutropenia.

Diabetes mellitus increases the risk of zygomycosis, and the risk is increased in patients with a prior history of treatment with voriconazole [160]. Newer azoles (voriconazole, posaconazole), echinocandins (micafungin, caspofungin, anidulafungin) and lipid preparations of amphotericin (Abelcet, Ambisome) have together tremendously improved the treatment of difficult fungal infections [161].

The most common virus causing infections in the pre-engraftment period was HSV, though acyclovir prophylaxis has significantly reduced HSV-associated morbidity. Community respiratory viruses are quite common in healthy adults and can cause significant morbidity or even mortality after HCT. Such viruses include RSV, parainfluenza, influenza, rhinoviruses, coronaviruses, adenoviruses, and metapneumovirus. It is important to prohibit transplant unit access to individuals with evidence of respiratory infection or recent contact with sick persons. Any suspicion for influenza should trigger the use of antiviral therapy (e.g., using oseltamivir or zanamivir). Intravenous immunoglobin may help with serious cases of other respiratory viruses where specific antivirals are lacking. Ribavirin is used frequently for RSV infections, but it has also been used as a desperate attempt to improve the course of other respiratory viral illnesses. Cidofovir may be effective against adenovirus infections [162].

Early post-engraftment infections are usually caused by quantitative and functional deficiencies in antigen-specific T cells, defective opsonization, and also by functional hyposplenism. A subset of infections is most likely to occur between engraftment and three months after HCT, with risk largely due to the immunosuppressive medications that are used for prevention and/or treatment of GVHD. Invasive fungal infections, including fluconazole-resistant *Candida*, *Aspergillosis*, *Zygomycosis*, *Fusariosis*, and *Scedosporiasis* are very serious especially in the context of corticosteroid use. *Candida albicans* and *Cryptococcal* infections are rare because of the prophylactic use of azoles. Posaconazole has decreased invasive fungal infections in patients with GVHD [163], though the original formulation is available only orally and dependent on oral food intake for absorption. Both posaconazole and voriconazole require gastric acidity to be absorbed, and most allo-HCT take proton pump inhibitors or H2-antagonists, which may limit absorption. Azoles can cause hepatotoxicity, which occasionally can be serious, and both voriconazole and posaconazole interact with calcineurin inhibitors (CNI, cyclosporine and tacrolimus) so that the dose of CNI is usually decreased empirically by 50%. Co-administration of sirolimus with newer azoles is very problematic because the sirolimus level may increase dramatically. After engraftment and especially the second and third month post-HCT, the incidence of *Pneumocystis jirovecii* pneumonia increases and most HCT patients are advised to take prophylaxis with trimethoprim/sulfomethoxazole (TMP/SMX), or if they are allergic to it, with pentamidine or atovaquone [164]. Bacterial infections besides catheter infections do not represent significant problems in the early post-engraftment period, with the exception of Listeria and Legionella. Steroids use can also trigger parasitic infections in certain areas like strongyloidosis, but the most common one in severely immunosuppressed recipients is toxoplasmosis. The use of TMP/SMX usually prevents toxoplasmosis, which otherwise can cause severe CNS damage. Mycobacterial infections can also develop in this early post-HCT period, either fast-growing mycobacteria (M. Abscessus) or slow-growing ones (Mycobacterium avium intracellulare, Mycobacterium tuberculosis). It seems that one of the reasons for the relative low incidence of mycobacterial infections post-transplant is the previous use of fluoroquinolones. Similarly, Nocardia infections are rare because of the use of TMP/SMX prophylaxis.

Viral infections are very important in the early post-engraftment period. Acyclovir usually prevents HSV and VZV infections, but much less CMV (if at all). CMV infection can be serious with interstitial pneumonia and colitis and without treatment, it is usually fatal. Other manifestations of CMV infections include myelosuppression, hepatitis, retinitis, and encephalitis. CMV sero-discordance between recipient and donor and TCD, as well as GVHD and use of steroids, are risk factors for the development of CMV viremia. CMV proto-infection in the seronegative recipient deteriorates immunosuppression and decreases overall survival. Post allo-HCT monitoring and preemptive anti-CMV therapy has decreased morbidity and mortality. EBV, HHV-6, and adenovirus infections can happen around the same period, mostly after TCD allo-HCT, cord allo-HCT, and in the context of GVHD that requires significant doses of immunosuppressive therapy. EBV proto-infection can cause pneumonia and severe mononucleosis syndrome, as well as hepatitis syndrome, and is the main cause of post-transplant lymphoproliferative disorder (PTLD), which can lead to a frank aggressive lymphoma. Adenovirus can cause gastrointestinal, respiratory, and liver problems, and HHV-6 can cause encephalitis with predilection for temporal lobe involvement, hepatitis, rash, interstitial pneumonia, and myelosuppression.

BK virus causes severe hemorrhagic cystitis, as well as nephritis. The treatment of BK viral cystitis/nephritis is problematic and usually involves decreasing the immunosuppression. In difficult cases, cidofovir may help. Ciprofloxacin may be preventive and Leflunomide has a probable anti-BK activity [165–167] [168, 169]. Viral gastroenteritis during the same period can be due to infections with coxackie, rotavirus, adenovirus, and norovirus, and must be recognized early, otherwise patients may be assumed to have GVHD and be given steroids.

Community respiratory viruses are frequent. Para-influenza infections can be very serious and may trigger chronic broncho-pulmonary inflammation. Patients with active HBV infection need to be covered with anti-viral treatment during immunosuppression. The same applies for patients who are HBcAb+ even if they are HBcAg-negative, since immunosuppression may trigger HBV re-activation, which can be very serious and lead to liver failure. Tenofovir, lamivudine, or entecavir can prevent HBV re-activation and have been used safely in the context of HCT.

Late post-engraftment infections (those happening later than three months post-HCT) are less common and are more frequent after allo-HCT and especially in recipients of TCD grafts or in patients with chronic GVHD. The main reasons for late post-engraftment infections are hypogammaglobulinemia and late T cell reconstitution. Hypogammaglobulinemia and hyposplenism predispose patients to infections with encapsulated bacteria (S. pneumonia, H. influenzae, N. meningitidis, and Capnocytophaga canimorsus). During the first year post-HCT, the incidence of pneumonia is high. The second types of infections that happen during this period are viral, especially VZV, which can manifest with atypical skin distribution and may disseminate, and EBV, which can cause PTLD. Patients are also at risk for childhood infections like measles, mumps, rubella, and parvovirus infections, which can cause significant graft dysfunction, especially pure red cell aplasia. BK virus often gives late infections, which can manifest as hemorrhagic cystitis. Patients on steroids during the late post-engraftment period are still at risk for CMV and fungal infections.

Multiple strategies are employed to reduce the incidence of infections after HCT [170]. In the pre-engraftment period, recipients are usually kept in a single patient room that has high efficiency particulate air filter (HEPA filter) and they have a low bacteria diet. Sterile techniques are applied during the use of central catheters and surgical interventions are kept to the minimum necessary. Meticulous personal hygiene is emphasized and patients are strongly discouraged to be close to patients with communicable infections. Multiple antibiotics are prescribed prophylactically. Newer fluoroquinolones like levofloxacin have a very broad spectrum of activity against Gram-positive and Gram-negative bacteria and can also help in bowel decontamination if they are started few days before the onset of neutropenia. After engraftment, fluoroquinolones are usually discontinued to avoid resistance, even though some centers continue them for few more weeks and some re-institute them during treatment of GVHD with systemic immunosuppression. Recipients of auto-HCT do not require any bacterial prophylaxis after engraftment; however, after allo-HCT, most centers prescribe antibiotics that have good activity against encapsulated bacteria for at least as long as immunosuppression continues. TMP/SMX that is usually prescribed for Pneumocystis prophylaxis has in general good coverage against encapsulated bacteria; however, some patients who cannot tolerate it are covered with penicillin or azithromycin. Prophylaxis against pneumocystis is usually started after engraftment and is given for approximately three months after auto-HCT or until withdrawal of immunosuppression after allo-HCT. Because Pneumocystis pneumonia risk is higher if CD4 is <200/µl, many advocate to continue such prophylaxis till CD4 count is >200/µl, even if patients have discontinued immunosuppressive medications after allo-HCT. The most effective prophylaxis is TMP/SMX, which prevents toxoplasmosis, Listeria, and Nocardia infections, as well as encapsulated bacteria. Alternatives to TMP/SMX (which is usually given at a dose of 160/800 mg three times a week) are monthly intravenous pentamidine, oral atovaquone, and dapsone. Atovaquone and dapsone can prevent toxoplasmosis as well. Before starting dapsone, patients should be screened for G6PD deficiency. Acyclovir or valacyclovir is prescribed to prevent HSV and VZV post-HCT.

Acyclovir at a dose of 800 mg twice daily has very good efficacy and myelosuppression is minimal; some believe that may decrease the incidence of CMV viremia as well. Acyclovir is usually given for six months after autologous HCT and until immunosuppression is withdrawn after allo-HCT (but not earlier than six months). Some others do not discontinue acyclovir prophylaxis until CD4>200/µl. CMV infections are usually managed with a preemptive strategy, wherein CMV DNA (or antigen expression within lymphocytes) is measured usually every week during the period that allo-HCT recipients are at greatest risk (e.g., typically at least 100 days after allo-HCT) or if they have received TCD grafts. Preemptive treatment (e.g., using intravenous ganciclovir or oral vaganciclovir) is given upon detection of even asymptomatic CMV reactivation, though the thresholds for intervention and the duration of therapy vary widely. For patients who cannot take oral medications reliably, or those who develop symptomatic infection, intravenous ganciclovir or foscarnet are typically administered. Cidofovir is typically reserved only for resistant cases. Both foscarnet and cidofovir are nephrotoxic, whereas ganciclovir and valganciclovir are myelosuppressive [171]. Cidofovir has broader antiviral activity, and can be useful in resistant cases of BK cystitis and adenovirus infections, as well. Recently the new medication Letermovir was FDA-approved for the prevention of CMV reactivation after allo-HCT in high-risk patients.

For high-risk patients, some centers switch from a preemptive strategy to prophylaxis, e.g., administering valganciclovir to seropositive recipients who undergo highly immunosuppressive GVHD treatment. When CMV disease occurs, CMV-Ig or IVIg may help, especially in cases of CMV pneumonia. Immunosuppressed patients are periodically monitored for EBV DNA and when viral replication is documented, patients are monitored closely and immunosuppression may be lowered to reduce the incidence of post-transplant lymphoproliferative disease (PTLD), which may result from the direct transforming effects of EBV on human B cells. Rituximab may be used when high levels of EBV viremia are detected and when PTLD is suspected, as rituximab may eliminate clonally expanded EBV-infected B cells. In PTLD, rituximab is often combined with chemotherapy. For resistant EBV cases, some institutions administer EBV-specific lymphocytes, or can administer small doses of DLI [172]. For fungal prophylaxis, fluconazole is usually given after allo-HCT for as long as immunosuppression is administered. Fluconazole does not cover molds, and for that reason, posaconazole is given when high levels of immunosuppression are employed. Voriconazole is an alternative, but does not cover *Zygomycetes* species, potentially favoring their selection. For high-risk patients, screening for fungal infection may be aided by measurement of the fungal products β-glucan or galactomannan [173]. Galactomannan production is suggestive of infection with *Aspergillus*, and may be falsely positive in patients receiving piperacillin/tazobactam.

The prognosis of invasive fungal infections has improved significantly with the successive approval of important classes of antifungal medications, including liposomal formulations of amphotericin, voriconazole, posaconazole, and echinocandins, including caspofungin and micafungin. In resistant fungal infections, immunosuppression is lowered; white blood cell transfusions have anecdotally been demonstrated to have value in neutropenic patients. To prevent post-transplant infection in allo-HCT recipients, IVIg is also given if IgG level is <400 mg/dL, though meta-analyses have failed to demonstrate benefit from routine (e.g., weekly) IVIg infusions after allo-HCT, a practice that was formally widespread. Post-HCT patients are immunized to facilitate the recovery of recall responses, including antigen-specific T cells and protective humoral responses. These vaccinations usually are started at six months post-HCT and include vaccines to prevent diphtheria, tetanus, pertussis (acellular), influenza, pneumococcus (Pneumococcal conjugate vaccine, PCV), hepatitis B, poliomyelitis (IPV), Haemophilus type B, and meningococcus. The combined MMR (measles, mumps, rubella) vaccine is typically administered two years after transplant when cellular immunity has improved [170] [174, 175].

Specific Complications of HCT

Sinusoidal Obstruction Syndrome

Radiation and alkylating agents used for conditioning before HCT can injure the endothelium of venules. This can lead to an obstruction of small venules and perivascular fibrosis, which can in turn lead to hepatocellular toxicity, liver failure, and death, and constitute the syndrome of hepatic veno-occlusive disease (VOD), now usually referred to as sinusoidal obstruction syndrome (SOS). Clinically, patients present with the triad of weight gain, tender hepatomegaly, and ascites. Doppler of the liver shows increased resistance index in the hepatic artery and later in the course of severe illness, may demonstrate a reversal in the portal flow. Hepatic veins are patent. Ascites and gallbladder wall thickening can be observed in the U/S, but they are not specific. High level of the N-terminal of procollagen type III is one of the most sensitive and specific markers for hepatic SOS, but is not widely available. A hypercoagulable state characterized by low levels of protein C and antithrombin-III and/or high plasminogen activator inhibitor 1 (PAI-1) levels is frequently seen, but its specificity has been questioned. Liver biopsy is diagnostic, but rarely performed due to the bleeding risk, though this is decreased by performing transjugular, rather than percutaneous, liver biopsy. Pathologic findings include venular narrowing caused by subendothelial trapped erythrocytes. Sinusoidal dilation filled with red cells is frequently seen. Later thickening of the small venules with obliteration of their lumens and fibrosis of the sinusoids are followed by factor VIII accumulation and collagen deposition [176] [177].

Many factors may increase the risk of developing SOS. Pre-transplant elevation of transaminases and of ferritin are associated with an increased rate of SOS. Factors associated with increased SOS include chronic hepatitis C infection, decreased lung diffusion capacity, the use of progestins, conditioning using oral busulfan (combined with high-dose cyclophosphamide), acetaminophen toxicity, and the presence of active infections early after transplant. The advent of intravenous busulfan [178], due to the lack of first pass metabolic effects and much more consistent drug levels across subjects (particularly when dosed according to measured pharmacokinetics), was associated with a significantly decreased risk (~one-third), compared to the historically high risk in the era of oral busulfan. Use of high doses of pre-transplant gemtuzumab ozogamicin or inotuzumab ozogamicin significantly increases the risk. The use of UDCA (ursodiol) has been shown to decrease cholestasis after conditioning and, due to the excellent safety profile of this agent, is now widely used [179–182].

Defibrotide is an adenosine receptor agonist, which improves endothelial function without causing systemic anticoagulation and with only minimal risk for bleeding. A phase III study in a pediatric population receiving myeloablative transplantation has shown that defibrotide decreases SOS, as well as the risk for renal dysfunction. The prognosis of SOS is contingent upon the severity of the syndrome. Although mild and moderate cases of SOS usually resolve spontaneously, patients with severe SOS (significant weight gain and very high bilirubin with or without coagulopathy) have a very high mortality rate due to liver failure, hepatorenal syndrome, hepatic encephalopathy, and bleeding.

Thrombotic Microangiopathy

Thrombotic microangiopathy (TMA) is an infrequent but important syndrome that may occur after allo-HCT. Patients may present thrombocytopenia, microangiopathic hemolytic anemia (MAHA), and may also present with acute kidney injury (AKI) and/or renal failure. The classic pentad of thrombotic thrombocytopenic purpura (TTP) is often incomplete, with the most common findings including a high LDH (typically higher than twice the upper limit of normal), thrombocytopenia, and a peripheral smear showing evidence of MAHA (red cell fragmentation with at least two schistocytes per high power field). Renal insufficiency and confusion are more variably present, as is fever. Use of calcineurin inhibitors (especially in combination with sirolimus), TBI before HCT, aGVHD, older age, and SOS are risk factors for TMA. Pathologically, there is thrombus formation in the small arterioles and the capillaries. In the glomeruli of the kidney, there is a loss of endothelial cells and amorphous non-immune deposits in the subendothelium which occludes the capillary loops. Endothelial cells look swollen and the glomeruli frequently have a "bloodless appearance." The main pathophysiologic event is endothelial damage that activates coagulation, leading to thrombin generation and fibrin clots. The natural anti-fibrinolytic molecule PAI-1 is elevated. Anti-ADAMTS13 antibodies are usually absent. Treatment is usually oriented to relieve the underlying cause, including the discontinuation of drugs (e.g., sirolimus or calcineurin inhibitors) that are suspected to have triggered TMA. Many patients die or develop chronic renal failure. The role of plasma exchange is not clear, but has been demonstrated anecdotally to have value, though has been questioned in the absence of a demonstrated pathologic antibody [183–186].

Pulmonary Complications of HCT

In addition to infections, which are the most common causes of lung injury after HCT, there are many other causes of pulmonary dysfunction post-transplant [187]. About ten days after the stem infusion and around the time of neutrophil engraftment or just before that, an engraftment syndrome may be characterized by a syndrome consisting of fever (often low grade) and an erythematous rash. Fluid retention and weight gain, as well mild-to-severe non-cardiogenic pulmonary edema, with or without pleural effusion, may be present. The constellation of these findings around the time of engraftment has been associated with increased levels of inflammatory cytokines (IL-2, IL-6, IL-8, TNFα) that spike with engraftment and cause a capillary leak; the syndrome is also likely mediated by recovering neutrophils that may adhere abnormally to the walls of capillaries and venules. It is usually self-limited, though the short-term administration of pulse steroids may relieve symptoms.

Some studies have shown increase in cGVHD rates after *engraftment syndrome*, but most believe that there is no effect on survival. The use of growth factors (especially GM-CSF) and high cell dose transplant have been reported to increase the incidence of engraftment syndrome. Pathologically, analysis of bronchoalveolar lavage fluid may reveal increased neutrophils and lung biopsy (though rarely performed) may reveal diffuse alveolar damage. Skin biopsy may demonstrate edema, especially at the dermal/epidermal junction and the presence of white cells in the small venules and capillaries. The absence of interface dermatitis, dermal lymphocytes, and apoptotic keratinocytes distinguishes it from hyper-acute GVHD.

In the first three to four months after transplantation (with a peak incidence at about three weeks post-HCT), some patients may develop a pneumonia picture with multiple alveolar infiltrates without identification of infectious agents even with invasive procedures, including BAL or lung biopsy. This is called "Idiopathic Pneumonia Syndrome" (IPS). Radiation and prior exposure to high doses of alkylating agents (especially carmustine or busulfan) seem to increase the incidence and the IPS is believed to be caused by alveolar epithelial cell damage by the conditioning regimen, followed by lymphocyte recruitment leading to the production of cytokines (including IL-6, TNFα) and chemokines (e.g., RANTES). The prognosis is serious, and steroids and respiratory supportive care, which may include mechanical ventilation, are the main elements of therapy. TNF blockade, via the addition of etanercept to steroid therapy, has had encouraging results in phase II studies, though later stage trials were not definitive [188–190].

One of the most feared complications occurring early (i.e., within the first few weeks after HCT) is the syndrome of "Diffuse Alveolar Hemorrhage" (DAH), which is rare but carries a very high mortality rate (greater than 80% in early series). The diagnosis is based on recovery of progressively "bloodier" fluid during BAL, with cytological analysis of BAL fluid demonstrating the presence of high proportions of macrophages that are hemosiderin-laden. The etiology and pathogenesis are unknown and the diagnosis requires exclusion of infections. The treatment is based on the empiric use of high doses of steroids and mechanical ventilation with precautions to minimize infections. Given the presence of pulmonary bleeding that acutely impairs gas exchange, typical management often includes platelet transfusion and anti-fibrinolytic agents, such as infusion of aminocaproic acid. Other conditions (e.g., vitamin K deficiency and hypofibrinogenemia) that may exacerbate the coagulopathy should be corrected with hemostatic equilibrium followed closely. Although infusions of activated factor VII has been demonstrated to have anecdotal value, the absence of phase III level evidence, the very high cost of the medication, and the associated risk of thrombosis have not supported its widespread use in DAH [191–193].

Cryptogenic organizing pneumonia (COP, previously known as BOOP) can be occasionally seen in allo-HCT recipients. It may be part of chronic GVHD or present without apparent cause or in association with conditioning injury or previous infections. Radiographically, areas of airspace consolidation or ground-glass opacities are mainly seen in the peripheral lung fields with a predilection for lower lobes. These changes are much better appreciated in CT scans than in plain films. COP usually responds dramatically to steroids [194].

Pulmonary cytolytic thrombi (PCT) syndrome is a rare complication, mostly reported in children who have received an allo-HCT. Patients present with dyspnea, cough, and/or fever, and CT scan shows peripheral nodules. The main differential is fungal infection, so tissue biopsy is essential. Pathologically, small vessel clots with associated hemorrhagic infarcts are seen and stains for fungi are negative. Steroids may be helpful since there is a possible association with GVHD [195].

Pulmonary veno-occlusive disease (PVOD) has been reported, but is rarer and less well-characterized than hepatic SOS. Patients present with dyspnea and dry cough and radiographic findings are suggestive of lung congestion, including Kerley B lines. Echocardiography reveals a normal left ventricular ejection fraction with increased pulmonary pressures. Right heart catheterization reveals findings suggestive of pulmonary hypertension, though the pulmonary artery wedge pressure is not elevated. Pulmonary function tests (PFT) usually disclose very low lung diffusion capacity (DLCO). Chest CT rules out the possibility of thromboembolic disease, but definitive diagnosis requires a lung biopsy. Treatment has not been standardized, but many use steroids in combination with anticoagulation and a trial of pulmonary vasodilators (calcium channel blockers, phosphodiesterase inhibitors, endothelin receptor antagonists, or prostaglandins), although the prognosis is usually very poor. For non-responders, lung transplantation is a heroic and often unrealistic option [196].

Chemotherapy or radiation-induced lung injury may present subacutely weeks or even months after conditioning. Nitrosureas (including carmustine, a frequent agent in autologous conditioning), busulfan, and cyclophosphamide are the alkylators mostly associated with lung injury. Patients present with dyspnea on exertion and dry cough. The diagnosis is usually one of exclusion after eliminating the possibility of infections and treatment is usually supportive in combination with a trial of at least a month of glucocorticoids.

Bronchiolitis Obliterans (BO) is a very serious complication of allo-HCT frequently associated with other manifestations of chronic GVHD (which is a risk factor for the development of BO). BO onset can be delayed (even months or years after transplant) and can be triggered by a respiratory infection. Dyspnea and dry cough with occasional wheezes or normal but diffusely decreased breath sounds characterize the syndrome clinically. Pulmonary function tests characteristically reveal mid-expiratory severe obstruction (FEF 25%–75% is very low, usually <30%) that is typically not reversible by bronchodilators. Chest CT scans may reveal air-trapping with some bronchiectasis. Treatment is usually accomplished through immunosuppression, as for other manifestations of chronic GVHD (e.g., CNI or sirolimus, typically in combination with steroids) [197]. Azithromycin and monteleukast have been associated with treatment responses after allo-HCT or lung transplantation. A retrospective analysis revealed that inhaled corticosteroids were able to stabilize the typical progression of lung function often observed [198]. Special care, including adequate infectious prophylaxis medication, vaccines, and IVIG infusions, should be taken to avoid infections that can be lethal. As with other chronic GVHD syndromes, extracorporeal photopheresis (ECP) may be employed, as it is associated with clinical responses with apparently little increase in the risk of opportunistic infections, although clinical trial data are lacking. In severe cases, lung transplantation has been successfully performed [199–201].

Mucositis

Mucositis is one of the most common complications after high dose chemotherapy. Older age, a history of extensive prior therapy, and poor nutritional status (including vitamin deficiency) at the time of transplant are risk factors. Total Body Irradiation (TBI) and high doses of melphalan, busulfan, and etoposide increase the risk, especially if they are given in combination (for example the Busulfan-Melphalan or the TBI-etoposide regimen). Mucositis can affect any of the mucosal surfaces, but gastrointestinal (GI) mucositis is the most clinically relevant and depending on the portion of the GI tract affected, may cause stomatitis, nausea, abdominal cramping, and/or diarrhea. Usually mucositis manifests five to ten days after chemotherapy or radiation. The mucosa becomes thinner and pale and leukoplakia or erythema may be present. Later, ulcerative lesions may develop that may be hemorrhagic and painful, and may interfere with the ability to maintain oral intake. Conditioning-induced damage to the basal epithelial cells is the main insult to the mucosa, leading to their apoptosis and inability to regenerate the upper epithelium strata. Epithelial stem cells can be injured and bacterial translocation and/or proliferation may play a major factor, consistent with the worsening typically seen once absolute neutropenia occurs. Pro-inflammatory mediators are secreted (through NFκB activation) by tissue macrophages and lymphocytes following epithelial damage. Bacterial periodontal disease, as well as *Candida* and HSV infection, can exacerbate the problem. Xerostomia, which is common after conditioning, may result in the loss of antibacterial benefits of saliva.

Poor oral hygiene predisposes to stomatitis, and peroxide solutions are used to keep the mouth clean. Dental work should be done before conditioning, and some centers use hypertonic solutions with salt and/or baking soda or glutamine solutions, in an attempt to limit mucositis. Palifermin (keratinocyte growth factor, KGF) has been shown to decrease the grade and duration of mucositis following TBI-based conditioning and has been approved by FDA [202], although no survival benefit or reduction of GVHD has been shown. Amifostine has also been shown to decrease mucositis in a retrospective analysis after Melphalan conditioning for auto-HCT in myeloma patients [203, 204]. Oral cryotherapy (typically accomplished by dissolving ice chips in the mouth and/or the consumption of popsicles or ice water) during and after melphalan infusion appears to decrease stomatitis, though the effects on esophagitis are more minimal. Systemic glutamine is of low benefit, if any, as well as allopurinol; however, an oral suspension (Saforis) that makes glutamine more bioavailable at the oral mucosa may be beneficial. Filgrastim facilitates more rapid neutrophil recovery (and therefore resolution) and supportive rinses with hydrogen peroxide or those containing a high concentration of calcium phosphate (Caphosol) appear to have benefit [205, 206].

Once mucositis develops, pain control is usually achieved with systemic opioids, though topical analgesics may benefit some patients, while others will experience only transient relief. In cases with significant injury resulting in bleeding, topical aminocaproic acid may limit oral bleeding. Intravenous hydration is important to avoid dehydration. Prolonged mucositis prompts the use of total parenteral nutrition to maintain nutritional status, although benefits related to overall survival are questionable [206, 207].

Graft-versus-Host Disease

Graft-versus-Host Disease remains one of the most common and vexing complications of allo-HCT, and is a major cause of morbidity, mortality, and impaired quality of life. GVHD is mediated by donor immune cells that recognize recipient major and minor antigens (i.e., those encoded by immunologic loci that differ from donor to host, as well as other antigenic differences). There is an acute form (aGVHD) that is commonly characterized by manifestations that may include skin rash (a maculopapular rash that can progress to erythroderma and exfoliation); gastrointestinal problems (diarrhea, abdominal pain, anorexia, nausea, vomiting, or GI bleeding); and liver function abnormalities (jaundice, bleeding diathesis, hypoalbuminemia, ascites, and encephalopathy). While often not mentioned along with the cardinal manifestations in the skin, GI tract, and liver, the hematolymphoid system is also a direct target of aGVHD, with direct injury to lymphoid organs including lymph nodes and the thymus that may further compromise recipient immune recovery.

There is also a chronic form of GVHD (cGVHD) with pleiotropic manifestations that may overlap with those seen

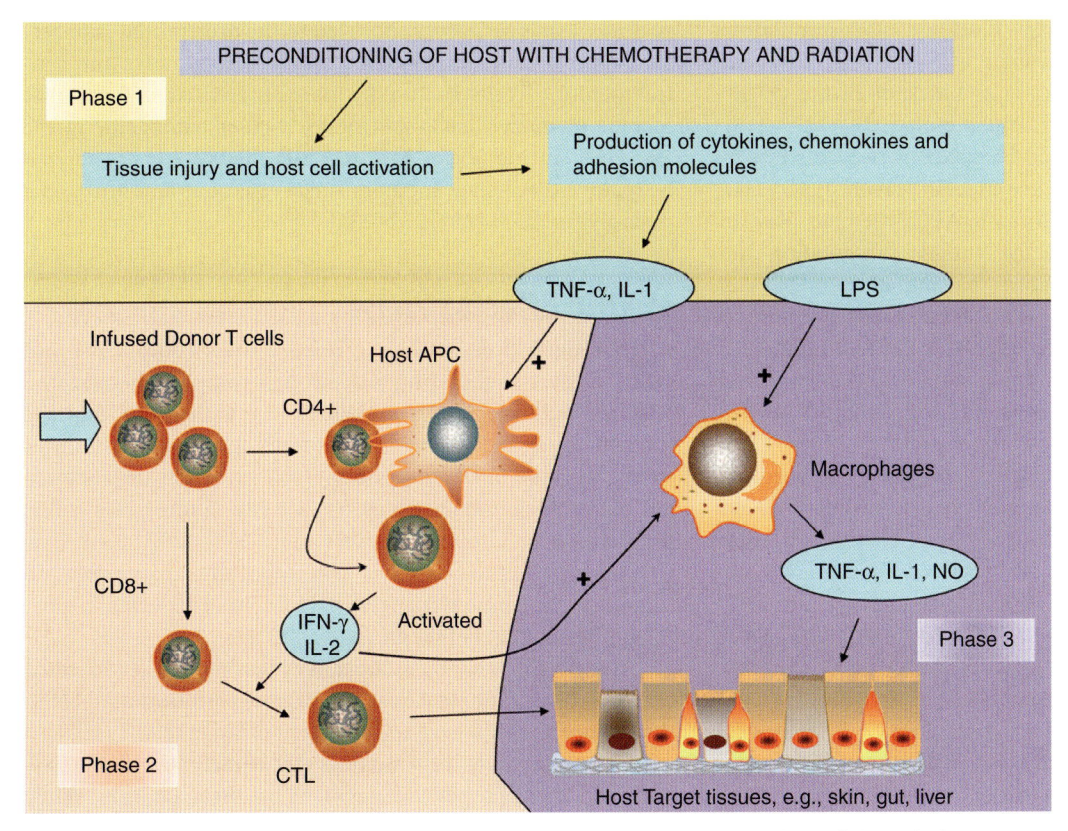

Figure 8.1 Pathogenesis of acute GVHD: tissue injury from conditioning regimen induces release of chemicals that activate antigen presenting cells (APCs, mainly of host origin) (phase 1). Then activated APCs prime T cells (phase 2). T cells and other immune cells (macrophages, NK cells) that are activated via T cell-produced cytokines induce target tissue damage (phase 3).

in a broad range of human autoimmune diseases in non-transplanted patients. Patients develop inflammation of the mouth (dryness, erythema, oral lichen planus, ulcers), eyes (keratoconjunctivitis sicca), and skin (lichenification, poikiloderma, systemic sclerosis, eosinophilic fasciitis) with or without arthalgias/arthritis or polyomyositis. They can also develop liver dysfunction and cholestasis, anorexia, nausea, pancreatic insufficiency, emesis, weight loss, malnutrition, bronchiolitis obliterans (BO), or cryptogenic organizing pneumonia (COP, formerly BOOP). Vaginal manifestations may be associated with sexual dysfunction. Other less common manifestations include glomerulonephritis with or without nephrotic syndrome, hypogonadism, and other hormonal deficiencies. Serosal inflammation with pleural effusions or ascites and nervous system involvement are very rare. Day +100 after the infusion of the allogeneic graft was the arbitrary cut-off to distinguish aGVHD from cGVHD; we now appropriately recognize that cGVHD can happen earlier (early onset cGVHD) and aGVHD can happen beyond day +100 (late onset aGVHD). Sometimes patients can have manifestations of both aGVHD and cGVHD simultaneously, and we call this "overlap syndrome." In up to 20% of patients with aGVHD, manifestations may occur very early (e.g., before day +15 and/or prior to the resolution of neutropenia). This is defined as hyperacute GVHD and may be associated with adverse outcomes [208–211].

aGVHD Pathogenesis: Antigen Presentation

In the initiation phase of aGVHD (see Figure 8.1), recipient antigens are presented to donor T cells. Although it was thought initially that antigens are presented only by "professional" recipient antigen presenting cells (APCs) that survive conditioning [212], especially myeloid dendritic cells (mDCs), more research has shown that antigens can be presented by recipient macrophages, B cells, plasmacytoid dendritic cells (pDCs), and also donor APCs. More recent studies have demonstrated that recipient antigens may be presented by non-hematopoietic recipient tissues, especially myofibroblasts and even intestinal epithelial cells themselves that, in conditions of stress and inflammation, express MHC-II and present antigens under the influence of IFNγ [213, 214]. The antigens that are presented are usually minor histocompatibility antigens (miHA), since the majority of allo-HCT is performed using HLA-matched donor-recipient pairs, as opposed to those encoded by the HLA loci that are discordant in mismatched transplantation. miHA disparity can cause significant allo-immune reactivity and GVHD [215] and is usually secondary to gene polymorphisms. HA-1, H-Y antigens, HA-2, HPA-3, and PANE-2 are examples of proteins that can be presented to the donor T cells as foreign antigens and induce GVHD.

Costimulation of lymphocytes is critical to activation, and is very important during antigen presentation; the absence of costimulation can cause anergy. Blockade of costimulatory molecule interactions can attenuate aGVHD (e.g., blockade of CD80 and CD86 by CTLA4-Ig or blockade of the OX40-OX40L axis, or of CD137, CD40L, etc.) [216, 217, 218]. Experimental data show that co-blockade of two co-stimulatory receptors can have an additive effect in preventing GVHD. Innate immune system receptors on APCs seem to play an equally important role in effective antigen presentation and priming of T cells. It is well-known that immature mDCs can be tolerogenic and increase the numbers of Tregs.

Following tissue damage resulting from conditioning, APC may be activated through multiple innate immune system receptors, the so-called pattern recognition receptors (PRR). Such receptors include the toll-like receptors (TLRs) [219, 220], the NOD-like receptors (NLRs) [221], and the receptors for damage-associated molecular patterns (DAMPs). DCs are also activated by cytokines and through the CD40 receptor that is activated by the CD40L expressed on T cells. Following tissue damage resulting in bacterial translocation, microbial products can reach DCs and activate their TLRs; for example, TLR4 is activated by bacterial lipopolypolysaccharide (LPS), TLR7 by single stranded RNA (ssRNA), and TLR9 is activated by CpG (cytosine paired with guanine) repeats. P2X7 is a DAMP receptor for ATP, which potentiates GVHD through DC activation [222]. Experimentally, selective inhibition of P2X7 ameliorates aGVHD, as well as bowel decontamination with oral antibiotics, whereas activation of TLR4, TLR7, and TLR9 potentiates alloreactivity. Specific polymorphisms of the NOD2 receptor (receptor for the cell wall component muramyl dipeptide) increase the risk of GVHD and increase treatment-related mortality (TRM) [223]. Signaling through the PRR receptors induces intracellular signaling through MyD88 or NFκB that activate the APCs, which then upregulate presentation molecules in their surface and secrete pro-inflammatory cytokines like IL-12 and TNFα that polarize appropriately the primed T cells (mainly to a T helper-1, Th1 phenotype).

Following production of naïve T cells in the thymus, cells that encounter antigens may progress through multiple memory stages that are characterized by functional differentiation and varying utilization of signaling pathways. Multiple studies have confirmed that alloreactivity is broader in the naïve T cell repertoire (TCR), in part due to the greater diversity of the TCR repertoire in naïve cells and also due to functional differences between naïve and progressively differentiated memory cells. Multiple studies have now demonstrated that the bulk of alloreactivity appears to reside in cells that are at the naïve and early (e.g., central memory) T cell stages [224–228]. Based on these observations derived from murine transplant models, multiple investigators are assessing whether depletion of naïve T cells (e.g., based on expression of the naïve surface marker CD45RA) may decrease aGVHD in the setting of human allo-HCT [224, 225, 229, 230]. In human preclinical studies and also in a murine model of mismatched allo-HCT, we confirmed that TCR signaling depends in part on activation of the mitogen activated protein kinase (MAPK) pathway, and that this pathway is most active in naïve and early memory T cells. We then confirmed that downstream suppression of this pathway using MEK inhibitors led to the preferential suppression alloreactivity and cytokine production by naïve and central memory T cells, but not by more differentiated T cells that include memory T cells specific for viruses pathogenic in the allo-HCT setting (e.g., CMV and EBV) that are characterized by relatively late-stage memory surface markers and functional phenotypes [231] [138, 232–234].

aGVHD: Effector Phase

After antigen presentation, primed T cells (both CD4 and CD8) migrate to target organs through complex chemokines, selectins, and integrins interactions. One of these molecules is the α4β7 integrin, which mediates homing of the lymphocytes to the gut and liver and is targetable with the monoclonal antibody vedolizumab, which has activity in ulcerative colitis and less so in Crohn's enteritis [235, 236] [237, 238]. The chemokine receptor CCR5 is also important for lymphocyte migration, and maraviroc (CCR5 inhibitor) has shown promising results in GVHD prevention [239].

After T cells reach their target, they become further activated and secrete effectors like FasL, granzyme, perforins, and TNFα that induce tissue damage and apoptosis of target cells. T cells also produce cytokines and chemokines that attract more T cells, NK cells, and macrophages that augment the tissue damage. While effector T cells express CD30 [240], an attempt to use brentuximab vedotin to kill them was proven toxic. Both Th1 and Th17 cells play a role in the effector phase of GVHD. Th17 cells produce IL-17 and IL-21 that contribute to tissue damage [241–243]. The intestinal crypts contain lymphoid cells (ILC) that produce IL-22, thereby contributing to the survival and proliferation of intestinal stem cells (ISCs) that have abundant IL-22 receptors. In severe intestinal aGVHD, ILC number and IL-22 production decrease and this results in a reduction of the number of ISCs and subsequent loss of intestinal epithelial integrity [244].

Regulatory T cells (Treg) and especially the CD4+CD25+Foxp3+ population are essential regulators of human adaptive immune responses and are critical to the prevention of autoimmunity. In murine transplantation models, it has been shown that Tregs may decrease the severity of GVHD without compromising GvL [245] or the ability to fight infections. Multiple recent and ongoing studies are attempting to manipulate (ex vivo or in vivo) the numbers of Tregs in an attempt to prevent or treat GVHD. Di Ianni et al. infused donor Tregs (CD4+ CD25+ CD127-) before the infusion of conventional T cells in the haploidentical setting with encouraging results in a pilot study [150]. Koreth et al. successfully treated steroid-refractory chronic GVHD by giving low dose IL-2 to expand residual Tregs, since these cells have high density of IL-2 receptors (CD25) that mediate their proliferation [246]. NKT cells play a role in the Treg expansion, and stimulation of NKT cells by administration of liposomal α-galactosylceramide has been shown to suppress GVHD in murine models.

Since severe aGVHD can be associated with substantial morbidity and a high risk of mortality, multiple groups have tried to use serum markers to predict severe aGVHD with the goal of tailoring prevention or treatment to those at greatest

Table 8.1 Stage and Overall Grading of aGVHD According to Keystone 1994 Criteria

	Stage 0	Stage 1	Stage 2	Stage 3	Stage 4
Skin	No rash	Rash <25% BSA	25%–50%	>50% Generalized erythroderma	Plus bullae and desquamation
Gut (for pediatric patients)	<500 mL diarrhea/day	501–1000 mL/day 5cc/kg-10cc/kg/day	1001–1500 mL/day 10cc/kg-15cc/kg/day	>1500 mL/day >15 cc/kg/day	Severe abdominal pain and ileus
UGI		Severe nausea/vomiting			
Liver	Bilirubin 2mg/dl	2.1–3 mg/dl	3.1–6 mg/dl	6.1–15 mg/dl	>15 mg/dl

Grade	Skin		Liver		Gut		KPS
I	1–2	&	0	&	0		
II	3	or	1	or	1		
III	0–4	or	2–3	or	2–4		
IV	4	or	4	or	0–4	or	KPS score ≤30% or decrease ≥40% from baseline KPS score

KPS: Karnofsky performance status, UGI: upper gastrointestinal tract

risk. Measurement of four biomarkers (hepatocyte growth factor, IL-8, soluble TNFR1, and soluble CD25) was found to be predictive of the severity of aGVHD [247–250]. Recently, another marker, ST2 (suppressor of tumorigenicity 2), the soluble receptor of IL-33, was found predictive not only of steroid-refractory aGVHD, but also of overall mortality, and multicenter validation studies are underway [251]. Gene polymorphisms (NOD2, IL-10 promoter) can also be predictive of aGVHD, but serum marker measurements may prove clinically more practical [252].

aGVHD: Clinicopathologic Findings (Table 8.1)

The most commonly affected organ in aGVHD is the skin. Initially, patients present with a maculopapular rash that may appear initially on the scalp, trunk, and back, and also may lead to early changes on the palms and the soles of the feet. The lesions are red or violaceous. In more serious cases, generalized erythroderma may be observed, with progression characterized by formation of vesicles and bullae, and eventually to epidermal necrosis and desquamation. Histologically, a perivascular dermatitis is followed by interface dermatitis where dyskeratotic cells of the basal and spinosum layers are infiltrated by lymphocytes. In later stages, extensive apoptosis of keratinocytes can be followed by bullae formation and skin ulceration [253] (see Figures 8.2, and 8.3).

The gastrointestinal tract is the second most common clinical target of aGVHD. When involving the lower GI tract, watery diarrhea is common. Mucus and fecal casts may be seen.

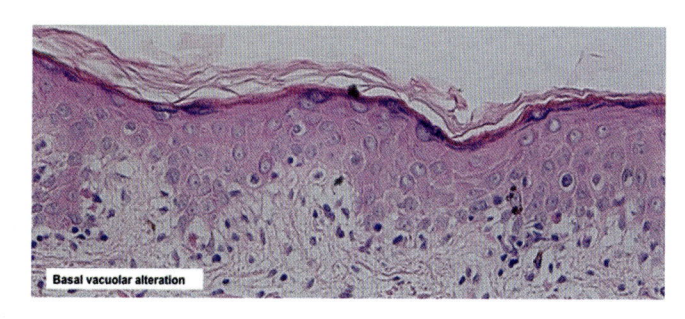

Figure 8.2 Skin GVHD: dyskeratotic and apoptotic keratinocytes.

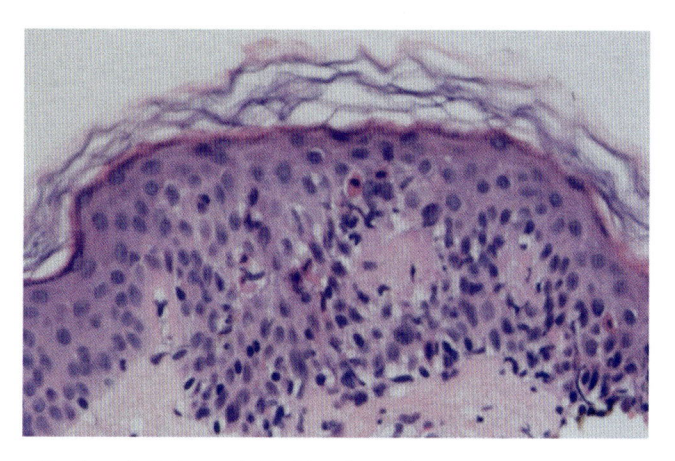

Dyskeratotic/apoptotic keratinocytes

Figure 8.3 Skin GVHD: vacuolar degeneration of the basal layer of the epidermis.

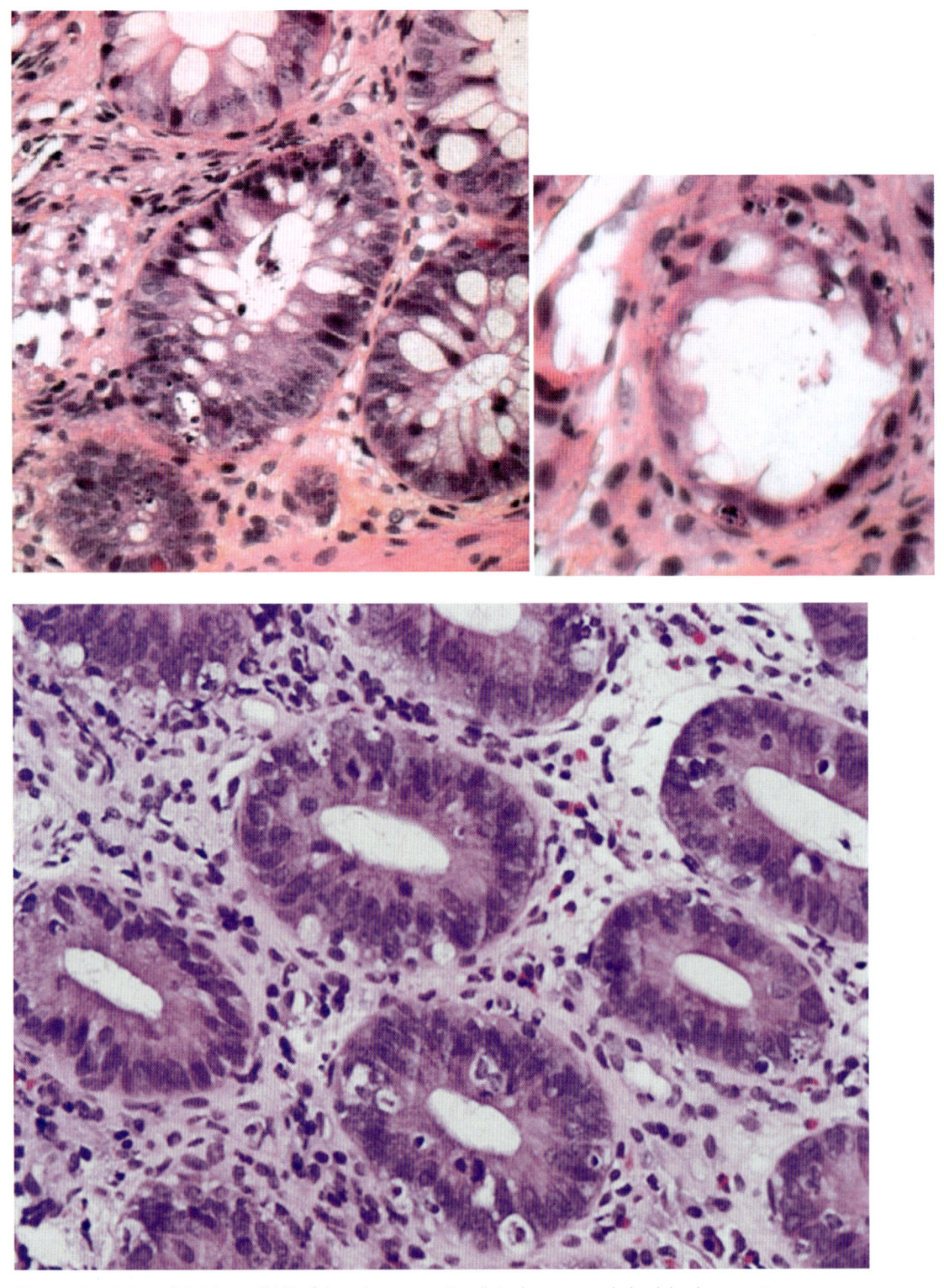

Figures 8.4, 8.5, and 8.6 Acute GVHD of the colon: apoptotic cells in the crypts and glandular degeneration.

Patients usually have crampy abdominal pain, but later can present with hematochezia or paralytic ileus. Severe dehydration and electrolyte abnormalities can follow the diarrhea, which can be of high volume (>3–4 liters/day). Although anorexia, nausea, and vomitus may accompany lower GI symptoms, upper GI symptomatology may be the only indication of GI involvement by GVHD. CT scans, although not routinely performed except to rule out perforation or abscess formation, may reveal significant edema of the bowel wall and, rarely, pneumatosis coli (in severe cases). Sloughing of the mucosa and erythema are the most common endoscopic findings. Histologically, the most characteristic initial finding is apoptosis of crypt cells with or without an associated lymphocytic infiltrate (see Figures 8.4, 8.5, and 8.6). As the process

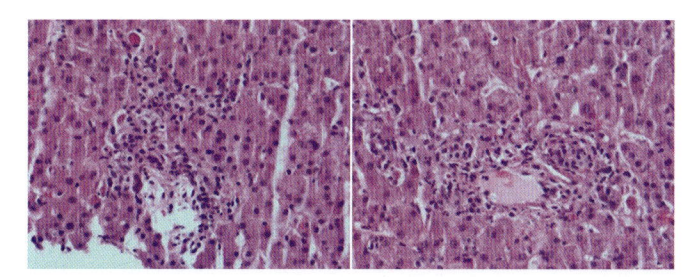

Figures 8.7 and 8.8 Hepatic GVHD: periportal lymphocytic infiltrates.

progresses, more apoptotic cells are seen in the crypts, which may fill with apoptotic debris and become infiltrated by lymphocytes, neutrophils, and eosinophils. Loss of crypts with mucosa denudation and ulceration follows [254]. Sometimes the diagnosis of GI GVHD is a diagnosis of exclusion after ruling out infections (CMV, *Clostridium difficile*, and other viral and parasitic infections, as well as damage from chemotherapy or other drugs like mycophenolate).

Liver aGVHD involvement may be asymptomatic, with isolated elevation of transaminases, or can manifest in a more fulminant fashion with cholestatic jaundice, ascites, coagulopathy, and hepatic encephalopathy. The most characteristic histologic change is the destruction of the interlobar small bile ducts with subsequent cholestasis. With more advanced involvement, a portal and periportal lymphocytic infiltrate can cause lobular necro-inflammatory changes with the hepatocytes being damaged by FasL produced by the inflammatory cells (see Figures 8.7 and 8.8). Cirrhotic changes are very rare [255, 256] [257].

aGVHD: Prevention and Treatment

At this point, the standard prophylaxis for GVHD remains the administration of a calcineurin inhibitor (CNI, tacrolimus, or cyclosporine) for several months (e.g., maintained in the fully therapeutic range until around post-HCT day +100, tapering thereafter depending on clinical status) with low doses of methotrexate early after transplant (typically administered for three to four doses, e.g., on days +1, +3, +6, and +11 after HCT). Pre-transplant antithymocyte globulin (ATG, from either equine or rabbit sources) is frequently added in the MUD setting. While a primary reason for the inclusion of ATG is to eliminate residual host lymphocytes to decrease the likelihood of graft rejection, the long circulating half-life of ATG preparations (typically, weeks) results in effective partial depletion of donor lymphocytes that are infused with the HCT graft. Thus, ATG has beneficial effects in lowering the incidence of graft rejection and aGVHD, but likely also may compromise beneficial (e.g., pathogen-specific and GvL) properties of the donor graft. Recently, high-dose cyclophosphamide post-transplant has been used as an alternative prophylactic method in the high-risk setting (e.g., haploidentical HCT where it is used in combination with a CNI), based on the rationale that the alloreactive T cells mediating GVHD are more susceptible to its effects than other T cells, potentially achieving somewhat selective inhibition of alloreactivity. Recent studies have dissected the recovery of non-host-reactive and regulatory T cells following post-transplant cyclophosphamide administration [258, 259].

Treatment of aGVHD consists mainly of high doses of corticosteroids and continuation of the CNI; if the disease is refractory to steroids, more immunosuppression is given and in light of the lack of standard therapies, clinical trials should be considered [260]. Examples of such additional immunosuppressives are: sirolimus, pentostatin, mycophenolate mofetil, infliximab or etanercept (inhibitors of TNFα), denileukin diftitox (an immunotoxin targeting CD25), alemtuzumab (anti-CD52), and thymoglobulin. Some physicians use extra-corporeal photophoresis (ECP), although the best evidence for ECP exists in the cGVHD setting. The prognosis of steroid-refractory aGVHD is dismal, and most patients succumb to infections [248, 250]. Recently the Jak 1/2 inhibitor ruxolitinib has shown significant promise in the treatment of steroid-refractory aGVHD.

Chronic GVHD (cGVHD): Pathogenesis and Its Impact on Treatment (Table 8.3)

Despite the prevalence (approximately 50% of all allo-HCT recipients) and significance of cGVHD, we understand much less about its pathogenesis. The use of PBSCs instead of bone marrow and the use of a female donor for a male recipient both increase its incidence. Although conventional T cells play a significant role in inducing cGVHD and Tregs ameliorate its manifestations, B cells are also important for its pathogenesis. This has been indirectly proven by the fact that rituximab has been successfully used for cGVHD treatment. Antibodies frequently found in autoimmune diseases (anti-nuclear, anti-mitochondrial, etc.) can be seen in cGVHD. Phenomena characteristic of autoimmune diseases mediated by autoantibodies are also seen in cGVHD, with sicca symptoms and sclerodermatous changes being the most characteristic examples. Anti-male (anti-H-Y) and agonistic anti-PDGFR antibodies are occasionally found as well [261, 262] [263]. Patients with cGVHD have high levels of B cell activating factor (BAFF) and low numbers of naïve B cells [133]. Elevated levels of BAFF promote Th17 differentiation [264], which is also important for the survival of plasma cells that also play a role in cGVHD [265]. Belimumab is an anti-BAFF humanized antibody approved for the treatment of systemic lupus [266] and this or other approaches might eventually be considered in trials of prevention or treatment of cGVHD. Since the proteasome inhibitor bortezomib has activity against both B cells and plasma cells, both of which play a role in cGVHD, its use as first-line treatment of cGVHD (in combination with steroids) is currently being studied. Bortezomib has been tested in trials of prevention of aGVHD in the mismatched setting, with encouraging results [267].

Multiple investigators are testing therapies that are aiming to increase the relative frequency of Tregs. Sirolimus, IL-2 [246], and ECP [268] have demonstrated promising results in cGVHD treatment, and all of them have been proposed to increase Tregs. The standard first-line therapy of cGVHD is corticosteroids, and although most patients initially respond, the majority of them become dependent on steroids, with many side effects, including serious infections, muscle atrophy, osteoporosis, mood instability, aseptic osteonecrosis of the hip, and disfiguring fat re-distribution. cGVHD relapses after withdrawal of steroids are very common. Recently FDA approved the Btk inhibitor ibrutinib for the treatment of chronic GVHD since it showed promising activity and steroid-sparing properties in a phase 2 clinical trial. Jak 1/2 inhibitors like ruxolitinib also show activity but they increase significantly the rate of opportunistic infections when they are added to high dose steroids. Some of the cGVHD symptoms (e.g., oral pain and severe scleroderma limiting mobility) can severely interfere with quality of life and many manifestations (e.g., bronchiolitis obliterans) for a significant proportion of subjects do not have an effective treatment. Second-line treatments for cGVHD are often combined with prednisone in an attempt to lower the steroid dose. Such medications include: rituximab [269, 270], sirolimus, ECP, pentostatin, mycophenolate, imatinib (mainly for sclerodermatous cGVHD), cyclosporine, thalidomide, hydroxychloroquine, clofazimine, and TNFα inhibitors (infliximab, etanercept). For pulmonary cGVHD, monteleukast and azithromycin may be considered [271]. Most of the evidence for the above approaches is relatively limited, with little consensus and significant heterogeneity in institutional practice strategies.

It is important to prevent and/or treat infections in patients who receive GVHD treatment. The use of posaconazole has demonstrated benefits compared to other azoles for the prevention of invasive fungal infections during treatment of GVHD with steroids. If immunoglobulins are low, replenishment is important. Most patients are covered against herpesviruses with acyclovir, though activity against CMV and EBV is limited, and against *Pneumocystis* with Bactrim. Screening for viruses (CMV, EBV, usually by quantitative PCR) and for fungal infections (via assessment of galactomannan or β-glucan, though neither is ideally sensitive or specific) may facilitate preemptive therapy. Usually, therapy with steroids or subsequent agents requires antiviral or extended antifungal prophylaxis (rather than preemptive management), given the much higher risk of life-threatening infections due to CMV and mold infections than in patients receiving CNI alone. Vaccinations with influenza, pneumococcus, and pediatric vaccines are essential and can save lives.

cGVHD: Clinicopathologic Findings

As noted previously, cGVHD is very pleiotropic, but the most common organs involved are skin, oral cavity, and eyes (Table 8.2). Severe cGVHD impairs survival both by direct effects on

Table 8.2 NIH Diagnostic Criteria for cGVHD [286]

Organ or Site	Diagnostic (Sufficient to Establish the Diagnosis of Chronic GVHD)	Distinctive (Seen in Chronic GVHD, but Insufficient Alone to Establish a Diagnosis of Chronic GVHD)	Other Features*	Common (Seen with Both Acute and Chronic GVHD)
Skin	Poikiloderma Lichen planus-like features Sclerotic features Morphea-like features Lichen sclerous-like features	Depigmentation	Sweat impairment Ichthyosis Keratosis pilaris Hypopigmentation Hyperpigmentation	Erythema Maculopapular rash Pruritus
Nails		Dystrophy Longitudinal Ridging, splitting, or brittle features Onycholysis Pterygium unguis Nail loss (usually symmetric; affects most nails)†		
Scalp and body hair		New onset of scarring or nonscarring scalp alopecia (after recovery from chemoradiotherapy) Scaling papulosquamous lesions	Thinning scalp hair, typically patchy, coarse, or dull (not explained by endocrine or other causes) Premature gray hair	
Mouth	Lichen-type features Hyperkeratotic plaques Restriction of mouth opening from sclerosis	Xerostomia Mucocele Mucosal atrophy Pseudomembranes† Ulcers†		Gingivitis Mucositis Erythema Pain

Table 8.2 (cont.)

Organ or Site	Diagnostic (Sufficient to Establish the Diagnosis of Chronic GVHD)	Distinctive (Seen in Chronic GVHD, but Insufficient Alone to Establish a Diagnosis of Chronic GVHD)	Other Features*	Common (Seen with Both Acute and Chronic GVHD)
Eyes		New onset dry, gritty, or painful eyes‡ Cicatricial conjunctivitis Keratoconjunctivitis sicca‡ Confluent areas of punctate keratopathy	Photophobia Periorbital hyperpigmentation Blepharitis (erythema of the eyelids with edema)	
Genitalia	Lichen planus-like features Vaginal scarring or stenosis	Erosions‡ Fissures‡ Ulcers‡		
GI tract	Esophageal web Strictures or stenosis in the upper-to-mid-third of the esophagus†		Exocrine pancreatic insufficiency	Anorexia Nausea Vomiting Diarrhea Weight loss Failure to thrive (infants and children)
Liver				Total bilirubin, alkaline phosphatase >2 × upper limit of normal† ALT or AST >2 × upper limit of normal†
Lung	Bronchiolitis obliterans diagnosed with lung biopsy	Bronchiolitis obliterans diagnosed with PFTs and radiology‡		BOOP
Muscles, fascia, joints	Fasciitis Joint stiffness or contractures secondary to sclerosis	Myositis or polymyositis‡	Edema Muscle cramps Arthralgia or arthritis	
Hematopoietic and immune			Thrombocytopenia Eosinophilia Lymphopenia Hypo- or hypergammaglobulinemia Autoantibodies (AIHA and ITP)	
Other			Pericardial or pleural effusions Ascites Peripheral neuropathy Nephrotic syndrome Myasthenia gravis Cardiac conduction Abnormality or cardiomyopathy	

target organs and as a result of its treatment, given the resulting immunosuppression, which is often profound. In the skin, cGVHD can cause lichen planus, poikiloderma, and sclerosis, which may be either superficial or deep (see Figures 8.9 and 8.10). Both hypo- and hyper-pigmentation can occur. Nails can become dystrophic and brittle, and onycholysis or even nail loss can happen. Patients note that their scalp hair (which may have just recovered from previous chemotherapy) may thin,

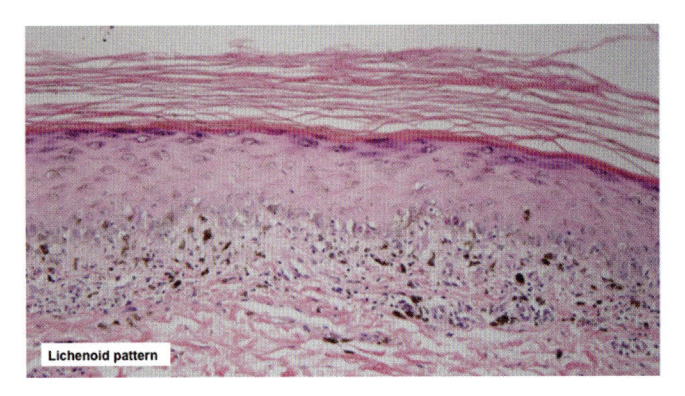

Figure 8.9 Skin GVHD: lichenification and pigment incontinence.

and alopecia with or without scarring can occur. Histologically, there is initially skin infiltration by lymphocytes and plasma cells that can also affect simultaneously the eccrine, lacrimal, and salivary glands, causing their destruction. Hyperkeratosis with irregular acanthosis is seen initially. Later, in the sclerotic phase, fibrosis and atrophy predominate. The sclerosis usually starts from the papillary dermis and progresses downwards, in contrast to systemic sclerosis, which typically evolves in an upward fashion. In patients who develop eosinophilic fasciitis, there is a cellulitic appearance of the skin with painful grooving. Biopsies may demonstrate edema and fibrosis of the fascia with lymphocytic and eosinophilic infiltration [272].

Patients with oral cGVHD [254, 273, 274] may develop painful erythematous lesions or ulcerations in the mouth with frequent development of oral lichen planus changes. Mucosal atrophy, mucoceles, dental caries, and later on, restriction of mouth opening can occur. Histologically, there is interface inflammation and apoptosis in the mucosa. Lymphocytic and plasma cell infiltration of the salivary glands can progress to fibrosis. cGVHD of the oral cavity increases the risk of oral squamous cancer. Similar changes can be found in the eyes where xerophthalmia and pain can be associated with keratoconjunctivitis sicca. Blepharitis, photophobia, and periorbital inflammation are frequently seen [275, 276]. cGVHD in the vagina may cause significant dryness, tenderness, and dyspareunia, and subsequent scarring and stenosis [277].

Patients occasionally develop symptoms of dyspnea and dry cough with or without fever. In these patients, lung biopsy may reveal either COP or BO, as discussed previously. In the former, there are areas of consolidation characterized mainly of monocytic infiltration and granulomatous tissue starting at the small bronchioles and extending to the alveoli and the interstitium. In cases of BO, there is constrictive stenosis or obstruction of the lumen of small bronchioles by subepithelial dense fibrosis that is often associated with lymphocytic bronchiolitis. FEV1 and, more impressively so, FEF (25%–75%), are reduced and residual volume is usually increased [278, 279].

cGVHD patients frequently have an elevation of cholestatic markers or of transaminases. Liver biopsy demonstrates ductopenia, chronic cholestasis, and periportal fibrosis [280]. Anti-mitochondrial or antinuclear antibodies may be elevated. The GI tract is infrequently involved, usually in the form of

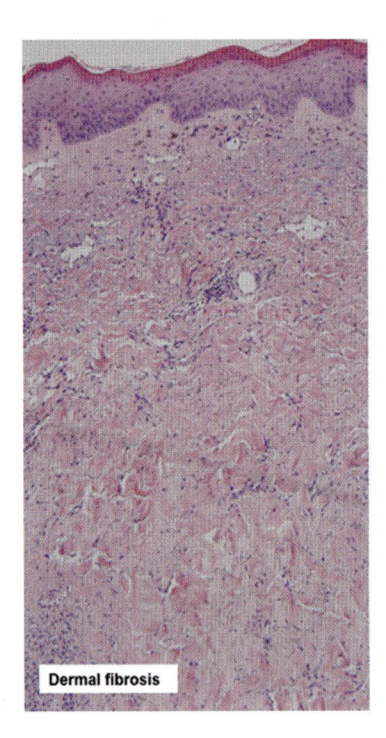

Figure 8.10 Skin GVHD: dermal fibrosis.

esophageal strictures. Diarrhea can be associated with exocrine pancreatic insufficiency. Rarely, patents may present with polymyositis, with significant elevation of creatine kinase and aldolase and characteristic findings by muscle biopsy [281]. Membranous nephritis with albuminuria [282] and serositis with ascites, pleural, and paricardial effusions are rare [283]. Myocarditis, myasthenia gravis, and peripheral neuropathy have been reported, but are not commonly manifestations of cGVHD.

Most patients with cGVHD have hypogammaglobulinemia and lymphopenia. In most serious cases, anemia and thrombocytopenia can occur and are mostly related to decreased marrow function due to inflammation rather than frank immune hemolytic anemia or immune thrombocytopenia. Eosinophilia may be seen. Most patients complain of fatigue and arthralgias. Quality of life decreases in non-steroid responsive cases of cGVHD and patients may develop significant depression. Because of the use of steroids, many patients suffer opportunistic infections and osteopenia or osteoporosis. Finally, the direct and indirect immunologic consequences of cGVHD in lymphoid organs may result in the dysregulation of germinal center formation in lymph nodes promoting B cell autoreactivity and delays in thymopoietic recovery that impair the regeneration of a diverse TCR repertoire (including the generation of Tregs, which are naturally produced in the thymus) and potentially lead to the loss of central tolerance, further promoting autoimmunity.

Conclusions

Over the past fifty years, HCT has dramatically improved the prognosis for a number of hematologic diseases, evolving as the standard of care for many patients with high-risk or

Table 8.3 Selected Novel Immune Manipulations for Prevention or Treatment of GVHD

Target	Method	Aim
↑Treg	Infusion of CD4+CD25+CD127(-) cells (before HCT)	Prevent aGVHD
	Low-dose IL-2 post-HCT.	Prevent aGVHD or treat cGVHD
	Photopheresis (preferential expansion of Treg)	Treatment of cGVHD
↑iNKT	Total lymphoid irradiation (0.8 Gy x 10) before HCT	Prevention of aGVHD
	Liposomal a-galactosylceramide (REG-2001) after HCT	
↓Th17	Ustekinumab (anti IL-12 and IL-23)	Prevent or treat aGVHD by preventing expansion of Th17
	Tocilizumab (anti IL-6)	
↓Tnaïve	Anti-CD45RA before HCT	Prevention of aGVHD through depletion of naïve CD4 cells
Gut flora	Rifaximin, metronidazole peritransplant	Prevention of a GVHD through decreasing TLR stimulation
CD80	CTLA-4 Ig (Abatacept, Belatacept)	Prevent aGVHD by blocking co-stimulation and inducing anergy
CD86		
α4β7	Vedolizumab	Prevent homing of T cells to gut
CCR5	Maravicor (oral drug inhibiting RANTES-CCR5 interaction)	Prevent homing of T cells
CD30	Brentuximab vedotin	Kills alloreactive T cells
Proteasome	Bortezomib, Carfilzomib	Prevent cGVHD
		Prevent aGVHD
BAFF	Belimumab	Prevent, treat cGVHD
HDAC	Vorinostat, romidepsin, panobinostat.	Prevent aGVHD, HDAC inhibitors decrease the efficiency of antigen presentation

Abbreviations: aGVHD: acute Graft-versus-Host Disease; cGVHD: chronic Graft-versus-Host Disease; HDAC: histone deacetylase; BAFF: B cell activating factor; Treg: regulatory T cells; iNKT: invariant natural killer T cells; TLR: toll-like receptor; IL: interleukin; HCT: hematopoietic stem cell transplantation

relapsed malignancies. Improvements in conditioning regimens and supportive care, as well as better understanding of the pathogenesis of complications, have significantly decreased mortality and improved outcomes over the last two decades, while facilitating a dramatic expansion in the number of potential candidates for treatment, particularly in older individuals. The main complication that remains frequent and problematic is GVHD, particularly the chronic form. Much research in murine models has shed light into the mechanisms underlying GVHD, and further advances in preclinical and early phase clinical human studies have resulted in more advanced clinical trials that aim to improve outcomes and standards of care that have evolved little despite our expanding understanding of GVHD pathophysiology.

The other primary challenge, especially for high-risk patients, remains the problem of relapse despite the combined effects of conditioning and adoptive immunotherapy that forms the modern basis of allo-HCT therapy. Use of targeted therapies (e.g., emerging classes of therapies that include ibrutinib, neddylation inhibitors, proteasome inhibitors, and DNA methyltransferase inhibitors) before or after HCT and use of further immunotherapy (e.g., checkpoint inhibition using anti-CTLA4 and anti-PD-1 targeting; cancer-specific transduced chimeric antigen receptor T cells) at the right time and at the right dose are destined to improve outcomes (Table 8.4) [284, 285].

We should not forget that ongoing research is needed in antimicrobial chemotherapy. We still have many patients dying from infections due to viruses, invasive fungi, or multi-resistant bacteria, but very few antibiotics have been approved in the last few years. Finally, better understanding of the interactions between certain neoplasms (prostate cancer, melanoma, renal cell carcinoma) and the immune system, along with disease-tailored conditioning regimens, may allow the expansion of the use of HCT in solid tumors as well.

Table 8.4 Selected Approaches to Decrease Relapse after Allogeneic Hct

APPROACH	RATIONALE	POTENTIAL PROBLEMS
Lenalidomide	Augment NK and T cell attack against myeloma MRD	Myelosuppression, GVHD
Abl-TKIs (imatinib, dasatinib, nilotinib, bosutinib, ponatinib)	Target MRD in CML and Ph+ ALL	Myelosuppression, immunosuppression
Ibrutinib	Minimize MRD in CLL and B-NHL by targeting Btk	GI symptoms, fatigue, hypogammaglobulinemia
5-azacytidine	Decrease relapse of myeloid malignancies	Myelosuppression
Rituximab	Decrease relapse of CD20+ malignancies, may reduce cGVHD	Hypogammaglobulinemia, myelosuppression
Ipilimumab	Inhibit immunologic tolerance by inhibiting CTLA-4	Aggravation of GVHD, immune endocrinopathies
CT-011	Inhibit anergy by blocking PD1	GVHD?
IL-2, IL-7, IL-21	Boost T cell function	Capillary leak syndrome, fever, arthralgia, GVHD?
Peptide vaccines (WT-1, PR1)	Educate the immune system to attack antigens over-expressed in malignant cells	Low immunogenicity
Dendritic cell vaccines +/- TLR7/TLR9 agonists	Enhance cancer cell antigen presentation	Complicated production of the vaccine
CARs	Join an immunoglobulin recognizing a cancer antigen to the TCR signaling cascade	Difficult production, decreased survival of engineered T cells, requires costimulatory receptors and a virus as a vehicle of the genes
NK cell infusion	Augment innate immunity	May need cytokine treatment for enhanced efficacy
Preemptive DLI	Augment GvL	GVHD
Donor with KIR ligand mismatch and/or donor with activating KIR receptors (e.g., KIR2DS1)	Increase NK activity against mainly myeloid malignancies	Difficult to find such donors

Abbreviations: NK=natural killer cells; MRD=minimal residual disease; GVHD=Graft-versus-Host Disease; TKI=tyrosine kinase inhibitor; CML=chronic myeloid leukemia; ALL=acute lymphoblastic leukemia; NHL=non-Hodgkin lymphoma; CLL=chronic lymphocytic leukemia; Btk=Bruton kinase; Ph=Philadelphia; GI=gastro-intestinal; PD1=programmed death-1; TLR=toll-like receptor; TCR=T cell receptor; CAR=chimeric antigen receptor; GvL=Graft-versus-Leukemia; KIR=killer immunoglobulin-like receptor; WT-1=Wilms tumor antigen 1; Abl=Abelson kinase

References

1. Kolb, H.J., Graft-versus-Leukemia Effects of Transplantation and Donor Lymphocytes. Blood, 2008. **112**(12): p. 4371–83.
2. Miller, J.S., et al., NCI First International Workshop on The Biology, Prevention, and Treatment of Relapse after Allogeneic Hematopoietic Stem Cell Transplantation: Report from the Committee on the Biology Underlying Recurrence of Malignant Disease following Allogeneic HSCT: Graft-versus-Tumor/Leukemia Reaction. Biol Blood Marrow Transplant, 2010. **16**(5): p. 565–86.
3. Mielcarek, M., et al., Outcomes among Patients with Recurrent High-risk Hematologic Malignancies after Allogeneic Hematopoietic Cell Transplantation. Biol Blood Marrow Transplant, 2007. **13**(10): p. 1160–8.
4. Porter, D.L. and J.H. Antin, Donor Leukocyte Infusions in Myeloid Malignancies: New Strategies. Best Pract Res Clin Haematol, 2006. **19**(4): p. 737–55.
5. Matte-Martone, C., et al., Graft-versus-Leukemia (GVL) against Mouse Blast-crisis Chronic Myelogenous Leukemia (BC-CML) and Chronic-phase Chronic Myelogenous Leukemia (CP-CML): Shared Mechanisms of T Cell Killing, but Programmed Death Ligands Render CP-CML and Not BC-CML GVL Resistant. J Immunol, 2011. **187**(4): p. 1653–63.
6. Foley, B., et al., NK Cell Education after Allogeneic Transplantation: Dissociation between Recovery of Cytokine-producing and Cytotoxic Functions. Blood, 2011. **118**(10): p. 2784–92.
7. Ruggeri, L., et al., Role of Natural Killer Cell Alloreactivity in HLA-mismatched Hematopoietic Stem Cell Transplantation. Blood, 1999. **94**(1): p. 333–9.
8. To, L.B., J.P. Levesque, and K.E. Herbert, How I Treat Patients Who Mobilize Hematopoietic Stem Cells Poorly. Blood, 2011. **118**(17): p. 4530–40.
9. Kumar, S., et al., Mobilization in Myeloma Revisited: IMWG Consensus Perspectives on Stem Cell Collection Following Initial Therapy with Thalidomide-, Lenalidomide-, or Bortezomib-containing Regimens. Blood, 2009. **114**(9): p. 1729–35.

10. Champlin, R.E., et al., Blood Stem Cells Compared with Bone Marrow as a Source of Hematopoietic Cells for Allogeneic Transplantation. IBMTR Histocompatibility and Stem Cell Sources Working Committee and the European Group for Blood and Marrow Transplantation (EBMT). Blood, 2000. **95**(12): p. 3702–9.

11. Attal, M., et al., A Prospective, Randomized Trial of Autologous Bone Marrow Transplantation and Chemotherapy in Multiple Myeloma. Intergroupe Francais du Myelome. N Engl J Med, 1996. **335**(2): p. 91–7.

12. Attal, M., et al., Single versus Double Autologous Stem-cell Transplantation for Multiple Myeloma. N Engl J Med, 2003. **349**(26): p. 2495–502.

13. Attal, M., et al., Lenalidomide Maintenance after Stem-cell Transplantation for Multiple Myeloma. N Engl J Med, 2012. **366**(19): p. 1782–91.

14. McCarthy, P.L., et al., Lenalidomide after Stem-cell Transplantation for Multiple Myeloma. N Engl J Med, 2012. **366**(19): p. 1770–81.

15. Bruno, B., et al., A Comparison of Allografting with Autografting for Newly Diagnosed Myeloma. N Engl J Med, 2007. **356**(11): p. 1110–20.

16. Jaccard, A., et al., High-dose Melphalan versus Melphalan plus Dexamethasone for AL Amyloidosis. N Engl J Med, 2007. **357**(11): p. 1083–93.

17. Schouten, H.C., et al., High-dose Therapy Improves Progression-free Survival and Survival in Relapsed Follicular Non-Hodgkin's Lymphoma: Results from the Randomized European CUP Trial. J Clin Oncol, 2003. **21**(21): p. 3918–27.

18. Philip, T., et al., Autologous Bone Marrow Transplantation as Compared with Salvage Chemotherapy in Relapses of Chemotherapy-sensitive Non-Hodgkin's Lymphoma. N Engl J Med, 1995. **333**(23): p. 1540–5.

19. Tam, C.S., et al., Mature Results of the M. D. Anderson Cancer Center Risk-adapted Transplantation Strategy in Mantle Cell Lymphoma. Blood, 2009. **113**(18): p. 4144–52.

20. Geisler, C.H., et al., Long-term Progression-free Survival of Mantle Cell Lymphoma after Intensive Front-line Immunochemotherapy with in Vivo-purged Stem Cell Rescue: A Nonrandomized Phase 2 Multicenter Study by the Nordic Lymphoma Group. Blood, 2008. **112**(7): p. 2687–93.

21. Ghielmini, M. and E. Zucca, How I Treat Mantle Cell Lymphoma. Blood, 2009. **114**(8): p. 1469–76.

22. Vose, J.M., et al., Phase III Randomized Study of Rituximab/Carmustine, Etoposide, Cytarabine, and Melphalan (BEAM) Compared with Iodine-131 Tositumomab/BEAM with Autologous Hematopoietic Cell Transplantation for Relapsed Diffuse Large B-cell Lymphoma: Results from the BMT CTN 0401 trial. J Clin Oncol, 2013. **31**(13): p. 1662–8.

23. Horning, S.J., et al., High-dose Therapy and Autologous Hematopoietic Progenitor Cell Transplantation for Recurrent or Refractory Hodgkin's Disease: Analysis of the Stanford University Results and Prognostic Indices. Blood, 1997. **89**(3): p. 801–13.

24. Lazarus, H.M., et al., Autotransplants for Hodgkin's Disease in Patients Never Achieving Remission: A Report from the Autologous Blood and Marrow Transplant Registry. J Clin Oncol, 1999. **17**(2): p. 534–45.

25. Schmitz, N., et al., Treatment and Prognosis of Mature T-cell and NK-cell Lymphoma: An Analysis of Patients with T-cell Lymphoma Treated in Studies of the German High-grade Non-Hodgkin Lymphoma Study Group. Blood, 2010. **116**(18): p. 3418–25.

26. Weisenburger, D.D., et al., Peripheral T-cell Lymphoma, Not Otherwise Specified: A Report of 340 Cases from the International Peripheral T-cell Lymphoma Project. Blood, 2011. **117**(12): p. 3402–8.

27. Einhorn, L.H., et al., High-dose Chemotherapy and Stem-cell Rescue for Metastatic Germ-cell Tumors. N Engl J Med, 2007. **357**(4): p. 340–8.

28. Matthay, K.K., et al., Treatment of High-risk Neuroblastoma with Intensive Chemotherapy, Radiotherapy, Autologous Bone Marrow Transplantation, and 13-cis-retinoic Acid. Children's Cancer Group. N Engl J Med, 1999. **341**(16): p. 1165–73.

29. Ladenstein, R., et al., Primary Disseminated Multifocal Ewing Sarcoma: Results of the Euro-EWING 99 Trial. J Clin Oncol, 2010. **28**(20): p. 3284–91.

30. Kushner, B.H. and P.A. Meyers, How Effective Is Dose-intensive/Myeloablative Therapy against Ewing's Sarcoma/Primitive Neuroectodermal Tumor Metastatic to Bone or Bone Marrow? The Memorial Sloan-Kettering Experience and a Literature Review. J Clin Oncol, 2001. **19**(3): p. 870–80.

31. Koreth, J., et al., Allogeneic Stem Cell Transplantation for Acute Myeloid Leukemia in First Complete Remission: Systematic Review and Meta-analysis of Prospective Clinical Trials. JAMA, 2009. **301**(22): p. 2349–61.

32. Andersson, B.S., et al., Once Daily I.V. Busulfan and Fludarabine (I.V. Bu-Flu) Compares Favorably with I.V. Busulfan and Cyclophosphamide (I.V. BuCy2) as Pretransplant Conditioning Therapy in AML/MDS. Biol Blood Marrow Transplant, 2008. **14**(6): p. 672–84.

33. Andersson, B.S., et al., Clofarabine +/- Fludarabine with Once Daily I.V. Busulfan as Pretransplant Conditioning Therapy for Advanced Myeloid Leukemia and MDS. Biol Blood Marrow Transplant, 2011. **17**(6): p. 893–900.

34. Goldstone, A.H., et al., In Adults with Standard-risk Acute Lymphoblastic Leukemia, the Greatest Benefit Is Achieved from a Matched Sibling Allogeneic Transplantation in First Complete Remission, and an Autologous Transplantation Is Less Effective than Conventional Consolidation/Maintenance Chemotherapy in All Patients: Final Results of the International ALL Trial (MRC UKALL XII/ECOG E2993). Blood, 2008. **111**(4): p. 1827–33.

35. Saber, W., et al., Impact of Donor Source on Hematopoietic Cell Transplantation Outcomes for Patients with Myelodysplastic Syndromes (MDS). Blood, 2013.

36. Ludwig, W.D., et al., Immunophenotypic and Genotypic Features, Clinical Characteristics, and Treatment Outcome of Adult pro-B acute Lymphoblastic Leukemia: Results of the German Multicenter Trials GMALL 03/87 and 04/89. Blood, 1998. **92**(6): p. 1898–909.

37. Jeannet, R., et al., Oncogenic Activation of the Notch1 Gene by Deletion of Its Promoter in Ikaros-deficient T-ALL. Blood, 2010. **116**(25): p. 5443–54.

38. Dail, M., et al., Mutant Ikzf1, KrasG12D, and Notch1 Cooperate in T Lineage Leukemogenesis and Modulate Responses to Targeted Agents. Proc Natl Acad Sci U S A, 2010. **107**(11): p. 5106–11.

39. Portell, C.A. and A.S. Advani, Novel Targeted Therapies in Acute

40. Porter, D.L., et al., Chimeric Antigen Receptor-modified T Cells in Chronic Lymphoid Leukemia. N Engl J Med, 2011. **365**(8): p. 725–33.
41. Grupp, S.A., et al., Chimeric Antigen Receptor-modified T Cells for Acute Lymphoid Leukemia. N Engl J Med, 2013. **368**(16): p. 1509–18.
42. Kebriaei, P., et al., Clofarabine Combined with Busulfan Provides Excellent Disease Control in Adult Patients with Acute Lymphoblastic Leukemia Undergoing Allogeneic Hematopoietic Stem Cell Transplantation. Biol Blood Marrow Transplant, 2012. **18**(12): p. 1819–26.
43. O'Brien, S.M., H. Kantarjian, and J. Radich, Update: Chronic Myelogenous Leukemia Clinical Practice Guidelines. J Natl Compr Canc Netw, 2003. **1** Suppl 1: p. S29–40.
44. Zelenetz, A.D., et al., Non-Hodgkin's Lymphomas, Version 1.2013. J Natl Compr Canc Netw, 2013. **11**(3): p. 257–72; quiz 273.
45. Scheinberg, P. and N.S. Young, How I Treat Acquired Aplastic Anemia. Blood, 2012. **120**(6): p. 1185–96.
46. Taniguchi, T. and A.D. D'Andrea, Molecular Pathogenesis of Fanconi Anemia: Recent Progress. Blood, 2006. **107**(11): p. 4223–33.
47. Cutler, C.S., et al., A Decision Analysis of Allogeneic Bone Marrow Transplantation for the Myelodysplastic Syndromes: Delayed Transplantation for Low-risk Myelodysplasia Is Associated with Improved Outcome. Blood, 2004. **104**(2): p. 579–85.
48. Kroger, N., Allogeneic Stem Cell Transplantation for Elderly Patients with Myelodysplastic Syndrome. Blood, 2012. **119**(24): p. 5632–9.
49. Greenberg, P.L., et al., Myelodysplastic Syndromes: Clinical Practice Guidelines in Oncology. J Natl Compr Canc Netw, 2013. **11**(7): p. 838–74.
50. Gupta, V., P. Hari, and R. Hoffman, Allogeneic Hematopoietic Cell Transplantation for Myelofibrosis in the Era of JAK Inhibitors. Blood, 2012. **120**(7): p. 1367–79.
51. Tefferi, A., How I Treat Myelofibrosis. Blood, 2011. **117**(13): p. 3494–504.
52. Rachmilewitz, E.A. and P.J. Giardina, How I Treat Thalassemia. Blood, 2011. **118**(13): p. 3479–88.
53. Hsieh, M.M., et al., Allogeneic Hematopoietic Stem-cell Transplantation for Sickle Cell Disease. N Engl J Med, 2009. **361**(24): p. 2309–17.
54. Cavazzana-Calvo, M., I. Andre-Schmutz, and A. Fischer, Haematopoietic Stem Cell Transplantation for SCID Patients: Where Do We Stand? Br J Haematol, 2013. **160**(2): p. 146–52.
55. Hutter, G., et al., Long-term Control of HIV by CCR5 Delta32/Delta32 Stem-cell Transplantation. N Engl J Med, 2009. **360**(7): p. 692–8.
56. Wynn, R., Stem Cell Transplantation in Inherited Metabolic Disorders. Hematology Am Soc Hematol Educ Program, 2011. **2011**: p. 285–91.
57. Prasad, V.K. and J. Kurtzberg, Cord Blood and Bone Marrow Transplantation in Inherited Metabolic Diseases: Scientific Basis, Current Status and Future Directions. Br J Haematol, 2010. **148**(3): p. 356–72.
58. Dick, J.E., Stem Cell Concepts Renew Cancer Research. Blood, 2008. **112**(13): p. 4793–807.
59. Papayannopoulou, T. and D.T. Scadden, Stem-cell Ecology and Stem Cells in Motion. Blood, 2008. **111**(8): p. 3923–30.
60. Li, L. and H. Clevers, Coexistence of Quiescent and Active Adult Stem Cells in Mammals. Science, 2010. **327**(5965): p. 542–5.
61. Moore, K.A. and I.R. Lemischka, Stem Cells and Their Niches. Science, 2006. **311**(5769): p. 1880–5.
62. Bigas, A. and L. Espinosa, Hematopoietic Stem Cells: To Be or Notch to Be. Blood, 2012. **119**(14): p. 3226–35.
63. Zon, L.I., Intrinsic and Extrinsic Control of Haematopoietic Stem-cell Self-renewal. Nature, 2008. **453**(7193): p. 306–13.
64. Reya, T. and H. Clevers, Wnt Signalling in Stem Cells and Cancer. Nature, 2005. **434**(7035): p. 843–50.
65. Blank, U., G. Karlsson, and S. Karlsson, Signaling Pathways Governing Stem-cell Fate. Blood, 2008. **111**(2): p. 492–503.
66. Doan, P.L., et al., Epidermal Growth Factor Regulates Hematopoietic Regeneration after Radiation Injury. Nat Med, 2013. **19**(3): p. 295–304.
67. Lucas, D., et al., Norepinephrine Reuptake Inhibition Promotes Mobilization in Mice: Potential Impact to Rescue Low Stem Cell Yields. Blood, 2012. **119**(17): p. 3962–5.
68. Katayama, Y., et al., Signals from the Sympathetic Nervous System Regulate Hematopoietic Stem Cell Egress from Bone Marrow. Cell, 2006. **124**(2): p. 407–21.
69. Adams, G.B., et al., Therapeutic Targeting of a Stem Cell Niche. Nat Biotechnol, 2007. **25**(2): p. 238–43.
70. Selleri, C., et al., The Metastasis-associated 67-kDa Laminin Receptor Is Involved in G-CSF-induced Hematopoietic Stem Cell Mobilization. Blood, 2006. **108**(7): p. 2476–84.
71. Hoggatt, J. and L.M. Pelus, Many Mechanisms Mediating Mobilization: An Alliterative Review. Curr Opin Hematol, 2011. **18**(4): p. 231–8.
72. Kawamori, Y., et al., Role for Vitamin D Receptor in the Neuronal Control of the Hematopoietic Stem Cell Niche. Blood, 2010. **116**(25): p. 5528–35.
73. Goldschmidt, H., et al., Mobilization of Peripheral Blood Progenitor Cells with High-dose Cyclophosphamide (4 or 7 g/m2) and Granulocyte Colony-stimulating Factor in Patients with Multiple Myeloma. Bone Marrow Transplant, 1996. **17**(5): p. 691–7.
74. DiPersio, J.F., et al., Plerixafor and G-CSF versus Placebo and G-CSF to Mobilize Hematopoietic Stem Cells for Autologous Stem Cell Transplantation in Patients with Multiple Myeloma. Blood, 2009. **113**(23): p. 5720–6.
75. Ramirez, P., et al., BIO5192, a Small Molecule Inhibitor of VLA-4, Mobilizes Hematopoietic Stem and Progenitor Cells. Blood, 2009. **114**(7): p. 1340–3.
76. Zohren, F., et al., The Monoclonal Anti-VLA-4 Antibody Natalizumab Mobilizes CD34+ Hematopoietic Progenitor Cells in Humans. Blood, 2008. **111**(7): p. 3893–5.
77. de Nigris, F., et al., CXCR4 Inhibitors: Tumor Vasculature and Therapeutic Challenges. Recent Pat Anticancer Drug Discov, 2012. **7**(3): p. 251–64.
78. Juarez, J.G., et al., Sphingosine-1-Phosphate Facilitates Trafficking of Hematopoietic Stem Cells and Their Mobilization by CXCR4 Antagonists in Mice. Blood, 2012. **119**(3): p. 707–16.
79. Alousi, A.M., et al., Who Is the Better Donor for Older Hematopoietic Transplant Recipients: An Older-aged Sibling or a Young, Matched Unrelated Volunteer? Blood, 2013. **121**(13): p. 2567–73.
80. Kanda, J., et al., Related Transplantation with HLA-1 Ag Mismatch in the GVH

81. Pietersma, F.L., et al., Influence of Donor Cytomegalovirus (CMV) Status on Severity of Viral Reactivation after Allogeneic Stem Cell Transplantation in CMV-seropositive Recipients. Clin Infect Dis, 2011. **52**(7): p. e144–8.
82. Confer, D.L., et al., Selection of Adult Unrelated Hematopoietic Stem Cell Donors: Beyond HLA. Biol Blood Marrow Transplant, 2010. **16**(1 Suppl): p. S8–S11.
83. Lee, S.J., et al., High-resolution Donor-recipient HLA Matching Contributes to the Success of Unrelated Donor Marrow Transplantation. Blood, 2007. **110**(13): p. 4576–83.
84. Costa, L.J., et al., Overcoming HLA-DPB1 Donor Specific Antibody-mediated Haematopoietic Graft Failure. Br J Haematol, 2010. **151**(1): p. 94–6.
85. Spellman, S., et al., The Detection of Donor-directed, HLA-specific Alloantibodies in Recipients of Unrelated Hematopoietic Cell Transplantation Is Predictive of Graft Failure. Blood, 2010. **115**(13): p. 2704–8.
86. Horowitz, M.M., Does Matched Unrelated Donor Transplantation Have the Same Outcome as Matched Sibling Transplantation in Unselected Patients? Best Pract Res Clin Haematol, 2012. **25**(4): p. 483–6.
87. Chakraverty, R., et al., Impact of in Vivo Alemtuzumab Dose before Reduced Intensity Conditioning and HLA-identical Sibling Stem Cell Transplantation: Pharmacokinetics, GVHD, and Immune Reconstitution. Blood, 2010. **116**(16): p. 3080–8.
88. Soiffer, R.J., et al., Impact of Immune Modulation with Anti-T-cell Antibodies on the Outcome of Reduced-intensity Allogeneic Hematopoietic Stem Cell Transplantation for Hematologic Malignancies. Blood, 2011. **117**(25): p. 6963–70.
89. Luznik, L., et al., High-dose Cyclophosphamide as Single-agent, Short-course Prophylaxis of Graft-versus-Host Disease. Blood, 2010. **115**(16): p. 3224–30.
90. Aversa, F., et al., Treatment of High-risk Acute Leukemia with T-cell-depleted Stem Cells from Related Donors with One Fully Mismatched HLA Haplotype. N Engl J Med, 1998. **339**(17): p. 1186–93.
91. Venstrom, J.M., et al., HLA-C-dependent Prevention of Leukemia Relapse by Donor Activating KIR2DS1. N Engl J Med, 2012. **367**(9): p. 805–16.
92. Barker, J.N., C. Byam, and A. Scaradavou, How I Treat: The Selection and Acquisition of Unrelated Cord Blood Grafts. Blood, 2011. **117**(8): p. 2332–9.
93. Eapen, M., et al., Effect of Donor-recipient HLA Matching at HLA A, B, C, and DRB1 on Outcomes after Umbilical-cord Blood Transplantation for Leukaemia and Myelodysplastic Syndrome: A Retrospective Analysis. Lancet Oncol, 2011. **12**(13): p. 1214–21.
94. Cutler, C., et al., Donor-specific Anti-HLA Antibodies Predict Outcome in Double Umbilical Cord Blood Transplantation. Blood, 2011. **118**(25): p. 6691–7.
95. de Lima, M., et al., Cord-blood Engraftment with ex Vivo Mesenchymal-cell Coculture. N Engl J Med, 2012. **367**(24): p. 2305–15.
96. Delaney, C., et al., Notch-mediated Expansion of Human Cord Blood Progenitor Cells Capable of Rapid Myeloid Reconstitution. Nat Med, 2010. **16**(2): p. 232–6.
97. Liu, H., et al., Reduced-intensity Conditioning with Combined Haploidentical and Cord Blood Transplantation Results in Rapid Engraftment, Low GVHD, and Durable Remissions. Blood, 2011. **118**(24): p. 6438–45.
98. Peled, T., et al., Nicotinamide, a SIRT1 Inhibitor, Inhibits Differentiation and Facilitates Expansion of Hematopoietic Progenitor Cells with Enhanced Bone Marrow Homing and Engraftment. Exp Hematol, 2012. **40**(4): p. 342–55 e1.
99. Porter, R.L., et al., Prostaglandin E2 Increases Hematopoietic Stem Cell Survival and Accelerates Hematopoietic Recovery after Radiation Injury. Stem Cells, 2013. **31**(2): p. 372–83.
100. North, T.E., et al., Prostaglandin E2 Regulates Vertebrate Haematopoietic Stem Cell Homeostasis. Nature, 2007. **447**(7147): p. 1007–11.
101. Xia, L., et al., Surface Fucosylation of Human Cord Blood Cells Augments Binding to P-selectin and E-selectin and Enhances Engraftment in Bone Marrow. Blood, 2004. **104**(10): p. 3091–6.
102. Xu, H., et al., A Critical Role for the TLR4/TRIF Pathway in Allogeneic Hematopoietic Cell Rejection by Innate Immune Cells. Cell Transplant, 2012.
103. Joffre, O., et al., Prevention of Acute and Chronic Allograft Rejection with CD4+CD25+Foxp3+ Regulatory T Lymphocytes. Nat Med, 2008. **14**(1): p. 88–92.
104. Scheffold, C., et al., Cytokines and Cytotoxic Pathways in Engraftment Resistance to Purified Allogeneic Hematopoietic Stem Cells. Biol Blood Marrow Transplant, 2005. **11**(1): p. 1–12.
105. Ciurea, S.O., et al., Donor-specific Anti-HLA Abs and Graft Failure in Matched Unrelated Donor Hematopoietic Stem Cell Transplantation. Blood, 2011. **118**(22): p. 5957–64.
106. Jabbour, E., et al., Treatment of Donor Graft Failure with Nonmyeloablative Conditioning of Fludarabine, Antithymocyte Globulin and a Second Allogeneic Hematopoietic Transplantation. Bone Marrow Transplant, 2007. **40**(5): p. 431–5.
107. Curley, C., et al., Outcomes after Major or Bidirectional ABO-mismatched Allogeneic Hematopoietic Progenitor Cell Transplantation after Pretransplant Isoagglutinin Reduction with Donor-type Secretor Plasma with or without Plasma Exchange. Transfusion, 2012. **52**(2): p. 291–7.
108. Worel, N., et al., Prophylactic Red Blood Cell Exchange for Prevention of Severe Immune Hemolysis in Minor ABO-mismatched Allogeneic Peripheral Blood Progenitor Cell Transplantation after Reduced-intensity Conditioning. Transfusion, 2007. **47**(8): p. 1494–502.
109. Helbig, G., et al., Pure Red-cell Aplasia Following Major and Bi-directional ABO-incompatible Allogeneic Stem-cell Transplantation: Recovery of Donor-derived Erythropoiesis after Long-term Treatment Using Different Therapeutic Strategies. Ann Hematol, 2007. **86**(9): p. 677–83.
110. Hirokawa, M., et al., Efficacy and Long-term Outcome of Treatment for Pure Red Cell Aplasia after Allogeneic Stem Cell Transplantation from Major ABO-incompatible Donors. Biol Blood Marrow Transplant, 2013. **19**(7): p. 1026–32.
111. Booth, G.S., et al., Clinical Guide to ABO-Incompatible Allogeneic Stem Cell Transplantation. Biol Blood Marrow Transplant, 2013. **19**(8): p. 1152–8.
112. Pavenski, K., et al., Efficacy of HLA-matched Platelet Transfusions for Patients with Hypoproliferative

Thrombocytopenia: A Systematic Review. Transfusion, 2013.

113 Rebulla, P., A Mini-review on Platelet Refractoriness. Haematologica, 2005. **90**(2): p. 247–53.

114 Radia, R. and D. Pamphilon, Transfusion Strategies in Patients Undergoing Stem-cell Transplantation. Expert Rev Hematol, 2011. **4**(2): p. 213–20.

115 Storek, J., et al., Reconstitution of the Immune System after Hematopoietic Stem Cell Transplantation in Humans. Seminars in Immunopathology, 2008. **30**(4): p. 425–437.

116 Gress, R.E., et al., Lymphoid Reconstruction and Vaccines. Biol Blood Marrow Transplant, 2007. **13**(1 Suppl 1): p. 17–22.

117 Cham, B.P., et al., Neutrophil Function in Pediatric Patients after Bone Marrow Transplantation. International Journal of Pediatric Hematology/Oncology, 1996. **3**(1): p. 75–82.

118 Barczyk, A., et al., Decreased Levels of Myeloperoxidase in Induced Sputum of Patients with COPD after Treatment with Oral Glucocorticoids. Chest, 2004. **126**(2): p. 389–393.

119 Orciuolo, E., et al., Effects of Aspergillus Fumigatus Gliotoxin and Methylprednisolone on Human Neutrophils: Implications for the Pathogenesis of Invasive Aspergillosis. J Leukoc Biol, 2007. **82**(4): p. 839–48.

120 Boeckh, M., et al., Cytomegalovirus in Hematopoietic Stem Cell Transplant Recipients: Current Status, Known Challenges, and Future Strategies. Biol Blood Marrow Transplant, 2003. **9**(9): p. 543–58.

121 Mullighan, C.G., et al., Mannose-binding Lectin Status Is Associated with Risk of Major Infection Following Myeloablative Sibling Allogeneic Hematopoietic Stem Cell Transplantation. Blood, 2008. **112**(5): p. 2120–2128.

122 Bochud, P.Y., et al., Toll-like Receptor 4 Polymorphisms and Aspergillosis in Stem-cell Transplantation. New England Journal of Medicine, 2008. **359**(17): p. 1766–1777.

123 Peggs, K.S., Immune Reconstitution Following Stem Cell Transplantation. Leuk Lymphoma, 2004. **45**(6): p. 1093–1101.

124 Lowdell, M.W., Natural Killer Cells in Haematopoietic Stem Cell Transplantation. Transfusion Medicine, 2003. **13**(6): p. 399–404.

125 Morris, E.S., et al., Induction of Natural Killer T Cell-dependent Alloreactivity by Administration of Granulocyte Colony-stimulating Factor after Bone Marrow Transplantation. Nat Med, 2009. **15**(4): p. 436–41.

126 Zeng, S.G., et al., Human Invariant NKT Cell Subsets Differentially Promote Differentiation, Antibody Production, and T Cell Stimulation by B Cells in Vitro. J Immunol, 2013. **191**(4): p. 1666–76.

127 Ly, D., et al., An Alpha-galactosylceramide C20:2 N-acyl Variant Enhances Anti-inflammatory and Regulatory T Cell-independent Responses that Prevent Type 1 Diabetes. Clin Exp Immunol, 2010. **160**(2): p. 185–98.

128 Talarn, C., et al., Kinetics of Recovery of Dendritic Cell Subsets after Reduced-intensity Conditioning Allogeneic Stem Cell Transplantation and Clinical Outcome. Haematologica, 2007. **92**(12): p. 1655–63.

129 Komanduri, K.V., et al., Delayed Immune Reconstitution after Cord Blood Transplantation Is Characterized by Impaired Thymopoiesis and Late Memory T-cell Skewing. Blood, 2007. **110**(13): p. 4543–51.

130 Chang, Y.J., et al., Immune Reconstitution Following Unmanipulated HLA-Mismatched/Haploidentical Transplantation Compared with HLA-identical Sibling Transplantation. J Clin Immunol, 2012. **32**(2): p. 268–80.

131 Corre, E., et al., Long-term Immune Deficiency after Allogeneic Stem Cell Transplantation: B-cell Deficiency Is Associated with Late Infections. Haematologica, 2010. **95**(6): p. 1025–9.

132 Kalwak, K., et al., Immune Reconstitution after Haematopoietic Cell Transplantation in Children: Immunophenotype Analysis with Regard to Factors Affecting the Speed of Recovery. Br J Haematol, 2002. **118**(1): p. 74–89.

133 Allen, J.L., et al., B Cells from Patients with Chronic GVHD Are Activated and Primed for Survival via BAFF-mediated Pathways. Blood, 2012. **120**(12): p. 2529–36.

134 Hazenberg, M.D., et al., T-cell Receptor Excision Circle and T-cell Dynamics after Allogeneic Stem Cell Transplantation Are Related to Clinical Events. Blood, 2002. **99**(9): p. 3449–53.

135 Storek, J., et al., Immune Reconstitution after Allogeneic Marrow Transplantation Compared with Blood Stem Cell Transplantation. Blood, 2001. **97**(11): p. 3380–9.

136 Storek, J., et al., Improved Reconstitution of CD4 T Cells and B Cells but Worsened Reconstitution of Serum IgG Levels after Allogeneic Transplantation of Blood Stem Cells Instead of Marrow. Blood, 1997. **89**(10): p. 3891–3.

137 Parmar, S., et al., Ex Vivo Expanded Umbilical Cord Blood T Cells Maintain Naive Phenotype and TCR Diversity. Cytotherapy, 2006. **8**(2): p. 149–57.

138 Ozdemir, E., et al., Cytomegalovirus Reactivation Following Allogeneic Stem Cell Transplantation Is Associated with the Presence of Dysfunctional Antigen-specific CD8+ T Cells. Blood, 2002. **100**(10): p. 3690–7.

139 Escalon, M.P. and K.V. Komanduri, Cord Blood Transplantation: Evolving Strategies to Improve Engraftment and Immune Reconstitution. Curr Opin Oncol, 2010. **22**(2): p. 122–9.

140 Della Chiesa, M., et al., Phenotypic and Functional Heterogeneity of Human NK Cells Developing after Umbilical Cord Blood Transplantation: A Role for Human Cytomegalovirus? Blood, 2012. **119**(2): p. 399–410.

141 Poulin, J.F., et al., Direct Evidence for Thymic Function in Adult Humans. Journal of Experimental Medicine, 1999. **190**(4): p. 479–86.

142 Douek, D.C., et al., Changes in Thymic Function with Age and during the Treatment of HIV Infection. Nature, 1998. **396**(6712): p. 690–5.

143 Clave, E., et al., Acute Graft-versus-Host Disease Transiently Impairs Thymic Output in Young Patients after Allogeneic Hematopoietic Stem Cell Transplantation. Blood, 2009. **113**(25): p. 6477–84.

144 Chung, B., et al., Combined Effects of Interleukin-7 and Stem Cell Factor Administration on Lymphopoiesis after Murine Bone Marrow Transplantation. Biol Blood Marrow Transplant, 2011. **17**(1): p. 48–60.

145 Andre-Schmutz, I., et al., IL-7 Effect on Immunological Reconstitution after HSCT Depends on MHC Incompatibility. Br J Haematol, 2004. **126**(6): p. 844–51.

146 Okamoto, Y., et al., Effects of Exogenous Interleukin-7 on Human

Thymus Function. Blood, 2002. **99**(8): p. 2851–8.

147 Min, D., et al., Sustained Thymopoiesis and Improvement in Functional Immunity Induced by Exogenous KGF Administration in Murine Models of Aging. Blood, 2007. **109**(6): p. 2529–37.

148 Goldberg, G.L., et al., Luteinizing Hormone-releasing Hormone Enhances T Cell Recovery Following Allogeneic Bone Marrow Transplantation. J Immunol, 2009. **182**(9): p. 5846–54.

149 Brunstein, C.G., et al., Infusion of ex Vivo Expanded T Regulatory Cells in Adults Transplanted with Umbilical Cord Blood: Safety Profile and Detection Kinetics. Blood, 2011. **117**(3): p. 1061–70.

150 Di Ianni, M., et al., Tregs Prevent GVHD and Promote Immune Reconstitution in HLA-haploidentical Transplantation. Blood, 2011. **117**(14): p. 3921–8.

151 Hanley, P.J., et al., Functionally Active Virus-specific T Cells that Target CMV, Adenovirus, and EBV Can Be Expanded from Naive T-cell Populations in Cord Blood and Will Target a Range of Viral Epitopes. Blood, 2009. **114**(9): p. 1958–67.

152 Harter, C., et al., Piperacillin/Tazobactam vs Ceftazidime in the Treatment of Neutropenic Fever in Patients with Acute Leukemia or Following Autologous Peripheral Blood Stem Cell Transplantation: A Prospective Randomized Trial. Bone Marrow Transplant, 2006. **37**(4): p. 373–9.

153 Koya, R., et al., Analysis of the Value of Empiric Vancomycin Administration in Febrile Neutropenia Occurring after Autologous Peripheral Blood Stem Cell Transplants. Bone Marrow Transplant, 1998. **21**(9): p. 923–6.

154 Clutter, D.S., et al., Fidaxomicin versus Conventional Antimicrobial Therapy in 59 Recipients of Solid Organ and Hematopoietic Stem Cell Transplantation with Clostridium Difficile-associated Diarrhea. Antimicrob Agents Chemother, 2013. **57**(9): p. 4501–5.

155 Dubberke, E.R., et al., Severity of Clostridium Difficile-associated Disease (CDAD) in Allogeneic Stem Cell Transplant Recipients: Evaluation of a CDAD Severity Grading System. Infect Control Hosp Epidemiol, 2007. **28**(2): p. 208–11.

156 Arango, J.I., et al., Incidence of Clostridium Difficile-associated Diarrhea before and after Autologous Peripheral Blood Stem Cell Transplantation for Lymphoma and Multiple Myeloma. Bone Marrow Transplant, 2006. **37**(5): p. 517–21.

157 Hogenauer, C., et al., Klebsiella Oxytoca as a Causative Organism of Antibiotic-associated Hemorrhagic Colitis. N Engl J Med, 2006. **355**(23): p. 2418–26.

158 Al-Anazi, K.A., et al., Klebsiella Oxytoca Bacteremia Causing Septic Shock in Recipients of Hematopoietic Stem Cell Transplant: Two Case Reports. Cases J, 2008. **1**(1): p. 160.

159 Bhatt, A.S., et al., Sequence-based Discovery of Bradyrhizobium Enterica in Cord Colitis Syndrome. N Engl J Med, 2013. **369**(6): p. 517–28.

160 Trifilio, S.M., et al., Breakthrough Zygomycosis after Voriconazole Administration among Patients with Hematologic Malignancies Who Receive Hematopoietic Stem-cell Transplants or Intensive Chemotherapy. Bone Marrow Transplant, 2007. **39**(7): p. 425–9.

161 Person, A.K., D.P. Kontoyiannis, and B.D. Alexander, Fungal Infections in Transplant and Oncology Patients. Infect Dis Clin North Am, 2010. **24**(2): p. 439–59.

162 Lindemans, C.A., A.M. Leen, and J.J. Boelens, How I Treat Adenovirus in Hematopoietic Stem Cell Transplant Recipients. Blood, 2010. **116**(25): p. 5476–85.

163 Ullmann, A.J., et al., Posaconazole or Fluconazole for Prophylaxis in Severe Graft-versus-Host Disease. N Engl J Med, 2007. **356**(4): p. 335–47.

164 Fishman, J.A., Prevention of Infection Caused by Pneumocystis Carinii in Transplant Recipients. Clin Infect Dis, 2001. **33**(8): p. 1397–405.

165 Koskenvuo, M., et al., BK Polyomavirus-associated Hemorrhagic Cystitis among Pediatric Allogeneic Bone Marrow Transplant Recipients: Treatment Response and Evidence for Nosocomial Transmission. J Clin Virol, 2013. **56**(1): p. 77–81.

166 Raval, M., et al., Evaluation and Management of BK Virus-associated Nephropathy Following Allogeneic Hematopoietic Cell Transplantation. Biol Blood Marrow Transplant, 2011. **17**(11): p. 1589–93.

167 Miller, A.N., et al., Efficacy and Safety of Ciprofloxacin for Prophylaxis of Polyomavirus BK Virus-associated Hemorrhagic Cystitis in Allogeneic Hematopoietic Stem Cell Transplantation Recipients. Biol Blood Marrow Transplant, 2011. **17**(8): p. 1176–81.

168 Chen, X.C., et al., Efficacy and Safety of Leflunomide for the Treatment of BK Virus-associated Hemorrhagic Cystitis in Allogeneic Hematopoietic Stem Cell Transplantation Recipients. Acta Haematol, 2013. **130**(1): p. 52–6.

169 Lekakis, L.J., et al., BK Virus Nephropathy after Allogeneic Stem Cell Transplantation: A Case Report and Literature Review. Am J Hematol, 2009. **84**(4): p. 243–6.

170 Tomblyn, M., et al., Guidelines for Preventing Infectious Complications among Hematopoietic Cell Transplantation Recipients: A Global Perspective. Biol Blood Marrow Transplant, 2009. **15**(10): p. 1143–238.

171 Boeckh, M. and P. Ljungman, How We Treat Cytomegalovirus in Hematopoietic Cell Transplant Recipients. Blood, 2009. **113**(23): p. 5711–9.

172 Heslop, H.E., How I Treat EBV Lymphoproliferation. Blood, 2009. **114**(19): p. 4002–8.

173 Maertens, J., et al., Screening for Circulating Galactomannan as a Noninvasive Diagnostic Tool for Invasive Aspergillosis in Prolonged Neutropenic Patients and Stem Cell Transplantation Recipients: A Prospective Validation. Blood, 2001. **97**(6): p. 1604–10.

174 Savani, B.N., et al., How I Treat Late Effects in Adults after Allogeneic Stem Cell Transplantation. Blood, 2011. **117**(11): p. 3002–9.

175 Meisel, R., et al., Pneumococcal Conjugate Vaccine Provides Early Protective Antibody Responses in Children after Related and Unrelated Allogeneic Hematopoietic Stem Cell Transplantation. Blood, 2007. **109**(6): p. 2322–6.

176 Coppell, J.A., et al., Hepatic Veno-occlusive Disease Following Stem Cell Transplantation: Incidence, Clinical Course, and Outcome. Biol Blood Marrow Transplant, 2010. **16**(2): p. 157–68.

177 Cutler, C., et al., Prediction of Veno-occlusive Disease Using Biomarkers of Endothelial Injury. Biol Blood

178. Ryu, S.G., et al., Randomized Comparison of Four-Times-Daily versus Once-Daily Intravenous Busulfan in Conditioning Therapy for Hematopoietic Cell Transplantation. Biol Blood Marrow Transplant, 2007. **13**(9): p. 1095–105.

179. Hassan, Z., Optimal Approach to Prevent Veno-occlusive Disease Following Hematopoietic Stem Cell Transplantation in Children. Pediatr Transplant, 2010. **14**(6): p. 683–7.

180. Lakshminarayanan, S., et al., Low Incidence of Hepatic Veno-occlusive Disease in Pediatric Patients Undergoing Hematopoietic Stem Cell Transplantation Attributed to a Combination of Intravenous Heparin, Oral Glutamine, and Ursodiol at a Single Transplant Institution. Pediatr Transplant, 2010. **14**(5): p. 618–21.

181. Tay, J., et al., Systematic Review of Controlled Clinical Trials on the Use of Ursodeoxycholic Acid for the Prevention of Hepatic Veno-occlusive Disease in Hematopoietic Stem Cell Transplantation. Biol Blood Marrow Transplant, 2007. **13**(2): p. 206–17.

182. Ruutu, T., et al., Ursodeoxycholic Acid for the Prevention of Hepatic Complications in Allogeneic Stem Cell Transplantation. Blood, 2002. **100**(6): p. 1977–83.

183. Laskin, B.L., et al., Small Vessels, Big Trouble in the Kidneys and Beyond: Hematopoietic Stem Cell Transplantation-associated Thrombotic Microangiopathy. Blood, 2011. **118**(6): p. 1452–62.

184. Rosenthal, J., et al., Transplant-associated Thrombotic Microangiopathy in Pediatric Patients Treated with Sirolimus and Tacrolimus. Pediatr Blood Cancer, 2011. **57**(1): p. 142–6.

185. Kennedy, G.A., et al., Transplantation-associated Thrombotic Microangiopathy: Effect of Concomitant GVHD on Efficacy of Therapeutic Plasma Exchange. Bone Marrow Transplant, 2010. **45**(4): p. 699–704.

186. Uderzo, C., et al., Risk Factors and Severe Outcome in Thrombotic Microangiopathy after Allogeneic Hematopoietic Stem Cell Transplantation. Transplantation, 2006. **82**(5): p. 638–44.

Marrow Transplant, 2010. **16**(8): p. 1180–5.

187. Wingard, J.R., J.W. Hiemenz, and M.A. Jantz, How I Manage Pulmonary Nodular Lesions and Nodular Infiltrates in Patients with Hematologic Malignancies or Undergoing Hematopoietic Cell Transplantation. Blood, 2012. **120**(9): p. 1791–800.

188. Frangoul, H., T. Koyama, and J. Domm, Etanercept for Treatment of Idiopathic Pneumonia Syndrome after Allogeneic Hematopoietic Stem Cell Transplantation. Blood, 2009. **113**(12): p. 2868–9; author reply 2869.

189. Yanik, G.A., et al., The Impact of Soluble Tumor Necrosis Factor Receptor Etanercept on the Treatment of Idiopathic Pneumonia Syndrome after Allogeneic Hematopoietic Stem Cell Transplantation. Blood, 2008. **112**(8): p. 3073–81.

190. Hildebrandt, G.C., et al., Donor T-cell Production of RANTES Significantly Contributes to the Development of Idiopathic Pneumonia Syndrome after Allogeneic Stem Cell Transplantation. Blood, 2005. **105**(6): p. 2249–57.

191. Shenoy, A., B.N. Savani, and A.J. Barrett, Recombinant Factor VIIa to Treat Diffuse Alveolar Hemorrhage Following Allogeneic Stem Cell Transplantation. Biol Blood Marrow Transplant, 2007. **13**(5): p. 622–3.

192. Majhail, N.S., et al., Diffuse Alveolar Hemorrhage and Infection-associated Alveolar Hemorrhage Following Hematopoietic Stem Cell Transplantation: Related and High-risk Clinical Syndromes. Biol Blood Marrow Transplant, 2006. **12**(10): p. 1038–46.

193. Wanko, S.O., et al., Diffuse Alveolar Hemorrhage: Retrospective Review of Clinical Outcome in Allogeneic Transplant Recipients Treated with Aminocaproic Acid. Biol Blood Marrow Transplant, 2006. **12**(9): p. 949–53.

194. Yoshihara, S., et al., Bronchiolitis Obliterans Syndrome (BOS), Bronchiolitis Obliterans Organizing Pneumonia (BOOP), and Other Late-onset Noninfectious Pulmonary Complications Following Allogeneic Hematopoietic Stem Cell Transplantation. Biol Blood Marrow Transplant, 2007. **13**(7): p. 749–59.

195. Bernard, D., et al., CBX7 Controls the Growth of Normal and Tumor-derived Prostate Cells by Repressing the Ink4a/Arf Locus. Oncogene, 2005. **24**(36): p. 5543–51.

196. Dandoy, C., et al., Pulmonary Hypertension after Hematopoietic Stem Cell Transplantation. Biol Blood Marrow Transplant, 2013.

197. Sakaida, E., et al., Late-onset Noninfectious Pulmonary Complications after Allogeneic Stem Cell Transplantation Are Significantly Associated with Chronic Graft-versus-Host Disease and with the Graft-versus-Leukemia Effect. Blood, 2003. **102**(12): p. 4236–42.

198. Bashoura, L., et al., Inhaled Corticosteroids Stabilize Constrictive Bronchiolitis after Hematopoietic Stem Cell Transplantation. Bone Marrow Transplant, 2008. **41**(1): p. 63–7.

199. Sengsayadeth, S.M., et al., Time to Explore Preventive and Novel Therapies for Bronchiolitis Obliterans Syndrome after Allogeneic Hematopoietic Stem Cell Transplantation. Biol Blood Marrow Transplant, 2012. **18**(10): p. 1479–87.

200. Au, B.K., M.A. Au, and J.W. Chien, Bronchiolitis Obliterans Syndrome Epidemiology after Allogeneic Hematopoietic Cell Transplantation. Biol Blood Marrow Transplant, 2011. **17**(7): p. 1072–8.

201. Chien, J.W., et al., Bronchiolitis Obliterans Syndrome after Allogeneic Hematopoietic Stem Cell Transplantation—An Increasingly Recognized Manifestation of Chronic Graft-versus-Host Disease. Biol Blood Marrow Transplant, 2010. **16**(1 Suppl): p. S106–14.

202. Spielberger, R., et al., Palifermin for Oral Mucositis after Intensive Therapy for Hematologic Cancers. N Engl J Med, 2004. **351**(25): p. 2590–8.

203. Phillips, G.L., 2nd, et al., A Phase I Trial: Dose Escalation of Melphalan in the "BEAM" Regimen Using Amifostine Cytoprotection. Biol Blood Marrow Transplant, 2011. **17**(7): p. 1033–42.

204. Spencer, A., et al., Prospective Randomised Trial of Amifostine Cytoprotection in Myeloma Patients Undergoing High-dose Melphalan Conditioned Autologous Stem Cell Transplantation. Bone Marrow Transplant, 2005. **35**(10): p. 971–7.

205. Hensley, M.L., et al., American Society of Clinical Oncology 2008 Clinical Practice Guideline Update: Use of Chemotherapy and Radiation Therapy Protectants. J Clin Oncol, 2009. **27**(1): p. 127–45.

206. Keefe, D.M., et al., Updated Clinical Practice Guidelines for the Prevention and Treatment of Mucositis. Cancer, 2007. 109(5): p. 820–31.
207. Bensinger, W., et al., NCCN Task Force Report. Prevention and Management of Mucositis in Cancer Care. J Natl Compr Canc Netw, 2008. 6 Suppl 1: p. S1–21; quiz S22–4.
208. Ferrara, J.L., et al., Graft-versus-Host Disease. Lancet, 2009. 373(9674): p. 1550–61.
209. Shlomchik, W.D., Graft-versus-Host Disease. Nat Rev Immunol, 2007. 7(5): p. 340–52.
210. Blazar, B.R., W.J. Murphy, and M. Abedi, Advances in Graft-versus-Host Disease Biology and Therapy. Nat Rev Immunol, 2012. 12(6): p. 443–58.
211. Saliba, R.M., et al., Hyperacute GVHD: Risk Factors, Outcomes, and Clinical Implications. Blood, 2007. 109(7): p. 2751–8.
212. Shlomchik, W.D., et al., Prevention of Graft versus Host Disease by Inactivation of Host Antigen-presenting Cells. Science, 1999. 285(5426): p. 412–5.
213. Koyama, M., et al., Recipient Nonhematopoietic Antigen-presenting Cells Are Sufficient to Induce Lethal Acute Graft-versus-Host Disease. Nat Med, 2012. 18(1): p. 135–42.
214. Koyama, M., et al., Plasmacytoid Dendritic Cells Prime Alloreactive T Cells to Mediate Graft-versus-Host Disease as Antigen-presenting Cells. Blood, 2009. 113(9): p. 2088–95.
215. Maier, T., J.H. Holda, and H.N. Claman, Graft-vs-Host Reactions (GVHR) across Minor Murine Histocompatibility Barriers. II. Development of Natural Suppressor Cell Activity. J Immunol, 1985. 135(3): p. 1644–51.
216. Guinan, E.C., et al., Transplantation of Anergic Histoincompatible Bone Marrow Allografts. N Engl J Med, 1999. 340(22): p. 1704–14.
217. Prigozhina, T.B., et al., CD40 Ligand-specific Antibodies Synergize with Cyclophosphamide to Promote Long-term Transplantation Tolerance across MHC Barriers but Inhibit Graft-vs-Leukemia Effects of Transplanted Cells. Exp Hematol, 2003. 31(1): p. 81–8.
218. Li, J., et al., Roles of CD28, CTLA4, and Inducible Costimulator in Acute Graft-versus-Host Disease in Mice. Biol Blood Marrow Transplant, 2011. 17(7): p. 962–9.
219. Cooke, K.R., et al., LPS Antagonism Reduces Graft-versus-Host Disease and Preserves Graft-versus-Leukemia Activity after Experimental Bone Marrow Transplantation. J Clin Invest, 2001. 107(12): p. 1581–9.
220. Calcaterra, C., et al., Critical Role of TLR9 in Acute Graft-versus-Host Disease. J Immunol, 2008. 181(9): p. 6132–9.
221. Penack, O., et al., NOD2 Regulates Hematopoietic Cell Function during Graft-versus-Host Disease. J Exp Med, 2009. 206(10): p. 2101–10.
222. Wilhelm, K., et al., Graft-versus-Host Disease Is Enhanced by Extracellular ATP Activating P2X7 R. Nat Med, 2010. 16(12): p. 1434–8.
223. Holler, E., et al., Both Donor and Recipient NOD2/CARD15 Mutations Associated with Transplant-related Mortality and GvHD Following Allogeneic Stem Cell Transplantation. Blood, 2004. 104(3): p. 889–94.
224. Anderson, B.E., et al., Memory CD4+ T Cells Do Not Induce Graft-versus-Host Disease. J Clin Invest, 2003. 112(1): p. 101–8.
225. Anderson, B.E., et al., Memory T Cells in GVHD and GVL. Biol Blood Marrow Transplant, 2008. 14(1 Suppl 1): p. 19–20.
226. Zhang, Y., et al., Host-reactive CD8+ Memory Stem Cells in Graft-versus-Host Disease. Nat Med, 2005. 11(12): p. 1299–305.
227. Chen, B.J., et al., Transfer of Allogeneic CD62L- Memory T Cells without Graft-versus-Host Disease. Blood, 2004. 103(4): p. 1534–41.
228. Chen, B.J., et al., Inability of Memory T Cells to Induce Graft-versus-Host Disease Is a Result of an Abortive Alloresponse. Blood, 2007. 109(7): p. 3115–23.
229. Zheng, H., et al., Central Memory CD8 + T Cells Induce Graft-versus-Host Disease and Mediate Graft-versus-Leukemia. J Immunol, 2009. 182(10): p. 5938–48.
230. Zheng, H., et al., Effector Memory CD4 + T Cells Mediate Graft-versus-Leukemia without Inducing Graft-versus-Host Disease. Blood, 2008. 111(4): p. 2476–84.
231. Shindo, T., et al., MEK Inhibitors Selectively Suppress Alloreactivity and Graft-versus-Host Disease in a Memory Stage-dependent Manner. Blood, 2013. 121(23): p. 4617–26.
232. Kim, T.K., et al., Co-engagement of Alpha(4)Beta(1) Integrin (VLA-4) and CD4 or CD8 is Necessary to Induce Maximal Erk1/2 Phosphorylation and Cytokine Production in Human T Cells. Hum Immunol, 2010. 71(1): p. 23–8.
233. Kim, T.K., et al., Human Late Memory CD8+ T Cells Have a Distinct Cytokine Signature Characterized by CC Chemokine Production without IL-2 Production. Journal of Immunology, 2009.
234. Martins, S.L., et al., Functional Assessment and Specific Depletion of Alloreactive Human T Cells Using Flow Cytometry. Blood, 2004. 104(12): p. 3429–36.
235. Petrovic, A., et al., LPAM (Alpha 4 Beta 7 Integrin) Is an Important Homing Integrin on Alloreactive T Cells in the Development of Intestinal Graft-versus-Host Disease. Blood, 2004. 103(4): p. 1542–7.
236. Murai, M., et al., Peyer's Patch Is the Essential Site in Initiating Murine Acute and Lethal Graft-versus-Host Reaction. Nat Immunol, 2003. 4(2): p. 154–60.
237. Sandborn, W.J., et al., Vedolizumab as Induction and Maintenance Therapy for Crohn's Disease. N Engl J Med, 2013. 369(8): p. 711–21.
238. Feagan, B.G., et al., Vedolizumab as Induction and Maintenance Therapy for Ulcerative Colitis. N Engl J Med, 2013. 369(8): p. 699–710.
239. Reshef, R., et al., Blockade of Lymphocyte Chemotaxis in Visceral Graft-versus-Host Disease. N Engl J Med, 2012. 367(2): p. 135–45.
240. Chen, Y.B., et al., Expression of CD30 in Patients with Acute Graft-versus-Host Disease. Blood, 2012. 120(3): p. 691–6.
241. Jankovic, D., et al., The Nlrp3 Inflammasome Regulates Acute Graft-versus-Host Disease. J Exp Med, 2013.
242. Ratajczak, P., et al., Th17/Treg Ratio in Human Graft-versus-Host Disease. Blood, 2010. 116(7): p. 1165–71.
243. Iclozan, C., et al., T Helper17 Cells Are Sufficient but Not Necessary to Induce Acute Graft-versus-Host Disease. Biol Blood Marrow Transplant, 2010. 16(2): p. 170–8.
244. Hanash, A.M., et al., Interleukin-22 Protects Intestinal Stem Cells from

244 ... Immune-mediated Tissue Damage and Regulates Sensitivity to Graft versus Host Disease. Immunity, 2012. **37**(2): p. 339–50.

245 Edinger, M., et al., CD4+CD25+ Regulatory T Cells Preserve Graft-versus-Tumor Activity while Inhibiting Graft-versus-Host Disease after Bone Marrow Transplantation. Nat Med, 2003. **9**(9): p. 1144–50.

246 Koreth, J., et al., Interleukin-2 and Regulatory T Cells in Graft-versus-Host Disease. N Engl J Med, 2011. **365**(22): p. 2055–66.

247 Levine, J.E., et al., Acute Graft-versus-Host Disease Biomarkers Measured during Therapy Can Predict Treatment Outcomes: A Blood and Marrow Transplant Clinical Trials Network Study. Blood, 2012. **119**(16): p. 3854–60.

248 Harris, A.C., et al., Plasma Biomarkers of Lower Gastrointestinal and Liver Acute GVHD. Blood, 2012. **119**(12): p. 2960–3.

249 Ferrara, J.L., Advances in the Clinical Management of GVHD. Best Pract Res Clin Haematol, 2008. **21**(4): p. 677–82.

250 Paczesny, S., et al., A Biomarker Panel for Acute Graft-versus-Host Disease. Blood, 2009. **113**(2): p. 273–8.

251 Vander Lugt, M.T., et al., ST2 as a Marker for Risk of Therapy-resistant Graft-versus-Host Disease and Death. N Engl J Med, 2013. **369**(6): p. 529–39.

252 Lin, M.T., et al., Relation of an Interleukin-10 Promoter Polymorphism to Graft-versus-Host Disease and Survival after Hematopoietic-cell Transplantation. N Engl J Med, 2003. **349**(23): p. 2201–10.

253 Goddard, D.S., et al., Clinical Update on Graft-versus-Host Disease in Children. Semin Cutan Med Surg, 2010. **29**(2): p. 92–105.

254 Washington, K. and M. Jagasia, Pathology of Graft-versus-Host Disease in the Gastrointestinal Tract. Hum Pathol, 2009. **40**(7): p. 909–17.

255 Shulman, H.M., et al., Histopathologic Diagnosis of Chronic Graft-versus-Host Disease: National Institutes of Health Consensus Development Project on Criteria for Clinical Trials in Chronic Graft-versus-Host Disease: II. Pathology Working Group Report. Biol Blood Marrow Transplant, 2006. **12**(1): p. 31–47.

256 Ma, S.Y., et al., Hepatitic Graft-versus-Host Disease after Hematopoietic Stem Cell Transplantation: Clinicopathologic Features and Prognostic Implication. Transplantation, 2004. **77**(8): p. 1252–9.

257 Deeg, H.J. and J.H. Antin, The Clinical Spectrum of Acute Graft-versus-Host Disease. Semin Hematol, 2006. **43**(1): p. 24–31.

258 Kanakry, C.G., et al., Aldehyde Dehydrogenase Expression Drives Human Regulatory T Cell Resistance to Posttransplantation Cyclophosphamide. Sci Transl Med, 2013. **5**(211): p. 211ra157.

259 Ross, D., et al., Antigen and Lymphopenia-driven Donor T Cells Are Differentially Diminished by Post-transplantation Administration of Cyclophosphamide after Hematopoietic Cell Transplantation. Biol Blood Marrow Transplant, 2013. **19**(10): p. 1430–8.

260 Martin, P.J., et al., First- and Second-line Systemic Treatment of Acute Graft-versus-Host Disease: Recommendations of the American Society of Blood and Marrow Transplantation. Biol Blood Marrow Transplant, 2012. **18**(8): p. 1150–63.

261 Wolf, D., et al., Novel Treatment Concepts for Graft-versus-Host Disease. Blood, 2012. **119**(1): p. 16–25.

262 Lee, S.J., New Approaches for Preventing and Treating Chronic Graft-versus-Host Disease. Blood, 2005. **105**(11): p. 4200–6.

263 Arai, S., et al., Global and Organ-specific Chronic Graft-versus-Host Disease Severity According to the 2005 NIH Consensus Criteria. Blood, 2011. **118**(15): p. 4242–9.

264 Zhi, L., et al., Enhanced Th17 Differentiation and Aggravated Arthritis in IEX-1-Deficient Mice by Mitochondrial Reactive Oxygen Species-mediated Signaling. J Immunol, 2012. **189**(4): p. 1639–47.

265 Sarantopoulos, S., et al., High Levels of B-cell Activating Factor in Patients with Active Chronic Graft-versus-Host Disease. Clin Cancer Res, 2007. **13**(20): p. 6107–14.

266 Navarra, S.V., et al., Efficacy and Safety of Belimumab in Patients with Active Systemic Lupus Erythematosus: A Randomised, Placebo-controlled, Phase 3 Trial. Lancet, 2011. **377**(9767): p. 721–31.

267 Koreth, J., et al., Bortezomib-based Graft-versus-Host Disease Prophylaxis in HLA-Mismatched Unrelated Donor Transplantation. J Clin Oncol, 2012. **30**(26): p. 3202–8.

268 Biagi, E., et al., Extracorporeal Photochemotherapy Is Accompanied by Increasing Levels of Circulating CD4+CD25+GITR+Foxp3+CD62L+ Functional Regulatory T-cells in Patients with Graft-versus-Host Disease. Transplantation, 2007. **84**(1): p. 31–9.

269 Cutler, C., et al., Rituximab Prophylaxis Prevents Corticosteroid-requiring Chronic GVHD after Allogeneic Peripheral Blood Stem Cell Transplantation: Results of a Phase 2 Trial. Blood, 2013. **122**(8): p. 1510–7.

270 Cutler, C., et al., Rituximab for Steroid-refractory Chronic Graft-versus-Host Disease. Blood, 2006. **108**(2): p. 756–62.

271 Wolff, D., et al., Consensus Conference on Clinical Practice in Chronic GVHD: Second-line Treatment of Chronic Graft-versus-Host Disease. Biol Blood Marrow Transplant, 2011. **17**(1): p. 1–17.

272 Chavan, R. and R. el-Azhary, Cutaneous Graft-versus-Host Disease: Rationales and Treatment Options. Dermatol Ther, 2011. **24**(2): p. 219–28.

273 Imanguli, M.M., et al., Oral Graft-versus-Host Disease. Oral Dis, 2008. **14**(5): p. 396–412.

274 Schubert, M.M. and M.E. Correa, Oral Graft-versus-Host Disease. Dent Clin North Am, 2008. **52**(1): p. 79–109, viii-ix.

275 Perez, R.L., et al., Limbus Damage in Ocular Graft-versus-Host Disease. Biol Blood Marrow Transplant, 2011. **17**(2): p. 270–3.

276 Mohty, M., et al., Chronic Graft-versus-Host Disease after Allogeneic Blood Stem Cell Transplantation: Long-term Results of a Randomized Study. Blood, 2002. **100**(9): p. 3128–34.

277 Spiryda, L.B., et al., Graft-versus-Host Disease of the Vulva and/or Vagina: Diagnosis and Treatment. Biol Blood Marrow Transplant, 2003. **9**(12): p. 760–5.

278 Xu, L., et al., Histologic Findings in Lung Biopsies in Patients with Suspected Graft-versus-Host Disease. Hum Pathol, 2013. **44**(7): p. 1233–40.

279 Hildebrandt, G.C., et al., Diagnosis and Treatment of Pulmonary Chronic GVHD: Report from the Consensus Conference on Clinical Practice in Chronic GVHD. Bone Marrow Transplant, 2011. **46**(10): p. 1283–95.

280 Demetris, A.J., Immune Cholangitis: Liver Allograft Rejection and Graft-versus-Host Disease. Mayo Clin Proc, 1998. **73**(4): p. 367–79.

281 Couriel, D.R., et al., Chronic Graft-versus-Host Disease Manifesting as Polymyositis: An Uncommon Presentation. Bone Marrow Transplant, 2002. **30**(8): p. 543–6.

282 Lin, J., et al., Membranous Glomerulopathy Associated with Graft-versus-Host Disease Following Allogeneic Stem Cell Transplantation. Report of 2 Cases and Review of the Literature. Am J Nephrol, 2001. **21**(5): p. 351–6.

283 Seber, A., S.P. Khan, and J.H. Kersey, Unexplained Effusions: Association with Allogeneic Bone Marrow Transplantation and Acute or Chronic Graft-versus-Host Disease. Bone Marrow Transplant, 1996. **17**(2): p. 207–11.

284 Hamid, O., et al., Safety and Tumor Responses with Lambrolizumab (Anti-PD-1) in Melanoma. N Engl J Med, 2013. **369** (2): p. 134–44.

285 Fong, L. and E.J. Small, Anti-cytotoxic T-lymphocyte Antigen-4 Antibody: The First in an Emerging Class of Immunomodulatory Antibodies for Cancer Treatment. J Clin Oncol, 2008. **26**(32): p. 5275–83.

286 Filipovich, A.H., et al., National Institutes of Health Consensus Development Project on Criteria for Clinical Trials in Chronic Graft-versus-Host Disease: I. Diagnosis and Staging Working Group Report. Biol Blood Marrow Transplant, 2005. **11** (12): p. 945–56.

Dermatological Complications in Transplant Patients and Composite Tissue Allotransplant Pathology

Emma Lanuti, Mohammed Sharaf, Brian Keegan, Ingrid Wolf, Marco Romanelli, Phillip Ruiz, and Paolo Romanelli

Introduction

Transplant recipients are susceptible to a number of well-described complications that include drug reactions, organ rejection, organ dysfunction, infection, and cancer. The type and severity of these complications is often determined by the method and the degree of immunosuppression [1, 2]. Cutaneous complications, including aesthetic alterations, infections, precancerous lesions, and malignancies have been reported in over 70% of transplant recipients [3]. Therefore, it is useful to review the common cutaneous manifestations observed in recipients of organ transplantation and to describe several unusual observations.

Drug Reactions in Transplant Patients

Drug rashes are common in transplant patients, given that these patients are exposed to multiple drugs, including antibiotics, antiviral medications, and immunosuppressive agents. Attributing a cutaneous drug reaction to a particular drug may be difficult due to the complexity of many immunosuppressive regimens. The drugs responsible for most cutaneous adverse drug reactions are the beta-lactams, sulfonamides, and non-steroidal anti-inflammatory drugs. Chemotherapeutic medications reported to cause a morbilliform drug exanthem include chlorambucil, cytarabine, etoposide, 5-fluorouracil, hydroxyurea, melphalan, and procarbazine [4]. Skin biopsies may help differentiate skin lesions of a drug rash from other causes such as cutaneous small-vessel vasculitis, but they are rarely helpful in identifying the causative medication. Histologically, features of drug eruptions can be heterogeneous and often include: interface dermatitis with basal vacuolar alteration, dyskeratotic keratinocytes, and a mild perivascular inflammatory infiltrate [5]. Eosinophil counts have sensitivity ranging from 22%–36% and thus are unlikely to be very useful for diagnosing drug reactions. *Acral erythema* is a localized cutaneous response to chemotherapeutic drug. It presents as painful erythema mainly of palms and soles that may evolve to blistering and desquamation. Histology may show vacuolar degeneration of the basal layer, spongiosis, dyskeratotic keratinocytes, papillary dermal edema, and a mild perivascular lymphohistiocytic infiltrate [5–7].

Common aesthetic alterations and cutaneous side effects of immunosuppressive drugs include hypertrichosis, stretch marks, skin atrophy, telangiectasia, acne, hyperpigmentation, and gingival hypertrophy [8]. Diffuse gingival enlargement can be seen with cyclosporine and the dosage and duration of immunosuppression with cyclosporine correlates with the incidence of this complication [9]. Diffuse gingival enlargement tends to be less severe with tacrolimus compared to cyclosporine [10]. The most prevalent cutaneous side effects of sirolimus are pathologies of the pilosebaceous apparatus, chronic edemas, angioedemas, and mucous membrane involvement [11–14]. It has been reported that recipients of renal transplantation taking sirolimus have an unusually high frequency of acne (45%), erupting soon after sirolimus initiation. In sirolimus-induced acne, only inflammatory lesions have been observed [15]. Sebaceous areas may be involved, but the lesions frequently extend to the forearms, internal surface of the arm, cervical area, and scalp. In some patients, severe unusual, painful, nodular, edematous lesions on the neck and face may be noted. Bacteriologic and histologic examinations suggest a nonspecific folliculitis [15]. In patients receiving sirolimus, it is important to be aware that this drug is associated with *mucositis* that can be difficult to distinguish from HSV infection. Everolimus is commonly used for prophylaxis of organ rejection in adult renal and heart transplant recipients. Acne and angioedema represent typical side effects early after everolimus initiation (see Figures 9.1A, 9.1B, 9.2A, 9.2B, and 9.3). Everolimus acne tends to be temporary and usually improves within a few weeks [16].

Nephrogenic Systemic Fibrosis

Nephrogenic systemic fibrosis (NSF) is a rare condition seen in patients with renal diseases, many of whom are hemodialysis or renal transplant patients. Skin involvement is common and it was once considered a purely cutaneous disorder [17]. Clinically, patients with skin involvement present with marked induration, peau d'orange changes, joint contractures, patterned plaques, cobblestoning, and scleral plaques. Histological features include increased dermal cellularity, CD34+ cells with tram-tracking, thick and thin collagen bundles, preserved elastic fibers, septal involvement, and osseous metaplasia. For superficial lesions, a 4 mm or greater punch biopsy extending to the subcutaneous fat is recommended. For deeper lesions, a wedge biopsy down to and including fascia can help with diagnosis. A scoring system based on the above clinical and histological features has recently been proposed to provide a standardized method of diagnosing NSF [18]. Patients often report pruritus, burning, and sharp pains in the affected areas and joint contractures may develop very rapidly and be debilitating [19]. NSF is distinguishable from scleromyxedema by its distribution pattern on the trunk and extremities and sparing of the face, absence of paraproteinemia, and absence of pools of

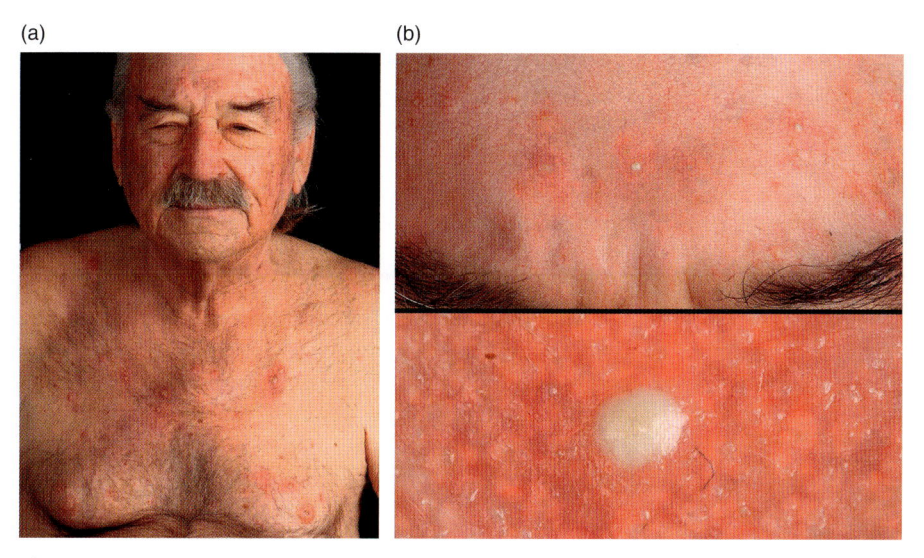

Dermatological Complications in Transplant Patients and Composite Tissue Allotransplant Pathology

Figures 9.1A, 9.1B Renal transplant patient with acneiform eruption – induced by everolimus (Certican). Note erythematous papules and pustules without comedomes.

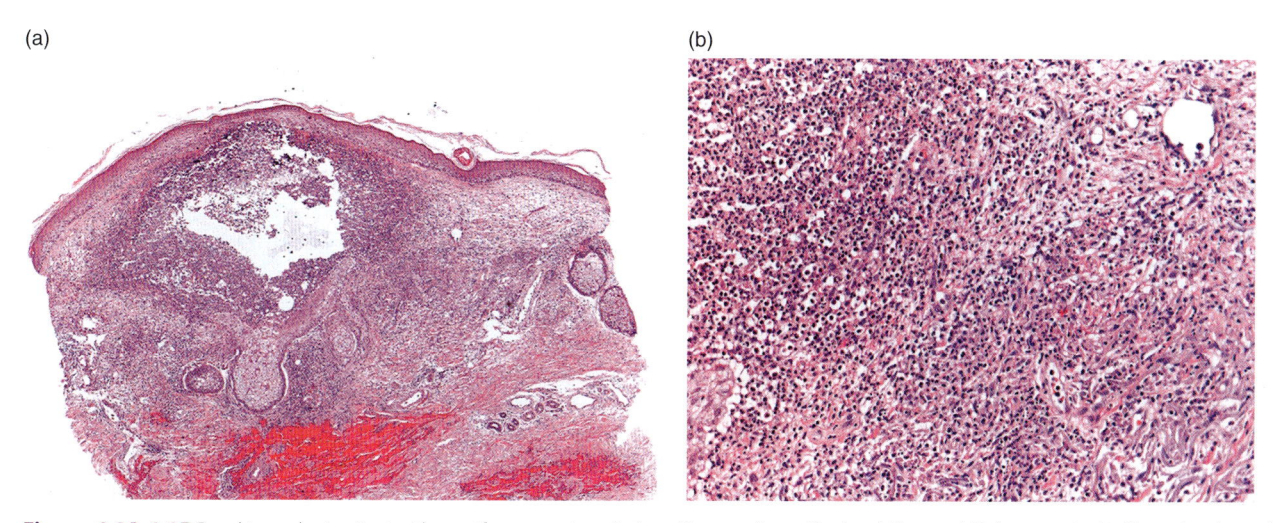

Figures 9.2A, 9.2B Renal transplant patient with acneiform eruption – induced by everolimus (Certican). Neutrophilic (suppurative) infiltrate (involving the follicular infundibula). Direct effect of everolimus on the follicle leads to the rupture of the follicle.

dermal mucin and plasma cell infiltrate. Chronic graft-versus-host disease is more likely to show lichenoid papules, erosive indurated plaques, and involvement of the trunk.

Graft-versus-Host Disease

Graft-versus-host disease (GVHD) is a multisystem disease initiated by allogeneic T lymphocytes that recognize foreign tissue antigens in the host. Conventionally, GVHD was divided into acute and chronic forms that have distinct disease patterns and were differentiated by whether onset was before or after 100 days following transplantation. Due to advances in hematopoietic cell transplantation, the current consensus is that clinical manifestations, and not the number of days after transplant, determine acute versus chronic GVHD. The broad category of acute GVHD includes (1) classic acute GVHD within 100 days after transplantation or donor lymphocyte infusions (DLI) and (2) persistent, recurrent, or late acute GVHD occurring beyond 100 days of transplantation or DLI, but without diagnostic or distinctive manifestations of chronic GVHD [20]. Acute GVHD beyond 100 days is often seen after withdrawal of immunosuppression. Diagnostic signs sufficient to establish the diagnosis of chronic GVHD include poikiloderma, lichen planus-like features, sclerotic features, morphea-like features, and lichen sclerosus-like features. Distinctive signs insufficient alone to establish a diagnosis include cutaneous depigmentation, new onset alopecia, nail dystrophy, onycholysis, pterygium unguis, nail loss, and nail ridging, splitting, or brittle features. The broad category of chronic GVHD includes (1) classic chronic GVHD without features characteristic of acute GVHD and (2) an overlap syndrome in which features of chronic and acute GVHD appear together [20].

Acute Graft-versus-Host Disease

Acute GVHD follows a graft-versus-host reaction targeted against epithelia of skin, gastrointestinal tract, and liver and is manifested with rash, diarrhea, and abnormal liver function

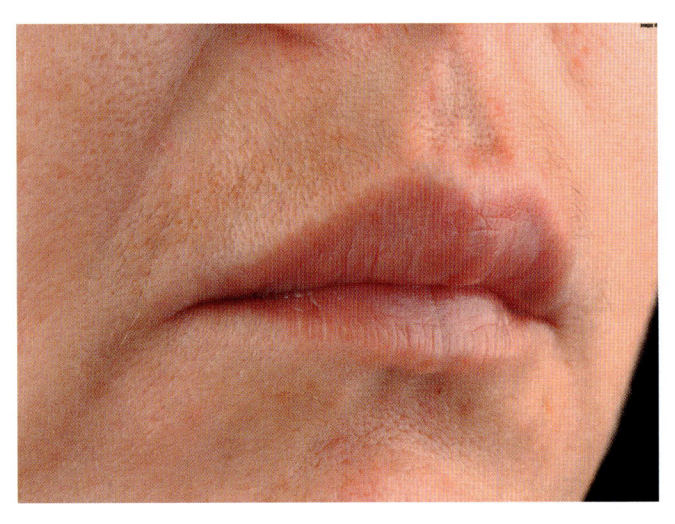

Figure 9.3 Renal transplant patient. Angioedema induced by everolimus (Certican).

test results. In the absence of histologic or clinical signs or symptoms of chronic GVHD, the persistence, recurrence, or new onset of characteristic skin, GI tract, or liver abnormalities should be classified as acute GVHD regardless of the time after transplantation. Early lesions of acute GVHD are often folliculocentric blanching erythematous macules or papules or scarlatiniform eruption often with acral accentuation. These lesions may develop bullae and extend to erythroderma and epidermal necrosis [21, 22] (see Figure 9.6). Histologically, cutaneous acute GVHD is characterized by varying degrees of damage to the epidermal keratinocytes. Since 1974, skin biopsies of acute GVHD are classified by the Lerner grading system, which was modified by Horn in 1994 [23, 24]. In *Grade I*, there is vacuolization of the basal keratinocytes (see Figures 9.4A and 9.4B); in *Grade II*, there are dyskeratotic keratinocytes in the epidermis and/or follicle, dermal lymphocytic infiltrate, and basal cell vacuolization is evident; in *Grade III*, there are numerous necrotic keratinocytes and focal clefting of the basal layer is formed; and in *Grade IV*, necrosis of the entire epidermis and complete separation from the dermis occurs [21] (see Figure 9.5). The lymphocytic infiltration and cytopathic changes of keratinocytes are the major features of acute GVHD. Characteristically, the clustered lymphocytes around dyskeratotic and/or dead keratinocytes are referred to as *satellite cell necrosis*. This sign usually has been considered illustrative of the pathogenesis of GVHD, with the presence of an activated donor lymphocyte recognizing a host cell. Focal or diffuse spongiosis may occur. Adnexal involvement – specifically, damage to upper portions of sweat glands and follicular structures – can aid in the diagnosis [25]. Direct immunofluorescence labeling of skin biopsy specimens from patients with acute GVHD has demonstrated granular deposits of IgM and/or C3, similar to a lupus band test [26].

Many studies have been conducted to determine which lymphocyte subpopulations are found in the skin of patients with acute GVHD. The patterns can be variable. For example, the infiltrate can be composed of a mixture of CD4+ and CD8+ T cells, or with one of these subsets predominating. Two reports indicated that natural killer (NK) cells were present in acute GVHD skin lesions [27, 28].

The use of skin biopsies in GVHD can be controversial and the interpretation of the skin biopsy may be difficult because large doses of cytotoxic drugs and irradiation can produce histopathologic changes that are indistinguishable from acute GVHD even in clinically normal skin [29–31]. Elafin, (also known as peptidase inhibitor-3, skin-derived antileukoproteinase or trappin-2) is a useful biomarker of skin GVHD. Plasma elafin levels are higher in patients with skin GVHD as well as overexpressed in GVHD skin biopsies. Plasma elafin levels and elafin protein expression by immunohistochemistry in skin biopsies can help discriminate between GVHD of the skin and from rashes of other etiologies [32].

Chronic Graft-versus-Host Disease

Chronic GVHD occurs in 25%–50% of patients and is frequently preceded by the acute form of GVHD, although it may occur *de novo* [33, 34]. Chronic GVHD develops after a mean delay of onset of four months, but manifestations resembling chronic GVHD can appear as early as day 40 following transplantation. The skin is involved in almost all cases of chronic GVHD and the mouth in 90% of patients. Both can develop spontaneously or be triggered by several events, notably ultraviolet irradiation, physical trauma, zoster, or even Borrelia infections. Traditionally, chronic cutaneous GVHD has been classified as lichenoid or sclerodermatous lesions. Clinical manifestations include poikiloderma (e.g., atrophic and pigmentary changes) (see Figures 9.11A, 9.11B, 9.11C, and 9.11D), lichen planus-like eruption (e.g., erythematous/violaceous flat-topped papules or plaques with or without surface reticulations or a silvery or shiny appearance on direct light), deep sclerotic features (e.g., smooth, waxy, indurated skin – "thickened or tight skin," caused by deep and diffuse sclerosis over a wide area), morphea-like superficial sclerotic features (e.g., localized patchy areas of moveable smooth or shiny skin with a leathery-like consistency, often with dyspigmentation), or lichen sclerosus-like lesions (e.g., discrete to coalescent gray to white moveable papules or plaques, often with follicular plugs, with a shiny appearance and leathery consistency)[20]. Depigmentation, sweat impairment, and intolerance to temperature change from loss of sweat glands are features also seen in chronic GVHD. Other subtypes of GVHD have been reported, including psoriasiform, keratosis pilaris-like, and asteatotic forms and rarely, GVHD variants occur that exhibit the features of autoimmune connective tissue diseases such as dermatomyositis and lupus erythematosus [35, 36]. Reports cite an aggressive form of eczema-like GVHD recently referred to as eczematoid GVHD, which is discussed separately [37–39].

The so-called *early phase* of chronic GVHD is seen in lichenoid lesions. Lichenoid phase may precede the sclerodermatous phase. However, others have found that lichenoid and sclerodermatous GVHD occur independently and dermal induration with no previous lichenoid phase may develop

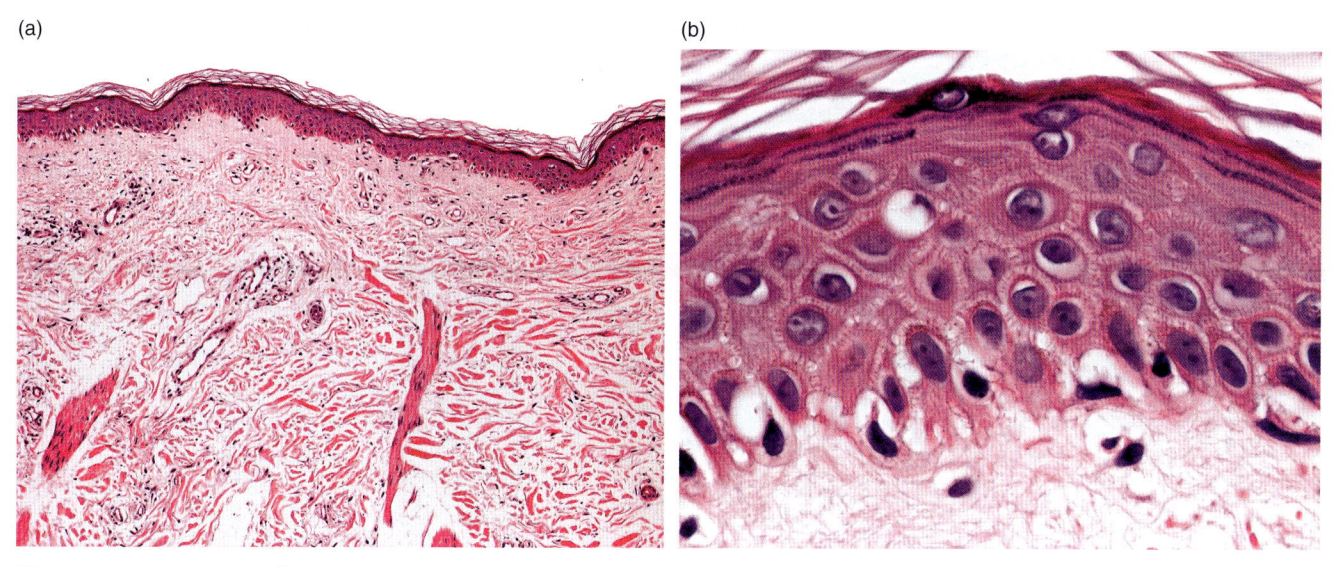

Figures 9.4A, 9.4B Acute graft-versus-host-disease. Grade I: Basal vacuolization. Higher magnification of Figure 9.4A.

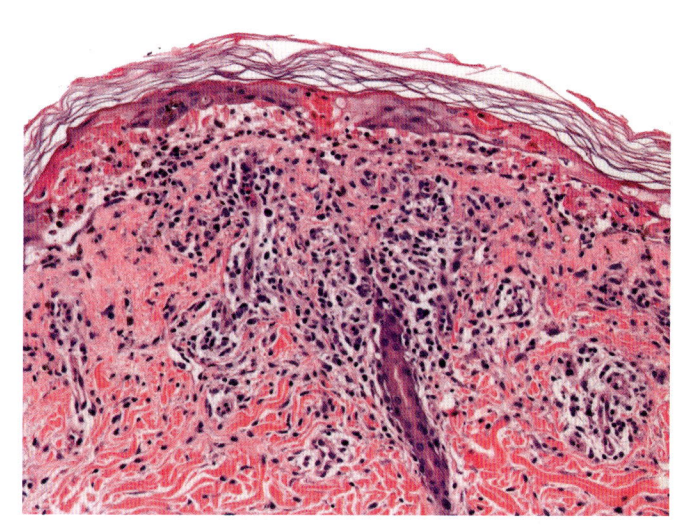

Figure 9.5 Acute graft-versus-host-disease. Grade IV: Beginning separation of necrotic epidermis from dermis. Lymphocytic infiltration.

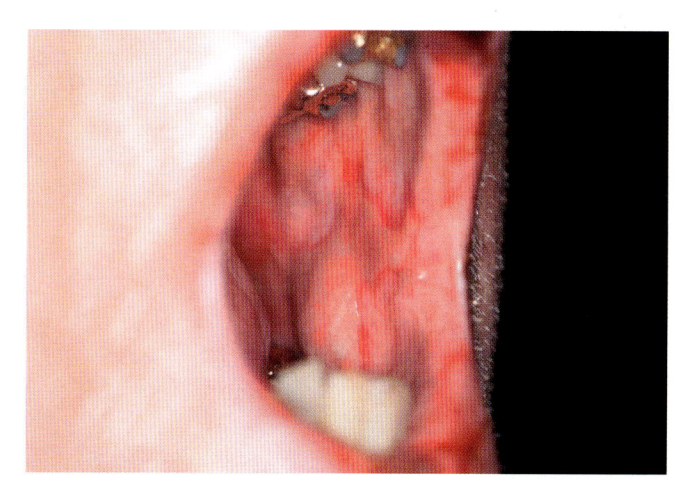

Figure 9.6 Acute graft-versus-host-disease. Erosions on lips and buccal mucosa.

[40–42]. The course starts as a generalized erythematous or violaceous rash, and progresses to poikiloderma with sclerotic hidebound skin (see Figures 9.7A and 9.7B). These lesions are erythematous or violaceous papules or plaques, with a squamous surface, sometimes forming larger confluent areas. These characteristic violaceous, indurated papules and plaques resemble lichen planus. The periorbital region, ears, palms, and soles are the typically affected sites [21]. In some cases, lichenoid papules can occur around hair follicles or be restricted to a dermatome [43]. Occasionally, the center blisters, leading to a vesicle, resembling dyshidrosis when present on the hands. Lichen planus-like GVHD can also affect the nails, with onychatrophia and pterygium and the genital organs, with a risk of phimosis and vaginal strictures [21]. Histologically, there is epidermal thickening by acanthosis (hyperplasia) with orthokeratosis and parakeratosis, hypergranulosis, a bandlike infiltrate along the dermal-epidermal junction, extensive apoptosis and vacuolization of basilar keratinocytes, sawtoothed (short blunted) rete ridges, and inflammation around the dermal adnexa. A variable degree of keratinocyte necrosis, sometimes with satellite cell necrosis, can be seen (see Figures 9.8A and 9.8B). The lymphocytic infiltrate of the superficial dermis with moderate exocytosis can resemble acute GVHD. In the dermis, the infiltrate is sometimes perineural. Melanophages can be found in variable numbers. The absence of wedge-shaped hypergranulosis and the presence of parakeratosis can distinguish chronic GVHD from lichen planus. It has been shown that patients with all the histological criteria of lichenoid GVHD were more likely to die of GVHD [21].

The so-called *late phase* corresponds to sclerodermatous lesions. Sclerodermoid GVHD has many clinicopathologic patterns, including cases resembling lichen sclerosus, morphea, and eosinophilic fasciitis (see Figure 9.9). Sclerosis in sclerodermoid GVHD can start and affect any level of the skin and can extend to involve the entire dermis, the subcutis, and even the fascia [44]. In sclerotic lesions, there is homogenization of most of the papillary dermis or reticular dermis. In the morpheic variant, sclerosis is seen in the reticular dermis or

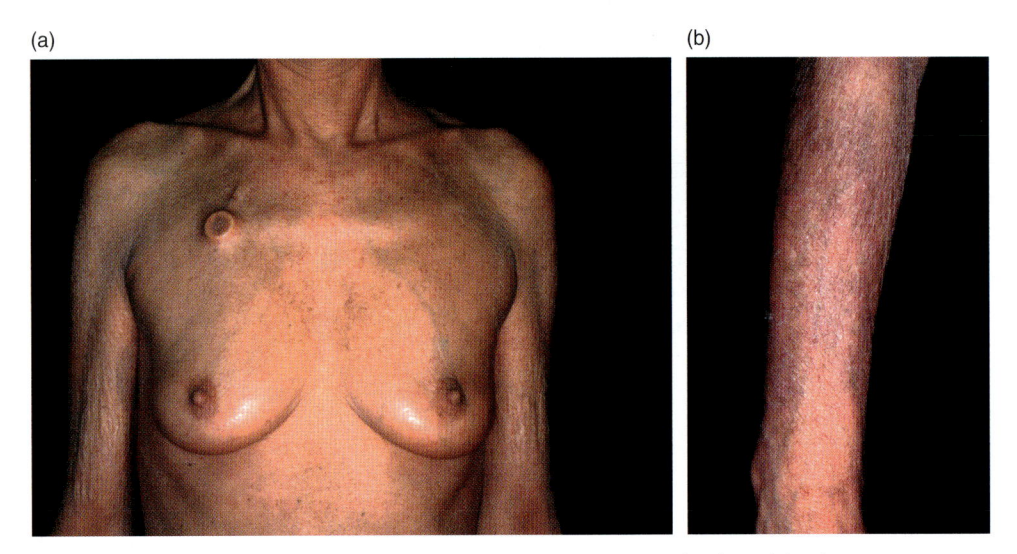

Figures 9.7A, 9.7B Chronic graft-versus-host-disease. Hyperpigmentation and scaling of the skin.

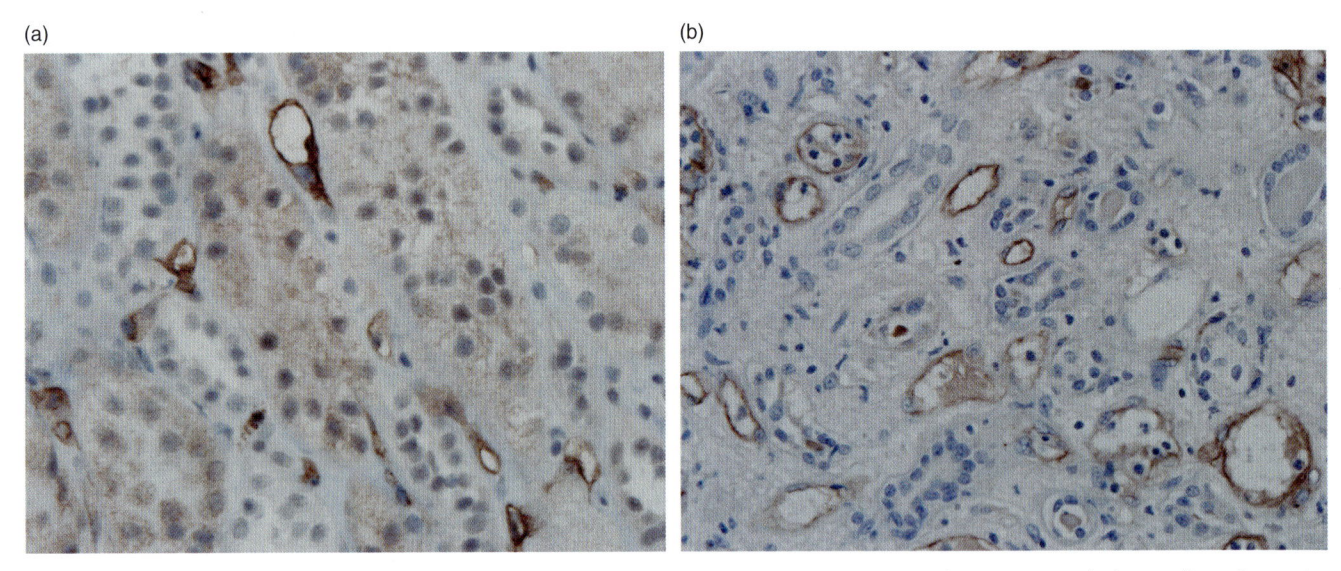

Figures 9.8A, 9.8B Chronic graft-versus-host-disease. Lichenoid interface dermatitis. Note numerous necrotic keratinocytes, including satellite cell necrosis.

along the dermal-hypodermal border with little or no epidermal involvement. The fasciitis variant may show fibrous thickening only in the fascia, with adjacent inflammation, but without any epidermal or dermal involvement [45]. This histological finding can be missed if the biopsies are not made deep enough. Follicular involvement has been described more commonly in patients with lichenoid chronic GVHD, but follicular keratosis can be found in the first phases of the sclerodermoid GVHD.

A leopard-skin eruption (widespread, hyperpigmented macules) may occur in patients with sclerodermoid GVHD and these pigmentary changes precede, almost constantly, the development of apparent sclerosis and are very distinctive [44–46]. Histology reveals sclerosis in the reticular dermis and slight vacuolar degeneration of the epidermis, with no other findings suggestive of a lichenoid eruption.

Oral manifestations are observed in the majority of patients with chronic GVHD. Oral manifestations include lichen planus-like lesions, leukoplakia, and the inability to open the mouth fully. Xerostomia, mucoceles, mucosal atrophy, pseudomembranes, and ulcers are also commonly seen [20]. Manifestations common to both acute and chronic GVHD include gingivitis, mucositis, erythema, and pain. Lichenoid lesions commonly affect all mucosal surfaces with predominant reticular and papular forms; tongue lesions usually are plaque-like. Ulcers are localized mainly in the buccal mucosa, palate, and dorsal part of the tongue. A lip biopsy specimen frequently is used to diagnose and determine the stage of the GVHD, and it has been noted that lip biopsy specimens should include both mucosal and salivary gland tissue [47]. Salivary gland biopsy findings have been correlated with the presence and clinical severity of GVHD, as well as being useful for evaluating the efficacy of therapeutic approaches.

Eczematoid GVHD is an aggressive, chronic dermatosis that requires substantial immunosuppression therapy to achieve

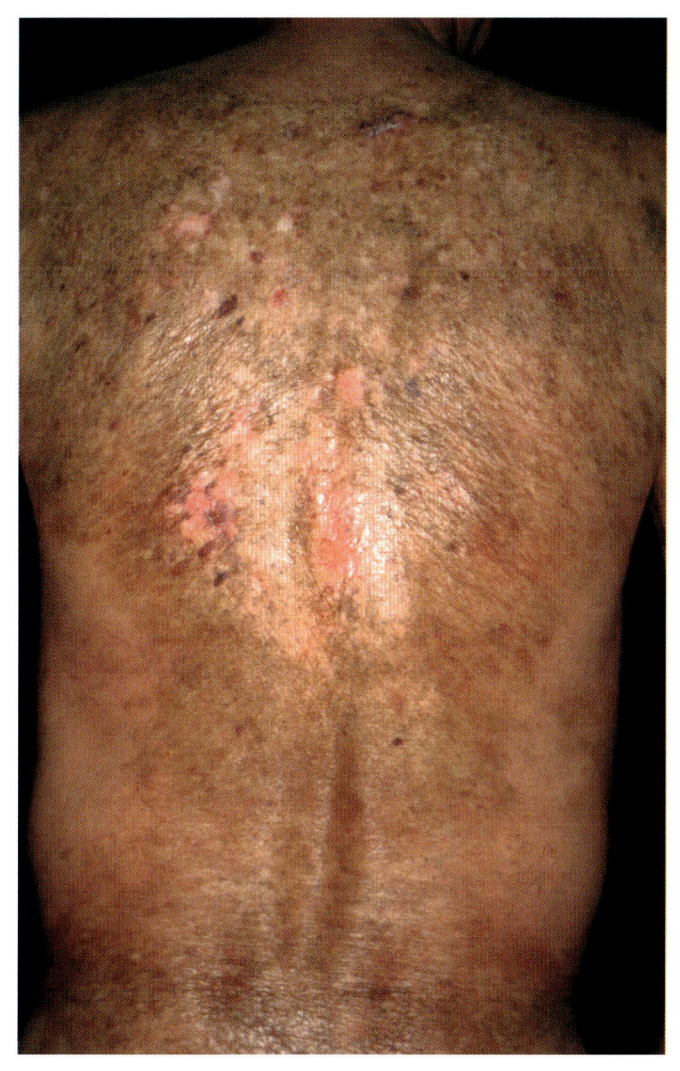

Figure 9.9 Chronic graft-versus-host disease. Papules and sclerodermatous changes.

control and is associated with a poor prognosis. Histologically, there are satellite cell necrosis, parakeratosis, lymphocyte exocytosis, and epidermal spongiosis reflecting the clinical appearance of eczema [37]. Dermal changes are less marked, often showing a sparse perivascular lymphocytic infiltrate with eosinophils [37].

Infections in Transplant Patients

Advances in immunosuppressive medications and treatment protocols have extended the survival of transplant recipients. However, there is a close relationship between the degree of immunosuppression and the severity of infection in transplant patients. Cutaneous infections are a high cause of morbidity and mortality in transplant patients and can be caused by viruses, bacteria, or fungi. Dermatologic infections after transplantation can be challenging and often need prompt treatment.

Viral Skin Infections in Transplant Patients

Viral skin infections are common findings in organ transplant recipients. Viral exanthems present as macular or papular eruptions. Many viral exanthems have no distinguishing histologic features. Often, vacuolar alteration of the basal layer, occasional dyskeratotic keratinocytes, and a sparse lymphohistiocytic perivascular infiltrate are seen. Dermal hemorrhage is usually not seen in drug-induced reactions, but may be present in some viral exanthems.

Varicella zoster virus (VZV) (aka, herpes zoster) occurs in approximately 10% of solid organ recipients and tends to be self-limited [48] (see Figures 9.12A and 9.12B). The incidence of VZV in immunosuppressed patients is increased 20- to 100-fold, and the severity of the disease is also increased. In one review, the overall incidence of VZV following solid-organ transplantation was 8.6% with a median time to onset of nine months; VZV in these patients was also associated with high rates of cutaneous scarring (18.7%) and post-herpetic neuralgia (42.7%) [49]. Although rare, untreated primary VZV infection in transplant patients can disseminate and cause hemorrhagic pneumonia, hepatitis, or encephalitis [48]. Disseminated zoster can occur in multiple dermatomes with crusts and scarring (see Figures 9.14A, 9.14B, and 9.14C). The diagnosis of VZV can be made clinically and confirmed with laboratory tests, including a Tzanck smear, skin biopsy, or viral cultures. Histologically, there are ballooned keratinocytes in the epidermis and lymphoid infiltrates in the dermis (see Figures 9.13A, 9.13B, and 9.13C). Immunofluorescent staining with monoclonal antibodies can also be used to confirm VZV infection or reactivation. Serologic tests can provide a retrospective diagnosis of VZV infection.

Reactivation of *herpes simplex virus (HSV)* is a common problem in transplant patients. Common manifestations of HSV infection in organ transplant recipients are orolabial and anogenital lesions. HSV viral shedding can be detected within 5–14 days after transplantation in 50%–66% of seropositive renal allograft recipients, although symptomatic vesicles or ulcers develop in only 15%–45% of recipients [50] (see Figure 9.16). Typically, herpetic vesicles break down to form shallow, grouped erosions and ulcers. In immunosuppressed patients, however, these ulcers may become large, confluent, chronic, granulating, and slow-healing. Infections may be complicated by severe esophagitis, bronchopneumonia, and encephalitis. Widespread disseminated HSV infection of the skin is not common, but is associated with high mortality rates. HSV infections can also trigger erythema multiforme, characterized by lesions with concentric color change *(target lesions)* that are symmetrically distributed predominantly over the extremities and acral areas. Diagnosis of HSV infection can usually be made by direct observation of the characteristic lesions, but the definitive diagnosis of active infection relies on culture of vesicular fluid, mucosal swabs, cerebrospinal fluid, or urine. Direct immunostaining of cells from these specimens with monoclonal antibodies specific for HSV-1 and HSV-2 antigens can be used. The Tzanck smear would show ballooned keratinocytes or giant cells. Molecular-based techniques such as polymerase chain reaction (PCR) have been used to detect HSV in herpes encephalitis, corneal infections, and skin lesions, including HSV-associated erythema multiforme.

Sources of cytomegalovirus (CMV) infection in organ transplant recipients include reactivation of latent virus or donor

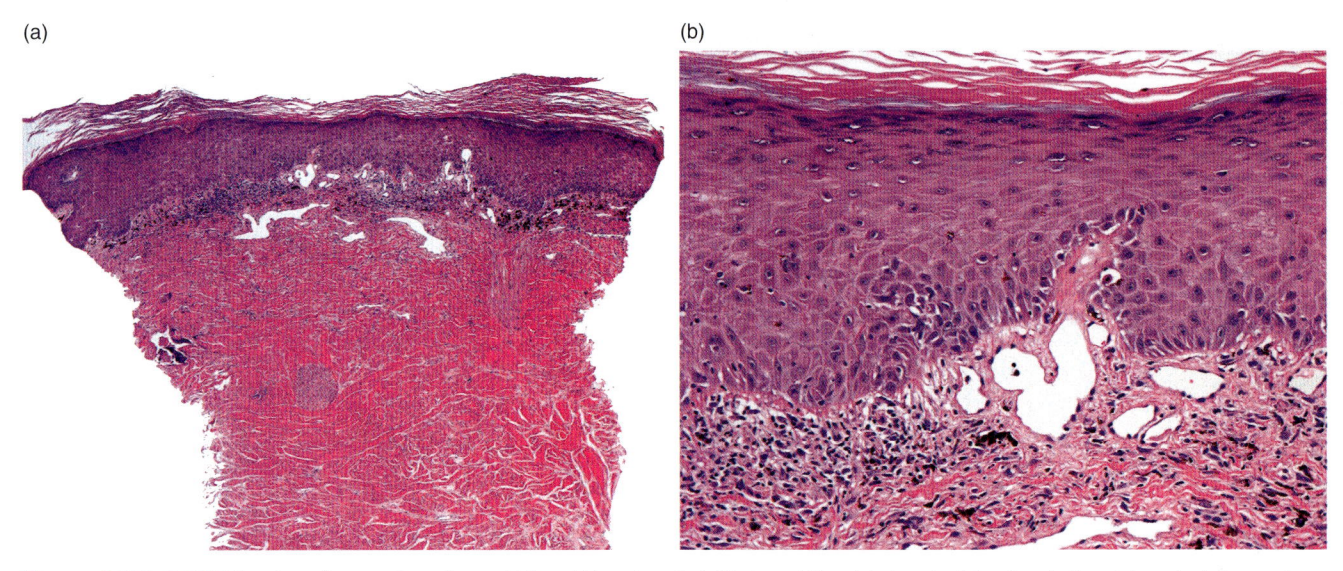

Figures 9.10A, 9.10B Chronic graft-versus-host-disease. Lichenoid lymphocytic infiltrate and fibrosis/sclerosis of the dermis. Note teleangiectatic vessels, melanophages, and necrotic keratinocytes.

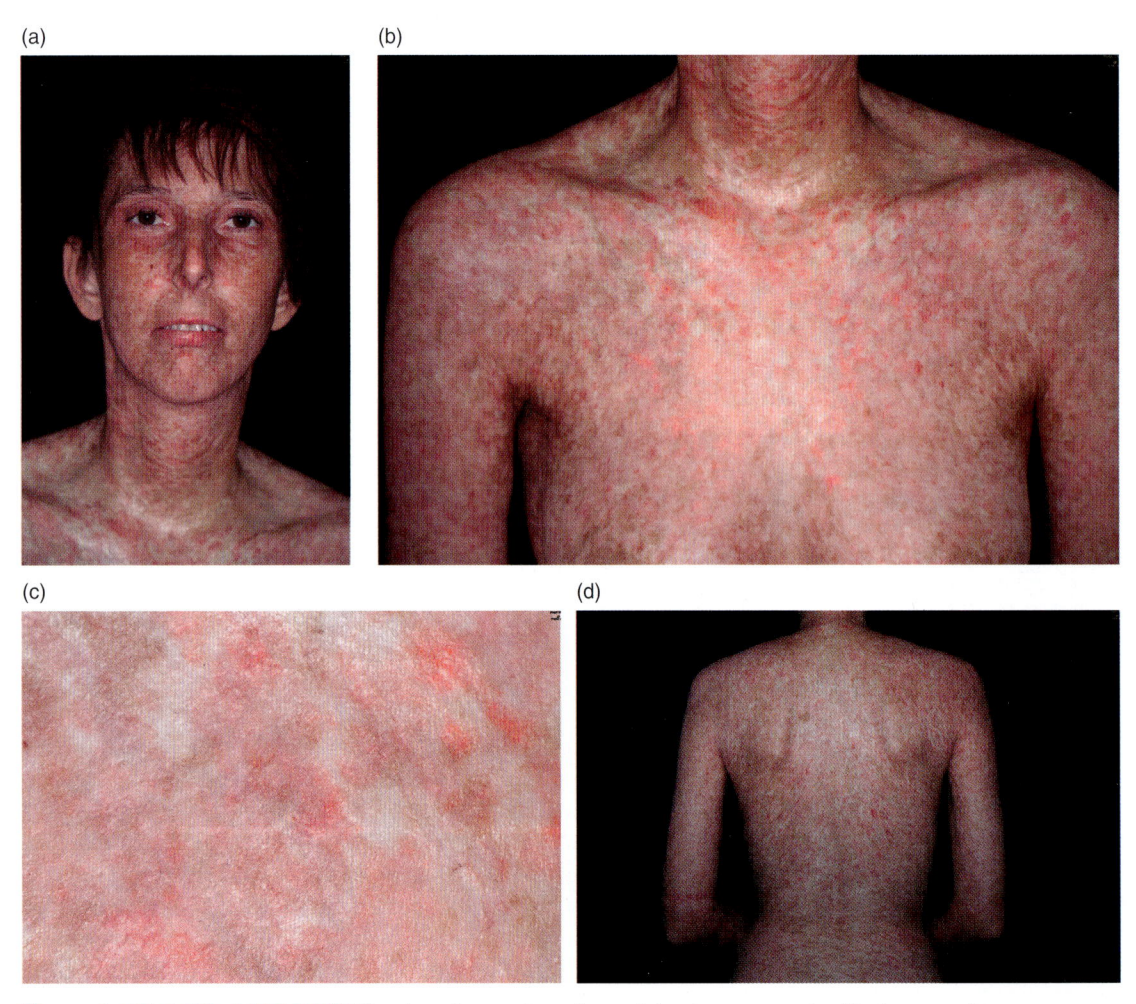

Figures 9.11A, 9.11B, 9.11C, 9.11D Chronic graft-versus-host-disease. Sclerodermatous and poikilodermatous features.

transmitted virus. Symptomatic CMV infection occurs in 20%–60% of all transplant recipients and is a significant cause of mortality and morbidity. The patient at highest risk of symptomatic disease is a seronegative recipient matched with a seropositive donor. A primary infection or reactivation of CMV can result in asymptomatic viral shedding to life-threatening multi-organ involvement. The patient may present with a mononucleosis-type syndrome with fever, malaise, leukopenia, and a

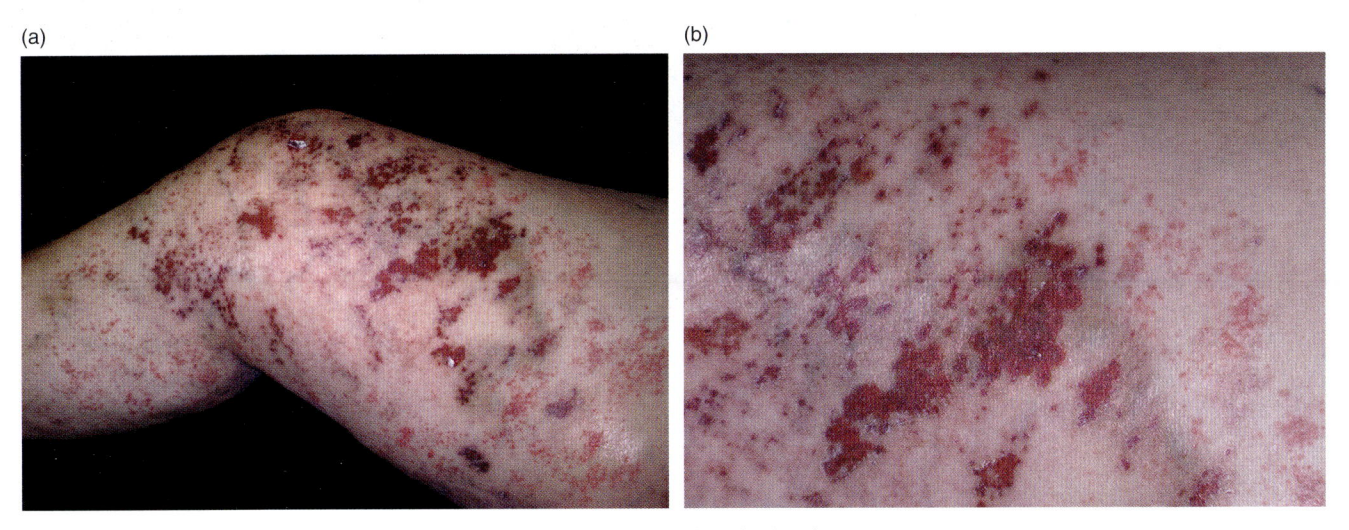

Figures 9.12A, 9.12B Renal transplant patient. Severe hemorrhagic zoster involving lumbar dermatomes.

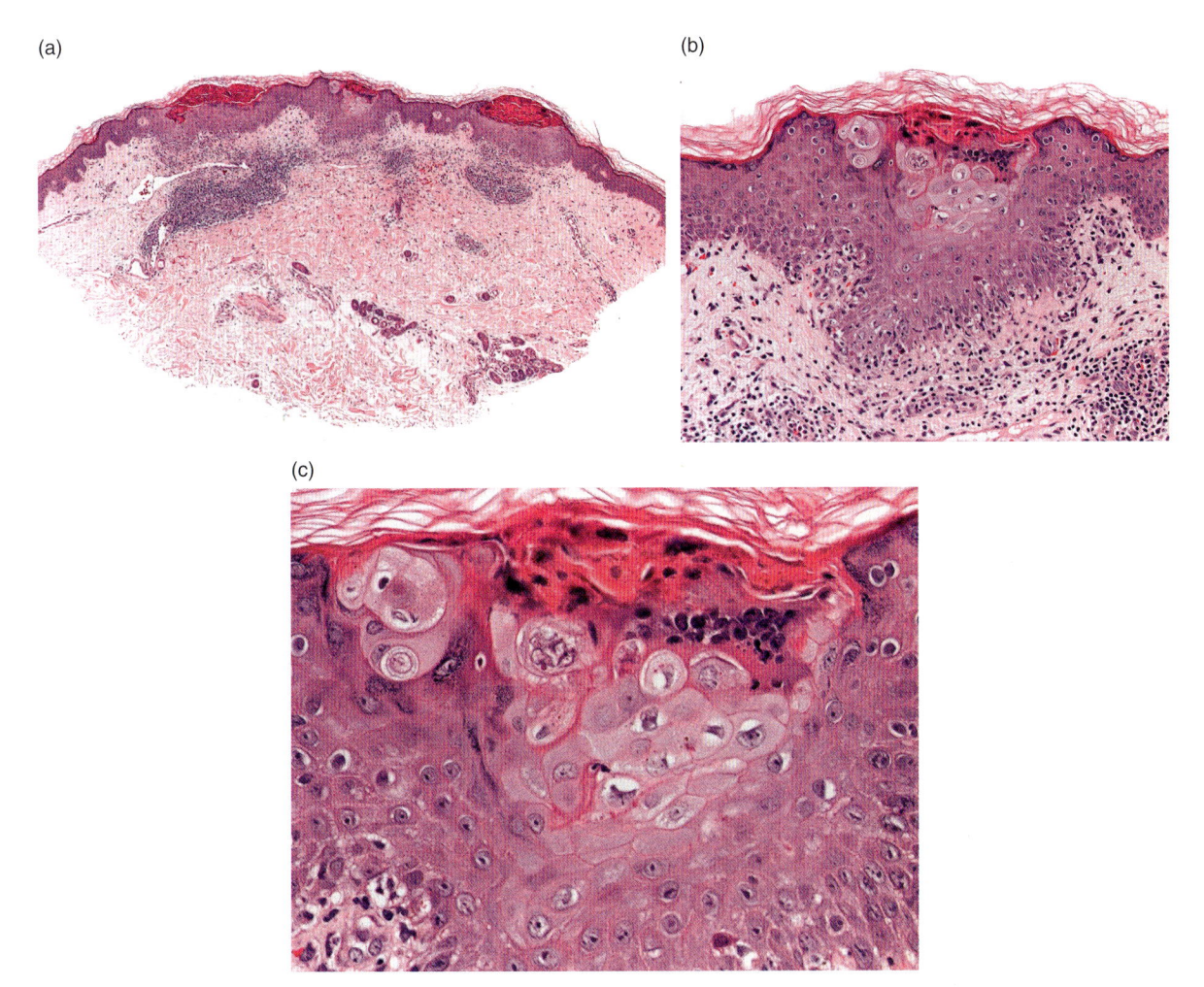

Figures 9.13A, 9.13B, 9.13C Renal transplant patients. Zoster presenting ballooned keratinocytes in the epidermis. Note lymphoid infiltrates in the dermis.

macular rash or progress to develop pneumonia, hepatitis, gastroenteritis, and retinitis. Cutaneous involvement is present in 10%–20% of patients with systemic CMV infection and is a sign of a poor prognosis. Cutaneous lesions are nonspecific and may include ulcers, morbilliform rashes, petechiae, purpuric eruptions, necrotic papules, and vesiculobullous eruptions. Chronic CMV infections are associated with risk of organ rejection, and also predispose the transplant recipient to higher risk of bacterial and fungal infections. Histology shows large intranuclear inclusions with a surrounding halo in endothelial cells. Confirmation of the diagnosis requires demonstration of the virus from skin, urine, throat washings, and buffy coat. Serologies are also helpful

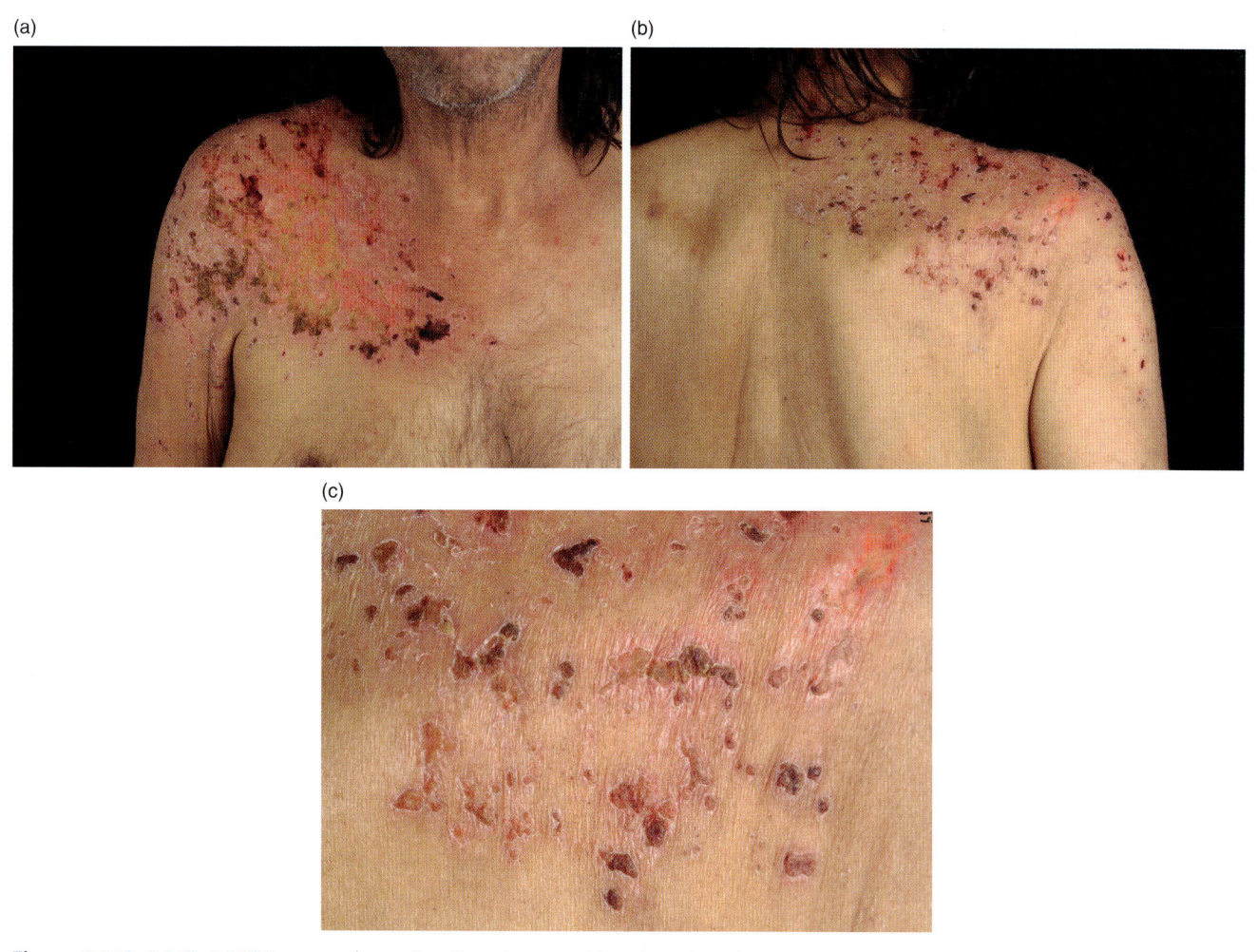

Figures 9.14A, 9.14B, 9.14C Liver transplant patient. Necrotic zoster with crusts and scarring.

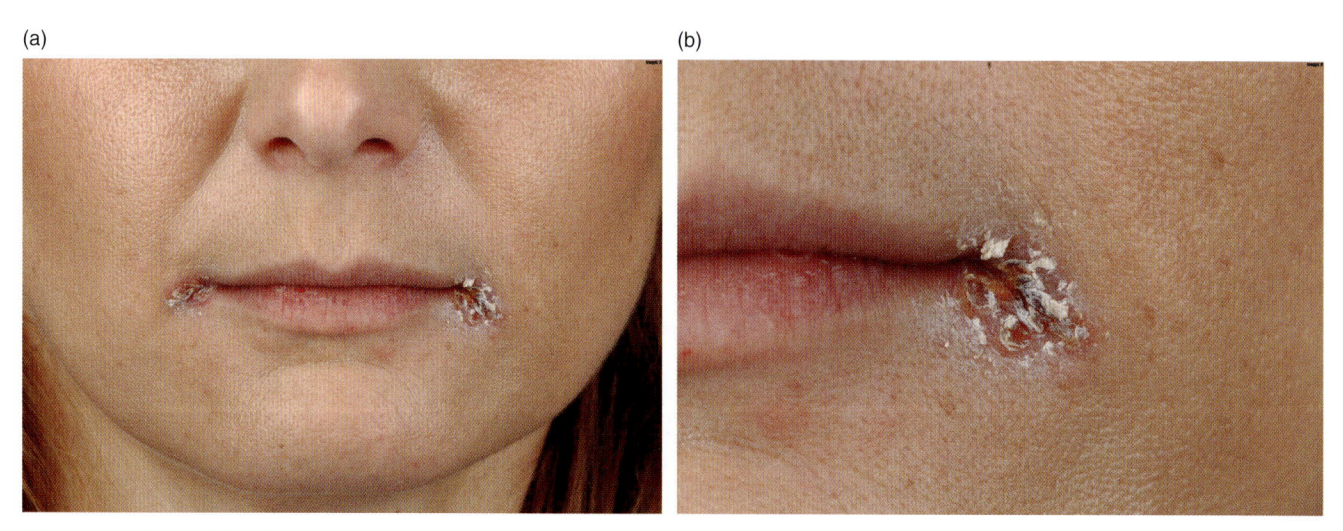

Figures 9.15A, 9.15B Renal transplant patient with cheilitis angularis.

in determining past exposure to CMV infection, but the transplant recipient's ability to mount an increasing antibody response may be blunted. Qualitative CMV polymerase chain reaction (PCR) assays are very sensitive in detecting CMV DNA and are used routinely in many transplant centers to diagnose active disease CMV disease, to screen patients for the use of preemptive therapy, and to monitor response to antiviral therapy.

Although transplant patients may develop a primary human herpes virus 6 (HHV-6) infection from transplanted tissue, the most common cause of active HHV-6 infection in

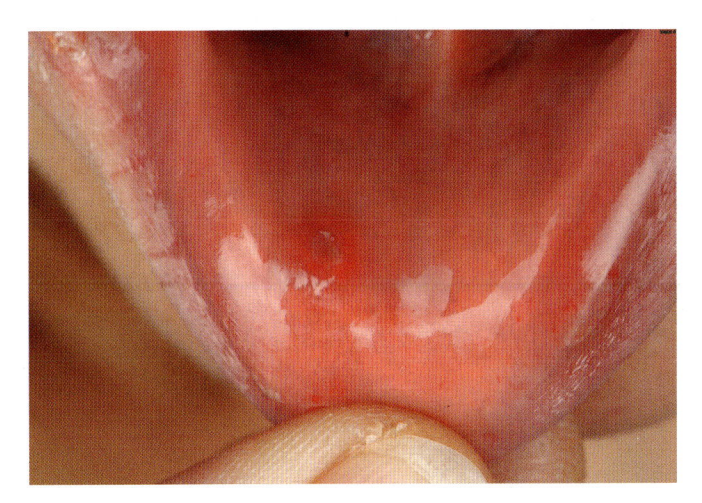

Figure 9.16 Renal transplant patient. Oral herpes simplex infection.

the transplant patient is reactivation of the latent virus. It has been reported in 38%–60% of bone marrow transplant recipients and in 31%–55% of solid-organ transplant recipients. It has been associated with *exanthem subitum* in children and is probably one of the viral causes of a mononucleosis syndrome in adults [51]. One study showed that after allogeneic bone marrow transplant, there is an increased risk of developing graft-versus-host disease, in which HHV-6 DNA is found in rectal and/or skin biopsy specimens [52].

Epstein-Barr virus (EBV) (HHV-4) is responsible for infectious mononucleosis, Burkitt lymphoma, oral hairy leukoplakia, and nasopharyngeal carcinoma. EBV is excreted in saliva and spread by close contact, often infecting hosts at a young age. Oral hairy leukoplakia lesions present as poorly demarcated keratotic areas with a corrugated or "hairy" appearance on the lateral borders of the tongue and are a sign of strong immunosuppression. The most severe complication of EBV is post-transplant lymphoproliferative disease (PTLD). PTLD is a well-known complication of organ transplantation (see Chapter 10). Although most post-transplant lymphomas are of B-cell origin, post-transplant primary cutaneous T-cell lymphoma has been described, presenting as tumors on the face and chest.

Human Papilloma Virus (HPV) is a frequent infection in transplant recipients. Verrucae can appear up to several years after transplantation and continue to grow and multiply over that time (see Figures 9.17A and 9.17B). HPV infection in transplant recipients is also important because of its link to the development of certain skin cancers, in particular, squamous cell carcinoma (see Figures 9.18A, 9.18B, 9.19A, and 9.19B).

Cutaneous Bacterial Infections in Transplant Patients

Systemic bacterial infections are a major cause of morbidity and mortality in transplant patients. Wound infections during the first month post-transplant are increasingly being caused by antibiotic-resistant strains (vancomycin-resistant enterococci and methicillin-resistant *Staphylococcus aureus*, MRSA) [53, 54]. Apart from wound infections, the spectrum of clinical lesions caused by bacteria includes impetigo, folliculitis, abscesses, cellulitis, and furuncles. Group A streptococci and *Staphylococcus aureus* are the most common causative organisms, similar to normal subjects. *Staphylococcus aureus* infections can manifest as pyoderma, but staphylococcal scalded skin syndrome as well as toxic epidermal necrolysis has been reported following liver transplantation [55, 56].

Less commonly, *E. coli*, *Legionella*, *Nocardia*, and *Salmonella* species have been reported in transplant patients [55–58]. Atypical mycobacteria infection (*M. kansasii*, *M. chelonae*, *M. fortuitum*, *M. marinum*) is an infrequent complication that can present months to years after transplantation with lesions affecting the skin, tenosynovium, and/or joints of the extremities [59, 60]. Cutaneous lesions are most common on the extremities.

Cutaneous Fungal Infections in Transplant Patients

Fungal infections typically develop within two months of transplantation and common sites of infection include surgical suture lines, skin, esophagus, and the urinary tract. The predominant organisms included *Candida* species and *Aspergillus* species. Although fungal infections are decreasing with the practice of prophylaxis, they are still are a large cause of morbidity and mortality.

The incidence of invasive candidiasis has declined, but *Candida* species remains the most frequent cause of fungal infections, with *Candida albicans* accounting for most cases [54]. Oral candidal infections may appear in one of several forms, most frequently as pseudomembranous candidacies (removable white plaques). Other less common clinical presentations include chronic hyperplastic candidacies (leukoplakia-like plaques that do not rub off), erythematous candidiasis (patchy or diffuse erythema), median rhomboid glossitis, and angular cheilitis (see Figures 9.15A and 9.15B). Skin lesions, usually erythematous and maculopapular in nature, can be the first evidence of disseminated candidiasis.

After *Candida albicans*, *Aspergillus* species are the second most common cause of opportunistic fungal infections in humans [61]. The lungs are the predominant site of infection, and cutaneous aspergillosis may be primary or secondary. Secondary cutaneous aspergillosis occurs as a result of hematogenous dissemination or by extension to skin from contiguous anatomic structure, and presents as eruptive maculo-papules; whereas in the rare type, primary cutaneous aspergillosis, manifestations are hemorrhagic bullae or an indurated, erythematous, violaceous plaque that progresses to a necrotic ulcer with a black eschar. The emergence of a new opportunistic *Aspergillus* infection, *Aspergillus ustus*, in solid-organ transplant recipients has recently been reported [62–64].

Only rarely have cutaneous manifestations of other fungi such as *Cryptococcus neoformans*, *Exophiala jeanselmei*, *Wangiella dermatitidis*, or *Alternaria species* been reported [55]. In organ transplant recipients, cutaneous cryptococcosis most commonly presents as bacterial cellulitis [65]. Cutaneous

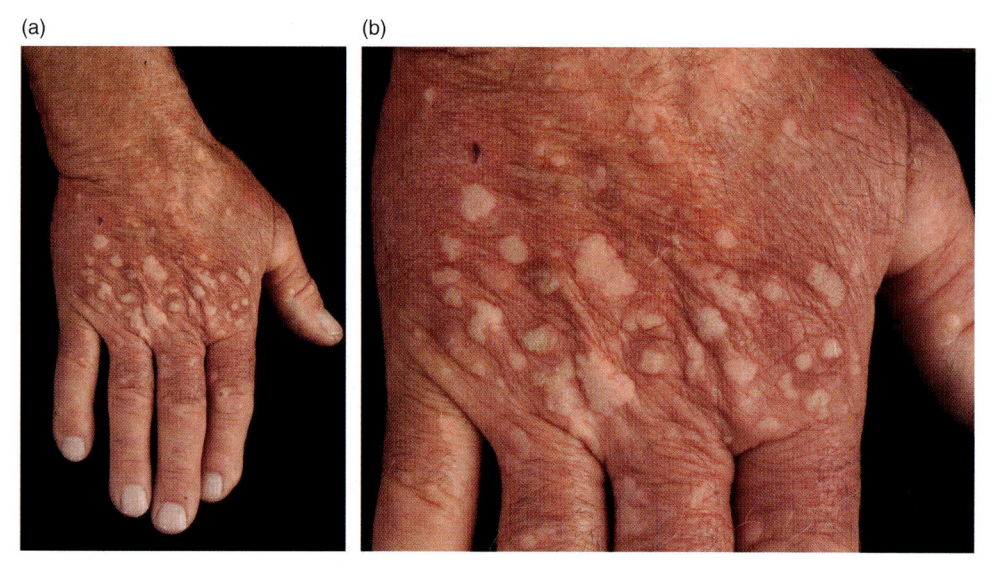

Figures 9.17A, 9.17B Large number of verrucae vulgares in a renal transplant patient.

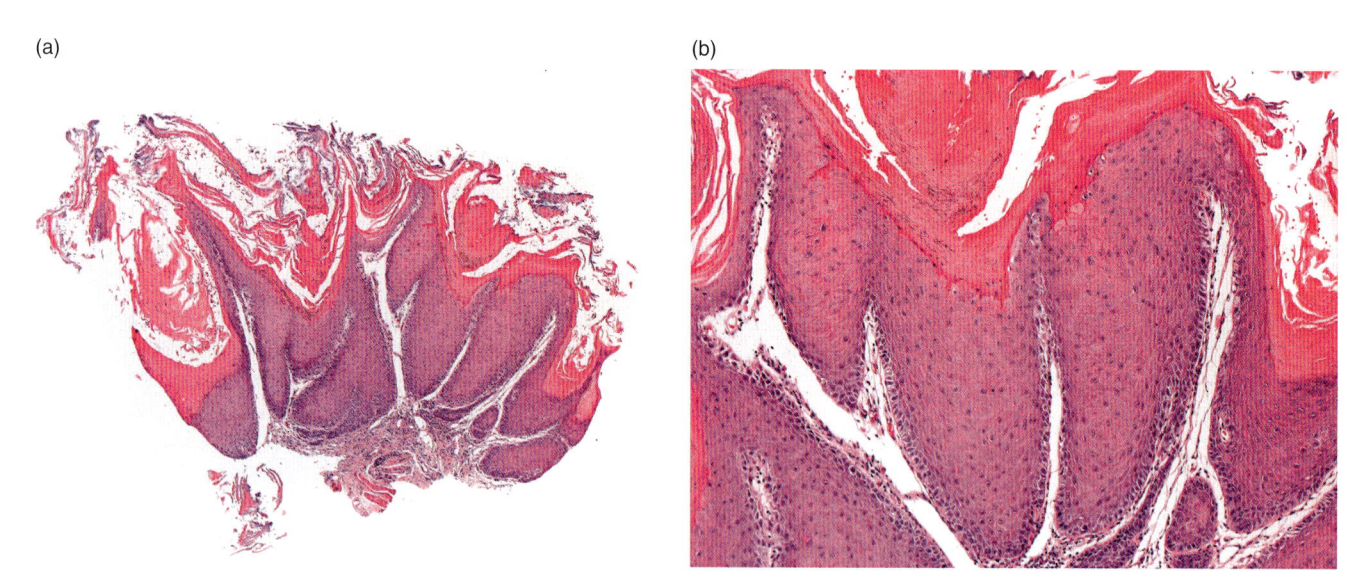

Figures 9.18A, 9.18B Bone marrow transplant patient. Verruca vulgaris on the tongue.

cryptococcosis represents disseminated infection and may also present itself as erythematous swellings, nodular firm, cystic-appearing excrescences, granulomas, acneiform papules or pustules, crusted or infiltrating plaques, or ulcers. Organ recipients living in areas of endemic histoplasmosis, coccidiomycosis, and blastomycosis infections are at risk of primary infection or reactivation following immunosuppression. Cutaneous involvement is most often a sign of dissemination and should be treated promptly in these patients.

Dermatophytes can cause several skin lesions in transplant recipients, including *Tinea corporis*, *Tinea pedis*, *Tinea cruris*, scalp infections, and nail infections. Localization is commonly on the face and buttocks, and diagnosis can be confirmed with periodic acid-schiff staining. Fingernail infections and involvement of multiple nails have been seen more commonly in immunocompromised patients than in other subjects. *Pityriasis versicolor* also has higher rates of infection in transplant patients [66].

Skin Cancer

The increased incidence of skin cancers in transplant patients is well-documented [1, 67] with squamous cell carcinoma (SCC), basal cell carcinoma (BCC), melanoma, Kaposi's sarcoma (KS), and post-transplantation lymphoproliferative disorders (PTLD) being the most commonly identified malignancies. In addition, it has been shown that these malignancies have more aggressive profiles in immunosuppressed patients leading to higher morbidity [68]. This increase in rate and aggressiveness of cutaneous malignancy is due in part to infection by oncogenic organisms, loss of immune surveillance and direct damage of DNA [69] [70].

A notable proportion (25%) of patients will develop their first *SCC* within five years of transplantation and usually in sun-exposed areas of the body with an increase in incidence of 60–100 fold over non-transplanted patients [71] (see Figures 9.20A, 9.20B, 9.21A, and 9.21B). The transplant patients at the

Dermatological Complications in Transplant Patients and Composite Tissue Allotransplant Pathology

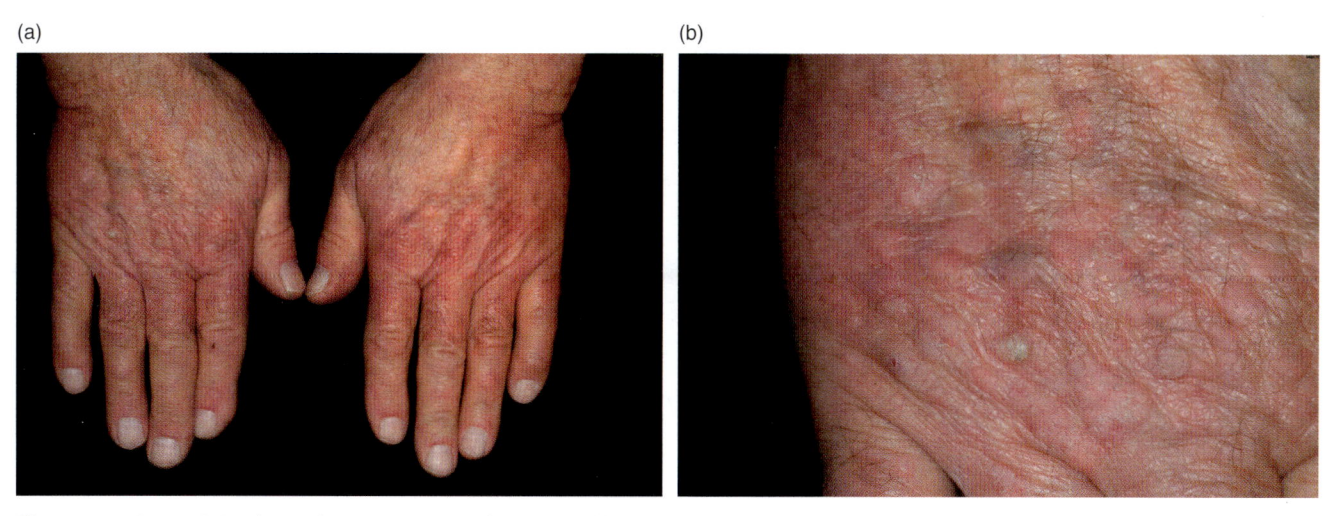

Figures 9.19A, 9.19B Renal transplant patient. Actinic keratoses and human papilloma-virus induced plane warts.

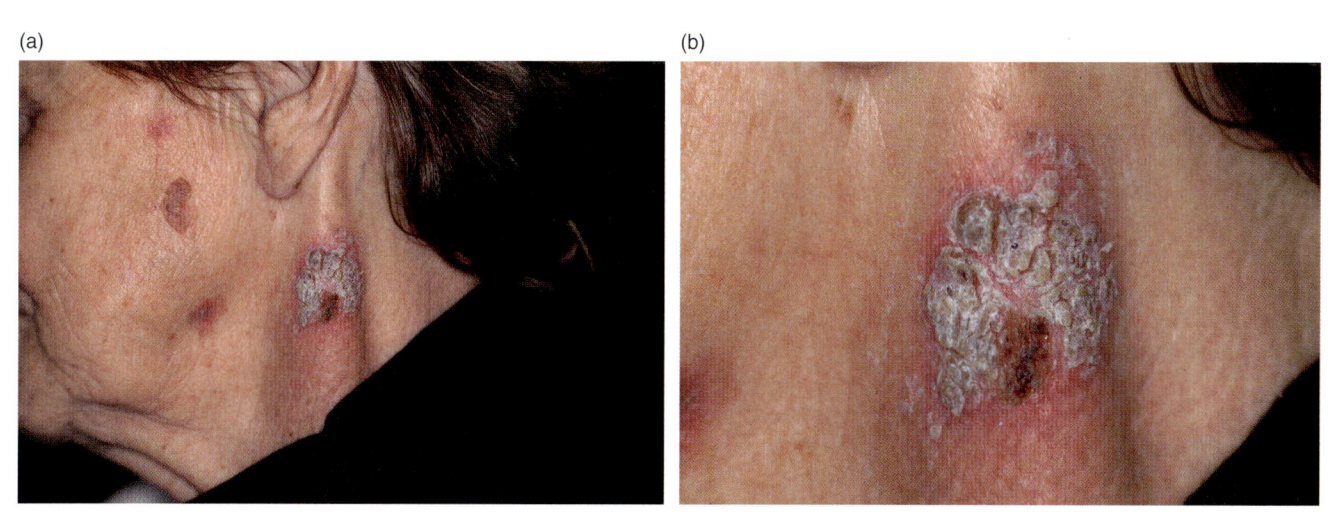

Figures 9.20A, 9.20B Renal transplant patient. Actinic keratoses and progression into invasive squamous cell carcinoma.

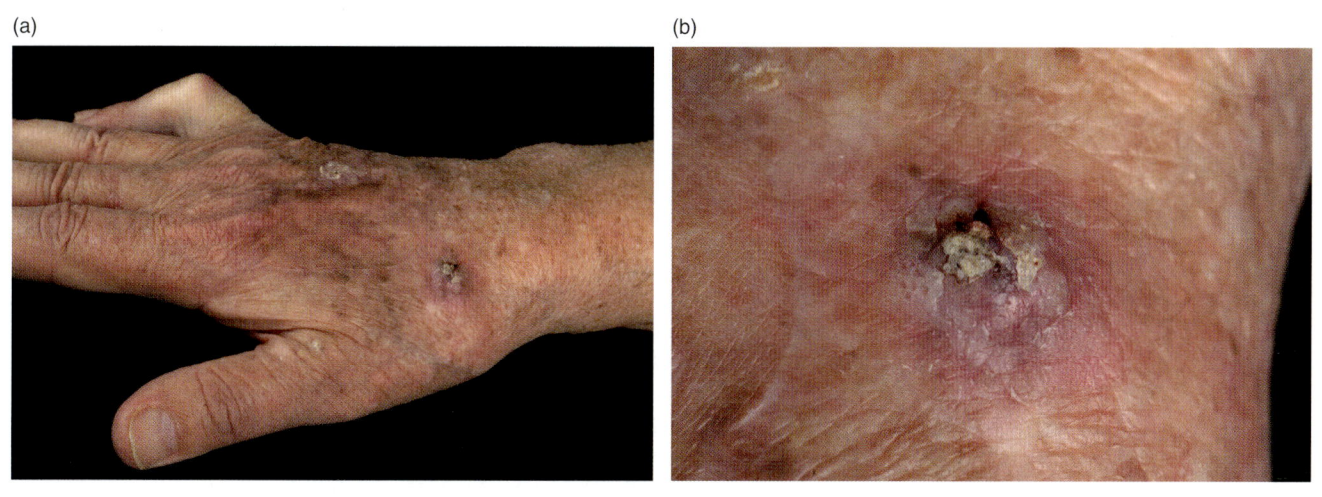

Figures 9.21A, 9.21B Renal transplant patient. Squamous cell carcinoma on sun-exposed skin.

highest risk are heart, kidney, and liver recipients [69]. Risk factors for development of SCC include: past history of SCC, Fitzpatrick skin type I, II, or III, increased age, HPV infection (HPV-5, HPV-8, HPV-16, and HPV-18), and history of UV exposure [1]. It is interesting to note that there may be some negative interaction between these last two factors, as UV exposure has been shown to inactivate the E6 protein of HPV, thus limiting its oncogenic potential [72], an interesting observation that requires more research. Given the time required to progress to SCC [73], it is therefore likely that the aforementioned chain of events is initiated soon after transplantation. Histologically, SCC is more aggressive in transplant recipients compared with non-immunosuppressed persons. Features of aggressive tumors include: poor differentiation, more than 5 mm tumor thickness and deep invasion of the nerves, muscle, bone, cartilage, and subcutis [74]. The histological features of SCC in organ transplant patients is similar to other SCC as they demonstrate nests of squamous epithelial cells arising from the epidermis and extending into the dermis. Minor differences that have been reported include: an increase in spindle cell morphology, acantholytic changes, early dermal invasion, an infiltrative growth pattern with or without desmoplasia, Bowen's disease with carcinoma, and a deeper invasion at diagnosis. Higher rates of metastasis to the parotid gland have been blamed on the combination of high incidence on the head and neck region, deeper invasion, and immunologic suppression. The management of SCC in organ transplant patients has been described in detail, with the emphasis being a requirement for more aggressive treatment, more frequent examinations, lower thresholds for biopsy, and the addition of imaging studies.

The rate of basal cell carcinoma (BCC) formation is about ten-fold higher in transplantation recipients [75]. This increase is not as substantial as some of the other cutaneous malignancies, leading the authors to suggest that the immune system is not as essential in regulation of this malignancy. One difference that was recently described demonstrated that there is an increased superficial component to BCC in transplant patients [76]. Histopathologically, there are few differences in the presentation, as the basal cell carcinomas are composed of nests or islands of basaloid cells with periphery of palisading cells [77]. The nuclei are hyperchromatic and sometimes atypical with numerous mitotic figures and little cytoplasm. A high rate of apoptosis and cell death is also noted. As with SCC, the management of BCC is generally more aggressive in organ transplant patients.

A 3.8–8 fold increase in the incidence of melanoma has been described in transplant patients [78]. It is interesting to note that a higher than expected proportion of these cancers developed in dysplastic nevi, which leads to the postulation that this was primarily a function of loss of immune suppression [79]. The histopathologic diagnosis of melanoma is both complex and evolving and differences in melanoma histology have not been specifically described in organ transplant patients; a detailed review of melanoma is provided by van Dijk, et al. [80]. Reducing the degree of immunosuppression has been suggested in the management of melanoma in organ transplant patients [81]; however, this is a complex clinical question requiring extensive analysis and discussion with the patient.

Kaposi's sarcoma (KS) is associated with HHV-8 infection and is a relatively common malignancy after kidney transplantation [82] with a recent report showing incidence nearly 500–1000 times higher than the non-transplanted patients [83], often developing approximately 16 months after transplantation. This is classified as iatrogenic KS and is thought to be secondary to the choice of immunosuppressive regimen [84]. Histopathologically, iatrogenic KS is not significantly different than other forms of KS consisting of interwoven bands of vascular cleft-like spaces between spindle cells in a network of collagen fibers [85]. Extravasated erythrocytes and hemosiderin-laden macrophages are commonly present. Patients with superficial disease respond to withdrawal of immunosuppression without serious renal dysfunction [86].

Post-transplant Lymphoproliferative Disease (PTLD) is a known complication of solid organ and bone marrow transplantation. The overall incidence of PTLD in allograft recipients varies depending on the type of organ transplanted, the degree of immunosuppressive therapy, and the age of the patient. Cutaneous lesions, which have a relatively better prognosis than internal lesions, may present as ulcers, nodules, or erythematous plaques. Most commonly, PTLD manifesting itself in the skin represents an Epstein-Barr virus (EBV)–driven proliferation of B lymphocytes, which histologically is represented as hyperplasia or malignant lymphoma [87–89]. Although most PTLD results from an abnormal growth of EBV-transformed B cells, EBV-negative PTLD and PTLD of T cell origin [90] do occur, particularly in PTLD that develops more than one year after transplantation.

Merkel cell carcinoma [91], angiosarcoma [92], fibroxanthoma [93], verrucous carcinoma [94], and metastatic disease have also been reported in transplant patients; however, since large-scale studies have not been performed, we will only mention their observation.

Pathology of Composite Tissue Allotransplantation

Composite Tissue Allotransplantation (CTA) is a relatively new area of allotransplantation [95] that encompasses surgical therapy of a variety of severe tissue or limb defects, including hand transplantation [96], abdominal wall transplantation [97], and face transplants [98]. CTAs typically include skin which is utilized to monitor signs of graft dysfunction and/or rejection. Macroscopic "classical" features of skin rejection include a diffuse, patchy, or focal maculopapular erythematous rash over the dorsal and volar aspects of the forearm and wrist and the dorsum of the hand; an "atypical" pattern of hand rejection has been described involving palmar skin and nail beds in patients exposed to repetitive and persistent mechanical stress of the palm. The skin may also display desquamation, ulceration, or necrosis.

Skin biopsies are utilized to monitor Acute Cellular Rejection and to date, there have been several grading schemes that have been proposed to assess this complication [99–101]. The incidence of acute rejection exceeds 80% in hand and face transplantation. At the 2007 BANFF Conference in La Coruna, Spain, a worldwide consortium of pathologists and clinicians with experience in clinical CTA met to define a universally accepted histological classification (*BANFF Score*) [102] [103]. Histologically, the skin biopsies demonstrate

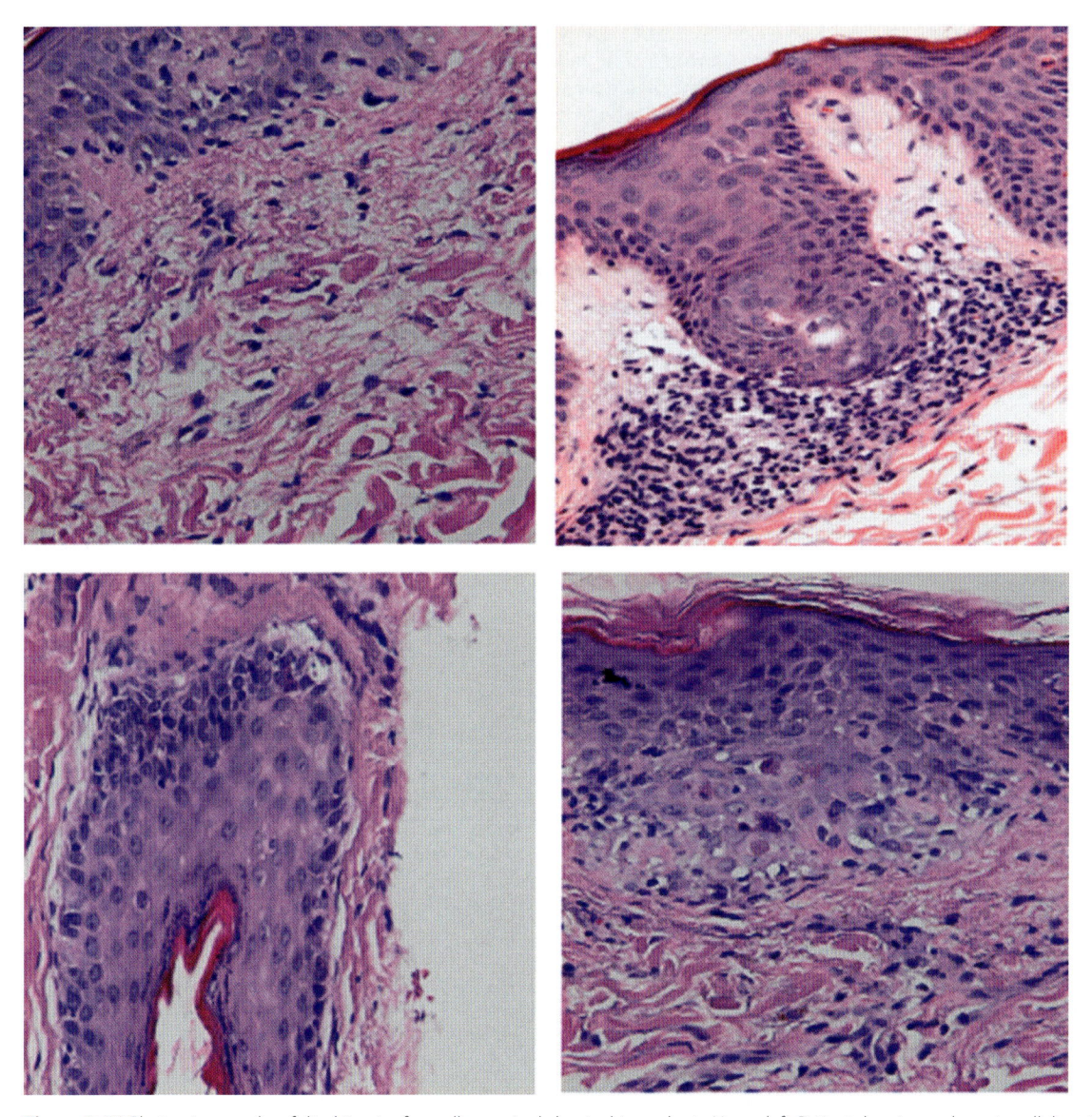

Figure 9.22 Photomicrographs of skin biopsies from allogeneic abdominal transplants. Upper left: Patient showing early acute cellular rejection (Grade 1, mild) with mild lymphocytic infiltrate; Patient showing Grade 2 (moderate) acute rejection showing more intense infiltrate in subepidermal region (upper right) with appendage involvement (lower left); Patient with focal necrosis of keratinocytes (lower right) – acute rejection (Grade 3, severe). All pictures were H&E, 200x.

mononuclear cell (small or large lymphocytes, macrophages) infiltration often with neutrophils (see Figure 9.22). The infiltrate may involve epidermis, adnexal structures, and dermis in a perivascular and/or interstitial pattern of involvement (see Figure 9.22). There may also be spongiosis, keratinocyte apoptosis, dyskeratosis, and necrosis (see Figure 9.22). Eosinophils may be present, but this cell population is not considered in grading.

Acute Humoral Rejection as of yet has not been consistently described in CTA rejection and is thus not present in the BANFF classification. Cases with donor-HLA specific antibodies and histological evidence of vasculitis, neutrophilic margination, and necrosis should be evaluated for the presence of C4d deposition.

Chronic Rejection is not currently defined in CTA. To date, chronic injury to skin and appendages in skin of CTA have been observed, but the underlying cause(s) of the fibrotic changes, injury, and atrophy to the allograft are not well-defined or readily distinguishable. Concurrent immune and non-immune etiologies overlap in causing chronic injury to the skin. Changes that may be seen are fibrosis of dermis and subcutaneum, vascular narrowing with myointimal proliferation, loss of adnexa, muscle atrophy, and nail changes. Reports about antibody-mediated rejection and chronic rejection remain scarce [104].

References

1 Kuijken I, B. 2000. Skin Cancer Risk Associated with Immunosuppressive Therapy in Organ Transplant Recipients: Epidemiology and Proposed Mechanisms. BioDrugs, **14** (5): 319–29.

2 Ulrich C, Hackethal M, Meyer T, Geusau A, Nindl I, Ulrich M, Forschner T, Sterry W, Stockfleth E. 2008. Skin Infections in Organ

Transplant Recipients. JDDG, **6**: 98–104.

3. Belloni-Fortina A, Piaserico S, Bordignon M, Gambato M, Senzolo M, Russo FP, Peserico A, De Matteis G, Perissinotto E, Cillo U, Vitale A, Alaibac M, Burra P. Skin Cancer and Other Cutaneous Disorders in Liver Transplant Recipients. Acta Derm Venereol, 2012 Jul;**92**(4): 411–5.

4. Mays SR, K.J., Truong E, Kontoyiannis DP, Hymes SR. 2007. Approach to the Morbilliform Eruption in the Hematopoietic Transplant Patient. Seminars in Cutaneous Medicine and Surgery, **26**: 155–162.

5. Kohler S, H.M., Chao NJ, Smoller BR. 1997. Value of Skin Biopsies in Assessing Prognosis and Progression of Acute Graft-versus-Host Disease. Am J Surg Pathol, **21**: 988–996.

6. Baack BR, B.W. 1991. Chemotherapy-induced Acral Erythema. Journal of American Academy of Dermatology, **24**: 457–61.

7. Bauer DJ, H.A., Horn TD. 1993. Histologic Comparison of Autologous Graft-vs-Host Reaction and Cutaneous Eruption of Lymphocyte Recovery. Archives of Dermatology, **129**: 855–8.

8. Sandoval M, Ortiz M, Díaz C, Majerson D, Molgó M. Cutaneous Manifestations in Renal Transplant Recipients of Santiago, Chile. Transplant Proc, 2009 Nov;**41**(9): 3752–4.

9. Radwan-Oczko M, Boratynska M, Klinger M, Zietek M. Risk Factors of Gingival Overgrowth in Kidney Transplant Recipients Treated with Cyclosporine A. Ann Transplant, 2003;**8**(4): 57–62.

10. Güleç AT, Haberal M. Lip and Oral Mucosal Lesions in 100 Renal Transplant Recipients. J Am Acad Dermatol, 2010 Jan;**62**(1): 96–101.

11. Aboujaoude W, M.M., Govani MV. 2004. Lymphedema Associated with Sirolimus in Renal Transplant Recipients. Transplantation, **77**(7): 1094–6.

12. Mahé E, M.E., Lechaton S, Sang KH, Mansouri R, Ducasse MF, Mamzer-Bruneel MF, de Prost Y, Kreis H, Bodemer C. 2005. Cutaneous Adverse Events in Renal Transplant Recipients Receiving Sirolimus-based Therapy. Transplantation, **79**(4): 476–82.

13. Mohaupt MG, V.B., Frey FJ. 2001. Sirolimus-associated Eyelid Edema in Kidney Transplant Recipients. Transplantation, **72**(1): 162–4.

14. van Gelder T, T.M.C., Hené R, Weimar W, Hoitsma A. 2003. Oral Ulcers in Kidney Transplant Recipients Treated with Sirolimus and Mycophenolate Mofetil. Transplantation, **75**(6): 788–91.

15. Mahé E, M.E., Lechaton S, Drappier JC, de Prost Y, Kreis H, Bodemer C. 2006. Acne in Recipients of Renal Transplantation Treated with Sirolimus: Clinical, Microbiologic, Histologic, Therapeutic, and Pathogenic Aspects. Journal of American Academy of Dermatology, **55**(1): 139–42.

16. Lehmkuhl H, R.H., Eisen H, Valantine H. 2005. Everolimus (Certican) in Heart Transplantation: Optimizing Renal Function through Minimizing Cyclosporine Exposure. Transplantation Proceedings, **37**(10): 4145–9.

17. Cowper SE, S.L., Bhawan J, Robin HS, LeBoit PE. 2001. Nephrogenic Fibrosing Dermopathy. American Journal of Dermatopathology, **23**(5): 383–93.

18. Girardi M, Kay J, Elston DM, Leboit PE, Abu-Alfa A, Cowper SE. Nephrogenic Systemic Fibrosis: Clinicopathological Definition and Workup Recommendations. J Am Acad Dermatol, 2011 Dec;**65**(6): 1095–106.

19. Levine JM, T.R., Elman LB, Bird SJ, Lavi E, Stolzenberg ED, McGarvey ML, Asbury AK, Jimenez SA. 2004. Involvement of Skeletal Muscle in Dialysis-associated Systemic Fibrosis (Nephrogenic Fibrosing Dermopathy). Muscle Nerve, **30**(5): 569–77.

20. Filipovich AH, Weisdorf D, Pavletic S, Socie G, Wingard JR, Lee SJ, Martin P, Chien J, Przepiorka D, Couriel D, Cowen EW, Dinndorf P, Farrell A, Hartzman R, Henslee-Downey J, Jacobsohn D, McDonald G, Mittleman B, Rizzo JD, Robinson M, Schubert M, Schultz K, Shulman H, Turner M, Vogelsang G, Flowers ME. National Institutes of Health Consensus Development Project on Criteria for Clinical Trials in Chronic Graft-versus-Host Disease: I. Diagnosis and Staging Working Group Report. Biol Blood Marrow Transplant, 2005 Dec;**11**(12): 945–56

21. Aractingi S, C.O. 1998. Cutaneous Graft-versus-Host Disease. Archives of Dermatology, **134**(5): 602–12.

22. Johnson ML, F.E. 1998. Graft-versus-Host Reactions in Dermatology. Journal of American Academy of Dermatology, **38**(3): 369–92.

23. Lerner KG, Kao GF, Storb R, Buckner CD, Clift RA, Thomas ED. Histopathology of Graft-vs-Host Reaction (GvHR) in Human Recipients of Marrow from HL-A Matched Sibling Donors. Transplant Proc, 1974 Dec;**6**(4): 367–71.

24. Horn TD. Acute Cutaneous Eruptions after Marrow Ablation: Roses by Other Names? J Cutan Pathol, 1994 Oct;**21**(5): 385–92.

25. Häusermann P, Walter RB, Halter J, Biedermann BC, Tichelli A, Itin P, Gratwohl A. Cutaneous Graft-versus-Host Disease: A Guide for the Dermatologist. Dermatology, 2008;**216**(4): 287–304.

26. Tsoi MS, S.R., Jones E, Weiden PL, Shulman H, Witherspoon R, Atkinson K, Thomas ED. 1978. Deposition of IgM and Complement at the Dermoepidermal Junction in Acute and Chronic Cutaneous Graft-vs-Host Disease in Man. Journal of Immunology, **120**(5): 1485–92.

27. Gilliam A, W.-M.D., Korngold R, Murphy G. 1996. Apoptosis is the Predominant Form of Epithelial Target Cell Injury in Acute Experimental Graft versus Host Disease. Journal of Investigative Dermatology, **107**: 377–383.

28. Leskinen R, T.E., Volin L, Ruutu T, Häyry P. 1992. Immunohistology of Skin and Rectum Biopsies in Bone Marrow Transplant Recipients. APMIS, **100**: 1115–22.

29. Drijkoningen M, D.W.-P.C., Tricot G, Degreef H, Desmet V. 1988. Drug-induced Skin Reactions and Cutaneous Graft-versus-Host Reaction: A Comparative Immunohistochemical Study. Blut, **56**: 69–73.

30. Sale GE, L.K., Barker EA, Shulman HM, Thomas ED. 1977. The Skin Biopsy in the Diagnosis of Acute Graft-versus-Host Disease in Man. American Journal of Pathology, **89**(3): 621–35.

31. Zhou Y, B.M., Rivers JK. 2000. Clinical Significance of Skin Biopsies in the Diagnosis and Management of Graft-vs-Host Disease in Early Postallogeneic Bone Marrow Transplantation. Archives of Dermatology, **136**(6): 717–21.

32. Paczesny S, Braun TM, Levine JE, Hogan J, Crawford J, Coffing B, Olsen S, Choi SW, Wang H, Faca V, Pitteri S, Zhang Q, Chin A, Kitko C, Mineishi S, Yanik G, Peres E, Hanauer D, Wang Y, Reddy P, Hanash S, Ferrara JL. Elafin is a Biomarker of Graft-versus-Host

33. Atkinson, K. 1990. Chronic Graft-versus-Host Disease. Bone Marrow Transplant, **5**(2):69–82.
34. Rouquette-Gally AM, B.D., Gluckman E, Abuaf N, Combrisson A. 1987. Autoimmunity in 28 Patients after Allogeneic Bone Marrow Transplantation: Comparison with Sjögren Syndrome and Scleroderma. British Journal of Haematology, **66**(1): 45–7.
35. Leber B, W.I., Rodriguez A, McBride JA, Carter R, Brain MC. 1993. Reinduction of Remission of Chronic Myeloid Leukemia by Donor Leukocyte Transfusion Following Relapse after Bone Marrow Transplantation: Recovery Complicated by Initial Pancytopenia and Late Dermatomyositis. Bone Marrow Transplantation, **12**(4): 405–7.
36. Ollivier I, W.P., Gherardi R, Wechsler J, Kuentz M, Cosnes A, Revuz J, Bagot M. 1998. Dermatomyositis-like Graft-versus-Host Disease. British Journal of Dermatology, **138**(3): 558–9.
37. Creamer D, M.-S.C., Osborne G, Kenyon M, Salisbury JR, Devereux S, Pagliuca A, Ho AY, Mufti GJ, du Vivier AW. 2007. Eczematoid Graft-vs-Host Disease: A Novel Form of Chronic Cutaneous Graft-vs-Host Disease and Its Response to Psoralen UV-A Therapy. Archives of Dermatology, **143**(9): 1157–62.
38. Sloane JP, T.J., Imrie SF, Easton DF, Powles RL. 1984. Morphological and Immunohistological Changes in the Skin in Allogeneic Bone Marrow Recipients. Journal of Clinical Pathology, **37**(8): 919–30.
39. Tanasescu S, B.X., Thomine E, Boullie MC, Vannier JP, Tron P, Joly P, Lauret P. 1999. Eczema-like Cutaneous Graft versus Host Disease Treated by UV-B Therapy in a 2-Year-Old Child. Annals of Dermatology and Venereology, **126**(1): 51–3.
40. Andrews ML, R.I., Weedon D. 1997. Cutaneous Manifestations of Chronic Graft-versus-Host Disease. Australasian Journal of Dermatology, **38**(2): 53–62.
41. Farmer, E. 1985. Human Cutaneous Graft-versus-Host Disease. Journal of Investigative Dermatology, **85**(1, suppl): 124S–8S.
42. White JM, C.D., du Vivier AW, Pagliuca A, Ho AY, Devereux S, Salisbury JR, Mufti GJ. 2007. Sclerodermatous Graft-versus-Host Disease: Clinical Spectrum and Therapeutic Challenges. British Journal of Dermatology, **156**(5): 1032–8.
43. Beers B, K.R., Kaye V, Dahl M. 1993. Unilateral Linear Lichenoid Eruption after Bone Marrow Transplantation: An Unmasking of Tolerance to an Abnormal Keratinocyte Clone? Journal of American Academy of Dermatology, **28**: 888–92.
44. Peñas PF, J.-C.M., Aragüés M, Fernández-Herrera J, Fraga J, García-Díez A. 2002. Sclerodermatous Graft-vs-Host Disease: Clinical and Pathological Study of 17 Patients. Archives of Dermatology, **138**(7): 924–34.
45. Shulman HM, Kleiner D, Lee SJ, Morton T, Pavletic SZ, Farmer E, Moresi JM, Greenson J, Janin A, Martin PJ, McDonald G, Flowers ME, Turner M, Atkinson J, Lefkowitch J, Washington MK, Prieto VG, Kim SK, Argenyi Z, Diwan AH, Rashid A, Hiatt K, Couriel D, Schultz K, Hymes S, Vogelsang GB. Histopathologic Diagnosis of Chronic Graft-versus-Host Disease: National Institutes of Health Consensus Development Project on Criteria for Clinical Trials in Chronic Graft-versus-Host Disease: II. Pathology Working Group Report. Biol Blood Marrow Transplant. 2006 Jan;**12**(1):31–47.
46. Roujeau JC, R.J., Touraine R. 1980. Graft versus Host Reactions. In: Rook A, Savin J, eds. Recent Advances in Dermatology, **5**: 131–57.
47. Nakhleh RE, Miller W, Snover DC. Significance of Mucosal vs Salivary Gland Changes in Lip Biopsies in the Diagnosis of Chronic Graft-vs-Host Disease. Arch Pathol Lab Med, 1989 Aug;**113**(8): 932–4.
48. Rubin R. 1994. Clinical Approach to Infection in the Compromised Host, 3rd ed. Plenum Medical Book Company. New York, N.Y.
49. Gourishankar S, M.J., Jhangri GS, Preiksaitis JK. 2004. Herpes Zoster Infection Following Solid Organ Transplantation: Incidence, Risk Factors and Outcomes in the Current Immunosuppressive Era. American Journal of Transplantation, **4**(1): 108–15.
50. Smith SR, B.D., Alexander BD, Greenberg A. 2001. Viral Infections after Renal Transplantation. American Journal of Kidney Diseases, **37**: 659–76.
51. LaRocco MT, B.S. 1997. Infection in the Bone Marrow Transplant Recipient and Role of the Microbiology Laboratory in Clinical Transplantation. Clinical Microbiology Reviews, **10**(2):277–97.
52. Appleton AL, S.L., Peiris JS, Taylor CE, Wilkes J, Green MA, Pearson AD, Kelly PJ, Malcolm AJ, Proctor SJ, et al. 1995. Human Herpes Virus-6 Infection in Marrow Graft Recipients: Role in Pathogenesis of Graft-versus-Host Disease. Bone Marrow Transplantation, **16**(6).
53. Bakir M, B.J., Newell KA, Millis JM, Buell JF, Arnow PM. 2001 Epidemiology and Clinical Consequences of Vancomycin-resistant Ente-Rococci in Liver Transplant Patients. Transplantation, **72**(6): 1032–7.
54. Singh N, P.D., Chang FY Gayowski T, Squier C, Wagener MM, Marino IR. 2000. Methicillin-resistant Staphylococcus Aureus: The Other Emerging Resistant Gram-positive Coccus among Liver Transplant Recipients. Clinical Infectious Disease, **30**(2): 322–7.
55. Schmied E, D.J., Euvrard S. 2004. Nontumoral Dermatologic Problems after Liver Transplantation. Liver Transplantation, **10**(3): 331–9.
56. Strauss G, M.A., Rasmussen A, Kirkegaard P. 1997. Staphylococcal Scalded Skin Syndrome in a Liver Transplant Patient. Liver Transplantation Surgery, **3**(4): 435–6.
57. Fishman JA, R.R. 1998. Infection in Organ-transplant Recipients. New England Journal of Medicine, **338**(24):1741–51.
58. Varon NF, A.G. 2004 Emerging Trends in Infections among Renal Transplant Recipients. Expert Rev Anti Infect Ther, **2**(1): 95–109.
59. Nathan DL, S.S. Kestenbaum TM, Casparian JM. 2000. Cutaneous Mycobacterium Chelonae in a Liver Transplant Patient. Journal of American Academy of Dermatology, **43**: 333–6.
60. Patel R, R.G. Keating MR, Paya CV. 1994. Infections Due to Nontuberculous Mycobacteria in Kidney, Heart, and Liver Transplant Recipients. Clinical Infectious Disease, **19**: 263.
61. Paya, C. 1993. Fungal Infections in Solid-organ Transplantation. Clinical Infectious Disease, **16**(5): 677–88.
62. Panackal A, I.A., Hanley EW, Marr KA. 2006. Aspergillus Ustus Infections among Transplant Recipients. Emerging Infectious Diseases, **12**(3): 403–8.
63. Stiller MJ, T.L., Rosenthal SA, Riordan A, Potter J, Shupack JL, Gordon MA. 1994. Primary Cutaneous Infection by Aspergillus Ustus in a 62-Year-Old Liver Transplant Recipient. Journal of

64. Vagefi PA, Cosimi AB, Ginns LC, Kotton CN. 2008. Cutaneous Aspergillus Ustus in a Lung Transplant Recipient: Emergence of a New Opportunistic Fungal Pathogen. The Journal of Heart and Lung Transplantation, 27: 131–134.
65. Husain S, Wagener MM, Singh N. 2001. Cryptococcus Neoformans Infection in Organ Transplant Recipients: Variables Influencing Clinical Characteristics and Outcome. Emerging Infectious Diseases, 7: 375–81.
66. Virgili A, Z.M., La Malfa V, Strumia R, Bedani PL. 1999. Prevalence of Superficial Dermatomycoses in 73 Renal Transplant Recipients. Dermatology, 199(1): 31–4.
67. Greenlee RT, Murray T, Bolden S, Wingo PA. 2000. Cancer Statistics, 2000. CA: A Cancer Journal for Clinicians, 50: 7–33.
68. Ulrich C, S.T., Nindl I, Meyer T, Sterry W, Stockfleth E. 2003 Cutaneous Precancers in Organ Transplant Recipients: An Old Enemy in a New Surrounding. Br J Dermatol, 149(Suppl 66): 40–2.
69. Berg D, Otley CC. 2002. Skin Cancer in Organ Transplant Recipients: Epidemiology, Pathogenesis, and Management. Journal of the American Academy of Dermatology, 47: 1–17; quiz 18–20.
70. Herman S, Rogers HD, Ratner D. 2007. Immunosuppression and Squamous Cell Carcinoma: A Focus on Solid Organ Transplant Recipients. SKINmed, 6: 234–8.
71. Perrem K, L.A., Conneely M, Wahlberg H, Murphy G, Leader M, Kay E. 2007. The Higher Incidence of Squamous Cell Carcinoma in Renal Transplant Recipients Is Associated with Increased Telomere Lengths. Human Pathology, 38(2): 351–8.
72. Dang C, Koehler A, Forschner T, Sehr P, Michael K, Pawlita M, Stockfleth E, Nindl I. 2006. E6/E7 Expression of Human Papillomavirus Types in Cutaneous Squamous Cell Dysplasia and Carcinoma in Immunosuppressed Organ Transplant Recipients. British Journal of Dermatology, 155: 129–36.
73. Fuchs A, Marmur E. 2007. The Kinetics of Skin Cancer: Progression of Actinic Keratosis to Squamous Cell Carcinoma. Dermatologic Surgery, 33: 1099–101.
74. Euvard S, Kanitakis J, Claudy A. 2003. Skin Cancers after Organ Transplantation. The New England Journal of Medicine, 348: 1681–91.
75. Boukamp, P. 2005. Non-melanoma Skin Cancer: What Drives Tumor Development and Progression? Carcinogenesis, 26(10): 1657–67.
76. Harwood CA, P.C., McGregor JM, Sheaff MT, Leigh IM, Cerio R. 2006. Clinicopathologic Features of Skin Cancer in Organ Transplant Recipients: A Retrospective Case-control Series. Journal of American Academy of Dermatology, 54(2): 290–300.
77. McGibbon, D. 1985. Malignant Epidermal Tumours. Journal of Cutaneous Pathology, 12(3–4): 224–38.
78. Penn, I. 1996. Malignant Melanoma in Organ Allograft Recipients. Transplantation, 61(2): 274–8.
79. Kubica AW, Brewer JD. 2012. Melanoma in Immunosuppressed Patients. Mayo Clinic Proceedings. Mayo Clinic, 87(10):991–1003.
80. van Dijk MC, A.K., van Hees F, Klaasen A, Blokx WA, Kiemeney LA, Ruiter DJ. 2008. Expert Review Remains Important in the Histopathological Diagnosis of Cutaneous Melanocytic Lesions. Histopathology, 52(2): 139–46.
81. Neuburg, M. 2007. Transplant-associated Skin Cancer: Role of Reducing Immunosuppression. Journal of the National Comprehensive Cancer Network, 5: 541–9.
82. Sampio MS, Cho YW, Qazi Y, Bunnapradist S, Hutchinson IV, Shah T. 2012. Posttransplant Malignancies in Solid Organ Adult Recipients: An Analysis of the U.S. National Transplant Database. Transplantation, 94(10): 990–8.
83. Marcelin AG, C.V., Dussaix E. 2007. KSHV after an Organ Transplant: Should We Screen? Current Topics in Microbiology and Immunology, 312: 245–62.
84. Campistol JM, Schena FP. 2007. Kaposi's Sarcoma in Renal Transplant Recipients–The Impact of Proliferation Signal Inhibitors. Nephrology Dialysis Transplantation, 22(Suppl 1): i17–22.
85. Chow JW, L.S. 1990. Endemic and Atypical Kaposi's Sarcoma in Africa–Histopathological Aspects. Clinical and Experimental Dermatology, 15(4): 253–9.
86. Nagy S, G.R., Kemeny L, Szenohradszky P, Dobozy A. 2000. Iatrogenic Kaposi's Sarcoma: HHV8 Positivity Persists but the Tumors Regress Almost Completely without Immunosuppressive Therapy. Transplantation, 69(10): 2230–1.
87. Gonthier DM, Hartman G, Holley JL. 1992. Posttransplant Lymphoproliferative Disorder Presenting as an Isolated Skin Lesion. American Journal of Kidney Diseases, 19: 600–3.
88. Schumann KW, Oriba HA, Bergfeld WF, Hsi ED, Hollandsworth K. 2000. Cutaneous Presentation of Posttransplant Lymphoproliferative Disorder. Journal of the American Academy of Dermatology, 42: 923–6.
89. Takahashi S, Watanabe D, Miura K., Ozawa H, Tamada Y, Hara K, Matsumoto Y. 2007. Epstein-Barr Virus-associated Post-transplant Lymphoproliferative Disorder Presenting with Skin Involvement after CD34-selected Autologous Peripheral Blood Stem Cell Transplantation. European Journal of Dermatology, 17: 242–4.
90. Coyne JD, Banerjee SS, Bromley M, Mills S, Diss TC, Harris M. 2004. Post-transplant T-cell Lymphoproliferative Disorder/T-cell Lymphoma: A Report of Three Cases of T-anaplastic Large-cell Lymphoma with Cutaneous Presentation and a Review of the Literature. Histopathology, 44: 387–93.
91. Dreno B, Mansat E, Legoux B, Litoux P. 1998. Skin Cancers in Transplant Patients. Nephrol Dial Transplant, 13: 1374–9.
92. O'Connor JP, Quinn J, Wall D, Petrie JJ, Hardie JR, Woodruff PW. 1986. Cutaneous Angiosarcoma Following Graft Irradiation in a Renal Transplant Patient. Clinical Nephrology, 25: 54–5.
93. Kanitakis J, Euvrard S, Montazeri A, Garnier JL, Faure M, Claudy A. 1996. Atypical Fibroxanthoma in a Renal Graft Recipient. Journal of the American Academy of Dermatology, 35: 262–4.
94. Kolker AR, Wolfort FG, Upton J, Tahan SR, Hein KD, Zewert TE. 1998. Plantar Verrucous Carcinoma Following Transmetatarsal Amputation and Renal Transplantation. Annals of Plastic Surgery, 40: 515–9.
95. Lanzetta M, Petruzzo P, Dubernard JM, Margreiter R, Schuind F, Breidenbach W, Nolli R, Schneeberger S, van Holder C, Gorantla VS., et al. 2007. Second Report (1998–2006) of the International Registry of Hand and Composite Tissue Transplantation. Transplant Immunology, 18: 1–6.

96 Gabl M, Pechlaner S, Lutz M, Bodner G, Piza H, Margreiter R. 2004. Bilateral Hand Transplantation: Bone Healing under Immunosuppression with Tacrolimus, Mycophenolate Mofetil, and Prednisolone. Journal of Hand Surgery – American Volume, **29**: 1020–7.

97 Levi DM, Tzakis AG, Kato T, Madariaga J, Mittal NK, Nery J, Nishida S, Ruiz P. 2003. Transplantation of the Abdominal Wall. Lancet, **361**: 2173–6.

98 Devauchelle B, Badet L, Lengele B, Morelon E, Testelin S, Michallet M, D'Hauthuille C, Dubernard JM. 2006. First Human Face Allograft: Early Report. Lancet, **368**: 203–9.

99 Kanitakis J, Petruzzo P, Jullien D, Badet L, Dezza MC, Claudy A, Lanzetta M, Hakim N, Owen E, Dubernard JM. 2005. Pathological Score for the Evaluation of Allograft Rejection in Human Hand (Composite Tissue) Allotransplantation. European Journal of Dermatology, **15**: 235–8.

100 Cendales LC, Kirk AD, Moresi JM, Ruiz P, Kleiner DE. 2006. Composite Tissue Allotransplantation: Classification of Clinical Acute Skin Rejection. Transplantation, **81**: 418–22.

101 Bejarano PA, Levi D, Nassiri M, Vincek V, Garcia M, Weppler D, Selvaggi G, Kato T, Tzakis A. 2004. The Pathology of Full-thickness Cadaver Skin Transplant for Large Abdominal Defects: A Proposed Grading System for Skin Allograft Acute Rejection. American Journal of Surgical Pathology, **28**: 670–5.

102 Cendales LC, K.J., Schneeberger S, Burns C, Ruiz P, Landin L, Remmelink M, Hewitt CW, Landgren T, Lyons B, Drachenberg CB, Solez K, Kirk AD, Kleiner DE, Racusen L. 2008. The BANFF 2007 Working Classification of Skin-containing Composite Tissue Allograft Pathology. American Journal of Transplantation, **8**(7): 1396–400.

103 Morelon E, Kanitakis J, Petruzzo P. 2012. Immunological Issues in Clinical Composite Tissue Allotransplantation: Where Do We Stand Today? Transplantation, **93**(9):855–9.

104 Weissenbacher A, et al. (2013). Vascularized Composite Allografts and Solid Organ Transplants: Similarities and Differences. Curr Opin Organ Transplant, **18**(6): 640–644.

Chapter 10

Malignancies of Transplantation

Michael A. Nalesnik

Introduction

Transplantation and malignancy intersect at multiple levels, resulting in clinical problems that require the skills of the pathologist. Historically, the most enigmatic of these complications have involved neoplasms that arise in the setting of iatrogenic immunodeficiency. However, the pathologist also plays an important role in the management of tumors in the transplant candidate and additionally bears responsibility for determining whether a post-transplant tumor represents a donor transmitted malignancy.

This chapter discusses neoplastic conditions that affect each of these patient populations with emphasis placed on the most commonly encountered conditions.

Cancer in Transplant Recipients

Risk of Cancer in Transplant Recipients

Epidemiological studies estimate the cancer risk in the transplant population to be two to four times that of a matched non-transplant population. A large-scale study linked data from over 175,000 U.S. organ recipients to cancer registry data and found an overall standardized incidence ratio (SIR) of 2.10 [1] with an increased risk for 33 different malignancy categories (excluding typical squamous or basal cell carcinomas, which are not reported to registries) (Table 10.1). Although registry-based analysis is generally limited to organ locations rather than individual tumor types, this provides a global overview of cancer risk for these patients.

An infectious link is known for many post-transplant tumors, whereas in other cases (e.g., salivary gland, thyroid, eye and orbit), only weak links or no links have been established to date. The latter tumors may be worth additional study. Curiously, a minor but significant decrease in breast cancer is seen in transplant recipients. It is not apparent whether this relates to the post-transplant background or to other factors such as recipient screening prior to transplant.

Recipients of specific organ types are at higher risk for tumors involving those individual organs. For example, post-transplant liver cancer risk is increased only in liver recipients, perhaps representing previously undiscovered or recurrent disease [1]. Moreover, lung or kidney cancer frequency is highest in recipients of these organs, but can occasionally arise in recipients of other allograft types.

In contrast to most registries, the Israel Penn International Transplant Tumor Registry (IPITTR), based at the University of Cincinnati, relies on voluntary reporting of detailed individual patient data. A study from this Center reported that melanomas or cancers of colon, breast, or bladder were more likely to be diagnosed at an advanced stage in transplant patients relative to baseline, despite the fact that organ recipients have close medical monitoring [2]. Further, these cancers were associated with poorer outcomes compared to cancers in non-immunosuppressed patients; raising the intuitive possibility that immunosuppression may facilitate cancer growth and/or aggressiveness.

The risk of post-transplant cancer is compounded by the possibility of donor-transmitted neoplasms, which will be discussed after considering some of the more common de novo cancers that arise in this patient population.

Epstein-Barr Virus (EBV)-associated Tumors and EBV-negative PTLD

PTLD Background

Lymphoid tumors in organ transplant recipients were first described in 1968 [3], evoking discussion as to whether they represented true neoplasms or aberrant lymphoid growths. By 1981, a strong association with EBV was discovered [4] and a range of lymphoid hyperplasias and neoplasias defined [5]. Regression of some tumors following lightening of immunosuppression was reported [6] and major pathologic categories of these growths based on this behavior were classified under the general term of post-transplant lymphoproliferative disorder (PTLD) [7]. Additional case accrual and pathologic refinements uncovered relationships between major categories and clonality, as well as, to a lesser extent, genetic alterations [8]. Efforts at diagnostic standardization led to the World Health Organization PTLD Classification, with the current (as of October 2013) version published in 2008 [9].

Frequency, Risk Factors, and Clinical Presentation

Analysis of UNOS data from 1988 through 1999 inclusively showed an overall 1.2% frequency of PTLD [10]. Intestinal and heart-lung recipients were most commonly affected, with PTLD in <1% of kidney, pancreas, kidney-pancreas, or liver transplant patients. A separate analysis based on Scientific Registry of Transplant Recipients (SRTR) data showed an overall cumulative incidence of 0.5% at five years and 1.4% by ten years after transplant. A more recent breakdown of SRTR data by lymphoma subtype (see Figure 10.1) showed a higher SIR in pediatric versus adult and in non-renal versus renal transplant patients [11].

Table 10.1 Standardized Incidence Ratios (Sir) for Cancer Development in 175,732 US Solid Organ Transplant Recipients (1987–2008) (Data from Engels et al.) [1]

	Cancer Type or Site	SIR	95% CI	Infection-Associated	p<0.001
1	Kaposi's sarcoma	61.46	50.95–73.49	Yes	Yes
2	Lip	16.78	14.02–19.92	No	Yes
3	Skin (non-melanoma non-epithelial)	13.85	11.92–16.00	No	Yes
4	Liver	11.56	10.83–12.33	+/−	Yes
5	Non-Hodgkin lymphoma, extra nodal	10.72	9.93–11.56	Yes	Yes
6	Vulva	7.6	5.77–9.83	Yes	Yes
7	Non-Hodgkin lymphoma, all	7.54	7.17–7.93	Yes	Yes
8	Non-Hodgkin lymphoma, nodal	6.08	5.68–6.51	Yes	Yes
9	Anus	5.84	4.70–7.18	Yes	Yes
10	Intra-hepatic bile duct	5.76	4.08–7.91	No	Yes
11	Kidney	4.65	4.32–4.99	No	Yes
12	Salivary gland	4.55	3.44–5.91	No	Yes
13	Penis	4.13	2.59–6.26	Yes	Yes
14	Hodgkin lymphoma	3.58	2.86–4.43	Yes	Yes
15	Chronic myeloid leukemia	3.47	2.46–4.77	No	Yes
16	Acute myeloid leukemia	3.01	2.45–3.65	No	Yes
17	Thyroid	2.95	2.58–3.34	No	Yes
18	Eye and orbit	2.78	1.72–4.24	No	Yes
19	Other oral cavity and pharynx (excluding lip)	2.56	2.17–3.01	No	Yes
20	Other biliary (excluding intra-hepatic, gallbladder)	2.45	1.74–3.35	No	Yes
21	Small intestine	2.43	1.80–3.20	No	Yes
22	Melanoma	2.38	2.14–2.63	No	Yes
23	Acute monocytic leukemia	2.35	0.64–6.01	No	No
24	Vagina	2.35	0.94–4.84	Yes	No

Table 10.1 (cont.)

	Cancer Type or Site	SIR	95% CI	Infection-Associated	p<0.001
25	Soft tissue including heart	2.25	1.74–2.87	No	Yes
26	Other acute leukemia	2.2	0.71–5.13	No	No
27	Acute lymphocytic leukemia	2.06	1.20–3.30	No	No
28	Renal pelvis	2.05	1.20–3.29	No	No
29	Oropharynx inc. tonsil	2.01	1.64–2.43	Yes	Yes
30	Gallbladder	2	1.25–3.02	No	No
31	Bones and joints	1.98	1.09–3.33	No	No
32	Lung	1.97	1.86–2.08	No	Yes
33	Testis	1.96	1.40–2.67	No	Yes
34	Plasma cell neoplasms	1.84	1.52–2.20	No	Yes
35	Stomach	1.67	1.42–1.96	Yes	Yes
36	Larynx	1.59	1.29–1.95	No	Yes
37	Esophagus	1.56	1.26–1.91	No	Yes
38	Urinary bladder	1.52	1.33–1.73	No	Yes
39	Pancreas	1.46	1.24–1.71	No	Yes
40	Mesothelioma	1.3	0.73–2.15	No	No
41	Colorectal	1.24	1.15–1.34	No	Yes
42	Cervix	1.03	0.75–1.38	Yes	No
43	Nasopharynx	0.96	0.42–1.90	Yes	No
44	Ovary	0.95	0.72–1.24	No	No
45	Prostate	0.92	0.87–0.98	No	No
46	Uterine corpus	0.86	0.70–1.05	No	No
47	Breast	0.85	0.77–0.93	No	Yes
48	Brain	0.76	0.55–1.01	No	No
49	Chronic lymphocytic leukemia	0.59	0.38–0.89	No	No

There is general consensus that pre-transplant recipient EBV seronegativity is the most important risk factor for PTLD [12]. Pediatric or elderly recipient ages are associated with increased risk. The likelihood of developing PTLD varies with the type of organ allograft (incidence estimates: bowel 6%, heart-lung 5.5%, heart 3.9%, lung 3.7%, liver 0.9%, kidney-

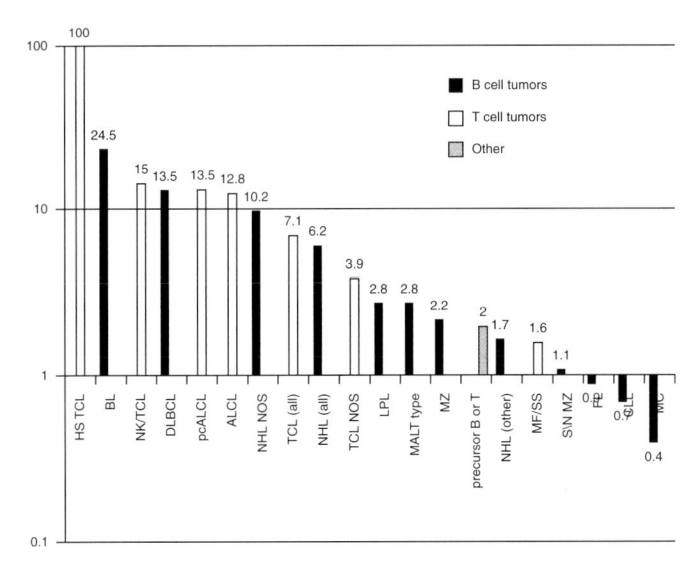

Figure 10.1 Standardized incidence ratios (SIRs) of lymphoma subtypes in solid organ transplant recipients. Abbreviations: ALCL: anaplastic T cell lymphoma; BL Burkitt lymphoma; CLL: chronic lymphocytic lymphoma; DLBCL: diffuse large B cell lymphoma; FL: follicular lymphoma; HS TCL: hepatosplenic T cell lymphoma; LPL: lymphoplasmacytic lymphoma; MALT: mucosal associated lymphoid tumor; MC: mantle cell lymphoma; MF/SS: mycosis fungoides/Sezary syndrome; MZ: marginal zone lymphoma; NHL: non-Hodgkin lymphoma; NK/TCL: NK/ T cell lymphoma; NOS: not otherwise specified; pcALCL: primary cutaneous anaplastic T cell lymphoma; TCL: T cell lymphoma; S/N MZ: splenic/nodal marginal zone lymphoma. Data derived from Clarke et al. [11].

pancreas or pancreas 0.8%, kidney 0.6%) [10]. There is agreement that the total immunosuppressive load increases PTLD risk, although it is not known whether this relates to total amount or drug levels at certain critical time points. Data on individual agents are variable and may be limited by extant clinical practice at time of report. Prior CMV disease is reported to predispose to PTLD [13]. Additional less well-established risk factors include HLA type or degree of HLA mismatch, underlying autoimmune hepatitis, history of prior malignancy, HCV infection, and donor source.

Clinical onset is variable with many cases occurring within the first post-transplant year. Median onset times for adults range from 25 to 72 months with a shorter median of 5.5 to 25 months in pediatric patients [14]. EBV-negative PTLDs can occur at any time, but typically occur late with median onset of four to five years post-transplant. T/NK cell PTLDs also have variable onset times with median interval of six years post-transplant.

The clinical presentation of PTLD can be divided into infectious mononucleosis-like (IM-like), lymphomatous, or systemic. Patients with IM-like syndrome have varying signs and symptoms that can include exudative pharyngitis and adenotonsillitis, hepatitis, airway obstruction, and splenomegaly. This is more common in the pediatric population early after transplant or after post-transplant primary EBV infection. Lymphomatous presentation results from one to multiple synchronous tumors and can occur early, but predominates in the later transplant years. It is the most common syndrome with manifestations dependent upon the site(s) of involvement. Early post-transplant PTLD more frequently involves the allograft and may simulate rejection. CNS involvement can occur in isolated form or as part of multifocal disease. Gastrointestinal involvement, often presenting as GI hemorrhage, abdominal pain, obstruction, or perforation, is common and can be strikingly multicentric within the gut. Skin PTLD tumors are occasionally seen, sometimes arising at sites of previous surgery. Solitary ocular involvement, as well as involvement of other unusual sites such as epididymis, is also described. In short, no location is immune from PTLD and a high level of suspicion should be maintained.

The fulminant presentation is extremely rare and progresses rapidly to sepsis and multiple organ failure. These patients can also have generalized lymphadenopathy and manifestations such as hemophagocytic syndrome. Discrete tumor formation is not a feature of this usually fatal form.

EBV Infection of B Cells

EBV is a double-stranded DNA gammaherpesvirus that infects B lymphocytes mainly via an interaction between the viral envelope glycoprotein gp350/220 and the B cell surface membrane molecule CD21 (complement receptor 2). The virus expresses a series of latency associated genes (latency III) (see Table 10.2) described functionally as the "growth" program" [15], leading to activation and proliferation of B cells with expression of viral proteins [16]. During normal infection, this occurs in lymphoid tissues, but not in peripheral blood. Following this proliferative burst, the virus downregulates several of its proteins, consequently reducing its immunogenicity, as it enters a separate latency stage (Latency II) termed the "default program." According to one current model, several viral proteins expressed at this time provide survival signals normally supplied by antigenic stimulation and T cell help. Specifically, viral latent membrane protein (LMP)-1 mimics a constitutively active tumor necrosis factor receptor (CD40) and LMP-2 downregulates B cell receptor activity while providing survival signals normally transduced by CD40. This model is oversimplified, but is useful to convey the concept that the virus does not normally promote endless B cell proliferation, but follows a sequence of events to first expand the infected B cell pool and then facilitate survival of these cells. After the B cell follows its normal differentiation pathway by rearranging its immunoglobulin genes and maturing into a memory cell via the germinal center reaction, EBV once again switches latency programs to downregulate almost all viral protein production (Latency 0), thereby effecting a "stealth" mode and allowing long-term persistence. Occasional physiologic cell division occurs in memory B cells, and at this time, the virus adapts by upregulating expression of a nuclear protein (EBNA-1) that distributes viral episomes between daughter cells (Latency I). Since EBV at this time no longer controls activity of the B cell receptor, stimulation of the memory B cell with transition into a plasma cell can occur and be accompanied by activation of the lytic program with viral replication and continued reinfection.

Table 10.2 Life Cycle Stage-specific Gene Expression of Epstein-Barr Virus

*Protein or RNA	Latency 0 (Latency Program)	Latency I (EBNA-1 Only Program)	Latency II (Default or Rescue Program)	Latency III (Growth Program)	Lytic Program	Comment
EBNA1	-	+	+	+	+	Associates with chromosomes during cell division to allow long-term viral persistence
EBNA2	-	-	-	+	+/-**	Notch mimic necessary for B cell transformation
EBNA3 (3a)	-	-	-	+	+?	
EBNA4 (3b)	-	-	-	+	+?	Facilitates EBNA2 activity, anti-apoptotic
EBNA6 (3c)	-	-	-	+	+?	
EBNA5 (LP)	-	-	-	+		Facilitates EBNA2 action
LMP1	-	-	+	+	+	Major viral oncogene, mimics CD40 signals, induces B cell growth, survival, and maturation via NF-κB, others
LMP2a	+	+?	+	+		Blocks and substitutes for B cell receptor signaling; LMP2b negatively regulates LMP2a
LMP2b	-	-	+?	+		
EBERs 1,2	+	+	+	+		May interfere with innate immunity, other actions
BZLF1	-	-	-	-	+	Induces lytic viral cycle
BART miRNAs	+	+	+	+	+	Multiple miRNAs with likely anti-apoptotic, other functions

See text for functional roles of Latency Programs in EBV life cycle.
* Not a complete listing of viral products; **Variable

Host Response to EBV Infection

The earliest host response to EBV infection involves conventional dendritic cells (DCs) likely stimulated by an interaction between viral RNA (EBER) and toll-like receptor (TLR) 3 in the DC [17]. This stimulates IL-12 production with activation of NK cells and production of interferon-γ, which can limit viral cell activation. Monocyte-derived DCs also prime adaptive T cell immune responses to the virus. Activation of plasmacytoid DCs via interaction of viral DNA with TLR9 leads to production of interferon-α/β, which further increases NK cytotoxicity [18].

These responses are insufficient to eradicate the virus, and adaptive immunity characterized by T cell and antibody activity soon predominates. CD8+ T cells, with lesser numbers of CD4+ cells and activated NK cells, comprise the bulk of circulating atypical lymphocytes in uncomplicated IM. Immunodominant latency-associated viral antigen targets of CD8+ cells differ from those of CD4+ cells and include Epstein-Barr nuclear antigens (EBNAs) 3–6 (or EBNAs 3a, 3b, LP, and 3c by alternate nomenclature), with subdominant targets of EBNA-1, latent membrane protein (LMP)-1, and LMP-2. T cells also target lytic viral antigens, in particular BZLF1 and BRLF1. These are actually major antigens in the acute phase and likely play a significant role in limiting primary infection.

The antibody response is directed against a variety of antigens, of which attention has focused primarily on antibody to the viral envelope gp350/220 because of potential virus neutralizing capability. This antibody, along with several others, typically persists for the life of the host.

As the infection evolves into a chronic stage, the immune response targets mainly latency-associated antigens. However, intermittent reactivation of the lytic viral cycle occurs and likely elicits a commensurate CD8-mediated immune response against early lytic antigens. Virions that escape destruction can re-infect additional B cells and induce cell transformation, resulting in destruction of at least some, but not all, of these cells due to T cell activity against latency-associated antigens. In this fashion, the cycle repeats intermittently and endlessly, typically at a subclinical level [15].

Altered Immune Response in Immunosuppressed Transplant Patients

Iatrogenic immunosuppression partially inhibits the T cell response to EBV and establishes a new "set point" equilibrium in which the genomic EBV load and viral shedding from the throat are both higher than in non-immunosuppressed individuals. Immune inhibition is not complete, as EBV seronegative transplant patients who sustain primary infection can mount a T cell response and patients seropositive for EBV at transplant continue to have CD8$^+$ cells specific for latent and lytic viral antigens. However, this cell population may be partially deficient as effector cells [19].

The altered equilibrium can lead in some cases to the development of hyperinfected B cells that lack surface immunoglobulin and contain multiple viral episomes. The fate of these abnormal B cells is unclear.

The simple concept that functional over immunosuppression of the antiviral T cell response predisposes to aberrant B cell proliferation and hence to PTLD finds support in the facts that a) most of these tumors express viral antigens associated with the growth program (latency III) and b) virus-specific effector T cells can induce disease remission. The clinical situation may be more complicated, with additional factors contributing to host-virus disequilibrium. For example, serial EBV genomic measurements in a heart transplant patient treated with anti-EBV T cells for PTLD showed a secondary rise in EBV levels coincident with an episode of trauma [20]. Since this occurred at a time of enhanced antiviral T cell activity, it suggests that separate mechanisms predisposing to viral growth may exist.

Pathogenetic Factors Contributing to PTLD

Several related pathways of PTLD development likely exist [16]. The major process (see Figure 10.2c) supported by current evidence invokes EBV infection of a naïve B cell, followed by cell maturation and progression through the germinal center reaction, which includes somatic hypermutation (SHM) of immunoglobulin genes [16, 21]. Since the B cell surface immunoglobulin (sIg) pathway is downregulated by viral LMP-2, these changes are not antigen-related as in normal B cells, but are driven by the virus directly. In some cases, SHM is successful and the virus-infected cells express sIg. In other cases, it is unsuccessful, in which case the cells would normally undergo apoptosis. However, EBV, with the CD40 pathway replaced by LMP-1 and B cell receptor stimulation replaced by LMP2a proteins, respectively, provides survival signals. The result is a proliferation of EBV$^+$ sIg$^-$ B cells. In either case, the virus continues to express latency type III proteins and survival of most infected cells is permitted by the weakened host response. This can eventuate in a monoclonal or polyclonal EBV$^+$ PTLD expressing Latency III viral proteins.

Uncommonly, separate pathways identical or closely related to those described for EBV associated Burkitt or Hodgkin lymphoma in non-immunosuppressed individuals may be followed (see Figures 10.2a and b).

Parallel virus induced activities may also amplify this process. Viral IL10, a cytokine with the potential to interfere with T cell response, is produced in the lytic phase and when the virus enters latency, LMP-1 upregulates cellular IL10 via the p38/MAPK and Akt/mTOR pathway [22].

The frequent presence of CD4$^+$ T cells within PTLD has suggested that regulatory cells may also be contributory. Genes associated with tolerance (VSIG4, CD274, IDO1) are upregulated locally, possibly mediated by EBV. This could create an "immune privileged" site allowing for growth despite T cell infiltration and account in part for the fact that EBV$^+$ PTLDs typically arise at an earlier time point than do EBV-negative tumors [23].

In contrast to the above, genes of the innate immune response are upregulated in EBV$^+$ PTLD. Conceivably, this could relate to the confluent necrosis often seen in polymorphic PTLDs [23].

Expression of viral latency III proteins in individual tumors may be modified, presumably as additional cell mutations make them superfluous for cell survival [16]. Increased numbers of chromosomal fragile site abnormalities in EBV-positive PTLDs relative to lymphomas in non-transplant patients suggests an active viral role in promoting cellular genomic instability [24].

The above scenarios may not necessarily apply to EBV-negative PTLD and the mechanisms operative in these tumors are largely undefined. Direct evidence for continued accrual of genetic abnormalities in EBV- tumors is limited to anecdotal reports of recurrent tumors. For example, in one series, a heart transplant patient developed an EBV- PTLD with three mutations considered due to aberrant SHM [25]. 14 years later, a recurrent EBV- tumor contained identical genetic changes along with nine additional mutations.

Morscio et al. found no difference in gene expression profiles between EBV- PTLD and diffuse large B cell lymphoma arising in non-transplant patients [23]. Further, they did not find upregulation of innate immune response or tolerance-associated genes as found in EBV$^+$ PTLD and concluded that EBV- PTLDs likely represent sporadic lymphomas arising in transplant patients. An alternate, although not mutually exclusive, hypothesis is that EBV may precipitate lymphoproliferation, but over time become a superfluous passenger in a tumor overtaken by a non-infected clone, the so-called "hit and run" hypothesis [21]. In the series cited above, a second heart transplant patient developed a monomorphic EBV$^+$ PTLD that expressed IgAκ and contained two point mutations

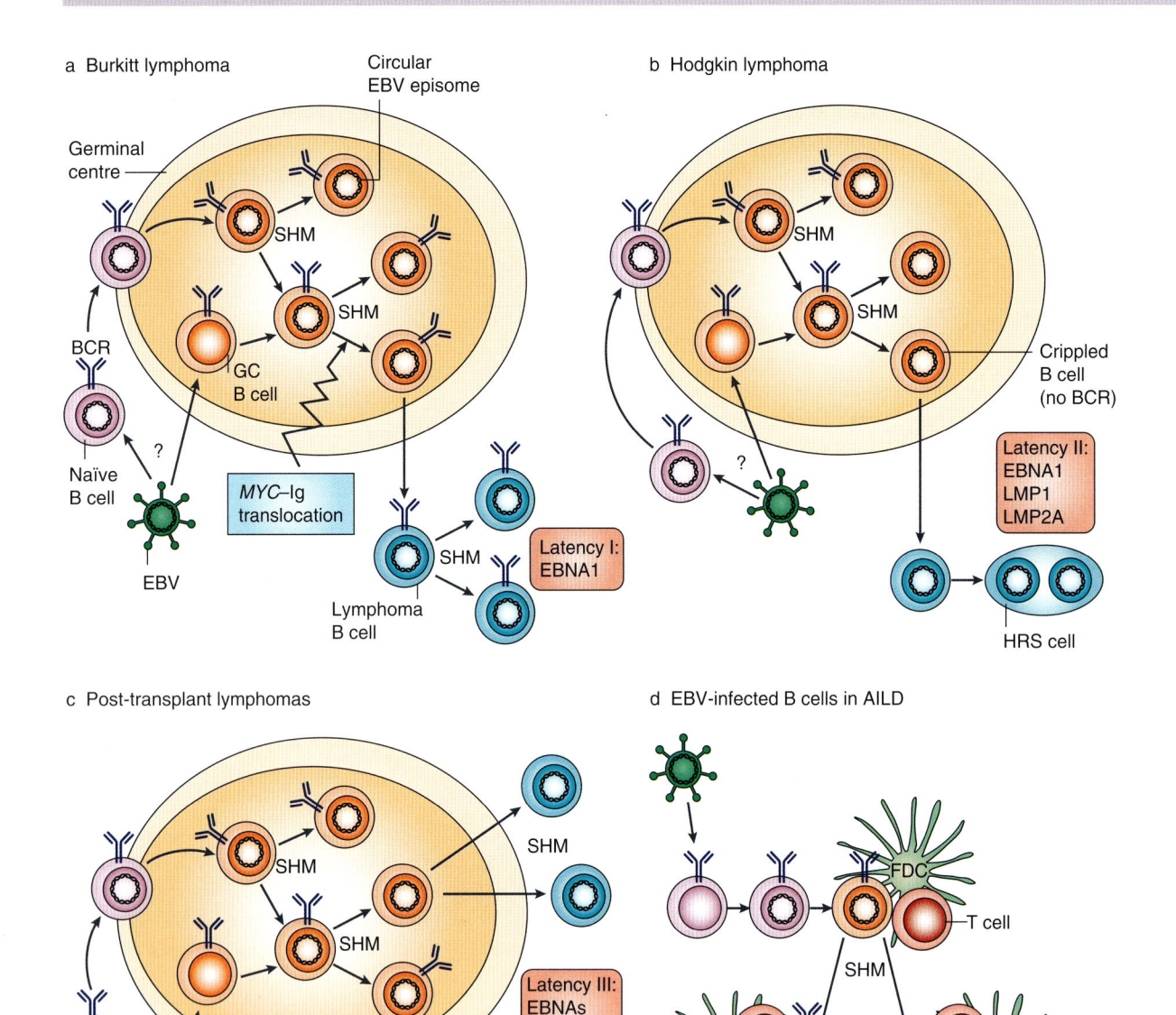

Figure 10.2 Pathogenetic models of EBV-associated B cell tumors. a) Burkitt lymphoma: infection of a naïve or germinal center B cell is followed by MYC translocation during somatic hypermutation or immunoglobulin class switch. This locks the cell into a germinal center centroblast form and facilitates cell proliferation. MYC can also induce apoptosis, but it is likely that EBV, possibly via EBER, interferes with that process. The virus is thus a cofactor and shows the limited protein expression of latency I. b) Hodgkin lymphoma: infection of the B cell is followed by progression through the germinal center reaction. In some cases, somatic hypermutation normally leads to deleterious genetic changes and marks the cell for apoptosis. EBV replaces survival signals of the B cell receptor with LMP 2a and of CD40 with LMP-1. Further loss of B cell-specific genes may allow the Hodgkin Reed-Sternberg (HRS) cell to avoid other normal physiologic B cell controls. c) Post-transplant lymphoma (PTLD): B cell infection by EBV is followed by a germinal center reaction that can either result in productive or defective somatic hypermutation. Continued production of EBV proteins of latency type III provides survival signals and continues to drive B cell proliferation. Continued mutations may occur in the B cell during clonal evolution, potentially leading to more malignant tumors. In occasional cases, direct stimulation of naïve B cells may occur, or in other cases, the pathways of Burkitt or Hodgkin lymphoma may be paralleled. d) Angioimmunoblastic lymphadenopathy with dysproteinemia (AILD): in this T cell lymphoma, EBV infected B cells are exposed to a non-physiologic environment of neoplastic T cells and frequent follicular dendritic cells that could drive a germinal center reaction. EBV may provide survival signals to the B cell regardless of whether somatic hypermutation is productive or nonproductive. This results in one or more clones of EBV infected B cells. It is possible that a similar process may lie behind rare composite T cell and B cell neoplasms that arise in the transplant setting, although this has not been demonstrated. (figure reprinted by permission from Macmillan Publishers Ltd: Nat Rev Immunol 3:809, copyright 2003) [21].

[25]. Approximately two years later, recurrent IgAκ PTLD showed the same two mutations with two additional mutations. However, this time, the tumor was EBV-.

WHO Classification

Many articles state that the histopathology of PTLD has historically been poorly defined when in fact each proposed classification has systematically built upon the preceding one(s) in a logical fashion, incorporating additional entities as they have been discovered and described (Table 10.3).

The seminal description by Frizzera et al. introduced the concept of a spectrum of lymphoproliferations and laid the foundation for subsequent work [5]. Shortly thereafter, uniform application of reduced immunosuppression showed regression in some lesions [6]. Because the relationship of high-grade EBV$^+$ tumors to standard lymphomas was not clear, and since these tumors differed as a group from the polymorphic appearing lesions that were more likely to undergo regression, the term "monomorphic" was introduced to distinguish such neoplasms [7]. Later studies of heart transplant patients showed a similar distribution of lesions that was now correlated with differences in molecular findings [8]. High-grade tumors were described on the basis of histologic similarity to standard lymphomas, limited to the types seen. In 2001, the WHO, expanding on a prior workshop report of the Society of Hematopathology [26], included additional lymphoma subtypes, retaining the term monomorphic as a general category with subdivision into T and B cell lymphomas. Polymorphic PTLD remained a distinct category and the term "early lesion" was introduced not as a temporal description, but as a category to contain conditions such as infectious mononucleosis or reactive plasmacytic hyperplasia, considered to represent early steps in the progression to lymphoma. Hodgkin and Hodgkin-like lymphomas were introduced as a separate category. Although lymphoid tumors not containing EBV were now known to occur, no distinction was made between tumors that did versus those that did not contain the virus.

The 2008 WHO classification represents the current standard for PTLD diagnosis and contains minor updates from the previous version [9]. Specifically, hepatosplenic T cell lymphoma is now included with T cell neoplasms and the Hodgkin category is restricted to classical Hodgkin lymphoma, with lesions showing only a resemblance to Hodgkin lymphoma incorporated into other categories (see below). Florid follicular hyperplasia is recognized as a reactive post-transplant growth, but is not formally included under the PTLD umbrella at present.

Pathology of PTLD

The pathology of PTLD is considered in line with the 2008 WHO classification in the following sections. Useful points to consider during workup of PTLD are presented in Table 10.4.

Early Lesions

Infectious Mononucleosis (IM)-like Lesion

For practical purposes, this may be considered to represent IM in an immunosuppressed patient. The process typically arises in tonsils/adenoids or lymph nodes and is characterized by lymphoproliferation with architectural preservation. Lymph node sinuses, tonsillar crypts, and follicles are evident. In some cases, follicular hyperplasia may be obvious, whereas in others, a few residual follicles are present, with identification facilitated by detection of B cells (CD10, CD20) or follicular dendritic cells (CD21).

Paracortical expansion is present and comprised mainly of immunoblasts, T cells, and plasma cells (see Figure 10.3a and b). Small necrotic foci may occur, but do not approach the size or confluence often seen with polymorphic PTLD. A trivial amount of lymphocyte "spillover" beyond the capsule can occur without destruction of underlying architecture. Cellular atypia is not present, although, similar to typical IM, rare cells resembling Hodgkin Reed-Sternberg (HRS) cells may occur and do not represent a reason to abandon the diagnosis.

Immunocytochemical evaluation shows polyclonal B cells and no evidence of aberrant T cell phenotype. EBV is demonstrable with EBER stain and, to a lesser extent, with immunocytochemical stain for LMP1.

Reactive Plasmacytic Hyperplasia

Reactive plasmacytic hyperplasia is a diffuse process containing numerous mature plasma cells in the setting of intact nodal/tonsillar architecture (see Figure 10.3c–d). A background of small T lymphocytes and occasional immunoblasts is also present. Cellular atypia is absent. Binucleate plasma cells and Russell bodies may be seen. Some examples contain features of both IM-like PTLD and reactive plasmacytic hyperplasia.

Immunocytochemistry demonstrates polyclonal plasma cells. EBV is detectable in most cases, and otherwise histologically typical examples that are EBV-negative are also included in this category at present.

Polymorphic PTLD

Polymorphic PTLD (see Figure 10.4) is a diffuse lymphoproliferation that effaces and frequently destroys underlying architecture, regardless of whether it is nodal or extranodal. It is comprised of B lymphocytes with a heterogeneous appearance due to the fact that all stages of B cell activation are represented. Additionally, numerous T cells and macrophages can be present, possibly representing an ineffectual host response. This combination is the basis of the polymorphic appearance and also precludes assignment to any of the standard lymphoma categories.

Two characteristic features not required for diagnosis include necrosis and atypical immunoblasts. Necrosis may be massive and consists of multiple irregular confluent areas. Large B cells with irregular vesicular nuclei and occasional prominent nucleoli with occasional resemblance to HRS cells are termed atypical immunoblasts and may be scattered in small numbers, typically in proximity to necrotic regions.

Table 10.3 Chronological Listing and Interrelationships of PTLD Classification Systems (1981–2014)

1981 (University of Minnesota) [5]	1988 (University of Pittsburgh) [7]	1995 (New York University) [8]	2001 (World Health Organization)		2008 (World Health Organization) [9]	
Reactive hyperplasia	Infectious mononucleosis	—	Early lesions	Infectious mononucleosis	Early lesions	Infectious mononucleosis-like lesion
		Plasma cell hyperplasia		Reactive plasmacytic hyperplasia		Plasmacytic hyperplasia
Polymorphic diffuse B cell hyperplasia	Polymorphic PTLD	Polymorphic diffuse B cell hyperplasia	Polymorphic PTLD		Polymorphic PTLD	
Polymorphic diffuse B cell lymphoma		Polymorphic diffuse B cell lymphoma				
Immunoblastic sarcoma	Monomorphic PTLD	Immunoblastic lymphoma	Monomorphic PTLD	B cell neoplasms	Monomorphic PTLD	B cell neoplasms	Diffuse large B cell lymphoma
				Diffuse large B cell lymphoma			Burkitt lymphoma
				Burkitt/Burkitt-like lymphoma			
				Plasma cell myeloma			Plasma cell myeloma
		Plasmacytoma		Plasmacytoma like lesions			Plasmacytoma-like lesion
							Other
				T cell neoplasms	Peripheral T cell lymphoma NOS		T cell neoplasms	Peripheral T cell lymphoma NOS
							Hepatosplenic T cell lymphoma
				Other types			Other
—	—	—	Hodgkin and Hodgkin-like lymphomas		Classical Hodgkin lymphoma type PTLD	

Table 10.4 Points to Consider during PTLD Workup

Context	Comment
Sample selection	Sampling of the largest tumor is preferred In the case of multiple tumors, it is useful to sample more than one site if possible to assess metastatic versus multiple independent tumors Tissue should be received fresh for optimum processing
Sample processing	With sufficient tissue, process as per standard lymphoma protocol; however, the basic histologic and immunohistochemical workup is most valuable With a limited sample (biopsy, cytology) CD3, CD20 (and additional B cell markers), and EBER offer the highest yield for diagnosis and should be prioritized Flow cytometry can be helpful in assessing cell type; when dividing tissue, remember that PTLD can have massive necrosis
Histology	Diagnosis requires attention to cell heterogeneity, cytologic features, and status of underlying architecture (see text for details) In the case of massive necrosis, exclusively mononuclear cell ghosts suggest the presence of PTLD Lymphomatous (monomorphic) PTLD can have significant cell heterogeneity, but the cells have similar (malignant) cytologic features PTLD can have an infiltrative rather than tumorous growth pattern, esp. in the allograft. Irregular distribution of heavy infiltrates alternating with areas of relatively sparse inflammation raises suspicion of PTLD
Immunophenotype	CD20 is particularly important if antibody therapy is being considered Immunoglobulin stains have limited use to resolve clonality. In some cases, molecular studies will show monoclonality even if immunostain looks mixed; other B cell PTLDs may not produce immunoglobulin at all B cell PTLD (esp. polymorphic) can have numerous infiltrating T cells CD15, CD20, and CD45 are useful to distinguish HRS from pseudo-HRS cells EBER is the best approach to detect EBV except in areas of massive necrosis where LMP1 stain may be useful EBER is particularly useful to distinguish PTLD from rejection
Molecular studies	Monoclonality, always seen in monomorphic PTLD, does not preclude the diagnosis of polymorphic PTLD. Both IgH and T cell receptor studies should be considered Clonal pattern may distinguish metastatic from multiple synchronous tumors or recurrent from metachronous de novo tumors Oncogene analysis is optional; positive results (e.g. MYC translocation) imply high-grade tumor
Karyotypic studies	Optional for clinical evaluation
Pathology report	Should include cell and PTLD type by WHO classification, status of CD20, EBV, and clonal assessment at a minimum

Although molecular studies show an underlying clonal proliferation in most cases, immunophenotype is variable and often shows a mixture of B cells interpreted as polyclonal. On occasion, clonal B cell populations may be identified by flow cytometry or immunohistochemistry. In the latter case, the finding may be focal. Clear-cut flow or immunohistochemical demonstration of a clonal B cell population does not preclude the diagnosis, but raises the possibility of (monomorphic) diffuse large B cell lymphoma PTLD variants (see below). A high proliferation index by Ki-67 immunostain or mitotic count is common and is also consistent with polymorphic PTLD.

EBV is detectable in almost all cases by EBER stain and, to a lesser extent, by detection of LMP1. Although EBER is typically more sensitive, tumors with massive necrosis may retain LMP-1-positivity even when EBER becomes undetectable (see Figure 10.5).

Monomorphic PTLD

Monomorphic PTLDs comprise those lymphoid tumors with features identical to accepted diagnostic categories of B or T/NK lymphomas. Notably, some tumors are not specifically included at present in this category and these include follicular lymphoma, small lymphocytic lymphoma/chronic lymphocytic leukemia, MALToma, or splenic marginal zone lymphoma (and neoplasms of the myeloid, histiocytic, or dendritic cell lines by definition).

Terminological confusion can be avoided if it is recalled that the term "monomorphic" was introduced at a time when the few cases of observed high-grade lymphomas in transplant patients were restricted to diffuse large B cell lymphomas with uniform immunoblastic features or to Burkitt lymphomas. As more entities were encountered, some fully developed lymphomas were characterized by cellular pleomorphism. Thus,

Malignancies of Transplantation

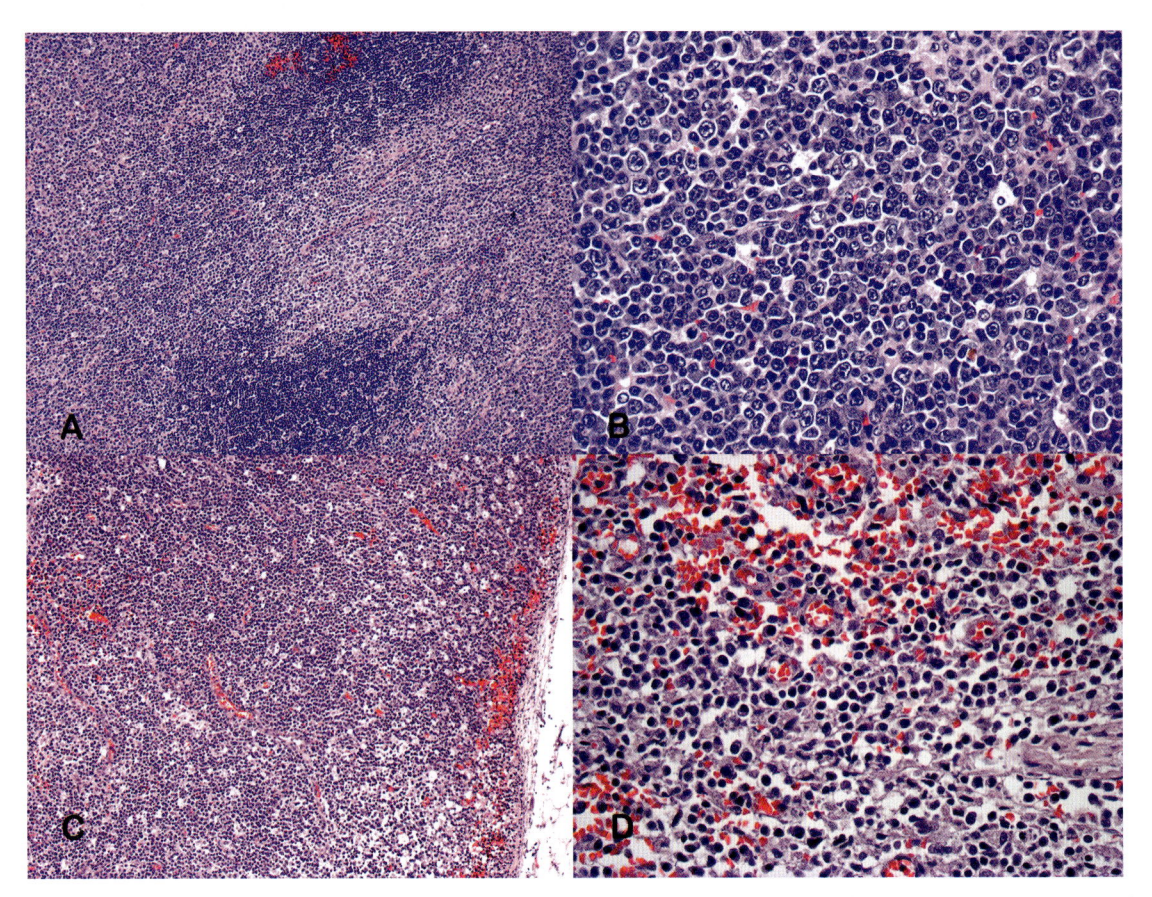

Figure 10.3 A) IM-like PTLD. Two follicles separated by paracortical expansion (x10). B) Paracortical cells include immunoblasts, transformed lymphocytes, small lymphocytes, and plasma cells (x40). C) Plasma cell hyperplasia showing diffuse cellular overgrowth without transgression of the capsule and with sinusoid retention (x10). D) Most cells are mature plasma cells (x40).

monomorphism in the sense of extreme cellular monotony is not a requirement for inclusion. However, the pleomorphic cells in monomorphic PTLD subtypes are also cytologically malignant (i.e., "cut from the same cookie cutter"), thus differing from the polymorphic PTLD, in which heterogeneity is generated by a combination of B cells at varying stages of activation and numerous infiltrating T cells and macrophages.

Diffuse Large B Cell (DLBCL) and Burkitt Lymphomas (BL)

DLBCL (see Figure 10.6b and c) represents the most common form of PTLD and appears as a diffuse proliferation of medium-to-large lymphoid cells with vesicular nuclei, variably prominent nucleoli, and variable amounts of cytoplasm. Any of the known subtypes of DLBCL are placed into this category, with centroblastic and immunoblastic forms most common. The latter may show significant plasmacytoid differentiation.

BL (see Fig 10.6a) may occur with a prototypic appearance. In some cases, there is heterogeneity due to coexistent slightly larger cells. Similar tumors in non-immunosuppressed patients are considered unclassifiable B cell lymphoma with features intermediate between DLBCL and BL [9].

B cell-associated antigens (CD19, CD20, CD79A) are usually highly expressed and immunoglobulin expression is variable. EBV stains are usually positive. It is possible to estimate the B cell maturation stage, but this does not have clinical applicability at present. Successful immunocytochemical staining or flow cytometry will show a monoclonal pattern, although some tumors do not express immunoglobulins. Clonal rearrangement of immunoglobulin genes is demonstrable in almost all cases.

Plasma Cell Neoplasms

Both multiple myeloma and extramedullary plasmacytoma (see Figure 10.7) exist as forms of PTLD, typically arising late post-transplant. Histologic features are similar to those described in the non-transplant setting, with sheets of mature or immature plasma cells, the latter with looser chromatin, more prominent nucleoli, and a higher nuclear: cytoplasmic ratio. Plasmablastic lymphoma may rarely arise in the transplant setting as a diffuse proliferation of cells ranging from immunoblasts to immature and occasionally mature plasma cells.

These clonal growths express plasma cell markers such as CD138 and IRF4/MUM1. CD20 is negative in myeloma and plasmacytoma, and absent or weak uptake of this antibody helps to distinguish plasmablastic lymphoma from DLBCL variants with plasmacytic features.

Many of these tumors are negative for EBV. The virus, if present, is more reliably detected by EBER stain than by LMP-1, which is weak or absent. A clonal immunoglobulin population is detectable by immunohistochemistry.

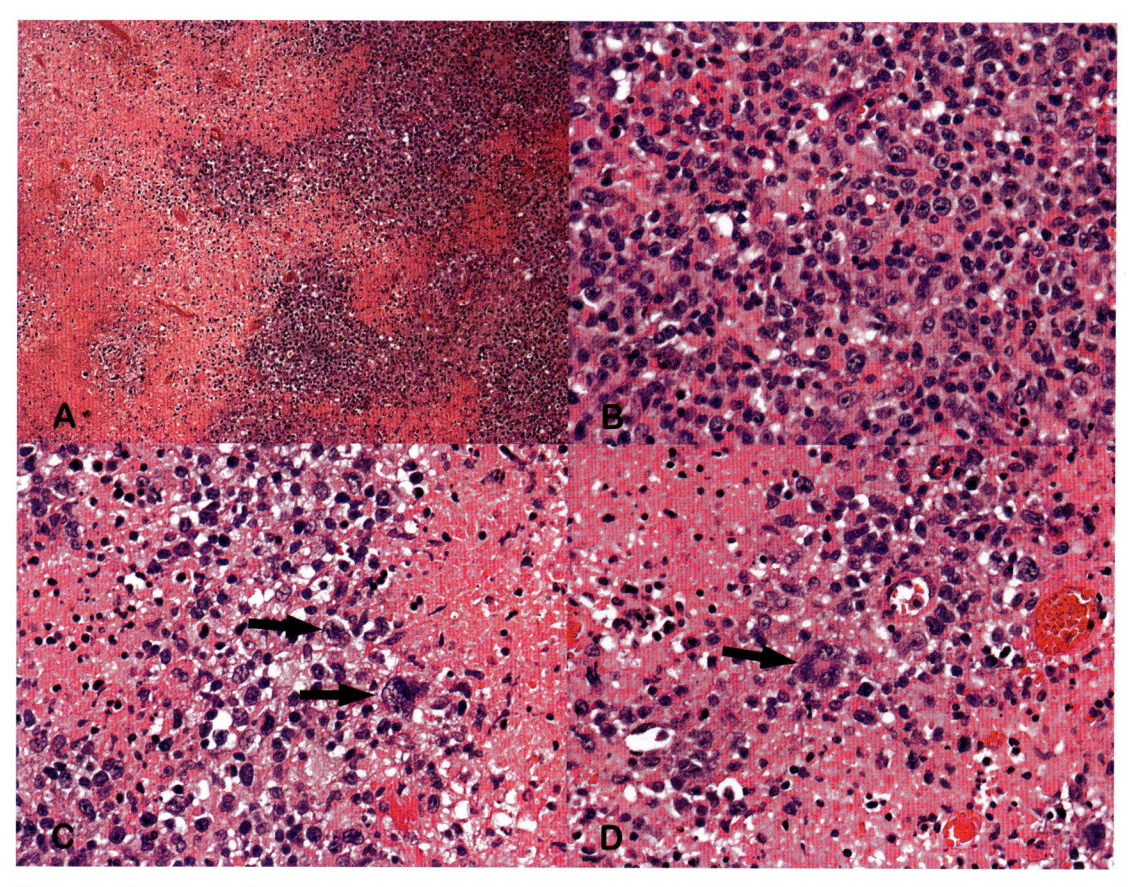

Figure 10.4 Polymorphic PTLD. A) Diffuse lymphoid infiltrate with confluent "geographic" necrosis (x10). B) Polymorphism is due to B cells in various stages of transformation, infiltrating T cells, and macrophages. Cells lack malignant features (x40). C) Enlarged B immunoblasts with irregular nuclear membranes ("atypical immunoblasts") (x40). D) Polylobated atypical immunoblast (x40).

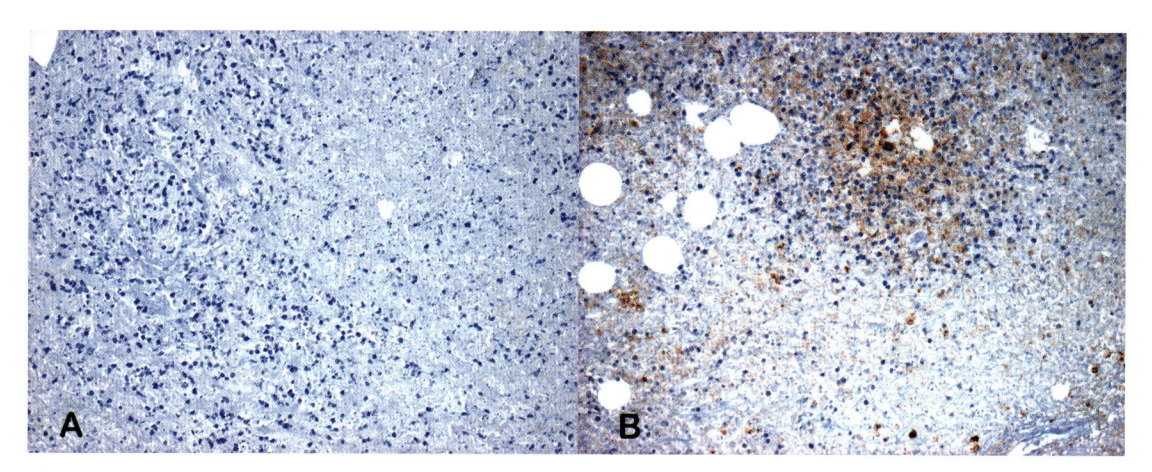

Figure 10.5 EBER and EBV immunostains in necrotic PTLD. In situ hybridization for EBER is normally much more sensitive than immunocytochemistry for LMP-1, except in necrotic regions. A) EBER stain (x20). B) LMP-1 immunocytochemistry in the same tumor (x20).

T/NK Cell PTLD

T/NK PTLD is a rare disorder with less than 150 cases reported. The most common subtypes include peripheral T cell lymphoma NOS (see Figure 10.8), hepatosplenic T cell lymphoma, and primary cutaneous or systemic anaplastic large cell lymphoma (ALCL) either ALK$^+$ or ALK$^-$. The morphologies of these tumors are identical to those described in the non-transplant population. In addition to the above subtypes, any of the T cell or NK cell neoplasms are included in this category.

The immunophenotype is dependent upon the particular variant. Aberrant expression of T cell antigens and evaluation of αβ and γδ T cell receptors are helpful in supporting the diagnosis and particularly helpful in lesions of liver or spleen. CD30-positivity is present in ALCL, but is not specific for this condition. Likewise, CD56 uptake occurs in both T and NK cell PTLD.

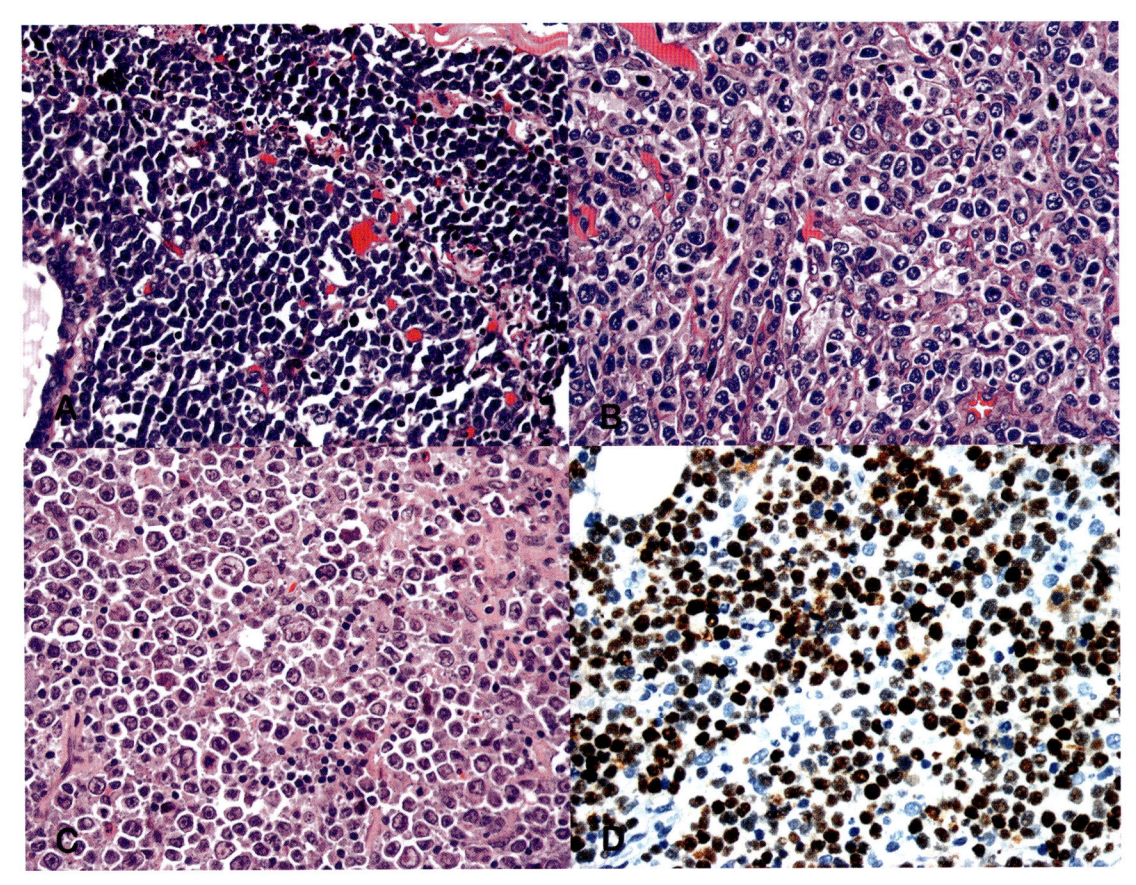

Figure 10.6 Representative B cell lymphoma subtypes categorized under the generic heading of monomorphic PTLD. A) Burkitt (x40). B) Diffuse large B cell lymphoma (x40). C) Diffuse large B cell lymphoma with plasmacytoid features (x40). D) EBER stain. Most but not all cells show strong positivity (x40).

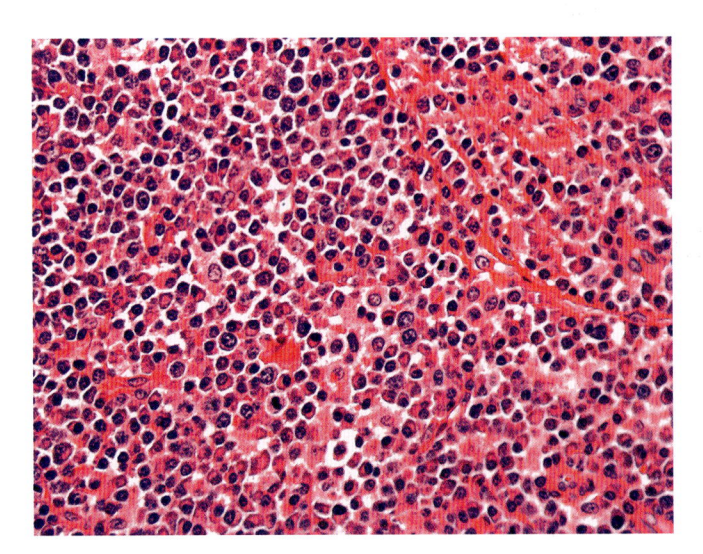

Figure 10.7 Extramedullary plasmacytoma. A diffuse proliferation of mature plasma cells, as well as those with more open nuclei, is evident (x40).

These are distinguishable since NK cells lack CD3 expression and do not show clonal T cell receptor gene rearrangement.

EBV is uniformly present in nasal type NK/T cell lymphomas and in approximately 36% of peripheral T cell lymphomas NOS [27, 28]. Establishing viral presence is not necessary for diagnosis.

Hodgkin Lymphoma (HL) PTLD

The existence of Reed-Sternberg-like cells in IM, as well as atypical immunoblasts in polymorphic PTLD, have historically complicated the diagnosis of HL in the transplant setting. The WHO has separated true HL from related EBV-associated conditions. Hodgkin-like lymphoma is no longer recognized and such lesions are typed as either polymorphic or monomorphic PTLD dependent upon overall morphology.

The diagnosis of HL PTLD is based upon diagnostic Hodgkin Reed-Sternberg (HRS) cells in the appropriate inflammatory setting (see Figure 10.9a). True HL is more likely to contain numerous small lymphocytes with eosinophils and more frequent HRS cells. A background of transformed lymphocytes of varying sizes is more suggestive of polymorphic PTLD according to the WHO (see Figure 10.9b), and a background of cells with malignant cytologic features or uniform large size is more consistent with monomorphic PTLD. Regardless of classification, cases resembling HD should be closely managed, as they may not respond to minimal therapeutic interventions.

Immunophenotypic studies are important for diagnosis. True HRS cells are classically CD15$^+$ and CD30$^+$ with absent-to-weak CD20 and CD45 expression. RS-like cells of poly/monomorphic PTLD are typically CD20$^+$, CD45$^+$, and CD30$^+$, but CD15 expression is absent. Occasional HRS cells may also lack CD15, but a cautious approach in diagnosing true HL in this setting has been recommended [9].

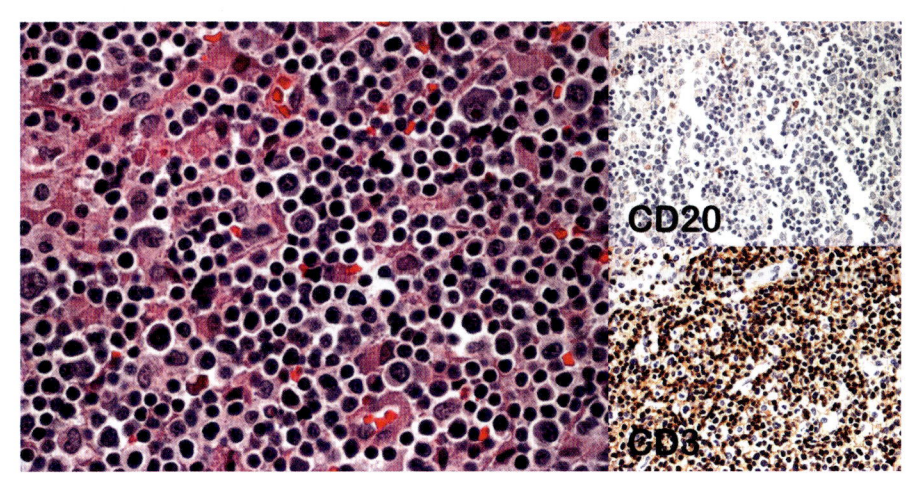

Figure 10.8 PTLD, T cell type (NOS). The morphologic spectrum of peripheral T cell lymphoma is quite broad and any variant can occur in the transplant patient (x60). Immunophenotype (CD3, CD20) confirms the T cell origin of the tumor. (Slide courtesy of Steven Swerdlow, M.D.).

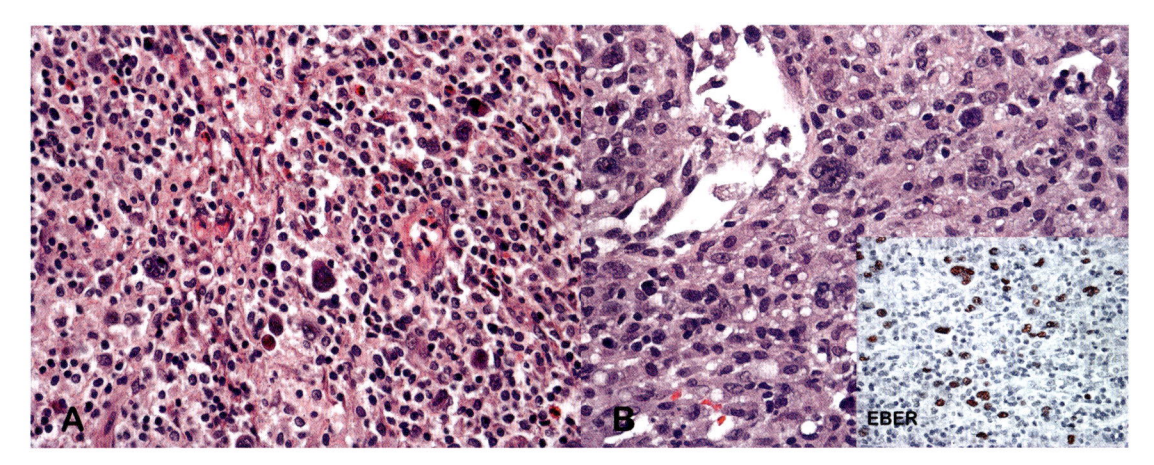

Figure 10.9 A) PTLD, Hodgkin subtype. Scattered HRS cells in a background of small lymphocytes and scattered eosinophils (x40) B) "Hodgkin-like" polymorphic PTLD. The background contains "activated" centroblastic B cells (x40). Inset) Scattered background cells in addition to larger HRS-like cells are EBER+.

In situ hybridization for EBER is also helpful, as true HRS cells are the main positive cells in HL PTLD, whereas frequent scattered background lymphoid cells in addition to RS-like cells are positive in poly/monomorphic PTLD (see Figure 10.9b inset).

Cytogenetic and Molecular Features

Molecular analysis of IM-like PTLD or reactive plasmacytic hyperplasia shows a polyclonal or usually minor oligoclonal pattern regardless of whether immunoglobulin heavy chain gene or EBV terminal repeat analysis is examined. Nonclonal or rarely clonal cytogenetic abnormalities can be present in some cases, whereas no anomalies are found in others.

Various cytogenetic abnormalities have been described in monomorphic PTLDs including breaks within 1q11-q21, 3q27, 8q24.1, 11q23–4, 14q32, and 16p13, as well as trisomies of chromosomes 2, 7, 9, 11, 12, and X [9]. A common defect is not known. BCL6 mutation is not uncommon, perhaps related to somatic hypermutation. One small study associated this with a worse prognosis, but this has not been confirmed [8].

Rearrangements of MYC gene are seen most frequently in the BL form, but are not specific for this subtype. Mutations of RAS and TP53 have also been described in individual DLBCL PTLDs [8].

Post-transplant Smooth Muscle Tumor

Background and Clinical

Post-transplant smooth muscle tumor (PTSMT) is a rare EBV-associated neoplasm with fewer than 100 reported cases. It arises from vascular smooth muscle, but the mechanism by which EBV infects this cell is unknown. PTSMT arises at a median of 48 months post-transplant, with individual cases reported a few months to 29 years after transplant, with earlier onset more typical in the pediatric population [29]. Approximately 20% of patients have had PTLD prior to the onset of PTSMT. The tumor is typically slow-growing, but progressive with symptoms related to location. Involvement of the allograft liver is common and intracranial involvement is a poor prognostic sign. Patients with multiple tumors do worse

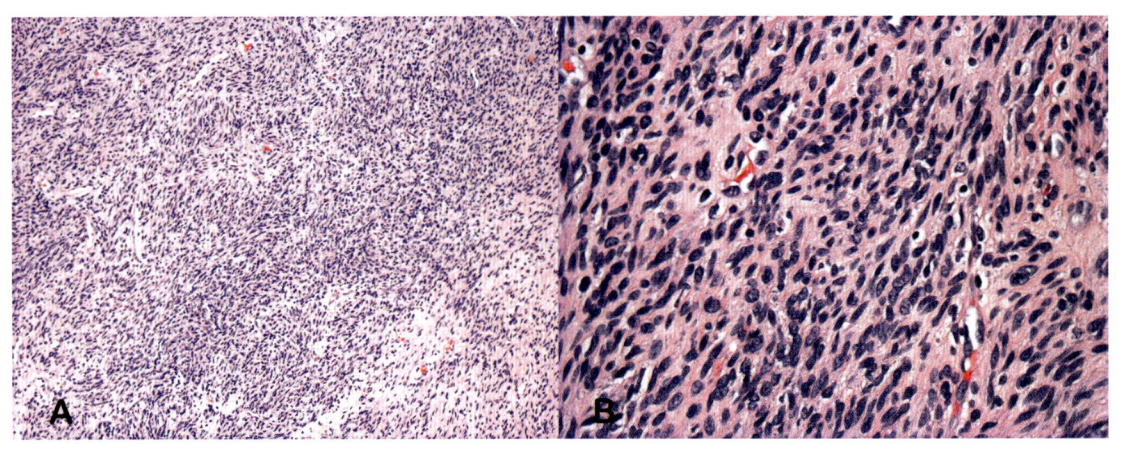

Figure 10.10 Post-transplant smooth muscle tumor A) Tumor cell fascicles show mild variation in density with focal storiform pattern (x10). B) Nuclei are plump without high-grade malignant features (x40). The tumor was strongly EBER-positive (not shown).

than those with an isolated mass. Multiple approaches to treatment have been employed, but no specific therapy has shown clear-cut superiority.

Histopathology, Immunocytochemical, and Molecular Features

PTSMT is characterized by a proliferation of spindle cells with elliptical nuclei arranged in intersecting fascicles (see Figure 10.10). Nuclei may be plump but without general indicators of high-grade sarcoma such as prominent atypia, frequent mitoses, or necrosis. These features, if present, are focal only. No histologic correlate to tumor aggressiveness has been uncovered.

Immunohistochemistry shows positivity for muscle markers such as desmin and smooth muscle actin. EBV is demonstrable by EBER stain, but LMP-1 is either poorly demonstrable or absent.

Clonal EBV is present within tumor cells, indicating a likely etiologic role [30]. Although viral LMP-1 is poorly expressed if at all, positivity for EBNAs 2 and 3 suggests a variant form of type III viral latency [31].

Tumors Associated with HHV8

Kaposi Sarcoma

HHV8 and KS

KS virus or Human Herpesvirus 8 (HHV8) is a double-stranded linear DNA virus discovered in 1994 [32]. Primary infection is spread by saliva, but hematogenous transfer is also possible. Prevalence is <10% in North America, Asia, and North Europe and rises to 30% in the Mediterranean, Middle East, and Caribbean while exceeding 50% in Africa and parts of South America.

Primary oral epithelial cells and a subset of tonsillar B cells are susceptible to infection, but most work analyzing the virus has employed primary effusion lymphoma cell cultures. Following infection, the virus enters a latent state with occasional entry into an abortive or full lytic phase.

Coordinated interactions between latent and lytic viral products generate the complex neovascular and inflammatory mixture that comprises KS [33]. Latency associated genes appear mainly responsible for transformation events which also require paracrine support by viral lytic and induced host proteins. Proposed roles for these products in the development of KS are shown diagrammatically in Figure 10.11.

Latency associated nuclear antigen (LANA-1) helps to maintain the viral genome during cell division and can partially inactivate the tumor suppressors Rb and p53. It also binds glycogen synthase kinase 3 beta, causing beta-catenin accumulation [34].

V-cyclin is a viral latency associated homologue of cyclin D1 that may play a role in cellular proliferation and genome destabilization. A third latent protein, v-FLIP, is the viral homologue of cellular FLIP (Fas-associated death domain [FADD]-like IL-1 beta converting enzyme), which has anti-apoptotic function, stimulates production of chemokines, and may promote spindle cell change of endothelial cells.

Kaposins are a group of three proteins differentially translated from a single viral mRNA. Kaposin A can induce cell transformation, whereas Kaposins B and C have pro-inflammatory activity. Viral micro-RNAs likely play a role in maintaining viral latency and influencing angiogenesis. The virus also upregulates cellular micro-RNAs linked to immune suppression and angiogenesis.

Several viral lytic proteins might also contribute to KS. For example, the early lytic protein vIL-6 can promote angiogenesis through stimulation of vascular endothelial growth factor and angiopoietin 2 and also upregulates IL6 and IL8 production.

The cell of origin of KS is in dispute, but is thought to be a precursor endothelial cell skewed toward lymphatic differentiation by viral effects. This is potentially a circulating cell, since post-transplant KS of donor origin has been described [35]. Lesions may be single or multiple and arise as hyperplastic foci of inflammation and neo-angiogenesis that can undergo regression if host immune function is reconstituted [36]. Conversely, uninterrupted immunodeficiency allows continued progression and some late tumors can demonstrate clonal growth with associated cytogenetic abnormalities [33].

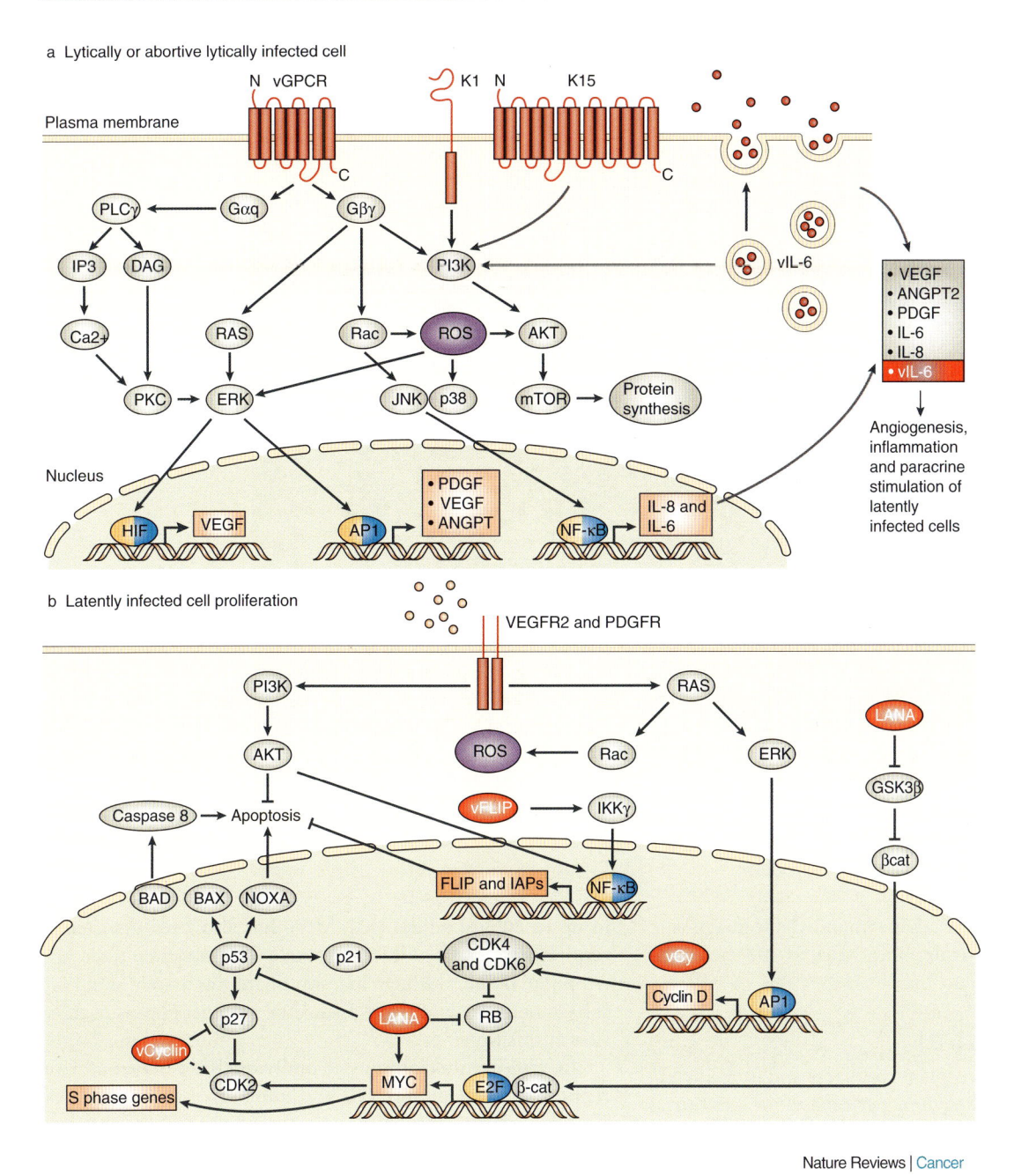

Figure 10.11 Proposed interactions between HHV8 lytic and latently infected cells in Kaposi's sarcoma. a) Lytic infected cell. The lytic viral membrane proteins G protein coupled receptor (vGPCR), K-1, and K 15, as well as viral IL-6 (v-IL6), converge to activate the Pi3k/Akt/mTOR pathway, inducing protein synthesis including vascular endothelial growth factor (VEGF) (not shown). Additionally, vGPCR upregulates the MAP kinase pathway (shown as RAS/ERK) and NFκB production, resulting in generation of VEGF, angiopoietin 2 (ANGPT), and platelet derived growth factor (PDGF), as well as cellular IL-6 and IL 8. These stimulate vasculogenesis and have paracrine effects on inflammatory and latently infected cells. b.) Latent infected cell. In addition to stimulation of NFκB and AP1-mediated transcription by paracrine products, the cell is also subject to alterations by viral latent proteins. Viral FLICE inhibitory protein (vFLIP) stimulates production of anti-apoptotic proteins and chemokines that likely facilitate tumor development. The latency associated nuclear antigen (LANA) interferes with the p53 and Rb tumor suppressor pathways and stimulates MYC activity. It also facilitates nuclear translocation of β-catenin by binding glycogen synthase kinase 3β (GSK3β). Viral cyclin (vCyclin) promotes polyploidy, which would normally activate p53. VCyclin interaction with cdk6 has been suggested as a separate cause of genomic instability. Additional viral latency factors such as kaposins and miRNAs also play a role in production of the inflammatory and angiogenic microenvironment (not illustrated) (Figure reprinted by permission from Macmillan Publishers Ltd: Nat Rev Cancer 10:713, copyright 2010) [33].

Histopathology of Kaposi Sarcoma

Early lesions contain a prominent mononuclear inflammatory infiltrate with fewer spindle cells and occasional epithelioid cells. Spindle cells and vascular slits containing erythrocytes predominate as the lesion progresses (see Figure 10.12). Significant pleomorphism is not present, although mitoses can be seen. PAS+ inclusions can occur in the spindle cells, but are not pathognomonic.

Tumor cells are usually positive for endothelial markers such as CD31 or CD34 and lymphatic antigens, e.g., D2–40 and podoplanin. Some cells may express CD68, smooth muscle actin, or the dendritic marker Factor XIII [33]. The availability

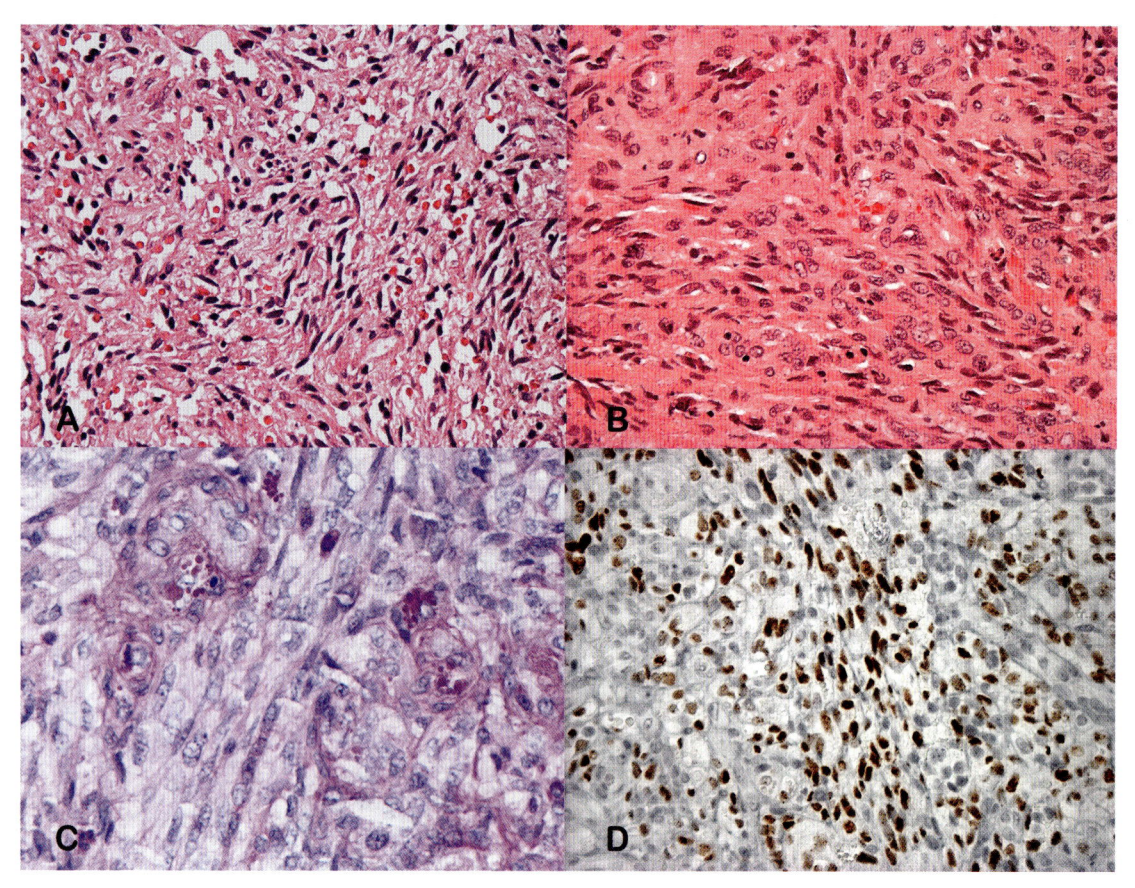

Figure 10.12 Kaposi sarcoma. A) Spindle cells exist within loose stroma containing scattered erythrocytes (x40). B) More solid area of spindle cells with occasional vascular slits (x40). C) Intracytoplasmic PAS+ bodies in KS (PAS x60). D) Immunostain for HHV8 latency associated nuclear antigen (LANA-1 x40).

of immunostaining for HHV8 has simplified the diagnostic separation of these lesions from other vascular and mesenchymal proliferations.

Primary Effusion Lymphoma (PEL)

PEL is extremely rare in transplant recipients and is characterized by a lymphomatous pleural, pericardial, or peritoneal effusion almost always without an accompanying discrete tumor, although in some cases, secondary tumors can arise [34]. PEL cells carry multiple copies of HHV8 and have a variable cytologic appearance that ranges from immunoblastic to plasmablastic to anaplastic with frequent mitoses. RS-like cells can also be seen in small numbers. PEL represents a monoclonal B cell proliferation and appears to have a post-germinal center immunophenotype positive for CD138, but not CDs 20, 19, or 79a. Aberrant T cell antigen expression can occur. Presence of the virus can be confirmed with LANA-1 stain. A number of these tumors are coinfected with EBV, but in this case, HHV8 downregulates LMP1 production, which will give a false negative result.

Merkel Cell Carcinoma (MCC)

The Merkel cell polyomavirus (MCV) is a non-enveloped double-stranded DNA virus that is a normal skin commensal in up to 80% of adults [37]. MCV has also been detected in respiratory secretions, blood, urine, gastrointestinal tract, and lymphoid tissue, although in lesser quantities than in skin [38]. It has not been definitively associated with neoplasms of those sites at this time.

In non-immunosuppressed individuals, episodes of viral replication elicit both T cell and antibody responses against viral capsid antigens. Immunosuppression weakens this surveillance, producing a more permissive environment for lytic viral infection (see Figure 10.13). In some cases, mutation of the viral T antigen allows nonspecific integration into the host genome by unknown mechanisms [39]. Activation of the integrated viral origin of replication does not cause formation of independent virus particles, but leads to generation of viral proteins, particularly T antigen itself, resulting in abnormal DNA replication, breakage, and cell death. In rare cases, the virus circumvents this with a second mutation of the T antigen gene (and several other genes) that inhibits DNA changes, but retains other properties of this protein, such as interaction with the tumor suppressor gene RB1 and upregulation of the BIRC5 gene leading to activation of cell survivin. Thus, in contrast to other cancers, MCC is actually dependent on mutations occurring in the viral, not the human, genome.

Although the viral T antigen is important in tumor development, the small t antigen is likely the main transforming

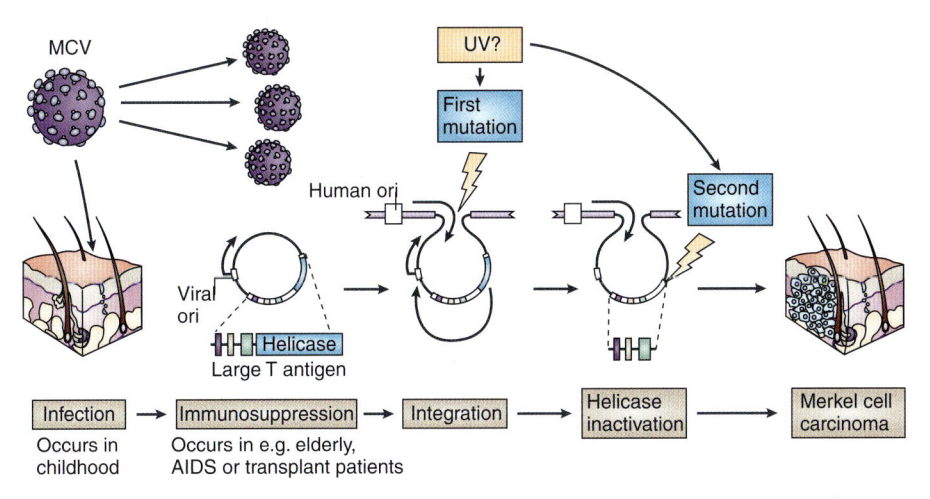

Figure 10.13 Basic pathogenesis of Merkel cell carcinoma. A viral T antigen gene mutation allows integration into the host genome. In rare cases, a second T mutation can avoid cell injury but preserve functions predisposing to malignancy (See text for details). (Figure reprinted by permission from Macmillan Publishers Ltd: Nat Rev Cancer 10:883, copyright 2010) [39].

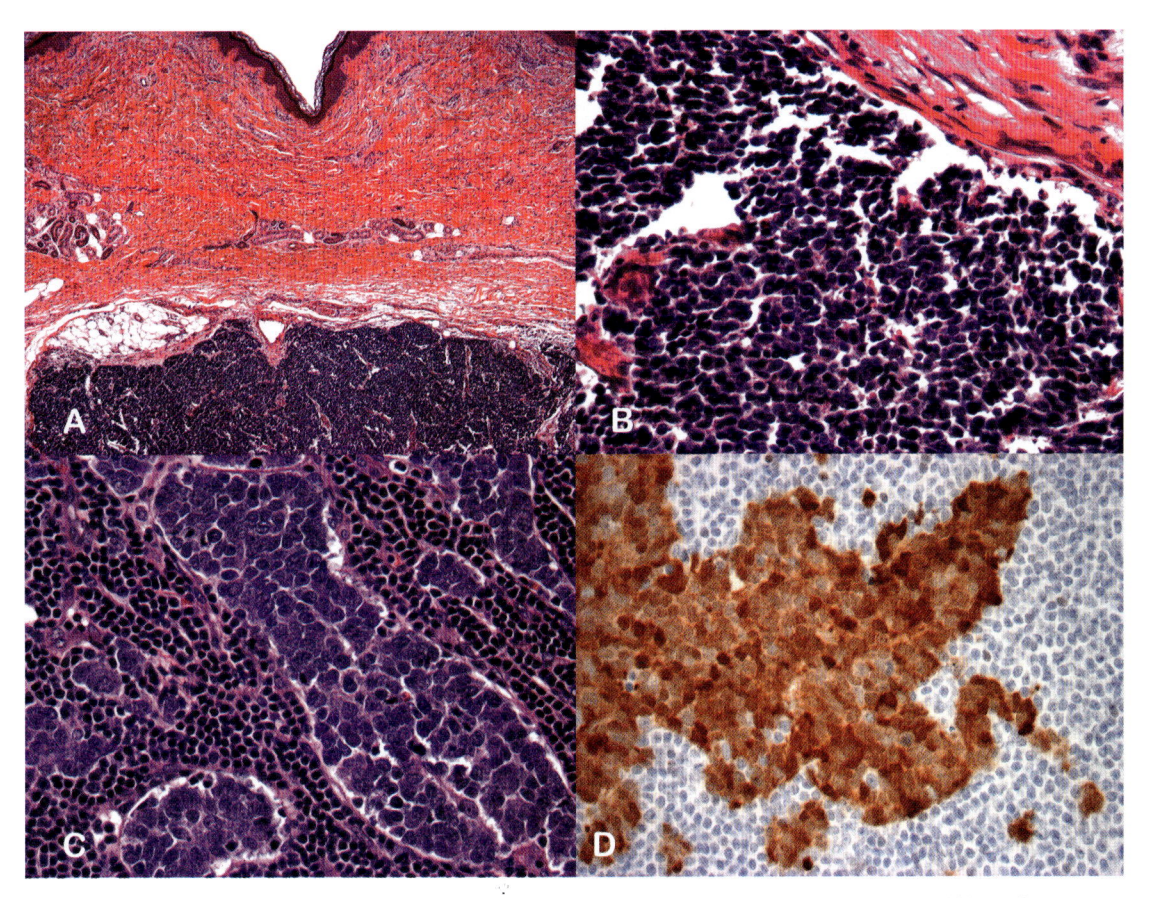

Figure 10.14 Merkel cell carcinoma. A) skin lesion with dermal/subcutaneous localization (x4). B). "Small round blue cell tumor" appearance (x40). C) Metastatic Merkel cell carcinoma in lymph node (x40). D). Immunostain for viral T antigen (x40). (Slides courtesy of Yuan Chang, M.D.).

protein. This small t antigen hyperphosphorylates the cellular translation factor eIF4E- binding protein 1 in a fashion dependent upon the Akt-mTOR pathway, which is also upregulated. In line with this, mTOR inhibitors show some activity against Merkel cell carcinoma.

MCC Pathology

MCC (see Figure 10.14) is a relatively rare neuroendocrine skin cancer that has been steadily increasing in frequency and has mortality in excess of 30%. It presents as a rapidly growing skin nodule that preferentially occurs in fair skinned individuals in areas of ultraviolet exposure. The tumor appears as a skin-colored to violaceous plaque or papulonodular lesion comprised of small cells with frequent mitoses, generally scant cytoplasm, and round nuclei with small nucleoli. It is centered in the dermis, often with a Grenz zone, although occasional epidermotropism may occur. The cells form sheets or trabeculae with frequent angiolymphatic involvement. In some cases, spindle or "oat cell"-like appearance may occur. The tumor may rarely coexist with other tumor types.

The usual differential diagnosis includes small cell variant of melanoma, metastatic neuroendocrine carcinoma, lymphoma, and leukemia. Merkel cell carcinoma shows punctate perinuclear uptake of CK20 and is negative for CK7. Neuroendocrine markers such as synaptophysin, chromogranin, and neuron-specific enolase are also positive. The tumor stains with antibody to c-kit, and S100 protein can be weakly positive (in contrast to the strong positivity of melanomas). Approximately 75% of MCC show positivity for T and/or t viral antigens.

Tumors Associated with Human Papillomavirus (HPV)

There are over 180 known human papillomaviruses, of which approximately 40 can infect squamous and mucosal epithelium. This DNA virus targets the basal epithelial layer, obtaining access in areas of injury, although injury is likely not necessary in certain areas, such as squamo-columnar junctions (e.g., cervical and anal transitional zones) or hair follicles. The virus replicates as extrachromosomal episomes along with the cells and produces low levels of viral proteins E1 and E2 that are necessary for survival, stimulate cell proliferation, and maintain viral presence below immunologic recognition [40]. As the epithelial cells mature, the virus produces additional proteins E4–7 that continue to stimulate the cell, inhibit apoptosis, and initiate amplification of the viral genome. In the upper layers of the epidermis, the virus produces two capsid proteins (L1 and L2) necessary for packaging of viral DNA and virion assembly. Infectious virus is then released when cells are shed. The entire life cycle occurs within epithelial cells and is not accompanied by viremia.

In the case of cervical infection, approximately 90% of individuals clear the virus within three years (although it is possible that viral DNA may persist without active infection in some cases). Of the remainder (in the non-transplant setting), approximately 1% will go on to cervical cancer if untreated [41].

Although the complete sequence of events leading to carcinogenesis remains to be defined, it is accompanied by aberrant increase in viral E6 and E7 proteins [42]. E6 expression degrades p53 in an E7-dependent fashion, inhibits apoptosis and anoikis, activates telomerase, degrades PDZ proteins thereby disturbing cell polarity, and inhibits interferon activity. E7 additionally inhibits Rb and activates E2F responsive genes, facilitating entry into the cell cycle and also causing centrosome formation, leading to increased genomic instability [43]. This process entails overexpression of cellular p16, which is a diagnostically useful marker for transcriptionally active HPV [44]. Continued protein production is aided by eventual integration of viral DNA into the host genome. Viral stimulation of host cell proliferation alone is not sufficient for development of carcinoma and, over time, accumulation of mutations in host DNA provides the final components necessary for neoplasia [43].

Cancer of the Skin and Epidermal Surfaces

Papillomavirus infection is associated with neoplasia in a number of sites, with most, but not all, of these representing squamous cell carcinoma (see Figure 15). Virus-associated cancers have been reported from the cervix, anus, oral cavity, penis, bronchus, larynx, middle ear, sinonasal region, urethra, vagina, and vulva. The histologic lesions include verruca vulgaris, condyloma acuminatum, bowenoid papulosis, verrucous carcinoma (giant condyloma of Buschke Lowenstein), (anal) intraepithelial neoplasia, and squamous cell carcinoma, including basaloid variants. Some cases of cervical or endocrine carcinoma and endocervical adenocarcinoma have also shown evidence of HPV presence.

The virus can be detected by in situ hybridization for viral DNA and immunohistochemical detection of p16 in tumor cells can also serve as a surrogate marker for the virus [44].

Donor Cancer Transmission

Recipient Cancers of Donor Origin

The diagnosis of donor origin cancer in a transplant patient has significance not only for the recipient, but also for others who may have received organs or tissues from that donor. For this reason, current US policy requires reporting such suspected tumors to UNOS immediately upon discovery, and does not require definitive proof of donor origin at the outset. This places the pathologist into the role of gatekeeper and the question arises as to when a donor-transmitted tumor in the transplant patient may reasonably be suspected.

There are no hard and fast rules but, in general, tumors that arise shortly after transplant or seem inappropriate for the patient's demographics should alert the pathologist to this possibility. For example, tumors inappropriate for patient age or sex, metastatic carcinomas with no evident site of primary tumor, CNS tumors occurring outside of the central nervous system, or tumors arising in the allograft itself should raise suspicion.

Two notable exceptions are PTLD and KS, which may be of donor cell origin but are not typically grouped with other donor-transmitted tumors, since they involve post-transplant events in the individual recipient.

Penn originally distinguished between "donor-transmitted" and "donor-derived" tumors, with the former present at transplant and the latter developing from donor cells and arising late after transplantation [45, 46]. This is a useful construct, but an objective cutoff time between these two categories is impossible to determine without knowledge of the number of tumor cells present at transplant and the doubling time of the specific tumor. It is reasonable to have a high suspicion for the possibility of donor tumor transmission with any cancer that arises within the first three post-transplant years, although tumors of donor origin may also occasionally arise after this time.

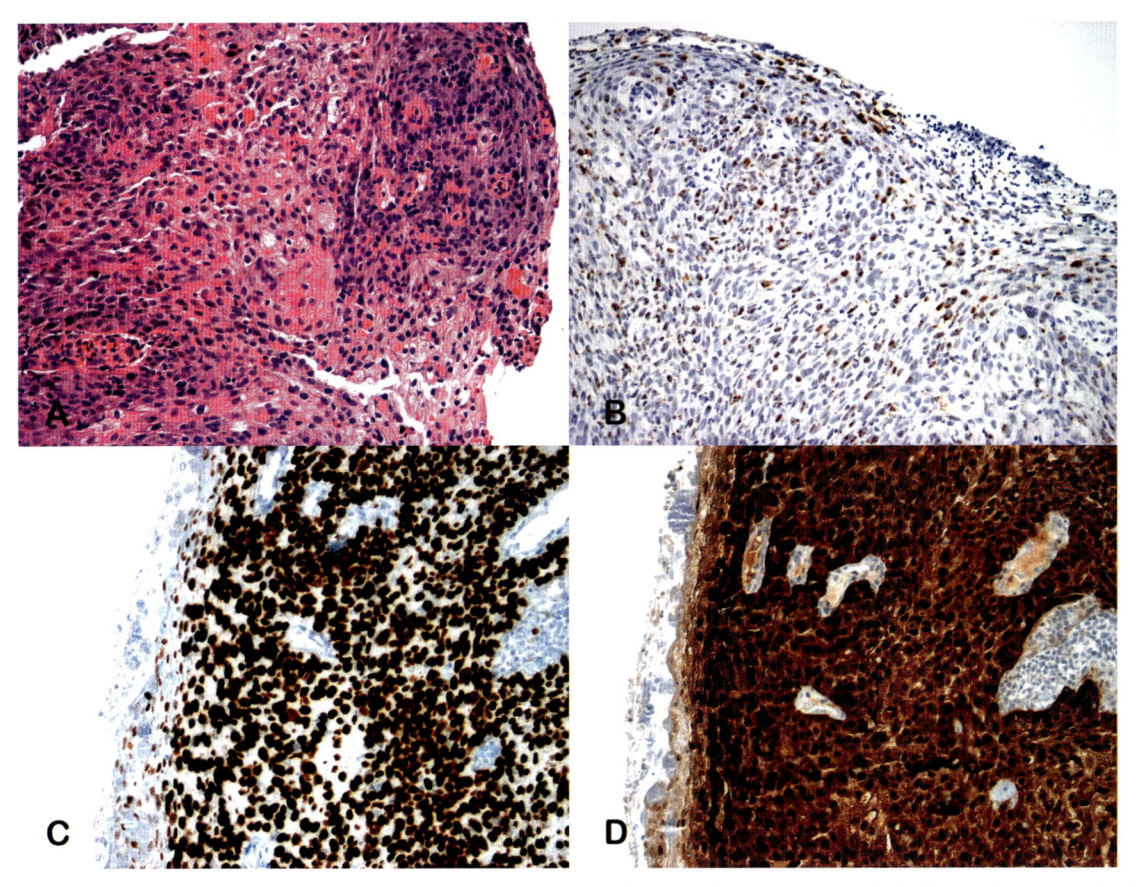

Figure 10.15 HPV-associated squamous cell carcinoma (SCC). A). Well-differentiated SCC (x20). B) In situ hybridization for HPV DNA (x20). C) p63 in tumor cells (x20). D) Diffuse p16 uptake. In these tumors, p16 is a surrogate marker for transcriptionally active HPV (x20).

Cancer in Organ Donors

There are several circumstances that involve the pathologist when a question of cancer in the organ donor arises. In some cases, active or historical cancer is known to be present and the surgeon may seek advice regarding the use of organs for transplant. In other cases, a suspicious lesion may be found during donor operation and a request for frozen section made. In yet other cases, the surgeon may consider use of a donor kidney with a small renal cell carcinoma and the pathologist is asked to evaluate the tumor to determine whether the kidney can be used for transplant. Finally, the pathologist may uncover a neoplasm at donor autopsy or on permanent section of tissue previously submitted for frozen section analysis at the time of organ donation. These issues are addressed in the following sections.

Known Active or Historical Donor Cancer at the Time or Organ Donation

The pathologist does not normally play a role in patient care when there is known active or historical cancer in a potential organ donor. The decision of whether to transplant the organs lies with the transplant surgeon in consultation and with informed consent of the patient and/or legal representatives. On occasion, the opinion of the pathologist may be sought for information regarding the likelihood of tumor transmission.

In 2011, a UNOS committee published a resource document estimating transmission risks of various tumors in this setting (Tables 10.5A and B) [47]. These estimates and recommended courses of action do not constitute OPTN policy, but provide a useful framework to guide discussion.

Recently, the Italian National Transplant Center in conjunction with the WHO has provided a database of reports documenting transmission events that have arisen as a consequence of transplantation. The database can be accessed at www.notifylibrary.org/notifylibrary/search/incident/ and represents the largest single source of information on this subject.

Lesions Submitted for Frozen Section Analysis at the Time of Organ Donation

The pathologist may infrequently be requested to perform frozen section on a mass lesion discovered at time of organ procurement. Full consideration of all potential tumors is beyond the scope of this chapter. However, some of the more common lesions are discussed in the following sections.

Mass Lesions in the Donor Kidney

Assessment of a mass discovered in the donor kidney differs from lesions of other sites because some surgeons may elect to resect the tumor and transplant the kidney even if renal cell carcinoma (RCC) is found. Therefore, it is important not only

Malignancies of Transplantation

Table 10.5A Estimated Transmission Risk Frequencies of Donor Cancer Present at Time of Organ Donation [47]

Minimal (>0 to ≤0.1%)*	Low (0.1 to ≤1%)*	Intermediate (1 to ≤10%)*	High (>10%)*
Bladder carcinoma, papillary noninvasive (T0 N0 M0) (non-renal transplant only)	CNS tumor, low-grade (WHO I or II)	Breast carcinoma, Stage 0 (carcinoma in situ)	Active cancer not listed elsewhere
Cervical carcinoma in situ	CNS tumor, mature teratoma	**CNS tumor, high-grade (WHO III or IV)	Breast carcinoma, >Stage 0
Kidney, renal cell carcinoma, completely resected and solitary, Fuhrman 1–2, 1.0 cm or smaller	Kidney, renal cell carcinoma, completely resected and solitary, Fuhrman 1–2, >1.0–2.5 cm	Colon Carcinoma, Stage 0 (carcinoma in situ)	Choriocarcinoma
Skin, basal cell carcinoma	Thyroid carcinoma, follicular, minimally invasive, 1.0–2.0 cm	Kidney, renal cell carcinoma, completely resected and solitary, Fuhrman 1–2, Stage 1 T1b	CNS tumor with shunt, surgery, irradiation, or extra CNS metastases
Skin, carcinoma in situ (non-melanoma)	Thyroid carcinoma, solitary, papillary, 0.5–2.0 cm		Colon carcinoma >Stage 0
Skin, squamous cell carcinoma without metastases			Kidney, renal cell carcinoma >7 cm or Stage II-IV
Thyroid carcinoma, follicular, minimally invasive, 1.0 cm or smaller			Leukemia
Thyroid carcinoma, solitary, papillary, 0.5 cm or smaller			Lung cancer (Stages I-IV)
Vocal cord carcinoma in situ			Lymphoma
			Metastatic carcinoma
			Neuroendocrine carcinoma (small cell), any site
			Sarcoma
			Skin, melanoma
			Small cell carcinoma, any site

* Transmission frequency risk estimate based on available data and expert opinion
** Recent studies suggest that these tumors may have low risk of transmission

Table 10.5B Estimated Transmission Risk of Historical Cancers [47]

Minimal (>0 to ≤0.1%)*	Historical cancers that would be considered to be of minimal transmission risk if active
Low (0.1 to ≤1%)*	Historical cancer treated five or more years earlier with >99% probability of cure
Intermediate (1 to ≤10%)*	Historical cancer treated five or more years earlier with 90%–99% probability of cure
	Historical cancer considered incurable
	Historical cancer treated five or more years earlier with <90% probability of cure
	Historical cancer with insufficient follow-up to predict behavior
High (>10%)*	History of leukemia
	History of lymphoma
	History of melanoma
	History of small cell/neuroendocrine carcinoma

* Transmission frequency risk estimate based on available data and expert opinion

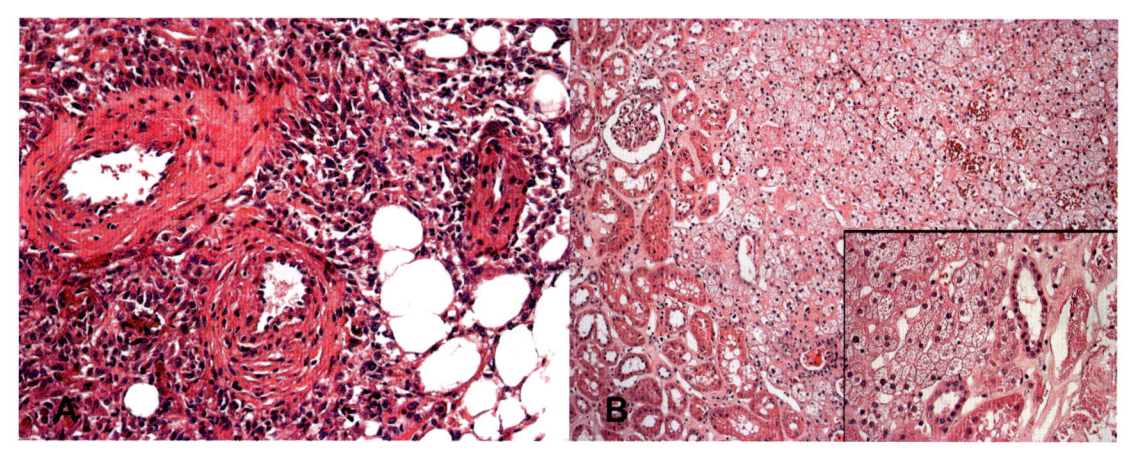

Figure 10.16 Selected masses other than renal cell carcinoma in donor kidneys. A) Angiomyolipoma (x20). B) Adrenal rest (x10). Inset) Characteristic bubbly cytoplasm of adrenal cortical cells. Adrenal cortical zonation, when present, is a helpful feature (x40).

to distinguish this cancer from other entities, but also to evaluate specific tumor characteristics to determine potential suitability for transplant.

Several lesions may mimic renal cell carcinoma, including oncocytoma, angiomyolipoma, xanthogranulomatous pyelonephritis, adrenal rests, and adenomas. On occasion, urothelial carcinoma may resemble RCC. The possibility of metastatic tumor should also be considered.

Oncocytoma classically has a mahogany brown macroscopic appearance and a central scar. The cells are uniform and well-differentiated with hypereosinophilic cytoplasm. Unless there is absolute certainty as to the diagnosis, it is best to defer or emphasize that the diagnosis is provisional and proceed as though the tumor could represent RCC.

Angiomyolipoma is the most common benign renal tumor and may reach large size. It contains varying amounts of blood vessels, myoid cells with a spindled appearance, and mature adipose tissue (see Figure 10.16a). Difficulty may occur in lesions with an abundance of myoid cells and additional sections from different areas may resolve this issue. Angiomyolipomas can on occasion show atypia of the spindle cells or contain atypical epithelial cells. These are more likely to behave in a malignant fashion.

Xanthogranulomatous pyelonephritis may form a mass lesion mimicking renal cell carcinoma. Microscopically, foamy macrophages can resemble clear cells of RCC. Although this is a non-neoplastic condition, we are unaware of donor kidneys with this condition being used for transplant.

Adrenal rests are small encapsulated lesions with architecture resembling normal adrenal cortex (see Figure 10.16b). If these features are not well-developed, it is best to defer the diagnosis and proceed with the possibility that this may represent a well-differentiated RCC. A similar approach is suggested for the rare intrarenal adrenal adenoma [48].

Urothelial carcinoma and RCC may both be papillary and difficult to differentiate on frozen section. If any doubt remains, it is better to take a conservative approach and defer the diagnosis, since urothelial carcinoma is more frequently multicentric and transplantation of such kidneys is not recommended even if all visible disease is completely excised.

The pathologist should provide a diagnosis of RCC and also assess tumor size, estimate histologic grade according to the Fuhrman classification, and determine adequacy of the resection margin. The tumor should be sampled sufficiently for grading purposes since heterogeneity may exist. In some cases, tubular distortion in the peritumoral region may resemble RCC, but the presence of other structures, such as glomeruli, may assist in defining true tumor extent. Information regarding resection margin should be directly communicated to the surgeon. Since renal cell carcinoma can be cystic, the entire wall of such lesions should be examined closely for tumor.

Mass Lesions in the Donor Liver

Common nodular masses in the donor liver include bile duct adenoma, focal nodular hyperplasia (FNH), hepatocellular adenoma (HA), von Meyenberg complexes, and granulomas.

Bile duct adenomas are typically small white subcapsular nodules containing numerous biliary type glands with unremarkable cuboidal to columnar epithelium in a fibrous or fibroinflammatory stroma. This lesion frequently incorporates portal tracts. Bile is not produced, but glands may contain mucin, raising concern for adenocarcinoma. Distinction is based on architectural features and bland cytologic appearance. Cautery may distort the tissue, rendering definitive diagnosis problematic, and should be avoided if possible. This lesion does not represent a contraindication to transplantation.

FNH may be single or multiple. In the latter case, there is no guarantee that each unsampled lesion is a separate FNH, since some may represent hepatocellular adenomas or, rarely, hepatocellular carcinomas. The features of FNH are discussed in the section below on small hepatocellular nodules. FNH does not preclude transplantation.

Von Meyenberg complexes are typically small (usually 5 mm or less) lesions comprised of bland cuboidal epithelial cells forming ducts or small cysts with irregular shapes in fibrous stroma often adjacent to a portal tract. The lumens of these structures may contain bile or proteinaceous material. They can rarely have an acute inflammatory component causing reactive atypia, raising the possibility of adenocarcinoma. Rarely, multiple von Meyenberg complexes have been reported in association with cholangiocarcinoma. However, this lesion itself does not contraindicate transplantation.

Recent advances in the classification of hepatocellular adenomas have revealed specific subtypes with differing risks of progression to hepatocellular carcinoma [49]. Unfortunately, this distinction relies upon immunohistochemistry, rendering it irrelevant for frozen section diagnosis. HA consists of normal appearing hepatocytes and trabecular architecture with isolated arterial vessels and typically without evidence of portal tracts. Although the clinical context is statistically important in determining the likelihood that a hepatocellular lesion represents an adenoma, frozen section cannot distinguish HA from a very well-differentiated hepatocellular carcinoma and this should be communicated to the surgeon. Additionally, the possibility of multiple lesions and additional new post-transplant growths exists. We are not aware that livers with HA have been used for transplant in our center.

In many cases, small white nodular lesions may represent granulomas. In our practice, one or a few granulomas do not normally represent a contraindication to transplant, in contrast to miliary disease that would disqualify the organ. The possibility of tuberculosis should also be considered from a clinicopathologic perspective.

Mass Lesions in the Donor Lung

Requests for frozen section of donor pulmonary lesions are uncommon and usually due to palpation of a firm area at time of donor operation or ordered on the basis of a prior radiograph with questionable findings. In our experience, these are invariably due to intra-pulmonary lymph nodes or granulomas. However, expanded criteria have led to increased numbers of elderly donors and the possibilities of primary tumors, particularly in donors with a history of smoking, or metastatic tumors (such as from colon) more common in the older age group should be remembered. These diagnoses should pose no difficulties on frozen section analysis. The diagnosis of bronchioloalveolar carcinoma/in situ adenocarcinoma should be made with extreme caution, because this may underestimate the ability of the tumor to recur and metastasize in the recipient. Differentiation between lymphoma and small cell neuroendocrine carcinoma is not necessary, as either of these conditions would preclude organ donation.

Mass Lesions from Sites Other than Donor Organs

Rarely, suspicious lesions from other areas are discovered and frozen section requested. In our experience at the University of Pittsburgh, many of these are benign cystic lesions of the ovary, or even atrophic ovaries, in female donors.

In some countries, it has been practice for the surgeon to excise the prostate and submit the organ for sectioning and frozen section analysis. Diagnosis of early prostate carcinoma by frozen section is fraught with difficulty and there is no good evidence that organ donation from older individuals, many of whom can be presupposed to have early prostate carcinoma, results in increased tumor transmission. Therefore, we do not recommend that the pathologist undertake this effort unless there is specific cause such as palpation of a mass lesion in the prostate.

Donor Cancer Discovered after Transplantation

On occasion, an autopsy performed on an organ donor will disclose cancer not detected at time of transplant. It is imperative that the pathologist transmits this as soon as reasonably possible to the surgeon so that appropriate patient management decisions can be made. Clinical transplant personnel will also forward the information to the Disease Transmission Advisory Committee of the OPTN/UNOS so that other recipients can be identified and receive appropriate care. The pathologist should not delay communication until the autopsy report is finalized. It is not even necessary that the tumor be fully characterized before the surgeon is informed. As the interval between transplant and therapy increases, so does the likelihood of tumor growth and/or metastatic seeding.

The same principle applies when a tumor is discovered on permanent section of material previously submitted for frozen section at the time of transplant.

Cancer in Transplant Candidates

Solid organ transplantation is rarely used as a form of cancer therapy with the notable exception of hepatocellular carcinoma (HCC), for which 1,155 transplants were performed in the year 2012 alone. Specific criteria exist for transplant eligibility of individuals with HCC and reporting of the pathologic status of the explant liver is required in the United States. Because of the specialized handling of these cases, this properly falls under the domain of the transplant pathologist.

Liver Cancer in Organ Transplant Candidates and Pretransplant Staging

In 1996, a report from the Milan group [50] showed that patients with a single HCC 5 cm or less in diameter or two to three tumors each less than 3 cm diameter by radiologic imaging had post-transplant survival similar to liver transplant patients without HCC. These criteria were adopted by the OPTN/UNOS to determine eligibility for liver transplant in patients with HCC. In February 2002, the OPTN introduced the more general Model for End-stage Liver Disease (MELD) as a basis for prioritizing liver transplant candidacy, which, however, did not account for patients with HCC. Current policy awards additional priority MELD points to patients with Stage II/T2 tumors by OPTN/UNOS criteria, but not to those with Stage I/T1 tumors (who have three-month survival similar to that of non-tumor candidates) or those with Stage III/T3 tumors or above (who exceed Milan criteria).

The pre-transplant HCC staging system used to determine candidacy relies upon radiologic imaging only [51]. This can cause confusion for the pathologist who uses the American Joint Cancer Commission (AJCC) classification [52], since the two systems use different criteria (Table 10.6). It is therefore useful to be familiar with and know the proper application of both systems.

Characteristic radiologic findings in the appropriate context are sufficient for the diagnosis of HCC [53]. However, other cases are problematic and biopsy is required for diagnosis. Since many

Table 10.6 AJCC [52] versus AASLD [51] (UNOS) Staging Systems for Hepatocellular Carcinoma

Tumor Stage	AJCC	AASLD
I	Solitary tumor without vascular invasion	1 nodule ≤1.9 cm
II	Solitary tumor with vascular invasion OR multiple tumors not more than 5 cm	1 nodule 2.0–5.0 cm OR 2–3 nodules each ≤3.0 cm
III	–	1 nodule >5.0 cm OR 2–3 nodules with any >3.0 cm
IIIA	Multiple nodules more than 5 cm	–
IIIB	Single tumor or multiple tumors of any size involving a major branch of the portal vein or hepatic vein	–
IIIC	Tumor(s) with direct invasion of adjacent organs other than the gallbladder or with perforation of visceral peritoneum	–
IVA	Regional lymph node metastases	–
IVA1	–	≥4 nodules of any size
IVA2	–	Stage II, III, or IVA1 AND gross intrahepatic portal or hepatic vein involvement on imaging
IVB	Distant metastases	Lymph node or distant metastases OR extrahepatic or portal involvement
Primary Application	Pathologic staging of explant liver	Pretransplant staging incorporating Milan criteria

examples involve small lesions, the differential diagnosis of such lesions is discussed.

Differential Diagnosis of Small Hepatocellular Nodules

There are seven main categories of hepatocellular mass lesions, including regenerative nodules, focal nodular hyperplasia, low-grade and high-grade dysplastic nodules, hepatocellular adenomas, early HCC, and "progressed" HCC [54]. These are generally distinguishable based on a combination of morphologic and immunocytochemical studies, although in some cases, diagnosis may be problematic or impossible due to inadequate sample or limitations of the needle biopsy.

Regenerative Nodules

Regenerative nodules are hyperplastic lesions comprised of benign hepatocytes with intact trabeculae and normal intralesional portal tracts (see Figure 10.17a). Sinusoidal compression may occur due to the expansile regenerative process. There can be a mild increase in cell density without atypia. Occasional isolated artery branches can occur and likely contribute to radiographic uncertainty.

Immunostains are usually not necessary. Glutamine synthetase shows a focal distribution in centrilobular locations (see Figure 10.17c). Cytokeratins 7 and 19 decorate bile ducts, ductules, and ductular hepatocytes, with CK19 more specific for bile ducts and ductules. Antigens suggestive or indicative of malignancy, such as alpha-fetoprotein (AFP) or glypican 3, are absent. One potential pitfall lies in the fact that occasional granular uptake of glypican 3 can occur in livers with underlying hepatitis C virus infection.

Focal Nodular Hyperplasia

FNH or lesions resembling FNH within a cirrhotic liver may occur. True FNH contains fibrous bands and isolated arterial vessels with vascular dysplasia, i.e., irregular muscular thickening (see Figure 10.17b). Ductular proliferation without true bile duct presence is typical, but may be variable in intralesional fibrotic regions. Dysplasia is not seen.

Glutamine synthetase is the single most useful stain for the diagnosis of FNH, as it shows a so-called "map-like" pattern (see Figure 10.17d). FNH-like lesions do not show this pattern and represent regenerative nodules.

Low-grade Dysplastic Nodule

Low-grade dysplastic nodules usually have a distinctly nodular appearance because of condensation of fibrous stroma similar to that of cirrhotic nodules, but on occasion may be only vaguely nodular [54]. There is a mild increase in cell density generally with a monotonous pattern (see Figure 10.18a). Large cell change may be present. Isolated arteries can be present, but atypical architectural features such as markedly thickened trabeculae or pseudogland formation are not seen. These lesions do not show evidence of stromal invasion (see below) and do not have a nodule in nodule appearance. It is difficult or

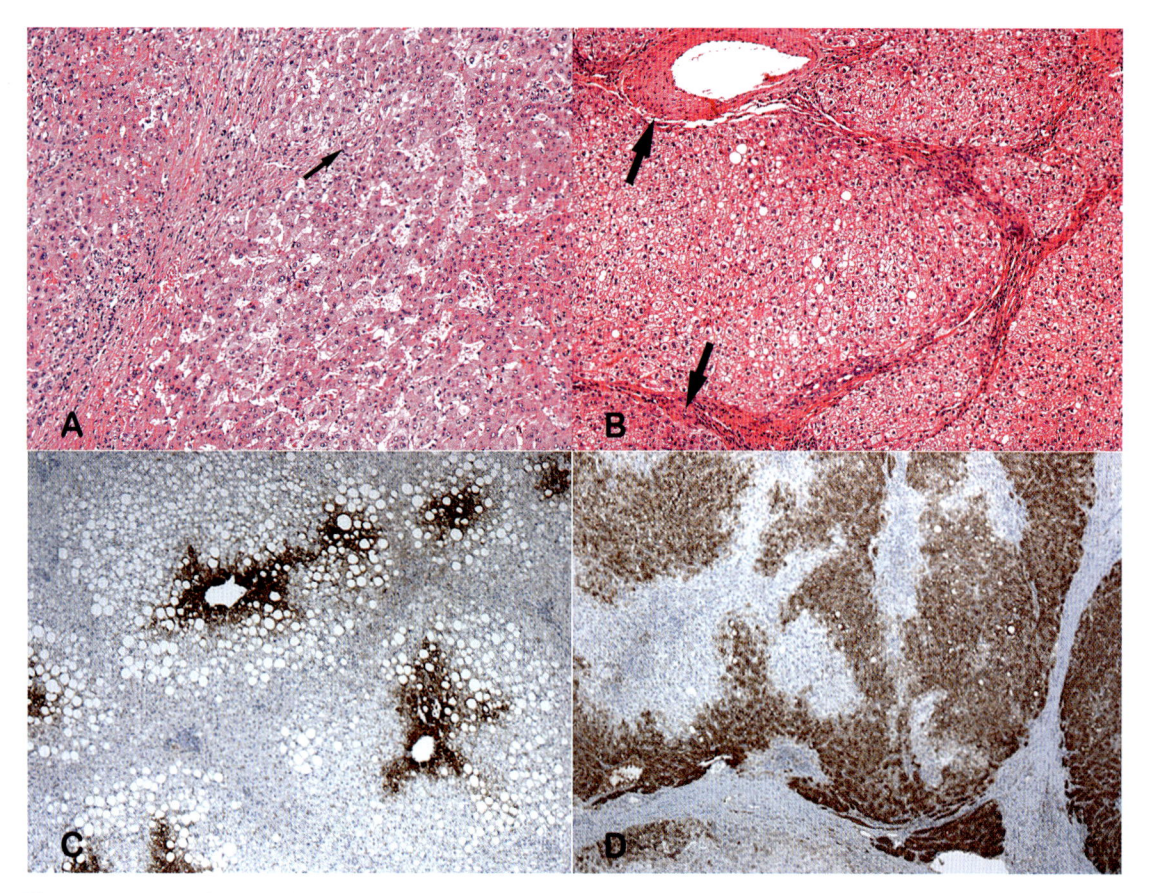

Figure 10.17 Benign hepatocellular lesions in explant livers. A) Regenerative nodule (right) and cirrhotic liver (left). Occasional isolated arteries are seen (arrow) (x10). B) Focal nodular hyperplasia with intersecting fibrosis and dystrophic arteries showing irregular thickening (arrows) (x10). C) Glutamine synthetase in regenerative nodules (x10). D) In contrast, glutamine synthetase in focal nodular hyperplasia shows a geographic or "map-like" configuration (x10). (Slides C and D courtesy of Eizaburo Sasaatomi, M.D., Ph.D.).

sometimes impossible to distinguish these nodules from large regenerative nodules, but this does not appear to have any significant consequences.

CD34 stain highlights the vascular endothelium and sinusoids, the latter in a heterogeneous or diffuse fashion. Immunostains suggestive of malignancy should be negative in this category.

High-grade Dysplastic Nodule

High-grade dysplastic nodules can be distinctly or vaguely nodular with increased cell density up to twice that of surrounding liver. Cytologic atypia is present and most often consists of small cell dysplasia (large cell change may also be present, but is insufficient for this diagnosis). There can be an irregular trabecular pattern and pseudogland formation can be seen. However, the cytologic and architectural changes are not sufficient for the diagnosis of HCC. Most lesions contain unpaired arteries in small numbers. Stromal invasion is not present by definition [54]. A nodule-in-nodule appearance may occasionally be seen (see Figure 10.18b). In such cases, the entire lesion is classified by the worst component, which typically is represented by the sub-nodule.

The presence of glypican 3 uptake raises suspicion for malignancy. Further, a high-grade dysplastic lesion that is also beta-catenin-positive or shows diffuse glutamine synthetase uptake has a high likelihood of malignant progression and in such cases, early hepatocellular carcinoma cannot be excluded even if stromal invasion is not identified, in our opinion.

Hepatocellular Adenoma

Hepatocellular adenomas are vanishingly rare in cirrhotic livers and liver resection rather than transplantation is the usual surgical intervention. Therefore, they are not further considered in this discussion.

Early Hepatocellular Carcinoma

"Early hepatocellular carcinoma" (see Figure 10.18c and d) is one of two subdivisions of small HCC, i.e., a tumor less than 2 cm in diameter. Early HCC by definition shows stromal invasion, defined as "tumor cell invasion into the portal tracts or fibrous septa within vaguely nodular lesions" [54]. It also shows varying combinations of the following: a) increased cell density more than twice that of surrounding tissue with an increased nuclear to cytoplasmic ratio and irregular thin trabecular pattern; b) intratumoral portal tracts (helpful in evaluating stromal invasion); c) pseudoglandular pattern; d) diffuse fatty change; and e) varying numbers of unpaired arteries [54].

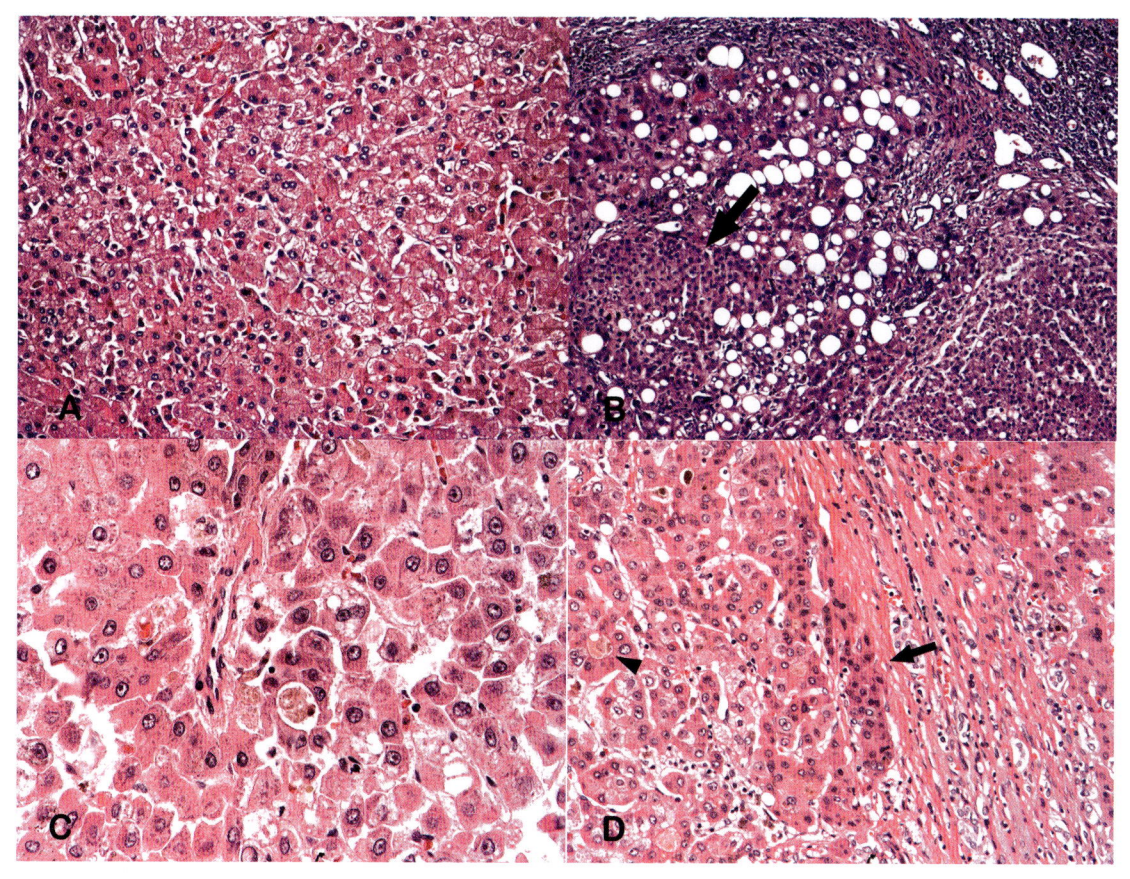

Figure 10.18 A) Low-grade dysplasia with mild increase in cell density (x20). B) High-grade dysplasia with more prominent alterations such as a nodule-in-nodule pattern (arrow) (x10). C) Early HCC. The criteria for diagnosis are listed in the text (x40). D) Early HCC with stromal invasion (arrow) and pseudogland formation (arrowhead) (x20).

Any of these features may also be individually found in high-grade dysplastic nodules, emphasizing the importance of stromal invasion to differentiate early HCC.

Diffuse positivity for any two of the three-stain combination of glypican 3, heat shock protein 70, and glutamine synthetase is considered to represent evidence of HCC [55]. Alpha-fetoprotein-positivity, if present, would lead to the same conclusion and uptake of glypican-3 would support the diagnosis. Cytokeratins 7 or 19 are useful in assessing stromal invasion (see Figure 10.19 A and B).

"Progressed" Hepatocellular Carcinoma

"Progressed" HCC is by definition less than 2 cm, but is distinctly nodular and generally represents a moderately differentiated hepatocellular carcinoma [54]. This form is not difficult to distinguish from the other above listed lesions. The features of hepatocellular carcinoma are considered in the following section discussing assessment of the explant liver.

Cancer in the Explant Organ

Reporting Requirments for HCC

As of 2013, the OPTN/UNOS requires each transplant center to report specific data derived from pathologic examination of liver explants from patients with MELD scores influenced by the presence of HCC. Pathologic evidence of HCC in the explant, either viable or nonviable, is reportable along with the number of tumors found. Annotation should be made as to whether or not the tumor was infiltrative, i.e., diffuse as opposed to well-defined. For example, so-called "cirrhotomimetic" HCC with innumerable small nodules indistinguishable in size from surrounding cirrhotic nodules would be considered infiltrative, whereas micro-penetration through one aspect of the tumor pseudo-capsule would not.

Additional variables are optional at this time, but may become required in the future. These include the macroscopic sizes of up to the five largest tumors, along with right/left lobe location and assessment regarding absent, incomplete or complete tumor necrosis, worst grade of tumor differentiation, and status of micro/macrovascular invasion. Presence or absence of satellite lesions is also targeted. A satellite lesion is defined as a tumor nodule less than 4 cm in diameter, less than 2 cm from the primary tumor, and less than 50% of the primary tumor diameter.

It is not the direct responsibility of the pathologist to report this to the OPTN/UNOS, but it is helpful to tailor the pathology report so that the clinical coordinators can easily gather the information. Since this data will be used to inform policy and

Malignancies of Transplantation

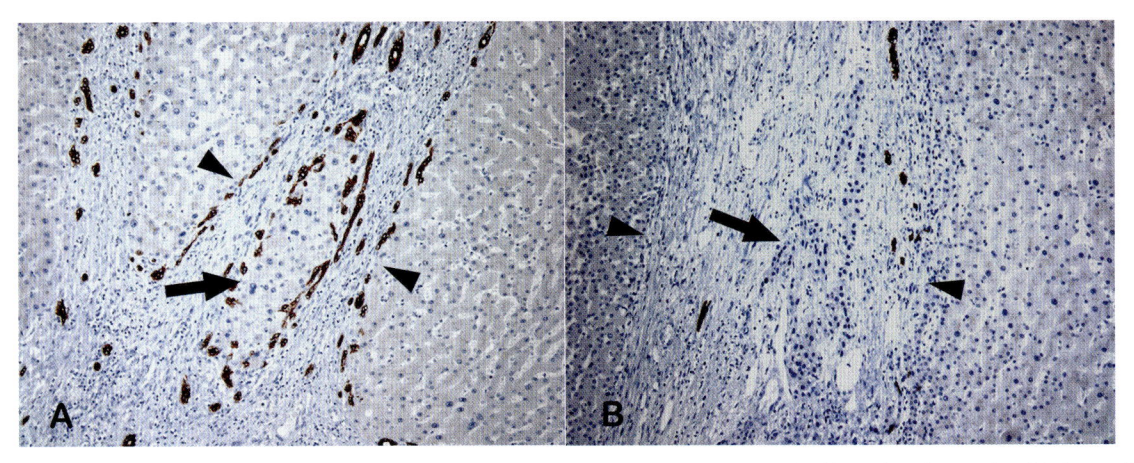

Figure 10.19 A) Pseudo-stromal invasion. Hepatocytes (arrow) may appear to be isolated within fibrous bands (arrowheads). CK19 will show a complete or nearly complete rim of ductular cells adjacent to fibrous regions (CK19 x10). B) In stromal invasion, malignant hepatocytes (arrow) directly infiltrate fibrous tissue (arrowheads) without this pattern (CK19 x10). (Slide courtesy of Eizaburo Sasatomi, M.D., Ph.D.).

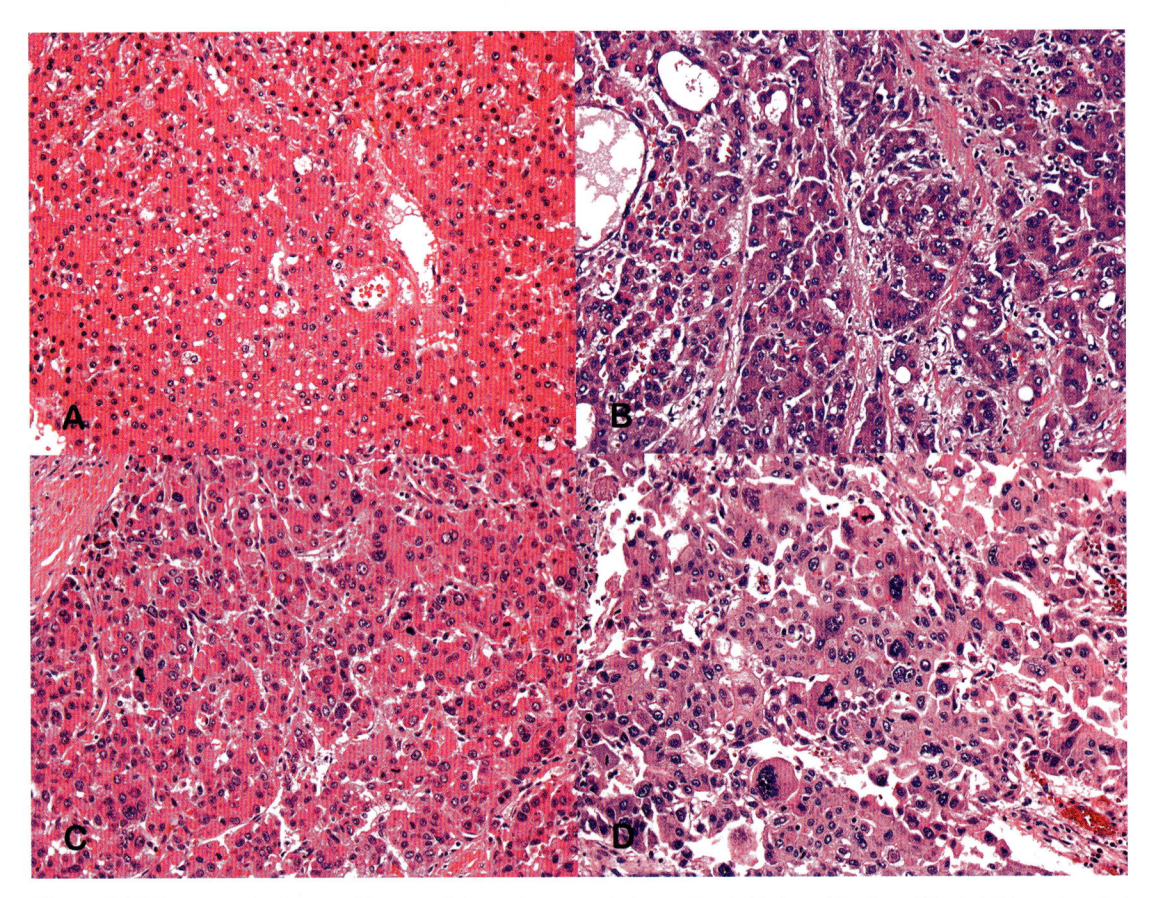

Figure 10.20 Representative images of hepatocellular carcinoma graded according to Ishak modification of the 1–4 Edmondson Steiner scale (see text for details). A) Grade 1. B) Grade 2. C) Grade 3. D) Grade 4 (all H&E x20).

maintain center compliance, accuracy and attention to detail are important.

Grading of Hepatocellular Carcinoma

Histologic grading of hepatocellular carcinoma has a statistically significant correlation with patient survival [56]. Most pathologists claim to use the classification of Edmondson and Steiner [57], but in fact, they are more likely to employ the later update of Ishak et al. [58] based exclusively on nuclear details. This approach is illustrated in Figure 10.20 and summarized as follows:

Grade 1 HCC contains cells with minimal nuclear irregularities and abundant cytoplasm, similar to hepatocellular adenoma. The diagnosis of HCC relies upon architectural features including trabecular abnormalities, pseudo-gland formation, and vascular invasion or metastatic disease. To this, we would

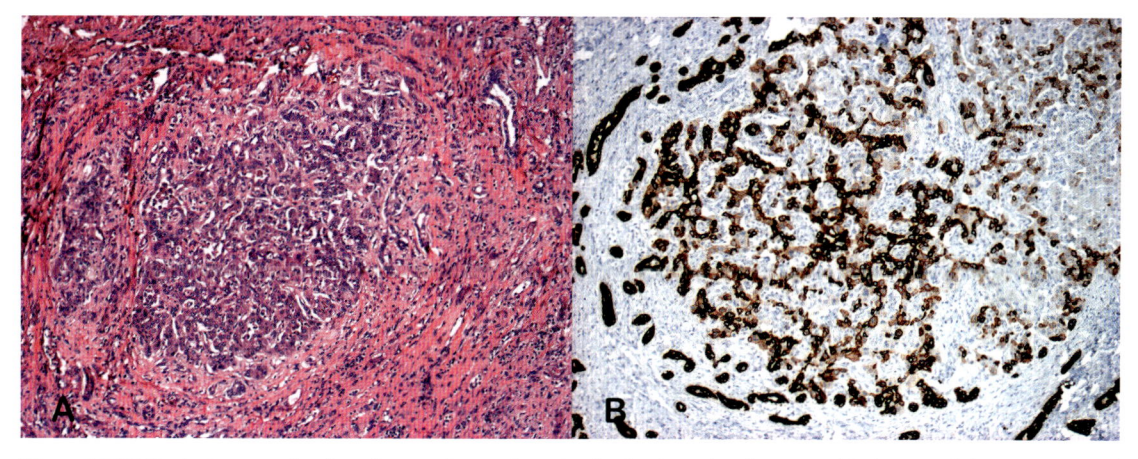

Figure 10.21 Atypical regenerative focus in area of parenchymal extinction in explant liver treated for hepatocellular carcinoma with radioactive microspheres. A) Atypical focus of regenerative ductular hepatocytes and ductules (x10). B) Immunostain with a biliary marker such as CK19 will confirm that these represent early attempts at parenchymal regeneration (CK19 x10).

add the presence of stromal invasion. In practice, HCC with Grade 1 features usually contains areas with more prominent cytologic abnormalities.

Grade 2 HCC shows more prominent nuclear hyperchromatism with fairly uniform round or ovoid nuclei and a mild but regular pattern of nuclear membrane irregularities. Grades 1 and 2 are often combined as Grade 1 when a three-grade system is used.

Grade 3 tumors have angulated nuclei with greater nuclear pleomorphism. The degree of atypia is distinctly higher than that of Grade 1 or 2 tumors and these can informally be considered as moderately or moderately-to-poorly differentiated HCC.

Grade 4 tumors show prominent nuclear pleomorphism and hyperchromatism and usually contain anaplastic giant cells. Multinucleated tumor cells without high-grade nuclear features would not be included in this category. Informally, the tumor appears to be a poorly differentiated to anaplastic carcinoma.

The Cancer Staging Manual of the AJCC, 7th edition [52], gives the option of using a two (2) grade, three (3) grade, or four (4) grade system. The number of grades in the system used at the individual center should be specified.

Effects of Ablation

Liver cancer transplant candidates may undergo tumor ablation procedures while on the wait list and the pathologist will encounter sequelae of this in the explant liver. Partial or complete necrosis of small tumors is the rule, and there is usually a rim of histiocytes beneath the tumor pseudocapsule, although on occasion ancillary stains may be necessary to exclude residual carcinoma.

Some forms of loco-regional ablation use therapeutic microspheres that preferentially accumulate in the tumor, but may also be seen within and outside of vascular branches, sometimes eliciting a foreign body response. In the case of radioactive microspheres, there can be a localized sinusoidal obstruction syndrome that evolves into parenchymal extinction with more prominent regional fibrosis and small regenerative nodules comprised of ductular hepatocytes (see Figure 10.21). It is necessary to be aware of this change, as the irregularity of these cells may suggest dysplasia or carcinoma, particularly if comparison to the original tumor cannot be made due to previous complete tumor destruction.

References

1 Engels EA, Pfeiffer RM, Fraumeni JF, Jr., et al. Spectrum of Cancer Risk among US Solid Organ Transplant Recipients. JAMA: The Journal of the American Medical Association. 2011;**306**:1891–901.

2 Miao Y, Everly JJ, Gross TG, et al. De novo Cancers Arising in Organ Transplant Recipients Are Associated with Adverse Outcomes Compared with the General Population. Transplantation. 2009;**87**:1347–59.

3 Murray JE, Wilson RE, Tilney NL, et al. Five Years' Experience in Renal Transplantation with Immunosuppressive Drugs: Survival, Function, Complications, and the Role of Lymphocyte Depletion by Thoracic Duct Fistula. Annals of Surgery. 1968;**168**:416–35.

4 Hanto DW, Frizzera G, Purtilo DT, et al. Clinical Spectrum of Lymphoproliferative Disorders in Renal Transplant Recipients and Evidence for the Role of Epstein-Barr Virus. Cancer Res. 1981;**41**:4253–61.

5 Frizzera G, Hanto DW, Gajl-Peczalska KJ, et al. Polymorphic Diffuse B-cell Hyperplasias and Lymphomas in Renal Transplant Recipients. Cancer Res. 1981;**41**:4262–79.

6 Starzl TE, Nalesnik MA, Porter KA, et al. Reversibility of Lymphomas and Lymphoproliferative Lesions Developing under Cyclosporin-steroid Therapy. Lancet. 1984;**1**:583–7.

7 Nalesnik MA, Jaffe R, Starzl TE, et al. The Pathology of Posttransplant Lymphoproliferative Disorders Occurring in the Setting of

Cyclosporine A-Prednisone Immunosuppression. American Journal of Pathology. 1988;133:173–92.

8. Knowles DM, Cesarman E, Chadburn A, et al. Correlative Morphologic and Molecular Genetic Analysis Demonstrates Three Distinct Categories of Posttransplantation Lymphoproliferative Disorders. Blood. 1995;85:552–65.

9. Swerdlow SH, Campo E, Harris NL, et al., editors. WHO Classification of Tumours of the Haematopoietic and Lymphoid Tissues. Lyon, France: IARC; 2008.

10. Dharnidharka VR, Tejani AH, Ho PL, et al. Post-transplant Lymphoproliferative Disorder in the United States: Young Caucasian Males Are at Highest Risk. American Journal of Transplantation: Official Journal of the American Society of Transplantation and the American Society of Transplant Surgeons. 2002;2:993–8.

11. Clarke CA, Morton LM, Lynch C, et al. Risk of Lymphoma Subtypes after Solid Organ Transplantation in the United States. British Journal of Cancer. 2013;109:280–8.

12. Dharnidharka VR, Lamb KE, Gregg JA, et al. Associations between EBV Serostatus and Organ Transplant Type in PTLD Risk: An Analysis of the SRTR National Registry Data in the United States. American Journal of Transplantation: Official Journal of the American Society of Transplantation and the American Society of Transplant Surgeons. 2012;12:976–83.

13. Manez R, Breinig MC, Linden P, et al. Posttransplant Lymphoproliferative Disease in Primary Epstein-Barr Virus Infection after Liver Transplantation: The Role of Cytomegalovirus Disease. The Journal of Infectious Diseases. 1997;176:1462–7.

14. Dharnidharka VR. Epidemiology of PTLD. In: Dharnidharka VR, Green M, Webber SA, editors. Post-Transplant Lymphoproliferative Disorders: Springer; 2010. p. 17–28.

15. Thorley-Lawson DA, Gross A. Persistence of the Epstein-Barr virus and the Origins of Associated Lymphomas. The New England Journal of Medicine. 2004;350:1328–37.

16. Young LS, Rickinson AB. Epstein-Barr Virus: 40 Years On. Nature Reviews Cancer. 2004;4:757–68.

17. Chijioke O, Azzi T, Nadal D, et al. Innate Immune Responses against Epstein Barr Virus Infection. Journal of Leukocyte Biology. 2013.

18. Aspord C, Laurin D, Richard MJ, et al. Induction of Antiviral Cytotoxic T Cells by Plasmacytoid Dendritic Cells for Adoptive Immunotherapy of Posttransplant Diseases. American Journal of Transplantation: Official Journal of the American Society of Transplantation and the American Society of Transplant Surgeons. 2011;11:2613–26.

19. Ning RJ, Xu XQ, Chan KH, et al. Long-term Carriers Generate Epstein-Barr Virus (EBV)-specific CD4(+) and CD8(+) Polyfunctional T-cell Responses which Show Immunodominance Hierarchies of EBV Proteins. Immunology. 2011;134:161–71.

20. Sherritt MA, Bharadwaj M, Burrows JM, et al. Reconstitution of the Latent T-Lymphocyte Response to Epstein-Barr Virus Is Coincident with Long-term Recovery from Posttransplant Lymphoma after Adoptive Immunotherapy. Transplantation. 2003;75:1556–60.

21. Kuppers R. B Cells under Influence: Transformation of B Cells by Epstein-Barr Virus. Nature Reviews Immunology. 2003;3:801–12.

22. Martinez OM, de Gruijl FR. Molecular and Immunologic Mechanisms of Cancer Pathogenesis in Solid Organ Transplant Recipients. American Journal of Transplantation: Official Journal of the American Society of Transplantation and the American Society of Transplant Surgeons. 2008;8:2205–11.

23. Morscio J, Dierickx D, Ferreiro JF, et al. Gene Expression Profiling Reveals Clear Differences between EBV-positive and EBV-negative Posttransplant Lymphoproliferative Disorders. American Journal of Transplantation: Official Journal of the American Society of Transplantation and the American Society of Transplant Surgeons. 2013;13:1305–16.

24. Rinaldi A, Capello D, Scandurra M, et al. Single Nucleotide Polymorphism-arrays Provide New Insights in the Pathogenesis of Post-transplant Diffuse Large B-cell Lymphoma. British Journal of Haematology. 2010;149:569–77.

25. Vakiani E, Basso K, Klein U, et al. Genetic and Phenotypic Analysis of B-cell Post-transplant Lymphoproliferative Disorders Provides Insights into Disease Biology. Hematological Oncology. 2008;26:199–211.

26. Harris NL, Ferry JA, Swerdlow SH. Posttransplant Lymphoproliferative Disorders: Summary of Society for Hematopathology Workshop. Seminars in Diagnostic Pathology. 1997;14:8–14.

27. George LC, Rowe M, Fox CP. Epstein-barr Virus and the Pathogenesis of T and NK Lymphoma: A Mystery Unsolved. Current Hematologic Malignancy Reports. 2012;7:276–84.

28. Tiede C, Maecker-Kolhoff B, Klein C, et al. Risk Factors and Prognosis in T-cell Posttransplantation Lymphoproliferative Diseases: Reevaluation of 163 Cases. Transplantation. 2013;95:479–88.

29. Jonigk D, Laenger F, Maegel L, et al. Molecular and Clinicopathological Analysis of Epstein-Barr Virus-associated Posttransplant Smooth Muscle Tumors. American Journal of Transplantation: Official Journal of the American Society of Transplantation and the American Society of Transplant Surgeons. 2012;12:1908–17.

30. Lee ES, Locker J, Nalesnik M, et al. The Association of Epstein-Barr Virus with Smooth-muscle Tumors Occurring after Organ Transplantation. The New England Journal of Medicine. 1995;332:19–25.

31. Ong KW, Teo M, Lee V, et al. Expression of EBV Latent Antigens, Mammalian Target of Rapamycin, and Tumor Suppression Genes in EBV-positive Smooth Muscle Tumors: Clinical and Therapeutic Implications. Clinical Cancer Research: An Official Journal of the American Association for Cancer Research. 2009;15:5350–8.

32. Chang Y, Cesarman E, Pessin MS, et al. Identification of Herpesvirus-like DNA Sequences in AIDS-associated Kaposi's Sarcoma. Science. 1994;266:1865–9.

33. Mesri EA, Cesarman E, Boshoff C. Kaposi's Sarcoma and Its Associated Herpesvirus. Nature Reviews Cancer. 2010;10:707–19.

34. Fukumoto H, Kanno T, Hasegawa H, et al. Pathology of Kaposi's Sarcoma-associated Herpesvirus Infection. Frontiers in Microbiology. 2011;2:175.

35. Barozzi P, Luppi M, Facchetti F, et al. Post-transplant Kaposi Sarcoma Originates from the Seeding of Donor-derived Progenitors. Nature Medicine. 2003;9:554–61.

36. Riva G, Barozzi P, Torelli G, et al. Immunological and Inflammatory Features of Kaposi's Sarcoma and Other Kaposi's Sarcoma-associated Herpesvirus/Human Herpesvirus 8-associated Neoplasias. AIDS Reviews. 2010;12:40–51.

37. Arora R, Chang Y, Moore PS. MCV and Merkel Cell Carcinoma: A Molecular

Success Story. Current Opinion in Virology. 2012;**2**:489–98.

38. Spurgeon ME, Lambert PF. Merkel Cell Polyomavirus: A Newly Discovered Human Virus with Oncogenic Potential. Virology. 2013;**435**:118–30.

39. Moore PS, Chang Y. Why Do Viruses Cause Cancer? Highlights of the First Century of Tumor Virology. Nature Reviews Cancer. 2010;**10**:878–89.

40. Connolly K, Manders P, Earls P, et al. Papillomavirus-associated Squamous Skin Cancers Following Transplant Immunosuppression: One Notch Closer to Control. Cancer Treatment Reviews. 2013.

41. Deligeoroglou E, Giannouli A, Athanasopoulos N, et al. HPV Infection: Immunological Aspects and Their Utility in Future Therapy. Infectious Diseases in Obstetrics and Gynecology. 2013;**2013**:540850.

42. Doorbar J. Papillomavirus Life Cycle Organization and Biomarker Selection. Disease Markers. 2007;**23**:297–313.

43. Moody CA, Laimins LA. Human Papillomavirus Oncoproteins: Pathways to Transformation. Nature Reviews Cancer. 2010;**10**:550–60.

44. Lewis JS, Jr. p16 Immunohistochemistry as a Standalone Test for Risk Stratification in Oropharyngeal Squamous Cell Carcinoma. Head and Neck Pathology. 2012;**6** Suppl 1:S75–82.

45. Penn I. Tumors Arising in Organ Transplant Recipients. Adv Cancer Res. 1978;**28**:31–61.

46. Penn I. The Problem of Cancer in Organ Transplant Recipients: An Overview. Transplant Sci. 1994;**4**:23–32.

47. Nalesnik MA, Woodle ES, Dimaio JM, et al. Donor-transmitted Malignancies in Organ Transplantation: Assessment of Clinical Risk. American Journal of Transplantation. 2011;**11**:1140–7.

48. Linder B, Hong Y, Jarrett T. Intra-renal Adrenal Adenoma: A Compelling Addition to the Differential Diagnosis of Renal Mass. International Journal of Urology: Official Journal of the Japanese Urological Association. 2009;**16**:912–4.

49. Bioulac-Sage P, Cubel G, Balabaud C, et al. Revisiting the Pathology of Resected Benign Hepatocellular Nodules Using New Immunohistochemical Markers. Seminars in Liver Disease. 2011;**31**:91–103.

50. Mazzaferro V, Regalia E, Doci R, et al. Liver Transplantation for the Treatment of Small Hepatocellular Carcinomas in Patients with Cirrhosis. The New England Journal of Medicine. 1996;**334**:693–9.

51. American Liver Tumor Study Group. A Randomized Prospective Multi-institutional Trial of Orthotopic Liver Transplantation or Partial Hepatic Resection with or without Adjuvant Chemotherapy for Hepatocellular Carcinoma. Investigators Booklet and Protocol. 1998.

52. Edge SB, Byrd DR, Compton CC, et al., editors. AJCC Cancer Staging Manual. 7th ed: Springer; 2010.

53. Bruix J, Sherman M, Practice Guidelines Committee AAftSoLD. Management of Hepatocellular Carcinoma. Hepatology (Baltimore, Md). 2005;**42**:1208–36.

54. International Consensus Group for Hepatocellular Neoplasia: The International Consensus Group for Hepatocellular N. Pathologic Diagnosis of Early Hepatocellular Carcinoma: A Report of the International Consensus Group for Hepatocellular Neoplasia. Hepatology (Baltimore, Md). 2009;**49**:658–64.

55. Bruix J, Sherman M, American Association for the Study of Liver D. Management of Hepatocellular Carcinoma: An Update. Hepatology (Baltimore, Md). 2011;**53**:1020–2.

56. Klintmalm GB. Liver Transplantation for Hepatocellular Carcinoma: A Registry Report of the Impact of Tumor Characteristics on Outcome. Annals of Surgery. 1998;**228**:479–90.

57. Edmondson HA, Steiner PE. Primary Carcinoma of the Liver: A Study of 100 Cases among 48,900 Necropsies. Cancer. 1954;**7**:462–503.

58. Ishak KG, Goodman ZD, Stocker JT, editors. Atlas of Tumor Pathology. Fascicle 31. Tumors of the Liver and Intrahepatic Bile Ducts. Washington, DC: American Registry of Pathology; 2001.

Chapter 11
Laboratory Medicine in Transplantation

Phillip Ruiz, Ana Hernandez, Emilio Margolles-Clark, Alexandra Amador, Valia Bravo, Jennifer McCue, and Casiana Fernandez-Bango

I The Histocompatibility Laboratory

Clinical laboratories offer highly specialized services that are essential for the clinical support of a transplant program. The histocompatibility laboratory provides a wide range of highly specialized clinical assays that allow for the analytical evaluation essential for the support of all transplant programs, both for solid organs and hematopoietic stem cell transplantation. In addition to the important role it plays in organ allocation, acceptance, and transplantation decision-making, the histocompatibility lab is intimately involved in the post-transplant monitoring and care of all transplant patients in an effort to facilitate both graft and recipient survival [1]. Moreover, the histocompatibility laboratory has the crucial responsibility of identifying and enabling reliable matching of HLA antigens between donor-recipient pairs of living donor transplant programs (both for related and unrelated donors), as well as for deceased unrelated donors. The advent of Kidney Paired Donation (KPD) [2, 3] in conjunction with desensitization programs [4] is revolutionizing renal transplantation by matching unrelated donors that are compatible when a designated living donor for a given recipient is incompatible. Center-specific, regional, and national KPD programs recognize and highlight the importance of a state of the art histocompatibility lab. They provide both the accurate, higher resolution molecular HLA typing and detailed allosensitization evaluation that guides proper organ allocation for this dynamic new field. In light of the increasing success of KPD programs and public awareness campaigns for transplantation, altruistic donation is becoming more accepted, allowing for regions and national "chains" of recipient-donor pairs, the largest with over 20 transplants occurring within a short time frame [5]. Throughout the entire process, the histocompatibility lab plays the primary role in ensuring that successful outcomes prevail [6].

The Human Leukocyte Antigen (HLA) Complex

The human Major Histocompatibility Complex (MHC), or HLA in humans, is composed of a group of genes that spans approximately 4.1 megabases and is located on the short arm of the chromosome 6 (6p21.3–22.2) (see Figure 11.1). There is extensive conservation of the human HLA region's genomic organization, gene sequence, and protein structure with the MHC of other mammals. More than 200 loci are included in this region and HLA regions are further subdivided into class I, class II, and class III regions, based upon their basic substructure. Class I and class II genes are the best characterized of the HLA complex.

Class I genes code for three globular domains, α1, α2, and α3, that comprise the heavy chain of the classical class I molecules known as HLA*A, HLA*B, and HLA*C [8]. These hetero-molecules also include a smaller non-covalently linked polypeptide, β-2 micro-globulin, which is encoded on chromosome 15 [9]. Class I HLA molecules are expressed on the membrane of most of the nucleated cells of the human body (see Figure 11.2). Their function is to present intracellular processed peptides, derived from protein synthesized in the cellular cytosol, to CD8+ cytotoxic T lymphocytes. This comprises the endogenous antigen presentation pathway. Additionally, the class I region encodes the non-classical genes HLA E, F, G, MICA and MICB, pseudogenes, and other genes with known and unknown functions.

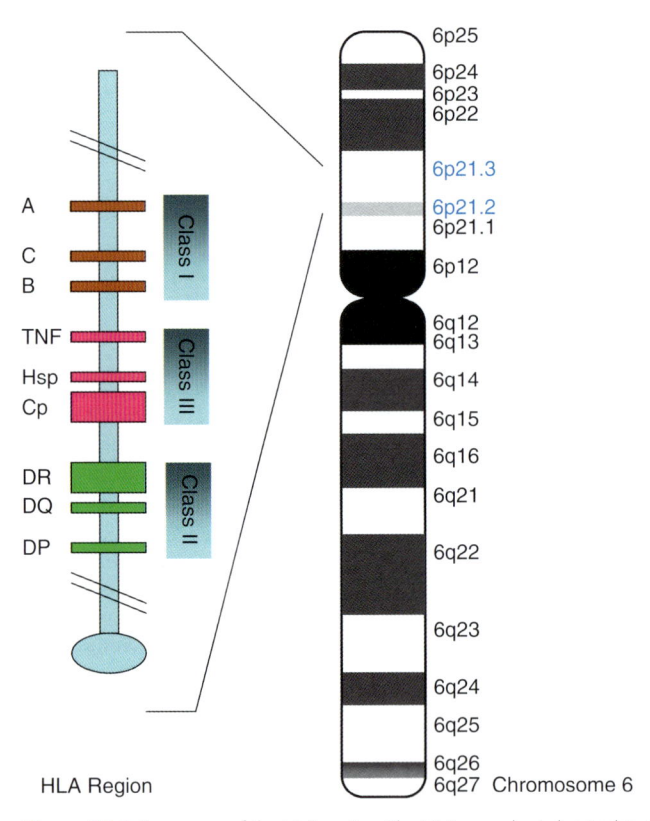

Figure 11.1 Gene map of the HLA region. The HLA complex is located in the chromosome 6. Class I, class II, and class III regions are shown. The relative positions of the genes encoding each region are represented by small boxes. Orange, pink, and green boxes show genes for classical class I, class III, and class II, respectively. Non-classical class I genes are represented in light orange.

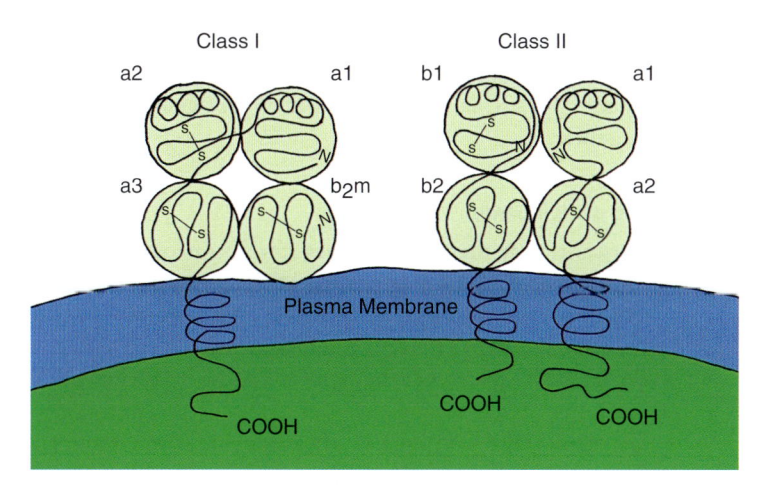

Figure 11.2 Schematic representation of the HLA molecules. HLA class I consists of a heavy chain (three globular domains, α1, α 2, and α 3), a transmembrane region, and a cytoplasmic tail. They are non-covalently associated to a β2-macroglobulin, which is the light chain. The HLA class II codes for two chains; α and β. Each chain has two extracellular domains (α 1 and α 2, and β 1 and β 2 respectively), a transmembrane region, and a cytoplasmic tail. S-S represents the disulfide bridges linking portions of each domain.

Class II HLA molecules code for genes of five molecules: HLA*DR, *DQ, *DP, *DM, and *DO. Each molecule has two α and β chains, and each of them has the same overall conformation consisting of two extracellular domains, α1 and α2, and β1 and β2 respectively [10] (see Figure 11.2). In contrast to class I, the class II HLA molecules are constitutively expressed on a more restricted range of cells, including antigen presenting cells (APC) such as dendritic cells, monocyte/macrophages, and B cells. In addition, expression can be upregulated in an inflammatory environment, i.e., activated T cells. These molecules present peptides derived from exogenous proteins contained in intracellular vesicles to CD4+ helper T cells, making up the exogenous presentation pathway.

It is well-established that HLA*A, *B, and *C class I molecules, in combination with HLA*DR, *DQ, and *DP class II molecules, play a key role in rejection of both solid organ allo-transplantation and stem cell transplantation. The role of non-classical class I HLA molecules in transplant rejection is not completely defined yet, but appears to have more limited involvement with transplant rejection events.

HLA class III genes are located between the class I and class II regions. Many of them have been directly or indirectly associated with the innate and acquired immune system, including complement molecules, tumor necrosis factor (TNF), lymphotoxin (LT), and Heat Shock Protein (HSP)-70. These molecules may be differentially expressed among the different cellular types, ranging from molecules highly expressed in many tissue types to others that are restricted to certain tissues or cell types.

The Role of the HLA Complex in Transplantation

The human Major Histocompatibility Complex (MHC), or HLA in humans, has one of the highest levels of polymorphism in the human genome and is critically involved in the immune response, disease defense, autoimmunity/neoplasia, and other disease susceptibility, in addition to variety of other physiological functions. The tremendous diversity or polymorphism in the number of HLA alleles presumably arose through evolution as a means to combat various infections and provide populations with heterogeneity and immune vigor. Due to the extensive genetic variability of the HLA genetic loci, the great majority of human transplantation combinations for donors and recipients will have some degree of MHC incompatibility between each other.

HLA proteins can be expressed at different levels and can be restricted to select cellular types. This phenomenon can translate into varying degrees of HLA molecule availability so that a transplanted organ (e.g., liver) may not be as immunogenic as another (e.g., kidney) for a particular donor-recipient pair. Regardless, a high level of HLA antigen compatibility or matching between the donor and recipient tends to augment the chances for a successful transplant acceptance by the recipient due to a lower level of immune response to the donor, which looks more like self than non-self. In contrast, the opposite scenario is true when there is a significant level of histocompatibility or mismatching. This makes MHC molecules the most important barriers in allo-transplantation within any species, as well as in xenotransplantation.

The cell membranes of each person express two different antigen molecules per HLA locus, one derived from the mother, the other from the father. An individual who is homozygous at an HLA locus inherited the same antigen molecule from both parents. Hence, the combination of ancestral alleles inherited by an individual is the result of the natural selection process and ultimately the phenotype and haplotype frequencies for HLA class I and class II that vary among different populations.

Adding to the complexity, the HLA region is inherited as a complete set of alleles or haplotypes due to strong linkage disequilibrium and the genes are characterized by a codominant expression where the incidence of some gene combinations are found more frequently than would be expected from existing gene frequencies in a population [7]. The degree of linkage disequilibrium varies within major ethnic and racial population groups such that certain combinations can be used to define the racial or ethnic origin of an individual. Additionally, not all HLA alleles show the same degree of linkage disequilibrium. These findings have strong implications when extensive matching of donor and recipient is essential, as in stem cell and most solid organ transplantation.

In general, cumulative mismatches at HLA*A, *B, *C, *DR, *DQ, and *DP are associated with poorer graft survival and will require more extensive immunosuppression. Thus, it is incumbent for a transplant program to be able to identify these major and, in many cases, minor mismatched differences and try to arrive at the best acceptable combination possible for the potential transplant recipient.

Allogeneic hematopoietic stem cell transplantation is a special case where the degree of HLA matching between the donor and the recipient is absolutely critical in order to minimize Graft-versus-Host Disease (GVHD) [11]. This condition occurs when the immune system of the graft (donor) recognizes the host (recipient) as foreign and attacks host cells. In this case, matching of donor with recipient at the allele level for at least the major loci (HLA*, HLA*B, HLA*C, and HLA*DRB1) is required and many programs match the HLA*DQB1 and HLA*DPB1 loci as well. Programs define the number of loci alleles matched and number of acceptable allele/antigen mismatches as part of their treatment algorithm with programs matching for HLA*A, B, C, and DRB1 considered as matching eight of eight possible alleles (8/8). Those that require DQB1 matching would be 10/10 and with DPB1, 12/12. Donors with more than one HLA allele/antigen mismatch as defined by the individual program are not acceptable due to the reported increased frequency of GVHD [11, 12].

Evolution of HLA Compatibility Assessment Techniques

Despite numerous advances in testing methods used to predict HLA compatibility between donor and recipient, their purpose remains the same: to provide a reliable assessment of the immunological risk for development of rejection/Graft-versus-Host Disease due to recognition of non-self HLA by the recipient/donor immune system. Initial techniques in the early 1960s only allowed discriminating between HLA identical, fully mismatched individuals and others. However, development of human T cell clones and molecular genetic techniques has led to a detailed understanding of the phenotypic polymorphism and diversity of HLA antigens [13]. Some centers still perform HLA typing and crossmatching by serological [14] and cellular assays. However, since the mid-1980s, more sensitive and specific tools such as molecular analysis and flow cytometry have been applied to pre-transplant HLA typing and crossmatching respectively [15, 16]. In addition, over the past two decades, a variety of highly sensitive and specific molecular-based assays have been developed for HLA typing. Currently, these are widely used and provide rapid and accurate HLA typing at low-resolution antigen level SSP PCR (single specific primer – polymerase chain reaction) typing as well as intermediate and high-resolution allele level typing sequence-specific oligonucleotide probes (SSOP PCR) and Sanger-based or Next Generation Sequencing (NGS) DNA sequencing respectively [17].

Despite the proven efficacy of these techniques for HLA typing, the latest implemented technologies such as NGS, together with the unprecedented progress of many data mining algorithms, will allow a reduction in the laborious nature of current techniques and reduce the time and the cost for histocompatibility testing. This topic will be discussed further in this chapter.

Typing of HLA Genes

Historically, two major techniques have been used for HLA typing: *serologic HLA typing* and more recently *molecular HLA typing*. The first technique is based on detection of the expressed phenotype of HLA proteins detected on cell surfaces, while the latter determines the genotype of the individual using DNA.

<u>Serologic HLA Typing.</u> As its name indicates, serologic typing requires a comprehensive group of antisera to encompass the broad variety of HLA specificities. In the past, these sera were usually prepared in the laboratory using multiparous female sera through differential adsorption and purification. Currently, monoclonal antibodies are regularly used and many antibodies to rare HLA types are commercially available. Serological HLA typing involves the use of these characterized antibodies and an individual's cells using a technique called the microlymphocytotoxicity assay [19]. The microlymphocytotoxicity assay uses lymphocytes as a cellular target to detect the expressed HLA proteins of an individual. The basis of this technique lies in the mixture of viable peripheral blood lymphocytes of the individual being typed with characterized antisera of known specificities. This cell-serum mixture is subsequently incubated with added rabbit complement, after which a vital dye is added. If specific antigen is present on the cell, antibody is bound, activating complement and damaging the cell membrane. Membrane damage results in cell permeability to the added vital dye and the reaction can be microscopically visualized. Typically a double stain (i.e., Ethidium Bromide and Acridine Orange) is used to allow simultaneous visualization of both living and dead cells. Since both T and B lymphocytes express class I antigens, either cell type or a mixture may be used for class I serological typing. However, B lymphocytes are required for class II serological typing since they express class II. Among the advantages of serological typing are the relative lack of required expensive equipment, simplicity to perform, and relatively quick results. However, the technique requires large volumes of blood and viable cells, with purity and viability greater than 90%. Moreover, it is very difficult to detect small differences in amino acids between the different HLA proteins that may be immunologically relevant and it is difficult to find antibodies to some rare HLA specificities.

Another significant drawback of this methodology is the cross-reactivity of HLA antigens and antisera that may cause the detection of "too many" antigens (i.e., more than two specific HLA antigens per locus) for an individual's HLA phenotype. Likewise, it is impossible to detect homozygosity at any locus and many individual typings will show these as a "blank" or unidentified type. While "blanks" may represent individuals truly homozygous for an HLA type at a particular locus, they could correspond to HLA types for which no antisera are present in the testing

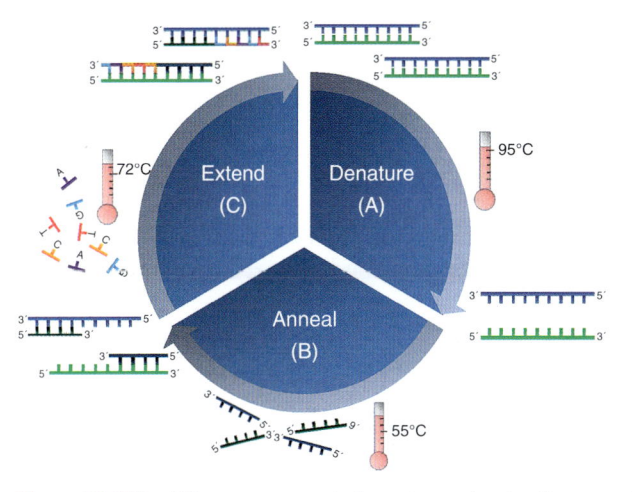

Figure 11.3 The PCR process occurs in three stages: denaturation, annealing, and extension. The process allows for millions of copies of a targeted area of DNA on the genome to be created. These targeted pieces of DNA allow for easier visualization of the DNA and/or to be utilized as a template for further testing, such as bead-based hybridization assays. (A) The first step of PCR is to *denature* the genomic DNA, breaking the hydrogen bonds of the complementary nucleotide bases. This is generally done by heating the sample to 95°C. (B) The second step of PCR is to *anneal* the targeted primers to the now single-stranded DNA. The primers are designed to bind to a specific location on the genomic DNA, allowing for targeted amplification of a region of interest. This is generally done by lowering the temperature of the reaction (the temperature for annealing is highly dependent on the primer and the targeted region, but generally are around 55°C. (C) The third step of the PCR reaction is to *extend* the DNA from the 3'-end of the primer. This rebuilding of the double-stranded DNA occurs at a slightly higher temperature (approximately 72°C) and with the presence of the nucleotides, a thermostable DNA polymerase, and buffers. This cycle then repeats multiple times, creating millions of copies of the region of interest.

panel or which are weakly expressed on the cell surface and cannot be detected using microcytotoxicity testing. For example, HLA C locus serologic typing is only able to detect certain antigen specificities (Cw1 through Cw7), while other specificities (Cw8 through Cw18) were not serologically detected. Today, we know that many "Cw blanks" were antigens that are now routinely tested for and reported.

Similar problems are found with serological typing for class II antigens. DR antigens, since more strongly expressed, can be typed with relative accuracy. However, DQ antigens are challenging, and many times, no clear typing can be obtained. The same scenario occurs with DRw antigens. As a result of these issues, serological typing is decreasing in its usage in HLA laboratories and is no longer accepted as a technique for HLA typing of donors by regulatory and professional organizations.

Molecular HLA Typing. The advent of PCR (see Figure 11.3) and the explosion of molecular biology in laboratory medicine have allowed the implementation of common molecular techniques for HLA typing. Currently, molecular-based HLA typing involves a group of techniques with different levels of resolution, ranging from low (antigen level) determination of HLA type to high-resolution discrimination of alleles found at a particular HLA locus – in other words, the varying degree to which either the antigen or allele found in a particular locus is identified. High-resolution HLA typing definitively identifies both alleles residing at a given locus, with certain caveats. Intermediate resolution typing lies between allele level typing and antigen level-low resolution typing, narrowing the allele string to fewer choices. Low-resolution typing is considered the same as original serologic typing and provides definition of the broad antigen found at a particular locus. Solid organ transplant programs can generally operate with low-resolution typing, although with the advent of well-defined antibody specificities, it is often necessary to perform higher resolution HLA typing with solid organ recipient-donor pairs. By comparison, stem cell transplantation programs demand the accuracy of high-resolution typing to minimize Graft-versus-Host Disease and promote long-term graft survival [20].

Four general steps are involved in molecular HLA typing: 1) isolation of the genomic DNA from nucleated cells; 2) PCR amplification of the region to be typed; 3) analysis of the PCR product either by gel electrophoresis, probe hybridization, or sequencing; and 4) interpretation of results.

Isolation of genomic DNA is performed using chaotropic salts, detergents, and proteolytic enzymes. These agents disrupt both the cellular and nuclear membrane releasing the super-coiled DNA. These agents also lyse and disrupt histone proteins that keep DNA in a super helix. Ethanol is added to the mixture, making the DNA sticky. The solution can be applied to a column or other solid matrix, the DNA sticks to the column, and the cell waste is centrifuged or vacuumed away. This is followed by a high-salt/ethanol wash and a low-salt/ethanol wash. Purified DNA is eluted with an aqueous solution. Solutions must be basic since acid solutions or water will hydrolyze the DNA. Commercial reagents based on individual matrix capture columns, magnetic beads, and/or fully automated systems are currently available. Although the use of these reagents can increase the cost per extraction, they significantly decrease the time and labor associated with the procedure and higher costs can be offset with higher throughput capabilities.

Molecular techniques were initially applied to HLA typing in 1987. At that time, the Southern Blot technique was used to identify *restriction fragment length polymorphisms (RFLPs)* associated with known serological DR/DQ and cellular Dw defined specificities. Each HLA allele or group of alleles has unique restriction enzyme cleavage patterns. This feature was used to determine the HLA typing. This method was cumbersome and had various disadvantages and is no longer in use. It was impossible to discriminate all of the class II alleles with this technique, and for class I, it was even more impractical due to the extremely complex patterns that resulted. The technique was also very costly, due to the large number of restriction enzymes required.

The introduction of the polymerase chain reaction (PCR) in the 1990s [21] allowed a remarkable enhancement to the histocompatibility laboratory's ability to detect new HLA alleles, as well as to better characterize those already known. Some of these are described below.

Sequence–specific Primers (SSP): Typing is based on the amplification of alleles at a locus using allele-specific primers [15]. Within the primer pair, one primer is specific to an area

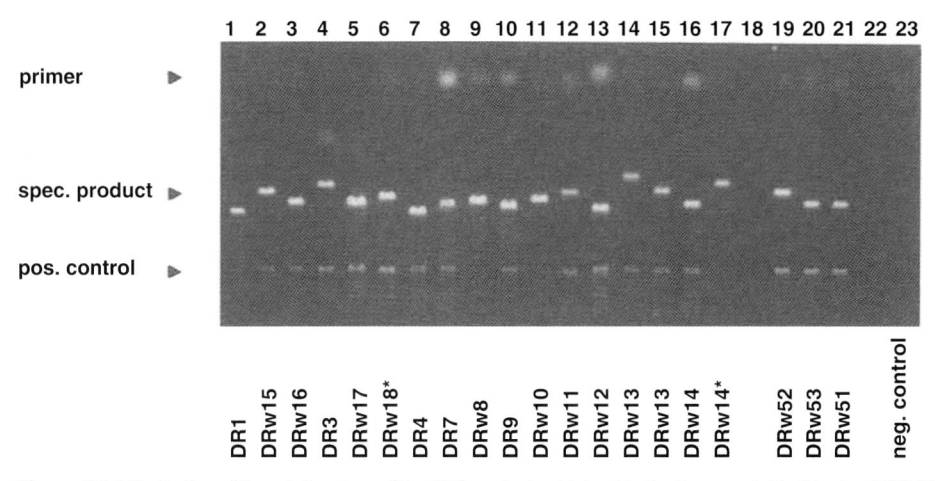

Figure 11.4 Illustration of the relative sizes of the PCR products obtained in the "low-resolution" typing (PCR-SSP) for the locus HLA-DR. PCR products are detected by agarose gel electrophoresis, where they are separated according to their fragment sizes. The lengths of the allele- and group-specific PCR products are visualized with ethidium bromide staining. Each PCR reaction includes an internal positive control primer (pos. control). PCR reaction mixtures containing primer pairs identifying allelic variants of DRB1 corresponding to the serologically defined series DR1-DRw18 (spec. product) are size separated in lines 1 to17. The external positive control reactions assigning the DRw52, DRw53, and DRw51 groups of alleles are in lines 19, 20, and 21, respectively. The negative amplification control is in line 23. Lines 18 and 23 are empty lines.* Denotes that the primer mix will amplify alleles belonging to more than one serological defined specificity.

conserved across many alleles (conserved primer), while the second primer is specific for a one-base pair difference that defines a specific allele. If the 3' end of the second primer binds to the complementary base in the target, primer extension occurs and a specific-size amplicon is produced. No amplification means a specific allele is not present. Product detection is usually via agarose gel electrophoresis with ethidium bromide staining (see Figure 11.4). SSP assays always include housekeeping gene control primers, at a much lower concentration, to demonstrate amplification efficiency for each reaction. If the control primer amplifies and the specific primer does not, the specific allele is ruled out.

The inherent advantage of using multiple primer sets to type for many alleles at a locus brought about different typing strategies. Currently, many SSP primers pairs are loaded on 96 well plates and when patient DNA is added, the electrophoretic pattern produced by the amplicon provides typing of several loci at one time. Currently, trays for low=resolution (antigen level) typing for class I (HLA*A, B, and C) or class II (HLA*DR, DQ, DRw) can be used to give accurate results for all six reported HLA loci in approximately four hours. Alternatively, SSP can resolve alleles at high-resolution levels (HR SSP), so a multiple reaction tray to define all alleles for A2 can also be used. Due to its manual nature, inability to automate or run multiple patients, and high reagent costs, SSP as a primary typing method is expensive and should be reserved when speed is necessary, as in cadaveric donor typing situations, or when ambiguity resolution is required, as when cis/trans ambiguities are encountered in sequence-based typing. Also, the technique requires large amounts of DNA, sometimes up to 500 nanograms. Therefore, the assay is not suitable for programs that type large numbers of patients. However, this is a well-established and reliable assay that can be performed rapidly with accurate and reproducible results.

Sequence-specific Oligonucleotide Probe (SSOP) Typing: Distinguishes the alleles using oligonucleotide DNA probes that bind complementary sequences unique for each allele when hybridized with PCR products amplified from the patient DNA and primers for the HLA locus being typed. PCR products are labeled with fluorescent primers or unlabeled, depending on the particular use. Variants of this technique include immobilization of either the probe (reverse SSO) or amplified patient DNA strands (SSO). DNA immobilization can be on filter paper, strips, or Luminex beads. Dot blot assays have immobilized amplified product with application of labeled probes, while slot blot assays have labeled probes added in a line over fixed product [22]. In the reverse probe hybridization assays, the probe is immobilized and the amplified target is labeled [22, 23]. SSOP probe hybridization steps use high stringency hybridization conditions. If the patient's DNA sequence matches the informative probe, it will bind in high stringency conditions. If mismatches exist, it will either not bind or be easily removed with washing under low-salt (high stringency) conditions. The labeled probes/amplicons are visualized using a reporter substrate to highlight where hybridization has occurred. For strip assays, using a template guide and a computer algorithm that resolves the individual's typing scores the result. Currently, SSOP typing utilizes probes bound to the polystyrene beads used in Luminex technology. Luminex SSOP HLA typing can be semi-automated and batching of many patients is possible, so high throughput can evaluate large numbers of samples. A 96 well PCR plate can simultaneously test 95 patients for a single locus. Six PCR plates are required to test all commonly typed loci. Results are scored using a program where positive beads are scored to resolve the individuals' HLA typing [24]. It can be performed in about four to six hours, depending on the number of samples tested. The resolution of the technique is considered intermediate because typing obtained is above the antigen level

DNA
↓
PCR Amplification
↓
Visualization of the Amplicons
↓
Enzymatic Amplicon Cleanup
↓
Cycle Sequencing Reaction
↓
Capillary Electrophoresis
in Genetic Analyzer
↓
Data Analysis

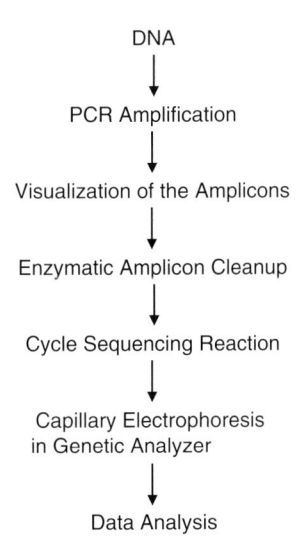

Figure 11.5 Sanger sequencing methodology. A high quality DNA is used for PCR amplification of each HLA locus. Presence of amplicons is visualized in gel electrophoresis following by enzymatic amplicon cleanup (ExoSAP-It). After product cleanup, forward and reverse sequencing primers for exons 2, 3, and 4 for class I (A, B, or C) loci, or exons 2 and 3 for DQB1 and \DRB1, are run using a short PCR protocol (cycle sequencing reaction) with fluorescently labeled bases. They are read on a genetic analyzer, a capillary electrophoresis instrument capable of detecting the multicolor fluorescent signals. The resultant sequence is analyzed using a program designed to identify HLA alleles that assign type by comparing to a known allele sequence.

obtained with SSP. Sometimes, SSOP will yield high-resolution results at certain loci, especially DQ typing [25]. SSOP can be combined with high-resolution SSP for additional resolution. It is important to mention that success of this technique depends on the quality of the DNA used, the degree of redundancy of the primers, and the technical proficiency of the laboratory analyst that performs the testing. It can be used as an adjunct to high-resolution typing strategies to rule out alleles that are not found. Its drawback is that additional probe sequences may be required to rule out new alleles as they are found and characterized.

Sequence-based Typing (SBT): Historically used Sanger sequencing methodology in the identification of MHC alleles found at particular loci for high-resolution HLA typing [20]. As with all DNA-based assays, isolation of high quality DNA is necessary, particularly for stem cell transplant patients who may have received chemotherapy, since inhibitors can cause sequencing reactions to fail. PCR amplification of each locus yields one or two large amplicons, some larger than one KB. Gel visualization of amplicon presence should be performed before proceeding with subsequent downstream steps. Enzymatic amplicon cleanup (ExoSapIt) is extremely important since "dirty" products can produce unreadable sequence products. After product cleanup, forward and reverse sequencing primers for exons 2, 3, and 4 for class I A, B, or C loci, or exons 2 and 3 for DQB1 and now DRB1, are run using a short PCR protocol (Cycle sequencing reaction) with fluorescently labeled bases. Cycle sequencing products are ethanol precipitated, washed, re-suspended, and formamide denatured. They are read on a genetic analyzer, a capillary electrophoresis instrument capable of detecting the multicolor fluorescent signals, and the resultant sequence is analyzed using a program designed to identify HLA alleles that assign type by comparing to a known allele sequence (see Figure 11.5). Several companies sell complete kits with most or all reagents. Currently, one company has obtained FDA approval for the technique and sells reagents as IVD. Although more laborious than SSOP, SBT by Sanger can produce high-resolution typing with reasonable throughput. One of the advantages of this technology is the possibility to detect new alleles. A drawback is that cis/trans ambiguous combinations cannot be resolved without further testing. This may require additional ambiguity resolution primers that will hybridize only to one or the other allele in a pair and give the base call needed to resolve the ambiguity. Another technique is to use HR-SSP trays that contain primers that will resolve these ambiguities.

Sequence-based Typing by Next Generation Sequencing (NGS): Sanger sequencing HLA typing has been the gold standard for high-resolution sequencing for more than 20 years. Very recently, Next Generation Sequencing (NGS) has opened a new frontier for DNA sequencing and is quickly becoming the new paradigm adopted for clinical implementation of high-resolution HLA typing. The NGS methodology combines molecular biology techniques and in-situ amplification of DNA with advanced microfluidics, digital signal detection instrumentation, and software development to allow massive parallel sequencing generating millions of reads. The assembly and alignment of these reads to a reference DNA renders reliable DNA sequences of long genomic regions.

Several NGS platforms have been developed for short and long reads, each of them utilizing different approaches to sequencing. Short read sequencing methods utilize two strategies; sequencing by ligation and sequencing by synthesis [28]. The two more commonly used NGS platforms for HLA typing fall in the category of short reads sequencing by synthesis; one developed by Ion Torrent (Thermo Fisher) and the other by Illumina, Inc. The Ion Torrent technology is based on detection of pH changes produced by the release of H^+ during DNA synthesis [29]. The synthesis process is carried out in a semiconductor chip containing millions of micro-wells, and in each well, a microsphere with a single DNA fragment attached clonally amplified *in-situ*. The instrument detects this massively parallel pH changes in each individual well and directly translates this chemically encoded information into digital information [30]. The principle of the Illumina technology is similar to Sanger sequencing, which is defined by the addition of dideoxy nucleotides (ddNTPs) in the sequencing reaction to stop DNA synthesis. The Illumina technology uses terminator dNTPs where the 3'-OH group is modified to prevent synthesis, but the modification is chemically reversible [31]. The sequencing process starts with a DNA template and a primer bound to the complementary region. The synthesis is initiated by adding polymerase and dNTPs, each labelled with a different fluorophore and 3'-blocked. After a single dNTP is incorporated, the unbound dNTPs are washed off and fluorescence is imaged. Then both fluorophore and blocking group are chemically removed, leaving the template ready for a new synthesis cycle. Before beginning sequencing cycles in the

Laboratory Medicine in Transplantation

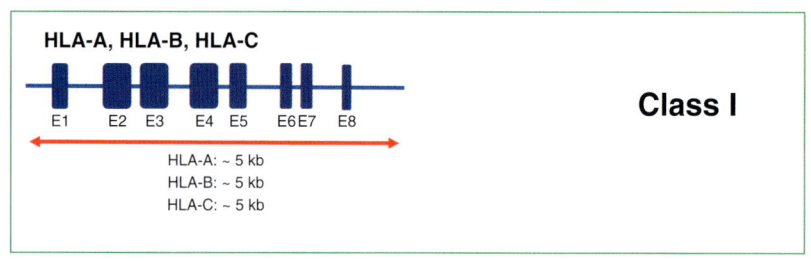

Figure 11.6 Coverage of HLA genes of class I and class II by NXType Next Generation Sequencing assays developed by OneLambda (ThermoFisher). Modified from the NXType product description on the One Lambda website.

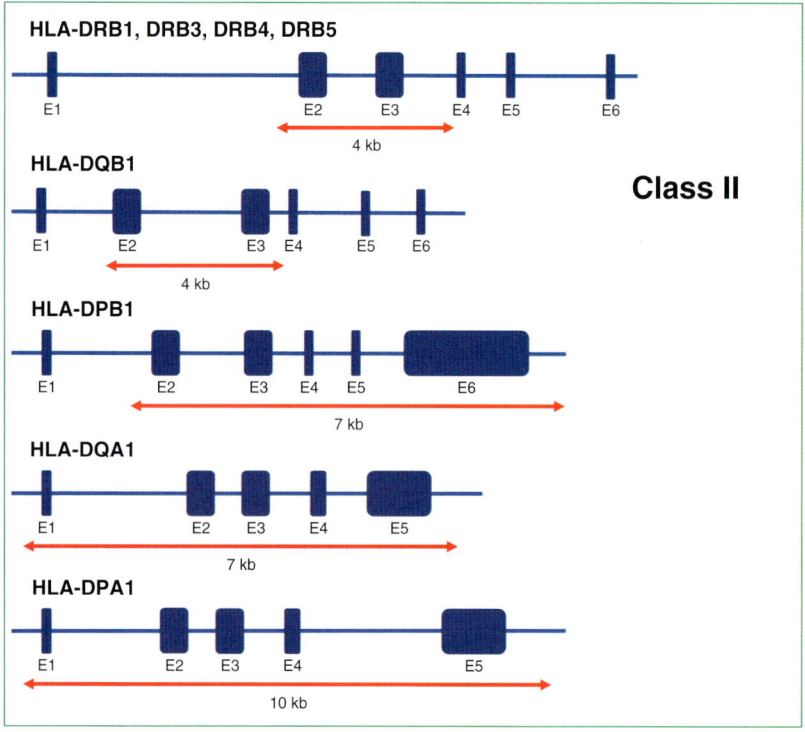

instrument, the templates are clonally amplified by solid-phase bridge amplification to increase signal output. This process starts by adding denatured templates containing two adapters (one at each end) to a flow cell that has two attached primers complementary to the adapters. The strands are captured by one primer and a polymerase synthesizes the complementary strand from this primer. The double strand is denatured and the original strand removed. The free end of the synthesized strand can interact with the other primer nearby, forming a bridge structure. Using PCR, the bridge amplification is carried out creating a cluster of the same template, and millions are created through the surface of the flow cell [32].

Regardless of the NGS platform, the current workflow for HLA typing requires i) library preparation which includes amplification of target genes from each sample, random fragmentation and attachment of adapter primers with a unique identifier or barcode, secondary amplification, and pooling of individual sample libraries; ii) template preparation by clonal amplification of fragments; and iii) sequencing and data analysis. The library preparation process is automatable and various liquid handler platforms have been adapted for this purpose. In the case of Ion Torrent technology, the template preparation and chip loading is fully automated using the Ion Chef system [33]. In the case of Illumina, Inc., the clonal amplification of templates occurs on the cell flow in the sequencer cell as part of the sequencing process.

Amplification of HLA genes has been particularly difficult because of the high levels of sequence homology between genes and pseudogenes present in the chromosome. The NGS HLA genotyping uses long-range PCR to acquire sufficient specific target genes from the specimen in question. Advances in primer design have allowed the development of multiplexing powerful primers to amplify large regions or entire genes (e.g., UTRs, exons and introns of all class I genes), significantly increasing gene coverage (see Figure 11.6). This is a great step forward compared to Sanger-based HLA typing that covers only key exons. In addition to large coverage, NGS renders continuous sequences of individual chromosomes generating ultra-high resolution (e.g. A*02:01:01:01/A*29:01:01:01). More importantly, this solves the vast majority of genotyping ambiguities previously unsolvable by Sanger typing, reducing the need for reflexing testing (e.g., SSP, GSSP, or Ambisolv). Furthermore, increase in coverage has revealed an increasing number of new alleles both in coding and non-coding regions with potential clinical relevance. The introduction of unique identifiers for each sample permits multiplexing of many samples, as well as several target regions in a single run, increasing greatly the through-put and reducing costs per sample (e.g., OneLambda NXType kit up to 96 samples and Illumina TruSight HLA v2 kit up to 24 samples). Software specifically developed for HLA typing automatically assembles the sequence of each targeted HLA gene using hundreds of thousands of sequencing reads and segregates each "barcoded" sample. The software also makes HLA typing calls for each locus comparing to known databases, which dramatically reduces time-consuming analyses of medical technologists.

The utility of NGS in the clinical laboratory is not limited to high-resolution HLA typing. The massive sequencing capacity together with the sensitivity, flexibility, and high throughput of the technology permits development of NGS-based clinical tests that are quickly being adopted. The scope includes custom genotyping tests for individual genes relevant to transplantation, like the APOL1 gene variants G1 allele (c.1024A>G (p.Ser342Gly, rs73885319), and c.1152 T>G (p.Ile384 Met, (rs60910145)) and G2 allele (c.1164_1169delTTATAA (rs71785313)), that are directly associated with specific forms of kidney diseases [34], as well as commercially available and custom panels designed for genotyping large groups of genes. Many current PCR- and RT-PCR-based tests are being actively transferred to NGS-based tests. For example, the PCR-based HID by STR test used to detect donor chimerism analyzes 16 markers. In comparison, the Ion-Torrent NGS HID test includes 165 autosomal markers and 24 samples can be multiplexed in one single run [35]. Furthermore, the use of NGS technology extends to gene expression profiling much like the RT-PCR approach, with the difference that NGS allows targeting tens of thousands of genes in a single reaction with minimal input RNA. This, together with the ability to multiplex samples in a single run and software developed for straightforward analysis, offers an affordable alternative method to examine large numbers of targets in large number of samples.

High-resolution allele-level HLA typing is a requirement for hematopoietic stem cell transplantation, since it has been reported that HLA compatibility is one of the most critical factors that affects recipient survival for this type of transplant. Initially, high-resolution typing meant that only two alleles, maternal and paternal, for each HLA locus typed were reported. With the finding and recording of ever more alleles, the probability that ambiguities will arise that need resolution also increased. The cost of resolving alleles to the initial definition of high-resolution would become astronomical, since more and more rule-outs would be required. In 2007, an international group of investigators published a landmark paper that analyzed all HLA alleles recognized for all typed loci and identified them as common alleles, well-documented alleles, and rare alleles [36]. Common alleles were found with a specified frequency in the population. Well-documented alleles must have been found at least three different times by different investigators in unrelated individuals. All the rest were defined as rare alleles. This definition of alleles brought about a new meaning for high-resolution HLA typing and in 2009, the National Marrow Donor Program (NMDP) in the U.S. issued its definition and criteria for high-resolution HLA typing based on the definition of common and well-documented alleles. It is important to note that there are problems with strict adherence to the CWD analysis for issuing high-resolution results. It did not take into account the fact that allele frequencies can vary in certain populations that may make non-required allele rule-outs a necessity as populations are further characterized. In 2013, a new analysis of the CWD list was issued [37] since the number of identified alleles has almost doubled in some loci. The NMDP is currently analyzing the new data and new guidelines are pending at this time. In the future, these limitations may be solved with the incorporation of next-generation sequencing technology, since single chromosomes are completely characterized and rule-outs will be unnecessary.

Special Considerations for Serologic Parent versus Split Antigens

As serologic HLA typing gained sophistication, more specific antisera were obtained using adsorption and elution and additional HLA specificities were defined. Historically, HLA antigens were defined taking into account the interactions between molecules based on the recognition of epitopes. The advent of more specific sera and eventually monoclonal antisera revealed that what were thought of as being one antigen by initial serological typing methods were actually groups of antigens with common epitopes. This process was called "splitting," since initial specificities were "split" into different antigens (e.g., A9 split into A23 and A24, A28 split into A68 and A69). The original antigen would be considered the "parent" antigen of these split specificities. Table 11.1 shows some examples of these splits.

Special Consideration for HLA Typing and Nomenclature Used in Solid Organ Transplantation: It is well-known that the correlation between serological and molecular nomenclature of HLA alleles is not always accurate. Since June of 2010, HLA typing of diseased donors in the U.S. was designated to be performed using molecular HLA typing. Since the HLA type in solid organ transplantation is still defined using serologic nomenclature, strict guidelines for assignment of serologic type are required when only molecular HLA typing is performed. In the U.S., the use of common nomenclature conventions for HLA typing is clearly defined and mandated by the Organ Procurement Transplantation Network (OPTN) policies. It is critical for the physician to be aware of which nomenclature is used by the HLA laboratory, whether molecular or serological. Table 11.1 provides a list with common HLA alleles with dissimilar serologic and molecular nomenclatures. Hence, communication with the HLA laboratory is essential to avoid errors in HLA typing assignment and erroneous recognition of donor-specific antibodies (DSA) due to these discrepancies. This problem does not involve stem cell transplantation, since serologic typing is not used and only high-resolution HLA typing is considered.

A particular case of nomenclature complications may occur for class II HLA molecules [38], since serologic nomenclature for these refers only to typing of class II beta chains. Serologic typing does not take into account the class II alpha chains, and as such, these important molecules cannot be reported using

Table 11.1 Broad Serological List of Splits

Original Broad Specificities	Splits and Associated Antigens
A2	A203, A210#
A9	A23, A24, A2403#
A10	A25, A26, A34, A66
A19	A29, A30, A31, A32, A33, A74
A24	A2403#
A28	A68, A69
B5	B51, B52, B5102#, B5103#
B7	B703#
B12	B44, B45
B14	B64, B65
B15	B62, B63, B75, B76, B77
B16	B38, B39, B3901#, B3902#
B17	B57, B58
B21	B49, B50, B4005#
B22	B54, B55, B56
B27	B2708#
B39	B3901#, B3902#
B40	B60, B61
B51	B5101#, B5103#
B70	B71, B72
Cw3	Cw9, Cw10
DR1	DR103#
DR2	DR15, DR16
DR3	DR17, DR18
DR5	DR11, DR12
DR6	DR13, DR14, DR1403#, DR1404#
DR14	DR1403#, DR1404#
DQ1	DQ5, DQ6
DQ3	DQ7, DQ8, DQ9
Dw6	Dw18, Dw19
Dw7	Dw11, Dw17

\#: associated antigens.

serology nomenclature. DQA antibodies have now been identified [39] and can be clinically relevant (i.e., DSA) in certain cases [40]; in these cases, only molecular nomenclature is used.

Finally, the clinician should be informed of the amount of mismatches considered and reported by the HLA laboratory, taking into consideration that up to 18 mismatches can be considered if typing of loci HLA-A, B, C, DRB1, DRB3/4/5, DQB1, DQA1, DPA1, and DPB1 is performed. Nevertheless, the most common approach considers only six antigen mismatches at loci HLA-A, B, C, DRB1, DRB3/4/5, and DQB1. The matching algorithm for UNOS Kidney and Kidney/Pancreas is currently based on matching of antigens for HLA*A, B, and DRB1 with added significance, and matching "points" for DRB1 matches.

Other PCR-based Techniques

Amplification refractory mutation system (ARMS) uses sequence-specific PCR primers; therefore, it is a special SSP. These primers allow amplification of DNA only if the sample contains the target allele. Hence, the presence or absence of the specific PCR product defines the presence or absence of the target allele. ARMS is able to detect any mutation involving single base change. Two different variations of the technique have been used; the first one tests the sample for a single mutation while multiplex ARMS variants are used for the analysis of two or more mutations.

Other PCR techniques are based on conformational modifications that determine the differential migration patterns which are resolved by electrophoresis. *Single strand conformational polymorphism (PCR-SSCP)* is based on the difference in conformational structure of the DNA encoding the HLA molecules even when a single nucleotide changes. In this case, DNA is denatured and rapidly cooled in order to minimize re-naturation, allowing the DNA molecule to adopt a specific secondary conformation. Hence, PCR-SSCP is suitable to detect minor nucleotide mutations between wild and mutant genes. *Heteroduplex analysis (PCR-HA)* is another technique where the single DNA molecule is allowed to cool in a gradual manner. The re-naturation process promotes the formation of homo- and hybrid-DNA double strands. These homo- and heteromolecules migrate differently. Usually, heteromolecules exhibit a delayed migration compared to the homomolecules due to incomplete hybridization.

Interestingly, both of these techniques have been used with crossmatching purposes. In these instances, the DNA of the patient and the potential donor are run at the same time. If the migration patterns are equal, it can be considered that both individuals have identical HLA type.

Donor Chimerism Analysis

An important molecular technique used in the histocompatibility laboratory is *Short tandem repeat (STR)* microsatellite testing for determination of donor chimerism [41]. It is well-established that at well-characterized microsatellite loci, the number of times certain short DNA sequences are repeated is different for individuals in the general population. Modern STR analysis groups many of these polymorphic loci (markers), whose repeat numbers (marker alleles) are known for many populations, into an easy-to-perform and sensitive assay to identify an individual genotype. STR analysis forms the basis of modern Human Identity Determination (HID) techniques today. This technique and these polymorphic loci are used around the world in forensic DNA testing. Therefore, not only is information widely available on the use of these STR loci, but there have been several ready-to-use kits that have been optimized to identify low-level mixtures in many sample types. In the transplant lab, these reagents or kits are instrumental in allowing the evaluation of the presence or absence of a post-transplant chimeric state in several different sample types. This testing can be performed on any biological specimen that contains DNA. Currently, testing of peripheral blood, bone marrow aspirates, fresh tissue, and formalin-fixed paraffin-embedded tissue biopsies are routinely performed; however, future applications of this technology may include testing urine, feces, or even hair.

Monitoring the chimeric state of patients post-hematopoietic stem cell transplantation has become routine. The post HSCT transplant patient should have the donor STR genotype in both the peripheral blood and bone marrow aspirate. The presence of recipient genotype in these samples can mean either graft loss or neoplastic disease recurrence.

Monitoring patients after certain solid organ transplants has also shown to be extremely informative for the physicians treating post-intestinal, multivisceral, or even liver patients. In the transplant of highly immunogenic organs, such as the intestines, Graft-versus-Host Disease (GVHD) is always a concern. One more tool in the physician's toolbox for monitoring post-transplant patients is chimerism analysis screening for the presence of donor genotype in the patient peripheral blood. The presence of donor genotype is indicative of the presence of donor white blood cells, indicating possible GVHD.

Since individual marker patterns are unique, pre-transplant analysis of recipient and donor DNA allows assignment of their unique marker/allele patterns. Subsequent post-transplant analysis facilitates the determination and proportion of DNA derived from donor, versus DNA derived from the recipient. The quantitative nature of the assay allows monitoring of levels of donor or recipient DNA levels, which relates directly to the levels of the cells in circulation – this may be useful in deciding whether therapeutic intervention is necessary in cases of possible Graft-versus-Host Disease in solid organ transplant patients (i.e., rising donor DNA levels) [42]. An increase in recipient genotype and concurrent reduction of donor genotype post HSCT may indicate neoplastic disease recurrence. In our laboratory, we have also developed techniques of using STR in paraffin-embedded biopsy specimens to identify the proportion of donor cells (i.e., DNA) in recipient tissues suspected of undergoing GVHD.

STR involves extracting DNA and amplification using commercially sold multiplex PCR reagents. Commonly used reagents use various numbers of markers, from 8 to 16, each amplified using fluorescently tagged primers. Labeled amplicons are separated by capillary electrophoresis and the amount of donor and recipient DNA is calculated using specialized programs. This method has sensitivity from one to five percent of either donor or recipient, thus it is not useful for establishing microchimerism (<1%). New techniques with higher sensitivity utilizing real time PCR have been developed, but are not currently the first choice for post-transplant monitoring since higher sensitivity has not been shown to offer clinical utility and the assays are often more time-consuming to perform. However, there have been studies linking the use of microchimerism testing to better outcomes when determining the choice between two parental donors [43, 44] (see Figure 11.7).

A variation of STR donor chimerism testing is called fractionated chimerism analysis [45, 46]. This technique combines the separation of different cell types in the post-transplant sample using CD marker antibodies labeled with magnetic beads or cell sorting. Routinely analyzed cells include B cells, T cells, and myeloid cells (see Figure 11.8). The advantage is relapse can be more quickly diagnosed if found in the original malignant cell compartment, since it would not be masked by the totality of the cells in circulation. For example, the finding of 10% recipient DNA in the myeloid compartment in a previous AML patient would indicate nascent relapse that may be missed since it would constitute less than 5% of the total percentage chimerism that would be mainly of donor origin.

Chimerism results are generally reported as percentage of *donor* chimerism, regardless of transplant type (bone marrow versus solid organ). After fully myeloablative HSCT, 100% donor cells should be found in the peripheral circulation. Current non-myeloablative regimens may transiently show some recipient genotype, but this mixed chimerism is eventually replaced by donor genotype. In certain situations, transplants are not geared to completely replace recipient genotype. This is the case in HSCT for sickle cell disease, where mixed chimerism remains long-term [47, 48]. For the majority of successful stem cell transplantation procedures, the donor chimerism proportion remains at 100%, implying complete engraftment. Unfortunately, 0% donor chimerism implies complete engraftment failure and has grave implications. Hence, determination of donor chimerism in the HSCT patient provides an important opportunity for medical intervention that can include adjustments in immunosuppression regimes, donor lymphocyte infusions, or additional chemotherapy.

Conversely, the analysis of chimerism for solid organ transplant patients, although still evaluating for *donor* chimerism, should be 0%. Any rise above 0% donor chimerism can be indicative of GVHD. Although most patients with indications of donor chimerism post-solid organ transplant are at high risk of losing the organ or eventually dying, there are some patients that maintain a chimeric state after transplant, with little or no effects. This phenomenon is not entirely understood, but may be related to some sort of immune tolerance [49].

HLA Antibody Testing

PRA, or *Panel Reactive Antibodies*, is a loosely-used term that signifies the measurement or presence of HLA antibodies in recipient serum. Historically, HLA antibodies were measured by microcytotoxicity testing with a panel of characterized

Laboratory Medicine in Transplantation

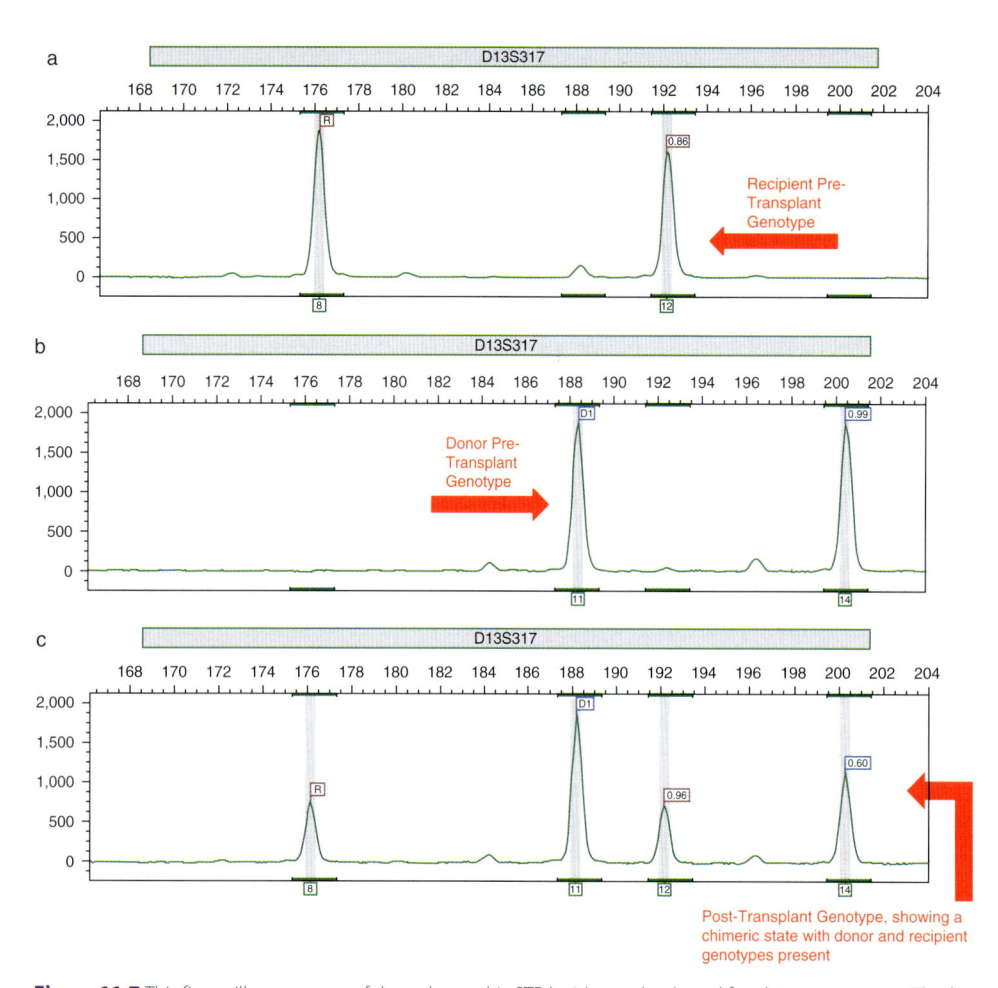

Figure 11.7 This figure illustrates one of the polymorphic STR loci (or markers) used for chimerism testing. This locus, D13S317, is a short tandem repeat located at 13q22-q31. This quad allelic STR ranges in repeats of 7–15. (A) Recipient D13S317 genotype *pre-transplant*. The recipient's two alleles are 8 and 12, indicating the inheritance of an 8 repeat STR from one parent and a 12 repeat STR from the other. (B) The Donor's D13S317 genotype is 11, 14. (C) This *post-transplant* analysis shows a mixture of both the recipient and donor genotype (8, 12 and 11, 14). For post-HSCT patients, this is indicative of recipient cells present in the peripheral blood or aspirate, likely due to neoplastic disease recurrence. For post-solid organ patients, this is indicative of donor cells present in the circulating peripheral blood, likely due to GVHD. The quantitative nature of this assay allows for the percent of donor chimerism to be calculated and monitored.

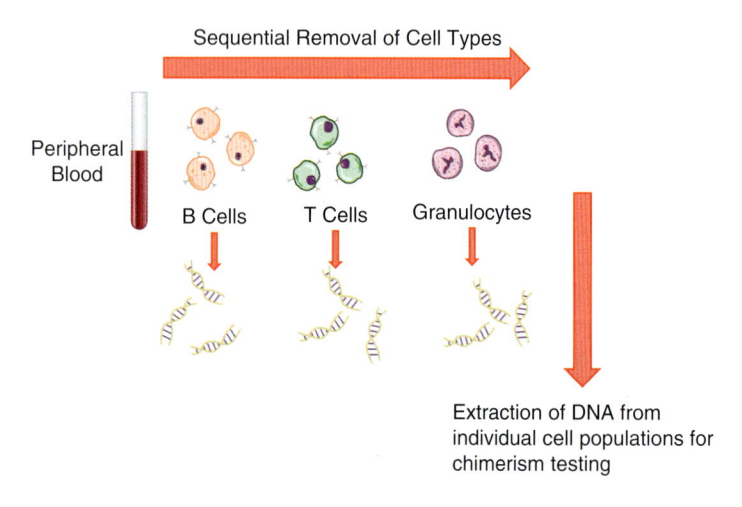

Figure 11.8 Monitoring the levels of donor chimerism present in certain cell populations allows for greater sensitivity and a more targeted approach. The process involves the sequential removal of cell types from peripheral blood or bone marrow aspirates using an immunomagnetic cell isolation procedure. B cells, T cells, and granulocytes are sequentially removed from the post-transplant sample. After separation, the individual cell groups are lysed and DNA is isolated. Analysis of percent donor chimerism on the whole blood and the cell subsets is performed.

donor cells. The analysis of patient serum samples involved laborious preparation of recipient serum trays and cell preparations from known HLA typed donors. A "panel" of 30 different cells, representing a majority of the HLA antigens in the local population, was tested with patient serum trays. The percent PRA referred to the percentage of panel cells that reacted with the patient's serum in the complement-mediated microcytotoxicity reaction. This number, a percentage of the number of positive reactions compared with the total number tested, gave clinicians an idea of the degree of sensitization of an individual patient. The importance of routine sensitization testing for renal patients on dialysis could determine if they would be quickly transplanted or would linger on dialysis for extended periods of time, since these patients were constantly being exposed to multiple HLA antigens due to their need for blood transfusions. Currently, the advent of erythropoietin therapy for dialysis patients has helped reduce the need for transfusions.

Screening cell panels had to be designed with certain features of the HLA system in mind: linkage disequilibrium between HLA loci, antibody cross-reaction between certain loci, and the variable representation of HLA antigens in different ethnic/racial populations. Common haplotypes (i.e., A1, B8) could not be over-represented in the panel, and as well, care was taken to avoid cells with known cross-reactive antigens (i.e., B35 and B53) or the percent of PRA would be under- or over-represented. Identification of anti-class II sensitization presented the unique challenge of requiring a fully characterized panel of B cells as well. Commercially prepared trays with frozen cells (LCT) [50] became available and were used extensively since the preparation of panels was tedious, expensive, and labor-intensive. However, even with careful panel selection or commercial tray availability, the complete identification of a patient's sensitization status was only an estimate and the answer of whether a particular donor would have a positive crossmatch with a sensitized patient was still elusive. While the information gained from such testing identified individuals which were not sensitized, important information on the antibody specificities found in highly sensitized individuals was not easily gained, even with a well-characterized panel. Also, 0% or negative PRA was only referring to levels of alloantibodies that would cause complement-mediated lysis in the microcytotoxicity assay, and thus AMR could still result since low-level sensitization that would flare up could still be present.

The arrival of *solid phase testing* for HLA sensitization changed solid organ transplantation in a dramatic way. The first solid phase assays used HLA antigens obtained from pooled cells and detected them in an ELISA-based assay [51–53] or using flow cytometry [54]. The use of ELISA represented the possibility of automation for HLA sensitization screening of waitlisted patients. Attempts to use HLA molecules from individual cells from culture gave the first antibody identification assays. These assays contained all antigens contained on the cell so that a variety of cells and the identification of reactivity patterns were required to crudely identify antibody specificities. The ELISA assays were slightly less sensitive than the AHG-complement-dependent cytotoxicity (CDC) assay (see below in Crossmatch for description). Assigning antibody specificity was sometimes difficult due to the innate problems with the use of HLA panels described above. Flow beads coated with an individual cell's antigens (haplotype beads) were more sensitive, but required more hands-on time. However, determining the specific sensitization status of a patient required multiple bead panels and all the problems with panel-based assays still applied.

Two technological changes brought about the current state of the art for HLA antibody testing: the purification of specific individual HLA antigens and the introduction of Luminex technology. The combination of both these innovations significantly changed the analysis of HLA antibodies. Luminex technology involves the use of a bead-based, multicolor flow cytometer [55, 56]. Polystyrene beads are coated with combinations of two fluorophors that create an individual identifying fluorescent signature for each bead. Up to 100 individual bead signatures can be identified by this system. However, recent advances in Luminex 3D technology will allow for up to 500 bead evaluations. The multiplexed beads are incubated with patient serum, washed, and a labeled anti-IgG is used as a reporter antibody. The degree of sensitization (screen) or specificity of the antibody is determined by the bead ID and the degree of fluorescence is proportional to the amount of antibody in the serum of the patient. Beads are coated with pooled purified protein from multiple cell lines (mixed screen) or individual identified beads coated with HLA specificities on one cell (phenotype beads), which could be used as a screening assay. More importantly, the purified *single HLA specificity or single antigen (SA)* on an identified bead can identify all antibodies found in a highly sensitized patient [57–60]. Multiplexing the 100 beads provides an assay that can identify the most commonly found HLA A, B, and C specificities for class I and DRB1, DQB1, DQA1, DPA1, and DPB1 specificities for class II (see Figure 11.9). Finally, the full characterization of patient antibody status is possible and allows accurate prediction of a positive crossmatch with a specific donor (virtual crossmatching) [61, 62].

There are many technical advantages of SA testing including that it allows for detection of HLA antibodies to all commonly found HLA alleles routinely found by previous methodologies as well as antibodies to antigens previously untested and unknown to elicit clinically significant sensitization such as Cw, DQA, and DPA antibodies. SA testing is sensitive and semi-quantitative, thereby allowing assignment of antibody levels (weak, intermediate, and strong). Testing is rapid and can be partly automated allowing for rapid high throughput testing. Since its implementation, it has allowed rapid detection of and monitoring for antibody-mediated rejection (AMR) as well as for detection of efficacy of therapy. Use of different secondary reporter antibodies and modifications of the assay allows for the detection of complement fixing and non-complement fixing antibodies (C1q Screen and Ig isotype testing). Some disadvantages of SA assays are occasionally high background levels that may require adsorption of serum with special beads. Positive results may also be due to antibodies to denatured HLA antigens [63]. False negative or weak positives may result from C1 or IgM inhibition of Ig binding to bead antigens, requiring serum pretreatment before analysis; prozone effects can also take place [64]. Also, there is no direct relation between the antigen density on Luminex beads and that found on a cell surface, so cell-based assays are still required to provide the correlation between SA results and both flow and CDC crossmatches. At this point, each individual laboratory must make these correlations and results

Laboratory Medicine in Transplantation

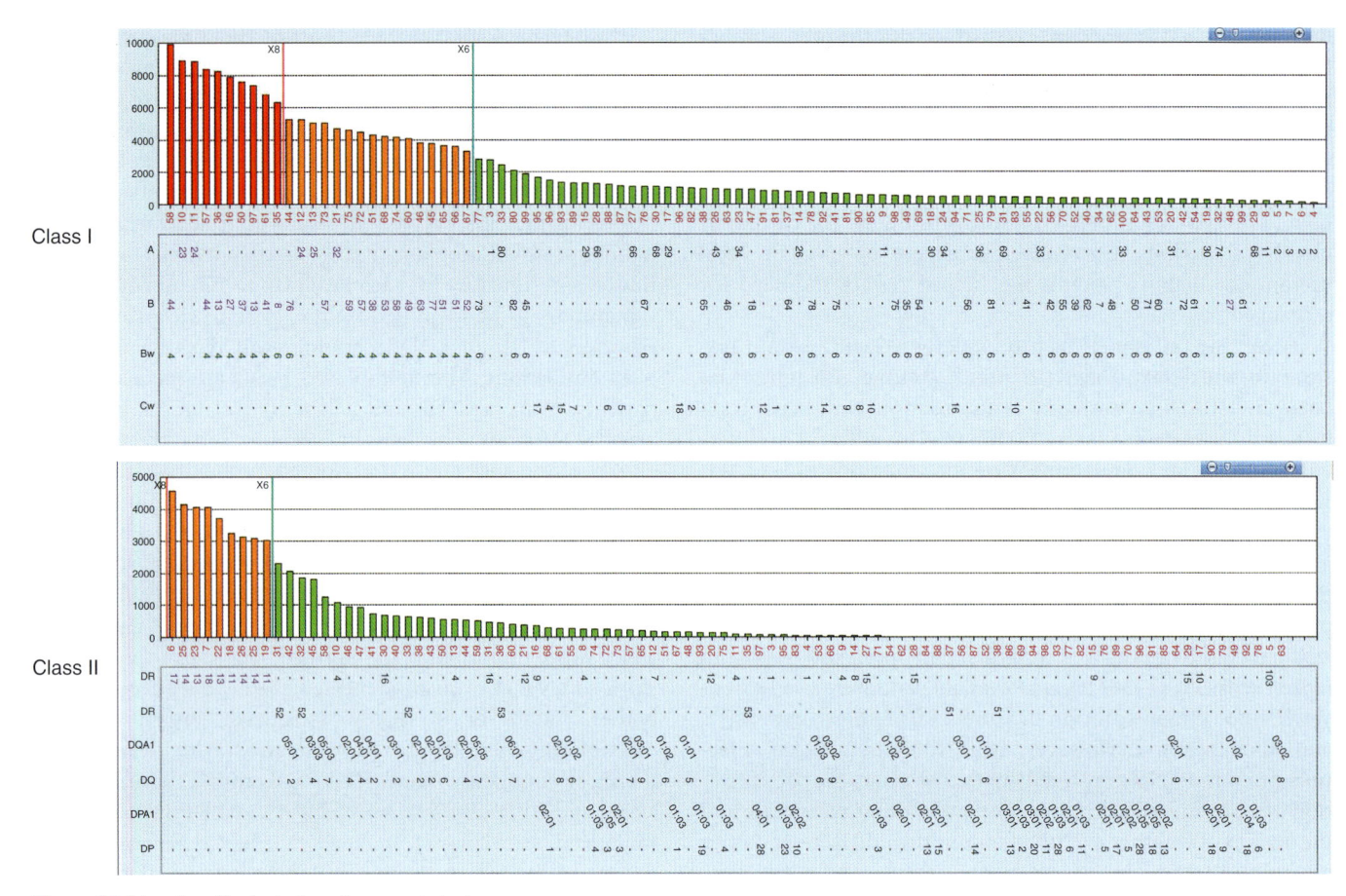

Figure 11.9 Luminex Single Antigen Assay analysis view.

are laboratory and center-based. Translation of results nationally will require much more intensive discussion to determine definitions of antibody strengths and what constitutes a positive crossmatch result [65].

SA testing in the U.S. since 2006 has provided ample information on the behavior of HLA antibodies and has assisted in predicting crossmatch results. Although standardization of the SA assay remains imperfect [66], its implementation has been pivotal in the current sensitization determination scheme used for the wait listing of renal allograft patients in the U.S., the cPRA or calculated PRA. cPRA is a value calculated by using the antibody specificities that would be expected to cause a positive crossmatch and the frequency of those specific antigens in the general population that become organ donors [67, 68]. These antibody specificities are listed in the cPRA calculator as Unacceptable Antigens, or UA. Certain antigens are strongly represented in the general population and would have a high probability of being found in a deceased donor. Antibodies to those antigens would give a higher value for cPRA. For example, a single antibody to the common antigen A2 gives a cPRA of 47% where a single antibody to less common A34 gives a cPRA of 2%. DQ specificities give a much higher cPRA because they are widely represented in the population and show strong linkage disequilibrium with multiple HLA DR types. Listing only DQ5 as an UA gives a cPRA of 59% most probably because of its strong association with certain alleles of DR1, 8, 10, 11, 12, 13, 14, 15, 16, and 17 and the high probability that a donor would have DQ5 in its HLA genotype. In essence, implementation of cPRA allows for initial elimination from a donor match run of recipients that would be expected to have a positive crossmatch with a specific donor. The corollary is that if a highly sensitized recipient does appear in a donor match run, that recipient would probably have an acceptable crossmatch result and could be transplanted. Current data shows that since the implementation of the cPRA in 2009, the proportion of highly sensitized patients receiving a transplant has increased significantly with a corresponding decrease of positive crossmatch organ refusals [67, 68]. In essence, the introduction of the cPRA implemented a preliminary "virtual crossmatch" for each recipient being considered for a donor.

The Virtual Crossmatch

The *virtual crossmatch (VXM)* is an algorithm used to predict the outcomes of a real crossmatch without actual mixing of cells and serum in a test tube [69–71]. It correlates the results of recipient antibody screening with the HLA typing of the donor, looking for the presence and levels of donor-specific antibodies (DSA). To fully implement this powerful tool in the transplant setting, it is essential to understand the possible limitations of this application. First, it is important to take into account that recipient antibody specificities and their titers often vary significantly over time. Consequently, it becomes critical to use recent antibody screening results for VXM purposes – in general, results older than six months should not be used, since they may not provide an accurate prediction of the recipient's current status. Furthermore, sensitizing events such as blood transfusions, transplants, infections, and pregnancies that happen after the antibody screening result was obtained may significantly change the specificities and titers of those antibodies.

Cases where low titer or non-complement fixing antibodies are present may result in negative actual XM. Also, if the technique used to detect the antibodies is more sensitive than the actual crossmatch technique or vice versa (i.e., Luminex SA testing and CDC XM, LCT tray, and flow XM respectively), results may not correlate. All these circumstances must be taken into account to ensure predictive accuracy and not exclude donors unnecessarily. A positive VXM result can result based on incorrect HLA antigen interpretation when donors have HLA-null alleles. In these cases, antigens are not expressed on cells, but unless accurate molecular typing is performed to identify null alleles, a donor may be excluded by VXM. A common example of this is the DR53 null allele (DRB4 01:03 N) found in association with DR7 and DQ9. A recipient with DR53 antibodies would not have a positive actual crossmatch with a donor with this typing. When patients develop allele-specific antibodies, donors may be also excluded if actual donor allele information is not available. In these instances, serological typing or assigned specificities are not sufficient and molecular typing information is necessary.

It is important to note that VXM results are dependent, as many areas within the histocompatibility laboratory on individual laboratory techniques and defined cut-offs. As mentioned above, the correlation between different MFI levels and crossmatch results for both flow cytometry and CDC must be performed by each laboratory to accurately define what results in a positive actual XM before VXM can be implemented [72]. Finally, a VXM must make sure a donor's specific alleles are fully represented on the solid phase panel in order to report a VXM as negative.

Special Considerations for HLA Antibody Analysis

Crossreactive HLA Antibodies and Crossreactive Groups (CREGs). Some decades ago, investigators first postulated the existence of "public" shared epitopes in HLA molecules, due to the observed serological cross-reactivity found in HLA alloantibodies from highly sensitized patients. This cross-reactivity was further studied, and in the 1980s, the existence of two types of epitopes, public and private, were demonstrated in HLA molecules [73, 74]. Public epitopes explained the strong reactions seen with dissimilar antigen specificities in panel screening or crossmatch reactions that could not be explained by the corresponding antigenic stimuli from a sensitizing event. Soon, class I cross-reactive epitopes were classified into major cross-reactive groups or CREGs (Table 11.2). Some CREGs are composed of antibodies to several public epitopes, but their pattern is distinctively observed in complex sensitized serum

Table 11.2 Serological Public Epitopes of HLA-A & HLA-B Molecules

CREG	Found on	Public Epitopes
1 C	A!, 3, 9 (23,24), 11, 29.30.31.36, 80	3–4, poorly defined
10 C	A10 (25,26,34,66), 11, 28 (68, 69), 32, 33, 43, 74	10. 28. 33 (10p)
2 C	2, 9 (23,24), 28 (68, 69), B17 (57, 58)	2, 28, 9 (9p)
		2, 28 (9p)
		2, 17 (17p)
5 C	B5 (51, 52), 15 (62, 63, 75, 76, 77, 78), 18, 21 (49, 50), 35, 46, 53, 70 (71, 72), 73, 4005, B17 (57, 58)	5, 35, 53, 18, 70 (5p)
		5, 15, 17, 21, 35, 70, 4005 (21p)
7 C	B7, 8, 13, 22 (54, 55, 56), 27, 40 (60, 61), 41, 42, 47, 48, 59, 67, 73, 81, 82	7, 27, 42, 46, 47, 54, 55, 56 (22p)
		7, 13, 27, 60, 61, 47 (27p)
		7, 8, 41, 42, 48, 60, 81 (7p)
8 C	8, 14 (64, 65), 16 (38, 39, 18, 51, 59, 67	8, 14, 16, 18, 51, 59, 67 (8p)
12 C	12 (44, 45) 13, 21 (49, 50), 37, 40 (60, 61), 41, 47, 4005, 48, 82	12, 13, 21, 37, 40, 41, 47 (12p)
4 C	B5 (51, 52, 5102, 5103), 0802, 0803, 13, 17 (57, 58), 1809, 27, 37, 38 (16), 44 (12), 47, 49 (21), 53, 5607, 59, 63, 67, 77, and A23, 24, 25, 32	Bw4
6 C	7, 703, 8, 1309, 18, 2708, 2712, 2718, 35, 39 (16), 3901, 3902, 4005, 4406, 4409, 45 (12), 46, 4702, 48, 50 (21), 54 (22), 55 (22), 56 (22), 60 (40), 61 (40), 62 (15), 64 (14), 65 (14), 67, 71 (70), 72 (70), 73, 75 (15), 76 (15), 78, 81	Bw5

samples. The definition of these epitopes has been closely studied [75]. Using current SA methodology, we see what could be CREG antibodies when analyzing sera from highly sensitized individuals. The extrapolation of a serum's reactivity panel with Luminex SA beads to a cell-based crossmatch must take this cross-reactivity into account. A patient with a 2CREG antibody may unexpectedly show positive crossmatch with cells carrying B57 or A68, even though the bead reactions for those specificities fall below the usual positive cut-off. A patient with a strong B53 antibody and no DSA antibodies may have a positive crossmatch with a donor carrying the B35 antigen due to the strong cross-reaction between those two specificities in the 5CREG. Also, the presence of cross-reactive antibodies and/or CREG specificities along with a weak

DSA may increase the strength of a positive crossmatch exponentially. Therefore, the reality of public epitopes and cross-reactive antibodies must be taken into account when performing VXM analysis.

The advent of SA testing has made it possible to define antibodies to individual HLA alleles. Today, epitope classifications are further refined and even "private" epitope alloantibodies have been further divided. "Group" epitopes define a family of closely related alleles such as A2 (A*02:01/02:02/02:03/02:06, etc.) and allele-specific epitopes define alloantibody to a specific HLA allele that does not cross-react with other members of the antigen family in question (i.e., allele-specific DRB1*04:01 antibody). Thus, it is possible for an individual to carry an HLA type (i.e., DR52) and also have alloantibody to a different allele in the same antigen family (anti-DRB3*01:01). These allele-specific antibodies provide a unique challenge for HLA antibody reporting, since serologic nomenclature only describes the broad antigen but allele-specific antibodies cannot be reported.

Crossmatch Testing

Crossmatch (XM) testing is a mandatory practice in the pre-transplant work up performed by the histocompatibility laboratory with the aim of identifying preformed cytotoxic alloantibodies in the prospective recipient that are identifying donor cells; this practice has been instrumental in the prevention of hyperacute rejection (HAR). In contrast to the simple detection of donor-specific HLA antibodies as described above, a positive cell-based CDC crossmatch is typically a true contraindication for transplant. Different scenarios can be encountered. For instance, a positive pre-transplant CDC crossmatch tends to be a contraindication to transplantation because it is associated with a high risk for AMR, unless DSA can be reduced with desensitization protocols. A positive pre-transplant flow cytometry crossmatch or a historically positive CDC crossmatch is associated with an intermediate risk for AMR. Therefore, a patient in these circumstances may need a more intense induction or maintenance immunosuppression. When negative current and positive flow or CDC crossmatch with historical sera are obtained, the patient can be treated with more conventional immunosuppression therapy, since this scenario is associated with a low risk for AMR. Finally, negative CDC crossmatches with current and historical sera tend to be associated with low risk for AMR, although the highly variable sensitivity of the CDC technique makes prediction somewhat difficult.

The complement-dependent cytotoxicity (CDC) crossmatch is a technique where the recipient serum is mixed with lymphocytes of the potential donor, in the presence of complement and a vital dye (see Figure 11.10). If the serum contains donor-specific alloantibodies of sufficient titer, complement will be fixed, causing cell lysis. The vital dye will enter the injured cells, allowing the technologist to distinguish and enumerate live and dead cells. The target cell used may be a mixture of B and T lymphocytes or lymphocyte populations enriched for T cells (used because they express class I HLA antigens) or B cells (used because they express both class I and

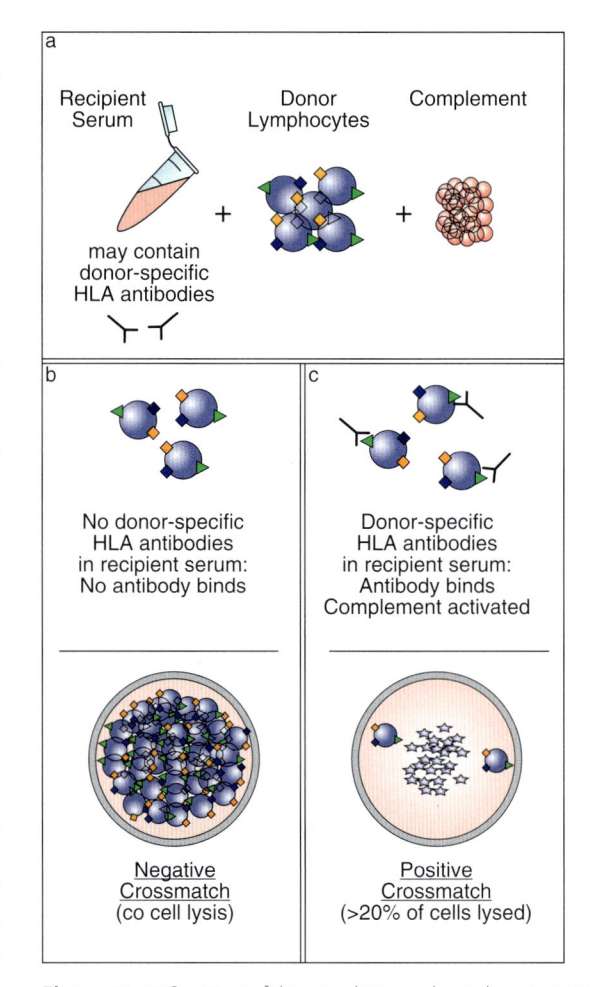

Figure 11.10 Overview of the complement- dependent cytotoxicity (CDC) crossmatch.

class II antigens). Thus, the lymphocytes serve as an *in vitro* surrogate of the actual allograft, since they express the same antigens on their surface as those expressed in the endothelium of the organ.

Although the antibody formed is usually specific for the immunizing antigen, antibodies that cross-react with the primary antigen may also be formed so that the presence of non-HLA antibodies, autoantibodies, and IgM antibodies may interfere with results, causing false positives. False negatives may be due to low titer of existing antibodies that may not activate complement. Historically, when cytotoxic antibodies were not detected, a crossmatch was interpreted as negative. However, graft loss still occurred in some of these "negative" cases. As a result, more sensitive complement-dependent assays were developed [76, 77]. These procedural improvements included a second wash step, extended serum/cell incubation time, or another reagent added to increase the sensitivity and assist in discovering these detrimental antibodies. The Amos test is a modification of the CDC procedure developed to eliminate anti-complementary factors that promote false-negative crossmatches. The procedure removes any unbound serum components from the lymphocyte suspension after the initial cell/serum incubation step, but before the addition of complement. It is used with both T cell and B cell

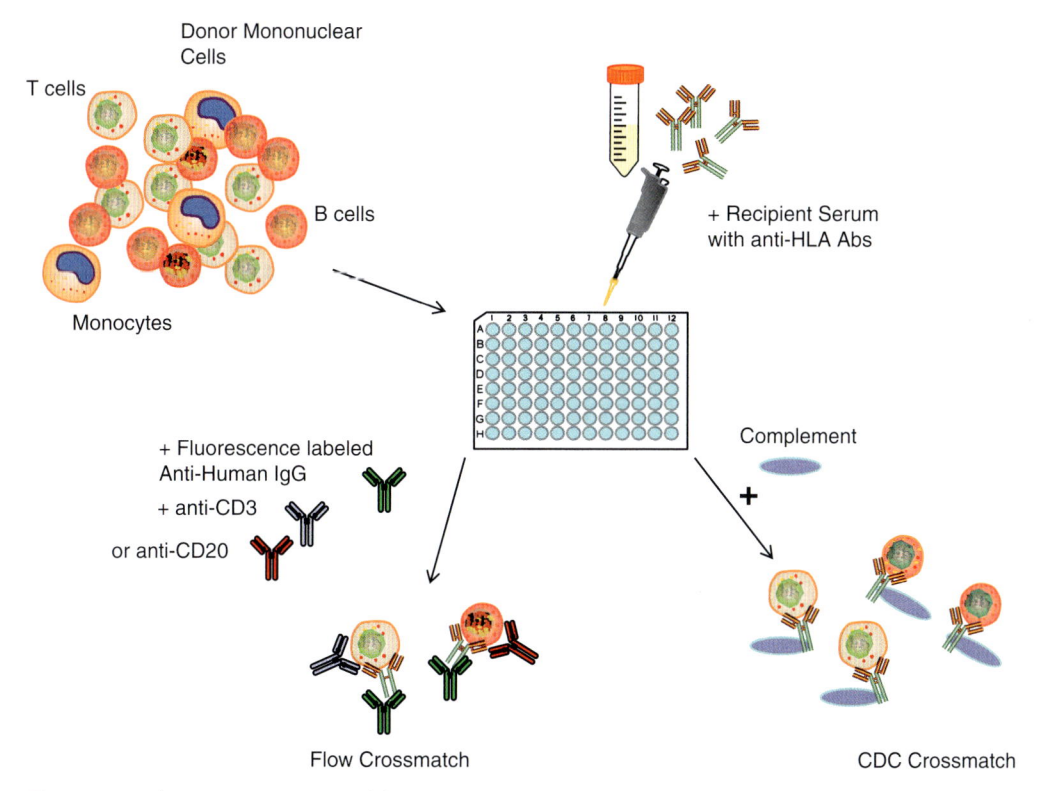

Figure 11.11 Flow cytometry crossmatch histograms.

targets to increase assay sensitivity. Another improvement is called the extended CDC in which the initial cell/serum incubation time is extended to increase sensitivity. The anti-human globulin (AHG)-CDC is a modification in which anti-human globulin is added after the initial cell/serum incubation to help identify DSA antibodies found at low titers that cannot fix complement in vitro, including the cytotoxicity-negative adsorption-positive (CyNAP) antibodies. In this assay, a second antibody, AHG (i.e., goat anti-human light chain), is added after the initial serum incubation, but before the addition of complement. This second antibody adds a second Fc receptor with close proximity that may be missing with low titer antibodies or with antibodies for low-density antigens. The AHG-CDC for B and T cells allows low-level antibodies to both class I and II to be detected more efficiently using B cells and T cells as targets.

The *flow cytometry crossmatch (FCXM)* is another widely used crossmatch technique in the HLA laboratory. The major difference between the FCXM and CDC crossmatch is the capability of flow cytometry to detect DSA in the absence of complement fixation [78–80] (see Figure 11.11). The technique has proven to be more sensitive than any of the CDC assays. After incubation of the patient serum with donor lymphocytes, several wash steps remove residual serum. Cells are then stained with a fluorochrome-conjugated secondary antibody, generally FITC-labeled antihuman IgG that is either monoclonal or polyclonal. Cells are subsequently stained with anti-CD3 and anti-CD19 monoclonal antibodies to identify T and B cells respectively and therefore identify class I and/or class II antibody reactivity (see Figure 11.12). The results of the flow crossmatch are usually expressed as number of channel shifts of mean fluorescence above the baseline or as ratios of mean fluorescence of the serum with respect to the negative control. However, the values that constitute a positive XM vary between laboratories and transplant programs tend to set center-specific thresholds for positivity. Since the flow crossmatch is a semi-quantitative technique, it provides an objective reading when compared to subjective approach of a technologist reviewing a CDC tray in a microscope to determine whether a reaction is negative or shows different grades of positivity.

A majority of laboratories perform the flow cytometry crossmatch, as well as the CDC assays, simultaneously. This approach helps to determine the ratio between complement binding and non-complement binding antibodies or low-level antibodies. Institutional differences influence the methodology used for solid organ transplantation crossmatches. Some programs use both FCXM and CDC XM when evaluating prospective living donor transplants, yet only perform CDC XM when evaluating cadaveric donors. There have been different studies to identify the ideal testing procedure for crossmatching for solid organ transplantation. There is not a clear consensus delineating which technique is the best, since significant variations in the methodology such as reagents, sera conditions, cell isolation, and numbers used as targets exist today. With CDC, care must be taken to review autologous XM results, as well as identify IgM antibodies that could be interpreted as positive yet are not a contraindication to transplantation.

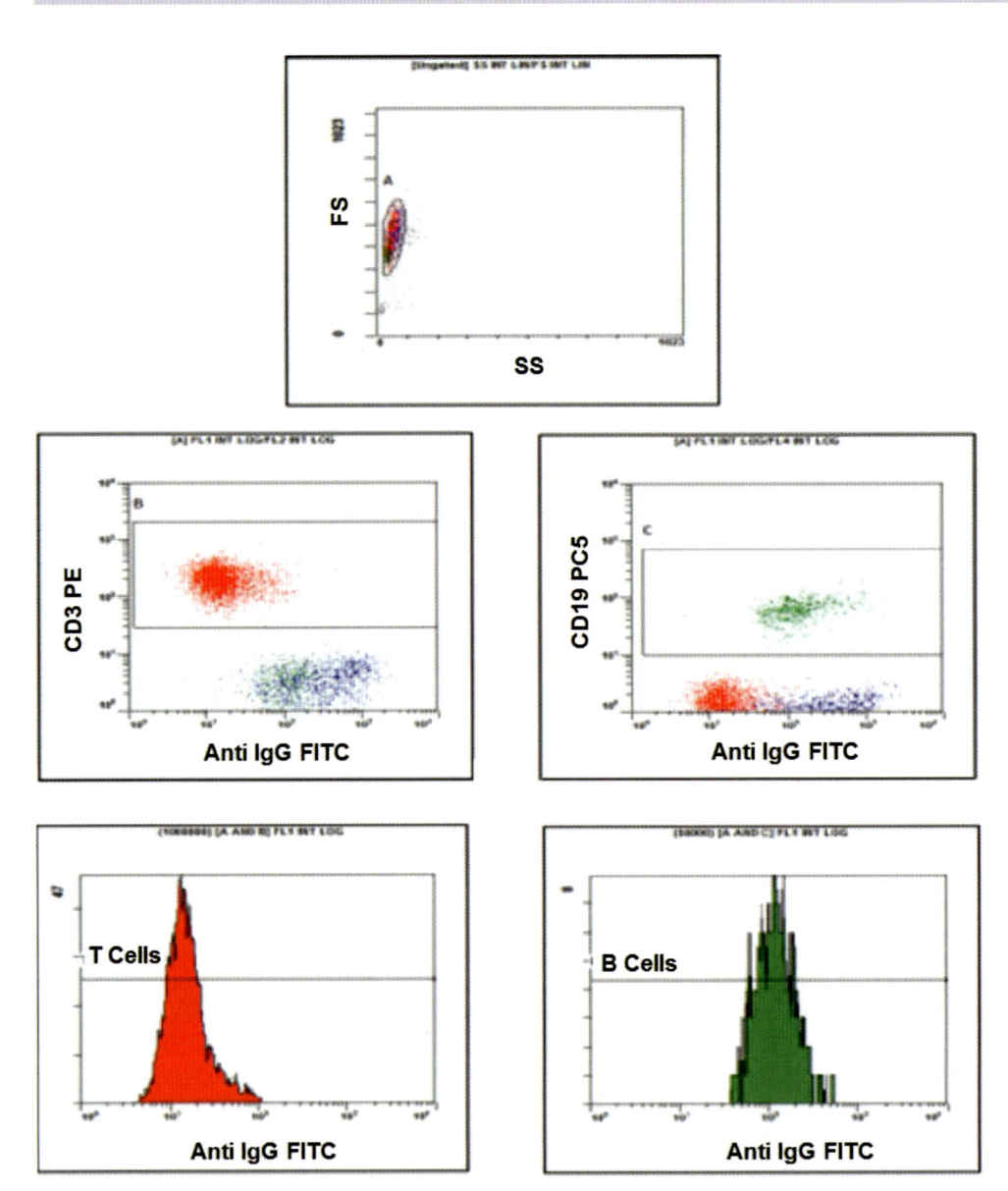

Figure 11.12 Representative flow cytometry histograms showing forward versus side scatter gating in top histogram, two-color histograms for the presence of IgG on T cells (CD3) or IgG on B cells (CD20) in the middle histograms, or single-color representations on the lower histograms.

Evaluation of Cellular Immunity in Transplantation

Pre- and post-transplant monitoring of cell-mediated immunity in transplant patients is desirable as an accompaniment to our assessment of humoral immunity as described above, since this allows for proper maintenance, via tailored immunosuppression, of a functional solid organ graft or cellular transplantation. Balancing the administration of immunosuppressant compounds helps to effectively avoid acute cellular rejection episodes while maintaining immune competence and graft function. Contrary to this, excessive immunosuppression could lead to toxicity that will damage the graft or predispose the patient to infectious or malignant complications.

Thus, the evaluation of cellular immunity status in transplantation and other patients with immune-based disorders is a growing area of the clinical laboratory. Three general types of measurements are possible: *in vivo*: immune activity is measured within the patient; *ex vivo*: cells from patient are put directly into an assay to measure activity; *in vitro*: cells, usually from peripheral blood mononuclear cells (PBMC), are cultured before activity assay. The source of cells is often from PBMC and some of the assays described below utilize *ex vivo* or *in vitro* measurements. Among the primary issues with the studies of the immune function assays is the establishment of test standardization, reproducibility, and determination of what phase of the complicated cellular response is in relation to the transplantation setting. Since there are many areas of the cellular immune response that can be measured, it is very important to correctly identify which phase is to be measured (e.g., assessment of naïve, effector, or memory T cell function; APC functions such as phagocytosis and antigen presentation; T cell recognition and activation). These tests are typically multi-step assays with complex readouts. Their high level of complexity can compromise data comparison between different sites and limit the ability for standardization of immune monitoring assays. The lack of standardization of these assays from lab to lab is reflected in the fact that only a few tests which are commercially available have clearance from the FDA and are offered as clinical tests. There are a variety of reasons for the difficulty in test standardization, but among them is the fact that whole cells are used, often with standard numbers versus phenotypically identical populations being used as the starting point in the assay. Thereafter, cells are usually cultured and it can be very difficult to obtain identical conditions between different lab environments; minor changes can profoundly affect the readout of these tests. Finally, the significant number of sequential steps that may be necessary and that can affect the test readout can be difficult to standardize.

Antigen-specific (or nonspecific) T cell or B cell responses can be measured by several techniques and each has its own limitations and advantages. *Lymphoid proliferation and cytotoxicity assays* are loosely based on the presumption that naïve and/or memory cells present in the patient's fluid or tissue sample will respond with primary or anamnestic (secondary) proliferation upon *in vitro* exposure to antigen. The antigen may be nonspecific (e.g., mitogens, antibody-crosslinking of receptors) or specific according to original immune stimulant within the recipient (e.g., alloantigens of the donor). The level of proliferation or cytotoxicity that subsequently occurs is a reflection of the level of stimulation that ensued following the antigen exposure and this is extrapolated to mirror the level of immune cell activation that is occurring *in vivo* in the host.

The *mixed lymphocyte culture (MLC)* is a test that has been utilized in transplantation for several decades in multiple configurations [81–83], but which is being used less often in its classical format than in previous years. The basic principle of the test is that lymphocytes from two different individuals with HLA mismatched antigens tend to proliferate against each other when placed in culture together within three to seven days. Typically, to single out a population response from the bidirectional reaction, one population (the donor cell population) is inhibited from proliferating by pre-culture treatment with irradiation or mitomycin C (and is named the stimulator population), while the other untreated population (from the recipient) is named the responder population. The degree of genetic disparity between the responder and stimulator as well as the level of memory cells specific to the stimulator, will often be proportional to the level of proliferation that ensues. The MLC can be very useful in pre-transplant determinations of living donor compatibility and/or sensitization. Among the limitations of this assay is the lack of standardization between institutions, the protracted amount of time for the readout (can be seven days), and the high level of complexity required for its performance. The measurement of proliferation can be performed with radioactive ^{3}H-tritium or with proliferation dyes (e.g., CFSE) that are non-radioactive and allow for simultaneous determination of the nature of the responding cells by flow cytometry as well as the extent of proliferation. Nevertheless, over the years, the MLC as described above has tended to be replaced by other forms of the assay.

The *mixed lymphocyte reaction (MLR)* is a test typically run parallel to the MLC and provides a measurement of the response potential of the cells placed in the MLC. The basic principle is to stimulate a single population of cells from the donor or recipient by mitogens (PHA, CoA, LPS, etc.) that do so independently of their genetic markup. Measurement of the response could also be done as in the MLC (with the same advantages and disadvantages). One test that is FDA-approved and which measures proliferation of peripheral CD4+ T cells in response to the mitogens PHA is the *Cylex ImmuKnow®* test [84]. This is a test based on the MLR previously mentioned, but with significant changes. It is performed without cell separation (done in whole blood) and after 17 hours of stimulation with the mitogens, CD4-positive cells are pulled out mechanically and assessed for the amount of ATP generated in relation to the immune cell activity in a luminometer. This test has a relationship in many studies with the level of immunosuppression present in the host; as such, several studies have demonstrated that monitoring serial levels of ImmuKnow® in transplant patients may be able to predict the onset of acute rejection or over-immunosuppression [85, 86].

Cytotoxic T lymphocyte (CTL) measurement is classically performed with a chromium release assay [87, 88]. The basic principle of the test starts with generating an MLC as described above. After seven days, the activated responder cells (primed responders) are then exposed to freshly prepared donor cells (same used as stimulator) now tested, not for proliferation, but for the ability to "kill" the targets [89–91] via direct cytotoxicity mechanisms. Target cells expressing antigen (e.g., alloantigen) on their surface are labeled with a radioactive isotope of chromium (^{51}Cr). The patient's primed cells are mixed with the target cell and incubated for several hours. Lysis of antigen-expressing cells releases ^{51}Cr into the medium. Specific lysis is calculated by comparing lysis of target cells in the presence or absence of patient effector primed cells, and is usually expressed as the % specific lysis.

CTL response can also be assessed by measuring cytokine production (e.g., IFN-γ by antigen-specific effector cells in an *ELISPOT (Enzyme Linked ImmunoSpot)* assay [92, 93]. In this assay, APC (e.g., donor PBMC depleted of T cells) are cultivated with effector cells (e.g., PBMC containing T cells) in a 96 well plate with a synthetic membrane at the bottom of the wells coated with a capture anti-IFN-γ (or whatever molecule is being measured) antibody. The plate is incubated for 18–24 hours to permit activation of alloreactive T cells and binding of subsequent released IFN-γ. Then the cells are washed off the plates, leaving behind only IFN-γ bound to the capture antibody. A second biotinylated anti-IFN-γ antibody is then added to the wells, which will only bind to the captured IFN-γ. Adding conjugated horseradish peroxidase (HRP) to streptavidin and later developing with a chromogen substrate will leave a precipitate on the membrane. These color spots on the membrane are the footprints of cells expressing IFN-γ. Once developed, the results are rapidly quantified by computer-assisted image analysis. Figure 11.13 demonstrates an example of a typical layout of an IFN-γ ELISPOT assay. This technique has been used in different variations to predict transplant outcome. One of the most common uses of IFN-γ ELISPOT is to assess the risk of acute rejection in kidney transplantation. A growing number of studies aimed at this purpose have found a negative correlation between increased frequencies of memory T cells expressing IFN-γ and graft function. Also, a direct correlation was found to exist between an elevated number of pre-transplant donor alloreactive memory T cells and acute rejection [92].

In hematopoietic stem cell transplantation (HSCT), ELISPOT has been used to predict acute Graft-versus-Host Disease (GVHD) [94]. In this case, PBMC from transplanted patients were cultivated without stimulation and the number of spot forming cells was determined for the cytokines IFN-γ, IL12, IL10, and IL4. The number of spots generated by cells producing IFN-γ and IL4 was significantly higher in patients with GVHD Grades II–IV compared to patients with Grades 0–I. This difference of cellular response could not be detected by measuring IFN-γ and IL4 in serum via ELISA [94].

The IFN-γ ELISPOT has been also used for measurement of alloreactivity of transplant recipients by culturing their cells with a pool of *in vitro* expanded purified B cells, instead of cells from a specific donor [95, 96]. This methodology allows selection of B cell lines expressing the desired repertoire of HLA alleles and it is an invaluable alternative when access to donor blood cells is not possible.

Measurement of cellular reactivity by the IFN-γ ELISPOT assay before transplantation has been used to help determine the choice of induction therapy in kidney transplant patients [97]. Pre-existing high levels of anti-donor reactive memory T cells have been effectively reduced in patients by treatment with antithymocyte globulin (ATG). Other induction treatments, such as IL-2 receptor blockers (basiliximab), were not as effective for these patients, but did offer adequate protection against immune-mediated injury to patients with low frequency of reactive memory T cells. Similarly, kidney transplant patients positive for anti-donor T cells, as determined via IFN-γ ELISPOT assay, that received induction therapy with basiliximab or ATG (all treated with calcineurin inhibitors) did not present symptoms of rejection 12 months after transplantation, while positive patients with no induction therapy (46%) experienced rejection episodes [98]. These memory T cells can proliferate without antigen re-exposure and they can mount effective rejection episodes in lymphopenic patients. Memory T cells are resistant to many immunosuppressant drugs, but their deleterious effects can be efficiently reduced with inhibitors of the calcineurin pathway [99]. The clinical use of measurements of donor-reactive memory T cells as a biomarker pre-and post-transplant is becoming a useful tool for risk assessment of acute rejection and for prediction of transplant outcome.

The IFN-γ ELISPOT is also useful for assessing the risk of viral infections and other opportunistic pathogens in immune compromised and immunosuppressed transplant patients. Infection with these common pathogens like polyoma virus, BK virus nephropathy (BKVN), and CMV disease in kidney transplant patients could have devastating effects on graft

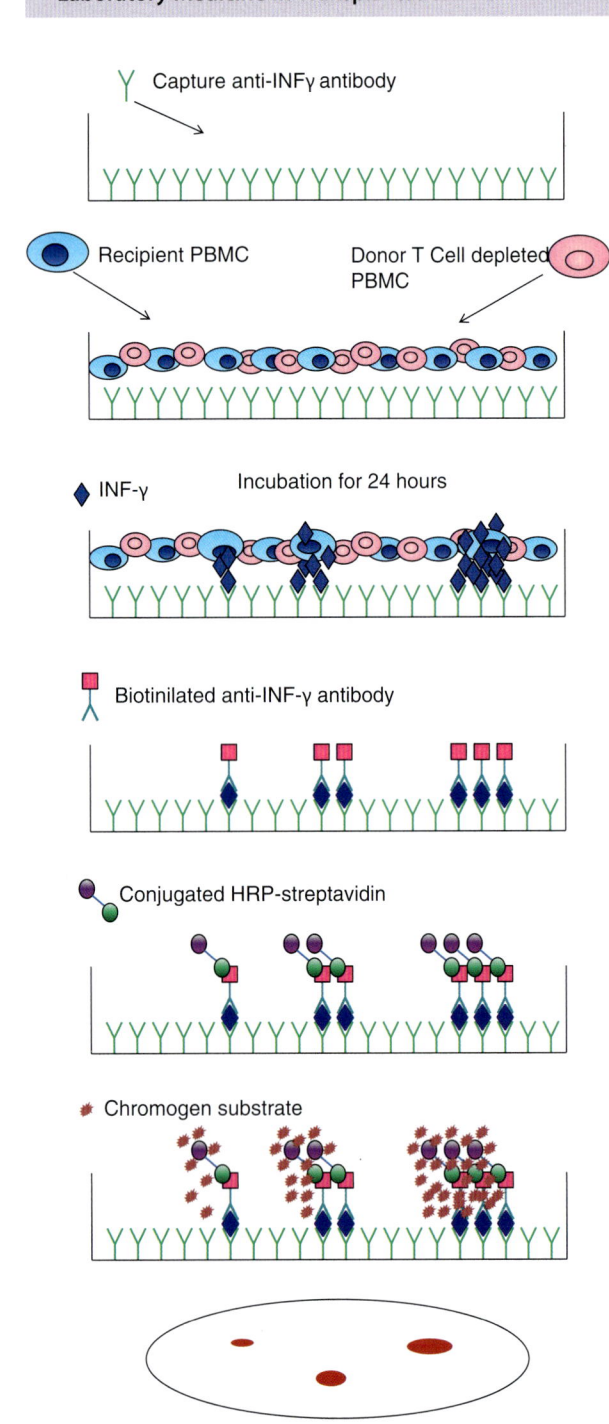

Figure 11.13 IFNγ ELISPOT. A. The assay resembles a sandwich ELISA. 96 well plates with a synthetic membrane as a floor are coated with a capture anti- IFNγ antibody. Responder and effector cells depleted of T cells are incubated for 18–24 hours to permit activation and release of IFNγ. The cells are washed off the plates and a second biotinylated anti- IFNγ antibody is then added to the wells. Conjugated horseradish peroxidase (HRP) to streptavidin is added to detect bound INFg and the plates are developed using a chromogen substrate that will precipitate on the membrane. The resulting spots at the site of IFNγ secretion indicate individual responder cells. B. Representative IFNγ ELISPOT assay of a transplant patient responding to donor cells. PBMC are cultivated in media alone to define the background. Phytohemagglutinin (PHA) is used to stimulate responder T cells as a positive control and stimulator cells as control for T cell depletion. Alloreactions of third party with donor and recipient with third party are included as background responses.

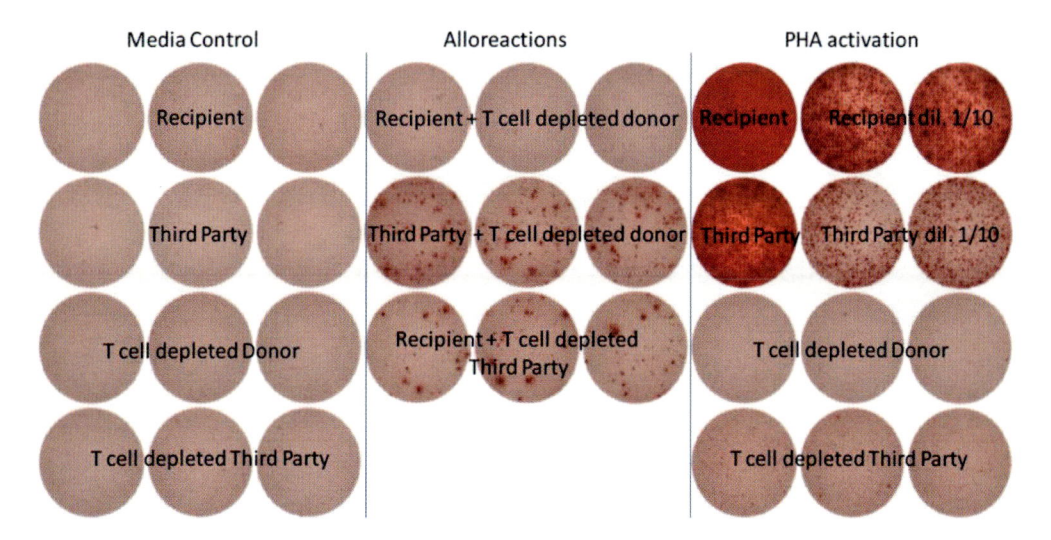

Figure 11.13 (Cont.)

function and can provoke graft loss at a high frequency. In this IFN-γ ELISPOT assay, PBMC isolated from patients are directly stimulated with a panel of common viral antigens added to the culture. Synthetic pools of overlapping peptides of viruses such as BK, CMV, and EBV are commercially available, as are extracts containing soluble antigens of common pathogens such as *Candida* and mumps (see Figure 11.2). Pre-transplant assessment of patients' response to these infectious pathogens with IFN-γ ELISPOT will determine their immune competence against these pathogens. Non-responsive patients with no or low number of memory T cells are at higher risk of becoming infected after transplant in general and specifically if transplanted with tissue or organ originating from a donor seropositive to these pathogens. Likewise, post-transplant monitoring of patients' response to these common antigens will determine their level of immune competence. Retention of an elevated number of reactive cells is associated with protection from infection [100, 101].

Another use of ELISPOT in transplantation is the B cell ELISPOT assay. This assay is aimed at measuring the number of circulating memory B cells in peripheral blood. We have previously described different methodologies, used in the clinical histocompatibility laboratory to identify anti-HLA antibodies in transplant recipients. However, it is possible to underestimate a humoral response in transplant patients due to adsorption of specific anti-donor antibodies to the organ graft [102]. Also, anti-donor antibodies might be undetectable during *de novo* humoral immune reactions due to low serum concentrations. Under such conditions, the B cell ELISPOT assay can be an important tool to estimate the humoral immune state of patients. A common approach with the B cell ELISPOT is to expose PBMC to polyclonal antigen, for 48 to 72 hours, to stimulate antibody secretion. Activation times are not sufficiently long for conversion of naïve B cells into lymphoblast or plasma cells that secrete antibodies. However, active circulating plasma cells will be detected in the non-activated control. The frequency of B cells expressing specific anti-HLA antibodies might be too low to be detected using PBMC, where they constitute 10%–15% of the total lymphocyte population. In this case, B cell concentration can be enriched by positive selection (anti-CD19[+]) or negative selection (anti-CD2[+], CD3[+], CD16[+], CD36[+], CD56[+], CD66b[+]) of the original PBMC preparation.

The B cell ELISPOT procedure is similar in principle to the IFN-γ ELISPOT assay. A capture anti-IgG is coated onto the ELISPOT plate and pre-activated PBMC are added onto the plate and incubated for 24 hours to allow expression of antibodies. Samples are divided and incubated in different wells for detection of total- or antigen-specific-IgG. After washing plates, secreted antibodies remain attached to capture antibodies. The total number of IgG-secreting cells can be detected with a secondary biotinylated anti-IgG antibody. To detect antigen-specific B cells, biotinylated specific antigens are added. Adding HRP-streptavidin conjugated and later developing with a chromogen substrate will reveal spots on the membrane. An alternative method to detect antigen-specific B cells, when antigen amounts are not limiting, is to coat the wells with streptavidin, followed by addition of biotinylated HLA antigens. In this case, the secreted specific anti-HLA antibodies will be "captured" by the antigen. Bound IgG is detected with an HRP-conjugated anti-IgG. Synthetic and recombinant specific HLA antigens have been generated in research studies to identify B cells secreting HLA-A and HLA-B antibodies [103]. Currently, there are no HLA antigens commercially available for this purpose.

Circulating antigen-specific CD8+ T cells and CD4+ T cells can also be identified by the *tetramer* assay. In this test, a specific epitope is bound to synthetic tetrameric forms of fluorochrome-labeled MHC class I or class II molecules [104, 105]. CD8+ T cells recognize antigen in the form of short peptides bound to class I molecules while CD4+ cells bind peptides on class II molecules; thus, cells with the appropriate T cell receptor will bind to the labeled tetramers and can be measured by flow cytometry. As compared to the CTL or ELISPOT assays, the tetramer assay measures only binding to the T cell receptor, not the functional status of the cells. This remains an important limitation of the tetramer assay, since all cells that bind a particular antigen do not necessarily become activated. Another limitation of the tetramer assay is that tetramers of all class I or class II subtypes are not

Laboratory Medicine in Transplantation

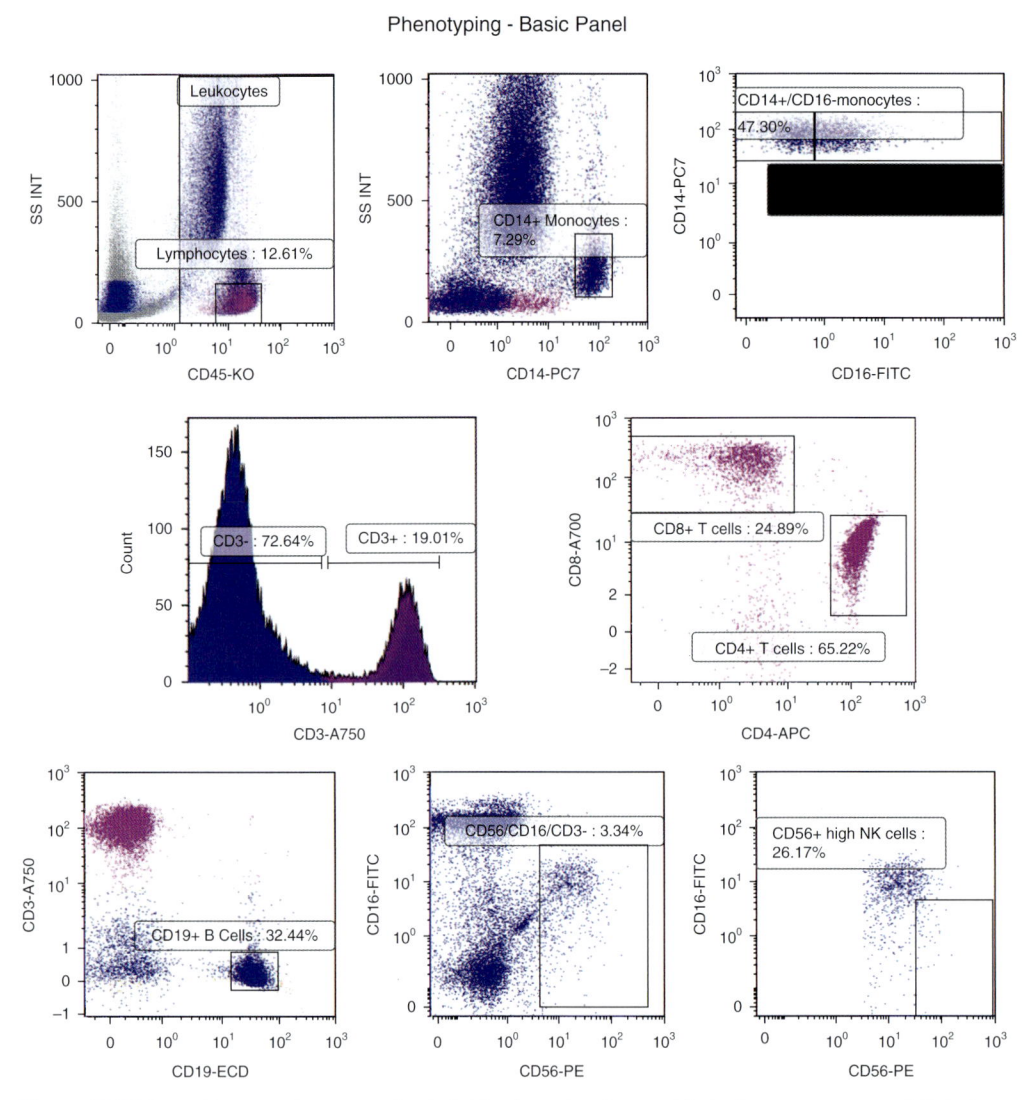

Figure 11.14 General immune phenotype of a whole blood sample using a multicolor flow cytometry panel. Only the most commonly studied subsets of immune cells are shown. T cells and their subsets, T helper cells and T cytotoxic cells, can be identified by the expression of cell surface markers CD3, CD4, and CD8, respectively. The activation status of each T cell subset can be obtained adding markers such as CD69. Another population of interest is the putative T regulatory cells (CD4+CD25High) analyzed from the T helper cells. To complete the delineation of the major cells classes, the addition of CD19 marker for the characterization of B cells and CD16/56 markers for the characterization of Natural Killer (NK) cells are included in this panel.

always available, so that some combinations may not be possible to test. Correlation between ELISPOT, tetramer, and cytotoxicity assays has not always been established.

Measuring the secretion or expression of the molecules associated or involved in cell-mediated killing has been used to assess the functional activity of cytotoxic lymphocytes. Among the mechanisms of cell-mediated cytotoxicity is exocytosis of cytoplasmic granules from the effector cell toward the target cell. These membrane-enveloped lysosomes are principally composed of granzymes and perforin. The lipid bilayer surrounding them contains lysosomal associated membrane glycoproteins (LAMPs) [106], including LAMP-1 (CD107a). As part of the fusion of membranes during the degranulation process, CD107a, once exclusive to granule membrane, is now expressed on the surface of effector cells [107]. Upon induction of apoptosis, phosphatidylserine (PS) is externalized resulting in its accessibility to the surface. This phospholipid can bind Annexin V. Thus, antibodies specific for CD107a and labeled Annexin V can be used by flow cytometry to identify effector cells and apoptotic target cells [108]. This assay may ultimately replace the more classical ^{51}CR assay.

Immunophenotypic analysis by flow cytometry can provide extremely useful immune status information of cellular populations following organ transplantation [109] – this technique can identify and monitor peripheral lymphocyte subpopulations that change in close relationship with the organ recipient's immune status during the principal complications (i.e., infections and rejections) in the post-transplant period. Multicolor flow cytometry is performed as a means of enumerating a variety of cell populations in the peripheral blood while simultaneously measuring their coexpression of many molecules that relate to activation status, maturation, and clonality (see Figure 11.14). T lymphocytes are critical for the initiation and maintenance of allograft rejection and cytofluorographic analysis of peripheral blood during rejection episodes reveals increases in CD4+ and CD8+ T lymphocytes expressing IL-2 receptors and/or HLA-DRw antigens, suggesting lymphocyte activation. Immunophenotyping by cytometry can also evaluate the presence of regulatory cells that may be associated with immunological quiescence and that may be leading to operational tolerance (e.g., FoxP3+ cells) [110], the effects caused by immunosuppressive drugs, monoclonal and polyclonal antibodies (whether depleting or non-depleting), and the magnitude of cellular depletion (e.g., CD52+ subpopulations following Campath® /alemtuzumab therapy). Infectious and malignant processes (e.g., clonality studies of B cells in PTLD) and antibody dependent injury (e.g., platelet antibody studies) can also be evaluated by flow cytometry. The most commonly used monoclonal antibody panels used to stain cells postoperatively aim to characterize T cells and their subsets (CD2, CD3, CD4, CD8, TcR alpha/beta, CD7), B cells (CD19, CD20, CD22, kappa, lambda), and NK cells (CD16/56), along with the coexpression of a variety of surface molecules (CD25, CD34, CD45, CD52, HLA-DRw, and CD138) and intracellular molecules (e.g., FoxP3), can also be evaluated [111].

The measurement of intracellular cytokines (ICC) along with coexpression of other lineage markers by flow cytometry or fluorescent microscopy has been a very useful tool to identify T cell subpopulations such as Th1 and Th2 cells [112, 113]. These cells have polarized cytokine gene expression and secretion (e.g., Th1 – IFN-γ; Th2 – IL-4, IL-5, IL-9, and IL-13). Indeed, heightened activity of either Th1 or Th2 cells has been associated with a variety of disease states (e.g., Th1 – sarcoidosis, graft rejection, some autoimmune conditions; Th2 – extracellular pathogens, antibody production, asthma), so that measurement of their levels often has some utility in assessing some conditions and in vaccine development [114, 115]. Th1 cell levels vary during transplant rejection or infectious disease in transplant patients and their measurement has generally been performed on the basis of the type of cytokine being expressed. Recently, other markers for T-Helper subset identification have emerged, such as GATA3 and T-bet. Future assays may be evaluating differential expression of these nuclear factors as a means of measuring these different effector T cell populations [116].

LDA (Limiting Dilution Assay): These assays measure precursor frequencies of different effector populations (e.g., T helper cells, T cytotoxic cells) within a sample to a specific antigen (e.g., alloantigen) and the readout can be proliferation or cytotoxicity. These tests are labor-intensive and time-consuming to perform and the numbers of donor and recipient cells available are often limited; as such, there is minimal current utility in the clinical lab. There are a variety of methods used for LDA analysis, with many based on the single-hit Poisson model or double-hit model [117–119].

II The Clinical Immunology and General Laboratories

Infectious Disease Screening

The presence of infectious agents endures as one of the principal causes of morbidity and mortality following transplantation, occurring to a great extent as a result of the profound immunosuppression these patients typically undergo. Infectious disease *serological* screening is a stalwart element of the clinical immunology laboratory, since it measures the presence of host antibody responses to bacterial, fungal, or viral antigens. There are a variety of means to measure antibodies in the clinical lab, including solid-phase ELISA (enzyme linked) assays, nephelometry, and immunofixation techniques. Microbial antigens may also be detected with these methods. Among the limitations of serological assessment are that some individuals have a poor antibody response or the measurement may be within the time period between initial infection and seroconversion. In addition to screening patients in the post-transplant period, these methods can also be used to screen potential donors for infectious pathogens.

Classical microbiological methodologies (e.g., culturing, identification, drug sensitivity testing) are essential maintenance tests of most transplant patients, but their description is beyond the focus and scope of this chapter.

Molecular methods for the identification of infectious agents identify the presence of the actual pathogen DNA or RNA sequence and these methods have become an indispensible part of the clinical laboratory. PCR is the typical method for many of these assays, although other molecular testing methods are also now becoming available. These molecular assays are used for detection and quantification, the latter often useful in immunocompromised transplant patients. Sequence-specific primers may be used for qualitative analysis and/ or a labeled oligonucleotide-probe to do quantitative analysis. In addition to being able to detect few molecules, this methodology is capable of rapid turnaround time (often two to four hours) to obtain a result. Several latent viruses, such as CMV and EBV, are monitored with these PCR quantitative methods [120]. The presence of HIV, HBV, HCV, and polyoma virus [121, 122] can be resolved without laborious and time-consuming culture methods. The sources of the measurements are often serum or plasma, but biopsy measurements are also now being performed.

The clinical laboratory also assists in the detection and monitoring of disease recurrence in allograft organs. Chronic HCV infection is a common cause of end-stage liver disease requiring liver transplantation. Although almost all patients that receive a liver allograft for HCV will have detectable HCV RNA levels post-transplant [123, 124], there is a wide variation in the severity of the clinical course and histological response. In this regard, investigators have focused on the levels of HCV viremia and the different HCV genotypes [122]. There are some laboratories that offer highly sophisticated PCR-based techniques to detect and quantitate HCV RNA and genotype the virus. HCV RNA levels performed monthly post-transplant are used in conjunction with surgical biopsies to evaluate the appropriateness of antiviral therapy.

Drug Monitoring in Organ Transplantation

The measurement of immunosuppressive drug levels is a critical test performed in the clinical transplant laboratory. Some of the standard immunosuppressive agents used in transplantation,

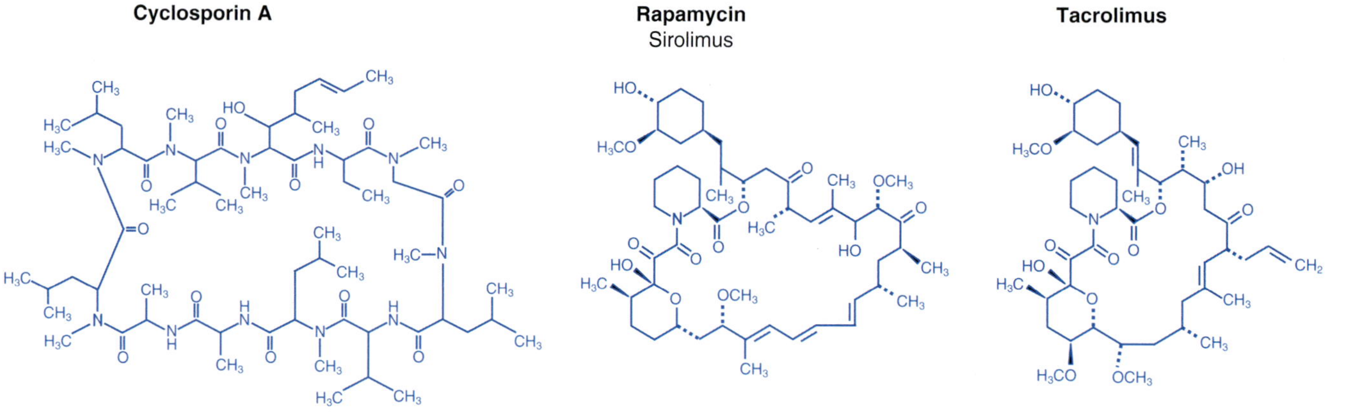

Figure 11.15 Chemical structures of common immunosuppressant agents.

particularly cyclosporine (CsA) and tacrolimus, have a very narrow therapeutic range and become ineffective at low concentrations and toxic at high concentrations [125]. Continuous monitoring of the dosage and trough level of immune suppressive drugs in organ transplantation therefore is critical in the management of the recipient's immune response to the allograft [126, 127]. Among the unfavorable side effects of immunosuppressive drugs are toxicity, cancer, and infection, and there is often a connection between acute complications and the elevated levels present in the recipient. Likewise, suboptimal levels of these drugs can have an association with rejection episodes occurring in the host, although the utility of post-transplant monitoring of immunosuppressive drugs to prevent rejection episodes remains inconclusive.

The optimal method to monitor these drugs has been a matter of debate [128]. There is extensive metabolizing in the liver of these compounds and an accumulation of metabolites may contribute to their toxicity, therefore determination of not only the parent drug, but also of its metabolites, is of clinical importance [129, 130]. High-pressure-liquid chromatography is considered the gold standard method for monitoring levels of many drugs [131]; however, this technique requires expensive instrumentation. Immunoassays utilizing monoclonal antibodies have also proved to be excellent alternatives for drug monitoring [132]. It is of paramount importance that these techniques demonstrate accuracy, precision, sensitivity, and specificity, since drug doses are taken at a specific time of the day and the sample should be taken before the next dose is due. The following drugs are among the most commonly monitored in a therapeutic drug-monitoring laboratory. These drugs often target cell activation pathways to inhibit immune cell populations [133, 134] and to a certain extent, there may be synergistic effects between them. Some of these drugs (see Figure 11.15) that are monitored by the lab are:

Tacrolimus (FK506, Prograf) inhibits the activation of T cells, and the active compound binds to the immunophilin, FKBP-12. A complex of tacrolimus-FKBP-12, calcium, calmodulin, and calcineurin is then formed and the phosphatase activity of calcineurin is inhibited [135]. Thereafter, dephosphorylation and translocation of nuclear factor of activated T cells (NF-AT), a nuclear component that initiates gene transcription and production of cytokines such as IL-2 and IFN-γ (see Figure 11.16), is transported. With this action, there is an inhibition of T lymphocyte activation (i.e., immunosuppression). There are many side effects associated with tacrolimus, since it can affect many organ systems, including gastrointestinal, nervous, and renal, and their incidence is high; the effects are typically dose-related [136]. The principal adverse reactions are tremor, headache, diarrhea, hypertension, nausea, and abnormal renal function. In some cases, tacrolimus can be used to reverse acute rejection episodes using higher doses. It is usually administered in the morning and the monitoring level is taken shortly before the morning dose. The optimal trough levels tend to be between 5 and 15 μg/L.

Cyclosporine (Neoral, CSA, Gengraf) is another potent immunosuppressive agent and also a calcineurin inhibitor, blocking IL-2 production that in turn downregulates T cell production and activation. Cyclosporine (CsA) binds to its immunophilin, cyclophilin (CpN), forming a complex between cyclosporine and CpN (see Figure 11.16). The cyclosporine–CpN complex binds and blocks calcineurin, inhibiting its phosphatase activity. As described above, CaN fails to dephosphorylate the cytoplasmic component of NF-AT, and its transport to the nucleus. There is no promoter of the interleukin 2 (IL-2) gene, a lack of IL-2 production, and no T cell activation. Therefore, though the pre-drugs cyclosporine and FK506 bind to different target molecules, both drugs ultimately inhibit T cell activation in the same fashion (see Figure 11.16). The principal adverse reactions can be similar to tacrolimus and include renal dysfunction, tremor, hirsutism, hypertension, and gum hyperplasia. Renal cyclosporine toxicity may be acute (e.g., glomerular capillary thrombosis) (see Figure 11.17) or chronic [137]. The target level for CSA is 100–400 μg/L. As with tacrolimus, there are a variety of oral and intravenous formulations.

Sirolimus (Rapamune) is a macrocyclic lactone produced by *Streptomyces hygroscopicus* that, in cells, binds to the immunophilin, FKBP-12, forming a complex that binds to and inhibits the activation of the mammalian Target of Rapamycin (mTOR), a key regulatory kinase (see Figure 11.18) [138]. The sirolimus: FKBP-12 complex has no effect on calcineurin activity. The mTOR inhibition suppresses cytokine-driven T cell proliferation, inhibiting the progression from the G_1 to the S phase of the cell cycle. It

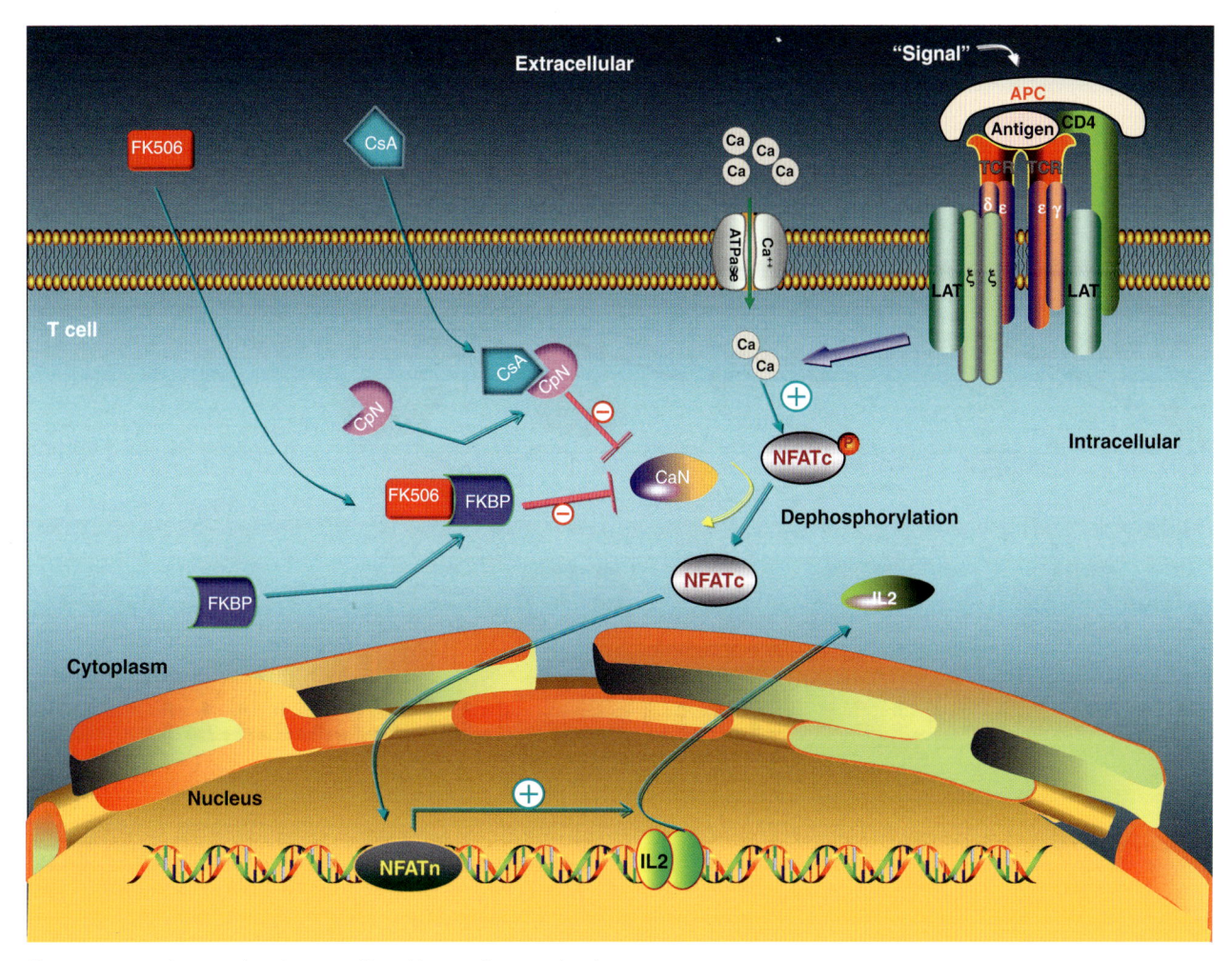

Figure 11.16 Pathways in lymphocytes affected by tacrolimus and cyclosporine.

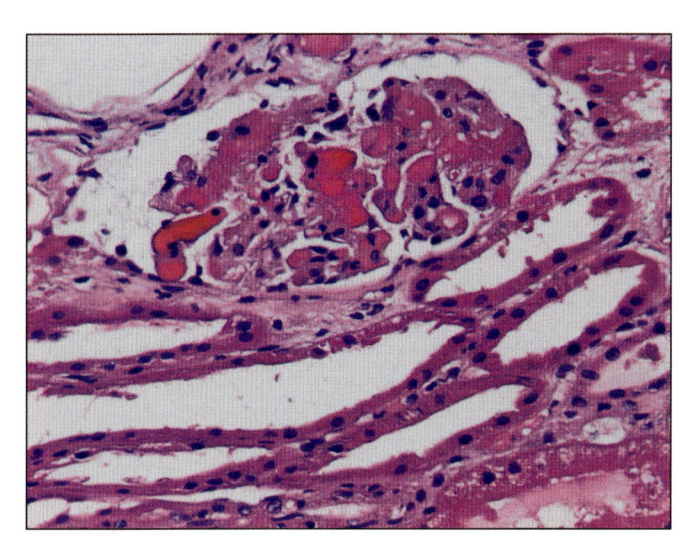

Figure 11.17 Renal biopsy showing glomerular thrombosis and isometric vacuolization (toxic tubulopathy) secondary to CsA toxicity (hematoxylin and eosin, 400X).

can be administered concomitantly with calcineurin inhibitors. Among the side effects of sirolimus are hypercholesterolemia, hyperlipemia, hypertension, rash, anemia, arthralgia, diarrhea, hypokalemia, and thrombocytopenia.

Everolimus (Zortress) is a 40-*O*-(2-hydroxyethyl) derivative of sirolimus and has a mechanism of action comparable to sirolimus as an inhibitor of mTOR [139]. Everolimus has been increasingly used as immunosuppression for several solid organ transplants [139, 140] and has been claimed to improve allograft vasculopathy in heart transplant patients [141]. This drug is also used as treatment for a variety of tumors [142, 143]. A number of side effects have been described [144].

Mycophenylate mofetil (MMF, Cellcept) is an inhibitor of inosine monophosphate dehydrogenase (IMPDH), affecting the *de novo* pathway of guanosine nucleotide synthesis without incorporation into DNA (see Figure 11.19) [145]. T cells and B cells are dependent on de novo synthesis of purines for their proliferation and have no salvage pathways, thus MMF has potent cytostatic effects on lymphocytes. MPA also suppresses antibody formation by B lymphocytes. MPA prevents the glycosylation of lymphocyte and monocyte glycoproteins involved in adhesion to endothelial cells and thus affects immune cell recruitment into sites of graft rejection.

Molecular Prognostic and Predictive, Systemic, and in Situ Biomarkers in Transplants

In addition to immune monitoring of transplant patients by measuring humoral and cellular alloreactivity, infectious

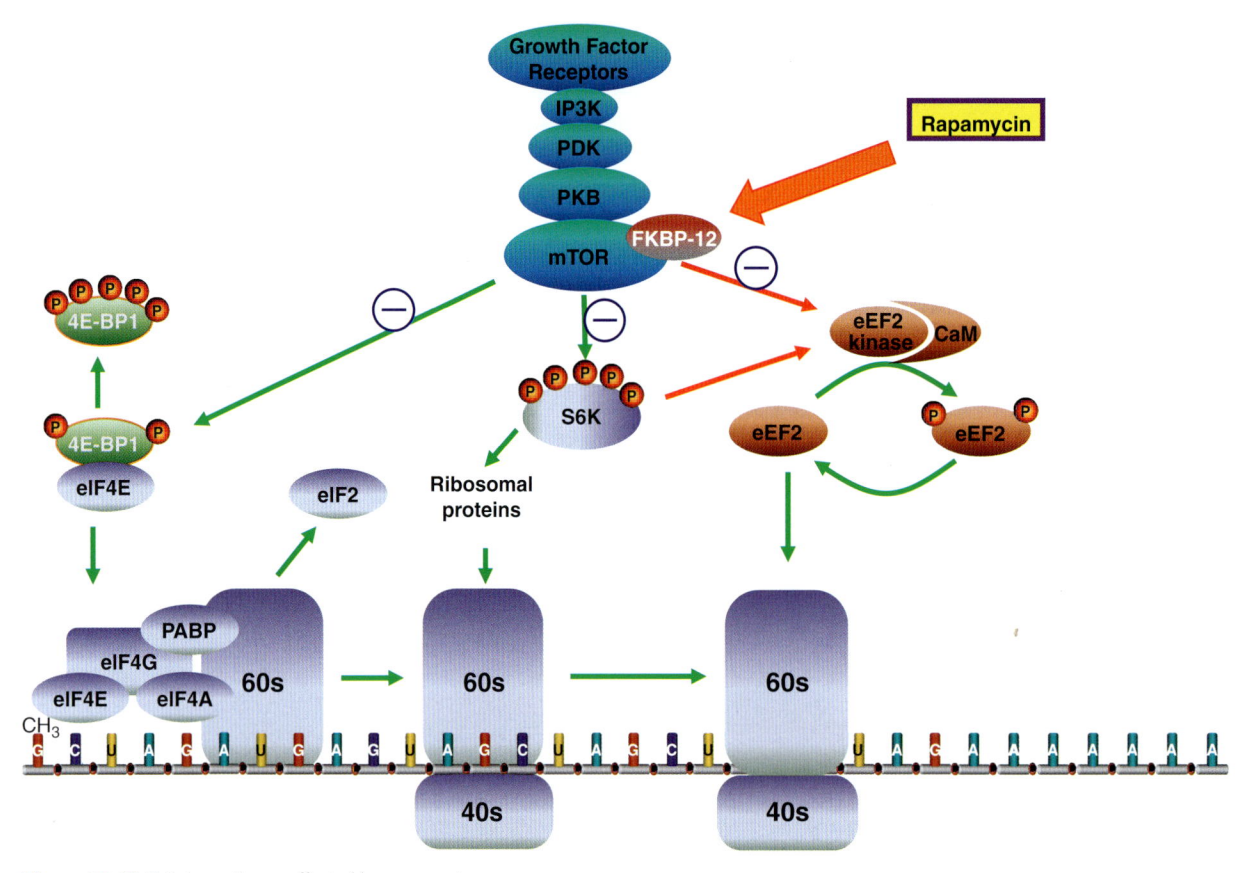

Figure 11.18 Cellular pathway affected by rapamycin.

monitoring, drug level determinations, and standard chemical measurements of end organ function, molecular markers are being steadily added to the toolbox that clinicians can use to determine the condition of grafts. Recent advances in molecular technologies, which have become more reliable and reproducible, have allowed the discovery of expression-based molecular markers that in the near future will be introduced as clinical assays in transplant laboratories. Expression analysis is a molecular method that measures the amount of messenger RNA (mRNA) of a specific gene within an individual's body fluids (urine and blood) or tissue. All cellular mRNA is isolated from the specimen and transcribed to complementary DNA (cDNA) by a reverse transcriptase and random decamer priming. Modern versions of natural reverse transcriptases have been engineered to reduced ribonuclease H activity and increase thermal stability to generate consistently high yields of full-length cDNA. To determine the copy number of specific mRNA, the cDNA is run on a real-time PCR machine, along with a negative control and four to five recombinant standards of known copy numbers from which a standard curve can be generated. The number of molecules of mRNA is calculated from this standard curve.

Gene expression profiling using DNA microarrays has become a powerful tool for analysis of gene expression changes in transplanted organs. Total RNA from samples can be directly labeled to use as probes or complementary DNA (cDNA). New microarray systems are constantly improving with updated definitions of mRNAs and annotations of the human genome. Today, high-density arrays can evaluate more than 60,000 genes and include non-coding RNA regions (miRNA, ncRNA, and lincRNA). This increase in the number of targets, together with improvement of dynamic range in several orders of magnitude, allows a more complete coverage of the human transcriptome. Simultaneous expression profiling of a large number of genes allows analyses of expression changes in specific pathways, giving a better understanding of the related pathological processes taking place. On the other hand, genome-wide profiling today is not practical as a rapid clinical test, given that microarray technology is not simple; it requires analysis of substantial amounts of data with software tools and is costly. The current utility of microarray falls on the discovery of specific transcripts that could be identified as potential biomarkers for molecular monitoring of transplant patients at risk of rejection.

An alternative technology to microarray is Real Time-PCR (RT-PCR). The RT-PCR technology was developed for detection of specific PCR amplification products using SYBR® Green or TaqMan probes. The technology can be applied to compare gene expression of two samples or to determine copy number of a specific mRNA. Measurements of differential gene expression are carried out by comparing a sample to a control, and the results are expressed as "fold change." A typical reaction will contain a forward and a reverse primer, and the detection label. These reactions are commercially available for expression

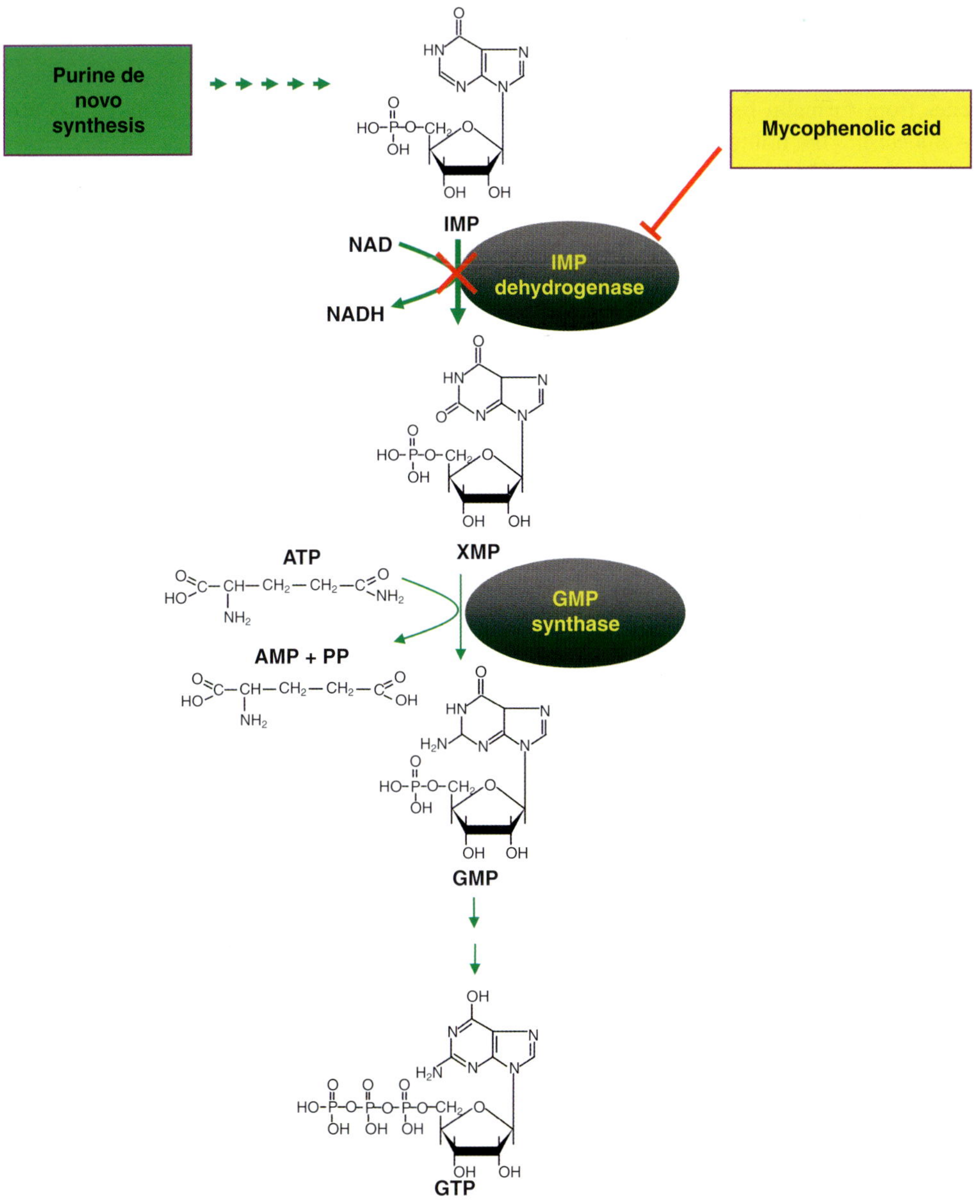

Figure 11.19 Cellular pathway affected by mycophenolate.

analysis of coding (mRNAs) and non-coding genes like microRNAs (miRNA), as a single assay or in array format containing many genes categorized in pathways. The technology is reliable and results are reproducible. In recent years, several studies have focused their efforts to identify mRNA and miRNA that could be used as molecular markers to monitor the functional status of transplanted grafts and rejection levels. Several genes involved in rejection, with potential to be used as biomarkers, have been uncovered using microarray- and RT-PCR–based expression studies. For example, a significant upregulation of genes involved in infiltration and activation of lymphocytes such as B cells, T cells, macrophages, and natural killer cells has been found in transplanted kidney biopsies of patients with acute kidney transplant rejection [146, 147]. Some of the genes involved in cellular rejection that have been nominated as potential markers are related to cytotoxic T cells (CD8, granzyme A and B, perforin, PD-1, and Fas ligand), T helper cells (CD4, CD28, and CTLA4), regulatory T cells (FOXP3), and antigen presenting cells such as B cells, dendritic cells, and macrophages (CD20, CD19, CD80, CD86, and CD14). Also, genes expressing chemokines (CXCL9, CXCL10, CXCL11, CCL2, CCL3, and CCL4) and chemokine receptors (CCR4, CCR5, and CCR7) are significantly overexpressed in infiltrated tissues. There are more than a thousand microRNAs in the human genome with predicted targets that exceed 60% of the expressed human genes. miRNAs are involved in downregulation of target genes and are expressed in specific cell types. They have been explored as a source of potential markers for monitoring graft status. miRNAs expressed in leukocytes (miR-142–5p, -142–3p, -886–3p, -155, -150, -223, and -132) are implicated in cellular rejection of kidney and small bowel grafts [148–150]. Strong correlations exist between the expression profiles of these candidate markers and their intra-graft expression detected by histology. Although these emerging biomarkers are promising, they will require multicenter validation. One large advance has been to be able to measure these genes from formalin-fixed, paraffin-embedded tissue; this greatly embellishes the utility of the biopsy. Recently, a molecular score was proposed for kidney transplant based on expression of relevant molecular markers. The aim of this diagnostic system is to help improve diagnosis based only on histology [151]. There has been also detection of expression variations of mRNAs and miRNAs in non-biopsy tissues such as serum, urine, sputum, or bronchoalveolar lavage (BAL) samples [152]; this may serve to be an adjunct or substitute for biopsies in some situations. These expression panels are becoming more refined and will ultimately permit accurate predictions of progression towards a rejection episode, differentiating between organ injury and cellular or humoral rejection.

References

1. Christiansen FT. HLA and Transplantation – The Role of the Histocompatibility Laboratory. Pathology – Journal of the RCPA. 2010;**42**:S46.
2. Becker LE, Susal C, Morath C. Kidney Transplantation across HLA and ABO Antibody Barriers. Curr Opin Organ Transplant. 2013;**18**(4):445–54.
3. Mierzejewska B, Durlik M, Lisik W, Baum C, Schroder P, Kopke J, et al. Current Approaches in National Kidney Paired Donation Programs. Ann Transplant. 2013;**18**:112–24.
4. Leffell MS, Zachary AA. The Role of the Histocompatibility Laboratory in Desensitization for Transplantation. Curr Opin Organ Transplant. 2009;**14**(4):398–402.
5. Leeser DB, Aull MJ, Afaneh C, Dadhania D, Charlton M, Walker JK, et al. Living Donor Kidney Paired Donation Transplantation: Experience as a Founding Member Center of the National Kidney Registry. Clin Transplant. 2012;**26**(3):E213–22.
6. Murphey CL, Bingaman AW. Histocompatibility Considerations for Kidney Paired Donor Exchange Programs. Curr Opin Organ Transplant. 2012;**17**(4):427–32.
7. de Bakker PI, Raychaudhuri S. Interrogating the Major Histocompatibility Complex with High-throughput Genomics. Hum Mol Genet. 2012;**21**(R1):R29–36.
8. Bjorkman PJ, Saper MA, Samraoui B, Bennett WS, Strominger JL, Wiley DC. Structure of the Human Class I Histocompatibility Antigen, HLA-A2. Nature. 1987;**329**(6139):506–12.
9. Gussow D, Rein R, Ginjaar I, Hochstenbach F, Seemann G, Kottman A, et al. The Human Beta 2-microglobulin Gene. Primary Structure and Definition of the Transcriptional Unit. J Immunol. 1987;**139**(9):3132–8.
10. Travers P, Blundell TL, Sternberg MJ, Bodmer WF. Structural and Evolutionary Analysis of HLA-D-region Products. Nature. 1984;**310**(5974):235–8.
11. Petersdorf EW. Genetics of Graft-versus-Host Disease: The Major Histocompatibility Complex. Blood Rev. 2013;**27**(1):1–12.
12. Shlomchik WD. Graft-versus-Host Disease. Nature Reviews Immunology. 2007;7(5):340–52.
13. Sheldon S, Poulton K. HLA Typing and Its Influence on Organ Transplantation. Methods in Molecular Biology (Clifton, NJ). 2006;**333**:157–74.
14. Mytilineos J, Lempert M, Scherer S, Schwarz V, Opelz G. Comparison of Serological and DNA PCR-SSP Typing Results for HLA-A and HLA-B in 421 Black Individuals: A Collaborative Transplant Study Report. Human Immunology. 1998;**59**(8):512–7.
15. Erlich H. HLA DNA Typing: Past, Present, and Future. Tissue Antigens. 2012;**80**(1):1–11.
16. Horsburgh T, Martin S, Robson AJ. The Application of Flow Cytometry to Histocompatibility Testing. Transpl Immunol. 2000;**8**(1):3–15.
17. Eng HS, Leffell MS. Histocompatibility Testing after Fifty Years of Transplantation. J Immunol Methods. 2011;**369**(1–2):1–21.
18. Lu Y, Boehm J, Nichol L, Trucco M, Ringquist S. Multiplex HLA-typing by Pyrosequencing. Methods in Molecular Biology (Clifton, NJ). 2009;**496**:89–114.
19. Terasaki PI, McClelland JD. Microdroplet Assay of Human Serum Cytotoxins. Nature. 1964;**204**:998–1000.
20. Petersdorf EW. The Major Histocompatibility Complex: A Model for Understanding Graft-versus-Host Disease. Blood. 2013;**122**(11):1863–72.
21. Gibbs RA. DNA Amplification by the Polymerase Chain Reaction. Analytical Chemistry. 1990;**62**(13):1202–14.
22. Schiffman MH. Validation of Hybridization Assays: Correlation of Filter in Situ, Dot Blot and PCR with Southern Blot. IARC Sci Publ. 1992 (**119**):169–79.
23. Stott DI. Immunoblotting, Dot-blotting, and ELISPOT Assays: Methods and Applications. Journal of Immunoassay. 2000;**21**(2–3):273–96.
24. Cao K, Chopek M, Fernandez-Vina MA. High and Intermediate Resolution DNA Typing Systems for Class I HLA-A, B, C Genes by Hybridization with Sequence-specific Oligonucleotide Probes (SSOP). Reviews in Immunogenetics. 1999;**1**(2):177–208.
25. Luo M, Blanchard J, Pan Y, Brunham K, Brunham RC. High-resolution Sequence Typing of HLA-DQA1 and -DQB1 Exon 2 DNA with Taxonomy-based Sequence Analysis (TBSA) Allele Assignment. Tissue Antigens. 1999;**54**(1):69–82.
26. Hosomichi K, Jinam TA, Mitsunaga S, Nakaoka H, Inoue I. Phase-defined Complete Sequencing of the HLA Genes by Next-generation Sequencing. BMC Genomics. 2013;**14**:355.
27. Trachtenberg EA, Holcomb CL. Next-generation HLA Sequencing Using the 454 GS FLX System. Methods in Molecular Biology (Clifton, NJ). 2013;**1034**:197–219.
28. Goodwin S, McPherson JD, McCombie WR. Coming of Age: Ten Years of Next-generation Sequencing Technologies. Nat Rev Genet. 2016;**17**(6):333–51.
29. Scientific TF. Ion Torrent™ Next-gen Sequencing Technology. 2014, May 19.
30. Rothberg JM, Hinz W, Rearick TM, Schultz J, Mileski W, Davey M, et al. An Integrated Semiconductor Device Enabling Non-optical Genome sequencing. Nature. 2011;**475**(7356):348–52.
31. Guo J, Xu N, Li Z, Zhang S, Wu J, Kim DH, et al. Four-color DNA Sequencing with 3'-O-modified Nucleotide Reversible Terminators and Chemically Cleavable Fluorescent

31. Dideoxynucleotides. Proc Natl Acad Sci U S A. 2008;**105**(27):9145–50.
32. Inc. I. Illumina Sequencing by Synthesis (Now in 3D). 2016, Oct 5.
33. Scientific. TF. The Workflow | Ion Chef System Enables Walk away Freedom. 2016 Jan 26.
34. Freedman BI, Pastan SO, Israni AK, Schladt D, Julian BA, Gautreaux MD, et al. APOL1 Genotype and Kidney Transplantation Outcomes from Deceased African American Donors. Transplantation. 2016;**100**(1):194–202.
35. Kidd KK1 KJ, Speed WC, Fang R, Furtado MR, Hyland FC, Pakstis AJ. Expanding Data and Resources for Forensic Use of SNPs in Individual Identification. Forensic Science International: Genetics. 2012;**6**(5):646–52.
36. Cano P, Klitz W, Mack SJ, Maiers M, Marsh SG, Noreen H, et al. Common and Well-documented HLA Alleles: Report of the Ad-Hoc Committee of the American Society for Histocompatiblity and Immunogenetics. Hum Immunol. 2007;**68**(5):392–417.
37. Mack SJ, Cano P, Hollenbach JA, He J, Hurley CK, Middleton D, et al. Common and Well-documented HLA Alleles: 2012 Update to the CWD Catalogue. Tissue Antigens. 2013;**81**(4):194–203.
38. Tambur AR, Leventhal JR, Zitzner JR, Walsh RC, Friedewald JJ. The DQ Barrier: Improving Organ Allocation Equity Using HLA-DQ Information. Transplantation. 2013;**95**(4):635–40.
39. Kaneku H. 2012. Annual Literature Review of Donor-specific HLA Antibodies after Organ Transplantation. Clin Transpl. **2012**:207–17.
40. Duquesnoy RJ, Awadalla Y, Lomago J, Jelinek L, Howe J, Zern D, et al. Retransplant Candidates Have Donor-specific Antibodies that React with Structurally Defined HLA-DR,DQ,DP Epitopes. Transpl Immunol. 2008;**18**(4):352–60.
41. Kristt D, Stein J, Yaniv I, Klein T. Assessing Quantitative Chimerism Longitudinally: Technical Considerations, Clinical Applications and Routine Feasibility. Bone Marrow Transplant. 2007;**39**(5):255–68.
42. Boeck S, Hamann M, Pihusch V, Heller T, Diem H, Rolf B, et al. Kinetics of Dendritic Cell Chimerism and T Cell Chimerism in Allogeneic Hematopoietic Stem Cell Recipients. Bone Marrow Transplant. 2006;**37**(1):57–64.
43. Kruchen A, Stahl T, Gieseke F, Binder TM, Ozcan Z, Meisel R, et al. Donor Choice in Haploidentical Stem Cell Transplantation: Fetal Microchimerism Is Associated with Better Outcome in Pediatric Leukemia Patients. Bone Marrow Transplant. 2015;**50**(10):1367–70.
44. van Besien K, Liu HT, Artz A. Microchimerism and Allogeneic Transplantation: We Need the Proof in the Pudding. Chimerism. 2013;**4**(3):109–10.
45. Kletzel M, Huang W, Olszewski M, Khan S. Validation of Chimerism in Pediatric Recipients of Allogeneic Hematopoietic Stem Cell Transplantation (HSCT) a Comparison between Two Methods: Real-time PCR (qPCR) vs. Variable Number Tandem Repeats PCR (VNTR PCR). Chimerism. 2013;**4**(1):1–8.
46. Taimur S, Askar M, Sobecks R, Rybicki L, Warshawsky I, Mossad S. Donor T-cell Chimerism and Early Post-transplant Cytomegalovirus Viremia in Patients Treated with Myeloablative Allogeneic Hematopoietic Stem Cell Transplant. Transpl Infect Dis. 2013.
47. Andreani M, Testi M, Gaziev J, Condello R, Bontadini A, Tazzari PL, et al. Quantitatively Different Red Cell/Nucleated Cell Chimerism in Patients with Long-term, Persistent Hematopoietic Mixed Chimerism after Bone Marrow Transplantation for Thalassemia Major or Sickle Cell Disease. Haematologica. 2011;**96**(1):128–33.
48. Hsieh MM, Kang EM, Fitzhugh CD, Link MB, Bolan CD, Kurlander R, et al. Allogeneic Hematopoietic Stem-cell Transplantation for Sickle Cell Disease. The New England Journal of Medicine. 2009;**361**(24):2309–17.
49. Pilat N, Wekerle T. Transplantation Tolerance through Mixed Chimerism. Nat Rev Nephrol. 2010;**6**(10):594–605.
50. Levin MD, de Veld JC, van der Holt B, van't Veer MB. Screening for Alloantibodies in the Serum of Patients Receiving Platelet Transfusions: A Comparison of the ELISA, Lymphocytotoxicity, and the Indirect Immunofluorescence Method. Transfusion. 2003;**43**(1):72–7.
51. Doughty R, James V, Magee J. An Enzyme Linked Immunosorbent Assay for Leucocyte and Platelet Antibodies. J Immunol Methods. 1981;**47**(2):161–9.
52. Okudaira K, Goodwin JS, Williams RC, Jr. Anti-Ia Antibody in the Sera of Normal Subjects after in Vivo Antigenic Stimulation. J Exp Med. 1982;**156**(1):255–67.
53. Bishara A, Nelken D, Bonavida B, Brautbar C. Enzyme-linked Immunosorbent Assay for Determination of HLA: Gene Dose Effect. Tissue Antigens. 1984;**23**(5):284–9.
54. Buican TN, Purcell A. 'Many-color' Flow Microfluorometric Analysis by Multiplex Labelling. Survey of Immunologic Research. 1983;**2**(2):178–88.
55. Keij JF, Steinkamp JA. Flow Cytometric Characterization and Classification of Multiple Dual-color Fluorescent Microspheres Using Fluorescence Lifetime. Cytometry. 1998;**33**(3):318–23.
56. Vignali DA. Multiplexed Particle-based Flow Cytometric Assays. J Immunol Methods. 2000;**243**(1–2):243–55.
57. Pei R, Lee JH, Shih NJ, Chen M, Terasaki PI. Single Human Leukocyte Antigen Flow Cytometry Beads for Accurate Identification of Human Leukocyte Antigen Antibody Specificities. Transplantation. 2003;**75**(1):43–9.
58. El-Awar N, Lee J, Terasaki PI. HLA Antibody Identification with Single Antigen Beads Compared to Conventional Methods. Hum Immunol. 2005;**66**(9):989–97.
59. Qiu J, Cai J, Terasaki PI, El-Awar N, Lee JH. Detection of Antibodies to HLA-DP in Renal Transplant Recipients Using Single Antigen Beads. Transplantation. 2005;**80**(10):1511–3.
60. Goodman RS, Taylor CJ, O'Rourke CM, Lynch A, Bradley JA, Key T. Utility of HLAMatchmaker and Single-antigen HLA-antibody Detection Beads for Identification of Acceptable Mismatches in Highly Sensitized Patients Awaiting Kidney Transplantation. Transplantation. 2006;**81**(9):1331–6.
61. Bray RA, Nolen JDL, Larsen C, Pearson T, Newell KA, Kokko K, et al. Transplanting the Highly Sensitized Patient: The Emory Algorithm. American Journal of Transplantation. 2006;**6**(10):2307–15.
62. Zachary AA, Sholander JT, Houp JA, Leffell MS. Using Real Data for a Virtual Crossmatch. Human Immunology. 2009;**70**(8):574–9.
63. Grenzi PC, de Marco R, Silva RZR, Campos ÉF, Gerbase-DeLima M. Antibodies against Denatured HLA Class II Molecules Detected in

64. Weinstock C, Schnaidt M. The Complement-mediated Prozone Effect in the Luminex Single-antigen Bead Assay and Its Impact on HLA Antibody Determination in Patient Sera. Int J Immunogenet. 2013;**40**(3):171–7.
65. Shenton BK, Bell AE, Harmer AW, Boyce M, Briggs D, Cavanagh G, et al. Importance of Methodology in the Flow Cytometric Crossmatch: A Multicentre Study. Transplantation Proceedings. 1997;**29**(1–2):1454–5.
66. Gandhi MJ, DeGoey S, Falbo D, Jenkins S, Stubbs JR, Noreen H, et al. Inter and Intra Laboratory Concordance of HLA Antibody Results Obtained by Single Antigen Bead Based Assay. Human Immunology. 2013;**74**(3):310–7.
67. Cecka JM. Calculated PRA (CPRA): The New Measure of Sensitization for Transplant Candidates. Am J Transplant. 2010;**10**(1):26–9.
68. Leffell MS. The Calculated Panel Reactive Antibody Policy: An Advancement Improving Organ Allocation. Curr Opin Organ Transplant. 2011;**16**(4):404–9.
69. Gebel HM, Bray RA. The Evolution and Clinical Impact of Human Leukocyte Antigen Technology. Curr Opin Nephrol Hypertens. 2010;**19**(6):598–602.
70. Chang D, Kobashigawa J. The Use of the Calculated Panel-reactive Antibody and Virtual Crossmatch in Heart Transplantation. Curr Opin Organ Transplant. 2012;**17**(4):423–6.
71. Campbell P. Clinical Relevance of Human Leukocyte Antigen Antibodies in Liver, Heart, Lung and Intestine Transplantation. Curr Opin Organ Transplant. 2013;**18**(4):463–9.
72. Ellis TM, Schiller JJ, Roza AM, Cronin DC, Shames BD, Johnson CP. Diagnostic Accuracy of Solid Phase HLA Antibody Assays for Prediction of Crossmatch Strength. Hum Immunol. 2012;**73**(7):706–10.
73. Kostyu DD, Cresswell P, Amos DB. A Public HLA Antigen Associated with HLA-A9, Aw32, and Bw4. Immunogenetics. 1980;**10**(5):433–42.
74. Parham P, McLean J. Characterization, Evolution, and Molecular Basis of a Polymorphic Antigenic Determinant Shared by HLA-A and B Products. Hum Immunol. 1980;**1**(2):131–9.
75. Hollenbach JA, Madbouly A, Gragert L, Vierra-Green C, Flesch S, Spellman S, et al. A Combined DPA1~DPB1 Amino Acid Epitope is the Primary Unit of Selection on the HLA-DP Heterodimer. Immunogenetics. 2012;**64**(8):559–69.
76. Gebel HM, Lebeck LK. Crossmatch Procedures Used in Organ Transplantation. Clinics in Laboratory Medicine. 1991;**11**(3):603–20.
77. Sandler SG, Abedalthagafi MM. Historic Milestones in the Evolution of the Crossmatch. Immunohematology / American Red Cross. 2009;**25**(4):147–51.
78. Bray RA, Tarsitani C, Gebel HM, Lee JH. Clinical Cytometry and Progress in HLA Antibody Detection. Methods Cell Biol. 2011;**103**:285–310.
79. Scornik JC. Detection of Alloantibodies by Flow Cytometry: Relevance to Clinical Transplantation. Cytometry. 1995;**22**(4):259–63.
80. Talbot D. Flow Cytometric Crossmatching in Human Organ Transplantation. Transpl Immunol. 1994;**2**(2):138–9.
81. Bach FH, Bach ML, Sondel PM, Sundharadas G. Genetic Control of Mixed Leukocyte Culture Reactivity. Transplant Rev. 1972;**12**:30–56.
82. DuPont B, Hansen JA. Human Mixed-lymphocyte Culture Reaction: Genetics, Specificity, and Biological Implications. Advances in Immunology. 1976;**23**:107–202.
83. Gordon J. The Mixed Leukocyte Culture Reaction. Med Clin North Am. 1972;**56**(2):337–51.
84. He J, Li Y, Zhang H, Wei X, Zheng H, Xu C, et al. Immune Function Assay (ImmuKnow) as a Predictor of Allograft Rejection and Infection in Kidney Transplantation. Clin Transplant. 2013;**27**(4):E351–8.
85. Ge S, Pao A, Vo A, Deer N, Karasyov A, Petrosyan A, et al. Immunologic Parameters and Viral Infections in Patients Desensitized with Intravenous Immunoglobulin and Rituximab. Transpl Immunol. 2011;**24**(3):142–8.
86. Schulz-Juergensen S, Burdelski MM, Oellerich M, Brandhorst G. Intracellular ATP Production in CD4+ T Cells as a Predictor for Infection and Allograft Rejection in Trough-level Guided Pediatric Liver Transplant Recipients under Calcineurin-Inhibitor Therapy. Therapeutic Drug Monitoring. 2012;**34**(1):4–10.
87. Klein E. Interpretation of Lymphocytotoxicity Assays and the Demonstration of Auto-tumor Reactive Lymphocytes in Patients: Central Issues of Present Day Tumor Immunology. The Tokai Journal of Experimental and Clinical Medicine. 1983;**8**(5–6):385–98.
88. Martz E, Heagy W, Gromkowski SH. The Mechanism of CTL-mediated Killing: Monoclonal Antibody Analysis of the Roles of Killer and Target-cell Membrane Proteins. Immunol Rev. 1983;**72**:73–96.
89. Biesecker JL, Fitch FW, Rowley DA, Scollard D, Stuart FP. Cellular and Humoral Immunity after Allogeneic Transplantation in the Rat. II. Comparison of a 51Cr Release Assay and Modified Microcytotoxicity Assay for Detection of Cellular Immunity and Blocking Serum Factors. Transplantation. 1973;**16**(5):421–31.
90. Bradley JA, Mason DW, Morris PJ. Evidence that Rat Renal Allografts Are Rejected by Cytotoxic T Cells and Not by Nonspecific Effectors. Transplantation. 1985;**39**(2):169–75.
91. Gurley KE, Lowry RP, Forbes RD. Immune Mechanisms in Organ Allograft Rejection. II. T Helper Cells, Delayed-type Hypersensitivity, and Rejection of Renal Allografts. Transplantation. 1983;**36**(4):401–5.
92. Augustine JJ, Hricik DE. T-cell immune Monitoring by the ELISPOT Assay for Interferon Gamma. Clin Chim Acta. 2012;**413**(17–18):1359–63.
93. Lehmann PV, Zhang W. Unique Strengths of ELISPOT for T Cell Diagnostics. Methods Mol Biol. 2012;**792**:3–23.
94. Hirayama M, Azuma E, Kumamoto T, Iwamoto S, Yamada H, Nashida Y, et al. Prediction of Acute Graft-versus-Host Disease and Detection of Distinct End-organ Targets by Enumeration of Peripheral Blood Cytokine Spot-forming Cells. Transplantation. 2005;**80**(1):58–65.
95. Poggio ED, Augustine JJ, Clemente M, Danzig JM, Volokh N, Zand MS, et al. Pretransplant Cellular Alloimmunity as Assessed by a Panel of Reactive T Cells Assay Correlates with Acute Renal Graft Rejection. Transplantation. 2007;**83**(7):847–52.
96. Zand MS, Bose A, Vo T, Coppage M, Pellegrin T, Arend L, et al. A Renewable Source of Donor Cells for Repetitive Monitoring of T- and B-cell Alloreactivity. Am J Transplant. 2005;**5**(1):76–86.
97. Cherkassky L, Lanning M, Lalli PN, Czerr J, Siegel H, Danziger-Isakov L, et al. Evaluation of Alloreactivity in Kidney Transplant Recipients Treated with Antithymocyte Globulin versus

IL-2 Receptor Blocker. Am J Transplant. 2011;11(7):1388–96.

98. Augustine JJ, Poggio ED, Heeger PS, Hricik DE. Preferential Benefit of Antibody Induction Therapy in Kidney Recipients with High Pretransplant Frequencies of Donor-reactive Interferon-gamma Enzyme-linked Immunosorbent Spots. Transplantation. 2008;86(4):529–34.

99. Pearl JP, Parris J, Hale DA, Hoffmann SC, Bernstein WB, McCoy KL, et al. Immunocompetent T-cells with a Memory-like Phenotype Are the Dominant Cell Type Following Antibody-mediated T-cell Depletion. Am J Transplant. 2005;5(3):465–74.

100. Abate D, Saldan A, Mengoli C, Fiscon M, Silvestre C, Fallico L, et al. Comparison of CMV ELISPOT and CMV Quantiferon Interferon-gamma Releasing Assays in Assessing Risk of CMV Infection in Kidney Transplant Recipients. J Clin Microbiol. 2013.

101. Prosser SE, Orentas RJ, Jurgens L, Cohen EP, Hariharan S. Recovery of BK Virus Large T-antigen-specific Cellular Immune Response Correlates with Resolution of BK Virus Nephritis. Transplantation. 2008;85(2):185–92.

102. Adeyi OA, Girnita AL, Howe J, Marrari M, Awadalla Y, Askar M, et al. Serum Analysis after Transplant Nephrectomy Reveals Restricted Antibody Specificity Patterns against Structurally Defined HLA Class I Mismatches. Transpl Immunol. 2005;14(1):53–62.

103. Heidt S, Roelen DL, de Vaal YJ, Kester MG, Eijsink C, Thomas S, et al. A NOVel ELISPOT Assay to Quantify HLA-specific B Cells in HLA-immunized Individuals. Am J Transplant. 2012;12(6):1469–78.

104. Altman JD, Davis MM. MHC-peptide Tetramers to Visualize Antigen-specific T Cells. Current Protocols in Immunology. Edited by John E Coligan [et al]. 2003;Chapter 17:Unit 17 3.

105. Nepom GT. MHC Class II Tetramers. J Immunol. 2012;188(6):2477–82.

106. Fukuda M. Lysosomal Membrane Glycoproteins. Structure, Biosynthesis, and Intracellular Trafficking. J Biol Chem. 1991;266(32):21327–30.

107. Zaritskaya L, Shurin MR, Sayers TJ, Malyguine AM. New Flow Cytometric Assays for Monitoring Cell-mediated Cytotoxicity. Expert Review of Vaccines. 2010;9(6):601–16.

108. Wlodkowic D, Skommer J, Darzynkiewicz Z. Cytometry of Apoptosis. Historical Perspective and New Advances. Experimental Oncology. 2012;34(3):255–62.

109. Mathew JM, Fuller L, Carreno M, Garcia-Morales R, Burke GW, 3rd, Ricordi C, et al. Involvement of Multiple Subpopulations of Human Bone Marrow Cells in the Regulation of Allogeneic Cellular Immune Responses. Transplantation. 2000;70(12):1752–60.

110. Takahashi H, Ruiz P, Ricordi C, Delacruz V, Miki A, Mita A, et al. Quantitative in Situ Analysis of FoxP3+ T Regulatory Cells on Transplant Tissue Using Laser Scanning Cytometry. Cell Transplant. 2012;21(1):113–25.

111. Setoguchi R, Hori S, Takahashi T, Sakaguchi S. Homeostatic Maintenance of Natural Foxp3+ CD25+ CD4+ Regulatory T Cells by Interleukin (IL)-2 and Induction of Autoimmune Disease by IL-2 Neutralization. Journal of Experimental Medicine. 2005;201(5):723–35.

112. Bleesing JJ, Fleisher TA. Cell Function-based Flow Cytometry. Semin Hematol. 2001;38(2):169–78.

113. Pala P, Hussell T, Openshaw PJ. Flow Cytometric Measurement of Intracellular Cytokines. J Immunol Methods. 2000;243(1–2):107–24.

114. De Rosa SC. Vaccine Applications of Flow Cytometry. Methods (San Diego, Calif). 2012;57(3):383–91.

115. Maecker HT, Nolan GP, Fathman CG. New Technologies for Autoimmune Disease Monitoring. Current Opinion in Endocrinology, Diabetes, and Obesity. 2010;17(4):322–8.

116. Afzali B, Lombardi G, Lechler RI, Lord GM. The Role of T Helper 17 (Th17) and Regulatory T Cells (Treg) in Human Organ Transplantation and Autoimmune Disease. Clinical and Experimental Immunology. 2007;148(1):32–46.

117. Dozmorov I, Eisenbraun MD, Lefkovits I. Limiting Dilution Analysis: From Frequencies to Cellular Interactions. Immunology Today. 2000;21(1):15–8.

118. Fazekas de St G. The Evaluation of Limiting Dilution Assays. J Immunol Methods. 1982;49(2):R11–23.

119. Sharrock CE, Kaminski E, Man S. Limiting Dilution Analysis of Human T Cells: A Useful Clinical Tool. Immunology Today. 1990;11(8):281–6.

120. Smith TF, Espy MJ, Mandrekar J, Jones MF, Cockerill FR, Patel R. Quantitative Real-time Polymerase Chain Reaction for Evaluating DNAemia due to Cytomegalovirus, Epstein-Barr Virus, and BK Virus in Solid-organ Transplant Recipients. Clinical Infectious Diseases. 2007;45(8):1056–61.

121. Hirsch HH, Randhawa P, the ASTIDCoP. BK Polyomavirus in Solid Organ Transplantation. American Journal of Transplantation. 2013;13(s4):179–88.

122. Manzia TM, Angelico R, Toti L, Lai Q, Ciano P, Angelico M, et al. Hepatitis C Virus Recurrence and Immunosuppression-free State after Liver Transplantation. Expert Review of Clinical Immunology. 2012;8(7):635–44.

123. Everhart JE, Wei Y, Eng H, Charlton MR, Persing DH, Wiesner RH, et al. Recurrent and New Hepatitis C Virus Infection after Liver Transplantation. Hepatology. 1999;29(4):1220–6.

124. Costes V, Durand L, Pageaux GP, Ducos J, Mondain AM, Picot MC, et al. Hepatitis C Virus Genotypes and Quantification of Serum Hepatitis C RNA in Liver Transplant Recipients. Relationship with Histologic Outcome of Recurrent Hepatitis C. American Journal of Clinical Pathology. 1999;111(2):252–8.

125. Wallemacq PE, Wallemacq PE. Therapeutic Monitoring of Immunosuppressant Drugs. Where Are We? Clinical Chemistry & Laboratory Medicine. 2004;42(11):1204–11.

126. Lin S, Cosgrove CJ, Lin S, Cosgrove CJ. Perioperative Management of Immunosuppression. Surgical Clinics of North America. 2006;86(5):1167–83.

127. Kirk AD. Induction Immunosuppression. Transplantation. 2006;82(5):593–602.

128. Armstrong VW, Schuetz E, Zhang Q, Groothuisen S, Scholz C, Shipkova M, et al. Modified Pentamer Formation Assay for Measurement of Tacrolimus and Its Active Metabolites: Comparison with Liquid Chromatography-tandem Mass Spectrometry and Microparticle Enzyme-linked Immunoassay (MEIA-II). Clinical Chemistry. 1998;44(12):2516–23.

129 Davis DL, Murthy JN, Gallant-Haidner H, Yatscoff RW, Soldin SJ. Minor Immunophilin Binding of Tacrolimus and Sirolimus Metabolites. Clinical Biochemistry. 2000;33(1):1–6.

130 Murthy JN, Davis DL, Yatscoff RW, Soldin SJ. Tacrolimus Metabolite Cross-reactivity in Different Tacrolimus Assays. Clinical Biochemistry. 1998;31(8):613–7.

131 Taylor PJ, Taylor PJ. Therapeutic Drug Monitoring of Immunosuppressant Drugs by High-performance Liquid Chromatography-mass Spectrometry. Therapeutic Drug Monitoring. 2004;26(2):215–9.

132 Andrews DJ, Cramb R. Cyclosporin: Revisions in Monitoring Guidelines and Review of Current Analytical Methods. Annals of Clinical Biochemistry. 2002;39(Pt 5):424–35.

133 Filler G. Calcineurin Inhibitors in Pediatric Renal Transplant Recipients. Paediatric Drugs. 2007;9(3):165–74.

134 Gustafsson F, Ross HJ, Gustafsson F, Ross HJ. Proliferation Signal Inhibitors in Cardiac Transplantation. Current Opinion in Cardiology. 2007;22(2):111–6.

135 Reichenspurner H. Overview of Tacrolimus-based Immunosuppression after Heart or Lung Transplantation. Journal of Heart & Lung Transplantation. 2005;24(2):119–30.

136 Bowman LJ, Brennan DC. The Role of Tacrolimus in Renal Transplantation. Expert Opin Pharmacother. 2008;9(4):635–43.

137 Chapman JR, Nankivell BJ. Nephrotoxicity of Ciclosporin A: Short-term Gain, Long-term Pain? Nephrology Dialysis Transplantation. 2006;21(8):2060–3.

138 Hartford CM, Ratain MJ. Rapamycin: Something Old, Something New, Sometimes Borrowed and Now Renewed. Clinical Pharmacology & Therapeutics. 2007;82(4):381–8.

139 de Pablo A, Santos F, Sole A, Borro JM, Cifrian JM, Laporta R, et al. Recommendations on the Use of Everolimus in Lung Transplantation. Transplant Rev (Orlando). 2013;27(1):9–16.

140 Beckebaum S, Cicinnati VR, Radtke A, Kabar I. Calcineurin Inhibitors in Liver Transplantation – Still Champions or Threatened by Serious Competitors? Liver International: Official Journal of the International Association for the Study of the Liver. 2013;33(5):656–65.

141 Eisen HJ, Tuzcu EM, Dorent R, Kobashigawa J, Mancini D, Valantine-von Kaeppler HA, et al. Everolimus for the Prevention of Allograft Rejection and Vasculopathy in Cardiac-transplant Recipients. New England Journal of Medicine. 2003;349(9):847–58.

142 Lebwohl D, Anak O, Sahmoud T, Klimovsky J, Elmroth I, Haas T, et al. Development of Everolimus, a Novel Oral mTOR Inhibitor, Across a Spectrum of Diseases. Ann N Y Acad Sci. 2013;1291:14–32.

143 Yao JC, Phan AT, Jehl V, Shah G, Meric-Bernstam F. Everolimus in Advanced Pancreatic Neuroendocrine Tumors: The Clinical Experience. Cancer Res. 2013;73(5):1449–53.

144 Pallet N, Legendre C. Adverse Events Associated with mTOR Inhibitors. Expert Opinion on Drug safety. 2013;12(2):177–86.

145 Allison AC, Eugui EM. Mechanisms of Action of Mycophenolate Mofetil in Preventing Acute and Chronic Allograft Rejection. Transplantation. 2005;80(2 Suppl):S181–90.

146 Ho J, Wiebe C, Gibson IW, Rush DN, Nickerson PW. Immune Monitoring of Kidney Allografts. Am J Kidney Dis. 2012;60(4):629–40.

147 Famulski KS, de Freitas DG, Kreepala C, Chang J, Sellares J, Sis B, et al. Molecular Phenotypes of Acute Kidney Injury in Kidney Transplants. J Am Soc Nephrol. 2012;23(5):948–58.

148 Anglicheau D, Sharma VK, Ding R, Hummel A, Snopkowski C, Dadhania D, et al. MicroRNA Expression Profiles Predictive of Human Renal Allograft Status. Proc Natl Acad Sci U S A. 2009;106(13):5330–5.

149 Sotolongo B, Asaoka T, Island E, Carreno M, Delacruz V, Cova D, et al. Gene Expression Profiling of MicroRNAs in Small-bowel Transplantation Paraffin-embedded Mucosal Biopsy Tissue. Transplant Proc. 2010;42(1):62–5.

150 Asaoka T, Sotolongo B, Island ER, Tryphonopoulos P, Selvaggi G, Moon J, et al. MicroRNA Signature of Intestinal Acute Cellular Rejection in Formalin-fixed Paraffin-embedded Mucosal Biopsies. Am J Transplant. 2012;12(2):458–68.

151 Reeve J, Sellares J, Mengel M, Sis B, Skene A, Hidalgo L, et al. Molecular Diagnosis of T cell-mediated Rejection in Human Kidney Transplant Biopsies. Am J Transplant. 2013;13(3):645–55.

152 Cravedi P, Heeger PS. Immunologic Monitoring in Transplantation Revisited. Curr Opin Organ Transplant. 2012;17(1):26–32.

Index

ABO-I AMR, 76, 77
ABO-incompatible liver, 78f
ABO-I transplants, 76
ABO-mismatch
    major or bidirectional, 267
    minor, 267
    transfusion of platelets or plasma, 267
accelerated graft arteriosclerosis. *see* cardiac allograft vasculopathy (CAV)
acinar atrophy/fibrosis, 229f
acinar cell injury, 218
acinar inflammation, 227f
    acute antibody mediated allograft rejection, 230f, 236f
    mild acute T-cell mediated rejection, 230, 236f
    multifocal, 231
acinar tissues in protocol biopsy, 232f
Actinomycetes-associated sulfur granule, 168, 169f
active enteritis, 205f, 205–6
active transplant arteriopathy, 222f, 238
acute allergic interstitial nephritides, 46, 47f
acute allograft rejection, pancreas transplants, 217–18
    CD3 stain, 223f
    immunological aspects, 220
    morphological features of, 221–4
    pathogenetic aspects of, 224
acute antibody mediated allograft rejection
    acinar inflammation in, 230f
    C4d stain, 230f
acute antibody-mediated rejection (AAMR), 10, 29, 39f–40f
    accelerated acute rejection, 35
    acute graft injury, 35
    alloantibodies, 10
    alloantibodies in, 10
    Banff classification scheme, 77
    biomarkers for, 10, 11f
C4d immunofluorescence staining, 37–8
C4d staining, 10, 37–8
clinical symptomatology of, 37
complement cascade activation, 10
DSA alloantibody, 37, 39f–40f
hyperacute rejection, 35, 39f
IgG in kidney undergoing, 10f
incidence of, 35
molecular gene profiling of grafts undergoing, 10
morphological presentations for, 37
acute antibody-mediated rejection (AAMR), liver transplant, 76
    Banff criteria for diagnosing, 77
    clinical presentation of, 77
    criteria for diagnosis of, 77t
    histopathologic features of, 77
    risk factors for, 77
acute antibody-mediated rejection (AAMR), pancreatic, 239f
    ACMR and, 237
    diagnosis of, 234–5, 236–7
    treatment of, 235
acute bacterial pyelonephritis, 52
acute bronchopneumonia, 168f, 168
acute cellular airway inflammation, 162–3
    grading basis of, 162
    interobserver variability, 162–3
    two-tier grading system of, 162, 163f
acute cellular rejection (ACR), 306, 307f
    ITx recipients. *see* acute T-cell mediated rejection in ITx recipients
    lung. *see* acute cellular rejection (ACR), lung transplants
    MVTx recipients. *see* acute T-cell mediated rejection in MVTx recipients
acute cellular rejection (ACR), heart transplants, 134t. *see also* acute T-cell mediated rejection (TCMR)
    effector cells, 135
    grading in endomyocardial biopsies, 135–6
    inflammatory infiltration, 135
    morphological features of, 135
    promoters and effectors of, 135
acute cellular rejection (ACR), lung transplants, 159–60
    acute cellular airway inflammation, 162–3
    acute cellular vascular rejection, 161–2
    BAL fluid analysis and, 163–4
    clinical presentation of, 159
    diagnostic tool for evaluating, 159–60
    immune reaction of recipient lymphocytes, 159
    incidence of, 159
    pathologic grading of, 160t, 160–1
    radiologic imaging of, 159
acute cellular vascular rejection, 161–2
    grade A0, 161
    grade A1, 161f, 161
    grade A2, 161f
    grade A3, 161–2, 162f
    grade A4, 162, 163f
    infiltrate, 161
acute graft injury, 35
acute humoral rejection and CTA, 307
acute ischemic tubular injury (ATI), 52
acute liver allograft rejection Banff grading of, 82t
acute lymphoblastic leukemia (ALL), 262
acute myeloid leukemia (AML), 262
acute promyelocytic leukemia (APL), 262
acute rejection (AR), 10, 47
    acute antibody-mediated rejection. *see* acute antibody mediated rejection (AAMR)
    antibody and cell mediated forms of, 43
    bowel, 187
    cell-mediated acute rejection. *see* cell-mediated acute rejection (CMAR)
    chronic rejection, 12–13
    definition of, 185
    drug toxicity, 15
    infection, 13–15
    kidney transplantation. *see* acute rejection in kidney transplantation
    molecular assays of, 43
    recurrent/de novo immune diseases, 15
acute rejection activity index (RAI), 82, 83t
acute rejection, in ITx and MVTx recipients, 185–6
    acute antibody-mediated rejection, 188f, 189f, 189t, 190f
    acute T-cell mediated rejection in. *see* acute T-cell mediated rejection in ITx recipients; acute T-cell mediated rejection in MVTx recipients
    clinical and endoscopic correlation of, 187
    histopathology associated with, 187
    hyperacute and accelerated, 187–8
    importance of diagnosing, 186–7
acute rejection (AR) in kidney transplantation, 30–43
    acute T-cell mediated rejection (TCMR), 30–5. *see also* acute T-cell mediated rejection (TCMR)
    definition, 30
    frequency of, 30
    grading scoring systems for evaluating, 30
    morphological interpretation of, 30

373

Index

acute rejection (cont.)
  pathological classification of, 30
  subclinical rejection, 30
  symptoms of, 30
acute rejection-mediated injury, 186–7
acute T-cell-mediated allograft rejection, 222f, 227f
  area of biopsy with, 229f
  epithelial damage, 238f
  inflammation in, 228f
  multifocal acinar inflammation and single cell acinar cell damage, 228f
  septal inflammation, 228f
acute T-cell mediated rejection (TCMR), 31f–3f
  arteritis in, 33f–4f
  Banff classification scheme, 36t–7t
  characterization of, 30–1
  ductitis, 237f
  etiology of, 31
  immunophenotypic evaluations, 31–2
  inflammatory response in, 32–3
  kidney with extensive tubulitis, 11f
  late onset. *see* late onset TCMR
  lymphocytic aggregates, 34
  mild, 229–30, 236f–8f
  moderate, 231–2, 236f
  response to immunosuppression, 32
  severe, 232–3
  stomach allograft, 11f
  transplant glomerulitis, 34–5, 37f–8f
  tubulitis, 31, 32–3
  variability in histological appearance of, 31
acute T-cell mediated rejection in ITx recipients, 190f
  bowel allograft, 191f
  classification schemes for grading. *see* small intestinal allograf, classification schemes for grading ACR in
  histological features associated with, 190
  pathophysiological processes of, 190
  susceptibility to, 190
acute T-cell mediated rejection in MVTx recipients
  colon allografts, 194, 195f–6f
  stomach allografts, 195, 197f, 198t
acute tubular injury (ATI), 28
  donor kidney, 27f, 27, 29
  donor kidney biopsies, 27f, 27
acute tubular necrosis (ATN), 28
  AAMR with, 37

acute tubulointerstitial rejection. *see* acute T-cell mediated rejection (TCMR)
acyclovir, 271
adaptive immune response, 9
adaptive immune system reconstitution after HCT, 268–9
adenocarcinoma in situ, 175
adenovirus (ADV) hepatitis, 91f
  differential diagnosis of, 92
  histopathologic findings, 91–2
  pathophysiology of, 91
adenovirus (ADV) infections, 251
  ADV hepatitis. *see* adenovirus (ADV) hepatitis
  ITx and MVTx, 200f–1f, 200
  pancreas transplantation complications, 251
adenovirus infections of renal allografts, 50–1
  adenovirus induced nephritis, 51
  diagnosis of, 50–1
  morphological features of, 50
  types of, 51
adipose tissue endomyocardial biopsy, 142f, 142–3
adjunct non-invasive lab and biomarker assays, 187
adrenal rests, 333
adverse drug reactions and toxic injury, 105
aGVHD (acute form of GVHD), 297f
  broad category of, 295
  cGVHD *vs.*, 275
  clinical manifestations of, 274, 295–6
  clinicopathologic findings of, 277t, 279
  early lesions of, 296
  effector phase of, 276–7
  gastrointestinal tract, 277, 278f
  hepatic, 279, 279f
  oral manifestations of, 298
  pathogenesis of, 275f, 276
  prevention and treatment of, 279
  skin, 277, 277f, 282f, 296
airway complications, lung transplantation, 159f, 159
airway inflammation. *see* acute cellular airway inflammation
alcoholic liver disease (ALD), 103
  clinical presentation of, 104
  histopathologic findings, 104
  pathophysiology of, 103–4
alcohol recidivism. *see* recurrent alcohol abuse
allelic mismatch and GVHD risk, 265–6

allergic type interstitial nephritides, 46–7
alloantibodies, 148
  AAMR, 10
  acute antibody mediated rejection, 10
  DSA, 37
alloantigen stimulation, chronic, 7
allogeneic donor selection, 265–6
  age criteria, 265
  allelic mismatch and GVHD risk, 265–6
  CMV serostatus, 265
  cord blood grafts, 266
  functional status, 149, 265, 361, 367
  GVHD prophylaxis, 266
  haplo-identical with recipient, 266
  immunosuppressive recipient conditioning, 266
  KIR/KIR-L mismatching, 266
  marrow as HSC source, 265
  MSD and MUD, 265, 266
  recipient screening for anti-HLA antibodies, 266
  sibling, 265
  UCBT and haplo-HCT, 265
allogeneic HCT (allo-HCT), 260
  acute lymphoblastic leukemia and, 262
  acute myeloid leukemia and, 262
  adaptive immune system reconstitution after, 268–9
  allogeneic donor selection, 265–6
  approaches to decrease relapse after, 283, 284t
  chronic lymphocytic leukemia and, 262
  chronic myelogenous leukemia and, 262
  GVL responses after, 260
  hemoglobinopathies and, 263
  immunodeficiencies and, 263–4
  inborn errors of metabolism and, 264
  indications for, 262–4
  lymphoproliferative disorders and, 263
  marrow failure syndromes and, 263
  myelodysplastic syndromes and, 263
  myeloproliferative neoplasms and, 263
  NK cell reconstitution after, 268, 269
  rationale in hematologic malignancy treatment, 260
  relapses occurring after, 260
allogeneic HCT (allo-HCT), infections after, 269
  adenovirus infections, 270
  antibiotic-responsive colitis syndrome, 269

  BK viral cystitis/nephritis, 270
  CMV infections, 270, 271
  community respiratory virus infections, 270
  diarrhea, 269
  early post-engraftment infections, 270
  EBV infections, 270
  fungal infections, 269–70
  gram-negative septicemias, 269
  gram-positive infections, 269
  HBV infection, 270
  HHV-6 infections, 270
  HSV and VZV infections, 270
  HSV infections, 270
  invasive fungal infections, 270, 271–2
  IVIg infusions for, 272
  late post-engraftment infections, 270–1
  mycobacterial infections, 270
  neutropenic fever, 269
  nocardia infections, 270
  parasitic infections, 270
  Pneumocystis jirovecii pneumonia, 270
  pneumocystis pneumonia, 271–2
  pneumonia, 271
  PTLD, 271
  strategies to reduce, 271–2
  vaccinations for, 272
  viral gastroenteritis, 270
allograft
  biopsies, 44
  histopathologic changes, 105
  immune response to, 135
  I/R injury to, 8–9
  preservation injury, 9
  recognition and rejection, antigen presentation mechanisms in, 3f
  rejection, thrombolytic and coagulation factors in, 148–9
  vasculopathy. *see* cardiac allograft vasculopathy (CAV)
allograft failure
  causes of, 70
  evaluation of, 68–70
allograft needle biopsy, 99
allograft re-infection, 93
allograft rejection
  cell types involved in, 4f
  thrombolytic and coagulation factors in, 148–9
alloimmune effector processes, 185
alloimmune responses, 10
  chronic rejection and, 12
alloimmunity
  definition, 2
  molecules involved in, 2t
AlloMap Molecular Expression Testing
  cardiac allograft biopsies, 110

Index

alloreactive responses, basis for, 2
alloreactivity, immune networks involved in, 4
  GVHD, 5–6
  HVG reactivity, 4–5
  immune tolerance, 6–8
allorecognition, 5
alveolar hemosiderosis, 176f, 176
aminoglycosides, 269
amiodarone, 174f
AMR signature, 110
amylase, 231f
amylasuria, 218
anaplastic large cell lymphoma (ALCL), 261, 323
anastomotic necrosis and dehiscence, 159
anastomotic strictures, 74
anergy and deletion, 7
angio-immunoblastic T cell lymphomas (AITL), 261
angiomyolipoma, 333
antibody-mediated rejection (AMR), 9
  heart transplant. see antibody-mediated rejection (AMR), heart transplant
  liver transplant. see antibody-mediated rejection (AMR), liver transplant
  lung transplant, 164–6
  pancreas. see antibody mediated rejection (AMR) in pancreas
antibody-mediated rejection (AMR), heart transplant, 134, 143–4, 145t
  clinical presentation, 147
  complement split products, immunostaining of, 144–5, 147
  complement staining artifacts, 148
  endomyocardial biopsies, immunostaining of, 145–6
  histopathologic features of, 144
  immunopathology, 147
  indications for immunostaining, 147
  ISHLT-WF-1990, 144
  ISHLT-WF-2005, 144, 147
  ISHLT-WF-AMR-2011, 147
  2013 ISHLT-Working formulation grades, 146–7
  long term outcome of, 144
  mixed acute cellular and, 147
  platelets and coagulation factors in, 148
  risk factors for, 144
  thrombolytic and coagulation factors in, 148–9
antibody mediated rejection (AMR) in pancreas
  acute. see acute antibody-mediated rejection (AAMR), pancreatic
  causes of, 233
  C4d staining of, 233–4
  chronic active, 237–8, 241f
  DSA studies, 233
  hyperacute rejection, 235–6
  mixed ACMR and, 238
antibody-mediated rejection (AMR), liver transplant, 76–9
  ABO-incompatible liver, 78f
  acute AMR, 76–7, 77t
  C4d staining, 79f
  chronic. see chronic antibody-mediated rejection (AMR)
  differential diagnosis of, 77–9
  lymphocytotoxic cross-match, 79f
antibody-mediated rejection (AMR), pancreas transplant
  early, mild, acute, 231f
  grading of, 226–7
  indeterminate for rejection, 228–9
  microvascular congestion and inflammation, 231f
  mild acute T-cell-mediated rejection, 229–30, 236f–8f
  moderate acute, 231f
  moderate acute T-cell mediated rejection, 231–2
  normal, 228, 232f–3f
  severe acute and chronic, 232f
  severe acute T-cell mediated rejection, 232–3
antigen presentation
  in allograft recognition and rejection, 3f
  direct and indirect, 6
antigen-presenting cells (APCs), MHC class I & class II molecules on, 2
antigen specific T-cell or B-cell responses, 359
anti-HBc+ livers, 67
anti-HLA antibodies, recipient screening for, 266
anti-human globulin (AHG)-CDC, 357
anti-mitochondrial antibodies (AMA), 99
antithymocyte globulin (ATG)
  aGVHD treatment, 279
  in vivo depletion with, 266
antiviral T cell response, 317
apoptosis of T cells, 7
apoptotic hepatocytes, 70
arterial capillary plexus, 75
arterial inflammation, 41, 238
arterial insufficiency, 73
arterial ischemia, 72
arterial ischemic injury, 72
arterial loss, 85
arterial vasodilator, 71
arteriolar hyalinosis, 45, 222f
arteriolosclerosis and arterial hypertension, 45
arteriosclerosis changes
  donor kidney, 26, 27f
  donor kidney biopsy, 26, 27f
arteritis
  intimal, 229f
  necrotizing, 230f
  transmural inflammation and, 230f
Aspergillus infection, 303
asymmetric narrowing of artery, 221f
asymptomatic long-term survivors, 105–9
atheroembolus, 222f
atovaquone, 271
autoantibodies, 98
autoimmune hepatitis (AIH), 98–9
  clinical presentation of, 99
  histopathology and differential diagnosis, 99
  risk factors, 98
"autoimmune" variant of HCV hepatitis, 96
autoimmunity, 3
autologous HCT (auto-HCT), indications for
  B-NHL, 261
  germ cell tumors, 262
  Hodgkin's lymphoma, 261
  mantle cell lymphoma, 261
  multiple myeloma, 261
  neuroblastoma, 262
  peripheral T cell lymphoma, 261
autologous HCT (auto-HCT), infections after, 269
autologous skin grafts, 1
azathioprine, 105
azoles, 270

bacterial infections, 141
  acute bacterial pyelonephritis, 52
  after liver transplantation, 86–7
  bacterial prophylaxis, 271
  cutaneous, 303
  mycobacterial, 270
  nontuberculous mycobacterial, 172
  systemic, 303
Banff category 2 chronic active antibody-mediated rejection. see sclerosing thrombotic microangiopathies
Banff classification scheme, 36t–7t
  acute antibody mediated rejection, 77
  acute T-cell mediated rejection, 36t–7t
  chronic rejection, 81–2, 82t, 83t
  donor kidney biopsies, 26
  TCMR, 81–2, 82t, 83t
basal cell carcinoma (BCC), 306
B cell, 279
  EBV infection of, 315
  recipient-derived, and T cells, 186
  reconstitution after HCT, 268
B-cell activating factor (BAFF), 279
B cell ELISPOT assay, 361
B cell lineage, 52
B cell lymphoma, 324f
B cell Non-Hodgkin Lymphoma (B-NHL), 261
BEC senescence, 99
belimumab, 279
bile duct adenomas, 333
bile duct complications, 74–6
  biliary tract reconstruction, 74
  clinical presentation of, 75
  differential diagnosis of, 76
  histopathologic findings, 75
  peribiliary capillary plexus, 75
  strictures. see strictures
bile duct loss, 85
biliary epithelial cells (BEC)
  loss and biliary strictures, 65
  senescence changes, 85
biliary stricture after transplantation
  BEC loss and, 65
  development of, 65
biliary tract obstruction/stricturing, 71
  chronic, 75f
  vs. TCMR, 76
biliary tract reconstruction, 74
biliary-vascular fistulas, 75
biopsy-negative allograft dysfunction, 143
biopsy-negative rejection, 143
bioptomes, 133f
BK virus positive tubular cells, 49f
bladder drainage. see pancreaticoduodenocystostomy
bone marrow (BM), 261, 265
bortezomib, 279
bowel acute rejection, 187
  diagnosis of, 187
  symptoms, 187
bowel allograf, apoptosis in, 191f
bronchiolitis obliterans (BO), 274, 282
bronchiolitis obliterans syndrome (BOS), 166
  and CMV infections, association between, 171
bronchoalveolar lavage (BAL)
  fluid analysis and ACR, 163–4
bronchoscopic biopsy, 159
Burkitt lymphomas (BL), 322
busulfan with cyclophosphamide (Bu-Cy), 262

Index

calcineurin, 43
calcineurin inhibitor complications
  calcineurin inhibitor induced early tubulopathy, 44f
  calcineurin inhibitor induced thrombotic glomerulopathy, 46f
  calcineurin inhibitor induced TMA, 45–6
  dose dependent, 43
  functional toxicity, 44, 45f
  morphologic changes, 44
  nephrotoxic side effect, 43, 44
  structural toxicity, 43–4
calcineurin inhibitor induced toxicity (CNIT), 44f
  definition, 43
  extended functional, signs of, 44
  glomerular alterations associable with, 45
  larger arteries in, 45
  pathognomonic for, 44
  structural, in arterioles, 44
calcineurin inhibitors (CNI), 43–6, 226, 270
  aGVHD treatment, 279
  complications. see calcineurin inhibitor complications
  outcomes in organ transplantation, 43
cancer in explant organ, 337–9
cancer in organ donors
  active or historical, 331
  discovered after transplantation, 334
  question of, 331
  transmission risks of, 331, 332t
cancer in transplant candidates, 334
cancer in transplant recipients, 312
  EBV infection of B cells, 315
  host response to EBV infection, 316–17
  PTLD. see post transplant lymphoproliferative disorders (PTLD)
  risk of, 312
  standardized incidence ratios for, 313t–14t
cancer, transmission risk of, 332t
Candida infections, 204f, 303
  lung transplant recipients, 169–70
capillaritis, AAMR with, 37
cardiac allograft biopsies
  AlloMap Molecular Expression Testing, 110
cardiac allograft rejection
  cellular rejection. see cellular rejection
  classification of, 134–5
  regulatory cells role in, 135
cardiac allograft vasculopathy (CAV)
  active vasculitis in, 149
  development of, 149
  epicardial coronary atherosclerosis, 149
  frank vasculitis, 149
  lesions of coronary arteries, 149, 150f
  thrombolytic and coagulation factors in AMR, 148–9
cardiac transplantation
  indications for, 133
  survival rate after, 133
  unresectable primary cardiac sarcomas, 149
cardiomyopathies, 133
C4d and CD68 staining, 145–6
CD4+ and CD8+ T cells, intestinal allografts, 190
CD49d inhibitors, 265
C3d immunofluorescence staining, 145, 146f, 147
C4d immunofluorescence staining, 79f, 145, 146f, 147, 234
  acute antibody mediated rejection, 37–8
  AMR in pancreas, 233–4
  AMR of liver transplant, 79f
  chronic antibody-mediated rejection and, 80
  IT samples, 251
CD3 stain, 223f, 227f
C4d stain
  acute antibody mediated allograft rejection, 230f
  increased serum amylase, 231f
cell-based CDC- recipients, 77
cell-mediated acute rejection (CMAR), 10–12
  cell populations causing, 10
  chemokines and, 12
  factors influencing, 10
  HLA class I and class II expression, 12
  identification of cell populations causing, 10–12
  inflammatory phenotype of, 10
cellular immune response, 358
cellular immunity in transplantation, evaluation of
  antigen specific T-cell or B-cell responses, 359
  B cell ELISPOT assay, 361
  cellular immune response, 358
  complexity of, 358–9
  CTL measurement, 359
  ELISPOT assay, 359–61
  exocytosis of cytoplasmic granules, 362
  ICC measurement, 363
  IFN-γ ELISPOT assay, 359–61
  immunophenotyping by cytometry, 362
  importance of, 358
  issues with, 358
  limiting dilution assay, 363
  lymphoid proliferation and cytotoxicity assays, 359
  methods for, 358
  mixed lymphocyte culture, 359
  mixed lymphocyte reaction, 359
  tetramer assay, 361–2
cellular proliferative processes, 175
cellular rejection, 137f
  acute. see acute cellular rejection
  classification of, 135
  hyperacute, 135
  non-rejection biopsy findings, 137–41
central deletional mechanisms, 6–7
central perivenulitis, 81, 82, 83t, 84f, 95, 96, 105
central tolerance, 6–7
centrilobular-based acute rejection, 99
cGVHD (chronic form of GVHD), 296, 300f
  aGVHD vs., 275
  broad category of, 295
  clinical manifestations of, 274–5, 279, 296
  clinicopathologic findings of, 280–82
  corticosteroids for, 279
  eczematoid, 298–9
  hyperpigmentation, 298f
  immunologic consequences of, 282
  lichenoid phase of, 296–7, 298f
  NIH diagnostic criteria for, 280t–1t
  oral manifestations of, 298
  pathogenesis of, 279
  sclerodermatous phase of, 297–8, 299f
  steroids for infection prevention in, 280
  treatment of, 279
cheilitis angularis, 302f
chemokines and cell-mediated acute rejection, 12
chemotherapy and HSC mobilization, 265
cholangiocarcinomas, 92
cholangiolar proliferation, 70
cholangitis, 76
cholestatic hepatitis, 71
cholestatic viral hepatitis, 76
chordae tendineae, 143
chronic active AMR, 237–8, 241f
chronic airway rejection, 166
  definition of, 166
  pathology of, 166
  subtotal, 166f
  total, 166f
chronic allograft arteriopathy, 197, 238
  with foam cells, 41f
  with minimal inflammatory component, 41f
  with prominent inflammatory component, 41f, 42f
chronic allograft enteropathy (CAE)
  chronic inflammatory cells, 197
  fibrosis, 197
  incidence of, 195
  mucosal biopsies, 197–8, 199f
  mucosal fibrosis, semiquantitative grading schema for, 199t
  myointimal hyperplasia, 199f
  pathognomonic microscopic lesion, 196
  pathophysiological process of, 195
  symptomology for, 195–6, 198f
chronic allograft nephropathy. see chronic rejection
chronic allograft rejection/graft sclerosis, pancreatic
  clinical diagnosis of, 224
  graft survival and, 243f
  histological grading of, 238, 242f
  morphological features of, 224–6
  pathogenetic aspects of, 224
chronically rejected livers, 76
chronic antibody-mediated rejection (AMR), 79–80
  C4d staining for, 80
  differential diagnosis for, 79–80
  pediatric liver allograft recipients, 79
  recurrence in adults, 79
chronic diarrhea, 250
chronic graft-versus-host disease (cGVHD), 260
chronic liver disease, 64
chronic lung allograft dysfunction (CLAD), 166
chronic lymphocytic leukemia (CLL), 262
chronic myelogenous leukemia (CML), 262
chronic obstructive pulmonary disease (COPD), 156
chronic rejection, 12–13, 76, 83, 84f, 85f, 85t, 86. see cardiac allograft vasculopathy (CAV)
  alloimmune responses and, 12
  banff grading schema for, 81–2, 82t, 83t
  causes of, 12
  classically-defined. see classically-defined chronic rejection
  CTA and, 307
  differential diagnosis of, 86

Index

early perivenular, 86
features favoring, 86
graft fibrosis, 12–13
histopathologic findings, 84, 85–6
interstitial scarring, 39
kidney allograft, 12f
late stage, 85, 86
molecular assays of, 43
progressive arteriopathy, 12
rejection-induced graft interstitial fibrosis, 39, 41f
risk factors for, 83–4
small bowel allografts. see chronic allograft enteropathy (CAE)
staging, 86
tissue injury, 38–9
transplant endarteritis, 39
chronic transplant glomerulopathy. see transplant glomerulopathy
chronic vascular injury, 224
chronic vascular rejection, 167f
cidofovir, 271
classical Hodgkin lymphoma-type PTLD, 174
classically-defined chronic rejection
  clinical presentation of, 83, 84
  histopathologic findings and staging, 84
clerosing transplant arteriopathy, 41–2
clofarabine, 262
clonal exhaustion after liver transplantation, 7
CMV hepatitis, 88f
  clinical presentation of, 87
  CMV-specific immunohistochemical stains, 87
  confused with EBV hepatitis, 88
  differential diagnosis of, 88
  histopathologic findings, 87–8
  medical therapy, 88
  prevalence of, 87
  risk factors for, 87
CMV infections. see cytomegalovirus (CMV) infections
CMV serostatus allogeneic donor selection, 265
CMV syndrome, 87
CNIT arteriolopathies, 44
  nodular protein deposits, 44
  quantitative scoring scheme of, 45
  regression of, 45
  severity of, 45
CNIT glomerulopathy, 45
coagulation factors in AMR, 148
cold ischemia, 70
collecting ducts, 48
colon allografts, acute T-cell mediated rejection in, 194, 195f–6f

combined heart-lung transplantation, 156
common rejection modules, 111
community acquired viral pneumonias, 172
compartmentalized disease, 87
complement cascade activation, 10
  detected by immunostains, 147
  MAC formation and, 147
  RCA and, 147
complement-dependent cytotoxicity (CDC) crossmatch, 356–7
complement split products
  diagnostic consideration in AMR, 147
  immunostaining of, 144–5, 147
complement staining artifacts, 148
composite tissue allotransplantation (CTA)
  acute cellular rejection monitoring, 306–7
  acute humoral rejection and, 307
  chronic rejection and, 307
  definition of, 306
  method for performing, 306
concurrent acute allograft rejection, 49
congenital heart disease, 133
contraction bands, 143
cord blood grafts
  allogeneic donor selection, 266
coronary vessels, 149
corrected count increment (CCI), 267
costimulatory signals, blockade of, 7
crossmatch (XM) testing, 356–7
crossreactive HLA antibodies and crossreactive groups (CREGs), 355t, 355–6
crypt epithelial cell apoptosis, 190
cryptogenic organizing pneumonia (COP), 273
cryptosporidium, 204f
cutaneous bacterial infections, 303
cutaneous complications, 294
  CTAs and, 306–7
  cutaneous bacterial infections, 303
  cutaneous fungal infections, 303–6
  drug reactions in transplant patients. see drug reactions, transplant patients
  graft-versus-host disease. see graft-versus-host disease (GVHD)
  nephrogenic systemic fibrosis, 294–5
  viral skin infections, 299–303

cutaneous cryptococcosis, 303–4
cutaneous fungal infections, 303–6
CXCR4 inhibitors, 265
cyclophosphamide
  aGVHD treatment, 279
  HSC mobilization and, 265
cyclosporine, 248, 364
  hyperglycemia and, 248–9
cyclosporine-A (CsA), 43
  structural toxicity, 43–4
cystic anomalies, 168
cystoscopic transduodenal pancreas biopsies, 219
cytologic atypia, 336
cytomegalovirus (CMV) infections, 13f, 49–50
  allo-HCT recipients, 271
  and BOS, association between, 171
  clinical manifestations of, 171
  CMV-glomerulopathy, 50
  CMV hepatitis. see CMV hepatitis
  CMV nephritis, 50
  CMV nephropathy, 50
  CMV pneumonitis, 171
  cytomegalovirus enteritis, 200–1, 202f
  definition of, 171
  detection methods, 171
  diagnosis of, 50
  immunohistochemistry staining, 171, 172f
  kidney allograft, 50f
  lesions induced by replication of, 49–50
  lung transplant recipients, 171
  nuclear inclusions, 171
  owls-eye appearance, 50
  skin infections, 299–302
  symptomatic, 49–50
  viral cytopathic changes, 50
cytotoxicity against graft, 5
cytotoxic T lymphocyte (CTL), 3
  GVL and, 260–1
cytotoxic T lymphocyte (CTL) measurement, 359
  B cell ELISPOT assay, 361
  ELISPOT (Enzyme Linked ImmunoSpot) assay, 359–61
  exocytosis of cytoplasmic granules, 362
  IFN-γ ELISPOT assay, 359–61
  immunophenotyping by cytometry, 362
  tetramer assay, 361–2

dapsone, 271
Dausse, Jean, 1
decoy cells, 48f
delayed graft function (DGF), 28
delayed-type hypersensitivity, 5

dendritic cells (DCs), 316
de novo AIH
  difficulty in establishing diagnosis for, 98
  pathophysiology of, 98–9
  risk factors, 98
dermatophytes, 304
diabetes mellitus (DM)
  causes of, 216
  complications associated with, 216
  recurrent autoimmune, 238–40
  treatment of, 216. see also islet transplantation; pancreas transplantation
  type 1. see diabetes mellitus type 1
  type 2. see diabetes mellitus type 2
diabetes mellitus type 1, 216
  complications, 216
  pancreas transplants in, 216
  recurrence in pancreas allograft, 246, 248f
  treatment, 216
diabetes mellitus type 2, 216
diabetic nephropathy, 53
diabetic nephropathy (DN), 53
diffuse acinar inflammation and multicellular acinar cell damage, 229f
diffuse alveolar damage, 171f
diffuse inflammatory process, 136
diffuse large B cell lymphoma (DLBCL), 322
  and EBV-negative PTLD, gene expression profiles between, 317
digital morphometric analysis, 111
digital pathology, 111–12
  digital morphometric analysis, 111
  laser scanning cytometry, 111
  metabolic array analyses, 111
  multiplex quantum dot staining, 111
  needle liver biopsies, 111
  telepathology, 111
direct antigen presentation pathways, 4–5
disseminated intravascular coagulation (DIC)
  donor kidney biopsy, 27f, 27
DNA microarrays, gene expression profiling using, 366
Doherty, Peter, 2
donated after circulatory death (DCD) donors, 64, 65
  characteristics, 66
  leukocyte and platelet sludging, 75
  peripheral core needle biopsy evaluation of, 66
donation after brain death (DBD) donors, 64, 65

Index

donor
  blood product screening and, 93
  DBD. *see* donation after brain death (DBD) donors
  DCD. *see* donated after circulatory death (DCD) donors
  definition of, 66
donor alloantigens and recipient immune system
  direct antigen presentation pathways, 4–5
  indirect antigen presentation pathways, 5
  semi-direct pathway, 5
donor antigens acquisition, processing and presentation of, 5
donor biopsy evaluation, deceased, 66–7
  anti-HBc+ livers, 67
  donor risk index, 66
  fatty donor liver evaluation, 67
  fibrosis, 67
  frozen section examination, 66
  gross and microscopic evaluation, 66
  histopathology, 66
  necrosis, 67
  neoplastic, infectious and metabolic diseases, 67
  pre-transplant frozen section evaluation, 67
donor biopsy evaluation, living, 67–8
  findings, 68
  macrovesicular steatosis, 68
donor cancer
  discovered after transplantation, 334
  transmission of, 330
  transmission risk frequencies of, 332t
donor dendritic cells, reconstitution of, 268
donor-derived "passenger" leucocytes, 5
donor kidney
  acute tubular injury and, 27f, 27, 29
  frozen section of mass lesions of, 331–3
donor kidney biopsies, 25
  BANFF criteria, 26
  categories of adequacy for, 26
  donor biopsies, 26
  indication biopsies, 26
  KDPI scores, 25
  needle biopsies, 25–6
  pre-existing lesions identification by. *see* donor kidney biopsies, pre-existing lesions identification by
  processing of, 26
  procurement, 25, 26
  protocol biopsies, 26
  wedge biopsies, 25
donor kidney biopsies, pre-existing lesions identification by, 26–8
  acute tubular injury, 27f, 27
  arteriosclerosis changes, 26, 27f
  ATI and ATN, 28
  glomerular sclerosis, 27f, 27–8
  microthrombi, 27f, 27
  renal cell carcinoma (RCC), 28f, 28
donor liver, frozen section of mass lesions of, 333–4
donor lungs
  frozen section of mass lesions of, 334
  pool, sources for expansion of, 158
  requirements for patient to qualify for, 156
  selection criteria for, 157
donor risk index, 66
donor specific antibodies (DSAs), 158, 233
donor T-cell
  activation of, 6
  proinflammatory changes in, 6
drug-associated effects in lungs, 174
  amiodarone, 174f
  sirolimus, 174
drug-induced acute tubulo-interstitial nephritis, 46–7
drug-induced liver injury (DILI)
  after liver replacement, 105
  histopathologic manifestations associated with, 105
drug monitoring in organ transplantation
  cyclosporine, 364
  everolimus, 365
  mycophenylate mofetil (MMF), 365
  optimal method for, 364
  significance of, 363–4
  sirolimus, 364–5
  tacrolimus, 364
drug reactions, transplant patients, 294
  acral erythema, 294
  diffuse gingival enlargement, 294
  drug rashes, 294
  everolimus, 294, 295f–6f
  sirolimus, 294
drug toxicities, 15, 43–7. *see also* immunosuppressives
  calcineurin inhibitors, 43–6
  drug-induced acute tubulo-interstitial nephritis, 46–7
  in kidney transplantation, 43–7
  sirolimus and everolimus, 47

DSA alloantibody, 37, 39f–40f
ductitis, 223f
  acute T-cell-mediated rejection, 237f
ductopenia, 85
duodenal graft pathology, 250
dysregulated immunity, disorders of
  autoimmune hepatitis. *see* autoimmune hepatitis (AIH)
  de novo AIH. *See* de novo AIH
  diagnosis, 98
  disease recurrence of, 98
  incidence of, 98
  primary biliary cirrhosis, 99–101
  recurrent AIH. *see* recurrent AIH
  recurrent PSC, 101
dystrophic calcification, 143

early lesions, 173
early perivenular chronic rejection, 86
early TCMR
  clinical presentation of, 80
  histopathologic findings and grading, 80–1, 81f
  risk factors for, 80
EBER probing, 90
EBV-associated B cell tumors, pathogenetic models of, 317–19, 318f
EBV-encoded nuclear RNA (EBER), 52
EBV encoded RNAs (EBER), 244
EBV hepatitis, 89f, 89
  confused with CMV hepatitis, 88
  differential diagnosis of, 90
EBV infections. *see* Epstein-Barr virus (EBV) infections
EBV-negative PTLDs
  and diffuse large B cell lymphoma, gene expression profiles between, 317
  genetic abnormalities in, 317
EBV positive PTLDs, 317
  chromosomal fragile site abnormalities in, 317
  monomorphic, 317, 319
  T cell infiltration, 317
  viral latency III protein expression, 317
EBV seronegative transplant patients, 317
eczematoid GVHD, 298–9
effector cell populations and cytokines, 5
efflux pumps, 264
electron microscopy of PVN, 48
ELISPOT (Enzyme Linked ImmunoSpot) assay, 359–61

endobronchial or transbronchial biopsy, 169
endocapillary hypercellularity. *see* transplant glomerulitis
endocardial lymphocytic infiltrates, 139, 140f
endocervical adenocarcinoma, 330
endocrine islets, 238
endomyocardial biopsy (EMB), 133–4
  acute cellular rejection grading in, 135f, 136f, 137f, 138f
  adipose tissue, 142f, 142–3
  biopsy-negative allograft dysfunction, 143
  chordae tendineae, 143
  contraction bands, 143
  dystrophic calcification, 143
  foreign bodies, 143
  gross examination, 134
  intussusception of small arteries, 143
  issues in interpretation of, 141–3
  lymphoid neoplasms, 143
  myocyte injury, 141
  opportunistic infections, 141f, 141–2
  pinching or forceps artifact, 143
  processing in pathology laboratory, 134
  pseudohemorrhage, 143
  sensitivity and specificity, 133
  telescoping, 143
  timing, 133
  tissue handling, 134
  tissue procurement, 133f, 133–4
  tissue samples, minimum numbers of, 134
  valvular tissue, 143
endomyocardial biopsy (EMB), immunostaining of, 145–6
  immunofluorescence staining, 145, 146f
  immunohistochemical staining, 145–6
  2013 ISHLT-Working formulation, 146–7
endothelial cell activation, 33f
engraftment syndrome, 273
enteric drainage, 217
enteropathy associated T cell lymphoma (EATL), 263
enteroscopic duodenal cuff biopsies, 219
eosinophilic colitis, 206f
eosinophilic esophagitis, 205f
eosinophilic infiltration, 206
epicardial coronary atherosclerosis, 149
epithelial damage, 238f
Epstein Barr Virus (EBV)
  altered T cell response to, 317

378

life cycle stage-specific gene expression of, 316t
survival signals, 317
Epstein-Barr virus (EBV) infections, 14–15, 51–2
B cells, 315
clinical presentation of, 89
differential diagnosis of, 90
EBV-associated tumors. see post transplant lymphoproliferative disorders (PTLD)
EBV hepatitis. see EBV hepatitis
histopathologic findings, 89, 90
host response to, 316–17
ITx and MVTx, 201
risk factors for, 88
skin infections, 303
everolimus, 47, 365
exfoliative rejection, 194
exocrine parenchyma, 243f
exocytosis of cytoplasmic granules, 362
exogenous antigens, 2
explant lung evaluation, 158
post-transplant pathologic diagnosis, 158
pre-operative pathologic evaluations, 158
explant organ, cancer in, 337–9
expression analysis, 366
extended criteria donors (ECD), 64, 66
extended functional CNIT signs of, 44

failed allografts, gross and microscopic evaluation of, 68–70
ancillary studies, 250
guidelines for, 250
failed allografts with obstructive cholangiography, 76
familial intra-hepatic cholestasis syndromes, 102
fatty donor liver evaluation, 67
FCH-associated liver damage, 97
FCH HCV, 95
FFPE tissues, molecular platforms for use with, 111
fibrinoid necrosis of microvasculature, 37
fibrosing cholestatic hepatitis (FCH), 95, 96–7
fibrosis, 67, 68, 197
mild /severe, 238
progression, 102
progression of, 238, 242f, 243f
filgrastim, 264, 268
fine microsurgery forceps, 134
flow cytometry crossmatch (FCXM), 357
fluconazole, 271
fludarabine and busulfan (Flu-Bu), 262

fluoroquinolones, 271
focal bile duct necrosis, 77
focal lymphocytic cholangitis, 95
focal nodular hyperplasia (FNH), 333, 335
focal segmental glomerulosclerosis (FSGS), 52, 53f
"for-cause" allograft biopsies, 110
foreign bodies, 143
forkhead/winged-helix transcription factor (FoxP3) expression, 7
frank vasculitis, 149
frozen section analysis of mass lesions
in donor kidney, 331–3
in donor liver, 333–4
in donor lung, 334
in donor prostate, 334
frozen section evaluation, pre-transplant, 67
frozen section examination, deceased donor biopsy, 66
findings, 67
tissue sampling for, 66
fungal exotoxins, 268
fungal hyphae, 169, 170f
fungal infections
after liver transplantation, 86–7
Aspergillus species, 303
Candida species, 303
cutaneous cryptococcosis, 303–4
dermatophytes, 304
development of, 303
explanted lungs, 168
invasive candidiasis, 303

ganglion cell clusters, 232f
gastric allograft. see stomach allografts
gastrointestinal allograft viral infection, 199–200
gastrointestinal tract GVHD, 277, 278f
gastrointestinal transplants
acute T-cell mediated rejection in. see acute T-cell mediated rejection in ITx recipients
susceptibility to ACR, 190
gene expression profiling using DNA microarrays, 366
germ cell tumors and autologous HCT, 262
giant cell interstitial pneumonia, 175
giant mitochondria, 44
glomerular capillary lumens, 45
glomerular endothelial cell injury, calcineurin inhibitor induced, 45
glomerular sclerosis, 27f, 27–8
donor kidney, 27f, 27–8

glomerular vasculature, 37
glomerulitis, AAMR with, 37
glomerulonephritis, 52
glomerulopathies following renal transplantation, 52–3
diabetic nephropathy, 53
focal segmental glomerulosclerosis, 52
membranoproliferative glomerulonephritis, 52
recurrent lupus nephritis, 53
thrombotic microangiopathy, 53
glucagon stain, 249f
glutamine synthetase, 335
graft, 1
failure and HCT, 266–7
fibrosis, 12–13
graft dysfunction after liver transplantation, see portal hyperperfusion
bile duct complications, 74–6
failed allograft evaluations, 68–70
hepatic artery thrombosis, 72
hepatic vein and vena caval complications, 74
operation, understanding, 68
portal vein thrombosis, 73
post-transplant allograft needle biopsies, 68
preservation/reperfusion injury. see preservation/reperfusion injury
small-for-size syndrome (SFSS). see small-for-size syndrome (SFSS)
timing of, 69t
vascular complications, 72
graft injury mechanisms, 8t, 15
acute rejection (AR). see acute rejection (AR)
adaptive immune response, 9
HSPs role in, 9
innate immune activation, 8–9
ischemia/reperfusion injury (I/R injury), 8, 9f
graft transmission of donor malignancy, 176
graft-versus-host disease (GVHD), 5–6, 261, 269, 283, 295
acute and chronic forms of, 6
acute form of. see aGVHD (acute form of GVHD)
after HLA-identical HSC, CTLs isolated from, 3
B cells role in, 268
chronic form of. see cGVHD (chronic form of GVHD)
clinical characterization of, 274, 295
frequency of, 5–6
immune manipulations for treatment of, 283t
mortality of patients diagnosed with, 6

native GI tissue, 206–7
NK cell role in, 6
pancreas transplantation complications, 250
prophylaxis and allogeneic donor selection, 266
regulatory T cells and, 269
use of steroids for, 268
graft-versus-leukemia responses and conditioning intensity, 260
GVL, 263
cytotoxic lymphocytes in, 260–1
hematologic malignancies sensitivity to, 260
responses after allogeneic HCT, 260
T-cell mediated process, 260

HBV hepatitis, 92, 93–4
allograft re-infection, 93
anti-viral treatment, 93
clinical presentation of, 93
differential diagnosis of, 94
donor and blood product screening, 93
histopathologic findings, 93–4
prevalence of, 93
HBV-induced cirrhosis, 93
HCT complications
bronchiolitis obliterans, 274, 282
cryptogenic organizing pneumonia, 273
engraftment syndrome, 273
graft-versus-host disease. see graft-versus-host disease (GVHD)
idiopathic pneumonia syndrome, 273
mucositis, 274
pulmonary cytolytic thrombi syndrome, 273
pulmonary veno-occlusive disease, 273
sinusoidal obstruction syndrome, 272
syndrome of "diffuse alveolar hemorrhage" (DAH), 273
thrombotic microangiopathy, 272
HCV hepatitis, 92, 94–7
after transplantation, 94
chronic, 94, 95
clinical presentation of, 95
differential diagnosis of, 97
disease progression, 95
FCH, 95, 96–7
HCV-induced cirrhosis, 94
plasma cell-rich or "autoimmune" variant of, 96
recurrent, 95f, 95, 96f
regimens for, 94
TCMR diagnosis in, 97
usual variant of, 95–6

Index

HDV hepatitis, 93–4
  acute form, 93
  histopathologic findings, 94
  infection patterns, 93
  treatment of, 93
heart allograft biopsies, 110–11
  molecular allograft biopsy analysis, 110–11
heart transplantation, pathology of, 133
  cardiac allograft rejection, 134–43
  endomyocardial biopsy. see endomyocardial biopsy (EMB)
heat shock proteins (HSPs), 9
hematologic neoplasms, post-HCT relapse of, 260
hematopoietic stem cells (HSC)
  cardinal properties of, 264
  delicate niches and, 264
  extracellular matrix role in retention of, 264
  factors influencing maintenance of, 264
  immunophenotype of, 264
  interactions, 264
  intracellular signals to, 264
  mobilization, 264–5
  regeneration of, 264
  sources of, 261
hematopoietic stem cell transplantation (HCT), 282
  allogeneic. see allogeneic HCT (allo-HCT)
  autologous, 260
  definition of, 260
  graft failure, 266–7
  graft-*versus*-leukemia responses and conditioning intensity, 260
  hematopoietic and immune reconstitution after, 268–9
  infections after, 269–72
  nonmyeloablative conditioning, 260
  transfusion support after, 267
hemoglobinopathies, 263
hemolytic-uremic-syndrome. see thrombotic microangiopathy
hepatic artery thrombosis (HAT), 72
  clinical presentation of, 72
  differential diagnosis of, 73
  histopathologic findings, 72, 73f
  pathophysiology of, 72
hepatic parenchymal health, 74
hepatic vein complications, 74
hepatitis A, 92–3
hepatitis B infection, 14
  hepatitis B virus (HBV)-induced cirrhosis, 64
  liver allograft, 14f
hepatitis B virus (HBV) vaccination, 64

hepatitis C infection, 14
hepatitis E virus, 92
hepatitis virus infections
  HBV hepatitis, 92, 93–4. see also HBV hepatitis
  HCV hepatitis, 92, 94–7. see also HCV hepatitis
  HDV hepatitis, 93–4. see also HDV hepatitis
  hepatitis A, 92–3
  hepatitis B. see hepatitis B infection
  hepatitis E virus, 92
  HEV, 97–8. see also HEV infection
hepatocellular adenoma (HA), 334, 336
hepatocellular carcinoma (HCC)
  ablation procedures effect on transplant candidates of, 339f
  differential diagnosis of, 335–7
  early, 336–7
  focal nodular hyperplasia, 335
  grading of, 338f, 339
  hepatic transplantation for, 92
  hepatocellular adenomas, 336
  high-grade dysplastic nodules, 336
  low-grade dysplastic nodules, 335–6
  organ transplant candidates and, 334
  progressed, 337
  regenerative nodules, 335
  reporting requirments for, 337–8
  staging systems for, 334, 335t
herpes simplex virus (HSV) infection
  HSV hepatitis. see HSV hepatitis
  ITx and MVTx, 201
  lung transplant recipients, 171–2
  skin infections, 299
heteroduplex analysis (PCR-HA), 350
HEV infection, 97–8
  acute and chronic, 98
  clinical presentation of, 98
  differential diagnosis of, 98
  histopathologic findings, 98
  pathophysiology, 97
HHV-7 infections in ITx and MVTx, 202
HHV-8, tumors associated with
  Kaposi sarcoma, 326–8
  primary effusion lymphoma, 328
high efficiency particulate air filter (HEPA filter), 271
high-grade dysplastic nodules, 336
high-resolution allele-level HLA typing, 349

high-throughput T-cell receptor sequencing, 98
histocompatibility 2 (H-2), 1
histocompatibility laboratory
  KPD programs and, 342
  roles and responsibilities of, 342
HLA typing. see human leukocyte antigen (HLA) typing
Hodgkin lymphoma (HL) PTLD, 324–5
Hodgkin Reed-Sternberg (HRS) cells, 324, 325f
Hodgkin's lymphoma and autologous HCT, 261
host DCs, maturation and activation of, 6
host *versus* graft (HVG)
  reactivity, 4–5
  organ rejection, 4
HSV hepatitis, 90
  clinical presentation of, 90
  differential diagnosis of, 90
  histopathologic findings, 90
HSV-induced hepatitis *vs.* CMV hepatitis, 88
human herpesvirus 8 (HHV8), 91, 326. see also HHV-8, tumors associated with
human herpes virus-6 (HHV-6) infection
  clinical diagnosis of, 91
  histopathologic findings of, 91
  ITx and MVTx, 201–2, 203f
  reactivation, 90–1
  skin infections, 302–3
human leukocyte antigen (HLA), 1–2, 159
  class I and HLA class II, 2
  molecules, baseline expression of, 5
human leukocyte antigen (HLA) antibody testing
  crossmatch (XM) testing, 356–7
  crossreactive HLA antibodies and crossreactive Groups (CREGs), 355t, 355–6
  panel reactive antibodies (PRA), 351–4
  virtual crossmatch (VXM), 354–5
human leukocyte antigen (HLA) compatibility assessment techniques
  amplification refractory mutation system (ARMS), 350
  donor chimerism analysis, 350–1
  history of, 344
  molecular-based assays, 344
  purpose of, 344
  short tandem repeat (STR) microsatellite testing, 350–1

human leukocyte antigen (HLA) complex
  class III molecules, 343
  class II molecules, 343
  class I molecules, 342, 343f
  genomic organization, 342f, 342
  role in transplantation, 343–4
human leukocyte antigen (HLA) typing
  molecular, 344, 345
  next generation sequencing (NGS), 347–9
  sequence-based typing (SBT), 347
  sequence-specific oligonucleotide probe (SSOP) typing, 346–7
  sequence-specific primers (SSP) typing, 345–6
  serologic, 344–5
  special consideration for, 349–50
human papillomavirus (HPV), 330
  skin infections, 303
human papillomavirus (HPV), tumors associated with
  cancer of skin and epidermal surfaces, 330
  cervical infection, 330
  sequence of events leading to, 330
humoral acute rejection. see acute antibody-mediated rejection (AAMR)
hyperacute rejection (HAR), 39f, 158–9
  clinical features of, 35
  histopathology of, 35
  immunofluorescence evaluations, 35
  transplant arteriopathy, 35
hyperdynamic portal circulation, 71
hyperglycemia
  acute pancreas rejection and, 218
  chronic rejection/graft sclerosis, 224
  cyclosporine and, 248–9
  drug toxicity and, 249
  islet amyloid polypeptide and, 249
  tacrolimus and, 248–9
hypervascular inflammatory lesion of bowel allograft, 206f
hypogammaglobulinemia, 282
hypothermic oxygenated machine perfusion (HOPE), 65

iatrogenic immunosuppression, 317
idiopathic pneumonia syndrome (IPS), 273

idiopathic post-transplant hepatitis (IPTH), 104–5
idiopathic pulmonary fibrosis (IPF), 156
IFN-γ ELISPOT assay, 359–61
IgG
  deposition in arteries, 240f
  kidney undergoing humoral acute rejection, 10f
immune effector cells and molecules, 186
immune ignorance, 7
immune reconstitution after HCT
  B cells, 268
  donor dendritic cells, 268
  factors influencing, 268
  NK cells, 268, 269
  plasmacytoid dendritic cells (pDCs), 268
  regulatory T cells, 269
  T cells, 268–9
immune response between recipient and donor, 1
immune responses, antigen-specific suppression of, 7
  regulatory cell populations, 7
  regulatory T cells. see regulatory T cells
immune tolerance, 6–8
  animal models, 6
  definition of, 6
  development of, 6
immune tolerance mechanisms
  anergy and deletion, 7
  central tolerance, 6–7
  classification of, 6t, 6
  immune ignorance, 7
  molecular phenotype of operational tolerance, 7–8
  peripheral tolerance, 6
  suppression of immune responses, 7
immunochemotherapy, 262
immunodeficiencies, 263–4
immunofluorescence microscopy of PVN, 48
immunologic constant of rejection, 111
immunomodulatory cytokines, 5
Immunoperoxidase stains, 249, 250
immunophenotyping by cytometry, 362
immunostaining
  complement split products, 144–5, 147
  indications for, 147
immunosuppressed transplant patients, altered immune response in, 317
immunosuppression (IS)
  calcineurin inhibitors and, 226
  lung transplantation, complications of, 175–6

managemen,pathologist role in, 109–10
regimen, 172
immunosuppressive recipient conditioning, 266
immunosuppressives. see also drug toxicities
  aGVHD treatment, 279
  effect on regulatory cells, 7
inadequate biopsy, 137–8
inborn errors of metabolism, 264
indication biopsies, 26
indirect antigen presentation pathways, 5
inducible lymphocyte costimulatory molecules, 11
infections, 13–15. see also adenovirus (ADV) infections; allogeneic HCT (allo-HCT), infections after; cytomegalovirus (CMV) infections; Epstein-Barr virus (EBV) infections; hepatitis virus infections; herpes simplex virus (HSV) infection; human herpes virus-6 (HHV-6) infection; opportunistic infections; viral skin infections; specific types
  after allogeneic HCT. see allogeneic HCT (allo-HCT), infections after
  bacterial. see also bacterial infections
  CMV, 13f
  EBV, 14–15
  factors influencing range of, 13
  hepatitis B, 14f, 14
  hepatitis C, 14
  opportunistic. see opportunistic infections
  PPV, 13f, 13–14
infections in ITx and MVTx, 198–9
  adenovirus infections, 200f–1f, 200
  bacterial, 203
  Calicivirus infections, 200
  Cytomegalovirus infection, 200–1, 202f
  EBV acute infection, 201
  HHV-6, 201–2, 203f
  HHV-7, 202
  HHV-8, 202–3, 203f
  HSV infection, 201
  Norovirus infections, 200
  Rotavirus infections, 200, 201f
  viral infection, 199–200
infections in kidney transplantation, 47–52
  Adenovirus, 50–1
  CMV, 49–50
  EBV, 51–2

Polyoma BK-virus nephropathy, 47–9
pyelonephritis, 52
infections in lung transplant recipients, 169t
  adenovirus infection, 172f, 172
  after one to six months, 168–9
  after six months, 172
  Aspergillus-associated lung disease, 169
  Candida, 169–70, 170f
  CMV infection, 171
  HSV infection, 171–2
  initial post-transplant period/first month, 168
  nontuberculous mycobacterial infections, 172
  peri-operative, 168
  Pneumocystis cysts, 170–1, 171f
  Pneumocystis jiroveci pneumonia, 170
  pulmonary, 167
  risk factors for, 167–8
  viral pneumonias, 172
infectious agents in endomyocardial biopsy, 141f, 141–2
infectious disease screening
  molecular methods for, 363
  PCR-based techniques, 363
  serological assessment, 363
infectious mononucleosis (IM), 173
infectious mononucleosis (IM)-like lesion, 319, 322f
inflammatory bowel disease (IBD), 204–5
inflammatory cell infiltrate, chronic, 190
inflammatory infiltrates, 228, 238
inflammatory lesions and processes, 205
innate immune activation, 8–9
innate immune response, polymorphisms of genes in, 268
insulin resistance, 248
insulin stain, 249f
insulin therapy for DM type 1, 216
interstitial fibrosis, 46, 49
interstitial scarring, 39, 46
intestinal donor organ procurement, 185
intestinal graft
  presentation, 184
  rejection, 184
intestinal (ITx) transplantation, 183
  complications of, 184t
  effective execution of, 183
  primary disease of patients receiving, 183t, 183
  variations in surgical procedure for, 183

intestinal (ITx) transplantation allografts
  acute T-cell mediated rejection in. see acute T-cell mediated rejection in ITx recipients
  histopathological evaluation of, 184–5
  ischemia reperfusion (I/R) injury to, 185, 186f
  transplant pathology of, 184
intestinal ulcers, 205
intimal arteritis, 221f, 229f
intracellular cytokine (ICC) measurement, 363
intussusception of small arteries, 143
invasive candidiasis, 303
iron overload, 149
ischemia reperfusion (IR injury), 8, 9f, 168
  definition of, 28
  ITx and MVTx allografts, 185, 186f
  mechanism, 28
ischemia reperfusion (IR injury), kidney transplantation, 28–9, 29f, 30f
  AAMR, 29
  acute tubular injury (ATI), 29
  alloreactive processes, 29
  DGF, 28
  gene changes and, 29
ischemic airway disease, 169
ischemic cholangiopathy, 72
ischemic cholangitis, 72
ischemic hepatitis, 72
ischemic injury
  late, 139
  perioperative, 138, 139f
islet amyloid polypeptide (IAPP), 249, 251
islet cell drug toxicity, 248–9, 249f
islet graft pathology
  islet amyloid, 249
  islet cell drug toxicity, 248–9, 249f
  nesidioblastosis, 249–50
  nonspecific, 245–6
  recurrence of type I diabetes mellitus, 246, 248f
islet inflammation, 245
islet pathology, 238–40
islet transplantation, 216
islet transplantation (IT)
  histological aspects of, 251
isohemagglutinins, 267
isometric vacuolization, 44
IVIg infusion after allo-HCT, 272

Jaffe's classification system, 101

Kaposins, 326
Kaposi sarcoma, 306, 326–8
  bowel, 202–3, 203f

Index

Kaposi sarcoma (cont.)
  cell of origin of, 326
  HHV8 lytic and latently infected cells, interactions between, 326, 327f
  histopathology of, 327, 328f
  prevalence of, 326
  viral lytic proteins in, 326
KDPI scores, 25
kidney allografts, 12f
  chronic rejection, 12f
  molecular signatures for, 110
kidney donor profile index (KDPI), 25
kidney transplant
  ischemia reperfusion injury, 9f
  recurrent/de novo immune diseases, 15
kidney transplantation, 25
  donor kidney biopsies. see donor kidney biopsies
  immunological and non-immunological variables influencing, 25
kidney transplantation complications, post transplant, 25
  acute rejection, 30–43
  drug toxicities, 43–7
  infections, 47–52
  IR injury, 28–9, 29f, 30f
  recurrent disease, 52–3
kidney with extensive tubulitis, acute TCMR of, 11f
killer cell immunoglobulin-like receptors (KIR), 266
KIR/KIR-L mismatching, 266
KS-associated herpesvirus (KSHV), 91

laparoscopic biopsy, 218
laser scanning cytometry, 111
latency associated nuclear antigen (LANA-1), 326
latent membrane protein (LMP)-1, 315
late-onset CMV disease, 171
late onset TCMR
  central perivenulitis, 82, 83t, 84f
  clinical presentation of, 80
  evolution of response, 82
  necrotizing arteritis, 81
LDA (limiting dilution assay), 363
Lerner grading system, 296
lichenoid GVHD, 296–7, 298f
lipase and acute pancreas rejection, 218
liver aGVHD, 279, 279f
liver allograft biopsies
  differential diagnosis, 68
  importance of, 68
  information needed for assessing, 68
  stains in, 68

liver allograft dysfunction, 105
  criteria used to diagnose, 109
  histopathologic features of, 106t–7t
  leading causes of, 105
liver allografts, 102
  biopsies. see liver allograft biopsies
  reduced size and living-related, 70
Liver Assist, 66
liver regeneration, 72
liver transplantation
  applications of, 64
  clonal exhaustion after, 7
  goal of, 102
  histopathology of, 64
  indications for, 64
  machine perfusion in. see machine perfusion in liver transplantation
  molecular allograft biopsy analysis, 111
  orthotopic, 64
Low-grade dysplastic nodules, 335–6
lung allocation score (LAS), 156–7
lung cancer, 175
lung, ischemia/reperfusion injury of, 9f
lung parenchyma, architectural abnormalities of, 168
lung transplantation
  causes of death in, 156
  explant lung evaluation, 158
  history of, 156
  incidence of, 156
  indications for, 156, 157t
  lung allocation for, 156–7
  median survival for, 156
lung transplantation, complications of, 174t, 174
  adenocarcinoma in situ, 175
  airway complications, 159f, 159
  alveolar hemosiderosis, 176f, 176
  amiodarone toxicity, 174f
  cellular proliferative processes, 175
  environmental exposures causing, 175
  giant cell interstitial pneumonia, 175
  graft transmission of donor malignancy, 176
  hyperacute rejection, 158–9
  immunosuppression, 175–6
  lung cancer, 175
  non-necrotizing granulomas, 175f, 175
  organizing pneumonia, 176f, 176
  post-transplant lymphoproliferative disorder. see post-transplant lymphoproliferative disorders (PTLD)

  primary graft dysfunction, 158
  pulmonary alveolar proteinosis, 175f
  pulmonary emboli, 175
  sarcoidosis, 174, 175
  sirolimus toxicity, 174
lung transplant patients, rejection in
  acute cellular. see acute cellular rejection (ACR), in lung
  surgical biopsies and, 160
lung volume resection surgery (LVRS), 156
lupus nephritis, recurrent, 53
lymphocytic and eosinophilic septal inflammation, 235f
lymphocytic cholangitis, 95, 100, 105
lymphocytotoxic cross-match, 79f
lymphoid neoplasms, 143
lymphoid proliferation and cytotoxicity assays, 359
lymphoproliferations, 319
lymphoproliferative disorders, 263

machine perfusion devices, 66
  Liver Assist, 66
  OrganOx metra, 66
  Transmedics Organ Care System, 66
machine perfusion in liver transplantation, 64–6
  challenges with portal vein/hepatic artery, 65
  definition of, 64
  HOPE, 65
  hypothermic, 65
  non-anastomotic biliary strictures, 65
  normothermic, 65
  organ preservation, 65
  subnormothermic, 65
  variables influencing, 64
macrosteatotic donor, 71
macrovesicular steatosis
  definition of, 67
  living donor biopsy, 68
  pre-transplant frozen section evaluation, 67
  severity estimation, 67
major histocompatibility complex (MHC), 1–2
  gene region products, 2
  research in mice and humans, 2
  restriction, 2
major histocompatibility complex (MHC) antigens
  APC and, 2
  archetypal function of, 2
  HLA class I and HLA class II, 2
  polymorphic diversity, 2
mantle cell lymphoma (MCL), 261

marrow failure syndromes, 263
Masson's trichrome, 228f
medullary inflammation, 47
membrane attack complex (MAC), 147
membranoproliferative glomerulonephritis (MPGN), 52
Merkel cell carcinoma (MCC), 328–9
  pathogenesis of, 328, 329f
  pathology of, 329f, 330
  viral T antigen mutation in, 328
Merkel cell polyomavirus (MCV), 328
mesangial regions, 45
mesangiolysis, 42
metabolic array analyses, 111
metabolic diseases after transplantation
  familial intra-hepatic cholestasis syndromes, 102
  Jaffe's classification system, 101, 102t
MHC-peptide complexes, 2
microcirculatory compromise, 70
microthrombi, 27f, 27
  donor kidney, 27f, 27
microvascular endothelial C4d staining, 80
microvascular endothelial cell HLA class II expression, 80
microvesicular steatosis
  definition of, 67
  high-grade, 67
  preservation/reperfusion injury, 70
mild TCMR
  clinical presentation of, 80
  histopathologic findings and grading, 80–1, 81f
  risk factors for, 80
minimal intimal arteritis, 231, 239f
minimal residual disease (MRD), 262
minor histocompatibility antigens (MiHA), 2–3
mixed acute cellular and antibody-mediated rejection, 147
mixed lymphocyte culture (MLC), 359
mixed lymphocyte reaction (MLR), 359
moderate or severe intimal arteritis, 232
moderate to severe acute cellular rejection, 81f
molecular allograft biopsy analysis, 110
  liver transplantation, 111
  renal and heart allograft biopsies, 110–11
molecular assays
  acute rejection, 43
  chronic rejection, 43

molecular HLA typing, 344, 345
molecular lab medicine, 43
molecular markers, 366
  expression analysis, 366
  gene expression profiling
    using DNA microarrays,
    366
  Real Time-PCR (RT-PCR),
    366–8
molecular phenotype of
  operational tolerance, 7–8
molecular platforms for FFPE
  tissues, 111
molecular signatures
  future applications of, 111
  kidney allografts, 110
monomorphic PTLD, 173,
  321–2, 325
mononuclear cuffing of vein, 223f
mTOR inhibitors, 47
mucosal fibrosis,
  semiquantitative grading
  schema for, 199t
mucositis, 274
multicellular acinar cell damage,
  229f
  diffuse acinar inflammation
    and, 229f
multifocal acinar inflammation,
  229f, 231
  single cell acinar cell damage
    and, 228f
multiple myeloma and
  autologous HCT, 261
multiple myeloma and
  extramedullary
  plasmacytoma, 322
multiplex quantum dot staining,
  111
multivisceral donor organ
  procurement, 185
multivisceral graft presentation,
  184
multivisceral transplantation
  (MVTx), 183, 216
  complications of, 184t
  effective execution of, 183
  primary disease of patients
    receiving, 183t, 183
  variations in surgical
    procedure for, 183
multivisceral transplantation
  (MVTx) allografts
  acute T-cell mediated
    rejection in. see acute T-cell
    mediated rejection in
    MVTx recipients
  histopathological evaluation
    of, 184–5
  ischemia reperfusion (I/R)
    injury to, 185, 186f
  transplant pathology of, 184
mycetoma, 168f, 168
mycobacteria infection, 303
mycophenylate mofetil (MMF),
  365
myelodysplastic syndromes
  (MDS), 263

myeloproliferative neoplasms,
  263
myocyte degeneration, 141
myocyte injury, 141
myocyte necrosis, 141
myofibroblast activation, 41
myointimal hyperplasia, 199f
myosin, 3

NAFLD, 103
Nanostring nCounter Digital
  Analysis System, 111
National Marrow Donor
  Program (NMDP), 349
necrosis, 67, 73
necrotic zoster, 302f
necrotizing arteritis, 81, 230f,
  232–3
needle biopsies, 25–6
needle core biopsies, 218
  adequacy of, 219
  cystoscopic transduodenal
    pancreas biopsies, 219
  enteroscopic duodenal cuff
    biopsies, 219
  laparoscopic biopsy, 218
  low power view of, 219f
  lymphoid infiltrates in
    expanded septal areas, 221f
  medium power view of, 222f
  open (surgical wedge)
    biopsies, 219
  percutaneous needle biopsy,
    218
needle core biopsy, 233f
needle liver biopsies, 111
neoadjuvant
  radiochemotherapy, 92
neoplasia, 251
neoplastic, infectious and
  metabolic diseases, 67
nephrogenic systemic fibrosis
  (NSF), 294–5
nephrotic syndrome, 44
nesidioblastosis, 249f, 249–50
neuroblastoma and autologous
  HCT, 262
neutrophilic reversible allograft
  dysfunction (NRAD), 166
neutrophils, 268
new onset chronic necro-
  inflammatory diseases
  inclusionary and exclusionary
    criteria for diagnosis of,
    108t
next generation sequencing
  (NGS), 347–9
NK cells, 266, 316
  CAMR by, 12
  graft failure by, 266, 267
  GVHD and, 6
  mechanisms inflicting injury
    on donor cells, 5f, 5
  reconstitution after HCT,
    268, 269
  role in GVHD, 6
NKT cells
  CAMR by, 12

mechanisms inflicting injury
  on donor cells, 5f, 5
role in GVHD, 6
nodular regenerative
  hyperplasia, 73
non-alcoholic steatohepatitis
  (NASH), 102–3
  clinical presentation of, 102–3
  differential diagnosis of, 103
  histopathology of, 103
  liver replacement for, 102
  recurrence of, 103
  risk factors, 103
  treatment of, 103
non-anastomotic biliary
  strictures post-
  transplantation,
  development of, 65
non-anastomotic strictures, 75
nonmyeloablative conditioning,
  260
non-necrotizing arteritis, 37
non-necrotizing granulomas,
  175f, 175
non-rejection biopsy findings,
  137–41, 138t
  biopsy adequacy, 137–8
  biopsy site, 141
  endocardial lymphocytic
    infiltrates, 139, 140f
  ischemic injury (late), 139
  ischemic injury
    (perioperative), 138, 139f
  quilty effect vs. lymphoid
    neoplasms, 140–1
  quilty effect vs. moderate
    rejection, 140
nonspecific islet graft pathology,
  245–6
nontuberculous mycobacterial
  infections, 172
normothermia, 65
normothermic machine
  perfusion, 65

obstructive cholangiopathy, 75f,
  76, 100
  features favoring, 86
oncocytoma, 333
open (surgical wedge) biopsies,
  219
operational tolerance
  definition of, 7
  molecular phenotype of, 7–8
opportunistic infections, 87,
  141f, 141–2
  CMV hepatitis, 88f
  EBV infections, 88–90
  vulnerability to, 87
oral cGVHD, 282
oral herpes simplex infection,
  303f
organizing pneumonia (OP),
  176f, 176
OrganOx metra, 66
organ rejection
  allorecognition and, 5
  classification of, 4

orthotopic heart
  transplantation, 133
osmotic nephrosis, 44
overlap syndrome, 275

pancreas after kidney (PAK))
  transplant, 216
  acute rejection in, 218
  graft survival rates, 216–17
pancreas allograft biopsies
  ganglion cell clusters in, 232f
  guidelines for processing, 219
  needle core biopsies. see
    needle core biopsies
  protocol biopsies, 219–20
pancreas allograft rejection
  banff grading schema, 224,
    225t–6t
  diagnostic categories, 226
  histological features, 226
pancreas fibrosis, 224
pancreas graft sclerosis. see
  chronic allograft rejection/
  graft sclerosis, pancreatic
pancreas graft surgical
  complications
  anastomotic leak, 242
  Cytomegalovirus infection,
    242–4, 246f
  EBV-related PTLD, 244, 247f,
    248f
  graft thrombosis, 240, 244f
  infectious peripancreatitis,
    241, 246f
  necrotizing infectious
    duodeno-pancreatitis, 242
  post transplantation
    (ischemic) pancreatitis,
    240–1, 245f
pancreas transplantation, 216
  acute allograft rejection,
    217–18. see acute allograft
    rejection, pancreas
    transplants
  chronic allograft rejection/
    graft sclerosis. see chronic
    allograft rejection/graft
    sclerosis, pancreatic
  graft survival rates, 216–17
  history of, 217
  indications for, 216–17
  pancreas and kidney rejection
    in, correlation between, 219
  segmental, 217
pancreas transplantation
  complications
  adenovirus infection, 251
  gastrointestinal drug toxicity,
    250
  graft versus host disease, 250
  neoplasia, 251
  polyomavirus infection, 250
  thrombotic microangiopathy,
    250
pancreas transplants, types of,
  216
pancreaticoduo-
  denocystostomy, 217

Index

panel reactive antibodies (PRA), 351–4
paracortical expansion, 319
PCR techniques
   Polyoma BK-virus nephropathy (PVN), 48
percutaneous needle biopsy, 218
perforin / granzyme family of molecules, 11
peribiliary capillary plexus, 75
pericholangitis, 101
periductal lamellar edema, 71
peripheral blood stem cells (PBSC), 261
peripheral deletion of immune cells, 7
peripheral T cell lymphoma and autologous HCT, 261
peripheral tolerance, 6
peritubular capillaries, 29, 30f
perivenular necro-inflammatory activity, 96
perivenular sinusoidal congestion, 74
phagocytosis and respiratory burst, 268
pinching or forceps artifact, 143
plasmablastic lymphoma, 322
plasma cell neoplasms, 322
"plasma cell rich" acute rejection (PCAR), 35
plasma cell-rich central perivenulitis, 99
plasma cell-rich variant of HCV hepatitis, 96
plasmacytic hyperplasia (PH), 173
plasmacytoid dendritic cells (pDCs) reconstitution, 268
plasma transfusion, 267
platelets and coagulation factors in AMR, 148
platelet transfusions post-HCT, 267
plerixafor and HSC mobilization, 265
Pneumocystis cysts, 170–1, 171f
Pneumocystis jiroveci pneumonia, 170
pneumocystis pneumonia, 271–2
polymorphic PTLD, 173f, 319
   diffuse lymphoproliferation, 319, 323f
   EBER and EBV immunostains in, 321, 323f
   heterogeneous appearance of, 319
   immunophenotype of, 321
   necrosis and immunoblasts, 319–21
polyoma BK-virus nephropathy (PVN), 47–9
   BK virus positive tubular cells in, 49f
   causes of, 47–8
   changes in kidney, 48
   histologic features of, 48

nuclear alterations in, 49f
polyomavirus activation and, 48
prevalence of, 48
stages of, 48–9
timing of, 48
polyoma BK-virus nephropathy (PVN), diagnosis of, 48
   electron microscopy, 48
   graft biopsy, 48
   PCR techniques, 48
   standard immunofluorescence microscopy, 48
polyoma virus (PPV)
   activation, 48f
   family, 47
   tissue sections, in, 48
polyoma virus (PPV) infection, 13f, 13–14. *see also* polyoma BK-virus nephropathy (PVN)
   changes in kidney, 48
   pancreas transplantation complications, 250
portal-based mononuclear inflammation, 109
portal hyperperfusion
   clinical presentation of, 71–2
   differential diagnosis of, 72
   histopathologic findings, 72
portal stromal C4d deposition, 77
portal vein flow, 71
portal vein thrombosis, 73
   clinical presentation of, 73
   differential diagnosis of, 73
   histopathologic findings, 73, 74f
portal venous blood flow, 71
posaconazole and voriconazole, 270
post-reperfusion, 70
post-reperfusion biopsies, 77
post-transplant allograft needle biopsies, 68
post-transplant diabetes mellitus, 248
post-transplant lymphoproliferative disorder, EBV related
   clinical manifestations of, 244, 247f
   diagnosis of, 244, 248f
   monomorphic, 247f
   polymorphous, 244, 247f
   time of occurrence, 244
   veins and arteries in, 244
post transplant lymphoproliferative disorders (PTLD), 51–2, 303, 306, 312–15
   all-HCT and, 271
   background of, 312
   Burkitt lymphomas, 322
   CD4+ T cells within, 317
   CHL-type, 174
   classification of, 319, 320t

clinical features of, 51f, 52
clinical presentation of, 89, 315
cytogenetic and molecular features of, 325
definition of, 51, 173
development of, 51
diagnosis of, 52, 173
differential diagnosis of, 90
diffuse large B cell, 322
early lesions, 173
EBV+. *see* EBV positive PTLDs
extrahepatic, 90
frequency of, 312
high-grade tumors, 319
histopathologic findings, 89
Hodgkin Lymphoma (HL), 324–5
infectious mononucleosis (IM)-like lesion, 319, 322f
ITx and MVTx patients, 207–8
monomorphic, 173. *see* monomorphic PTLD
morphologic categories of, 207t, 208f
pathogenetic factors contributing to, 317–19
pathologic categories of, 173t, 173
pathology of, 319
plasma cell neoplasms, 322
points to consider during workup of, 321t
polymorphic, 173f. *see* polymorphic PTLD
prevalence of, 51
reactive plasmacytic hyperplasia, 319
risk factor for, 314–15
risk factors for, 88, 89, 172–3
sinusoidal lymphocytosis to, 89
sites of occurence, 173
T/NK cell, 323–4, 325f
types of, 51
uncontrolled EBV replication, 89f
viral latency III protein expression, 317
post transplant smooth muscle tumor (PTSMT)
   histopathology of, 326f, 326
   immunohistochemistry of, 326
   incidence of, 325
   molecular features of, 326
pox-like granulomas, 91
preservation-associated injury, ITx and MVTx allografts, 185, 186f
preservation methods based on donor organ cooling, 65
preservation/reperfusion injury, 71f
   blood reperfusion, 70

clinical presentation of, 70
DCD donors, 70
definition of, 70
differential diagnosis of, 70–1
histopathologic findings, 70
pre-transplant frozen section evaluation, 67
pre-weaning biopsy and weaning, 110
primary biliary cirrhosis (PBC), 99–101
   clinical presentation of, 99–100
   definition of, 99
   differential diagnosis of, 100–1
   histopathologic findings, 100
   pathophysiology of, 99
primary effusion lymphoma (PEL), 328
primary graft dysfunction (PGD), 158
progressive arteriopathy, 12
prophylaxis against pneumocystis, 271
protocol biopsies, 26, 219–20
   asymptomatic long-term survivors, 105–9
   HCV-negative recipients, 105
   portal-based mononuclear inflammation, 109
pseudohemorrhage, 143
PTA recipients
   acute rejection in, 218
   protocol biopsies, 219–20
pulmonary allograft rejection. *see* acute cellular rejection (ACR), lung transplants
pulmonary alveolar proteinosis (PAS), 175f
pulmonary cytolytic thrombi (PCT) syndrome, 273
pulmonary emboli, 175
pulmonary veno-occlusive disease (PVOD), 273
pure red cell aplasia, 267
pyelonephritis, 52f

quilty effect
   lymphoid neoplasms *vs.*, 140–1
   moderate rejection *vs.*, 140
quilty effect infiltrates, 140
quilty lesions. *see* endocardial lymphocytic infiltrates

rapamune. *see* sirolimus
rapamycin. *see* sirolimus
reactive plasmacytic hyperplasia, 319
real time-PCR (RT-PCR), 366–8
recipient APC, 5
recipient cancers of donor origin, 330
recipient dendritic cells (DCs) and MHC molecules, 5
recipient-derived B cells and T cells, 186

Index

recipient RBC hemolysis, 267
recurrent AIH
  difficulty in establishing diagnosis for, 98
  risk factors, 98
recurrent alcohol abuse. see alcoholic liver disease
recurrent alcoholism
  differential diagnosis of, 103
recurrent autoimmune diabetes mellitus, 238–40
recurrent/de novo immune diseases, 15
recurrent disease following renal transplantation, 52–3
  diabetic nephropathy, 53
  focal segmental glomerulosclerosis, 52
  glomerulonephritis, 52
  glomerulopathies, 52
  membranoproliferative glomerulonephritis, 52
  recurrent lupus nephritis, 53
  thrombotic microangiopathy, 53
recurrent disease in lung allograft, 174t, 175
  adenocarcinoma in situ, 175
  cellular proliferative processes, 175
  environmental exposures causing, 175
  giant cell interstitial pneumonia, 175
  lung cancer, 175
  non-necrotizing granulomas, 175f, 175
  sarcoidosis, 174, 175
recurrent diseases
  allograft and patient, 149
  following renal transplantation. see recurrent disease following renal transplantation
  in kidney transplantation, 52–3
  in liver allografts, 92
  lung allograft. see recurrent disease in lung allograft
recurrent diseases in ITx and MVTx
  active enteritis, 205f, 205–6
  eosinophilic infiltration, 206
  GVHD, 206–7
  inflammatory bowel disease, 204–5
  inflammatory lesions and processes, 205
  PTLD, 207–8
recurrent lupus nephritis, 53
recurrent membranous glomerulonephritis, 14f
recurrent necro-inflammatory diseases, diagnosis of, 108t
recurrent primary biliary cirrhosis
  clinical presentation of, 99–100
  differential diagnosis of, 100f, 101
  progression, 100
recurrent PSC, 101
  differential diagnosis of, 101
  early stage, 101
  histopathologic findings, 101
  long-term mortality and graft loss, 101
  recurrence rate, 101
  risk factors, 101
regenerative nodules, 335
regulators of complement activation (RCA), 147
  complement activation cascade and, 147
  expression in heart transplantation, 148
  serum concentration of complement components and, 148f
  types of, 147–8
regulatory cells
  role in cardiac allograft rejection, 135
regulatory T cells (Treg cells), 7
  CD4/CD25 coexpression, 7
  heterogeneity among, 7
  immunosuppressive regime modification effects on, 7
  marker of, 7
  role in clinical transplantation tolerance, 7
rejection-associated portal inflammation, 100
rejection-induced graft interstitial fibrosis, 39, 41f
rejection induced transplant glomerulitis, 50
rejection, liver allograft, see antibody-mediated rejection (AMR)
  categorization of, 76
  chronic antibody-mediated injury, 79–80
  chronic rejection, 83, 84f, 85t, 86
  T cell-mediated rejection, 80–2
renal allograft
  PPV infection, 13f
  tacrolimus-associated nephropathy, 15f
renal allograft biopsies, 110–11
  grading scoring systems for evaluating, 30
  molecular allograft biopsy analysis, 110–11
renal allograft biopsy, 25
renal cell carcinoma (RCC), 28f, 28, 331
  diagnosis of, 333
  donor kidney, 28f, 28
  mass lesions of donor kidney, 331–3
  urothelial carcinoma and, 333
renal transplantation. see kidney transplantation

renal tubules, 48
restrictive allograft syndrome (RAS), 166
sarcoidosis, 174, 175
satellite cell necrosis, 296
sclerodermatous GVHD, 297–8, 299f
sclerosing thrombotic microangiopathy, 42
self-immunity, 3
septal area, fibrous expansion of, 222f
septal inflammation, 228, 233f, 234f
  acute T-cell mediated rejection, 236f
septal inflammatory infiltrate, 229
sequence-based typing (SBT), 347
sequence-specific oligonucleotide probe (SSOP) typing, 346–7
sequence-specific primers (SSP) typing, 345–6
serologic HLA typing, 344–5
severe acinar inflammation and acinar cell damage, 232
severe acute cellular rejection, 82f
Sezary syndrome, 263
simultaneous pancreas-kidney (SPK) transplant, 216
  graft survival rates, 216–17
  history of, 217
  pancreas and kidney rejection in, correlation between, 219
  renal function monitoring in, 218
single strand conformational polymorphism (PCR-SSCP), 350
sinusoidal lymphocytosis, 89
sinusoidal obstruction syndrome (SOS), 272
sirolimus, 47, 174, 364–5
skin cancers
  basal cell carcinoma (BCC), 306
  incidence in transplant patients, 304
  Kaposi's sarcoma, 306
  squamous cell carcinoma. see squamous cell carcinoma (SCC)
skin GVHD, 277, 278f, 282f, 296
skin infections, viral, 299–303
  Cytomegalovirus (CMV), 299–302
  Epstein-Barr virus (EBV), 303
  herpes simplex virus (HSV), 299
  human herpes virus 6 (HHV-6), 302–3
  human papilloma virus (HPV), 303
  varicella zoster virus, 299, 301f
skin rejection, 306

small-for-size syndrome (SFSS)
  clinical presentation of, 71–2
  differential diagnosis of, 72
  histopathologic findings, 72
small intestinal allograf,
  classification schemes for grading ACR in, 190, 191t
  grade IND, 192f, 192
  mild (grade 1), 192f–3f
  moderate (grade 2), 193f–4f, 193
  no evidence of acute rejection (grade 0), 191f, 192
  severe (grade 3), 193, 194f–5f
Snell, George, 1
solid organ transplantation, 159. see also specific types
  clinical tolerance in, 7
somatic hypermutation (SHM) of immunoglobulin genes, 317
Splendore-Hoeppli effect, 169f
splits, serological list of, 350t
squamous cell carcinoma (SCC)
  actinic keratoses and progression into, 305f
  histological features of, 306
  incidence of, 304
  risk factors for development of, 304–6
  sun-exposed skin, 305f
standardized incidence ratios (SIRs)
  lymphoma subtypes in solid organ transplant recipients, 315f
Staphylococcus aureus infections, 303
static cold storage, 65
steatohepatitis
  causes of, 103
  steatosis and, 103
steatosis, 67
  deceased donor biopsies, 67
  severity, 103
  steatohepatitis and, 103
sterile techniques, 271
stomach allografts
  acute T cell mediated rejection, 11f
  acute T-cell mediated rejection in, 195, 197f, 198t
strictures
  anastomotic, 74
  categorization of, 74
  non-anastomotic, 74–5
subclinical rejection (SCR), 187
subnormothermic machine perfusion, 65
suboptimal portal vein flow, 73
surgical biopsies rejection, 160
surgical hepatitis, 70
surveillance protocol biopsies, 133
syndrome of "Diffuse Alveolar Hemorrhage" (DAH), 273
Systemic bacterial infections, 303

Index

tacrolimus, 43, 248, 364
  hyperglycemia and, 248–9
  structural toxicity, 43–4
T antigen expression and polyomavirus replication, 48
T cell-mediated rejection (TCMR), 76, 80–2, 104, 110, 227f
  Banff Grading schema for, 81–2, 82t, 83t
  biliary tract obstruction/stricturing vs., 75
  definition of, 80
  differential diagnosis of, 82
  early. see early TCMR
  late onset, 82, 84f. see late onset TCMR
  mild. see mild TCMR
  moderate to severe acute cellular rejection, 81f
  severe acute cellular rejection, 82f
T cell receptor (TCR), 269
T cell receptor repertoire, 5
T cells, 279
  graft failure by, 266, 267
  reconstitution after HCT, 268–9
T cell subtypes within rejecting allografts
  CD103, 11, 12f
  CD4 and CD8, 11f, 11
telepathology, 111
telescoping, 143
terminal portal tracts, 85
tetramer assay, 361–2
thickened artery with active transplant arteriopathy, 221f
thrombocytopenia, 46, 47, 77, 78, 89, 263, 272, 282, 365
thrombolytic and coagulation factors in AMR, 148–9
thrombosed renal artery, 45f
thrombosis, 224
thrombotic microangiopathy (TMA), 37, 42, 44, 45–6, 53, 250, 272

calcineurin inhibitor induced, 45
thymopoiesis, 269
tissue specific antigens (TSA), 3–4
tissue triage, 68
T lymphocytes, 135
T-lymphocytes -main effectors CD3 stain, 227f
T/NK cell PTLD, 323–4, 325f
toll-like receptors (TLRs), immune cell responses activated by, 9
total body irradiation with cyclophosphamide (TBI-Cy), 262
toxic injury and adverse drug reactions, 105
transbronchial biopsy, 167
transfusion support after HCT, 267
  ABO-mismatch and, 267
  platelet transfusions, 267
transhepatic cholangiography, 75
Transmedics Organ Care System, 66
transmural arteritis/vasculitis, 233
transmural fibrinoid arterial necrosis, 233
transplant arteriopathy, 35
transplant-associated vasculopathy (TAV), 167
transplantation. see also specific types
  central tenets about, 1
  failure causes, 1
transplantation antigens recognition of, 5
transplantation, history of, 1, 2t
  Medawar's works, 1
  MHC concept, 1–2
  Saints Cosmas and Damian works, 1f, 1
  Snell's works, 1
transplant coronary artery disease. see cardiac

allograft vasculopathy (CAV)
transplant endarteritis, 39
transplant glomerulitis, 41
transplant glomerulopathy, 42f
  clinical presentation of, 42
  diagnosis of, 42
  immunohistochemistry of, 42
  prevalence of, 42
  ultrastructural evaluation of, 42, 43f
transplant nephrectomy, 40f
trimethoprim/sulfomethoxazole (TMP/SMX), 270, 271
tubular atrophy, 49
tubular calcifications, 44
tubular compartmen, morphologic changes in, 44
tubular epithelial cell atypia, 49
tubulo-interstitial rejection, 46
tubulopathy, sirolimus therapy for, 47f
tumor-associated antigens, 260–1
type 1 diabetes. see diabetes mellitus type 1
type 2 diabetes. see diabetes mellitus type 2
tyrosine kinase inhibitors (TKI), 262

umbilical cord blood transplantation (UCBT)
  haplo-HCT and, 265
unpaired arteries, 85–6
urine amylase and acute pancreas rejection, 218
usual interstitial pneumonia (UIP), 156

vaccinations
  post-HCT patients, 272
valvular tissue, 143
vancomycin, 269
varicella-zoster (VZ) hepatitis, 90
  clinical presentation of, 90

differential diagnosis of, 90
histopathologic findings, 90
varicella-zoster (VZ) virus skin infections, 299, 301f
vascular complications, 72
vascular compromise, 190
vascular endothelium, 5
vascular lesions, 46, 238
V-cyclin, 326
vena caval complications, 73–4
venulitis, 223f, 237f
verrucae vulgares, 304f
viral inclusion bodies, 48
viral infections, 141
virally induced epithelial cell injury, 49
viral pneumonias, 172
viral skin infections, 299–303
  CMV, 299–302
  EBV, 303
  HHV-6, 302–3
  HPV, 303
  HSV, 299
  varicella zoster virus, 299, 301f
viral exanthems, 299
virtual crossmatch (VXM), 354–5
von Meyenberg complexes, 333–4
voriconazole, 271

warm ischemia, 70
weaning
  clinical features associated, 109
  pre-weaning biopsy and, 110
wedge biopsies, 25
whole pancreas transplantation. see pancreas transplantation
wound infections, 303

xanthogranulomatous pyelonephritis, 333

Zinkernagel, Rolf, 2
zortress. see everolimus